Musculoskeletal Trauma in the Elderly

Musculoskeletal Trauma
in the **Elderly**

Edited by

Charles M Court-Brown, MD, FRCSEd(Orth)
University of Edinburgh, UK

Margaret M McQueen, MD, FRCSEd(Orth)
University of Edinburgh, UK

Marc F Swiontkowski, MD
University of Minnesota Minneapolis, MN, USA

David Ring MD, PhD
Dell Medical School, The University of Texas at Austin, USA

Susan M Friedman MD,MPH
University of Rochester School of Medicine and Dentistry, USA

Andrew D Duckworth, MSc, PhD, FRCSEd(Tr&Orth)
Edinburgh Orthopaedic Trauma Unit and University of Edinburgh, UK

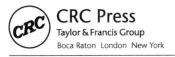

CRC Press
Taylor & Francis Group
Boca Raton London New York

CRC Press is an imprint of the
Taylor & Francis Group, an **informa** business

CRC Press
Taylor & Francis Group
6000 Broken Sound Parkway NW, Suite 300
Boca Raton, FL 33487-2742

© 2017 by Taylor & Francis Group, LLC
CRC Press is an imprint of Taylor & Francis Group, an Informa business

First issued in paperback 2020

No claim to original U.S. Government works

ISBN 13: 978-0-367-57465-9 (pbk)
ISBN 13: 978-1-4822-5202-6 (hbk)

Library of Congress Cataloging-in-Publication Data

Names: Court-Brown, Charles M., editor. | McQueen, Margaret M., editor.
Title: Musculoskeletal trauma in the elderly / editors, Charles Court-Brown, Margaret McQueen.
Description: Boca Raton : CRC Press/Taylor & Francis, 2016. | Includes bibliographical references and index. | Description based on print version record and CIP data provided by publisher; resource not viewed.
Identifiers: LCCN 2015045103 (print) | LCCN 2015043909 (ebook) | ISBN 9781482252033 () | ISBN 9781498715911 () | ISBN 9781482252026 (alk. paper)
Subjects: | MESH: Aged. | Musculoskeletal System--injuries. | Dislocations--therapy. | Fractures, Bone--therapy.
Classification: LCC RC925.53 (print) | LCC RC925.53 (ebook) | NLM WE 140 | DDC 618.97/67--dc23
LC record available at http://lccn.loc.gov/2015045103

Visit the Taylor & Francis Web site at
http://www.taylorandfrancis.com

and the CRC Press Web site at
http://www.crcpress.com

Contents

Preface

The last 20 to 30 years have seen a massive increase in the number of fractures and other injuries in the older population. Both the fracture morphology and overall health of the patients are very different from the fractures and the patients who were seen and treated in the heady days of expanding trauma systems in the 1970s and 1980s, which were developed mainly to treat high energy trauma. We believe that it is only now that surgeons are realizing that the techniques developed to cope with high energy injuries are not always appropriate for the older patient. However, there has also been a realization that high energy injuries in younger patients and low energy injuries in older patients have a number of similarities, the main one being that an interdisciplinary approach is required to treat both types of patients. As a result, orthogeriatric units are being established in many countries.

Medical literature has failed to keep pace with the rapid expansion of musculoskeletal trauma in the older patient. Studies of fragility fractures have concentrated mainly on proximal femoral fractures, and there is still a belief that the only musculoskeletal problems in the elderly are the common fragility fractures. This is clearly not the case and we are grateful to a distinguished group of orthopaedic authors from 11 different countries who have detailed the spectrum of musculoskeletal trauma in older adults together with appropriate treatment algorithms.

We have targeted the book at both geriatricians and orthopaedic surgeons. It will become increasingly important to utilize an orthogeriatric team approach when treating elderly patients in order to optimize the functional outcomes for the patients and their families. We therefore cover both medical and surgical issues, and are fortunate to have a group of experienced international physicians and surgeons on board. We are grateful for their industry and expertise. It is our hope that this book will facilitate communication between surgeons and geriatricians and will also be a stimulus for increased clinical research in this rapidly expanding area.

Charles M. Court-Brown
Margaret M. McQueen
Marc F. Swiontkowski
David C. Ring
Susan M. Friedman
Andrew D. Duckworth

Contributors

Paul A. Anderson MD
Department of Orthopedics and Rehabilitation,
University of Wisconsin, Madison, Wisconsin

George S. Athwal MD FRCSC
Hand and Upper Limb Center, University of Western
Ontario, London, Ontario, Canada

Roger M. Atkins MA MB BS DM FRCS
Consultant Orthopaedic Surgeon, Bristol Royal Infirmary,
Bristol, UK

Jarrad A. Barber MD
Department of Trauma and Orthopaedics,
The Hughston Clinic at Gwinnett Medical Center,
Atlanta, Georgia

Jan Bartoníček MD DSc
Department of Orthopaedic, 1st Faculty of Medicine of
Charles University Prague and Central Military Hospital
Prague, Czech Republic
Department of Anatomy, 1st Faculty of Medicine of
Charles University Prague, Czech Republic

Leela C. Biant FRCSEd MSres MFSTEd
Department of Trauma and Orthopaedics, Royal Infirmary
of Edinburgh, Edinburgh, Scotland

Derek Boersma MSc PT
Department of Geriatric Medicine, Nepean Hospital,
Kingswood, NSW, Australia
Musculoskeletal Ageing Research Program, Sydney
Medical School Nepean, The University of Sydney,
Penrith, NSW, Australia

Stig Brorson MD PhD DMSc
Department of Orthopaedic Surgery, Herlev University
Hospital, Herlev, Denmark

Kate E. Bugler BMBCh BA MRCS
Department of Trauma and Orthopaedics,
Royal Infirmary of Edinburgh,
Edinburgh, Scotland

Susan V. Bukata MD
Department of Orthopaedics, UCLA Health System,
David Geffen School of Medicine, Los Angeles,
California

Lisa K. Cannada MD
Department of Orthopaedic Surgery, Saint Louis
University, St. Louis, Missouri

Kevin C. Chung MD MS
Section of Plastic Surgery, Department of Surgery,
University of Michigan Health System, Ann Arbor,
Michigan

Nicholas D. Clement PhD MRCS Ed MBBS
Department of Trauma and Orthopaedics,
Royal Infirmary of Edinburgh,
Edinburgh, Scotland

Charles M. Court-Brown MD FRCS Ed
Department of Trauma and Orthopaedics,
University of Edinburgh, Edinburgh, Scotland

Eleanor Davidson MBChB Hons BSc Hons MRCS Ed
Department of Trauma and Orthopaedics,
Royal Infirmary of Edinburgh,
Edinburgh, Scotland

Oddom Demontiero MBSS PhD FRACP
Department of Geriatric Medicine, Nepean Hospital,
Kingswood, NSW, Australia
Musculoskeletal Ageing Research Program, Sydney
Medical School Nepean, The University of Sydney,
Penrith, NSW, Australia

Tina K. Dreger MD
Department of Orthopaedic Surgery,
Saint Louis University, St. Louis, Missouri

Andrew D. Duckworth BSc(Hons) MBChB MSc FRCSEd(Tr&Orth) PhD
Department of Trauma and Orthopaedics,
Royal Infirmary of Edinburgh,
Edinburgh, Scotland

Gustavo Duque MD PhD FRACP
Australian Institute for Musculoskeletal Sciences (AIMSS),
The University of Melbourne, Melbourne, Victoria,
Australia

Kenneth A. Egol MD
Department of Orthopedic Surgery,
Hospital for Joint Diseases, NYU Langone Medical Center,
New York, New York

David Fischer MD
Department of Orthopaedic Surgery,
University of Minnesota, Minneapolis, Minnesota
TRIA Orthopaedic Center, Bloomington, Minnesota

Susan M. Friedman MD MPH
School of Medicine and Dentistry, University of Rochester,
Rochester, New York

Alessio Giai Via MD
Department of Orthopaedic and Traumatology,
School of Medicine, University of Rome 'Tor Vergata',
Rome, Italy

Peter V. Giannoudis MD FRCS
Academic Department of Trauma & Orthopaedics, Leeds
General Infirmary, Leeds, UK

Jan-Erik Gjertsen MD PhD
Department of Orthopaedic Surgery, Haukeland
University Hospital, University of Bergen, Bergen, Norway

George Haidukewych MD
Department of Orthopaedic Surgery,
Orlando Regional Medical Center, Orlando, Florida

Mark Henry MD
Hand and Wrist Center of Houston, Houston, Texas

Patrick D. G. Henry MD
Department of Orthopaedic Surgery, Sunnybrook Health
Sciences Centre, Toronto, Canada

Dolfi Herscovici, Jr. DO
Florida Orthopaedic Institute, Tampa General Hospital,
Tampa, Florida

Adam G Hirschfeld MD
Department of Trauma and Orthopaedics,
The Hughston Clinic at Gwinnett Medical Center,
Atlanta, Georgia

Taylor A. Horst MD
Excel Orthopaedic Specialists, Woburn, Massachusetts

Tet Sen Howe MD
Department of Orthopaedic Surgery,
Singapore General Hospital, Singapore, Singapore

Sameer Jain MB ChB MRCS
Trauma and Orthopaedic Surgery, Academic Department
of Trauma and Orthopaedic Surgery, University of Leeds,
Leeds, UK

Houman Javedan MD
Department of Geriatrics, Brigham and Women's Hospital,
Harvard Medical School, Boston, Massachusetts

Jesse B. Jupiter MD
Department of Orthopaedics, Massachusetts General
Hospital, Boston, Massachusetts

Rishi Mugesh Kanna MS MRCS FNB
Department of Orthopaedics and Spine Surgery,
Ganga Hospital, Coimbatore, India

Matthew D. Karam MD
Department of Orthopaedics and Rehabilitation,
University of Iowa Hospitals & Clinics, Iowa City, Iowa

Stephen L. Kates MD
Department of Orthopaedic Surgery, Virginia
Commonwealth University, Richmond, Virginia

John Keating MPhil FRCS
Department of Trauma and Orthopaedics,
Royal Infirmary of Edinburgh,
Edinburgh, Scotland

Graham King MD MSc FRCSC
Roth | McFarlane Hand and Upper Limb Centre,
St. Joseph's Health Centre, London, Ontario, Canada

Joyce S. B. Koh MD FRCSEd
Department of Orthopaedics, Singapore General
Hospital, Singapore, Singapore

Patrick Kortebein MD
Novartis Institutes for Biomedical Research, East Hanover,
New Jersey

Paul M. Lafferty MD
Department of Orthopaedic Surgery,
University of Minnesota, Minneapolis, Minnesota
Department of Orthopaedic Surgery, Regions Hospital,
St. Paul, Minnesota

Olivia C. Lee MD
Department of Orthopaedic Surgery, Louisiana State
University School of Medicine, New Orleans, Louisiana

Nicola Maffulli MD PhD FRCP FRCS
Department of Musculoskeletal Disorders,
School of Medicine and Surgery, University of Salerno,
Salerno, Italy
Mary University of London, Barts and the
London School of Medicine and Dentistry, Centre
for Sports and Exercise Medicine, Mile End Hospital,
London, UK

Anupama Mahesh, MD FRCR
Department of Radiodiagnosis,
Ganga Hospital, Coimbatore, India

J. Lawrence Marsh MD
Department of Orthopedic Surgery and
Rehabilitation, University of Iowa Hospitals and
Clinics, Iowa City, Iowa

Kjell Matre MD PhD
Department of Orthopaedic Surgery, Haukeland
University Hospital, University of Bergen, Bergen,
Norway

Cyril Mauffrey MD FACS FRCS
Department of Orthopaedics,
Denver Health Medical Center, University of Colorado,
Denver, Colorado

Evan P. McGlinn BS
Department of Surgery, University of Michigan Health
System, Ann Arbor, Michigan

Michael D. McKee MD FRCS(C)
Division of Orthopaedics, Department of Surgery,
St. Michael's Hospital and the University of Toronto,
Toronto, Canada

Margaret M. McQueen MD FRCSEd
Department of Trauma and Orthopaedics,
University of Edinburgh, Edinburgh, Scotland

Joseph A. Nicholas MD MPH
Division of Geriatrics, School of Medicine and Dentistry,
University of Rochester, Rochester, New York

William T. Obremskey MD MPH MMHC
Department of Orthopedics, Vanderbilt University
Medical Center, Nashville, Tennessee

Francesco Oliva MD PhD
Department of Orthopaedics and Traumatology,
School of Medicine, University of Rome 'Tor Vergata',
Rome, Italy

Eleonora Piccirilli MD
Department of Orthopaedics and Traumatology,
School of Medicine, University of Rome 'Tor Vergata',
Rome, Italy

S. Rajasekaran MS DNB MCh (Liv) FRCS (Edin) FRCS (Lon) PhD
Department of Orthopaedics, Trauma and Spine Surgery,
Ganga Hospital, Coimbatore, India

Stuart H. Ralston MBChB MD FRCP FMedSci FRSE
Arthritis Research UK, Centre for Genomic and
Experimental Medicine, Institute of Genetics and
Molecular Medicine, University of Edinburgh, Western
General Hospital, Edinburgh, Scotland

David C. Ring MD PhD
Department of Surgery and Perioperative Care,
Dell Medical School—The University of Texas at Austin,
Austin, Texas

Nathan Sacevich MD FRCSC
Roth | McFarlane Hand and Upper Limb Centre,
St. Joseph's Health Centre, London, Ontario, Canada

Adam Sassoon MD
Department of Orthopaedics and Sports Medicine,
University of Washington, Seattle, Washington

Julia M. Scaduto ARNP
Foot and Ankle/Trauma Service, Tampa General Hospital,
Florida Orthopaedic Institute, Tampa, Florida

Lisa K. Schroder BSME MBA
Department of Orthopaedic Surgery, University of
Minnesota – Regions Hospital, St. Paul, Minneapolis,
Minnesota

Ajoy Prasad Shetty MS DNB
Department of Orthopaedics and Spine Surgery,
Ganga Hospital, Coimbatore, India

Sang-Jin Shin MD PhD
Ewha Shoulder Disease Center, Mokdong Hospital, Ewha
Womans University, Seoul, Korea

Cornel Christian Sieber MD PhD
Institute for Biomedicine of Aging, Friedrich-Alexander
University Erlangen-Nürnberg, Nürnberg, Germany

Robby Sikka MD
Department of Anesthesiology, TRIA Orthopaedic Center,
University of Minnesota, Minneapolis, Minnesota

Katrin Singler MD MME
Institute for Biomedicine of Aging, Friedrich-Alexander
University Erlangen-Nürnberg, Nürnberg, Germany

Richard D. Southgate MD
University of Rochester School of Medicine,
Rochester, NY, USA

Murray D. Spruiell MD
Department of Orthopaedics,
Denver Health Medical Center, University of Colorado,
Boulder, Colorado

Alexandra Stavrakis MD
Department of Orthopaedics, University of California,
Los Angeles, California

Marc F. Swiontkowski MD
Department of Orthopaedic Surgery,
University of Minnesota, Minneapolis, Minnesota

Julie A. Switzer MD
Geriatric Trauma Program, Regions Hospital,
University of Minnesota, St. Paul, Minneapolis,
Minnesota

Marc Tompkins MD
Department of Orthopaedics, TRIA Orthopaedic Center,
University of Minnesota, Minneapolis, Minnesota

Samir Tulebaev MD
Department of Geriatrics, Brigham and Women's Hospital,
Harvard Medical School, Boston, Massachusetts

Wakenda K. Tyler MD MPH
Division of Musculoskeletal Oncology,
Department of Orthopaedic Surgery, University of
Rochester, Rochester, New York

Mark S. Vrahas MD
Harvard Orthopaedic Trauma Service, Brigham and
Women's Hospital & Massachusetts General Hospital,
Harvard Medical School, Boston, Massachusetts

Amy S. Wasterlain MD
Department of Orthopedic Surgery, Hospital for Joint
Diseases, NYU Langone Medical Center,
New York, New York

Paul S. Whiting MD
Department of Orthopaedics and Rehabilitation,
University of Wisconsin Hospital and Clinics, Madison,
Wisconsin

Guang Yang MD
Department of Hand Surgery, China-Japan Union Hospital
of Jilin University, Changchun, China

Bruce H. Ziran MD FACS
Department of Trauma and Orthopaedics, The Hughston
Clinic at Gwinnett Medical Center, Atlanta, Georgia

Epidemiology of fractures in the elderly

CHARLES M. COURT-BROWN AND KATE E. BUGLER

Fractures in the elderly are increasing in incidence very rapidly and are becoming a major socio-economic problem in most countries. A rapid rise in life expectancy has meant that there are many more patients aged ≥65 years in the population than there were only two generations ago. It is forecast that this increase in the proportion of elderly in the population will continue to increase and there is no doubt that fractures in the elderly will become a more important health issue in the next 20–30 years.

The scope of the problem is highlighted by reviewing life expectancy over the past century. In the United States, life expectancy in 1900 was 46.3 years for males and 48.3 years for females.[1] In the United Kingdom, the equivalent figures in 1911 were 49.4 and 53.1 years, respectively.[2] By 2010, the figures were 78.7 and 81.3, respectively, in the United States[1] and 78.5 and 82.5, respectively, in the United Kingdom,[2] and by 2030, it is projected that life expectancy in the United States will average 78.3 years in males and 84.2 years in females[3] with the equivalent UK figures being 83.1 years and 86.4 years.[4] It has been forecast that the population of the United States aged ≥65 years will rise from 35 million in 2000 to 71 million in 2030.[5] In 2000, the population ≥65 years represented 12.4% of the whole population and this will rise to 19.6% by 2030.[5] Table 1.1 gives figures for the proportion of the population aged ≥65 years in 1950 and 2000 in different parts of the world. It also shows projected figures for 2050.[6] It can be seen that it is projected that there will be a significant rise in the elderly population throughout the world. The increase is projected to be highest in the less developed world. The analysis of the population aged ≥80 years in the United States shows an increase from 9.3 million in 2000 to 19.5 million in 2030. These figures emphasize the scope of the problem for the next 20–30 years.

HISTORY

The analysis of skeletons over the past seven millennia has shown signs of osteoporosis, particularly in females. Fractures which were possibly osteoporotic have been found in Egyptian mummies and in skeletons from the Middle Ages in England.[7] These latter skeletons revealed healed rib and vertebral fractures, particularly in women with a lower femoral neck bone mineral density. There were no femoral neck fractures, probably due to the limited life expectancy in the Middle Ages.

Malgaigne analysed 2377 fractures in the Hôtel-Dieu, Paris, between 1806–1808 and 1830–1839.[8] He found that fractures were commonly seen in patients between 25 and 60 years of age and recorded that there were very few fractures in patients >60 years of age, but he noted that there were very few people of that age in the population. He did observe that diaphyseal fractures tended to occur in adulthood, whereas intra-articular fractures occurred in the elderly. He also stated that fractures of the 'cervix femoris' and 'cervix humeri' tended to occur in old age and that women often sustained fractures of 'the carpal extremity of the radius'. Stimson in New York[9] and Emmet and Breck in El Paso, Texas,[10] analysed very large numbers of fractures in 1894–1903 and 1937–1956, respectively. They looked at fractures in children and adults of all ages and a comparison of their results with the prevalence of fractures in adults and children in the United Kingdom in 2000[11,12] is shown in Table 1.2. Allowing for differences in data collection, it is clear that the prevalence of fragility fractures of the proximal femur and distal radius has risen, whereas the prevalence of higher energy injuries such as fractures of the finger phalanges or the tibial and fibular diaphyses has fallen.

Table 1.1 Estimates of the prevalence of the population aged ≥65 years in different parts of the world between 1950 and 2050

Population aged ≥65 years	1950 %	2000 %	2050 %
World	5.2	6.9	15.9
North America	8.2	12.3	20.5
Europe	8.2	14.7	27.9
More developed world	7.9	14.3	25.9
Less developed world	3.9	5.1	14.3

The changing epidemiology of fractures is highlighted by a review of a study of fractures in the elderly undertaken in Dundee, Scotland, and Oxford, England, under the auspices of the Medical Research Council.[13] The Medical Research Council held a conference to discuss fractures in the elderly in 1956 and undertook a 5-year study. The medical and social changes between the 1950s and now are highlighted by the fact that they chose to study fractures in the elderly by analysing patients >35 years of age. The results of this study were compared with a prospective study of fractures in patients aged >35 years in Edinburgh, Scotland, in 2010/2011.[14] Edinburgh and Dundee are only 60 miles apart and have a very similar racial and social structure. The results highlighted the considerable changes in fracture epidemiology over a 60-year period. The overall prevalence of fractures increased by 50%, but the prevalence in males only increased by 5% compared with 85% in females. The analysis of the classic fragility fractures shows a 209% increase in the prevalence of proximal humeral fractures. This was mirrored in humeral diaphyseal fractures (129% increase), distal humeral fractures (267% increase), proximal ulnar fractures (220% increase), distal radial and ulnar fractures (39% increase), pelvic fractures (240% increase), proximal femoral fractures (186% increase), femoral diaphyseal fractures (92% increase) and distal femoral fractures (400% increase). There was an increased rate of fall related fractures in all age groups in both males and females. The study highlighted the considerable increase in fragility fractures in the last 60 years and the effect of socio-economic change on the incidence of fractures.[14]

FRACTURE INCIDENCE

Accurate analyses of fracture incidence are surprisingly difficult to find in the literature for a number of reasons.[15] In many parts of the world, there are no facilities to allow accurate analysis of what is a common medical condition. However, even in more affluent areas, little accurate information is available. In many countries, orthopaedic trauma is treated in different types of institutions, with severe trauma being treated in Level 1 trauma centres, or the equivalent, whereas less severe trauma is treated in community hospitals or by community surgeons in private practice. Thus very few large hospitals treat the whole range of orthopaedic trauma injuries and as there is very little communication between hospitals, accurate epidemiological information is hard to find. For this reason, a number of different methodologies have been used to try to assess fracture epidemiology. Not infrequently, information is gained from emergency department records. In many countries, emergency departments are mainly staffed by emergency doctors or surgeons in training who are very inexperienced in fracture diagnosis. This combined with the fact that information is not usually obtained from surgeons in private practice means that the epidemiological information is inaccurate. Surgeons have tried to obtain information by postal questionnaires asking patients if they have ever had a fracture. An analysis of the results of this method of obtaining fracture information has shown that reported fracture incidence is up to three times greater than the true incidence of fractures in the population.[15] This is because many patients may be told by paramedical professionals or others that they may have had a fracture because they have unexplainable pain.

In countries with privatized medical systems, insurance records have been used to assess fracture incidence. Again this method relies not only on the accuracy of data input but also on the prevalence of insured people in the population. The same problem occurs if only inpatient information is used. This is easier to obtain, but the data tend to be inadequate and do not represent the whole population.

The epidemiology of fractures in the elderly has unfortunately been largely ignored by orthopaedic surgeons who have concentrated mainly on high energy injuries in younger patients. Thus much of the epidemiological information has been collected by rheumatologists and other physicians whose main interest is in the diagnosis and management of osteoporosis or in the other comorbidities associated with fractures in elderly patients. Much excellent research has been done,[16,17] but understandably little information about many different types of fracture has been obtained. This problem has been complicated by the assumption that is often made that fragility fractures are simply those of the thoracolumbar spine, proximal humerus, distal radius, proximal femur and pelvis. Some comparative epidemiological data are available for these fractures, but there are many other fragility fractures in the elderly that we have very little information about. In a number of studies, fractures of the lower limb and upper limb are simply combined together and therefore little useful information is provided about many fragility fractures.

In this chapter, information about fractures in the older population has been mainly derived from two 1-year prospective studies of fracture incidence carried out in the Royal Infirmary of Edinburgh 2 years apart.[18] This is the only hospital treating a defined adult population of about 520,000. There is no private orthopaedic trauma clinic in the area. In the two 1-year studies, 13,507 consecutive non-spinal fractures were analysed in patients ≥16 years of age. Of these 4786 occurred in patients ≥65 years of age and

Table 1.2 A comparison of fracture incidence in New York (1894–1903), El Paso, Texas (1937–1956) and Edinburgh, Scotland (2000)

	Fracture prevalence (%)		
	1894–1903[3]	1937–1956[4]	2000[5,6]
Clavicle	5.9	6.2	4.3
Scapula	0.7	0.7	0.2
Proximal humerus	5.7*	2.6	4.8
Humeral diaphysis	5.7*	2	1
Distal humerus	5.7*	5.2	2.5
Proximal ulna	1.1	21.2*	0.8
Proximal radius	9*	21.2*	3.8
Radius and ulna diaphysis	9*	21.2*	2.3
Distal radius and ulna	11.2	21.2*	22.2
Carpus	0.2	2.4	2
Metacarpus	9.7	4.2	10.5
Finger phalanges	19.3	7.6	11.2
Pelvis	0.7	2.5	1.2
Proximal femur	4.7*	6.6	8.9
Femoral diaphysis	4.7*	2.5	0.9
Distal femur	4.7*	0.6	0.4
Patella	1.7	1.8	0.8
Proximal tibia	10.4*	7.3*	1
Tibia and fibula diaphyses	10.4*	7.3*	2
Distal tibia	10.4*	7.3*	1
Ankle	10.6	8.8	7.7
Tarsus	1.5	3.5	1.6
Metatarsus	2.8	4.1	6.4
Toe phalanges	3.1	4.4	2
Others	1.5	4.6	–
Fracture numbers	8962	9379	7760

Sources: From Stimson LA. *A Practical Treatise on Fractures and Dislocations.* 4th ed. New York: Lea, 1905; Emmett JE, Breck LW. *J Bone Joint Surg (Am)* 1958; 40-A: 1169–75; Court-Brown CM, Caesar B. *Injury* 2006; 30: 691–7; Rennie L, et al. *Injury* 2007; 38: 913–22.

Note: Where it was impossible to separate the prevalence of individual fracture types in the same body area, they have each been given the cumulative prevalence and marked with an asterisk.

these have been analysed to give information about the epidemiology of fractures in the elderly. Spinal fractures were not included in the analysis because comparatively few low energy spinal fractures in the elderly are actually reviewed by doctors and the epidemiology of these fractures is very difficult to determine.

For the purposes of defining fracture epidemiology in older patients, data about patients aged ≥65 and ≥80 years will be presented. It is accepted that age and gender have a significant effect on fracture epidemiology, and the fracture distribution curves of the adult population ≥16 years of age show that males have a bimodal distribution with an increased incidence of fractures in young and older males, and females have a unimodal distribution with a significant increase in fracture incidence in the post-menopausal years.[15]

Analysis of fracture incidence in the 65+ population shows that the incidence of fractures rises with increasing age in both males and females. In females, there is a steady rise from 65 years of age, which accelerates in the late 70s. In males, the increased incidence of fractures occurs about one decade later (Figure 1.1).

Overall, 34.6% of all adult fractures occur in patients ≥65 years of age.[18] The analysis shows that 77% occur in females and 23% occur in males (Table 1.3). A review of the group aged ≥80 years shows that 17.4% of all adult fractures occur in this group with 80% occurring in females and 20% occurring in males. Table 1.3 shows the overall basic epidemiology of fractures in patients aged 65+ and 80+. It can be seen that fractures of the proximal humerus, distal radius and ulna and proximal femur comprise about 65% of all fractures in patients aged 65+ and

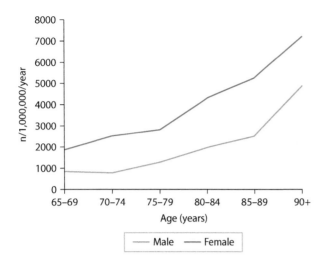

Figure 1.1 The age distribution curve for fractures in the 65+ population. (From Court-Brown CM, et al. *Bone Joint J* 2014; 96-B: 366–72.)

about 75% in patients aged 80+. However, it is important to observe that more fractures of the proximal humerus, distal humerus, pelvis, proximal femur, femoral diaphysis, distal femur and patella occur in patients aged ≥65 years than in younger patients. More than 50% of all pelvic and proximal femoral fractures occur in patients aged ≥80 years. In the 65+ group, only fractures of the tibia and fibula, talus and toes occur as commonly in males as in females. In the 80+ group, all fractures are more commonly seen in females.

Tables 1.4 and 1.5 show similar epidemiological data for both males and females, but they also show the incidence of each fracture type. In males, it can be seen that only fractures of the proximal femur and femoral diaphysis are seen predominantly in patients ≥65 years of age and that overall 16.9% of male fractures occur in this age group. The data show that 7.1% of fractures in males occur in patients ≥80 years of age. In this group, 56.4% of all fractures involve the proximal humerus, distal radius or proximal femur.

Table 1.3 The epidemiology of fractures in a 2-year period in patients 65+ years and 80+ years

	All patients					
	≥65 years			≥80 years		
	All fractures (%)	≥65 (%)	M/F (%)	All fractures (%)	≥80 (%)	M/F (%)
Clavicle	20.2	2.3	37/63	9.4	2.2	23/77
Scapula	34.8	0.6	26/74	15.7	0.6	7/93
Proximal humerus	58.3	12.1	21/79	24.8	10.2	20/80
Humeral diaphysis	42.3	1.1	29/71	19.2	1.0	32/68
Distal humerus	51.4	1.1	22/78	28.0	1.2	17/83
Proximal ulna	40.3	1.3	32/68	17.1	1.1	27/73
Proximal radius	12.6	1.5	17/83	2.5	0.6	14/86
Proximal radius/ulna	35.6	0.2	9/91	22.6	0.3	14/86
Radial diaphysis	18.4	0.1	40/60	13.1	0.2	20/80
Ulnar diaphysis	20.6	0.3	46/54	13.1	0.2	20/80
Radius/ulna diaphyses	21.4	0.1	17/83	10.7	0.1	33/67
Distal radius/ulna	42.9	21.7	12/88	18.1	18.2	9/91
Carpus	8.5	0.7	32/68	1.5	0.2	17/83
Metacarpus	7.5	2.4	29/71	2.5	1.6	32/68
Finger phalanges	13.4	3.9	38/62	5.4	3.1	36/64
Pelvis	69.8	3.6	23/77	52.0	5.4	19/81
Proximal femur	90.5	29.7	25/75	64.2	41.9	23/77
Femoral diaphysis	69.9	2.5	34/66	39.3	2.8	29/71
Distal femur	55.2	0.9	17/83	36.8	1.2	14/86
Patella	50.5	1.1	19/81	23.8	1.0	24/76
Proximal tibia	34.3	1.0	25/75	16.4	1.0	22/78
Tibia/fibula diaphyses	13.9	0.5	50/50	5.2	0.4	22/78
Distal tibia	17.4	0.3	19/81	5.4	0.2	20/80
Ankle	23.6	6.8	25/75	5.8	3.4	18/82
Talus	4.4	0.04	50/50	0	0	–
Calcaneus	9.2	0.2	36/64	2.5	0.1	0/100
Midfoot	13.8	0.2	33/67	1.5	0.04	0/100
Metatarsus	17.6	3.3	16/84	4.6	1.7	12/88
Toes	7.2	0.4	65/35	1.3	0.1	100/0
Total	34.6	100	23/77	17.4	100	20/80

Source: From Court-Brown CM, et al. *Bone Joint J* 2014; 96-B: 366–72.

Table 1.4 The epidemiology of male fractures in a 2-year period in patients 65+ years and 80+ years

	Males					
	≥65 years			≥80 years		
	All fractures (%)	≥65 (%)	n/10^5	All fractures (%)	≥80 (%)	n/10^5
Clavicle	10.3	3.8	49.4	3.0	2.5	61.2
Scapula	15.7	0.7	9.5	2.0	0.2	5.2
Proximal humerus	39.4	11.2	146.9	16.5	10.6	260.5
Humeral diaphysis	25.0	1.5	20.4	12.5	1.6	40.2
Distal humerus	23.8	0.9	10.7	11.9	1.0	25.0
Proximal ulna	27.4	1.8	24.1	9.6	1.4	35.5
Proximal radius	4.5	1.1	14.4	0.8	0.4	10.5
Proximal radius/ulna	9.1	0.1	1.2	9.1	0.2	5.2
Radial diaphysis	6.5	0.2	2.3	3.2	0.2	5.2
Ulnar diaphysis	13.0	0.6	7.3	2.2	0.2	5.2
Radius/ulna diaphyses	5.0	0.1	1.2	5.0	0.2	5.2
Distal radius/ulna	17.6	11.5	150.8	5.5	8.0	199.6
Carpus	6.4	1.0	13.2	0.6	0.2	4.8
Metacarpus	2.7	3.0	39.4	1.0	2.5	59.7
Finger phalanges	8.2	6.4	84.3	3.1	5.6	138.0
Pelvis	44.3	3.6	46.9	28.4	5.1	127.5
Proximal femur	85.1	33.1	434.5	54.7	47.8	1174.1
Femoral diaphysis	51.9	3.8	46.9	25.3	4.1	101.5
Distal femur	35.0	0.6	8.4	20.0	0.8	20.1
Patella	25.6	0.9	12.0	15.4	1.2	30.6
Proximal tibia	17.1	1.1	14.3	7.1	1.0	25.4
Tibia/fibula diaphyses	9.1	1.1	14.3	1.5	0.4	10.5
Distal tibia	5.1	0.3	3.5	1.7	0.2	5.2
Ankle	12.8	7.5	98.4	2.2	2.9	70.5
Talus	3.2	0.1	1.2	0	0	0
Calcaneus	4.4	0.4	4.8	0	0	0
Midfoot	8.6	0.3	3.6	0	0	0
Metatarsus	7.4	2.3	30.1	1.5	1.0	25.4
Toes	8.1	1.0	13.3	2.3	0.6	15.6
Total	16.9	100	1307.3	7.1	100	2467.4

Source: From Court-Brown CM, et al. Bone Joint J 2014; 96-B: 366–72.
Note: The prevalence of each fracture in the whole adult fracture population (≥16 years of age) is shown as is the prevalence in the 65+ or 80+ groups. The incidences of each fracture in the 65+ and 80+ groups are shown.

Only proximal femoral fractures show a predominance in patients aged ≥80 years compared with younger patients.

Table 1.5 shows that in females the situation is somewhat different. In females, 50.5% of all fractures occur in patients aged ≥65 years and 26.2% occur in patients ≥80 years of age. In 15 of the different fracture types listed in Table 1.5, there was a higher prevalence in patients aged ≥65 years compared with younger patients, and in patients aged ≥65 years proximal humeral, distal radial and proximal femoral fractures accounted for 66.6% of all fractures. Analysis of the 80+ group shows that 26.2% of fractures occurred in this group and in four fracture types at least 50% of the fractures occurred in patients aged 80+ years. These are fractures of the radial diaphysis, pelvis, proximal femur and femoral diaphysis.

Analysis of the incidence of fractures in 5-year intervals from 65 to 89 years and in those aged 90+ years shows that there are six patterns of fracture incidence in the older population (Figure 1.2).[18] In Type I fractures, there is a statistical correlation between increasing age and increasing fracture incidence in both males and females between 65–90 years of age. This occurs in fractures of the proximal humerus, distal radius and ulna, pelvis, proximal femur and femoral diaphysis. Type II fractures show an increasing incidence in females only. This is seen in fractures of the clavicle, distal humerus, radial diaphysis, ulnar diaphysis, distal femur and proximal tibia. In Type III fractures, there is an increased incidence in males, but not in females. This is seen in metacarpal fractures. In Type IV fractures, there is a decreasing incidence in males with

Table 1.5 The epidemiology of female fractures in a 2-year period in patients 65+ years and 80+ years

	Females					
	≥65 years			≥80 years		
	All fractures (%)	≥65 (%)	n/10^5	All fractures (%)	≥80 (%)	n/10^5
Clavicle	45.2	1.9	61.2	25.8	2.1	106.6
Scapula	60.5	0.6	19.8	34.2	0.7	34.6
Proximal humerus	66.8	12.3	391.5	28.7	10.2	520.3
Humeral diaphysis	59.1	1.1	33.6	25.8	0.9	45.4
Distal humerus	66.1	1.2	37.0	38.5	1.3	66.7
Proximal ulna	53.2	1.1	36.2	24.1	1.0	42.4
Proximal radius	19.8	1.6	50.0	4.1	0.6	32.0
Proximal radius/ulna	50.0	0.3	8.6	30.0	0.3	24.1
Radial diaphysis	75.0	0.2	5.1	50.0	0.2	10.5
Ulnar diaphysis	41.2	0.2	6.0	23.5	0.2	5.4
Radius/ulna diaphyses	62.5	0.1	4.3	25.0	0.1	13.2
Distal radius/ulna	53.4	24.7	787.0	23.4	20.8	1065.6
Carpus	10.0	0.6	19.8	2.2	0.3	13.3
Metacarpus	26.7	2.2	70.7	8.5	1.5	69.2
Finger phalanges	22.2	3.1	99.1	9.3	2.5	127.7
Pelvis	83.7	3.7	115.4	65.0	5.4	276.7
Proximal femur	92.4	28.6	913.0	67.7	40.4	2069.0
Femoral diaphysis	84.0	2.1	68.1	51.1	2.5	128.1
Distal femur	62.5	0.9	30.1	42.9	1.2	64.0
Patella	65.2	1.2	37.0	28.8	1.0	50.5
Proximal tibia	50.0	1.0	31.1	25.0	0.9	48.3
Tibia/fibula diaphyses	30.0	0.3	10.2	17.5	0.4	18.8
Distal tibia	39.4	0.4	11.2	12.1	0.2	10.6
Ankle	33.1	6.5	208.6	8.9	3.4	173.2
Talus	7.1	0.03	0.8	0	0	0
Calcaneus	24.1	0.2	5.9	10.3	0.2	7.9
Midfoot	28.6	0.2	5.1	4.8	0.05	2.7
Metatarsus	23.8	3.6	114.6	6.3	1.8	93.0
Toes	5.9	0.2	5.1	0	0	0
Total	50.5	100	3186.1	26.2	100	5119.8

Source: From Court-Brown CM, et al. Bone Joint J 2014; 96-B: 366–72.
Note: The prevalence of each fracture in the whole adult fracture population (≥16 years of age) is shown, as is the prevalence in the 65+ or 80+ groups. The incidences of each fracture in the 65+ and 80+ groups are shown.

increasing age. This is seen in fractures of the ankle and calcaneus. In Type V fractures, it is females who show evidence of a decreasing incidence with increasing age. This is seen in fractures of the midfoot and toes. All other fracture types have a Type VI pattern with no correlation between fracture incidence and increasing age. However, four of the fractures that showed a Type VI pattern showed evidence of increasing or decreasing incidence which failed to reach statistical significance. With an increasing population and increasing number of fractures in the elderly population, it is likely that these four fractures will need to be reclassified. Humeral diaphyseal fractures would be classified as a Type II fracture, proximal ulnar fractures would be reclassified as a Type III fracture, proximal radial fractures would become a Type IV fracture and carpal fractures would show a Type V pattern.

Surgeons will not be surprised by the Type I fractures, but when considering the Type II and III patterns, they may be surprised at the increasing incidence of clavicular, radial diaphyseal, ulnar diaphyseal and proximal tibial fractures in females and metacarpal fractures in males. Further analysis of clavicular fractures shows that both distal and diaphyseal clavicular fractures increase in incidence in females with increasing age and distal clavicle fractures increase in incidence in males, giving distal clavicle fractures a Type I pattern.

Some fractures continue to increase in incidence up to the mid-70s, but then decrease in incidence, particularly

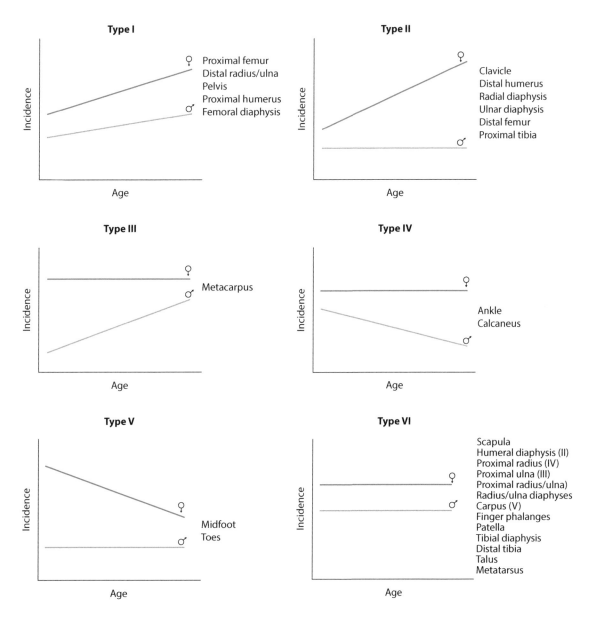

Figure 1.2 Six fracture patterns that are seen in patients aged ≥65 years. In the Type VI fractures four fracture patterns will probably change in the future. (From Court-Brown CM, et al. *Bone Joint J* 2014; 96-B: 366–72.)

in males. This is seen in ankle and calcaneal fractures. In a previous study,[11] it was stated that bimalleolar and trimalleolar ankle fractures should be considered as fragility fractures as the patients' average age was the same as that of patients presenting with distal radial fractures. Whereas the incidence of distal radial fractures increases after 80 years, the incidence of ankle fractures decreases, particularly in males. This is also seen in calcaneal fractures and presumably relates to increasing male frailty with increasing age when compared with females.

CAUSES OF FRACTURE

Review of different modes of injury that cause fractures in the elderly shows that falls from a standing height have a Type I pattern[18] with increasing fracture incidence in both males and females. Falls from a low height (<6 feet) or downstairs are unusual, in that there is a positive correlation with age in males, but not in females. This again may reflect male frailty. Falls from a height, direct blows or assaults, road traffic accidents and sports related fractures showed a Type VI pattern[18] with no correlation between increasing age and fracture incidence. However, spontaneous fractures showed a Type III pattern[18] with increasing fracture incidence in males.

Falls from a standing height

It is widely accepted that falls from a standing height cause most fractures in elderly patients. Table 1.6 presents an analysis of the prevalence of falls in each fracture type and it can be seen that overall 90.8% of fractures in

Table 1.6 The prevalence of fractures caused by falls from a standing height and high energy (HE) injuries is shown, as is the prevalence of open and multiple fractures

	≥65 years				≥80 years			
	Falls (%)	HE (%)	Open (%)	Multiple (%)	Falls (%)	HE (%)	Open (%)	Multiple (%)
Clavicle	83.9	5.3	0	7.4	92.3	1.9	0	4.0
Scapula	64.5	16.1	0	9.7	78.6	14.3	0	28.6
Proximal humerus	93.9	0.7	0	10.5	96.7	0.4	0	7.3
Humeral diaphysis	87.3	0	1.8	3.4	92.0	0	0	8.0
Distal humerus	96.2	1.9	0	17.8	93.3	3.3	0	10.0
Proximal ulna	88.7	1.6	6.5	18.7	96.2	0	3.8	11.5
Proximal radius	92.9	2.8	0	7.1	92.9	0	0	14.3
Proximal radius/ulna	100	0	9.1	0	100	0	14.3	0
Radial diaphysis	87.5	0	0	0	100	0	0	0
Ulnar diaphysis	61.5	7.1	7.1	7.1	83.4	0	0	16.7
Radius/ulna diaphyses	66.6	0	16.7	16.7	33.3	0	0	0
Distal radius/ulna	93.4	1.3	0.9	4.0	96.8	0.7	0.7	11.2
Carpus	100	0	0	5.9	100	0	0	0
Metacarpus	86.6	4.3	5.7	26.7	86.8	5.3	2.4	34.2
Finger phalanges	69.2	3.2	10.8	19.5	69.4	5.3	6.4	22.2
Pelvis	92.5	3.5	0	12.0	96.9	1.6	0	11.6
Proximal femur	95.7	0.4	0	5.0	95.9	0.1	0	4.1
Femoral diaphysis	84.2	0.8	0	3.6	94.1	0	0	2.9
Distal femur	95.2	0	2.4	4.8	96.4	0	0	3.6
Patella	90.6	1.9	1.9	13.2	100	0	0	12.0
Proximal tibia	68.7	18.7	2.1	12.0	65.2	26.1	0	26.1
Tibia/fibula diaphyses	68.8	31.2	43.8	25.0	85.7	14.3	42.8	14.2
Distal tibia	87.5	0	6.2	0	100	0	20.0	0
Ankle	87.3	2.8	1.5	2.8	89.7	1.3	5.1	6.4
Talus	100	0	0	0	–	0	–	–
Calcaneus	54.5	27.3	0	33.3	100	0	0	0
Midfoot	55.6	22.2	0	0	100	0	0	0
Metatarsus	89.9	3.2	0	12.6	83.7	10.0	0	20.0
Toes	31.6	0	17.6	5.9	0	0	0	0
Total	90.8	1.9	1.2	4.7	94.1	1.2	1.0	6.6

patients ≥65 years of age are caused by falls from a standing height. Falls cause 82.5% of fractures in males and 93.2% of fractures in females aged ≥65 years. In the 80+ group, 94.1% of fractures were caused by falls. In males, 89.5% of fractures were caused by falls and in females this rose to 95.3%. Table 1.6 shows that in 10 fracture types, at least 90% of all fractures were caused by falls in the 65+ group. This rose to 17 fracture types in the 80+ group emphasizing the importance of falls in the very elderly. The only fracture where less than 50% of fractures in the 65+ group were caused by falls was the toe fracture, where most were caused by direct blows. However, it should be noted that the prevalence of fall related fractures is less in the scapula and in the proximal tibia, tibial diaphysis, calcaneus and midfoot, than it is in other fractures. These fractures are more commonly seen in younger patients, particularly in males. Falls are discussed in detail in Chapter 12.

High energy fractures

In recent years, there has been considerable interest in high energy fractures[19] but virtually all studies have concentrated on younger patients. Table 1.6 shows that 1.9% of fractures in the 65+ group and 1.2% of fractures in the 80+ group were caused by high energy injuries, these being defined as road traffic accidents or falls from a height. Table 1.6 shows that in the 65+ group the fractures most likely to be caused by a high energy injury are those of the scapula, proximal tibia, tibial diaphysis, calcaneus and midfoot. In the 80+ group, fractures of the scapula, proximal tibia and tibial diaphysis had the highest likelihood of being caused by high energy injuries. In the 65+ group, 84.6% of high energy fractures were caused by a road traffic accident and 15.4% were caused by a fall from a height (>6 feet). In the 80+ group, the figures were 76.7% and 23.3%, respectively.

Analysis of the patients injured in road traffic accidents in the 65+ group showed that 57.5% of the fractures occurred in pedestrians, 18.2% in cyclists, 16.7% in vehicle occupants and 7.6% in motorcyclists. Further analysis showed that 31.8% presented with multiple fractures and 9.1% of the fractures were open. In the 80+ group, 73.9% of the fractures were in pedestrians, 17.4% in vehicle occupants and 8.7% occurred in motorcyclists. This older group were more severely injured with 76.9% of patients having multiple fractures and 15% presenting with open fractures. High energy fractures in the elderly are discussed in detail in Chapter 14.

MULTIPLE FRACTURES

Table 1.6 shows that the prevalence of multiple fractures in older patients[20] increases with age and analysis of the incidence of multiple fractures in 5-year age ranges shows that multiple fractures have a Type I pattern,[18] with increasing incidence in both males and females with increasing age. In younger patients, multiple fractures tend to occur as a result of high energy injuries, but in older patients increasing frailty means that multiple fractures can occur as a result of low energy trauma. This is the cause of the increased prevalence of multiple fractures in the group aged 80+ years. Multiple injuries are discussed in detail in Chapter 15.

OPEN FRACTURES

Table 1.6 shows that open fractures are uncommon in the elderly, but analysis of the prevalence of open fractures in the younger patients (<65 years) during a 2-year study showed that 3.2% of fractures in males were open, compared with 1.2% of fractures in females. Thus the proportion of fractures in the elderly that are open is not actually dissimilar to that in younger patients. The analysis shows that open fractures in the elderly have a Type VI distribution[18] with no correlation between increasing age and fracture incidence in patients ≥65 years of age.

Because of the rarity of open fractures in the elderly, a study was undertaken to examine the epidemiology of open fractures in the elderly over a 15-year period between 1995 and 2009.[21] During this period there were 484 open fractures in the elderly. The incidence of open fractures increased with age. In patients <65 years of age the incidence was $29.74/10^5$/year. This increased to $33.2/10^5$/year in the 65+ group and to $44.7/10^5$/year in the 80+ group. Thus despite the fact that Table 1.6 indicates that there is a low prevalence of open fractures in older patients, the incidence rises with age. The fracture distribution curves for open fractures are very different to those for closed fractures. Figure 1.3 shows the fracture distribution curves for open fractures in all age groups in males and females. It can be seen that in males the highest incidence is in the 15- to 19-year-old group where it was $53.7/10^5$/year. In males, the incidence of open fractures declines in an almost linear

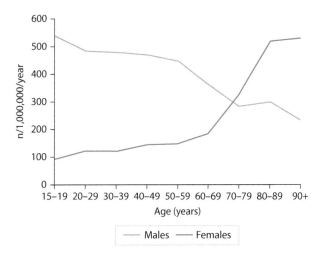

Figure 1.3 The fracture distribution curves for open fractures. (From Court-Brown CM, et al. *Injury* 2015; 46:189–94.)

fashion with age, so that in males aged ≥90 years the incidence is $23.2/10^5$/year. In females, the 15- to 19-year-old group has a very low incidence of open fractures at $9.3/10^5$/year. This gradually increases until the seventh decade of life when the incidence accelerates rising to $52.6/10^5$/year in the ≥90-year-old group.

The epidemiology of open fractures in the 65+ and 80+ groups is shown in Tables 1.7 and 1.8. These tables show that the incidence of many open fractures is similar in males and females, the major differences being the higher incidence of open distal radial and ankle fractures in females and a higher incidence of open finger phalangeal fractures in males. The situation is similar in both the 65+ and 80+ groups. It is important to remember that in all older patients the majority of open fractures are caused by low energy falls, but Tables 1.7 and 1.8 show that despite this there is a high prevalence of Gustilo type III[22] open fractures. This is particularly true of lower limb fractures in females. In fact, a comparison of open fractures of the tibia and fibula diaphyses in younger and older patients shows that in patients aged <65 years the incidence of open fractures was $3.4/10^5$/year and 46.1% of the fractures were a Gustilo type III. In the ≥65-year-old group, the incidence was $3.3/10^5$/year and 37.5% were Gustilo type III fractures. Most of the fractures in the younger patients were high energy fractures, but most of the fractures in the older group occurred as a result of simple falls. The fact that there is a high incidence of fractures in subcutaneous locations in the elderly, such as the distal radius and ulna, finger phalanges, tibia and fibula and ankle indicates that poor skin quality is probably a factor accounting for the high incidence of open fractures in the elderly.[21] It has been shown that aging alters the mechanical properties of skin and it seems likely that this accounts for the increased incidence of open fractures in elderly females which occurs about one decade after the post-menopausal

Table 1.7 The number and incidence of open fractures in males and females aged 65+ over a 15-year period. The prevalence of Gustilo III fractures is also shown

Fractures	Males ≥65 years			Females ≥65 years		
	n	n/10⁶/year	GIII (%)	n	n/10⁶/year	GIII (%)
Scapula	0	0	0	0	0	0
Clavicle	1	1.7	0	0	0	0
Proximal humerus	1	1.7	0	2	2.3	0
Humeral diaphysis	3	5.1	33.3	3	5.2	33.3
Distal humerus	3	5.1	33.3	3	3.4	0
Proximal radius/ulna	1	1.7	0	0	0	0
Proximal radius	0	0	0	0	0	0
Proximal ulna	5	8.5	0	10	11.5	10.0
Radial/ulna diaphyses	4	6.8	0	5	5.7	0
Radial diaphysis	1	1.7	0	0	0	0
Ulnar diaphysis	1	1.7	100	3	3.4	33.3
Distal radius/ulna	13	22.2	0	111	127.4	2.7
Carpus	0	0	0	0	0	0
Metacarpus	3	5.1	33.3	5	5.7	0
Finger phalanges	83	141.8	18.1	63	72.3	14.3
Pelvis	1	1.7	0	0	0	0
Proximal femur	0	0	0	0	0	0
Femoral diaphysis	1	1.7	0	1	1.7	0
Distal femur	0	0	0	5	5.7	60.0
Patella	2	3.4	0	3	3.4	33.3
Proximal tibia	1	1.7	0	6	6.9	66.6
Tibia/fibula diaphyses	13	22.2	7.7	35	40.2	48.6
Distal tibia	0	0	0	7	8.0	42.9
Ankle	10	17.1	30	44	50.5	56.8
Talus	0	0	0	0	0	0
Calcaneus	1	1.7	100	3	3.4	66.6
Midfoot	0	0	0	0	0	0
Metatarsus	3	5.1	33.3	4	4.6	50.0
Toes	17	29.0	11.7	3	3.4	0
Total	168	287.1	16.1	316	362.6	22.8

Source: From Court-Brown CM, et al. Bone Joint J 2014; 96-B: 366–72.

increase in fracture incidence (Figure 1.3). With increasing numbers of elderly females in the population over the next few decades it seems likely that this will have significant implications for orthopaedic surgeons and plastic surgeons.

EPIDEMIOLOGY OF DIFFERENT FRACTURE TYPES

Clavicle

Overall fractures of the clavicle have a Type II pattern[18] meaning that in females the incidence increases with increasing age. Lateral third clavicle fractures have a Type I pattern[18] with an increasing incidence being seen in both males and females with increasing age. Review of

the clavicle fractures treated in the 65+ and 80+ groups shows that lateral clavicle fractures accounted for 63.4% and 73.1%, respectively, of all clavicle fractures. The prevalence of middle third clavicle fractures was 33.9% and 25.0%, respectively. Standing falls caused most clavicle fractures in the elderly although Table 1.6 shows that clavicle fractures have the seventh highest prevalence of high energy injuries. Review of high energy clavicle fractures shows that 71.4% occurred in road traffic accidents and that 60% of these occurred in cyclists or motorcyclists. Tables 1.7 and 1.8 show that open fractures of the clavicle in the elderly are very rare and review of the multiple fractures associated with clavicle fractures in the 65+ group shows that they mainly involve the shoulder with 33.3% occurring in the scapula and 22.9% in the proximal humerus.

Table 1.8 The number and incidence of open fractures in females and females aged 65+ over a 15-year period. The prevalence of Gustilo III fractures is also shown

Fractures	Males ≥80 years			Females ≥80 years		
	n	n/10⁶/year	GIII (%)	n	n/10⁶/year	GIII (%)
Scapula	0	0	0	0	0	0
Clavicle	1	8.3	0	0	0	0
Proximal humerus	0	0	0	1	3.8	0
Humeral diaphysis	0	0	0	2	7.6	50.0
Distal humerus	0	0	0	2	7.6	0
Proximal radius/ulna	1	8.3	0	0	0	0
Proximal radius	0	0	0	0	0	0
Proximal ulna	0	0	0	4	15.1	25.0
Radial/ulna diaphyses	2	16.6	0	1	3.8	0
Radial diaphysis	0	0	0	0	0	0
Ulnar diaphysis	0	0	0	0	0	0
Distal radius/ulna	3	24.9	0	53	200.4	3.8
Carpus	0	0	0	0	0	0
Metacarpus	1	8.3	0	4	15.1	0
Finger phalanges	17	141.1	28.6	29	109.6	17.2
Pelvis	0	0	0	0	0	0
Proximal femur	0	0	0	0	0	0
Femoral diaphysis	1	8.3	0	0	0	0
Distal femur	0	0	0	3	11.3	66.6
Patella	0	0	0	2	7.6	50.0
Proximal tibia	0	0	0	3	11.3	33.3
Tibia/fibula diaphyses	3	24.9	0	15	56.7	46.7
Distal tibia	0	0	0	1	3.8	0
Ankle	3	24.9	33.3	15	56.7	73.3
Talus	0	0	0	0	0	0
Calcaneus	0	0	0	0	0	0
Midfoot	0	0	0	0	0	0
Metatarsus	0	0	0	2	7.6	50.0
Toes	3	24.9	33.3	0	0	0
Total	35	290.4	11.4	137	517.9	23.4

Source: From Court-Brown CM, et al. Bone Joint J 2014; 96-B: 366–72.

Scapula

The literature strongly suggests that scapula fractures result from high energy injuries and occur in young adults. However, Table 1.3 shows that over a third of scapula fractures occur in 65+ patients, this rising to 60% in females (Table 1.5). Even in elderly patients high energy injuries are important with 16% of scapula fractures in the 65+ group and 14% in the 80+ group being caused by a road traffic accident or fall from a height. This, together with increasing frailty, accounts for the fact that almost 30% of 80+ patients present with associated fractures (Table 1.6). As with clavicle fractures, the majority of fractures associated with scapula fractures are around the shoulder with 40% occurring in the proximal humerus and 30% in the clavicle. Tables 1.7 and 1.8 show that there were no open scapular fractures in the 15-year study.[21] It would seem

likely that in elderly patients open scapular fractures are associated with fatal injuries.

Proximal humerus

Proximal humeral fractures are one of the classic fragility fractures[17] and have a Type I pattern.[18] Table 1.3 shows that they account for about 12% of all fractures in patients ≥65 years of age and about 10% of all fractures in the 80+ group. There is evidence that their incidence is increasing and a study of proximal humeral fractures treated in the Royal Infirmary of Edinburgh shows an increasing incidence in the whole adult population (≥16 years) from 47.2/10⁵/year in 1993 to 92.4/10⁵/year in 2010/2011.[15] The increase was seen in both males and females.

In the elderly population the overwhelming majority of these fractures follow a simple fall and Table 1.6 shows that high energy fractures are very rare. In the 2-year period that was examined, 97.2% of all proximal humeral fractures in the 65+ group followed a standing fall or a fall from a low height. The equivalent figure for the 80+ group was 99.1%. A review of the fracture morphology showed that in the 65+ group 64.8% of the fractures were AO/OTA[23] Type A extra-articular unifocal fractures, 27.3% were Type B bifocal fractures and the remaining 7.2% were Type C articular fractures. The prevalences were very similar in the 80+ group (64.6%, 25.6% and 9.7%).

There is an association between the three common fragility fractures and in the 65+ group 53.6% of patients who presented with a proximal humeral fracture and an additional fracture presented with a proximal femoral fracture and 14.3% with a distal radial fracture. Equivalent figures for the 80+ group were 61.1% and 16.6%, respectively.

Humeral diaphyseal fractures

There is a high prevalence of humeral diaphyseal fractures in the elderly. Overall, 25% of all male humeral fractures and 60% of all female humeral fractures occur in the 65+ population, and this accounts for the fact that they have a Type II pattern.[18] The majority occur as a result of a fall, but 9.1% were pathological fractures and 3.6% occurred as a result of a low fall. There were no high energy fractures. Few patients presented with associated fractures. Of those that did 50% had a distal radial fracture and 25% had a proximal femoral fracture.

Distal humerus

Table 1.3 shows that distal humeral fractures are more commonly seen in older patients than in younger patients and 66% of female distal humeral fractures occur in older patients. They have a Type II pattern[18] with the incidence of distal humeral fractures in elderly females increasing with age. The analysis shows that in the 65+ group, 58.5% had extra-articular AO/OTA[23] Type A fractures, 28.3% had partial articular Type B fractures and 13.2% had complete articular Type C fractures. As one might expect in the 80+ group, the fracture morphology was less severe with 70% having a Type A fractures, 23.3% a Type B fracture and 6.6% a Type C fracture. Periprosthetic fractures were uncommon with only 1.9% of the fractures being periprosthetic.

Virtually all distal humeral fractures in the elderly follow a fall. There was a relatively high prevalence of multiple fractures in the 65+ group. Of these 33% involved the proximal radius or ulna, 25% were metacarpal and 16.7% were proximal femoral fractures.

Proximal ulna

Table 1.3 shows that about 40% of all proximal ulna fractures occur in the older population. Analysis shows that in males the incidence rises after 75 years of age and it is therefore likely that with an increasingly elderly population

proximal ulna fractures will have a Type III pattern[18] in the future. Proximal ulna fractures are mainly caused by falls and a review of the 65+ population shows that 98.1% were caused by a standing fall or a low fall with all of those in the 80+ population being so caused. Analysis of the fracture morphology in the 65+ group showed that 96.8% were AO/OTA[23] Type B unifocal olecranon fractures with the remaining 3.2% being Type A olecranon avulsion fractures. Morphology in the 80+ group was virtually identical (96.2% and 3.8%).

The subcutaneous location of the olecranon means that even low energy trauma will result in open fractures, and Tables 1.7 and 1.8 show a relatively high prevalence of open fractures in the frail 80+ group, although few are severe. There is also a high prevalence of multiple fractures and if one excludes those patients who presented with proximal radius and ulna fractures, analysis of the 65+ group shows that 33.3% presented with distal radial fractures, 22.2% with a proximal humeral fracture and 22.2% with a proximal femoral fracture.

Proximal radius

Proximal radial fractures are less commonly seen in older patients and Table 1.4 shows that they are very uncommon in older males. Review of their distribution in older males showed that they rarely occurred after the age of 80 and it is therefore likely that, in the future, they will have a Type IV pattern.[18] In the 65+ group, 68.6% were radial head fractures and 31.4% were radial neck fractures. In the 80+ group, the proportion was 50/50. Most proximal radial fractures in the older population follow a fall and open fractures are rare. In those patients aged 65+ who did not have an associated proximal ulna fracture, 23.1% had a distal radial fracture, 15.4% had a distal humeral fracture and 15.4% had a metacarpal fracture.

Proximal radius and ulna

Combined fractures of the proximal radius and ulna are worth considering separately because a previous study has shown that the fracture distribution curves for this fracture are the same as those of the proximal humerus and proximal femur, making it a fragility fracture.[11] Table 1.6 shows that all proximal radius and ulna fractures were caused by a standing fall, but there was a relatively higher prevalence of open fractures, particularly in the 80+ group, emphasizing the problems of a subcutaneous location in a frail patient.

In the AO/OTA[23] fracture classification, Type A fractures of the proximal radius and ulna are both extra-articular. In Type B fractures, one of the fractures is intra-articular, and in Type C fractures, both fractures are intra-articular. Review of the 65+ group shows that 18.2% were Type A, 36.4% were Type B and 45.5% were Type C. The equivalent figures for the 80+ group were 28.6%, 42.9% and 28.6%. No patient presented with multiple fractures.

Radius and ulna

The basic epidemiology of individual fractures of the radius and ulna and combined radial and ulna fractures is given in Tables 1.3 through 1.6. Radial diaphyseal fractures and ulnar diaphyseal fractures show an increasing incidence in older females and both have a Type II pattern,[18] although combined radius and ulna fractures have a Type VI pattern.[18] In the 65+ group, 29.6% of forearm fractures were isolated radial fractures, 51.9% were isolated ulna fractures and 18.5% were radius and ulna fractures. The fracture distribution in the 80+ group was very similar at 30.8%, 46.1% and 23.1%, respectively. Overall, 76.9% of forearm fractures resulted from a fall in the 65+ group with only 3.3% being caused by a high energy injury. The equivalent figures for the 80+ group were 78.6% and 0%.

In the 65+ group, 6.5% of the fractures were open, but Tables 1.6 through 1.8 show that it tends to be combined fractures of the proximal radius and ulna which have a higher prevalence of open fractures. However, they are relatively minor open fractures and there were no Gustilo type III[22] fractures in the 15-year study.[21] Multiple fractures are rare with only one ulna diaphyseal fracture being associated with a proximal tibial fracture and one radius and ulna fracture being associated with a proximal radius and ulna fracture.

Distal radius and ulna

Distal radial fractures are one of the classic fragility fractures,[24,25] but they are common in all ages and even in females, only 62.5% occur in the 65+ population (Table 1.5). They increase in incidence 65–90+ years giving them a Type I pattern.[18] In 65+ males, their prevalence is about the same as proximal humeral fractures and it is about one-third that of proximal femoral fractures. In 65+ females, they are twice as common as proximal humeral fractures and have almost the same prevalence as proximal femoral fractures.

The literature shows considerable variation in the incidence of distal radial fractures. In patients ≥50 years, the incidence in Texas, USA, was recorded as $78.2/10^5$/year in males and $256.9/10^5$/year in females.[24] This compares with $139.6/10^5$/year and $631.8/10^5$/year in Edinburgh, Scotland, and $141.6/10^5$/year and $676.7/10^5$/year in South Sweden.[25] It is unlikely that the incidences in Texas, Edinburgh and Sweden are so different and the reason for the differences is unknown. It would seem that the incidence of distal radial fractures is increasing and a review of the overall incidence in the whole population in Edinburgh (≥16 years of age) between 1990 and 2010/2011[15] shows that it increased from $158.3/10^5$/year to $235.9/10^5$/year with the increase being seen in both males and females.

Analysis of the severity of the distal radial fractures shows that in the 65+ group 65.6% were AO/OTA[23] Type A extra-articular fractures, 11.7% were Type B partial articular fractures and 22.7% were Type C complete articular fractures. The equivalent distribution in the 80+ group was very similar with 68.8% Type A, 11.2% Type B and 20% Type C fractures.

In most patients these fractures follow a simple fall and there are very few high energy injuries. However, the subcutaneous location of the distal radius and ulna means that in the 15-year study of open fractures, distal radial and ulna fractures had the highest incidence of all open fractures in 65+ and 80+ females. In the 65+ group, 26.2% of patients with multiple injuries had bilateral fractures, 40.5% had an associated proximal femoral fracture and 9.5% a proximal humeral fracture. The equivalent figures for the 80+ group were 25.9%, 44.4% and 11.1%.

Carpus

Table 1.3 shows that carpal fractures are unusual in 65+ patients and even in females only 10% of carpal fractures occur in this age group. Analysis showed that carpal fractures have a Type VI pattern,[18] but the declining incidence in older females indicates that in the future they may well have a Type V pattern.[18] In the 65+ group, 50% of the carpal fractures occurred in the scaphoid, 35.3% in the triquetrum, 5.9% in the pisiform and 2.9% in the lunate. In the 80+ group, all fractures were in the scaphoid (50%) or triquetrum (50%). All fractures occurred as a result of a simple fall, none were open and the only associated fractures occurred in the 65+ group with 50% of the patients having a distal radial fracture.

Metacarpus

Tables 1.4 and 1.5 show that metacarpal fractures are relatively unusual in 65+ males, but more common in 65+ females. Analysis of the incidence in males, however, shows that the incidence increases after the age of 65 and metacarpal fractures have a Type III pattern.[18] Analysis of the distribution of metacarpal fractures in the 65+ group shows that, as with younger patients, the prevalence of these fractures increases towards the ulnar border of the hand. In the 65+ group, 4.9% of the metacarpal fractures occurred in the thumb metacarpal, 5.7% in the index finger metacarpal, 10.6% in the middle finger metacarpal, 14.6% in the ring finger metacarpal and 64.2% in the little finger metacarpal. The equivalent figures for the 80+ group were very similar at 4.9%, 2.4%, 9.7%, 14.6% and 68.3%. Most metacarpal fractures followed falls, but 4–5% in each age group result from high energy injuries. Tables 1.7 and 1.8 show that there is a relatively high incidence of open fractures in the metacarpus and this increases in the 80+ group. There is a high prevalence of Gustilo type III[22] fractures compared with other fracture types, presumably because of the subcutaneous location of the finger phalanges in this frail group of patients. In the 65+ group, 16.2% of the patients had multiple metacarpal fractures, with a similar prevalence being seen in the 80+ group (17.1%).

Finger phalanges

Fractures of the finger phalanges are more commonly seen in younger patients with only 8.2% of 65+ males and 22.2% of 65+ females presenting with finger fractures (Tables 1.4 and 1.5). In both groups of patients, the thumb, ring and little fingers are more commonly involved. In the 65+ group, 18.0% of the fractures were in the thumb, 5.4% in the index finger, 11.2% in the middle finger, 22.4% in the ring finger and 38.0% in the little finger. The equivalent figures for the 80+ group were 23.1%, 6.4%, 10.3%, 24.4% and 35.9%. Tables 1.7 and 1.8 show that the incidence of open phalangeal fractures is high, particularly in males.

Falls caused fewer finger fractures than metacarpal fractures, but Table 1.6 shows that there was a relatively low prevalence of high energy injuries. However, 18.4% of finger fractures in the 65+ group and 12.5% of the 80+ group were caused by a direct blow or assault to the fingers. In the 65+ group, 14.6% of patients had multiple finger fractures, with 8.3% occurring in the 80+ group.

Pelvis

Tables 1.4 and 1.5 show that pelvic fractures are common in both elderly males and elderly females. They are acknowledged to be a fragility fracture[17,26] and they show a Type I pattern,[18] In younger patients, they tend to be high energy injuries, but in the elderly most pelvic fractures are caused by falls. Table 1.6 shows that high energy pelvic fractures do occur in the elderly, but they are rare.

Analysis of the changing incidence of pelvic fractures in Edinburgh, Scotland, between 1991 and 2010/2011[15] shows that the overall incidence has remained unchanged and this is true of males and females. However, the average age of males with pelvic fractures increased from 46 years in 1991 to 64.7 years in 2010/2011.[15] The increase in females was from 73.6 to 80.3 years. The fact that standing falls caused 28.9% of pelvic fractures in males and 73.9% in females in 1991 compared with 56.4% and 91.6% in 2010/2011 strongly indicates that, despite the overall incidence of pelvic fractures remaining unchanged, there is a declining incidence of pelvic fractures in younger patients and an increasing incidence of pelvic fractures in older patients.

Analysis of the type of pelvic fracture in the 65+ group shows that 85.6% were rami fractures, 9.2% were acetabular fractures and 5.2% involved the ilium or sacrum. The equivalent figures for the 80+ group were very similar at 86.7%, 7.1% and 6.2%. There were no open fractures. A review of the fractures associated with pelvic fractures shows that 20% were distal radial fractures, 16% were proximal humeral fractures and 12% were proximal femoral fractures. Similar figures were recorded in the 80+ group with 20% of patients having an associated proximal femoral fracture or proximal humeral fracture and 13.3% having a distal radial fracture.

Proximal femur

The epidemiology of proximal femoral fractures has been widely documented.[16,17,27-31] There are a number of studies which suggest that the incidence of proximal femoral fractures started to stabilize, or fall, after the mid-1990s, but this does not appear to be the case throughout the world. A review of studies which reported the incidence of proximal femoral fractures in patients ≥50 years of age who were either Caucasian or the results were age adjusted for the Caucasian population, showed that the incidence of proximal femoral fractures varied between $88/10^5$/year in males and $218/10^5$/year in females in Malaysia to $390/10^5$/year and $706/10^5$/year in Sweden.[15] Different studies have also showed different incidences of proximal femoral fractures in the same country in similar time periods.[15]

A review of proximal femoral fractures in Edinburgh between 1991 and 2010/2011[15] showed that overall there was no change in incidence, but the incidence in males had risen from $57.4/10^5$/year to $84/10^5$/year, and in females it had dropped from $220.8/10^5$/year to $200.4/10^5$/year. This probably reflects increasing male longevity. Further studies are clearly required to define the exact incidence of proximal femoral fractures and to see why there are differences in similar countries.

Analysis of the patients shows that in the 65+ group, 39.2% presented with a trochanteric fracture and 60.8% with a subcapital fracture. Overall, 0.5% of these fractures were periprosthetic. In the 80+ group, 41.6% were trochanteric and 58.4% were subcapital with 0.6% of the fractures being periprosthetic. Table 1.6 shows that virtually all proximal femoral fractures follow a standing fall, but in the 65+ group, 2.3% were caused by a low fall or fall downstairs and 1.4% were pathological or spontaneous. The equivalent figures for the 80+ group were 2.3% and 1.5%. None of the fractures were open and 29.3% of the 65+ patients who presented with multiple fractures had distal radial fractures with 26.8% presenting with a proximal humeral fracture.

Femoral diaphysis

There is a view among some orthopaedic surgeons that femoral diaphyseal fractures are high energy injuries. However, nowadays they are in fact a classic fragility fracture with a Type I pattern.[18] Table 1.6 shows that 84.2% of femoral fractures were caused by falls and in this older population there was only one femoral diaphyseal fracture that occurred as a result of a road traffic accident. There is no doubt that high energy femoral diaphyseal fractures do occur in younger patients, but overall the femoral diaphyseal fracture is now a fragility fracture. A review of the incidence of femoral diaphyseal fractures in Edinburgh, Scotland, between 1991 and 2010/2011[15] showed no change in incidence in males and females, but there was a significant change in the average age of the patient. In 1991 males and females with femoral fractures averaged 39.5 and 62.0 years of age, respectively, whereas in 2010/2011 the average ages were 63.4 and 75.6 years. There was also a higher prevalence of fractures from standing falls in both males and females in 2010/2011 compared with 1991.[15]

A review of the fracture morphology in the 2-year study shows that in 65+ patients 85.0% were AO/OTA[23] Type A simple fractures and 14.2% were Type B wedge fractures. Only 0.8% were Type C complex fractures in the 65+ group with no complex fractures occurring in the 80+ group. In this group, 87.5% of the fractures were Type A and 12.5% Type B. In the 65+ group, 93.6% of the fracture were either pathological or spontaneous or caused by a fall. The equivalent figure for the 80+ group was 95.6%. It should be noted that in the two patient groups 34.2% and 35.3%, respectively, of all femoral fractures were periprosthetic and it is likely that, with increasing prosthetic use in many parts of the world, the incidence of these fractures will rise in the next few decades. There were no open fractures and very few patients presented with multiple fractures.

Distal femur

Fracture of the distal femur, like femoral diaphyseal fracture, used to be assumed to be a high energy injury, but is now a fragility fracture, particularly in females. It has a Type II pattern[18] and its incidence increases with age in older females. In elderly patients, it is a low energy injury with all the patients in this study being injured in standing falls, low falls or falls downstairs. A review of the fracture morphology in the 65+ group shows that 81% were AO/OTA[23] Type A extra-articular fractures, 2.4% were Type B partial articular fractures and 16.7% were Type C complete articular fractures. The equivalent figures for the 80+ group were 85.7%, 0% and 14.3%. As with femoral diaphyseal fractures, there is a high prevalence of periprosthetic fractures with 26.2% occurring in the 65+ group and 35.7% in the 80+ group. Tables 1.7 and 1.8 show that open fractures tend to occur in females with a higher incidence being seen in the 80+ group. There was a high prevalence of Gustilo type III fractures[22] in both the 65+ and 80+ groups. Associated fractures are rare.

Patella

Table 1.3 shows that about 50% of patella fractures occur in older patients. In older females, this figure rises to 65%. In a previous study,[11] it was shown that the average age of patients who presented with patella fractures was actually higher than in those who presented with distal radial fractures and this indicated that the patella fractures should be regarded as fragility fractures. Using the AO/OTA[23] classification, 92.5% of the 65+ group presented with a Type C complete articular transverse patella fracture and all of the 80+ group presented with this fracture type. In the 65+ group, 5.7% of the patients presented with a Type A extra-articular avulsion fracture and 1.9% with

a Type B partial articular vertical fracture. Virtually all were caused by a standing fall, although 3.8% of the 65+ group were caused by a direct blow. Open fractures are very rare, but as with all subcutaneous fractures, Tables 1.7 and 1.8 show that they are more commonly seen in the 80+ group. In the 65+ group, 33.3% of patients presented with associated distal radial fractures. This rose to 50% in the 80+ group.

Proximal tibia

The epidemiology of proximal tibial fractures is similar to that of distal femoral fractures in that more older females are affected than older males and they show a Type II pattern[18] with an increasing incidence in 65+ females. However, there are some differences, the main one being that there is higher prevalence of high energy fractures in the proximal tibia. Analysis of these in the 65+ group shows that 87.5% were caused by a road traffic accident and that 66.6% occurred in pedestrians. Despite this, Tables 1.7 and 1.8 show that the prevalence of open fractures is relatively low, although it rises in the 80+ group, presumably because of increased frailty.

Examination of fracture morphology also shows some differences when compared with the distal femoral fracture. In the 65+ group with proximal tibial fractures, 22.9% were AO/OTA[23] Type A extra-articular fractures, 64.6% were Type B partial articular fractures and 12.5% were Type C complete articular fractures. The figures for the 80+ group were similar at 17.4%, 69.6% and 13.0%, respectively. Analysis shows that there was a high prevalence of multiple fractures. The most common associated fractures were metacarpal and pelvic fractures in both age groups. In the 65+ group, 28.6% were metacarpal fractures and 14.3% were pelvic fractures. In the 80+ group, both fracture types occurred in 25% of patients who presented with multiple fractures.

Tibia and fibula

Tibia and fibula diaphyseal fractures are unusual, in that their incidence is falling. This is partially due to improved work-place legislation for younger patients in first world countries, but also because they are not fragility fractures and the increased incidence of fragility fractures in the older population has not had the same effect on tibial diaphyseal fractures as it has had on femoral diaphyseal and other fractures. A previous study from Edinburgh has shown that in 1991, the overall incidence of tibial fractures in the whole population was 24.4/10⁵/year. The incidence fell to 13.3/10⁵/year in 2010/2011, the reduced incidence being seen in males and females. The average age of males rose from 32.8 to 41.0 years, but in females, it fell from 60.7 to 43.6 years.[15]

Table 1.3 shows that relatively few tibial fractures occur in older patients and even in 65+ females only 30% of fractures occur in this age group. However, the fractures that do occur are associated with a high prevalence of high energy injuries and open fractures. Tables 1.7 and 1.8 show that there is a high incidence of open fractures, particularly in 80+ females, again illustrating the problems of a subcutaneous location and increasing frailty.

Table 1.6 shows that all tibial diaphyseal fractures occurred as a result of a standing fall or a high energy injury. All of the high energy injuries were road traffic accidents and 80% of these fractures occurred in pedestrians. Assessment of the fracture morphology shows that despite a high incidence of open fractures there were very few AO/OTA[23] Type C complex fractures. In the 65+ group, 56.2% were Type A simple fractures, 37.5% were Type B wedge fractures and 6.3% were Type C fractures. The equivalent figures for the 80+ group were 57.1%, 42.9% and 0%. The most common associated fracture was the proximal humerus fracture which occurred in 40% of the 65+ group.

Distal tibia

Many orthopaedic surgeons associate distal tibial fractures with high energy injuries in young patients. Tables 1.4 and 1.5 indicate that this is the case in males but 39.4% of all distal tibial fractures in females occurred in the 65+ group. As with other elderly fractures, their morphology tends to be more benign than that seen in younger patients and in the 65+ group 87.5% were AO/OTA[23] Type A extra-articular fractures and 12.5% were Type B partial articular fractures. The equivalent figures for the 80+ group were 80% and 20%. Virtually all distal tibial fractures in the elderly are caused by falls, but as with other fractures, the subcutaneous location of the distal tibia means that there is a relatively high incidence of open fractures in the 80+ group (Table 1.6). It should, however, be noted that Tables 1.7 and 1.8 show that in the 15-year study the highest incidence of open fractures was seen in 65+ females[21] and that there was also a high prevalence of Gustilo type III[22] fractures in this group. No patients presented with associated fractures.

Ankle

Ankle fractures are very common but only 23.6% of all ankle fractures occurred in patients ≥65 years of age. However, Table 1.3 shows that ankle fracture accounted for 6.8% of all fractures in the 65+ group and they were the fourth most common elderly fracture. In females, the incidence stays constant from 65+ onwards, but in males, it decreases from 75 onwards and thus the fracture has a Type IV[18] pattern. A previous study has shown that bimalleolar and trimalleolar fractures present more commonly in older patients and these ankle fracture variants should be regarded as fragility fractures.

Analysis of fracture morphology shows that in the 65+ group 25.9% were AO/OTA[23] Type A infra-syndesmotic fractures, 67.6% were Type B trans-syndesmotic fractures and 6.5% were Type C supra-syndesmotic fractures. The equivalent figures in the 80+ group were 24.4%, 74.4%

and 1.3%, indicating that older patients tend to have more benign ankle fractures. In the elderly, most ankle fractures follow a fall, but despite this, like all fractures in the tibia, the subcutaneous location of the ankle means that older patients, with frailer skin, will have a higher prevalence of open fractures.[21] Tables 1.7 and 1.8 show that the incidence of open fractures is higher in females and in the 80+ group. Analysis of the fractures associated with ankle fractures in the 65+ group showed that 53.3% were in the foot with 26.7% being metatarsal fractures and 15.0% being calcaneal fractures.

Talus

Fractures of the talus very rarely occur in older patients. Only two occurred in the 2-year study. Both were lateral process fractures that followed standing falls. Neither were open and there were no associated injuries. In the 15-year study of open fractures,[21] there were no open talar fractures.

Calcaneus

Like distal tibial and talar fractures, calcaneal fractures are associated with high energy injuries in younger patients. This is undoubtedly the case, but Table 1.5 shows that 24.1% of all calcaneal fractures in females occurred in the 65+ group. As with ankle fractures, the incidence in males declines after 75 years of age giving them a Type IV fracture pattern.[18]

The epidemiology was different in the 65+ and 80+ groups. In the 65+ group, 36.4% were extra-articular and 63.6% were intra-articular. The high energy nature of the fracture morphology is confirmed by the fact that 18.2% occurred as a result of a fall from a height and 9.1% after a road traffic accident. All of the associated fractures were in the foot and 60% were ankle fractures.

In the 80+ group, all of the fractures followed standing falls, again implying patient frailty. Analysis showed that 66.6% were extra-articular and 33.3% were intra-articular. There were no associated fractures. Tables 1.7 and 1.8 show that open calcaneal fractures in the elderly are rare, but when they do occur they tend to be Gustilo type III[22] fractures.

Midfoot

Midfoot fractures, like other fractures of the foot, occur mainly in younger patients. Even in females only 28.6% occur in patients aged ≥65 years. However, in females the rate decreases after 75 years of age and consequently midfoot fractures have a Type V fracture pattern.[18] In the 65+ group, 44.4% of fractures were in the cuboid, 33.3% were cuneiform fractures and 22.2% were navicular fractures. There was only one cuneiform fracture in the 80+ group. Analysis shows that, like calcaneal fractures, there was a high prevalence of high energy injuries in the 65+ group.

Further review shows that 66.6% of the high energy fractures occurred in road traffic accidents and 33.3% in falls from a height. There were no open fractures and no associated fractures. Tables 1.7 and 1.8 show that in the 15-year study, there were no open midfoot fractures.[21]

METATARSUS

Metatarsal fractures are more commonly seen in younger patients, although Table 1.5 shows that 23.8% of female metatarsal fractures occur in the 65+ group. Analysis shows that fractures are more common in the lateral metatarsals in both 65+ and 80+ patients. In the 65+ group, 2.5% occurred in the hallux metatarsal, 10.2% in the second metatarsal, 10.7% in the third metatarsal, 15.7% in the fourth metatarsal and 60.9% in the fifth metatarsal. The equivalent figures in the 80+ group were 2.0%, 14.3%, 10.2%, 16.3% and 51.1%.

Table 1.6 shows that most metatarsal fractures in the elderly occur as a result of a standing fall, but in the 65+ group and 80+ group 5.1% and 6.1%, respectively, were caused by a direct blow. There were no open fractures in the 2-year study, but review of Tables 1.7 and 1.8 shows that when open fractures occur they tend to be in older females and there is a high prevalence of Gustilo type III[22] fractures. In the 65+ group, 12.6% of patients had multiple fractures, but 44.4% of these presented with multiple metatarsal fractures and 27.8% had ankle fractures. In the 80+ group, 28.6% had other metatarsal fractures and 28.6% also had ankle fractures.

Toes

Fractures of the toes are relatively rare in older patients. None occurred in 80+ females. Overall, 64.5% were caused by direct blows or crush injuries and the only associated fractures were other toe fractures which occurred in 5.9% of the 65+ group. Table 1.5 shows that toe fractures did not occur in 80+ females and Tables 1.7 and 1.8 show open toe fractures occur more commonly in males.

Spinal fractures

Spinal fractures were not recorded during the study period because the epidemiology of spinal fractures in the elderly is virtually impossible to assess. Grados et al.[32] analysed the prevalence of vertebral fractures in elderly French women and found that 22.8% of women, with an average age of 80.1 years, had a vertebral fracture. The prevalence and number of fractures increased with age such that 41.4% of women aged ≥85 years had vertebral fractures.

Recently, attempts have been made to assess the frequency of vertebral fractures in post-menopausal females using radiological techniques. A recent study[33] has shown that 30.7% of women ≥50 years of age had a previously undiagnosed vertebral fracture. This indicates that the incidence of vertebral fractures in women is extremely high and it suggests that vertebral fractures have a Type II pattern.[18]

The incidence of vertebral fractures in older males is essentially unknown, but it is perfectly possible that vertebral fractures actually have a Type I pattern.[18]

FRACTURE PROBABILITY

The probability of the 65+ and 80+ populations having a fracture has been assessed by analysing all patients treated in the Royal Infirmary of Edinburgh over three 1-year periods between 2000 and 2011. During these periods, about 7000 fractures were treated in patients aged ≥65 years and analysis of the number of fractures and size of the 65+ and 80+ populations has allowed the calculation of fracture probabilities in males and females. Some fractures, such as those of the scapula, talus and midfoot, are so rare in the elderly that the probability of fracture could not be calculated, but Table 1.9 shows the probability of most fractures in males and females aged ≥65 and 80 years. The overall fracture probability and the probability of upper and lower limb fractures are also shown.

THE FUTURE

By extrapolating the data gained from the 2-year study in Edinburgh[18] and adding fractures that have been previously shown to be fragility fractures,[11] it is possible to list all the fractures that are liable to increase in incidence in the elderly population over the next few decades. These fractures are shown in Table 1.10. Obviously, with increasing population size, all fractures are likely to become more common, but unless there are massive socio-economic changes in the population or osteoporosis is treated more effectively, it seems likely that the fractures listed in Table 1.9 will become more common, particularly in first world countries.

Analysis of the Edinburgh figures together with an assessment of life expectancy permits the calculation of fracture risk.[18] In 65+ patients, the lifetime risk of fracture is 18.5% for males and 52.0% for females. The equivalent figures for the 80+ group are 13.3% and 34.8%. If the results of the study are extrapolated to 2030, it is likely that there will be about 393,000 non-spinal fractures in the elderly in the United Kingdom. If one simply takes the projected population of people aged ≥65 years in the United States in 2030 and compares it with the projected population of the United Kingdom, it becomes clear that there will be about 1.8 million fractures in the 65+ group in the United States in 2030. Further extrapolation of the Edinburgh data shows that the classic fragility fractures of the proximal femoral, distal radius and ulna, proximal humerus and pelvis will account for 31.8%, 20.2%, 11.7% and 4.0%, respectively, but the other fractures listed in Table 1.9 will account for 32.3% of non-spinal fractures in the elderly. It is therefore clear that fractures in the elderly are going to become a major health issue and all countries should be planning how these fractures are going to be treated in 20 years time.

Table 1.9 The probability of males and females aged ≥65 years and ≥80 years getting different types of fractures

	≥65 years		≥80 years	
	Males	Females	Males	Females
Clavicle	2147-1	1875-1	1346-1	1016-1
Proximal humerus	720-1	288-1	358-1	199-1
Humeral diaphysis	5521-1	2683-1	2861-1	1920-1
Distal humerus	10539-1	3115-1	4578-1	1620-1
Proximal radius/ulna	2273-1	1044-1	1526-1	926-1
Radius/ulna diaphyses	10539-1	6977-1	5723-1	2880-1
Distal radius/ulna	637-1	131-1	440-1	91-1
Scaphoid	16562-1	8721-1	0	10368-1
Metacarpus	3864-1	1466-1	1761-1	1127-1
Finger phalanges	1247-1	1246-1	818-1	894-1
Pelvis	5797-1	13417-1	2289-1	6480-1
Proximal femur	229-1	113-1	71-1	46-1
Femoral diaphysis	2415-1	1571-1	954-1	720-1
Distal femur	14492-1	3876-1	5723-1	1571-1
Patella	6820-1	2769-1	3815-1	1058-1
Proximal tibia	6820-1	3792-1	3270-1	2469-1
Tibia/fibula diaphyses	7729-1	6977-1	7630-1	3703-1
Distal tibia	38644-1	9180-1	22890-1	8640-1
Ankle	1026-1	535-1	1205-1	524-1
Calcaneus	12881-1	15856-1	0	12960-1
Toes	8918-1	17442-1	5723-1	51840-1
Upper limb fractures	187-1	67-1	111-1	46-1
Lower limb fractures	139-1	68-1	54-1	32-1
Overall	77-1	33-1	36-1	19-1

Table 1.10 Fractures that are likely to become more common in elderly patients

Males	Females
Distal clavicle	Clavicular diaphysis
Proximal humerus	Distal clavicle
Proximal ulna	Proximal humerus
Distal radius and ulna	Humeral diaphysis
Metacarpus	Distal humerus
Pelvis	Proximal radius and ulna
Thoracolumbar spine	Radial diaphysis
Proximal femur	Ulnar diaphysis
Femoral diaphysis	Distal radius and ulna
	Pelvis
	Thoracolumbar spine
	Proximal femur
	Femoral diaphysis
	Distal femur
	Patella
	Proximal tibia
	Bimalleolar ankle
	Trimalleolar ankle

REFERENCES

1. United States Life Tables. www.cdc.gov/nchs/data/nusr/nusr63_07.pdf. Last reviewed 1/02/2016.

2. Office of National Statistics. www.ons.gov.uk/. Last reviewed 1/02/2016

3. Life expectancy-United States. www.data360.org. Last reviewed 1/02/2016

4. Life expectancies. www.ons.gov.uk. Last reviewed 1/02/2016

5. Population division. www.un.org/en/development/desa/population. Last reviewed 1/02/2016

6. World human population. https://en.wikipedia.org/wiki/World_human_population. Last reviewed 1/02/2016

7. Stride PJO, Patel N, Kingston D. The history of osteoporosis: Why do Egyptian mummies have porotic bones? *J R Coll Physicians Edinb* 2013; 43: 254–61.

8. Malgaigne JF. *A Treatise on Fractures.* Philadelphia, PA: Lippincott, 1859.

9. Stimson LA. *A Practical Treatise on Fractures and Dislocations.* 4th ed. New York: LEA, 1905.

10. Emmett JE, Breck LW. A review and analysis of 11,000 fractures seen in a private practice of orthopaedic surgery 1937–1956. *J Bone Joint Surg (Am)* 1958; 40-A: 1169–75.

11. Court-Brown CM, Caesar B. Epidemiology of adult fractures: A review. *Injury* 2006; 30: 691–7.

12. Rennie L, Court-Brown CM, Mok JY, Beattie TF. The epidemiology of fractures in children. *Injury* 2007; 38: 913–22.

13. Knowelden J, Buhr AJ, Dunbar O. Incidence of fractures in persons over 35 years of age. A report to the MRC working party on fractures in the elderly. *Br J Prev Soc Med* 1964; 18: 130–41.

14. Court-Brown CM, Biant LC, Bugler KE, McQueen MM. Changing epidemiology of adult fractures in Scotland. *Scott Med J* 2014; 59: 30–4.

15. Court-Brown CM. The epidemiology of fractures and dislocations. In: Court-Brown CM, Heckman JD, McQueen MM, Ricci W, Tornetta P (eds), *Rockwood and Green's Fractures in Adults.* 8th ed. Philadelphia, PA: Lippincott, Williams and Wilkins, 2014.

16. Kanis JA, Odén A, McCloskey EV, Johansson H, Wahl DA, Cooper C. A systematic review of hip fracture incidence and probability of fracture worldwide. *Osteoporos Int* 2012; 23: 2239–56.

17. Cooper C, Cole ZA, Holroyd CR, Earl SC, Harvey NC, Dennison EM, Melton LJ, Cummings SR, Kanis JA. Secular trends in the incidence of hip and other osteoporotic fractures. *Osteoporos Int* 2011; 22: 1277–88.

18. Court-Brown CM, Clement ND, Duckworth AD, Aitken S, Biant LC, McQueen MM. The spectrum of fractures in the elderly. *Bone Joint J* 2014; 96-B: 366–72.

19. Switzer JA, Gammon SR. High-energy skeletal trauma in the elderly. *J Bone Joint Surg (Am)* 2012; 94-A: 2195–204.

20. Clement ND, Aitken S, Duckworth AD, McQueen MM, Court-Brown CM. Multiple fractures in the elderly. *J Bone Joint Surg (Br)* 2012; 94-B: 231–6.

21. Court-Brown CM, Biant LC, Clement ND, Bugler KE, Duckworth AD, McQueen MM. Open fractures in the elderly. The importance of skin aging. *Injury* 2015; 46: 189–94.

22. Gustilo RB, Anderson JT. Prevention of infection in the treatment of 1035 open fractures of long bones: Retrospective and prospective analysis. *J Bone Joint Surg (Am)* 1976; 58: 453–8.

23. Müller ME, Nazarian S, Koch P, Schatzker J. *The Comprehensive Classification of Fractures of Long Bones.* Berlin: Springer, 1990.

24. Orces CH, Martinez FJ. Epidemiology of fall related forearm and wrist fractures among adults treated in US hospital emergency departments. *Inj Prev* 2011; 17; 33–6.

25. Brogen E, Petranek M, Atroshi I. Incidence and characteristics of distal radius fractures in a southern Swedish region. *BMC Musculoskelet Disord* 2007; 8: 48.

26. Prieto-Alhambra D, Avilés FF, Judge A, Van Staa T, Nogués X, Arden NK, Díez-Pérez A, Cooper C, Javaid MK. Burden of pelvis fracture: A population-based study of incidence, hospitalisation and mortality. *Osteoporos Int* 2012; 23: 2797–803.

27. Chevally T, Guilley E, Herrman FR, Hoffmeyer P, Rapin CH, Rizzoli R. Incidence of hip fracture over a 10-year period (1991–2000): Reversal of a secular trend. *Bone* 2007; 40: 1284–9.

28. Bergstrom U, Jonsson H, Gustavson Y, Pettersson U, Stenlund H, Svensson O. The hip fracture incidence curve is shifting to the right. A forecast of the age-quake. *Acta Orthop* 2009; 80: 520–4.

29. Rosengren BE, Alhborg HG, Gärdsell P, Sernbo I, Daly RM, Nilsson JA, Karlsson MK. Bone mineral density and incidence of hip fracture in Swedish urban and rural women 1987–2002. *Acta Orthop* 2010; 81: 453–9.

30. Lau EM, Lee JK, Suriwongpaisal P, Saw SM, Das De S, Khir A, Sambrook P. The incidence of hip fracture in four Asian countries: The Asian Osteoporosis Study (AOS). *Osteoporosis Int* 2001; 12: 239–43.

31. Chang KP, Center JR, Nguyen TV, Eisman JA. Incidence of hip and other osteoporotic fractures in elderly men and women: Dubbo Osteoporosis Epidemiology Study. *J Bone Miner Res* 2004; 19: 532–6.

32. Grados F, Marcelli C, Dargent-Molina P, Roux C, Vergnol JF, Meunier PJ, Fardellone P. Prevalence of vertebral fractures in French women older than 75 years from the EPIDOS study. *Bone* 2004; 34: 362–7.

33. Van den Berg M, Verdijk NA, van den Bergh JP, Geusens PP, Talboom-Kamp EP, Leusink GL, Pop VJ. Vertebral fractures in women aged 50 years and older with clinical risk factors for fractures in primary care. *Maturitas* 2011; 70: 74–9.

2

Age-related changes in the elderly

KATRIN SINGLER AND CORNEL CHRISTIAN SIEBER

INTRODUCTION

Changes associated with aging affect all organ systems and are associated with a decreased functional reserve capacity.[1] The changes are physiologic and do not represent a disease process but nevertheless accompany a loss of substance or functional decline.[2] The loss of functional reserve becomes particularly evident under the influence of internal and/or external stressors, leading to an increased risk of injury, such as falls and other traumas. In addition to physiologic age-related changes, many older patients have multiple comorbidities that signify an added risk for injuries, so in orthogeriatric patients, age-related changes as well as concomitant diseases play an important role in diagnosis, treatment and primary and secondary prevention. Important age-related changes in orthogeriatric patients and their consequences for patient care are discussed in this chapter.

DIVERSITY OF AGING AND FUNCTIONAL DECLINE

When people speak of older adults, they often mean a homogeneous group of individuals beyond the age of 65 years. This does not recognize the great differences between 65- and 75-year olds, and particularly those beyond the age of 80, the so-called 'oldest old'. In addition, even within a particular chronological age cohort of older adults, there is extensive diversity due to various factors such as genetic background and preventive measures as well as the presence of mono- or multimorbidity. As a

consequence, older adults need a customized diagnostic and treatment approach. This is also true for orthogeriatric patients.

Nearly all organ systems show signs of an aging process, what we usually mean by the term 'normal aging'. The term 'successful aging' means that these normal declines over the lifespan do not negatively interfere with functionality and thereby independence. By accepting aging as a normal process, geriatricians therefore view the 'anti-aging' hype with a certain reserve, as we usually do not start to treat as long as functionality in the activities of daily living (ADL) is preserved. When treatment is required, it is often carried out by interdisciplinary teams.

Another characteristic of orthogeriatric patients is the common co-existence of various chronic diseases. These have to be taken into account when dealing with such patients as they can directly or indirectly interfere with surgical procedures. Some examples include frequent treatment with anticoagulants, arterial hypertension, diabetes mellitus and kidney dysfunction. Comorbidities may also be risk factors for perioperative complications such as delirium (detailed below).

PRINCIPLES OF NUTRITIONAL AND FLUID INTAKE

The caloric demands of older adults are around 10% less than those of younger adults and are 25–30 kcal/kg body weight per day. This demand is only lower when mobility is decreased to a significant extent. Adequate protein intake is especially important in multimorbid patients with frailty (see below) who should consume 1.0–1.2 g/kg body weight per day.[3] Older persons show a good protein anabolism potential but reach an earlier ceiling effect. This means that protein intake has to be well distributed over all meals during the day. If such intake is not possible, food has to be fortified or oral protein-rich supplements given between meals.

Malnutrition is frequent in older adults, and in those admitted to hospital, the risk of overt malnutrition is above 50%. Nutritional state can be easily determined using the Mini Nutritional Assessment (MNA) instrument, the only nutritional screening tool especially developed for older adults.[4]

Weight reducing diets in older persons are nearly always contraindicated, as elderly individuals mainly lose muscle mass when their caloric intake is lower than their daily needs. If a diet is introduced, it must be accompanied by a physical activity program to preserve the – often already diminished – muscle mass. The loss of fat-free mass (mainly muscle) leads to sarcopenia (see below) and often causes falls with subsequent fragility fractures.

Regarding adequate fluid intake, a daily intake of 1500–2000 mL is considered necessary. A fluid intake history is important, as older women especially often do not achieve such volumes in daily life. This fluid volume includes fluid in foods. A frequent problem is the continuation of diuretic therapy which may lead to falls due to orthostatic dysregulation, as well as being an important risk factor for perioperative cognitive disturbance. This has to be balanced against the fear of cardiac decompensation due to the significant functional implications and possibilities for complications.

AGE AS A RISK FACTOR FOR DELIRIUM*

Delirium is the most frequent mental disorder in older individuals in the acute setting and the development of postoperative delirium is a common complication in geriatric patients. As age is one of the strongest risk factors for delirium, the likelihood of developing delirium increases with age. The incidence of delirium in hospitalized patients is affected by predisposing factors and the severity of the underlying cause of hospitalization. Older people undergoing surgery for a fracture are particularly prone to delirium.

Cognitive impairment and dementia are also strong risk factors for the development of delirium and present in more than 50% of surgical patients presenting with delirium. Cognitive impairment can last up to 1 year postoperatively.[5,6]

Delirium often shows a multifactorial causal mechanism. Several interacting biological factors result in disruption of the neuronal networks of the brain, resulting in acute cognitive dysfunction.[7] Current evidence suggests that neuroinflammatory processes, changes in the balance of neurotransmitters, physiological stressors, metabolic derangements as well as electrolyte disorders and genetic factors contribute to the development of delirium.[8,9]

Many transmitters are implicated in disturbed neurotransmission, but cholinergic deficiency and/or dopaminergic excess are of special importance as these systems are often influenced by medications known to interfere with synaptic transmission and therefore potentially cause delirium. Cytokines, such as IL-1, IL-2, IL-6, TNFα and interferon, which influence the permeability of the blood–brain barrier, disturb the process of neurotransmission. In addition, systemic inflammatory processes, trauma, hypoxia and even surgery cause an increase in cytokine levels, resulting in activation of the microglia and presenting a risk for delirium.

Risk factors for the development of delirium in orthopaedic patients, which should be assessed routinely in every patient, are as follows:

- Advanced age
- Pre-existing cognitive impairment
- Polypharmacy
- Development of delirium during/after surgery
- Small changes in fluid and food balance
- Decline in sight and/or hearing
- Functional impairment
- Pain
- Immobility
- Physical restraints including bladder catheters, infusions, etc.

IDENTIFICATION OF INFECTIONS

Infections are the main cause of mortality in older hospitalized patients and are a common complication in orthogeriatric patients. This applies both to patients living in long-term care facilities and to patients who before hospitalization lived independently in their own homes. Mortality risk due to infections rises with increasing age and is strongly influenced by the presence of comorbidities, such as diabetes, circulatory disturbances or chronic heart failure.[10] Immunological changes that accompany increasing age, functional impairment and changes in physiological barriers, such as the skin and the mucous membrane, favour infections in older individuals. In addition to prevention, early recognition and initiation of therapy are very important to reduce the impact of infections in geriatric patients.

Common infections in orthogeriatric patients are urinary tract infections (UTI), pneumonia, wound infections and catheter associated infections. UTIs are favoured by the presence of underlying incontinence, immobility and particularly urinary catheters. The incidence of bacteriuria due to urinary catheters is 3–10% and is considered a strong risk factor for the development of nosocomial UTIs.[11] Dysuria, one of the main symptoms of UTIs in younger patients, is often missing, presenting a challenge for the treating physician

* Also see Chapter 7.

to distinguish between an asymptomatic UTI and a bacteriuria. However, such differentiation is important as antibiotic treatment for a bacteriuria does not affect morbidity but often results in adverse drug events and other negative consequences. Therefore, diagnosis of a UTI requires thorough clinical evaluation and often urinary analyses and cultures.[12]

Pneumonia is encouraged by restricted clearing of the respiratory tract, and alterations in lung structure and respiratory mechanics.[13,14] Compared with younger individuals, up to 36% of older patients with pneumonia present without cough with/without expectoration and sometimes without fever.[15,16]

These examples demonstrate that avoidance of diagnostic delays in older patients is often difficult as symptoms of infection are frequently atypical and non-specific and the informative value of diagnostic tools differs from that in younger patients.

Very often, a non-specific presentation, such as a fall, or acute alterations in cognitive function (delirium) and/or mobility may herald an underlying infection in old age. Weakness and fatigue are common complaints in the older person, often resulting in emergency department visits. As recent literature has shown, pneumonia and UTIs are among the most common primary diagnoses causing weakness and fatigue.[17] Therefore it is vital that even subtle changes are recognized in the treatment of these vulnerable patients.

Careful interpretation of vital as well as laboratory parameters in older patients with infections reveals characteristic features that must be taken into account. Pathological results can be markedly reduced or even missing in infection.[18] For example, tachycardia, one of the trigger symptoms in severe infections, can be missing in older patients due to reduced heart rate variability and polypharmacy.[19]

Fever, one of the cardinal symptoms in bacterial infection, is missing in up to 30% of older patients.[20] This is due to a decline in basal body temperature (−0.15°C per decade), decreased thermoregulation, and reduced and inadequate production of endogenous pyrogens.[21,22] The cutoff temperature for 'fever' is defined inconsistently in clinical guidelines as between 38.0°C and 38.3°C. As these guidelines do not take into account the special characteristics of older patients, it is assumed that lower cutoff values have to be considered when evaluating for infections in older adults. First data from the emergency department show that a cutoff tympanal temperature of 37.3°C or rectal temperature of 37.8°C should trigger further diagnostic investigation for bacterial infection.[23]

In addition, pathological laboratory test results, for instance indicating leucocytosis or elevated C-reactive protein (CRP), can be missing or only slightly elevated at the beginning of an infection and therefore are unreliable parameters to identify infections in older patients.[16] Identification of infections without an inflammatory response is important in the treatment of older patients as it is associated with greatly increased mortality.[24]

Further diagnostic tools, such as chest X-rays for the identification of pneumonia, are diagnostically limited, as alterations in lung structure are often non-specific and infiltrates can persist for months.[25]

Identification of infections in older patients can be a big challenge. Therefore in older patients with non-specific clinical symptoms (weakness, fatigue, acute change in functional or cognitive status, falls, etc.) the diagnosis of an underlying infection should be considered even if vital or laboratory parameters are only slightly abnormal, and radiographic intervention does not show any obvious underlying causes of infection.

CHRONIC AND ACUTE PAIN

'Pain is an unpleasant sensory and emotional experience associated with actual or potential tissue damage, or described in terms of such damage'.[26] There are various definitions for the duration of chronic pain, but most describe chronic pain as lasting more than 3–6 months.

Inadequate pain management in the older patient is a common problem in both acute and chronic pain and is pronounced in cognitively impaired patients. This not only means discomfort for the patient but is also associated with negative effects on the patient's health, impaired functional abilities and increased healthcare costs.

Previous observational studies have found that postoperative pain in older adults undergoing lower extremity orthopaedic surgery is associated with an increased risk of delirium, prolonged hospital stay and rehabilitation, higher probability of a physiotherapy session being missed or shortened, delays in ambulation postoperatively, impaired functional recovery and greater pain at 6 months after the surgery (Figure 2.1).[27,28] The consequences of pain in older patients differ from those in younger patients, as functional decline is associated with diminished functional reserve (Figure 2.2).

Barriers to adequate analgesia (i.e. timely administration and effective pain control) are listed in Table 2.1. Despite these barriers there is a widespread misperception among

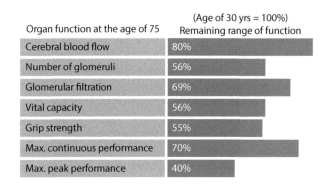

Figure 2.1 Organ function at the age of 75. (Adapted from Shock NW, et al. *Normal Human Aging: Baltimore Longitudinal Study of Aging.* Baltimore: NIH, 1984.)

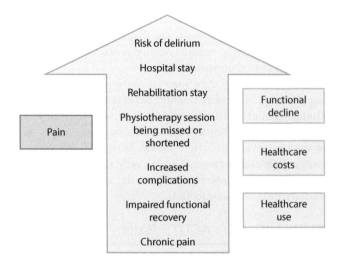

Figure 2.2 Consequences of inadequate pain management in older patients.

Table 2.1 Common causes of inadequate analgesic administration in the elderly

Under-reporting of pain
Inadequate knowledge of pain assessment and management
Missing pain assessment
Concerns about the use of analgesics in older comorbid and/or cognitively impaired patients

patients and physicians that pain is a physiological consequence of aging. However, pain is not an age-related change, but an unpleasant sensory experience that has to be assessed and treated. No physiological changes in pain perception in older adults have been demonstrated, but there is evidence that older adults experience more pain than younger individuals.[29]

Underreporting of pain is also a common problem in orthogeriatric patients. In addition to the fact that pain is often assumed to be associated with aging, under-reporting is caused by communication problems (hearing loss, problems with speaking, for example dry mouth, comorbidities such as Parkinson disease, etc.), fear of addiction and the side effects of pain treatment, and the incorrect assumption that the pain is related to a comorbidity rather than a trauma. As in infections, pain, especially in patients with cognitive impairment, often presents non-specifically and atypically. Delirium, an acute decline in function or an acute reduction in nutritional intake can all be caused by pain. Therefore it is important to look for subtle changes in patient behaviour, cognitive and functional status and use a standardized pain assessment instrument regularly.

In addition, pain management requires advanced knowledge of age-related changes regarding unspecific and/or atypical presentation of pain and changes affecting pharmacokinetics and pharmacodynamics.

METABOLIC CHANGES (RENAL, LIVER, GUT) AND THEIR IMPACT ON MEDICATION

Geriatric patients are characterized by multimorbidity that often results in polypharmacy. As age-related changes affect pharmacokinetics (what the body does to the drug) and pharmacodynamics (what the drug does to the body), such changes play an important role in the medication of older patients.[30] Pharmacokinetics includes the resorption, distribution, metabolism and elimination of drugs. Age-related changes are also important in the management of orthogeriatric patients, for example regarding pain medication.

Resorption

Gastric bicarbonate secretion decreases with age as does intestinal blood flow and mucosal function, while intestinal villus atrophy increases. As gastric emptying time is also increased, older patients have decreased stomach protection and an increased risk of developing intestinal ulcers and gastrointestinal bleeding while taking non-steroidal anti-inflammatory drugs (NSAIDs).

Distribution

Increasing age is associated with a significant change in drug volume and distribution. The proportion of body fat increases, while the proportion of lean body mass decreases. Consequently, the percentage of body water decreases with age (Figure 2.3). This increases the risk of dehydration and also influences the volume and distribution of hydrophilic (water soluble) and lipophilic (fat soluble) drugs. In particular, initial serum concentrations for a given dose of a water soluble drug, such as digoxin or hydrochlorothiazide, are higher than expected, while a fat soluble drug, such as amiodarone or NSAIDs, shows a longer half-life as expected due to the slow release from fatty tissue.[31]

Malnourished patients show reduced plasma protein levels (including albumin). This also has an impact on medication in older patients as malnutrition commonly causes increased levels of unbound drugs, as for example NSAIDs with strong protein binding.

Drug metabolism

Metabolism of medications occurs mostly in the liver. Liver size and function also decrease with age. Hepatic blood flow is reduced by up to 25%, and the number of functional hepatocytes and enzyme activity decline.[32] These changes result in altered first-pass metabolism and clearance of certain drugs, for example acetaminophen. Non-synthetic hepatic biotransformation reactions (e.g. oxidative) and synthetic enzymatic reactions (e.g. conjugation) also change with aging.[1] These age-related changes in hepatic metabolism and clearance are difficult to estimate.

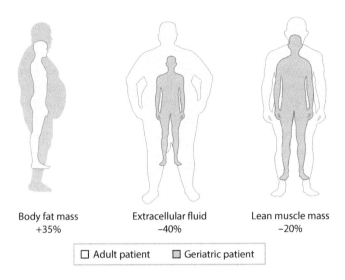

Body fat mass
+35%

Extracellular fluid
−40%

Lean muscle mass
−20%

☐ Adult patient　■ Geriatric patient

Figure 2.3 Changes in volume of distribution in old age.

Elimination

The kidneys are the most important organs for the elimination of drugs. Renal drug elimination in the older person is affected by a decrease in the glomerular filtration rate (GFR) of approximately 10% per decade after 20 years of age. Creatinine clearance also decreases due to diminished renal perfusion, atrophy of the glomeruli and decreased tubular efficiency.[1,31]

As lean body mass and therefore creatinine production decrease with age, serum creatinine is not a reliable parameter for the assessment of renal function as there is a risk of overestimation. Therefore the more reliable parameter of creatinine clearance should be calculated using, for instance, the Cockcroft–Gault formula to estimate GFR (Figure 2.4).[33]

Alterations in pharmacodynamics (what the drug does to the body) in older patients may even be more important than changes in pharmacokinetics, although they have not been studied to any great extent.[30] The response to a drug by its target organ may be increased, decreased or unchanged.[31]

One important target organ is the cardiovascular system. Physiological age-related changes include increasing arterial stiffness as well as a decreased adrenergic response of the cardiovascular system. Therefore it is difficult for the body to increase cardiac output and orthostatic (side)effects of medication will be more pronounced. Also, the aging central nervous system is influenced by altered pharmacodynamics. It shows a higher sensitivity to psychotropic drug effects due to a reduction and shift in neurotransmitters often resulting in delirium.

SARCOPENIA AND FRAILTY

Sarcopenia is the term for age-related loss of muscle mass. Muscle mass peaks at around 40 years of age and then steadily declines, a process which can be delayed and

$$eC_{cr} = \frac{(140 - age) \times mass\ (in\ kg) \times [0.85\ if\ female]}{72 \times serum\ creatinine\ (in\ mg/dL)}$$

Figure 2.4 The Cockcroft–Gault formula.

lowered through regular physical activity[34] and a well-balanced protein-rich diet.[3] *Sarcopenia* is defined as a measured loss of muscle mass in combination with a loss of strength (mainly determined by handgrip strength) or function (mainly measured by gait speed). Sarcopenia is relevant to older adults as it directly affects their functionality. It is closely linked to frailty syndrome, characterized by decreased tolerability and responsiveness to internal and external stressors.[35,36] Frailty can be separated into physical, psychological and social frailty. Physical frailty is central to orthogeriatrics and can quite easily be determined by the Fried criteria.[37]

Although most frail and sarcopenic patients are not seen before an accident occurs, they should be assessed for frailty and sarcopenia impact before specific strategies are implemented, not least in the postoperative period, including rehabilitation.

SKIN CHANGES

The skin is the largest organ of the body and accounts for approximately 7% of total body weight. It provides a barrier against external exposures and is also involved in thermoregulation of the body and hydration status as well as sensory and immunological functions and vitamin D synthesis. Like all other organs the skin shows significant age-related changes that have an impact on the management of older patients. These changes are partially provoked by exposure to the environment throughout life and include changes in neurosensory perception, permeability, response to injury and repair capacity.[38]

Structurally, the skin consists of the epidermis and the dermis. Skin thickness, especially of the epidermis, decreases over the lifespan by about 6.4% per decade, although the number of cell layers remains stable.[39,40] Subcutaneous fat also diminishes with age. It has an important role in thermoregulation and therefore older patients are at risk of becoming hypothermic. As the distribution of subcutaneous fat changes with age, a reduction in subcutaneous fat over bony areas increases the risk of pressure ulcers and fractures with advancing age.[41] Also, the decrease in the density of Pacinian and Meissner's corpuscles as well as the loss of sensory nerve endings in the epidermis and dermis with age fosters injuries due to environmental stimuli.[38]

Age-related changes in the skin are associated with an increase in reactive oxygen species (ROS) levels and a decreased antioxidant defense system as well as a reduction in hormones and chemical signals important for the repair capacity of the skin.[39] The amount of dermal blood vessels and the length of capillary loops are decreased with age, also contributing to the impaired thermoregulation in older age. As the repair capacity of the skin is diminished compared with younger individuals, wound healing is delayed and the risk of postoperative wound reopening is considerably increased.[38]

Vitamin D

The skin is the place where vitamin D3 and 1,25-dihydroxyvitamin D3 synthesis occurs. In the skin ultraviolet B radiation (UVB) converts 7-dehydrocholesterol to provitamin D3 which is then converted into vitamin D3. Vitamin D plays an important role in calcium homeostasis and bone integrity but is also essential for several other aspects of human health. With increasing age the dermis and epidermis lack epidermal 7-dehydrocholesterol and the release of vitamin D into the blood is reduced by up to 75%.[42,43]

PULMONARY READINESS

Chronic lower respiratory tract disease is the third leading cause of death in older people.[44] Age-related changes in the lung include structural changes, changes in muscle function and changes in pulmonary immunologic function.

One structural change is the narrowing of intervertebral disk spaces leading to deformation of the spine, such as kyphosis, and decreased space between the ribs, shortened intercostal muscles and a smaller chest cavity. Such structural changes affect both patient mobility and pulmonary function as they cause a decline in the fraction of exhaled volume in 1 second (FEV1) and vital capacity (VC).[45] In patients with osteoporotic vertebral fractures these parameters of pulmonary function are even more affected.[46]

Age-related decreased muscle strength affects inspiratory and expiratory muscles and results in reduced cough strength.[47] Also mucociliary clearance of the lung is diminished with increasing age. Therefore it is important to be attentive to pulmonary infections, to assess pulmonary status regularly and to involve physiotherapy in order to optimize pulmonary function perioperatively.

Older persons show reduced elasticity of the lung and reduced lung parenchyma.[48] In addition to the above structural and muscle function changes, immunological function also decreases with age. Immunosenescence dampens an adequate immune response to immunological threat, complicating the diagnosis of infections in the older person.

CHANGES IN BONE METABOLISM – OSTEOPOROSIS*

Other age-related changes are the loss of total bone mass and the decline in bone integrity resulting in a loss of bone strength. These changes result in increased bone fragility enhancing the risk of fractures and other orthopaedic trauma.[49]

* Also see Chapter 10.

Bone is a living tissue and is metabolically active throughout life. Osteoclasts, deriving from monocytic stem cells (MSC), and osteoblasts and osteocytes, deriving from mesenchymal precursor cells, interact and regulate bone mass, microarchitecture and bone quality. Osteoporosis in most cases is a multifactorial process influencing physiological bone renewal and leading to a loss in bone mass via an imbalance between bone construction and depletion (Figures 2.5 and 2.6).

Osteoporosis is a common condition affecting about 40% of Caucasian post-menopausal women.[50] The prevalence of osteoporosis is expected to increase steadily during the next decades as it is closely associated with increasing age and is influenced by genetic, epigenetic and environmental factors.[51] Osteoporosis is characterized by systemic impairment of bone mass and microarchitecture resulting in fragility fractures defined as fractures resulting from a low trauma event, such as falling from a standing height or less.[52,53] Peak bone mass is attained during the third decade of life, after which the physiological loss of total bone mass is approximately 0.5% per year.[54]

Secondary forms of osteoporosis due to underlying endocrinological problems also increase with age. As geriatric multimorbidity is often associated with polypharmacy, medications such as corticosteroids play an important role. Renal insufficiency and the long-term effects of diabetes and/or atherosclerosis lead to a decline in bone quality,[55] while geriatric syndromes together with cognitive as well as functional decline contribute to the development of gait disturbances with subsequent falls or immobility leading to fragility fractures, or enhance the risk of further bone loss.

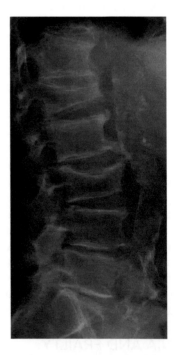

Figure 2.5 X-ray of osteoporotic spine. (Courtesy of Prof. Dr. F. Jakob, Orthopedic Center for Musculoskeletal Research, Experimental and Clinical Osteology, Orthopedic Department, University of Würzburg, Germany.)

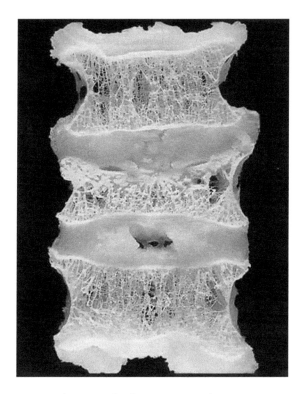

Figure 2.6 Photograph of osteoporotic bone. (Courtesy of Prof. Dr. F. Jakob, Orthopedic Center for Musculoskeletal Research, Experimental and Clinical Osteology, Orthopedic Department University of Würzburg, Germany.)

Cell differentiation and regeneration capacity

The number of MSC in relation to the number of myeloid cells decreases with age. Tissue regeneration is often affected by 'replicative senescence' to avoid proliferation of cells with DNA damage.[56] Senescent cells are still integrated in the tissue but do not take part in regeneration processes. On the other hand, mesenchymal precursor cells are able to produce adipose tissue. It is supposed that with advancing age MSC show an increased readiness to differentiate into adipose tissue.[54,57] Vitamin D has the capacity to inhibit bone marrow adipogenesis.[58]

Vitamin D and calcium

More than 60% of the daily demand of vitamin D is provided by endogenous production in the skin induced by sun exposure (wavelength 280–320 nm). The capacity of the skin to produce vitamin D decreases with skin aging. Therefore, general supplementation appears to be sensible.[59] As the serum level of vitamin D in older people very often is clearly below 75 nmol/L (30 ng/mL) guidelines recommend at least 800 IU vitamin D supplementation per day.[60] This recommended dose will most probably be increased up to 2000 IU per day in years to come when the results of several ongoing trials are published.

Additionally, gastrointestinal resorption of calcium is diminished with increasing age due to decreased production of gastric acid and the reduced vitamin D dependent resorption capacity of the small intestine. Long-term intake of proton-pump inhibitors (PPIs), anatomic changes due to surgery and atrophic gastritis are important factors causing hypochlorhydria. Therefore long-term PPIs should only be prescribed if there is a clear indication, and should be re-evaluated regularly.

Chronic vitamin D deficiency and reduced calcium intake lead to secondary hyperparathyroidism and subsequent decalcification of the bones,[55] so a general calcium intake of 1000 mg daily is recommended.

In addition to these well-known effects of vitamin D, recent evidence has shown other properties of vitamin D such as prevention of osteoblast apoptosis and enhancement of new bone formation by induction of osteoblastogenesis and osteoblastic activity in senescent animals.[61]

Immobilization as a risk factor

Immobilization leads to a decrease in bone and muscle mass as well as an increase in the risk of falling and fracture risk. Many geriatric patients have comorbidities, such as sarcopenia or musculoskeletal diseases, which in turn result in limited mobility and increase the risk of functional impairment.

As immobility is associated with a loss of bone and muscle mass as well as muscle strength, it is a risk factor for the development of osteoporosis and sarcopenia. It is therefore important to avoid any increase in immobilization (see Sarcopenia and frailty section above).

ELDER ABUSE

Elder abuse is a violation of human rights and a significant cause of illness, injury, loss of productivity, isolation and despair. Abuse occurs in people of all ages, but especially in vulnerable people and those dependent on others. An increase in the prevalence of elder abuse can be expected with demographic changes.

Elder abuse can be subdivided into physical abuse, psychological or emotional abuse, sexual abuse, financial or material exploitation, neglect, self-neglect and discriminatory abuse and abandonment.[62] It is associated with increased morbidity and mortality.[63,64] It is estimated to affect more than 6% of the older general population and up to 25% of vulnerable, dependent older people with a big variation across cultures and depending on differences in definitions and assessment tools used in the different studies.[64] Elder abuse and neglect is estimated to cost billions of dollars a year.[1] Despite this high prevalence elder abuse is still under-reported and under-recognized.

The definitions of elder abuse and neglect are highly variable. The WHO definition in the Toronto Declaration on Elder Abuse defines elder abuse as 'a single or repeated act, or lack of appropriate action occurring within any relationship, where there is an expectation of trust, which causes harm or distress to an older person'.[65] This is in accordance with a panel convened by the US National Academy of Sciences which defines elder abuse as '(a) intentional actions that cause harm or create a serious risk of harm (whether or not harm is intended), to a vulnerable elder by a caregiver or other person who stands in a trust relationship to the elder, or (b) failure by a caregiver to satisfy the elder's basic needs or to protect the elder from harm'.[66]

Elder abuse is often underreported due to fear, shame, guilt or cognitive problems. Consequently identification can be difficult. Visits to the general practitioner or the emergency department provide an opportunity to identify mistreated patients. Unexplained falls or unusual locations of bruises can suggest underlying mistreatment and should be followed by a thorough investigation. Further hints indicating elder abuse include a delay in seeking treatment, the presence of injuries in various stages of evolution, inconsistency between the injuries and the information given in the patient history, and contradictions in the history given by the patient and the caregiver, poor hygiene, malnutrition and pressure ulcers.

Mistreatment can be often detected by a direct non-judgmental approach. The American Medical Association recommends a routine enquiry about abuse and mistreatment in geriatric patients, even if signs are absent.[67] Thorough documentation of the history and all findings is essential.

Once elderly patients suffering from abuse are identified, intervention consists of several steps including immediate intervention, long-term intervention and prevention. During this process the balance between the patient's safety and their autonomy should always be kept in mind.[68] Healthcare professionals often need assistance with the reporting of identified cases of elder abuse. Contact with hospital social services is often very helpful. Useful advice can also be found on the website of the National Center on Elder Abuse (NCEA) (http://www.ncea.aoa.gov). Patients should be informed about possible interventions and institutions providing further help.

REFERENCES

1. Carpenter CR, Stern ME. Emergency orthogeriatrics: Concepts and therapeutic alternatives. *Emerg Med Clin North Am* 2010;28:927–949.
2. Peddi R, Morley JE. The physiology of aging. In: Meldon SW, Ma OJ, Woolard R, eds., *Geriatric Emergency Medicine*. New York: McGraw-Hill, 2004, pp. 4–12.
3. Bauer J, Biolo G, Cederholm T, et al. Evidence-based recommendations for optimal dietary protein intake in older people: A position paper from the PROT-AGE Study Group. *J Am Med Dir Assoc* 2013;14:542–559.
4. Kaiser MJ, Bauer JM, Ramsch C, et al. Validation of the Mini Nutritional Assessment short-form (MNA-SF): A practical tool for identification of nutritional status. *J Nutr Health Aging* 2009;13:782–788.
5. Saczynski JS, Marcantonio ER, Quach L, et al. Cognitive trajectories after postoperative delirium. *N Engl J Med* 2012;367:30–39.
6. Krogseth M, Wyller TB, Engedal K, et al. Delirium is an important predictor of incident dementia among elderly hip fracture patients. *Dement Geriatr Cogn Disord* 2011;31:63–70.
7. Inouye SK, Westendorp RG, Saczynski JS. Delirium in elderly people. *Lancet* 2014;383:911–922.
8. Cerejeira J, Firmino H, Vaz-Serra A, et al. The neuroinflammatory hypothesis of delirium. *Acta Neuropathol* 2010;119:737–754.
9. Flacker JM, Cummings V, Mach JR, et al. The association of serum anticholinergic activity with delirium in elderly medical patients. *Am J Geriatr Psychiatry* 1998;6:31–41.
10. Heppner HJ, Cornel S, Peter W, Philipp B, Katrin S. Infections in the elderly. *Crit Care Clin* 2013;29:757–774.
11. Kommission für Krankenhaushygiene und Infektionsprävention am Robert-Koch-Institut. Empfehlungen zur Prävention und Kontrolle Katheter-assoziierter Harnwegsinfektionen. *Bundesgesundheitsblatt Gesundheitsforschung Gesundheitsschutz* 1999;42:806–809.
12. Mody L, Juthani-Metha M. Urinary tract infections in older women: A clinical review. *JAMA* 2014;311:844–854.
13. Ho J, Chan K, Hu W, et al. Aging impacts nasal mucociliary clearance, beat frequency, and ultrastructure of respiratory cilia. *Am J Respir Crit Care Med* 2001;163:983–988.
14. Meyer K. The role of immunity in susceptibility to respiratory infection in the aging lung. *Respir Physiol* 2001;128:23–31.
15. Riquelme R, Torres A, El Ebiary, et al. Community-acquired pneumonia in the elderly. Clinical and nutritional aspects. *Am J Respir Crit Care* 1997;156:1908–1914.
16. Simonetti AF, Viasus D, Garcia-Vidal C, et al. Management of community-acquired pneumonia in older adults. *Ther Adv Infect Dis* 2014;2:3–16.
17. Bhalla MC, Wilber ST, Stiffler KA, et al. Weakness and fatigue in older ED patients in the United States. *Am J Emerg Med* 2014;32:1395–1398.
18. Hogan TM, Losmann ED, Carpenter CR, et al. Development of geriatric competencies for emergency medicine residents using an expert consensus process. *Acad Emerg Med* 2010;17:316–324.
19. Samaras N, Chevalley T, Samaras D, et al. Older patients in the emergency department: A review. *Ann Emerg Med* 2010;56:261–269.
20. Norman DC. Fever in the elderly. *Clin Infect Dis* 2000;31:148–151.

21. Waalen J. Is older colder or colder older? *J Gerontol A Biol Sci Med Sci* 2011;66:487–492.

22. Blatteis CM. Age-dependent changes in temperature regulation—A mini review. *Gerontology* 2012;58:289–295.

23. Singler K, Bertsch T, Heppner HJ, et al. Diagnostic accuracy of three different methods of temperature measurement in acutely ill geriatric patients. *Age Ageing* 2013;42:740–746.

24. Ahkee S, Srinath L, Ramirez J. Community-acquired pneumonia in the elderly: Association of mortality with lack of fever and leukocytosis. *South Med J* 1997;90:296–298.

25. Delerme S, Ray P. Acute respiratory failure in the elderly: Diagnosis and prognosis. *Age Ageing* 2008;37:251–257.

26. International Association for the Study of Pain (IASP). Definition of pain. www.iasp-pain.org (accessed 20 Dec 2014).

27. Morrison RS, Magaziner J, McLaughlin MA, et al. The impact of post-operative pain on outcomes following hip fracture. *Pain* 2003;103:303–311.

28. Shock NW, Greulich RC, Andres R, et al. *Normal Human Aging: Baltimore Longitudinal Study of Aging.* Baltimore, MD: NIH, 1984.

29. Kamel HK, Phlavan M, Malekgoudarzi B, et al. Utilizing pain assessment scales increases the frequency of diagnosing pain among elderly nursing home residents. *J Pain Symptom Manage* 2001;21:450–455.

30. Hilmer SN, Ford GA. General principles of pharmacology. In: Halter JB, Ouslander JG, Tinetti ME, et al., eds., *Principles of Geriatric Medicine and Gerontology,* 6th ed. New York: McGraw-Hill, 2009, pp. 103–123.

31. Terrell KM, Heard K, Miller DK. Prescribing to older ED patients. *Am J Emerg Med* 2006;24:468–478.

32. Blanda MP. Pharmacologic issues in geriatric emergency medicine. *Emerg Med Clin North Am* 2006;24:449–465.

33. Cockcroft DW, Gault MH. Prediction of creatinine clearance from serum creatinine. *Nephron* 1976;16:31–41.

34. Giné-Garriga M, Roque-Figuls M, Coll-Planas L, et al. Physical exercise interventions for improving performance-based measures of physical function in community-dwelling, frail older adults: A systemic review and meta-analysis. *Arch Phys Med Rehabil* 2014;95:753–769.

35. Cooper C, Dere W, Evans W, et al. Frailty and sarcopenia: Definitions and outcome parameters. *Osteoporos Int* 2012;23:1839–1848.

36. Cruz-Jentoft AJ, Landi F, Schneider SM, et al. Prevalence of and interventions for sarcopenia in ageing adults: A systemic review. Report of the International Sarcopenia Initiative (EWGSOP and IWGS). *Age Ageing* 2014;43:748–759.

37. Fried LP, Tangen CM, Walston J, et al. Frailty in older adults: Evidence for a phenotype. *J Gerontol A Biol Sci Med Sci* 2001;56:M146–M156.

38. Farage MA, Miller KW, Elsner P, et al. Functional and physiological characteristics of the aging skin. *Aging Clin Exp Res* 2008;20:195–200.

39. Farage MA, Miller KW, Elsner P, et al. Characteristics of the aging skin. *Adv Wound Care (New Rochelle)* 2013;2:5–10.

40. Grove GL. Physiologic changes in older skin. *Clin Geriatr Med* 1989;5:115.

41. Farage MA, Miller KW, Elsner P, et al. Structural characteristics of the aging skin: A review. *Cutan Ocul Toxicol* 2007;26:343–357.

42. Reichrath J, Lehmann B, Carlberg C, et al. Vitamins as hormones. *Horm Metab Res* 2007;39:71–84.

43. MacLaughlin J, Holick MF. Aging decreased the capacity of human skin to produce vitamin D3. *J Clin Invest* 1985;76:1536–1538.

44. Miniño AM. Death in the United States, 2011. *NCHS Data Brief* 2013;115:1–8.

45. Sharma G, Goodwin J. Effect of aging on respiratory system physiology and immunology. *Clin Interv Aging* 2006;1:253–260.

46. Lombardi I Jr, Oliveira LM, Mayer AF, et al. Evaluation of pulmonary function and quality of life in women with osteoporosis. *Osteoporosis Int* 2005;16:1247–1253.

47. Kim J, Davenport P, Sapienza C. Effect of expiratory muscle strength training on elderly cough function. *Arch Gerontol Geriatr* 2009;48:361–366.

48. Lowery EM, Brubaker AL, Kuhlmann E, et al. The aging lung. *Clin Interv Aging* 2013;8:1489–1496.

49. Lin JT, Lane JM. Osteoporosis: A review. *Clin Orthop Relat Res* 2004;425:126–134.

50. Rachner TD, Khosla S, Hofbauer LC. Osteoporosis: Now and the future. *Lancet* 2011;377:1276–1287.

51. Burge R, Dawson-Hughes B, Solomon DH, Wong JB, King A, Tosteson A. Incidence and economic burden of osteoporosis-related fractures in the United States, 2005–2025. *J Bone Miner Res* 2007;22:465–475.

52. Friedman SM, Mendelson DA. Epidemiology of fragility fractures. *Clin Geriatr Med* 2014;30:175–181.

53. Bouxsein ML, Kaufman J, Tosi L, et al. Recommendations for optimal care of the fragility fracture patient to reduce the risk of future fracture. *J Am Acad Orthop Surg* 2004;12:385–395.

54. Duque G, Troen BR. Understanding the mechanisms of senile osteoporosis: New facts for a major geriatric syndrome. *J Am Geriatr Soc* 2008;56:935–941.

55. Jakob F, Seefried L, Schwab M. Age and osteoporosis: Effects of aging on osteoporosis, the diagnostics and therapy. *Internist (Berl)* 2014;55:755–761.

56. Campisi J. Cancer, aging and cellular senescence. *In Vivo* 2000;14:183–188.

57. Duque G. Bone and fat connection in aging bone. *Curr Opin Rheumatol* 2008;20:429–434.

58. Duque G, Macoritto M, Kremer R. Vitamin D treatment of senescence accelerated mice (SAM-P/6) induces several regulators of stromal cell plasticity. *Biogerontology* 2004;5:421–429.

59. Jakob F, Seefried L, Ebert R. Pathophysiology of bone metabolism. *Internist (Berl)* 2008;49:1159–1160, 1162, 1164.

60. Bischoff-Ferrari HA, Shao A, Dawson-Hughes B, et al. Benefit-risk assessment of vitamin D supplementation. *Osteoporosis Int* 2010;21:1121–1132.

61. Duque G, Macoritto M, Dion N, et al. 1,25 (OH)2D3 acts as a bone-forming agent in the hormone-independent senescence-accelerated mouse (SAM-P/6). *Am J Physiol Endocrinol Metab* 2005;288:E723–E730.

62. National Center on Elder Abuse. Types of elder abuse in domestic settings. Available at http://www.ncea.aoa.gov/Resources/Publication/docs/fact1.pdf (accessed 15 Jul 2014).

63. Lachs MS, Williams CS, O'Brien S, et al. The mortality of elder mistreatment. *J Am Med Assoc* 1998;280:428–432.

64. Cooper C, Selwood A, Livingston G. The prevalence of elder abuse and neglect: A systematic review. *Age Ageing* 2008;37:151–160.

65. WHO. *The Toronto Declaration on the Global Prevention of Elder Abuse*. Geneva: WHO, 2002.

66. Bonnie R, Wallace R, eds. *Elder Mistreatment: Abuse, Neglect, and Exploitation in an Aging America*. Washington, DC: National Academies Press, 2002.

67. American Medical Association. *Diagnostic and Treatment Guidelines on Elder Abuse and Neglect*. Chicago, IL: American Medical Association, 1992, pp. 4–37.

68. Lachs MS, Pillemer K. Elder abuse. *Lancet* 2004;364:1263–1272.

3

Preoperative assessment and care of the elderly

JOSEPH A. NICHOLAS

INTRODUCTION

Like many other geriatric medical topics, preoperative assessment and care practices are heavily informed by the integration of geriatric principles with evidence extrapolated from other populations. There is a paucity of well-validated literature on preoperative risk assessment and management of geriatric surgical patients, and even less concerning the subset of patients undergoing urgent or emergent procedures, for instance following orthopaedic trauma. For these reasons, the existing literature in these areas can be best used as a starting point for practice recommendations and then further modified for the unique and varied physiologies and vulnerabilities of older adults.

The lack of explicit evidence-based guidelines for each preoperative clinical issue can be a source of frustration and skepticism for clinicians, especially for those hoping to access uniform and detailed algorithms for the preoperative assessment and optimization of fragility fracture patients. Despite this, centres using a standardized geriatric medicine approach to preoperative care have reliably demonstrated improved outcomes in mortality, length of stay and reduction in complications.[1-3] This chapter focuses on the strategies used by many of these centers and describe the unique physiologic considerations of the geriatric trauma patient, medical, cognitive and functional status assessment, preoperative risk assessment, preoperative testing and medical optimization for surgery.

MAJOR GOALS IN THE PREOPERATIVE PERIOD

In contrast to patients undergoing elective procedures, the preoperative care for older adults with acute trauma is additionally focused on pain control and preoperative hemodynamic stability and avoidance of functional decline (Table 3.1). Early surgery is typically the most important means to achieve these goals, and the preoperative medical assessment needs to prioritize early surgery and early mobility over most other clinical issues. For these reasons, high performing geriatric fracture centers have implemented clinical pathways that emphasize timely transition to operative repair, even in highly comorbid or frail older adults. Many notable comorbidities warranting more intensive preoperative testing and consultation prior to elective surgery are not vigorously pursued in the urgent surgical setting.

UNIQUE PHYSIOLOGIC CONSIDERATIONS

The older adult is prone to exaggerated hypotension in the perioperative period.[4] This is a predictable consequence of cardiovascular aging and often exacerbated by commonly used cardiovascular medications (including antihypertensive and antianginal medications) as well as opioid analgesic and other anaesthetic medications. The heart and vascular tree undergo significant losses in elasticity and compliance over time and result in secondary clinical problems including impaired ventricular

Table 3.1 Major goals of the preoperative period

Hemodynamic stabilization
Pain control
Perioperative risk assessment
Timely preoperative optimization

Table 3.2 Nottingham Hip Fracture Score

Variable	Value	Points
Age (years)	66–85	3
	≥86	4
Sex	Male	1
Admission hemoglobin	<10 g/dL	1
Mini-mental test score	<6/10	1
Living in an institution	Yes	1
Number of comorbidities	≥2	1
Malignancy	Yes	1

Source: Adapted from Maxwell MJ, et al. *Br J Anaesth* 2008;101:511–17.

filling, widened pulse pressure, diastolic hypotension and elevated atrial pressures. Even in patients without a demonstrated impairment on resting echocardiography, the older heart is less able to easily respond to blood loss, pain and vasodilation. The aging of the autonomic nervous and cardiac conduction systems also results in impaired neurocardioprotective reflexes, postural hypotension and limited ability to compensate for volume loss or vasodilation.[5] Large drops in intraoperative blood pressure can be common and severe, even in patients whose preoperative blood pressure is normal or elevated. While this is well known in the anesthesia literature, it may be underappreciated by medical physicians and surgeons.

In addition, older adults are more prone to a number of serious and potentially conflicting perioperative complications, including excessive bleeding and thrombosis, agitated delirium and lethargy. While not the focus of this chapter, the initial preoperative plan is important to minimize the development of these common complications. Further discussion of postoperative complications can be found in Chapter 7.

Many fragility fractures occur in patients with multiorgan age and disease-related impairments, producing a general state of *decreased physiologic reserve.*[6] This concept is useful as an overarching paradigm to explain the diversity of complications that can emerge in older adults, as well as to reinforce the central role of general strategies to minimize stress (including intravascular volume depletion), immobility and pain.

PREOPERATIVE RISK ASSESSMENT

For all but the most critically ill patients, the benefits of operative fracture repair (hemostasis, pain control, mobilization) will exceed the risks related to anesthesia and surgery. This is due both to advanced anesthetic and surgical techniques and to the excessive morbidity and mortality of the hip fracture patients in the absence of surgical repair. One of the major goals of the preoperative assessment is to estimate the risk of poor surgical outcomes, including cardiovascular complications, stroke and death. Patient specific risks can be roughly estimated with the careful and limited use of preoperative risk calculators.

Risk calculators

The Nottingham Hip Fracture Score[7] is the best-validated instrument for predicting 30-day and longer outcomes in the hip fracture population and incorporates measures

of comorbidity burden, functional status (type of residence), cognitive status (mini-mental test score) and key demographic factors (age, sex). Some elements (institutionalization, mini-mental test score) are not universally uniform across different international settings but likely can be approximated and remain useful for estimating perioperative risk and short-term outcomes (Table 3.2).

A number of additional calculators have been developed in an attempt to provide a reasonable estimate of serious complications in surgical patients; none are validated in older adults undergoing urgent orthopaedic surgery. Three calculators that were examined in the most recent American College of Cardiology/American Heart Association (ACC/AHA) guidelines include the Revised Cardiac Risk Index (RCRI),[8] the Myocardial Infarction or Cardiac Arrest (MICA) calculator[9] and the American College of Surgeons' National Surgical Quality Improvement Project (ACS NSQIP) risk calculator[10] (Table 3.3). Each calculator has strengths and weaknesses; the RCRI is by far the most common of these and has been incorporated into studies of older adults with hip fractures. Although they have outperformed the RCRI in initial studies, neither the MICA nor the NSQIP calculators have been well validated outside of a single center or cohort. While all three attempt to address procedure specific risk and comorbidity measures, the NSQIP and the MICA also incorporate a gross measure of functional status. The standard RCRI may be improved[11] by removing the diabetes criteria and substituting a glomerular filtration rate of less than 30 mL/min for the original creatinine criteria (serum creatinine greater than 2 mg/dL). In light of these considerations, any of the three calculators will likely give a reasonable estimate of risk that can be further adjusted based on patient specific trajectory and reserve.

Biomarkers

Patients with elevated biomarkers (B-type natriuretic peptide and troponin assays) have been shown to have a significantly increased risk of perioperative morbidity and mortality,[12,13] but the optimal ways to use these measures in this setting remain unclear. There is no evidence that treatment aimed at these biomarkers is helpful, and there is concern that abnormal findings may inappropriately delay

Table 3.3 Risk assessment calculators

Calculator	Predictor elements	Strengths	Weaknesses
RCRI	CAD history CHF history TIA/CVA history Diabetes CKD (creatinine >2 g/dL) High risk surgery (intrathoracic, intraperitoneal, suprainguinal vascular) ≤2 predictors, 6.6% perioperative event rate ≥3 predictors, 11% perioperative event rate	Validated in hip fracture population Simple	Does not incorporate functional status Does not incorporate procedure specific risks
MICA calculator	Age CKD (creatinine >1.5 g/dL) ASA class Preoperative functional status Procedure	Includes functional status Includes procedure specific risks Simple online calculators available May outperform RCRI	Not validated in multiple populations Not validated in urgent surgery
ACS NSQIP	Multiple patient and procedure specific factors	Most comprehensive assessment	Most cumbersome Not widely validated outside of original cohort

Note: ACS NSQIP, American College of Surgeons' National Surgical Quality Improvement Project risk calculator[10]; ASA, American Society of Anesthesiologists; CAD, coronary artery disease; CHF, congestive heart failure; CKD, chronic kidney disease; CVA, cerebrovascular accident; MICA, Myocardial Infarction or Cardiac Arrest calculator[9]; RCRI, Revised Cardiac Risk Index[8]; TIA, transient ischemic attack.

Table 3.4 Barthel Index of Activities of Daily Living

Activities	Scoring (range of responses), maximum score 20
Bowels	0–2 points (incontinent–fully continent)
Bladder	0–2 points (incontinent–fully continent)
Grooming	0–1 point (needs help–independent)
Toilet use	0–2 points (dependent–independent)
Feeding	0–2 points (dependent–independent)
Transfer	0–3 points (unable–independent)
Mobility	0–3 points (immobile–independent without device)
Dressing	0–2 points (dependent–independent)
Stairs	0–2 points (unable–independent)
Bathing	0–1 point (dependent–independent)

Source: Adapted from Mahoney F, Barthel D. Md Med J 1965;14:61–5.

surgery or prompt potentially harmful interventions (acute diuresis, antithrombotic treatment) in hemodynamically and hemostatically unstable patients. Further prospective studies will be needed.

Other assessments of prognostic importance

Despite the historical emphasis on comorbidity scoring for estimating surgical risk, there has been increasing recognition that other assessments may also play an important role in correctly stratifying patients and predicting outcomes. These assessments aimed at functional status, cognition, exercise capacity and nutritional status may provide significant predictive ability, and, in some cases (nutrition), stimulate helpful interventions. Functional and cognitive impairments have long been recognized in geriatric medicine to predict outcomes including mortality,[14] and measures of both function and cognition are beginning to be embedded in some preoperative risk assessments.

Functional assessments

Although the details are beyond the scope of this chapter, functional dependence is often evaluated by activities of daily living (ADL) scoring (e.g. the Barthel Index) (Table 3.4).[15] The Parker Mobility Score is a simple measure of function that has been derived and validated in the hip fracture setting and evaluated in multiple settings and for multiple important outcomes including mortality[16] and postsurgical independence[17] (Table 3.5).

Cognitive assessments

Impaired cognition is significantly associated with functional dependence and poor outcomes and by itself is often a marker of increased perioperative risks and postoperative dependency.[18] Patients with a pre-existing diagnosis of dementia have a significant risk of mortality at

Table 3.5 New Mobility Scale (Parker Mobility Scale)

Mobility	No difficulty	With a device	With assistance	Unable
Gets about within residence	3	2	1	0
Gets about outside residence	3	2	1	0
Able to go shopping	3	2	1	0

New mobility total score	1 year mortality
<5	51%
≥5	20%

Source: Adapted from Parker MJ, Palmer CR. J Bone Joint Surg 1993;75-B:797–8.

6 months. For patients without a pre-existing diagnosis, diagnostic assessment for dementia is often not possible during the preoperative period, in light of the high prevalence of delirium. In these situations historical features can often suggest underlying cognitive impairment; impairments in telephone use, handling of finances and medication self-administration best correlate with underlying dementia.[19]

Exercise capacity

Exercise capacity is used as a surrogate for functional capacity and physiologic reserve and has been incorporated into the ACC/AHA guidelines to distinguish between high and low risk patients, using a threshold of four metabolic equivalents of task (METs). Common activities that meet this threshold include walking up a flight of stairs, walking up a hill, walking on level ground at a minimum pace of 4 mph, or heavy housework (scrubbing floors, moving heavy furniture). For patients undergoing elective surgery, these guidelines suggest that patients who can perform this level of exertion do not require additional cardiovascular testing preoperatively.

Nutritional status

Malnutrition[20] is highly prevalent in hip fracture patients and is suggested by low body mass index, low serum albumin or significant unintentional weight loss.[21] It is independently associated with poor perioperative and postoperative outcomes and can further inform prognostication for older adults. Simple historical tools to identify patients with weight loss and routine albumin testing can both be incorporated into preoperative assessment practices.

PREOPERATIVE TESTING

In an attempt to minimize surgical delay, pain and delirium, the standard preoperative evaluation should consist of only essential radiographic studies, bedside clinical evaluation by medical, surgical and anesthesiology teams and basic serum blood work and electrocardiography. Observational studies suggest that excellent perioperative outcomes can be obtained with protocols that emphasize plain radiography of the fracture, hemoglobin levels and platelet counts, basic serum electrolytes and renal function and a resting electrocardiogram[22] (Table 3.6). Additional studies to identify contributors to metabolic bone disease (calcium and phosphorus, parathyroid hormone, thyroid hormone, vitamin D levels) or help identify malnutrition (albumin levels) can be obtained preoperatively as well, although the results of these studies are not essential prior to proceeding to surgical fixation. Order sets and protocols for fragility fracture patients can help streamline this preoperative testing process and help minimize inappropriate variation in care.[23]

Bedside clinical evaluation remains the cornerstone of preoperative assessment and should be focused on the assessment of intravascular volume status and the rapid identification of the small numbers of active medical conditions that would warrant surgical delay, including acute pulmonary oedema, acute coronary syndrome, sepsis, unstable arrhythmias or acute stroke.

For most fragility fracture patients there is no demonstrated benefit to routine advanced investigations such as echocardiography, non-invasive cardiovascular stress testing or prolonged preoperative cardiac rhythm monitoring. Retrospective studies suggest that routine intensive cardiovascular testing, including routine echocardiography, results in significant surgical delay without any clinically important changes in management.[24,25] In addition, the preoperative care teams should carefully avoid preoperative workup of otherwise stable chronic comorbidities (e.g. chronic renal failure, chronic stable coronary disease and chronic neurologic deficits); there is no known benefit to more intensive workup and consultation prior to fracture fixation. Other routine tests of uncertain preoperative impact include routine urinalysis, chest radiography and biomarker assays (BNP and troponin). The high incidence of asymptomatic bacteria in older adults (particularly women) can result in complications related to inappropriate antimicrobial use, and abnormal biomarker levels may prompt acute interventions that may promote hypotension, bleeding and surgical delay.

Table 3.6 Basic preoperative testing

Blood counts (hemoglobin, hematocrit, platelet counts)
Serum electrolytes
Renal function
Resting electrocardiogram
Plain radiography of fracture
Metabolic bone studies (vitamin D, calcium, phosphorus, parathyroid hormone, thyroid studies)

Until there are better prospective data supporting routine use of biomarker assays in fragility fracture patients, these should be limited in this setting to symptomatic patients.

PREOPERATIVE TREATMENTS

In addition to clinical assessments and risk stratification, preoperative optimization typically requires a small set of interventions to minimize surgical delay and intraoperative hypotension.

Intravascular volume restoration

Most older adults with femur fractures suffer from acute intravascular volume depletion. This is a predictable result of bleeding at the fracture site and decreased enteral intake surrounding the fracture workup. Signs often thought to be consistent with volume overload (elevated jugular venous pressure, peripheral oedema) are very non-specific findings in many older adults, and their presence should not limit an initial trial of volume restoration in most acutely fractured patients. In addition, adequate volume restoration may serve to mitigate the exaggerated intraoperative hypotension seen in older adults, that is a result of neurocardiovascular instability and anesthetic and analgesic induced vasodilation. Initial hemoglobin assessment prior to volume restoration can significantly underestimate the degree of anemia, and blood loss can continue until the fracture is reduced. Acute blood loss can be enhanced by antithrombotic and anticoagulant medications, many of which have a prolonged effect in older adults.

Most published reviews support the initiation of isotonic intravenous fluids as soon as possible for patients not in clinically significant acute pulmonary oedema. Geriatric fracture centers typically report preoperative hemoglobin targets of 10 mg/dL, in anticipation of further blood loss during the perioperative period.[26]

In general, it is easier to treat the consequences of pulmonary oedema from overhydration than to manage those related to volume depletion (hypotension, stroke and renal failure), justifying the routine use of intravenous fluids in the preoperative setting.

Pain control

Acute pain control is another cornerstone to acute preoperative care for fragility fracture patients. Inadequate pain control is associated with increased adrenergic drive and myocardial oxygen demand and can contribute to a number of perioperative complications including delirium, tachyarrhythmia and myocardial infarction.

Pain control is one of the reasons that early surgical fixation is associated with improved postoperative complications. In the preoperative phase, most published protocols use standard doses of intravenous opiates to achieve adequate pain control. Morphine sulfate, hydromorphone and oxycodone have all been shown to be effective and

safe when used in adjusted doses for frail older adults. In addition, there is a growing body of literature on the safety and efficacy of blocks of the femoral nerve and other local nerves, particularly with ultrasound guidance.[27] Successful nerve blocks can produce faster time to analgesia and result in less opiate use for the duration of the block. Intravenous acetaminophen/paracetamol has not been well studied in this population but is expected to be helpful as well, although its use may be limited by cost in many institutions.

Medication management

One of the most problematic and nuanced areas in preoperative and perioperative optimization is the management of chronic medications in older adults. Each medication should be evaluated for its potential efficacy or harm in the acute fracture setting, and the risk of continuation, acute cessation or, in the case of some anticoagulants, reversal, determined.

Antihypertensive medications

The high risk of perioperative hypotension in the elderly fracture patient makes the routine continuation of chronic blood pressure medications particularly dangerous in this setting. With the exception of beta blockers and clonidine, acute cessation of most other commonly used antihypertensive medications is not highly problematic.

Beta blockers

Perioperative beta blocker recommendations have undergone dramatic changes over the past 10 years, and the initiation of beta blockers in patients in this setting is no longer recommended in the most recent ACC/AHA and European Society of Cardiology (ESC) guidelines. This comes on the heels of several studies that failed to confirm the benefit of beta blockade initiated for non-vascular surgery, as well as a single large randomized controlled trial that demonstrated harm (hypotension and stroke) in excess of a reduction in myocardial ischemia.[28] In addition, a series of studies that supported the titration of perioperative beta blockers in elective non-cardiovascular surgery were retracted over integrity concerns.[29] The strongest applicable recommendations for geriatric fracture patients remain: continuation of chronic beta blocker therapy and avoidance of initiation of beta blockers in the perioperative setting. Dose attenuation of beta blockers may still be required in patients with perioperative hypotension.

Angiotensin converting enzyme inhibitors/receptor blockers

Angiotensin converting enzyme inhibitors/receptor blockers (ACEI/ARB) are known to cause hypotension and acute kidney injury in the perioperative setting,[30,31] as well as to contribute to acute kidney injury in haemodynamically unstable patients.[32] In stable patients undergoing elective surgical procedures, both the ACC/AHA and ESC guidelines allow for continuation or cessation of ACEI/ARB depending on patient specific risks and the ability to closely monitor blood pressure and renal function. In the typical fragility fracture patient with increased risks for hypotension and acute renal failure, routine cessation of ACE/ARBs in the preoperative period can be justified.

Statins

Both the ACC/AHA and the ESC guidelines support the continuation of statin therapy for patients already taking them. There is no evidence for the acute initiation of statin therapy in patients undergoing urgent non-vascular surgery.

Calcium channel blockers

The distinction between non-dihydropyridine (i.e. verapamil and diltiazem) and dihydropyridine calcium channel blockers (e.g. amlodipine and felodipine) is important, as the former often have a role in rate control of chronic or episodic tachycardias. Abrupt cessation of verapamil or diltiazem should be weighed against the risks of hypotension. Dihydropyridine agents do not produce clinically significant heart rate control and can be held with less risk for perioperative tachycardia.

Diuretics

In light of the concerns for intravascular volume depletion in the acute fracture patient, all diuretics are typically held in the preoperative period.

Noncardiovascular medications

Oral diabetic medications will typically need to be held preoperatively to avoid clinically significant hypoglycaemia in the perioperative phase. Patients using insulin chronically will also need attenuation of chronic insulin doses; the use of frequent blood sugar monitoring and short acting insulin is the safest approach in the dynamic perioperative period. Patients on chronic psychiatric medications will often need these continued, although dose attenuation or temporary cessation in the event of excessive sedation or other side effects may need to be considered. Patients on chronic opiate or benzodiazepine therapy are at risk for withdrawal with abrupt cessation, and parenteral replacement may be necessary if patients are not able to take oral medications in the perioperative setting. Patients on chronic opiate therapy may need to have augmented doses of opiates to overcome tolerance and achieve effective pain relief. Overall, patients require routine monitoring for acute toxicity and complications of chronic medications in the dynamic perioperative setting.

MANAGEMENT OF PREOPERATIVE ANTICOAGULATION AND THROMBOSIS

Older fracture patients are at increased risk for both thrombosis and excessive perioperative bleeding. In addition, many fragility fracture patients are managed with chronic antithrombotic and anticoagulant medications for a diverse number of conditions including coronary artery disease, cerebrovascular disease, peripheral arterial disease, atrial fibrillation and valvular heart disease. Management of anticoagulation in the perioperative setting is as much art as science, and the impact of the use or cessation of anticoagulant medication needs to be closely monitored until the patient has recovered. In the preoperative setting, almost all antithrombotic and anticoagulant medications should be held or reversed, with resumption depending on the attainment of adequate hemostasis and on the risk of thrombosis for particular indications.[33]

Management of chronic antithrombotic treatment

For patients on chronic antithrombotic treatment, there is no effective reversal agent for either aspirin or adenosine diphosphate (ADP) receptor inhibitors (clopidogrel, prasugrel, ticlopidine), and their antiplatelet effect can persist for 5–10 days, depending on the agent and the patient. Despite concerns about clinically significant bleeding related to the more potent ADP receptor inhibitors, retrospective reviews have failed to show significantly increased bleeding complications in patients undergoing urgent surgery.[34] Most high performing fracture centers stop aspirin and other antiplatelet agents in the preoperative setting and proceed to surgery within 24 hours.

Management of chronic warfarin therapy

Patients on chronic vitamin K antagonist (VKA) therapy (e.g. warfarin and coumarol) should be considered for urgent reversal of anticoagulation, both to promote hemodynamic stability by stemming fracture related blood loss and to allow for safe surgical reduction as soon as possible. Surgical delay until spontaneous resolution of anticoagulation is not typically recommended, mostly due to the extremely long half-life of VKAs in elderly patients.[35] Options for reversal include vitamin K and factor replacement.

Vitamin K administration (2.5–5 mg oral or IV) begins to take effect in 6–12 hours and may be all that is required if surgical repair is not possible in that time frame. Oral vitamin K has the advantage of enteral circulation to its hepatic site of action; intravenous administration is also rapidly available to the liver for synthesis of clotting factors. Vitamin K reversal will have a longer duration of action than reversal with plasma-derived factor replacement; this may further limit postoperative bleeding but may also make postoperative restoration of full anticoagulation with VKAs more problematic.

Plasma infusions have the advantage of more urgent reversal and can typically reverse VKA anticoagulation within hours. The amount of plasma required depends on the degree of anticoagulation and size of the patient, but its effect can be reliably determined with international normalized ratio (INR) monitoring and can reduce the INR to approximately 1.6 in most patients.[36] Risks include volume overload for hypervolemic patients and adverse reactions to plasma.

Prothrombin complex concentrate (PCC) is a combination of multiple plasma-derived factors (II, VII, IX, X, Protein C and Protein S) and is a highly effective and concentrated way to rapidly reverse anticoagulation.[37] Its expense limits more widespread and routine use, and it is typically reserved for emergency reversal of severe coagulopathy.

Patients at high risk for perioperative arterial and venous thrombosis (mechanical heart valves, intracardiac thrombosis, hypercoagulable disorders) will be candidates for 'bridging therapy' in the postoperative setting, using unfractionated heparins (UFH) or low-molecular weight heparins (LMWH) to achieve rapid anticoagulation until oral anticoagulants can be safely resumed. The dose and timing of bridging therapy should be individualized based on postoperative hemostasis and stability; consultation with hematology and cardiology during the preoperative phase may facilitate this planning.[33]

Management of non-vitamin K oral anticoagulants

The development of non-vitamin K oral anticoagulants (NOACs) further complicates the preoperative management of fracture patients, particularly in light of the current lack of effective antidotes, monitoring and the variable half-life of these medications in older adults. Both the direct thrombin inhibitors (dabigatran) and factor Xa inhibitors (e.g. rivaroxaban, apixaban and edoxaban) have variable clearance in patients with chronically or transiently impaired renal function; this is particularly problematic for dabigatran due to its high renal excretion rate. Hemodialysis (for dabigatran) and PCC administration (for all agents) may be partially effective, but will not reliably produce complete reversal of anticoagulation in a rapid time frame.[38] Most patients require at least a surgical delay of 48 hours to make surgical intervention reasonably safe. Close consultation with hematology is typically necessary to individualize safe surgical timing.

Prophylaxis against venous thromboembolism

In hemodynamically stable patients for whom surgical repair will occur more than 12 hours after presentation, it is reasonable to initiate deep vein thrombosis (DVT) prophylaxis with UFH or LMWH, particularly if non-pharmacologic methods are not well tolerated. Typical doses include enoxaparin 40 mg q 24 hours (further adjusted if significant renal impairment), UFH 5000 units q 8–12 hours or dalteparin 5000 units q 24 hours. Subcutaneous doses of UFH or LMWH should not be given later than 12 hours prior to surgery, to ensure adequate clearance prior to repair.[39] It is important to consider that frail elderly patients can achieve very high levels of anticoagulation on DVT prophylaxis dose LMWH, due to renal impairment and decreased lean body mass.

OTHER PREOPERATIVE ISSUES

There are a number of common perioperative medical complications that impact postsurgical outcomes; many of these develop or require intervention in the postoperative period. Co-management with a general medical service with experience with common geriatric syndromes is essential to optimal outcomes. Some of these issues emerge in the preoperative phase and will be introduced here.

Delirium

Delirium is an acute, waxing and waning change in mental status marked by deficits in attention and often complicated by agitation, lethargy or disorganized thinking. It is common in hospitalized older adults, particularly in those with underlying cognitive disorders including dementia. Delirium can be provoked by underlying medical issues (Table 3.7), which should always be sought. In the preoperative setting, uncontrolled pain should be strongly considered, particularly in patients with no other obvious cause. Initial attempts at management should include treating underlying clinical issues, optimizing pain control and attempting non-pharmacologic supports like reorientation, decreasing excessive stimulation and restoring eyeglasses and hearing aids. For severe agitation or distress, low dose haloperidol (0.5 mg IV or oral) can be administered safely in most patients. Delirium is not a contraindication to surgical fixation; fracture reduction and mobilization may be necessary to promote resolution.

Urinary retention

Urinary retention can be due to a number of contributing factors, including pain, delirium and prostatic hypertrophy and is a common side effect of opioid medications. Bedside physical exam and bladder scan can assist with

Table 3.7 Common causes of delirium

Pain
Medication toxicity (anticholinergics, benzodiazepines)
Withdrawal states (alcohol, illicit and prescription drugs)
Metabolic abnormalities (hypernatremia, hypercalcemia, renal failure, hypoxia)
Urinary retention
Severe constipation
Infection (urinary tract, pneumonia)
Sensory deprivation (hearing loss and visual loss)

the diagnosis. Urinary catheterization carries risks, such as infection, urinary bleeding and delirium and should be used judiciously.

Polypharmacy

In light of the number of competing acute and chronic issues faced by most older adults, polypharmacy and its effects can be viewed as a distinct clinical issue. Polypharmacy is associated with delirium, functional decline and poor surgical outcomes. In addition to avoiding poorly tolerated classes of medications (anticholinergic agents, benzodiazepines), careful reduction in the number and doses of other medications may be helpful in optimizing outcomes.

INDIVIDUALIZING CARE

This chapter has painted in broad strokes the most common issues and approaches encountered in the preoperative setting, but the medical management of almost all geriatric patients requires attention to the unique goals, physiologies and treatment responses of each patient. Osteoporotic fractures often occur in the frailest adults in the last stage of life and the presence of other degenerative diseases (e.g. dementia and end stage cardiomyopathy) warrants acknowledgement in this setting as well. Goals of care may differ widely for patients with similar fractures, depending on their functional potential, life expectancy and personal values. In addition to important communication between the medical, surgical and anesthesiology teams, interdisciplinary communication with nursing and social work as well as the patient and their family is often required to achieve appropriate outcomes for each patient.

CONCLUSION

Preoperative care of geriatric fracture patients is essential to ensuring optimal surgical and functional outcomes. Standardized practice that emphasizes intravascular volume restoration, pain control and early surgery while avoiding iatrogenic harm can best be achieved through informed medical co-management using geriatric principles.

REFERENCES

1. Ellis Folbert EC, Smit RS, van der Velde D, et al. Geriatric fracture center: A multidisciplinary approach for older patients with hip fracture improved quality of clinical care and short term outcomes. *Geriatr Orthop Surg Rehabil* 2012;3:259–67.
2. Fisher AA, Davis MW, Rubenach SE, et al. Outcomes for older patients with hip fractures: The impact of orthopedic and geriatric medicine cocare. *J Orthop Trauma* 2006;20(3):172–80.
3. Friedman SM, Mendelson DA, Bingham KW, et al. Impact of a comanaged geriatric fracture center on short-term hip fracture outcomes. *Arch Intern Med* 2009;169(18):1712–17.
4. Alecu C, Cuignet-Royer E, Mertes PM, et al. Pre-existing arterial stiffness can predict hypotension during induction of anaesthesia in the elderly. *Br J Anaesth* 2010;105(5):585–8.
5. Cheitlin MD. Cardiovascular physiology – changes with aging. *Am J Geriatr Cardiol* 2003;12(1):9–13.
6. Buchner DM, Wagner EH. Preventing frail health. *Clin Geriatr Med* 1992;8(1):1–17.
7. Maxwell MJ, Moran CG, Moppett IK. Development and validation of a preoperative scoring system to predict 30 day mortality in patients undergoing hip fracture surgery. *Br J Anaesth* 2008;101(4):511–17.
8. Lee TH, Marcantonio ER, Mangione CM, et al. Derivation and prospective validation of a simple index for prediction of cardiac risk of major noncardiac surgery. *Circulation* 1999;100:1043–9.
9. Gupta PK, Gupta H, Sundaram A, et al. Development and validation of a risk calculator for prediction of cardiac risk after surgery. *Circulation* 2011;124:381–7.
10. Bilimoria KY, Liu Y, Paruch JL, et al. Development and evaluation of the universal ACS NSQIP surgical risk calculator: A decision aid and informed consent tool for patients and surgeons. *Journal of the American College of Surgeons* 2013;217(5):833–842.
11. Davis C, Tait G, Carroll J, et al. The Revised Cardiac Risk Index in the new millennium: A single-center prospective cohort re-evaluation of the original variables in 9,519 consecutive elective surgical patients. *Can J Anaesth* 2013;60:855–63.
12. Karthikeyan G, Moncur RA, Levine O, et al. Is a pre-operative brain natriuretic peptide or N-terminal pro-B-type natriuretic peptide measurement an independent predictor of adverse cardiovascular outcomes within 30 days of non-cardiac surgery? A systematic review and meta-analysis of observational studies. *J Am Coll Cardiol* 2009;54:1599–606.
13. Chong CP, Lam QT, Ryan JE, et al. Incidence of post operative troponin I rises and 1-year mortality after emergency orthopedic surgery in older patients. *Age Ageing* 2009;38(2):168–74.
14. Penrod JD, Litke MA, Hawkes WG, et al. Heterogeneity in hip fracture patients: Age, functional status and comorbidity. *J Am Geriatr Soc* 2007;55(3):407–13.
15. Mahoney F, Barthel D. Functional evaluation: The Barthel index. *Md Med J* 1965;14:61–5.
16. Parker MJ, Palmer CR. A new mobility score for predicting mortality after hip fracture. *J Bone Joint Surg* 1993;75-B:797–8.
17. Kristensen MT, Foss NB, Ekdahl C, Kehlet H. Prefracture functional level evaluated by the New Mobility Score predicts in-hospital outcome after hip fracture surgery. *Acta Orthop* 2010;81(3):296–302.

18. Seitz, DP, Adunuri N, Gill SG, et al. Prevalence of dementia and cognitive impairment among older adults with hip fractures. *J Am Med Dir Assoc* 2011;12(8):556–64.

19. Cromwell DA, Eagar K, Poulos RG. The performance of instrumental activity of daily living scale in screening for cognitive impairment in elderly community residents. *J Clin Epidemiol* 2003;56(2):131–7.

20. Lumbers M, New SA, Givson S, et al. Nutritional status in elderly female hip fracture patients: Comparison with an age-match home living group attending day centers. *Br J Nutr* 2001;85:733–40.

21. Chow WB, Rosenthal RA, Merkow RP, et al. Optimal preoperative assessment of the geriatric patient: A best practices guideline from the American College of Surgeons national Surgical Quality Improvement Program and the American Geriatrics Society. *J Am Coll Surg* 2012;215(4):453–66.

22. Friedman SM, Mendelson DA, Bingham KW, et al. Impact of a comanaged geriatric fracture center on short-term hip fracture outcomes. *Arch Intern Med* 2009;169(18):1712–17.

23. Friedman SM, Mendelson DA, Kates SL, et al. Geriatric co-management of proximal femur fractures. *J Am Geriatr Soc* 2008;56:1349–56.

24. Ricci WM, Della Rocca GJ, Combs C, Borelli J. The medical and economic impact of preoperative cardiac testing in elderly patients with hip fractures. *Injury* 2007;38:S39–42.

25. O'hEireamhoin S, Beyer T, Ahmed M, Mullhall KJ. The role of preoperative cardiac testing in emergency hip surgery. *J Trauma* 2011;71(5):1345–7.

26. Nicholas JA. Preoperative optimization and risk assessment. *Clin Geriatr Med* 2014;30:207–18.

27. Brener S. *Nerve Blocks for Pain Management in Patients with Hip Fractures: A Rapid Review.* Toronto, ON: Health Quality Ontario, 2013.

28. Devereauz PJ, Yang H, Usef S, et al. Effects of extended-release metoprolol succinate in patients undergoing non-cardiac surgery (POISE) trial: A randomized controlled trial. *Lancet* 2008;371(9627):1839–47.

29. Notice of Concern. *J Am Coll Cardiol.* 2012;60(25):2696–2697.

30. Cittanova ML, Zubicki A, Savo C, et al. The chronic inhibition of angiotensin-converting enzyme impairs post operative renal function. *Anesth Analg* 2001;93:1111–15.

31. Arora P, Rajagopalam S, Ranjan R, et al. Preoperative use of angiotensin-converting enzyme inhibitors/ angiotensin receptor blockers is associated with increased risk for acute kidney injury and cardiovascular surgery. *Clin J Am Soc Nephrol* 2008;3(5):1266–73.

32. Onuigbo MA. Reno-prevention vs. reno-protection: A critical re-appraisal of the evidence-base from the large RAAS blockade trials after ONTARGET–a call for more circumspection. *QJM* 2009;102(3):155–67.

33. Douketis JD, Spyropoulos AC, Spencer FA, et al. Perioperative management of antithrombotic therapy: Antithrombotic Therapy and Prevention of Thrombosis, 9th ed: American College of Chest Physicians Evidence-Based Clinical Practice Guidelines. *Chest* 2012;141(4):1129.

34. Nydick JD, Farrell ED, Marcantonio AJ, et al. The use of clopidogrel (Plavix) in patients undergoing nonelective orthopedic surgery. *J Orthop Trauma* 2010;24(6):383–6.

35. Gleason LJ, Mendelson DA, Kates SL, Friedman SM. Anticoagulation management in individuals with hip fracture. *J Am Geriatr Soc* 2014;61(1):159–64.

36. Rashidi A, Tahhan HR. Fresh frozen plasma dosing for warfarin reversal: A practical formula. *Mayo Clin Proc* 2013;88:244–50.

37. Frumkin K. Rapid reversal of warfarin-associated hemorrhage in the emergency room by prothrombin complex concentrates. *Ann Emerg Med* 2013;62(6):616–26.

38. Lazo-Langner A, Lang ES, Douketis JD. Clinical review: Clinical management of new oral anticoagulants: A structured review with emphasis on the reversal of bleeding complications. *Crit Care* 2013;17:230.

39. Yngve FY, Francis CW, Johanson NA. Prevention of VTE in orthopedic surgery patients: American College of Chest Physicians Evidence Based Practice Guidelines. *Chest* 2012;141(2 Suppl):e278S–325S.

4

The orthogeriatric team approach to the management of the elderly

RICHARD D. SOUTHGATE AND STEPHEN L. KATES

INTRODUCTION

Hip fractures are a serious public health issue worldwide. There are an estimated 330,000 hip fractures annually in the United States.[1] Age is a major risk factor, with those over the age of 85 at greatest risk for hip fractures.[2] Since this age group is the fastest growing segment of the population,[3] the incidence of these injuries will assuredly increase in the coming decades.

Not only are hip fractures common, but these injuries carry with them a high incidence of complications, with studies consistently reporting a 3% inpatient mortality and a 21–23% 1-year mortality.[1,4,5] For those who survive the initial treatment, long-term disability is common. Half of these patients fail to regain their prefracture level of mobility,[6] and 25% of those who lived independently will require long-term nursing home care.[7]

Elderly hip fracture patients often have several comorbid conditions which affect the outcome of care. While almost all hip fractures require surgical treatment, medical physicians are most able to manage the patient's comorbid medical conditions. Geriatricians are expert at caring for medically complex hip fracture patients.[8] Aside from medical problems, geriatricians are skilled in dealing with polypharmacy, where more than six to nine different medications have been prescribed to a patient. Polypharmacy is common in the elderly hip fracture population.[9] Polypharmacy usually causes drug–drug interactions that can further affect geriatric hip fracture patients in the perioperative period and in the long term.

DIFFERENT MODELS OF CARE FOR HIP FRACTURES

There are five different models of care for hip fractures, which have been summarized well by Giusti et al.[10] These include the traditional model, consultant team, interdisciplinary care/clinical pathway model, geriatric-led fracture service and geriatric co-managed care.

Under the traditional model, a patient is admitted to an orthopaedic ward with an orthopaedic surgeon assuming responsibility for care. Questions regarding medical issues and complications are managed by consultant services. Different physicians might end up managing the patient during the inpatient stay. Early rehabilitation takes place on the orthopaedic ward with a hospitalization lasting up to 2 weeks. At discharge, the patient is transferred home, to a skilled nursing facility (SNF) or acute rehabilitation facility without substantial continuity of care. The discharge timing and destination heavily depend on the medical system and country in which the patient is treated.[10]

A consultant team model is a variation of the traditional model, in which a patient is admitted to the orthopaedic surgery service but with a medical consulting service regularly seeing the patient, frequently during the postoperative phase of care.

With interdisciplinary care/clinical pathway models, there are some differences in how the models are described. However, the defining aspect of this type of care is the absence of 'single true leadership' in the management of patients.[10] Additionally, several different healthcare professionals with different patient care duties are involved in patient care.

A geriatrician-led fracture service with an orthopaedic consultant has been described in which the patient is admitted to the geriatrics service. The admitting geriatrician coordinates timing of surgery, procedures, diagnostic testing, treatments and discharge planning.[10] Meanwhile, the orthopaedic surgeon is a consulting physician who performs surgery and follows the patient intermittently until complete wound healing.

In the co-management model for hip fracture, also known as the Rochester Model of Care, the patient is technically admitted to the orthopaedic surgery service but co-managed by both orthopaedics and geriatrics, meaning that the patient is seen by both teams every day. This chapter will focus on the Rochester Model of co-management developed to treat hip fracture patients.

ORTHOGERIATRIC CO-MANAGEMENT

Given the multiple comorbidities and propensity for poor outcomes in geriatric hip fracture patients, the involvement of geriatricians is desirable to assist with medical management. This type of care is referred to as orthogeriatric co-management and was first used in the United Kingdom during the 1950s but not widely adopted in the United States until recently.[11] Studies have demonstrated that co-management reduces in-hospital complications,[12,13] decreases the length of hospital stay,[14-17] reduces readmission rates,[13] lowers mortality,[12,13,18-21] lowers costs,[15] requires lower levels of care at discharge[15,20] and results in better function postoperatively.[22] Orthogeriatric co-management results in better satisfaction for patients and providers alike.[18] Orthogeriatric co-management has also rarely been described in the United States.[23-25] These factors led to the development of a comprehensive program combining orthogeriatric co-management with lean business principles to provide an improved model of care.[8,11]

HISTORY OF THE ROCHESTER MODEL OF CARE

The Rochester Model of Care for geriatric co-management of hip fractures has evolved over a 20-year period. It started with a 'lean business model', which has been used successfully in business but rarely applied to medicine.[26]

The Rochester Model was developed at Highland Hospital, a community hospital affiliated with a major teaching institution in western New York. A formal organized program was initiated in 2004 and was called the Geriatric Fracture Center (GFC). Since its inception, the GFC has become a tertiary referral centre in the region for patients with hip fractures as well as other fractures in the geriatric population. The program has grown and matured with time and this model has been adopted by an estimated 300 other hospitals in the United States, Europe, Latin America and Asia.

HISTORY OF LEAN BUSINESS PRINCIPLES

The Rochester Model of Care employs lean business principles. Lean business principles were developed in Japan during the 1950s by W. Edwards Deming, Taiichi Ohno, Eiji Toyoda and Kiichiro Toyoda.[27,28] Deming was an advisor for the United States Army who worked with the Toyoda family, industrialists who owned Toyota Motor Corporation. The goal of this collaboration was to produce motor vehicles with limited resources, less production space, faster changeover times and higher quality.[27] Dr. Deming implemented the Plan-do-check-act (PDCA) cycle as a fundamental method of continuous quality improvement. This approach resulted in fewer manufacturing defects and reduced waste. When applied in the automobile sector, the PDCA cycle further improved on the mass production model developed by Henry Ford earlier in the twentieth century. The end result was the spectacular rise of the Japanese motor industry, culminating with Toyota overtaking General Motors as the world's largest automaker in 2008.[29] Taking note of the benefits of this accomplishment, most industries use lean business models as the standard business model for production and service; healthcare is the one notable exception.[28,30]

Many lessons from the business world can be applied to healthcare, to achieve a reduction in adverse events and improved efficiency, ultimately leading to reduced costs.[31] It has been estimated that the percentage of waste is 30–60% in American healthcare.[28] This is especially important in the United States, where such a high proportion of the gross domestic product is spent on healthcare.

Lean business principles have been successfully applied to healthcare in the Rochester Model of Care.[5,8,11,31] The Rochester Model features standardized order sets, standardized care maps, early surgical intervention and many other standard work processes.[31] This standardized work process serves to reduce unwarranted variation and has been shown to improve outcomes at the same time as reducing costs.

THE ROCHESTER MODEL

The program is co-directed by an orthopaedic surgeon and a geriatrician, who share leadership responsibilities. In addition to the attending surgeons and physicians who are part of the program, orthopaedic surgery residents and geriatrics fellows are also involved. A key aspect of the Rochester Model is that, even though the patient is technically admitted to the orthopaedic team, both services have equal and full responsibility for each patient.[5] This approach fosters cooperation and avoids 'turf wars' about who will admit the patient or look after certain aspects of their care. Essential team members include anaesthesiologists, midlevel providers (nurse practitioners and physician assistants), nurses, physiotherapists, occupational therapists, social workers, nutritionists and patient care aides, in addition to the patient and family. Consulting providers from medical specialties such as cardiology or neurology are involved only when necessary. All care team members consistently set the same expectations and goals for the patient.

Six principles of care of the Rochester Model

The Rochester Model is based upon six principles of care, which were developed from the Acute Care for Elders model first reported by Covinsky et al.,[32] with adaptations for fragility fracture patients.[11] These have been updated as follows, based on the experience of the previous decade. The six principles of the GFC are shown in Table 4.1.

MOST HIP FRACTURES REQUIRE SURGERY

Non-ambulatory patients benefit from surgery because they can obtain pain relief and surgical repair facilitates nursing care.[33,34] Hip fractures are rarely managed non-operatively. Reasons for non-operative care include refusal to provide surgical consent, limited life expectancy or inability to medically tolerate surgery. Palliative care should be offered to non-operatively treated hip fracture patients.

EARLY SURGERY IS ESSENTIAL TO IMPROVE OUTCOMES

Numerous manuscripts published since 1995 have documented the benefits of early surgical intervention for hip fractures.[35–38] The most frequent cause for surgical delay is a poorly functioning system of care. Because this parameter is modifiable, physicians and surgeons should make every effort to promote early surgery. Early surgery lessens the risks of venous thromboembolism, skin breakdown, pulmonary decompensation and infection.[39] Surgical delay slows the return to full weight-bearing status and functional recovery.[40] Numerous studies have found a reduction in mortality with surgical repair within 48 hours.[35–38]

Hip fractures are treated as urgent cases, although not emergent. All patients are evaluated by the orthopaedics service in the emergency department. They are seen by a geriatrician on the same day in most cases. Both orthopaedists and geriatricians are available 7 days a week and

Table 4.1 The six principles of care for the Rochester Model of co-management

1. Most hip fractures require surgery.
2. Early surgery is essential to improve outcomes.
3. Co-management with frequent communication avoids adverse events and promotes collegiality.
4. Standardized protocols, order sets and care plans reduce variation and improve outcomes.
5. Discharge planning begins when the patient is admitted.
6. Surgeon and medical physician leadership is essential for program success.

Source: Courtesy of Stephen Kates, MD.

round on the patient on a daily basis. Surgeries are completed as soon as patients are medically stable and as facilities allow.

CO-MANAGEMENT WITH FREQUENT COMMUNICATION AVOIDS ADVERSE EVENTS AND PROMOTES COLLEGIALITY

The benefits of geriatric co-management have been well documented by Cohen et al.[41] Hospital complications have been frequently shown to be related to communication problems between healthcare providers. Daily communication between team members with shared responsibility for the patient's care enables providers to successfully manage the medical and surgical aspects of care in the most effective manner. The resulting sense of collegiality improves provider satisfaction and helps to retain providers in the system.

STANDARDIZED PROTOCOLS, ORDER SETS AND CARE PLANS REDUCE VARIATION AND IMPROVE OUTCOMES

Variability in healthcare, as in other businesses, results in unwanted errors, waste and increased costs. Variability can be reduced by using standardized orders and protocols. Standardized order sets enable 'usual care' to be a predictable, evidence based, high level standard of care for every hip fracture patient. Practitioners consider the individual circumstances of each patient and adapt the orders to the individual patient's circumstances and needs. Representatives from each department develop standardized order sets for each step in the process from the emergency department to the ward through the postoperative phases of care. Standard orders address all important topics including pain assessment and management, use of beta blockers, thromboembolic prophylaxis, urinary catheter use and rehabilitation.

DISCHARGE PLANNING BEGINS WHEN THE PATIENT IS ADMITTED

The early involvement of social workers shortens the length of hospital stay by setting goals and plans for the patient and their family. More than 90% of patients are discharged for rehabilitation to a SNF. Developing close relationships with SNFs and long-term care facilities can facilitate this process.

SURGEON AND PHYSICIAN LEADERSHIP IS ESSENTIAL FOR PROGRAM SUCCESS

The authors have learned from implementing the Rochester Model of Care and by helping other surgeons and physicians to develop their own version of the program, that committed surgeon and physician leadership is essential to successfully establish a program and maintain the program over time. Both surgeons and physicians have numerous commitments and responsibilities that require their attention on a daily basis. Only a fully committed leadership team will be successful in maintaining a successful geriatric fracture program in the long term. Needless to say, support from colleagues, nursing staff, therapists, social workers and hospital administration is also essential to establish and maintain a successful program.

STANDARDIZED CARE ACCORDING TO THE ROCHESTER MODEL

Patient-centred, protocol-driven care

All hip fracture patients in the Rochester Model navigate through a similar care pathway, which is patient-centred yet protocol-driven (Figure 4.1). In the emergency department, X-rays of the hip, pelvis and chest are ordered. Isotonic intravenous fluids are started for rehydration and preoperative laboratory tests sent. A urinary catheter is usually placed and urinalysis is performed to ensure that the patient does not have asymptomatic bacteriuria or urinary tract infection upon presentation. Pain is then assessed at regular intervals with a standard pain regimen. The patient is seen by orthopaedic surgery personnel to admit the patient. A geriatrics consultation is requested. Typically, geriatrics recommendations are provided the same day.

The patient is then admitted preferentially to a designated unit on the orthopaedics service where nursing care protocols are initiated per standardized order sets and care plans. Past medical records are obtained if the patient has no prior entries in the hospital system's record. The patient is made NPO (nothing by mouth), and intakes and outputs are monitored with pain assessment every 3 hours. If surgery is not expected to be performed within 24 hours, thromboembolic prophylaxis may be indicated. If a patient is taking beta blockers, these are usually continued, and, if not, a decision is made by the geriatrician as to whether a beta blocker is indicated. A bowel regimen is started. Certain medications are avoided, including hypnotics, antihistamines (especially diphenhydramine), anticholinergics and benzodiazepines. Antiemetics are ordered as needed.

Finally, a trifold brochure discussing the diagnosis and prognosis of hip fractures is given to the patient and their family. The patient goes to the operating room as early as possible, once they have been assessed and optimized by the geriatrics consultant.

Postoperatively, the patient is seen daily by orthopaedics and geriatrics, with frequent communication between the two teams. Prophylactic antibiotics are continued and a standardized, low-dose opiate pain regimen with around-the-clock acetaminophen is started; the bowel regimen is continued. Anticoagulation is started. Urinary catheters are routinely discontinued by 10:00 am on postoperative day 1 per the standard order set and only occasionally maintained past that time if the geriatrics service is especially concerned about fluid status and the patient is not able to orally rehydrate. Along those lines, intakes and outputs are measured and recorded to assess fluid balance. Oxygen is weaned as tolerated to keep pulse oximetry saturations greater than 89%. The patient is instructed to turn, cough and breathe deeply every 1–2 hours while awake to prevent development of atelectasis. With respect to activity, the patient is mobilized out of bed to a chair twice daily by postoperative day 1. Further activity level is determined by weight-bearing status and cognitive status of the patient. Physical and occupational therapy are also commenced on postoperative day 1, and social work finalizes discharge planning. Postoperative films are usually taken on the first postoperative day.

At discharge, detailed instructions include the names of the doctors involved in the patient's care, osteoporosis management, medical reconciliation, and follow-up instructions are given to the subsequent care facility.

Standard order sets, consultation forms and discharge forms should be evidence based whenever possible. This helps to reduce errors and minimize waste in the care of these patients. In creating order sets, the total quality management principle is employed so that every facet of care is provided in the safest, most efficient manner possible.[42]

Standardized Protocol for Hip Fracture Patients in the Rochester Co-Management Model		
Emergency Department	**Preoperative Management**	**Postoperative Management**
X-rays of hip/pelvis and chest	Admitted to orthopaedic floor	Patient seen daily by orthopaedics and geriatrics
Intravenous fluids started, preoperative labs drawn, urinary catheter placed	Nursing care per protocols, pain assessed at regular intervals, delirium avoidance	Standardized pain regimen, discontinue urinary catheter by 10 am postoperative day 1
Patient seen by orthopaedics, geriatrics notified	Hip fracture care brochure given to patient and family	Activity bed to chair twice a day by postoperative day 1; weight bearing as tolerated with PT
Goal is 2-hour stay in the emergency department	Geriatric assessment completed, goals of care established	Detailed discharge instructions and handoff to subsequent care facility

Figure 4.1 All hip fracture patients navigate through a similar patient-centred yet protocol-driven care pathway. The patient is admitted to the orthopaedic surgery service on preferentially designated floors. Geriatrics sees the patient to optimize them for their surgery. Postoperatively, both the orthopaedic surgery and geriatrics teams round on the patient daily, with frequent communication between the care teams. The patient is mobilized on postoperative day 1, and social work is consulted early on. Upon discharge, detailed discharge instructions are given to the subsequent care facility. (Adapted from Friedman SM, et al. *J Am Geriatr Soc*, 2008; **56**(7): 1349–56.)

Another important aspect of this protocol for management of hip fracture patients according to the Rochester Model is the preferential use of generic medications, to help achieve cost savings, and ensure its profitability.

PREOPERATIVE CONSIDERATIONS

There are many aspects of preoperative care of hip fracture patients that are crucial to enhance the likelihood of the patient successfully recovering from the fracture. Frequent communication between the geriatrician and the orthopaedic surgeon during the preoperative period is crucial.

The history and physical examination should try to clarify the circumstances related to the fall that led to the injury. Providers should ascertain the patient's functional status, as this allows 'demand matching' for implants, as an octogenarian patient with multiple comorbidities would be best served by a hemiarthroplasty, while a total hip arthroplasty might be indicated for a more active patient. In addition, functional status and general health immediately prior to the injury allow the treating physicians to comment on prognosis and goals of care. End-of-life issues are discussed and it is determined whether the patient desires intensive interventions such as cardiac resuscitation or intubation, or whether they would wish to receive a 'do-not-resuscitate' (DNR) and/or a 'do-not-intubate' (DNI) order.

Any associated injuries should be sought including other fragility fractures of the distal radius, proximal humerus, ribs and spine (compression fractures). A mental status examination is performed to look for signs of delirium and dementia. In addition, a detailed medication assessment is performed to eliminate harmful and troublesome medications. Another important aspect of medication history is use of anticoagulants. If on warfarin (Coumadin), the patient is given vitamin K by mouth and then fresh frozen plasma immediately before surgery, depending on the international normalized ratio (INR).[43] An antiplatelet agent such as clopidogrel (Plavix®) may preclude the use of neuraxial anesthesia. Both physicians must assess and correct hydration status and anemia to optimize the patient for the physiologic stress of the operating room and post-operative period.

To help counsel the patient and his or her family regarding the prognosis, the geriatrician risk-stratifies the patient. The rest of the treatment team, including the surgeon and anaesthesiologist, will benefit from classification into low, medium, high or very high risk categories. During this process, additional medicine specialty consultations are requested by geriatrics but are only rarely needed.[11] Supplementary tests such as echocardiograms are used only in certain instances which will change management of the patient. The American College of Cardiology and American Heart Association have published guidelines on the perioperative management of cardiac patients.[44] Familiarity with these can overcome the tendency to over-consult cardiology or request preoperative echocardiograms.

Only after all these aspects of care are complete, including communication between the treatment teams, may the patient proceed to the operating room.

OPERATIVE CONSIDERATIONS

Early surgery is a fundamental element of the Rochester Model of Care. At Highland Hospital (Rochester, NY), 78% of patients undergo operative stabilization within 24 hours with an average time to surgery of 17 hours. A designated trauma room available at the start of the day will help to improve time to surgery. Anesthesia is often administered via neuraxial blockade if possible, as this has been shown to decrease the risk of postoperative delirium.[45]

The goals of surgery are stable fixation of the fracture and immediate weight bearing. The procedure itself is as brief as possible, which helps to minimize blood loss. It is also important to avoid braces and drains, which can aggravate elderly patients and contribute to delirium.

POSTOPERATIVE CONSIDERATIONS

In the postoperative period, the hip fracture patient continues to be co-managed, using standardized postoperative order sets along with standard nursing care plans.[42] Following evaluation of the postoperative radiograph taken on postoperative day 1, weight bearing is started. Delirium must be avoided after surgery. The Rochester Model employs a restraint-free program, with the avoidance of braces and other tethers such as drains. Patients are encouraged to wear glasses and hearing aids to reduce the incidence of delirium.[46,47] Medications which affect mental status such as centrally acting antihistamines, H2 blockers, hypnotics, anticholinergics and benzodiazepines are best avoided. Pain is assessed regularly, and the nursing staff are experienced in caring for frail adults at risk for developing delirium. Families of those patients who are at risk are encouraged to provide support and reorientation to the patient.[42] Pain management uses around-the-clock acetaminophen and low-dose opiates to minimize the chances of developing delirium; nonsteroidal anti-inflammatory drugs (NSAIDs) are avoided to prevent the development of gastrointestinal bleeding, acute kidney injury, delirium, stroke and cardiovascular events.[42] Finally, anticoagulation is used to prevent deep vein thrombosis (DVT) or pulmonary embolism (PE).

Discharge usually occurs on postoperative day 3 to a SNF.[8,11] The patients are sent to the rehabilitation facility with a standardized discharge instruction set and a medication reconciliation that has been reviewed by both orthopaedics and geriatrics.

Follow-up with the orthopaedic surgeon and the patient's primary care provider is arranged as an outpatient. As low-energy hip fractures are fragility fractures, essentially all patients are considered to have osteoporosis. Metabolic bone laboratory studies (vitamin D, parathyroid hormone, thyroid hormone, serum albumin and ionized calcium) are ordered on all patients. All patients are discharged on vitamin D supplementation and anti-resorptive therapy is recommended upon discharge.

RESULTS OF THE MODEL

All geriatric fracture patients treated with this model are registered in a quality management registry. A dedicated program research nurse collects demographic, medical, surgical, functional and outcome measures; much of the information is obtained from the medical chart. Financial results are obtained from the finance department. Mortality information is gleaned from a query of social security database, the patient's medical record and follow-up phone calls with the patient/family or nursing facility.

Tables 4.2 and 4.3 show information on recent demographics and outcomes, respectively. The average age of patients at the GFC is 85 years of age, with 77% being female and the average Charlson Comorbidity Index being 2.9. In terms of outcomes, patients spend a mean of 2.8 hours in the emergency department prior to being brought

Table 4.2 Characteristics of hip fracture patients in the Geriatric Fracture Center, June 2013–June 2014

Number	195
Age (years), mean (±SD)	85 (±9.0)
Female	77%
Primary Residence Prior to Admission	
Home	61.0%
Assisted living	13.9%
Nursing home	25.1%
Type of Admission	
Emergency room	87.7%
Hospital transfer	11.3%
Direct admission	1.0%
Charlson Comorbidity Index, mean (±SD)	2.9 (±2.1)

Table 4.3 Outcomes of the Geriatric Fracture Center

Mean Time (±SD) to OR (hh:mm)	
From arrival in ER	21:03 (±12:04)
	18:22 (±12:00)
Time spent in ER	2:48 (±2:31)
To OR in <24 hours	75%[a]
To OR in <48 hours	98.5%
Overall complication rate	53%
Length of stay (days), mean (±SD)	4.98 (±2.67)
Readmission within 30 days	8.2%
In-hospital mortality	1.5%

Note: ER, emergency room; OR, operating room.

[a] 75% of patients were taken to the OR within 24 hours of arrival at the hospital. That figure rose to 82% for patients going to the OR within 24 hours from time of admission.

up to the hospital floor. Overall, 75% of patients undergo surgery within 24 hours of presenting to the hospital, a figure that rises to 82% when measuring from time of admission; 99% of patients are operated on within 48 hours of arrival at the hospital. In-hospital mortality was 1.5%.

The average length of stay in the United States is 6.4 days[1] with a 14.5% readmission rate[48]; this represents a significant use of hospital beds throughout the nation. Following implementation of the GFC, the average length of stay at Highland Hospital is 5 days and the 30-day readmission rate is 8.2%.[31] The total direct charge to payers is $15,188, which is substantially less than the average charges throughout the United States (~$42,000).[5] Efficient delivery of care for hip fractures in a cost-effective manner helps free up healthcare resources for other patients and decrease costs to society.

In addition to these economic gains, there are benefits for the patient. When compared with usual care, there are better outcomes with co-management, even after adjusting for baseline differences. Patients have surgery a half day sooner than they otherwise would and the complication rates are lower: 31% with co-management as opposed to 46% with usual care.[8] These improvements lead to a shorter length of stay and smoother recovery for the patient.

Adopting a Rochester-style co-managed program consisting of protocol-driven care and total quality management principles may help reduce the morbidity and functional decline that occurs in older patients with hip fractures.

OTHER TYPES OF FRACTURES

Principles used in this program are readily applicable to other types of fractures in older adults. In fact, the order sets in care maps are typically useful for any lower extremity fracture and major upper extremity fractures in the geriatric population. The principles are the same. However, the fracture management will differ. In some fractures, weight bearing may not be possible due to the lack of stability of the construct. Some examples are selected articular surface fractures and periprosthetic fractures where secure fixation is not possible. Nonetheless, the six principles above will serve patients and their care teams well if applied uniformly and thoughtfully.

IMPLEMENTING A ROCHESTER-STYLE PROGRAM

Several factors should be considered when deciding whether or not to implement the Rochester Model of Care. The first is that an institution must see a reasonable volume of hip fractures in order to develop expertise. While there is no precise figure, Kates et al. believe that 100 or so cases per year are sufficient to make this program cost effective.[42] In addition to having a sufficient number of hip fractures, there must be enough hospitalists or geriatricians willing to participate in the co-management program. Depending on the region, this may be a challenge, as there are a limited number of geriatricians relative to the growing patient population. At present, there are approximately 7100 geriatricians practicing in the United States.[49] The use of hospitalists in co-management might be an important variation on the model, as has been described previously.[50] Other studies have shown improved outcomes versus usual care when using internists or hospitalists to co-manage care.[51,52]

A strong desire to implement the program is required, as implementation will involve considerable effort. Strong leadership is essential, and a surgeon champion and a medical champion should be identified to lead the program; these individuals should communicate well and be committed to implementation of the program and resolution of any barriers that may arise.[42] It is critical that the relationship with the hospital administration be one of trust, honesty, community and mutual respect.[28] Along those lines, the leaders of this program must recognize that they are dealing with culture change at the hospital, which is at times met with some resistance. In addition to the departments of orthopaedic surgery and geriatrics, the geriatrician and surgeon will need buy-in from other departments and services, such as anaesthesiology, nursing, social work, physical therapy and medicine consulting services. When addressing other departments and services, emphasis on streamlining care, standardizing care and making efforts to simplify the process are important aspects of the discussion.

Common barriers include physician leadership issues, need for a clinical case manager, lack of operating room time, anesthesia department support, lack of hospital administration support and difficulty obtaining pre-surgical cardiac clearance. When discussing the program with hospital administration, it should be presented as a solution to an existing problem rather than making it a problem of its own. In the current fee-for-service reimbursement model, a well-organized and efficient program will almost assuredly result in improved net margin per case.[31] The same can also be said about bundled payments for care improvements that are on the horizon of American healthcare. Specific methods to mitigate the rest of these barriers have been previously published.[31,53]

Lean business models use data-driven performance for decision-making[27,30,54]; a comprehensive quality improvement database should be implemented to evaluate processes and clinical and financial outcomes. This will allow targeting of areas in need of improvement and reinforce the value of the program to hospital administrators. Basic data required include length of hospital stay, time from admission to surgery, inpatient mortality, 30-day readmission and mortality, costs of care, and provision of recommendation for managing the patient's osteoporosis after discharge from the hospital. Most of these data are generally available because they are already reported to the federal government as performance metrics.[31] Collecting and following these data allow for the performance of the program to be assessed once it is instituted. Using this database, the Rochester Model at Highland Hospital has demonstrated a shorter length of stay, which is significant because

hospital costs account for 44% of direct costs for hip fracture patients.[55] This impact combined with reduced readmission rates led to an increased profit margin for the hospital, which increased administrative support for implementing this program. The senior author of this chapter has helped other hospitals throughout North America and internationally to implement this model of care.

SUMMARY

The Rochester Model of Care for geriatric hip fracture offers many benefits for the patient, physicians and healthcare system as a whole. This highly replicable model results in improved care and reduced costs. It has been shown to lead to a shorter length of hospital stay, attributable to reductions in time required for surgical repair and early involvement of social work for discharge planning. The decreased time to surgery leads to fewer adverse outcomes of acute hospitalization and a decrease in overall complication rates.

Hip fracture patients are a homogeneous population that responds well to protocol-driven care. Wide application of this model of care could substantially improve the quality and cost of caring for frail elders with fragility fractures.

REFERENCES

1. Barrett, M., et al. *2007 HCUP Nationwide Inpatient Sample (NIS) Comparison Report.* HCUP Methods Series Report # 2010-03. 2010. Available from: http://www.hcup-us.ahrq.gov/reports/methods/2010_03.pdf (accessed 2013 June 15).
2. Dennison, E., et al. Epidemiology of osteoporosis. *Rheum Dis Clin North Am*, 2006; **32**(4): 617–29.
3. Federal Interagency Forum on Aging-Related Statistics. *Older Americans: Key Indicators of Well-Being.* 2008. Available from http://www.agingstats.gov/Main_Site/Data/2008_Documents/OA_2008.pdf (accessed 2008 December 2015).
4. Brauer, C.A., et al. Incidence and mortality of hip fractures in the United States. *JAMA*, 2009; **302**(14): 1573–9.
5. Kates, S.L., et al. Comparison of an organized geriatric fracture program to United States government data. *Geriatr Orthop Surg Rehabil*, 2010; **1**(1): 15–21.
6. Braithwaite, R.S., et al. Estimating hip fracture morbidity, mortality and costs. *J Am Geriatr Soc*, 2003; **51**(3): 364–70.
7. Magaziner, J., et al. Recovery from hip fracture in eight areas of function. *J Gerontol A Biol Sci Med Sci*, 2000; **55**(9): M498–507.
8. Friedman, S.M., et al. Impact of a comanaged Geriatric Fracture Center on short-term hip fracture outcomes. *Arch Intern Med*, 2009; **169**(18): 1712–17.
9. Baranzini, F., et al. Fall-related injuries in a nursing home setting: Is polypharmacy a risk factor? *BMC Health Serv Res*, 2009; **9**: 228.

10. Giusti, A., et al. Optimal setting and care organization in the management of older adults with hip fracture. *Eur J Phys Rehabil Med* 2011; **47**(2): 281–96.

11. Friedman, S.M., et al. Geriatric co-management of proximal femur fractures: Total quality management and protocol-driven care result in better outcomes for a frail patient population. *J Am Geriatr Soc*, 2008; **56**(7): 1349–56.

12. Vidan, M., et al. Efficacy of a comprehensive geriatric intervention in older patients hospitalized for hip fracture: A randomized, controlled trial. *J Am Geriatr Soc*, 2005; **53**(9): 1476–82.

13. Fisher, A.A., et al. Outcomes for older patients with hip fractures: The impact of orthopedic and geriatric medicine cocare. *J Orthop Trauma*, 2006; **20**(3): 172–8; discussion 179–80.

14. Hempsall, V.J., et al. Orthopaedic geriatric care— Is it effective? A prospective population-based comparison of outcome in fractured neck of femur. *J R Coll Physicians Lond*, 1990; **24**(1): 47–50.

15. Elliot, J.R., et al. Collaboration with orthopaedic surgeons. *Age Ageing*, 1996; **25**(5): 414.

16. Smith, D.L. The elderly in the convalescent orthopaedic trauma ward: Can the geriatrician help? *Health Bull (Edinb)*, 1984; **42**(1): 36–44.

17. Boyd, R.V., et al. The Nottingham orthogeriatric unit after 1000 admissions. *Injury*, 1983; **15**(3): 193–6.

18. Amatuzzi, M.M., et al. Interdisciplinary care in orthogeriatrics: A good cost-benefit model of care. *J Am Geriatr Soc*, 2003; **51**(1): 134–6.

19. Barone, A., et al. A comprehensive geriatric intervention reduces short- and long-term mortality in older people with hip fracture. *J Am Geriatr Soc*, 2006; **54**(7): 1145–7.

20. Thwaites, J.H., et al. Shared care between geriatricians and orthopaedic surgeons as a model of care for older patients with hip fractures. *N Z Med J*, 2005; 118(1214): U1438.

21. Thwaites, J., et al. Older patients with hip fractures: Evaluation of a long-term specialist orthopaedic medicine service in their outcomes. *N Z Med J*, 2007; **120**(1254): U2535.

22. Shyu, Y.I., et al. A pilot investigation of the short-term effects of an interdisciplinary intervention program on elderly patients with hip fracture in Taiwan. *J Am Geriatr Soc*, 2005; **53**(5): 811–18.

23. Khasraghi, F.A., et al. The economic impact of medical complications in geriatric patients with hip fracture. *Orthopedics*, 2003; **26**(1): 49–53; discussion 53.

24. Zuckerman, J.D., et al. Hip fractures in geriatric patients. Results of an interdisciplinary hospital care program. *Clin Orthop Relat Res*, 1992; (274): 213–25.

25. De Jonge, K.E., et al. Hip Fracture Service – An interdisciplinary model of care. *J Am Geriatr Soc*, 2001; **49**(12): 1737–8.

26. Graban, M. *Lean Hospitals: Improving Quality, Patient Safety, and Employee Satisfaction*. 1st ed. New York: Productivity; 2008.

27. Womack, J.P., et al., eds. *The Machine that Changed the World*. 1st ed. Vol. 1. New York: Rawson; 1990.

28. Chalice, R. *Improving Healthcare using Toyota Lean Production Methods*. 2nd ed. Vol. 1. Milwaukee, WI: ASQ Quality Press; 2007.

29. Chowdhury, S.D. Strategic roads that diverge or converge: GM and Toyota in the battle for the top. *Bus Horiz*, 2014; **57**(1): 127–36.

30. Zidel, T.G. *Lean Guide to Transforming Healthcare*. 1st ed. Vol. 1. Milwaukee, WI: ASQ Quality Press; 2006.

31. Kates, S.L. Lean business model and implementation of a geriatric fracture center. *Clin Geriatr Med*, 2014; **30**(2): 191–205.

32. Covinsky, K.E., et al. Improving functional outcomes in older patients: Lessons from an acute care for elders unit. *Jt Comm J Qual Improv*, 1998; **24**(2): 63–76.

33. Irvine, R.E. Rehabilitation in geriatric orthopaedics. *Int Rehabil Med*, 1985; **7**(3): 115–20.

34. Hay, D., and M.J. Parker. Hip fracture in the immobile patient. *J Bone Joint Surg Br*, 2003; **85**(7): 1037–9.

35. Novack, V., et al. Does delay in surgery after hip fracture lead to worse outcomes? A multicenter survey. *Int J Qual Health Care*, 2007; **19**(3): 170–6.

36. Zuckerman, J.D., et al. Postoperative complications and mortality associated with operative delay in older patients who have a fracture of the hip. *J Bone Joint Surg Am*, 1995; **77**(10): 1551–6.

37. Rogers, F.B., et al. Early fixation reduces morbidity and mortality in elderly patients with hip fractures from low-impact falls. *J Trauma*, 1995; **39**(2): 261–5.

38. Bottle, A., and P. Aylin. Mortality associated with delay in operation after hip fracture: Observational study. *BMJ*, 2006; **332**(7547): 947–51.

39. Creditor, M.C. Hazards of hospitalization of the elderly. *Ann Intern Med*, 1993; **118**(3): 219–23.

40. Morrison, R.S., and A.L. Siu. *Medical Consultation for Patients with Hip Fracture*. 2007. http://www.uptodate.com/contents/medical-consultation-for-patients-with-hip-fracture (accessed 2007 July 11).

41. Cohen, H.J., et al. A controlled trial of inpatient and outpatient geriatric evaluation and management. *N Engl J Med*, 2002; **346**(12): 905–12.

42. Kates, S.L., et al. Co-managed care for fragility hip fractures (Rochester model). *Osteoporos Int*, 2010; **21**(Suppl 4): S621–5.

43. Gleason, L.J., et al. Anticoagulation management in individuals with hip fracture. *J Am Geriatr Soc*, 2014; **62**(1): 159–64.

44. Fleisher, L.A., et al. 2009 ACCF/AHA focused update on perioperative beta blockade incorporated into the ACC/AHA 2007 guidelines on perioperative cardiovascular evaluation and care for noncardiac surgery. *J Am Coll Cardiol*, 2009; **54**(22): e13–18.

45. Sieber, F.E., et al. Sedation depth during spinal anesthesia and the development of postoperative delirium in elderly patients undergoing hip fracture repair. *Mayo Clin Proc*, 2010; **85**(1): 18–26.

46. Inouye, S.K. Delirium in older persons. *N Engl J Med*, 2006; **354**(11): 1157–65.

47. Marcantonio, E.R., et al. Reducing delirium after hip fracture: A randomized trial. *J Am Geriatr Soc*, 2001; **49**(5): 516–22.

48. Goodman, D.C., et al. *After Hospitalization: A Dartmouth Atlas Report on Post-Acute Care for Medicare Beneficiaries.* Hanover, NH: Dartmouth; 2011.

49. Retooling for an Aging America, *National Academies of Science*, 2008. http://iom.nationalacademies. org/~/media/Files/Report%20Files/2008/Retooling-for-an-Aging-America-Building-the-Health-Care-Workforce RetoolingforanAgingAmerica BuildingtheHealthCareWorkforce.pdf (accessed 2008 September 23).

50. Batsis, J.A., et al. Effects of a hospitalist care model on mortality of elderly patients with hip fractures. *J Hosp Med*, 2007; **2**(4): 219–25.

51. Phy, M.P., et al. Effects of a hospitalist model on elderly patients with hip fracture. *Arch Intern Med*, 2005; **165**(7): 796–801.

52. Watters, C.L. and W.P. Moran. Hip fractures— A joint effort. *Orthop Nurs*, 2006; **25**(3): 157–65; quiz 166–7.

53. Kates, S.L., et al. Barriers to implementation of an organized geriatric fracture program. *Geriatr Orthop Surg Rehabil*, 2012; **3**(1): 8–16.

54. Liem, I.S., et al. Literature review of outcome parameters used in studies of geriatric fracture centers. *Arch Orthop Trauma Surg*, 2014; **134**(2): 181–7.

55. Barrett-Connor, E. The economic and human costs of osteoporotic fracture. *Am J Med*, 1995; **98**(2A): 3S–8S.

5

The management of osteomyelitis

BRUCE H. ZIRAN, ADAM G. HIRSCHFELD AND JARRAD A. BARBER

INTRODUCTION

Medical care of the elderly will assume a greater proportion of most physicians' practice in the future and thus orthopaedists must have a better understanding of how to manage the unique ailments of the geriatric patient. Infection will continue to be a significant complication of all invasive surgical specialties. Unique to the geriatric population are both systemic and local physiologic changes that make care of geriatric infections much more challenging. Using the Cierny–Mader classification of osteomyelitis, the patient is characterized by both infection status and host status (Figures 5.1 and 5.2). The host status is reflective of systemic and local extremity influences that exist due to a variety of factors. The geriatric patient is almost always by definition a B-systemic and B-local host because of changes in the vascular and immunologic systems. Even though geriatric patients demonstrate healing capacity, their existing issues and postoperative demands and restrictions make the care of geriatric infections challenging.

Bacteria are an essential part of human existence with trillions of bacteria living within and on our bodies at any given moment. This normal flora represents a symbiotic relationship between the host and microbacterial world and demonstrates that the simple existence of bacteria does not equate to an infectious process. In fact, most bacterial–host interactions are beneficial for both entities and it is only when there is some imbalance in the relationship or introduction of a new or altered state that a potential problem may arise. Bacteria are needed for proper digestion as well as defence against certain more virulent strains. The host bacteria are often competing among themselves in this symbiotic relationship. Thus, a positive culture, which can easily be obtained from nearly any body part, does not necessarily equate to an infection or require treatment. A study conducted by Moussa et al. highlighted this phenomenon and found that nearly 50% of cultures taken during hardware removals were positive in patients who had no evidence or symptomatology of infection.[1] Our understanding of infection and the relationship between humans and bacteria continues to evolve, especially the geriatric population who continue to increase their life expectancy. This chapter addresses osteomyelitis in the geriatric population highlighting the various clinical, laboratory and imaging diagnostic methods and the multidisciplinary treatment approach needed to treat this difficult problem.

PATHOPHYSIOLOGY

Infections in orthopaedics typically result from some type of trauma or may have an iatrogenic cause after internal fixation or arthroplasty. Bacterial colonization is a necessary first step but may not be sufficient to cause infection. Colonization is typical of biofilm-forming bacteria and this section reviews the pathophysiologic processes involving the normal host defense mechanisms, the formation of colonies and the evolution from colonization to infection as well as the host response to infection.

Normal host defenses

The host immune system is constantly fighting against breaches that may threaten host existence. It is estimated that at any given moment there are millions of bacterial invasions being neutralized by host defense mechanisms. For example, there are over 180 different types of bacteria on our skin and over 400 bacterial species in one section of large intestine at any given moment.[2,3] These host defense mechanisms are

- A-host
  - Healthy physiology
  - Healthy tissue bed
- B-systemic host
  - Nutritional compromise
  - Immunosuppression
  - Nicotine use
  - Neoplasm/prior chemo
  - Advanced age
  - Poly-trauma
- B-local host
  - Previous surgery
  - Vascular disease
  - Prior infection
  - Radiation therapy
- C-host
  - ASA IV risk factors
  - Likelihood of peri-operative death
  - Multiple co-morbidities

Figure 5.1 Cierny–Mader classification of osteomyelitis showing the types of hosts.

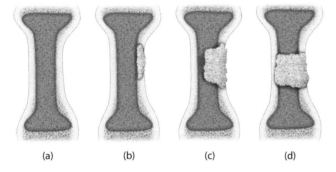

Figure 5.2 Cierny–Mader classification of osteomyelitis showing the types of bony lesions. (a) Medullary osteomyelitis. (b) Superficial osteomyelitis. (c) Invasive osteomyelitis with axial stability maintained. (d) Invasive osteomyelitis with loss of axial stability.

complex and outside the scope of this chapter. However in summary the host uses B cell defenses primarily against bacteria, T cell defenses primarily against viral invasions and the macrophage system against foreign bodies.[4] Healthy hosts are able to defend against most bacterial species that enter and exist in isolation (called the planktonic state and intended to be analogous to plankton floating in the ocean). As long as bacteria are in the planktonic state, they are susceptible to host defenses, which attack and neutralize the bacterial invasion through phagocytosis, oxidative enzymatic destruction and a number of other mechanisms. If the bacteria evade the host defenses, they must then find a suitable surface or location to begin adherence and initiate their reproductive cycle and form colonies which ensures their ongoing survival. Bacterial adhesion is the first step but can only occur on an inert surface, such as a foreign body, or on non-viable or necrotic tissue. Implants and traumatized tissues are very suitable surfaces that can harbor bacteria and allow colonization by virtue of being outside the normal vascular or living intercellular spaces. They are also remote from any antibiotic agent

that requires access to bacteria for efficacy. The presence of a foreign body decreases the minimal abscess-forming dose of *Staphylococcus aureus* by at least 10,000-fold in the animal model as well as in humans.[2] Numerous phenomena and interactions are involved with bacterial adhesion but the formation of a colony usually requires bacteria that have evaded host defenses long enough to begin a geometric reproductive cycle. Reproductive cycles of bacteria are geometric and have been reported to occur every 20 minutes and increase in an exponential manner.[5]

Host defenses will identify and attack bacteria and begin a systematic process of destruction (oxidative and enzymatic processes) as well as recruitment of other host cells (chemotaxis) to aid in the destruction of any invasion. As in wars of attrition, an imbalance that results in either a mitigated host response (immune suppression) or an overwhelming bacterial invasion (inoculation) may tip the balance in favour of bacterial species and allow reproduction and colony formation. Immunologic function in humans varies from birth to death and vulnerabilities exist in various ages. In the elderly, there is a known reduction in the immune response which will predispose the elderly to such imbalances between bacterial invasion and defense mechanisms. The immunologic changes in the elderly include a decline in the normal lymphoid cell activity known as immunosenescence. The hematopoietic stem cells diminish in capacity which in turn leads to a decrease in cell lines including phagocytes and lymphocytes.[6] This decline in the lymphocytic cell line affects both function and production. In addition to changes in immune responses, the usual beneficial effects of inflammation present earlier in life become detrimental to the elderly host. It should be further noted that changes in the lymphoid cell line are not solely responsible for the malfunctioning of the immune system in the elderly. Even though the myeloid cell line does not diminish with normal aging, macrophages can become improperly regulated as a consequence of environmental changes.[7] All of these changes in the elderly lead to a decreased immune response and a more advantageous environment for bacterial colonization and subsequent infection.

Adherence and colonization

Postsurgical or traumatized tissues are perfect environments for bacterial adherence and the initiation of colony formation. However, colony formation is not guaranteed because of one very important host defense mechanism, tissue integration. Concomitant with host defense systems fighting against bacterial invasion is the host response to the inert surface of dead tissue or an implant. Host cells will attempt to eradicate dead tissue through oxidative processes and replace the dead tissue with intact, living host tissue. Implants that are biocompatible will often be covered with a neo-membrane of tissue integration that is not inert and therefore resistant to bacterial adhesion. This is the first step. Vascular tissue can also provide a conduit for the delivery of antibiotics and more host immune cells and thus reduce the chances of colonization. Bacteria that are trapped or 'sequestered' are either slowly killed or become quiescent through adaptive metabolic changes. Such a phenomenon would explain the previous findings of Moussa et al. which showed that asymptomatic hardware retrievals resulted in culture positive specimens.[1] Thus the 'race for the surface' is the inciting event that will often determine whether colonization, and potential infection, or bio-integration occurs. The time period between injury and implantation may allow useful interventions to help favor the host versus bacterial infection.

Colony formation begins a complex process and bacteria can metastasize and form new colony forming units. Colonies have been found to have some ability to 'communicate' with primitive signaling mechanisms and develop their own defenses against the host response. Once colonization occurs, bacteria can begin to form a mucopolysaccharide glycocalyx protective film that is colloquially called 'slime'. This protective layer serves multiple purposes and helps maintain the colony while also protecting it against host defenses. The glycocalyx membrane will prevent penetration of host cells and their oxidative enzymes as well as serving as a diffusion barrier against antibiotics. This nearly impermeable matrix is so strong that antibiotic concentrations upwards of 1000 times normal may be required to just reach the bacteria encapsulated in the colony biofilm.[8] Even if antibiotics reach the bacteria, their main mechanism of function is either cell wall disruption or interference with the nuclease function required for reproduction.[2] One of the features of mature colonies is the lower metabolic state of encapsulated bacteria. The lower metabolic state may be thought of as a sort of hibernation that results in the appearance of so-called 'pseudo-resistance'. If bacteria are not actively reproducing or metabolically active, any effect on the cell wall such as transport of nutrients or nuclease production will not be realized and while the bacterial species may still be sensitive to the antibiotic in their active state, their lack of active reproduction will appear as resistance and allow antibiotic concentrations to lapse. Thus, in a short period of time after the cessation of antibiotic treatment, the antibiotic will diffuse away, and if the bacteria emerge into a more metabolically active state, the antibiotic will be perceived to have failed. This phenomenon helps explain the waxing and waning characteristic of chronic infections and osteomyelitis.

Another effect of biofilm interfering with the host response is auto-injury. As host immune cells react to local signaling proteins and begin to recruit other cells and begin their 'attack' on the encapsulated cells, the release of their oxidative enzyme can potentially result in harm to intact local host tissue. The accumulation of white cells and local tissue damage typically manifests as the purulence and inflammation of infection. While some bacteria also contain endotoxin and harmful agents that may be damaging in their effect, such as the toxins of necrotizing fasciitis, much of the local tissue damage in an active infection may actually be the result of the host attempting to eradicate encapsulated organisms. As the condition becomes more chronic, the host will 'sequester' the effort to localize it and prevent systemic spread. Sequestra and sinus tracts are the results of this effort and characterize chronic infectious states. However, despite host efforts to isolate infectious processes in the elderly, systemic spread may be difficult to prevent due to the compromised local and systemic state of the host.

CLASSIFICATION

The numerous osteomyelitis classification systems use time, aetiology, mechanism or management as the basis for classification. Osteomyelitis has been described as either acute or chronic based on the length or duration of symptoms. Acute osteomyelitis can be characterized as an infection presenting with oedema, small vessel thrombosis and vascular congestion within 2 weeks of onset. Chronic osteomyelitis is defined as osteomyelitis lasting more than 6 weeks or a recurring infection after appropriate treatment.[9] This type of osteomyelitis often occurs in conjunction with conditions of vascular compromise such as peripheral vascular disease or diabetes mellitus. It is not uncommon for both of these comorbidities to be present in an elderly patient with osteomyelitis. While the temporal definitions appear rather arbitrary, and not based on any true science, the intent is to help differentiate infectious processes that might require different treatment paradigms. Acute infections may potentially be eradicated with less invasive or regressive methods, whereas a more mature infection requires more aggressive or staged techniques.

Aetiologic classifications of osteomyelitis focus on the mechanism of occurrence, such as route of entry. Hematogenous causes are a result of a bacteremia from whatever cause. Oral procedures, trauma or surgical procedures can introduce an inoculum of bacteria into the blood stream. Any bacteria escaping host defense efforts may manifest themselves in another part of the body. This process is one of the main reasons empiric or prophylactic antibiotic treatment was advocated for patients with prostheses undergoing invasive dental procedures. While not absolutely proven or disproven, the known bacteremia from oral procedures and the occurrence of infection after such a procedure in the absence of other explanations remains an empiric, or non-evidence based, explanation for its occurrence and treatment. Iatrogenic and nosocomial infections are frequently caused by species of *Staphylococcus*, *Streptococcus* or enteric organisms. As it is commonly perceived that hospital acquired infection (HAI) and surgical site infection (SSI) are avoidable, there are numerous regulatory and financial efforts to mitigate their occurrence. In reality, the incidence of such infections will probably never be zero and some low, although acceptable, incidence of these infections should probably become the normative benchmark. Until regulatory agencies acquire such a reasonable understanding of infection, the efforts put forth towards mitigating such infections are well intended but potentially confusing to both provider and patient.

The most common classification of osteomyelitis is that of Cierny and Mader which focuses on describing bone pathology and the status of the host or patient (Figures 5.1 and 5.2). In this system there are four main considerations when classifying osteomyelitis: the host condition, the functional impairment caused by the insult, the involved site and the extent of bony necrosis. The most compelling finding of the Cierny–Mader study was that probably the most important factor for outcome was the physiologic status of the host.[10]

In the Cierny–Mader system, the 'type A' host has normal immune status, with healthy local and systemic physiology (Figure 5.1). The 'type B' host is immunocompromised to some degree and is further subclassified into B-systemic and/or B-local compromised groups. Examples of B-systemic compromise include vascular disease, malignancy, diabetes, poor nutritional status, renal or hepatic insufficiency, nicotine or substance abuse and immunocompromising diseases or treatments. Examples of B-local compromise include local or previous limb cellulitis, lymphedema, previous surgery, radiation treatment, peripheral vascular disease and any trauma including minor or major injury. The C host is a specific type of host that is compromised to such an extent that Cierny described it as someone where 'treatment to cure the infection was worse than the infection itself'. In these patients, chronic suppression, amputation or death is often the only choice. Taking this classification into consideration, the geriatric population will likely provide very few A hosts, and most will start as B-systemic and/or B-local hosts presenting as 'type C' hosts with few curative options available.

The Cierny–Mader system also describes the bone lesion as having four distinct types (Figure 5.2). Type I osteomyelitis is a medullary osteomyelitis with an endosteal nidus. The bone is axially stable and the cortex is infrequently permeated. Its cause has been proposed to be haematogenous spread or seeding. It is typically seen in children and adolescents where a bacteremia will seed the injured area of the hypovascular region of the growth plate. This lesion does not typically require any form of bone grafting procedure and many can be treated with either local treatment or antibiotics alone. Type II osteomyelitis is a superficial osteomyelitis that affects the outer surface of the bone. It does not permeate the cortex and is axially stable. It is typical of pressure ulcers or outside-in inoculations. Local treatment and soft tissue coverage will usually provide definitive cure. Type III osteomyelitis involves both cortical and medullary bone but is by definition an infection that maintains axial stability or continuity of the bone. This type of osteomyelitis is typically labeled after excision and may often be due to what appears as a type II lesion becoming a type III lesion after treatment. The axial stability is not necessarily sufficient to allow weight bearing, but it does not require osseous reconstruction to result in an axially stable limb that can eventually become weight bearing. Type IV osteomyelitis is a permeative destructive lesion that causes instability because of segmental cortical and medullary involvement. This lesion results in osseous discontinuity that will require some type of reconstruction either initially or in a staged manner. Frequently, what appears or presents as a type III lesion will become a type IV lesion after appropriate treatment. Both type III and type IV lesions are commonly seen after fracture or traumatic injuries (Figure 5.1).

One of the main benefits of this classification system is the data and outcomes provided by Cierny and Mader. They found that A hosts achieved up to a 98% success rate even with type III and type IV lesions. B hosts had success rates ranging from 79% to 92% and in such patients preparatory interventions such as improving disease states or nutrition had the greatest impact.[11] The take-away message from their work is that the host's physiologic condition plays just as integral a role, if not more, as proper treatment of the osteomyelitis. The physiologic importance of the host is magnified in the elderly population and the effect of physiologic optimization in geriatric patients with osteomyelitis cannot be overstated. In the elderly, systemic and prior local compromise is almost always present. Even in the very healthy elderly there is undoubtedly some systemic compromise in cardiovascular and immune function that must be taken into account. The most compelling intervention attributed to Cierny's work is improvement of the host status. We know this to be true when the elderly present with a fractured hip. They are frequently dehydrated with electrolyte abnormalities, and they often have diabetes, cardiac disease, neurocognitive dysfunction and poor physiologic reserve. Such patients are never really 'cleared for surgery'. Instead their physiologic status is optimized for the necessary surgical intervention. With infection the same process should occur as undertaken for hip fractures, but because the infection may not be as acute a condition there is opportunity to improve host status even further. Optimizing nutrition, normalizing serum protein, improving tissue oxygenation and withholding some cytotoxic agents are all relatively easy to achieve even in the elderly. Even though this is also done in the non-elderly population, the geriatric host provides an excellent opportunity to optimize a host that may benefit the most from preoperative intervention.

DIAGNOSIS

The diagnosis of osteomyelitis in the geriatric population can be made using existing clinical and laboratory tools in conjunction with imaging modalities. Symptoms can be vague and normal signs of overt infection can be absent due to a blunted host response. Patients may complain of generalized fatigue, malaise, fever and lethargy. Local signs like swelling, warmth, erythema and drainage may or may not be present in the affected area. A high index of suspicion should be present when an elderly patient has a history of infection at another site, such as cellulitis, pulmonary infection or urinary infection, in combination with an orthopaedic injury or disease. Specifically genito-urinary problems occur in the elderly that can result in transient bacteremia or the spread of infection through Batson's plexus into the spine. The literature supports an association between existing urinary tract infections and prosthetic infection.[12] The elderly may also have poor dentition that can result in infection. Patients with a history of prior trauma or who are immunocompromised should prompt the clinician to undertake further investigations.

The most common screening tests are the erythrocyte sedimentation rate (ESR), C-reactive protein (CRP) and complete blood count (CBC) to look for other potential conditions, such as hematologic neoplastic disorders, that mimic infection. Blood cultures are unlikely to be helpful unless systemic symptoms are present but they are usually undertaken in any workup for osteomyelitis. Elevations in the white blood cell (WBC) count, ESR and CRP are suggestive of an infection but remain non-specific markers of inflammation. When the CRP and ESR are combined, the specificity increases to 90–95%. If both are negative, it is unlikely that acute infection is present.[13] Greidanus et al. looked at ESR and CRP in assessing infected arthroplasties and found that these parameters were poor for screening but had high specificities and negative predictive values, which were helpful in making treatment decisions.[14] It is important to understand that the measurement of ESR and CRP is only one tool that clinicians should use as a part of their armamentarium for diagnosing osteomyelitis in the geriatric population. These values can and will be elevated for up to 6 months in a patient who has had recent surgery and they may be normal in a patient with a chronic infection. Additionally, both ESR and CRP are helpful once a diagnosis of osteomyelitis has been made since they provide a baseline value to monitor before, during and after treatment.

Once the decision has been made to proceed with operative treatment, biopsy and culture should be performed to try to identify the infective organism. Superficial cultures are not helpful and can even lead to inappropriate antibiotic selection and promotion of antibiotic resistance. Deep cultures and bone biopsy are the preferred diagnostic tools for osteomyelitis. Zuluaga et al. found that non-bone specimens produced 52% false negatives and 36% false positives.[15] This is not to say that superficial and non-bone specimens cannot be helpful. However, they should be evaluated critically relative to multiple bony specimens in order to maximize the potential for correct diagnosis. Even when bony specimens are obtained, no organism is recovered in up to 50% of cases. The low recovery and identification is most likely due to sampling error or partial treatment. Therefore, numerous cultures and specimens are recommended. *Staphylococcus aureus* remains the most common infecting agent that is recovered and represents 80–90% of all infections.[16] The clinician must also be aware that other potential pathogens exist concomitantly with the more common species. For instance, Gram-negative rods can occur in the same area and the same infection as the expected strains of *S. aureus*. Many bacteria can co-exist in a wound and in osteomyelitis, but polymicrobial infections without

a dominant organism may be especially challenging in the elderly because of their diminished host capacity.

Imaging studies

The use of imaging studies is evolving but they typically involve initial radiographs followed by another modality. Radiographs may take up to 10 days from the onset of acute osteomyelitis to manifest any visible signs of infection, which are typically a permeative lesion or periosteal reaction (Figure 5.3).[13] The earliest changes are usually seen in the adjacent soft tissues with swelling and potential loss of normal fat and muscle planes. It is not uncommon for an effusion to be present in adjacent joints as well. In order for bony changes on plain radiographs to be identified, the osteomyelitis must extend at least 1 cm and compromise 30–50% of the bone. Other specific changes include a periosteal reaction, bone lysis, loss of the osseous trabecular architecture, regional osteopenia, endosteal scalloping and eventual formation of a sequestrum and involucrum.[17] The permeative changes in the bone have also been described as a 'motheaten' appearance. All of these radiographic characteristics are more difficult to diagnose in the elderly due to their relative osteopenia. This is particularly true in the trauma setting where hardware and callus formation can make these osseous changes more difficult to assess.

Computerized tomography (CT) remains superior to plain films and magnetic resonance imaging (MRI) is probably the best investigative modality for demonstrating signs of infection. Both tests can help identify the bony margins of a sequestrum and surrounding involucrum. CT scans are

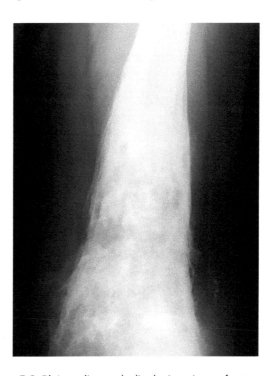

Figure 5.3 Plain radiograph displaying signs of osteomyelitis with characteristic changes of periosteal reaction and permeative 'motheaten' bone.

useful during staged debridements of osteomyelitis, especially for identifying an infected non-union after trauma. Software manipulation programs for both CT and MRI are making them more useful in the vicinity of metallic hardware and their use continues to evolve (Figures 5.4 and 5.5).

MRI has become an excellent modality to identify osteomyelitis and it can delineate between infected bone and adjacent soft tissue involvement. T1 weighted images will characteristically display a hypointense central component, whereas T2 weighted images will have a central hyperintense signal, relative to the surrounding anatomy. MRI also helps display cortical bone destruction, abscess margins and adjacent soft tissue and periosteal collections of fluid. MRI becomes less specific in identifying osteomyelitis when there is a fracture or in the vicinity of an implant but it can still be helpful for preoperative planning in assessing the degree of bony debridement needed. Recent advances in software have allowed MRI to be even more useful and the advent of carbon fiber implants (CarboFix, Israel) now allow even better diagnostic use of MRI (Figure 5.6). Ultrasound provides a cheap, fast examination of the soft tissues but is unable to visualize within bone. Where ultrasound can be utilized in the setting of osteomyelitis is in the assessment of soft tissue abscesses and adjacent joint effusions, especially in the presence of orthopaedic hardware that obscures

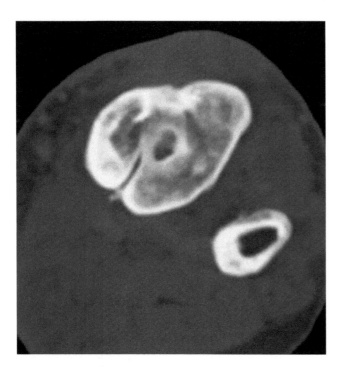

Figure 5.4 CT scan displaying osteomyelitis with a sequestrum and sinus tract.

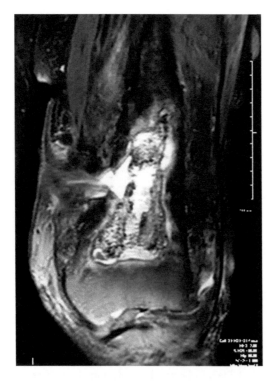

Figure 5.5 MRI reveals cortical destruction and abscess margins in a case of osteomyelitis.

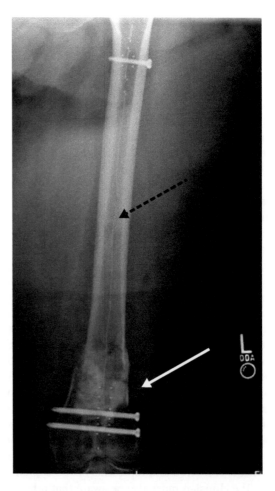

Figure 5.6 Radiograph of carbon fiber implant demonstrating its advantages with imaging. The dashed line is a radiographic marker in the nail. The solid line is antibiotic cement in the lesion. Carbon fiber markedly improves radiographic imaging without metal obscuration and allows use of CT and MRI.

MRI images. It is also a valuable tool in bedside evaluation both in the ER and ICU when a patient cannot have more time-consuming advanced imaging studies. The primary use of ultrasound is the identification of a fluid collection which may be aspirated for further diagnosis.

There are multiple nuclear medicine techniques that can be helpful in detecting osteomyelitis including technetium-99m bone scintigraphy, gallium-67 scintigraphy and indium-111 labelled WBC scanning. Studies to date have shown a wide variation in the sensitivities and specificities concerning the detection of osteomyelitis using these modalities. The technetium-99m scan is typically only useful to identify metabolically active bone. Osteomyelitis will present as a 'hot' or active area in all three phases of the scan, allowing it to sometimes differentiate a fracture from a loosening prosthesis, which should be 'cold' in the early phase. However, because of the many other conditions that can cause a 'hot' scan, this scan alone is rarely useful for diagnosis of osteomyelitis.

A labeled leukocyte cell scan demonstrates white cell activity that theoretically accumulates around an infectious nidus. These labeled leukocyte scans are able to reveal an abnormal accumulation of leukocytes in active osteomyelitis in patients who may have a 'cold' area of activity on the red cell bone scan. They are also very useful in detecting both vertebral and diabetic osteomyelitis, but again there is a very wide range of reported sensitivities and specificities. Unfortunately, older gallium labeled scans did not have as much success as anticipated so have been replaced by the indium-111 and technetium labeled leukocyte scans. With modern agents, results are reported to be 97% sensitive and 82% specific, and they have replaced gallium labeled scans for detecting infection.[18] However, patients who have an overlying soft tissue infection can still exhibit a false-positive result. Under these circumstances an accompanying bone scan is particularly useful and can help distinguish osteomyelitis from soft tissue infections. When the labeled agent scan is combined with the technetium-99m scan, their combined interpretation results in greater diagnostic specificity. A recent study by Stucken et al.[19] has cast some doubt on the use of any scintigraphy for the diagnosis of osteomyelitis. The study found that it was the least predictive method for revealing infection when used in the preoperative assessment of patients with non-unions and is consequently not cost effective. Since this isolated study has not been reliably reproduced, the authors feel that the use of scintigraphy remains a useful modality and provides additional information for a complex clinical condition, and as we discuss below, the use of other scintigraphic modalities can further improve the diagnosis.

The sulfur colloid scan is a measure of bone marrow activity and is typically positive with a myeloid lesion of the marrow but inactive with infection which usually suppresses hematopoietic and myeloid activity. Typically, the sulfur colloid scan is 'cold' in the presence of infection, while the red cell and white cell scans are 'hot.'[20] The authors have utilized all of the above studies and found that the most reliable combination is white cell and sulfur

scans but the difficulty has been finding a radiologic center that has appropriately trained people to interpret the scans and can also obtain the injection vehicle. The utility of such diagnostic testing is also dependent on the skill with which the scans are read and subjective interpretations undoubtedly affect results.

Finally, positron emission tomography (PET) scanning is a relatively new technique that is becoming more available and is currently thought to be the best modality for the diagnosis of infection.[21] The PET scan has demonstrated wide success in conditions such as sarcoid and neoplasm but due to cost it has been slow to be covered by insurers for infection. Yet it may have the highest diagnostic accuracy in confirming or excluding chronic osteomyelitis and it is considered superior in detecting chronic osteomyelitis in the axial skeleton.[22] PET scanning may become the preferred modality in detecting osteomyelitis in the geriatric population in the near future as more studies concerning its use become available. Unfortunately, the lack of payment coverage for this study has curtailed its use for the diagnosis of orthopaedic infections.

TREATMENT

The management of geriatric osteomyelitis requires a multidisciplinary approach with input and expertise from multiple groups of specialists including internal medicine, radiology, orthopaedics, plastics and infectious disease. Also, consideration should be given to involving the vascular surgery team for preoperative planning in patients with a micro- or macrovascular disease. Even with a thorough debridement, some patients may not have the capacity to heal their surgical wound and preoperative CT angiography or arterial Doppler ultrasound may be useful in minimizing trips to the operating theatre.

Generalizing a treatment algorithm is difficult and each patient should be treated on an individual basis to give them the best chance for cure, or remission, and ongoing quality of life. The first step of course is the successful diagnosis of osteomyelitis. Once the diagnosis has been made, the patient's nutritional and physiologic status should be optimized. An attempt should be made to identify the causative organism, ideally before initiation of antibiotic therapy. Then the appropriate surgical and medical interventions can be initiated to give the patient the best chance of cure or, in the instance of a C host, initiate suppressive therapy or limb amputation.

In an ideal world, the best treatment for geriatric osteomyelitis would be prevention of the infection in the first place. Meticulous, sterile operative technique accompanied by the administration of prophylactic antibiotics is essential for all elective and fracture procedures.[23] Boxma et al. showed that a single dose of ceftriaxone resulted in a 3.6% infection rate in comparison to a placebo group infection rate of 8.3%.[24] As the prevalence of MRSA increases in hospitals, consideration should also be given to incorporating vancomycin as a prophylactic antibiotic. Its use would be based on the nosocomial flora of each institution. In the treatment of an open fracture, the historic antibiotic choices are a first generation cephalosporin with the addition of an aminoglycoside for a more contaminated wound and/or penicillin for soil contamination. Often elderly patients will report a penicillin allergy which may or may not be real. If they do not report respiratory or systemic reactions but do report an upset stomach, or they cannot remember, the operative setting may be the best time to try a cephalosporin since the crossreactivity between pencillins and cephalosporins is extremely low, and if present can be readily treated. Furthermore, the alternative of clindamycin may precipitate colitis and gastrointestinal problems that may far exceed the infectious problem with regard to duration, management and patient happiness. Even cephalosporins can cause colitis in the elderly and should be used judiciously. The same is true for an aminoglycoside which can result in renal and ototoxicity and should thus be used at the appropriate dosage and for only the prescribed time period. More current regimens of once daily aminoglycosides should be used at the lower end of the dosage scale (3 mg/kg/day) to avoid a large single dose (7 mg/kg/day) that could cause renal or auditory complications. The authors have consulted with their institutional infectious disease specialists, who have recommended that in high risk patients who are MRSA carriers or who have an allergy, renal disease or heavy contamination, and hospitals with a higher than usual MRSA incidence, the use of vancomycin and a second generation or later cephalosporin is an excellent alternative to clindamycin because of its risk of colitis in the elderly. Antibiotic use is no substitute for appropriate and aggressive debridement and their use can be thought of as analogous to the use of chemotherapy in the setting of neoplasms requiring resection. Surgical resection is often marginal resection and subsequent chemotherapy is intended to treat the tumour load left behind.

Once geriatric osteomyelitis has been diagnosed, collaboration between the orthopaedist, the internist and infectious disease specialist is paramount. Infectious disease experts should facilitate treatment by selecting an effective antibiotic with the lowest complication and toxicity profile. At our institution, successful debridement of osteomyelitis is followed by 6–8 weeks of antibiotic therapy with continued observation of ESR and CRP. There is, of course, no general consensus supported in the literature for antibiotic duration, so consideration must be given on a case-by-case basis. No therapy is without consequences, however, as bacterial resistance, poor patient compliance and tolerance as well as financial issues must all be considered when selecting an antibiotic regimen. This is where the infectious disease specialist becomes an integral part of the team in treating geriatric osteomyelitis. With regard to oral versus intravenous antibiotics, there are few recommendations in geriatric osteomyelitis. While many new oral antibiotics make it possible to avoid some of the pitfalls of long-term intravenous therapy, this decision should be made based on each patient's unique situation.

The hallmark of surgical treatment for osteomyelitis remains a thorough debridement. Necrotic and non-viable tissue should be debrided to remove all infected material. The geriatric patient presents a unique risk/benefit scenario for the clinician in comparison to younger and healthier individuals. Large debridements may eradicate the infection and osteomyelitis but also may leave a very large defect. While younger patients can undergo extensive reconstructions, the elderly may not be able to endure the repetitive surgical procedures, and due to vascular disease, may not be able to undergo free tissue transfer.[25] Thus, in the older population, a more definitive approach to acute fracture care, such as amputation or staged arthroplasty, may be necessary. Open fractures remain a relative contraindication for arthroplasty but even the higher risk of infection should be weighed against the problems associated with extensive reconstructive procedures. If amputation is chosen, preoperative vascular studies such as skin oximetry or CT angiography may help determine the healing potential of tissues at the level of amputation. While arthroplasty is relatively contraindicated with infection, a staged arthroplasty with its added risk of ongoing infection may still be the best option in the advanced elderly who may have few years of life left. In these individuals, the ability to have functional mobility for transfers might provide a better end-of-life quality than the immobility resulting from amputation or extensive reconstruction. While there is little science in this area with regard to geriatric osteomyelitis, the experience in acute trauma has been encouraging.

Technical aspects of treatment remain the same in the elderly and are analogous to tumour surgery. While a wide resection with clean margins would be the ideal approach, the amount of tissue and bone resection may result in a destabilizing condition that is associated with even greater morbidity in the form of extensive reconstructive procedures. The next best option is a marginal resection which is nearly complete but may leave some affected tissues at the periphery. This type of resection may still be destabilizing but is probably the most commonly seen. Use of local modalities such as antibiotic beads along with systemic treatment will often result in successful treatment. In some circumstances, such as lesions near joints or neurovascular structures, even a marginal resection may not be possible. In such cases, an intra-lesional resection combined with long-term suppressive antibiotics may provide the patient with adequate treatment.

Effective debridement is ideally performed without completely destabilizing the bone and limiting any periosteal stripping. The involucrum can be preserved but the entire sequestrum must be removed. If the osteomyelitis is primarily intramedullary, as often occurs after intramedullary nailing of long bones, then hardware removal, intramedullary reaming with or without re-implantation depending on whether bone is healed or not, should be considered. The reamer–irrigator–aspirator (RIA) system cleans the medullary canal while aspirating contents and irrigating the length of the long bone. The RIA is very effective for such cases but requires some expertise to understand its assembly, select the correct reamer size and manage the complications. If such technology is not available, or affordable, then standard medullary reamers will be just as effective and there are numerous studies advocating the use of intramedullary reaming as a debridement technique.[26-28] Pommer et al. found that reaming an infected intramedullary canal resulted in 100% infection eradication, compared to 62% eradication in patients who had multiple surgeries prior to the reaming and nailing.[28] Ochsner and Brunazzi observed 40 patients with chronic osteomyelitis, who underwent intramedullary reaming, for an average of 4.4 years with only four patients suffering a recurrence of their infection.[26] When we treat post-nailing infections, we like to open a distal portal, where previous interlocking screws were placed, using a high speed burr and allow a portal of efflux for detritus. This portal can be used to extract medullary tissue and facilitate an adequate flow of antiseptic fluid from proximal to distal. We have found this technique to be very useful and cost effective (Figure 5.7).

Essential to the debridement process is the collection of sterile intraoperative cultures to properly identify the offending organism. This is particularly important in the elderly as they are more susceptible to infection from low virulence bacteria and have an increased susceptibility to the detrimental side effects of antibiotics. In an elderly patient with vertebral osteomyelitis this is of utmost importance because, if mismanaged, epidural spread can

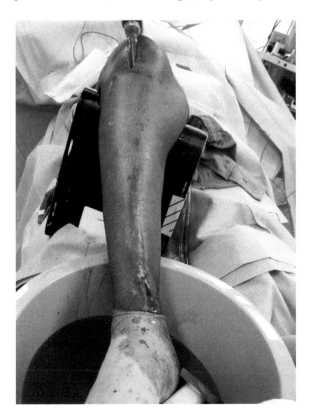

Figure 5.7 Clinical picture of a two portal technique after medullary reaming and use of medullary irrigation that allows efflux of material and fluid through the canal.

occur resulting in paraplegia. Peripheral cultures can be misleading in this age group as co-infection is not uncommon.[29] Once vertebral osteomyelitis has progressed to the point that neurologic changes such as myelopathy or epidural involvement occur, then surgical intervention in the form of debridement and/or fusion is required. Concomitant antibiotics should be initiated and curtailed with the help of a qualified infectious disease team.[25] Spinal osteomyelitis is unfortunately more common despite better health care. The tuberculous and syphilitic aetiology of the past has been replaced by other organisms that remain populous in the elderly host.

The topic of irrigation technique and method has recently been debated. Some studies have shown that pulsatile high-pressure irrigation systems, while capable of removing more bioluminescent bacteria in an animal model than a bulb syringe,[30] can also damage soft tissue and even force bacteria deeper into the surgical wound.[31-33] This can be potentiated in the already frail geriatric patient. Recent studies have tried to establish the usefulness of gravity flow of fluid through large bore tubing. While this obviously mitigates the theoretical injury caused by high-pressure flow, the benefit of using low pressure pulsatile irrigation is its ability to help 'detach' adhered bacteria without damaging tissue. The physical effect of low pressure on tissues has been found to be safe in recent studies and potentially better than simple gravity flow irrigation. From a common sense perspective, comparison of the fact that bacteria adhere to tissue with the theoretical damage to soft tissues with pulsed irrigation suggests that pulsed irrigation is the more sensible modality.

The use of iodine, betadine and most antiseptics directly in wounds is associated with known tissue toxicity to both soft tissue and bone.[34] In fact, use of such toxic chemicals probably causes more tissue damage than pulsatile lavage. The authors recommend the use of a low pressure pulsatile lavage with the addition of Clorpactin® (oxychlorosene; Guardian Laboratories, UK) in the irrigation solution and the strict avoidance of any tissue toxic chemicals in the wound. Clorpactin has a little to no tissue toxicity when dissolved in fluid and is most commonly used with interstitial cystitis. Its chemical characteristics are very similar to dilute Dakins® (sodium hypochlorite) solution used in exposed tissues and in burns. Only in the most severely contaminated wounds, such as those contaminated with cow manure or human excrement, or heavily contaminated freshwater, would we consider direct application of tissue toxic antiseptic to intact tissue, because in these situations, the problems associated with tissue damage are exceeded by the problems of severe contamination.

Just as important as systemic antibiotic therapy may be the local delivery of antibiotics in the wound bed and area of osteomyelitis in geriatric patients. Local antibiotic delivery systems provide a high concentration of antibiotic in the area of infection with minimal systemic absorption. Our institution utilizes vancomycin and gentamicin laden PMMA antibiotic beads in a ratio of 1–4 g to 1.2–4.8 g, respectively. The use of higher doses (>1.0 g and 1.2 g, respectively) will obviously result in 'caking' of the antibiotic setting but use of saline (not monomer) will help equalize the powder liquid ratio and result in a very porous and effective delivery system. These local cements can be made into various shapes including balls, oblong cylinders and disks and they can be placed on an 18 gauge wire depending upon the shape, size and character of the tissue planes they are being placed in (Figure 5.8). Similarly an antibiotic intramedullary rod can be fashioned utilizing the same combination. A recent article discussed the efficacy of a bioabsorbable gel as a vector for the delivery of antibiotics into a wound made in the laboratory. This animal model study suggested that gel delivery may be superior to antibiotic bead delivery and is resorbable so that a subsequent retrieval procedure would not be necessary.[31] These are early studies, with the emphasis being that new and better ways to deliver higher concentrations of antibiotics into wound beds or infected tissue are currently being developed.

If a large osseous defect is still present after a thorough debridement has been performed, some types of temporary stability are required until the secondary reconstruction can be undertaken. This situation is often seen after severe open fractures or in type III and type IV osteomyelitis. Typically the stabilization is undertaken within an external fixator. In complicated cases, or in those with segmental bone loss, distraction osteogenesis or bone transport can be used successfully for bone lengthening. The use of bone transport is not suitable for every patient because it is physically and psychologically taxing on the patient, hospital staff and family. Even though the elderly are often tougher and more resilient psychologically, they may not be able to endure such a complicated treatment regime. Other alternatives include a vascularized bone transfer or the Masquelet technique, which involves the creation of a neo-vascular sleeve around

a cement spacer which is often mixed with antibiotic. This provides a sort of cambium cell layer that promotes osteogenesis once the spacer is removed and replaced by osteoconductive and osteoinductive material in the form of bone graft. Approximately 4–6 weeks after placement of the spacer, a vascularized pseudomembrane is formed with high concentrations of growth factors including vascularized endothelial growth factor, transforming growth factor beta and bone morphogenic protein.[35] The patient returns to the operating room at a later date when the cement spacer is removed and the void replaced with bone graft.[36,37] Other techniques similar to this are the cylindrical mesh technique, which uses titanium wire cages, similar in construct to those used in spinal fusions, packed with cancellous autograft.[38] This can be supported with intramedullary nailing, internal fixation or external fixation.[31] However all of these procedures involve multiple surgeries and their risks and benefits in the elderly population must be considered.

Finally, arthroplasty may be the only non-amputation, non-suppression option. The typical scenario is the infected periarticular fracture in a B or C host, or the infected prosthetic joint in the B host. Most elderly patients will tolerate a two-stage procedure but not much more. In the case of open or infected periarticular fractures and infected total joints, the whole joint is resected at the metaphyseal level to achieve at least a marginal resection. An antibiotic spacer is placed and after a period of treatment, an aspiration and laboratory values can determine the effectiveness of treatment. Then, a tumour type or revision type of arthroplasty is performed with the knowledge that the risk of recurrent infection is elevated and may result in the need for amputation. In these cases, we supplement treatment with a suppressive antibiotic regime to allow time for biologic tissue integration. We also coat the exposed body of the implant surface with antibiotic cement (Figure 5.9). The literature concerning the success of these types of cases is sparse and not definitive but we believe that application of sound principles is a logical and prudent approach. In the C host, there are only two options, suppression and amputation. With prosthetic technology advancing tremendously after the recent Gulf War, which resulted in numerous amputations in soldiers, amputation is not entirely a bad option, but we must recognize that there is still a significant cardiovascular burden placed on the elderly which may be detrimental. For example, a below knee amputation has been shown to incur a 40% increased metabolic demand for gait, while an above knee amputation incurs a 68% increase. These are important issues in the elderly and should be taken into consideration. Suppression is also a possible treatment in patients who are not candidates for either amputation or staged treatment (C host). There is some literature that supports irrigation and debridement followed by very long-term antibiotic suppression. Rao et al. found an 86.2% success rate in their series.[39] Again, relevant studies are few and not definitive but they do provide an alternative in the management of difficult cases.

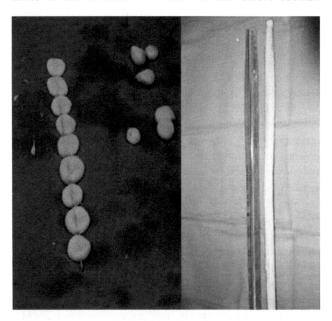

Figure 5.8 Several antibiotic bead configurations that are clinically useful.

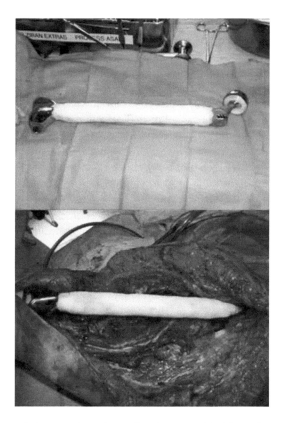

Figure 5.9 An arthroplasty that is 'coated' with antibiotic impregnated bone cement to reduce the available surface for bacterial adherence while simultaneously providing local antibiotic delivery.

SUMMARY

The geriatric population is a unique, complicated group of patients that will continue to grow in number. As 'baby boomers' age and modern medical advancements allow humans to live longer lives, all physicians, including orthopaedists, will continue to serve increasing numbers of elderly patients. Geriatric osteomyelitis presents an extremely difficult yet important part of that orthopaedic care. While the treatment principles may remain the same as in younger patients, careful consideration must be given to optimizing the geriatric host both pre- and postoperatively. Responsible surgical management and utilization of long-term suppressive therapy in lieu of large reconstructions should always be considered. At the same time, the healthy, active geriatric patient will be seen more frequently and they deserve the same attempts at reconstruction and salvage as given to younger patients if they can tolerate them. These difficult management decisions are best made through a multidisciplinary approach where expectations, goals and quality of life after intervention are thoroughly discussed between the managing physicians, the patient and their family. This will allow for the best care to be delivered while maximizing patient outcomes unique to each individual situation.

REFERENCES

1. Moussa FW, Anglen JO, Gehrke JC, Christensen G, Simpson WA. The significance of positive cultures from orthopedic fixation devices in the absence of clinical infection. *Am J Orthop.* 1997;26(9):617–20.
2. Zimmerli W, Moser C. Pathogenesis and treatment concepts of orthopaedic biofilm infections. *FEMS Immunol Med Microbiol.* 2012;65(2):158–68.
3. Gao Z, Tseng CH, Pei Z, Blaser MJ. Molecular analysis of human forearm superficial skin bacterial biota. *Proc Natl Acad Sci U S A.* 2007;104(8):2927–32.
4. Keller MA, Stiehm ER. Passive immunity in prevention and treatment of infectious diseases. *Clin Microbiol Rev.* 2000;13(4):602–14.
5. Novick A. Growth of bacteria. *Ann Rev Microbiol.* 1955;9:97–110.
6. Ito, K, Hirao A, Arai F, et al. Regulation of oxidative stress by ATM is required for self-renewal of haematopoietic stem cells. *Nature.* 2004;431(7011):997–1002.
7. Cambier J. Immunosenescence: A problem of lymphopoiesis, homeostasis, microenvironment, and signaling. *Immunol Rev.* 2005;205:5–6.
8. Jefferson KK. What drives bacteria to produce a biofilm? *FEMS Microbiol Lett.* 2004;36(2):163–72.
9. Cunha B. Osteomyelitis in elderly patients. *Aging Infect Dis.* 2002;35:287–93.
10. Cierny G 3rd, Mader JT, Penninck JJ. A clinical staging system for adult osteomyelitis. *Clin Orthop Relat Res.* 2003;(414):7–24.
11. Cierny G, Mader JT, Pennick JJ. A clinical staging system for adult osteomyelitis. *Contemp Orthop.* 1985;10:17–37.
12. Sousa R, Muñoz-Mahamud E, Quayle J, et al. Is asymptomatic bacteriuria a risk factor for prosthetic joint infection? *Clin Infect Dis.* 2014;59(1):41–7.
13. Wheat J. Diagnostic strategies in osteomyelitis. *Am J Med.* 1985;78(6B):218–24.
14. Greidanus NV, Masri BA, Garbuz DS, et al. Use of erythrocyte sedimentation rate and C-reactive protein level to diagnose infection before revision total knee arthroplasty. A prospective evaluation. *J Bone Joint Surg Am.* 2007;89(7):1409–16.
15. Zuluaga AF, Galvis W, Jaimes F, Vesga O. Lack of microbiological concordance between bone and non-bone specimens in chronic osteomyelitis: An observational study. *BMC Infect Dis.* 2002;2:8.
16. Kumar V, Abbas AK, Fausto N, et al. Robbins and Cotran pathologic basis of disease. Philadelphia, PA: WB Saunders, 2005.
17. Pineda C, Espinosa R, Pena A. Radiographic imaging in osteomyelitis: The role of plain radiography, computed tomography, ultrasonography, magnetic resonance imaging, and scintigraphy. *Semin Plast Surg.* 2009;23(2):80–9.

18. McCarthy K, Velchik MG, Alavi A, et al. Indium-111-labeled white blood cells in the detection of osteomyelitis complicated by a pre-existing condition. *J Nucl Med.* 1988;29(6):1015–21.

19. Stucken C, Olszewski DC, Creevy WR, Murakami AM, Tornetta P. Preoperative diagnosis of infection in patients with nonunions. *J Bone Joint Surg Am.* 2013;95(15):1409–12.

20. Palestro CJ, Mehta HH, Patel M, et al. Marrow versus infection in the Charcot joint: Indium-111 leucocyte and technetium-99m sulfur colloid scintigraphy. *J Nucl Med.* 1998;39(2):346–50.

21. Chacko TK, Zhuang H, Nakhoda KZ, et al. Applications of fluorodeoxyglucose positron emission tomography in the diagnosis of infection. *Nucl Med Commun.* 2003;24(6):615–24.

22. Pineda C, Vargas A, Rodríguez AV. Imaging of osteomyelitis: Current concepts. *Infect Dis Clin North Am.* 2006;20(4):789–825.

23. Cavanaugh DL, Berry J, Yarboro SR, et al. Better prophylaxis against surgical site infection with local as well as systemic antibiotics. An in vivo study. *J Bone Joint Surg Am.* 2009;91(8):1907–12.

24. Boxma H, Broekhuizen T, Patka P, et al. Randomised controlled trial of single-dose antibiotic prophylaxis in surgical treatment of closed fractures: The Dutch trauma trial. *Lancet.* 1996;347(9009):1133–7.

25. Mader J, Shirtliff M, Bergquist S, et al. Bone and joint infections in the elderly: Practical treatment guidelines. *Drugs Aging.* 2000;16(1):67–80.

26. Ochsner PE, Brunazzi MG. Intramedullary reaming and soft tissue procedures in treatment of chronic osteomyelitis of long bones. *Orthopedics.* 1994;17(5):433–40.

27. Pape HC, Zwipp H, Regel G, et al. Chronic treatment refractory osteomyelitis of long tubular bones—Possibilities and risks of intramedullary boring. *Unfallchirurg.* 1995;98(3):139–44.

28. Pommer A, David A, Richter J, et al. Intramedullary boring in infected intramedullary nail osteosyntheses of the tibia and femur. *Unfallchirurg.* 1998;101(8):628–33.

29. Velan G, Leitner J, Gepstein R. Pyogenic osteomyelitis of the spine in the elderly: Three cases of a synchronous non-axial infection by a different pathogen. *Spinal Cord.* 1999;37:215–17.

30. Svoboda S, Bice T, Gooden H, et al. Comparison of bulb syringe and pulsed lavage irrigation with use of a bioluminescent musculoskeletal wound model. *J Bone Joint Surg.* 2006;88(10):2167–74.

31. Penn-Barwell J, Murray C, Wenke J. Local antibiotic delivery by a bioabsorbable gel is superior to PMMA bead depot in reducing infection in an open fracture model. *J Orthop Trauma.* 2013;28(6):370–5.

32. Boyd JI 3rd, Wongworawat MD. High-pressure pulsatile lavage causes soft tissue damage. *Clin Orthop Relat Res.* 2004;(427):13–17.

33. Hassinger SM, Harding G, Wongworawat MD. High-pressure pulsatile lavage propagates bacteria into soft tissue. *Clin Orthop Relat Res.* 2005;439:27–31.

34. Sato S, Miyake M, Hazama A, et al. Povidone-iodine-induced cell death in cultured human epithelial HeLa cells and rat oral mucosal tissue. *Drug Chem Toxicol.* 2014;37(3):268–75.

35. Pelissier P, Masquelet AC, Bareille R, Pelissier SM, Amedee J. Induced membranes secrete growth factors including vascular and osteoinductive factors and could stimulate bone regeneration. *J Orthop Res.* 2004;22(1):73–9.

36. Karger C, Kishi T, Schneider L, et al. Treatment of posttraumatic bone defects by the induced membrane technique. *Orthop Traumatol Surg Res.* 2012;98(1):97–102.

37. Masquelet AC, Begue T. The concept of induced membrane for reconstruction of long bone defects. *Orthop Clin North Am.* 2010;41(1):27–37.

38. Cobos JA, Lindsey RW, Gugala Z. The cylindrical titanium mesh cage for treatment of a long bone segmental defect: Description of a new technique and report of two cases. *J Orthop Trauma.* 2000;14(1):54–9.

39. Rao N, Crossett LS, Sinha RK, et al. Long-term suppression of infection in total joint arthroplasty. *Clin Orthop Relat Res.* 2003;(414):55–60.

6

Other orthopaedic complications

MARGARET M. McQUEEN, ROGER M. ATKINS AND PETER V. GIANNOUDIS

ACUTE COMPARTMENT SYNDROME IN THE ELDERLY

MARGARET M. McQUEEN

Introduction

Acute compartment syndrome (ACS) occurs when the pressure inside a confined compartment rises to a level and for a duration beyond which there is a critical reduction in blood flow to the tissues contained within. Without urgent decompression tissue ischaemia, necrosis, functional impairment and sometimes loss of limb will result. This is one of the few true emergency situations in orthopaedic trauma practice.

It is important to differentiate ACS from other related conditions. Exertional compartment syndrome is raised intracompartmental pressure (ICP) during exercise, causing ischaemia, pain and rarely neurological symptoms and signs. It normally resolves with rest but may proceed to ACS if exercise continues. Volkmann's ischaemic contracture is the end stage of neglected ACS with irreversible muscle necrosis leading to contractures. The crush syndrome is the systemic result of muscle necrosis commonly caused by prolonged external compression of an extremity. In the presence of established muscle necrosis, ICP may rise as a result of intracellular and intracompartmental oedema, causing a superimposed ACS.

Epidemiology – who is at risk?

The incidence of ACS in a westernized population is 3.1 per 100,000 of the population per annum.[1] The annual incidence for males is 7.3 per 100,000 compared with 0.7 per 100,000 for females, a 10-fold increase in risk for males. The age and gender-specific incidences are illustrated in Figure 6.1, showing a type B pattern[2] or the L-shaped pattern described by Buhr and Cooke.[3] The mean age is 32 years; the median age for males is 30 years and for females 44 years. It is clear therefore that older patients are at less risk of ACS. This is thought to be due to a combination of smaller muscle bulk allowing more room for swelling within a compartment and a possible protective effect of hypertension. The only exception to youth being a risk factor in ACS is in cases with soft tissue injury only. These patients have an average age of 36 years and are significantly older than those with a fracture.[4]

The most common underlying condition causing ACS is a fracture in 69% of cases (Table 6.1). Tibial diaphyseal fracture is the most frequent, occurring in 36% of cases of ACS and with a prevalence of ACS being reported in up to 14% of cases of tibial fracture.[1,5,6] The second most common cause is soft tissue injury which accounts for almost one quarter of cases of ACS. The second most common fracture causing ACS is distal radius fracture. Other causes of ACS are listed in Table 6.2. Although most of these are uncommon, several are relevant to the older patient who may have comorbidities. The crush syndrome is probably more frequent than realized in the elderly who may lie in an obtunded state for many hours after a fall. In these circumstances creatinine kinase levels should be monitored. Comorbidities such as diabetes and treatment with anticoagulants are frequent in the older patient and treating surgeons should be aware that they may increase the risk of ACS developing.

Although there is a persistent belief that high energy injury is a risk factor for the development of ACS, there is no evidence to support this. In tibial diaphyseal fracture in adults complicated by ACS, the proportion of high compared with low energy injury shows a slight preponderance of low energy injury (59%).[1] In an analysis of 1,403 tibial diaphyseal fractures presenting to the Edinburgh Orthopaedic Trauma Unit over the period from 1995 to

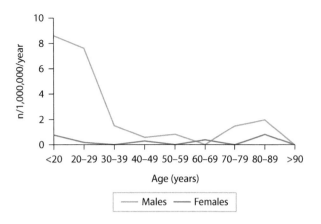

Figure 6.1 The age and gender related incidence of acute compartment syndrome showing a reduction in both genders with age.

Table 6.1 The underlying causes of acute compartment syndrome presenting to an orthopaedic trauma unit

Underlying condition	Percent of cases (%)
Tibial diaphyseal fracture	36.0
Soft tissue injury	23.2
Distal radius fracture	9.8
Crush syndrome	7.9
Diaphyseal fracture forearm	7.9
Tibial plateau/pilon fracture	5.5
Femoral diaphyseal fracture	3.0
Hand fracture(s)	2.5
Foot fracture(s)	1.8
Other (foot, ankle, pelvis, humerus)	2.4

2007 there was an increased risk of ACS in closed compared with open fractures (*P*<0.05). This suggests ACS may be more prevalent after low energy injury, possibly because in low energy injury the compartment boundaries are less likely to be disrupted and an 'autodecompression' effect is avoided.

Risk factors for the development or late diagnosis of ACS are listed in Table 6.3. As well as demographic risk factors, altered pain perception can delay diagnosis. This can occur if the patient has an altered conscious state, has cognitive difficulties or with the use of spinal or epidural anaesthesia or patient controlled analgesia. Comorbidities such as diabetes and treatment with anticoagulants are frequent in the older patient and treating surgeons should be aware that they may increase the risk of ACS developing.

Diagnosis

Prompt diagnosis of ACS is the key to a successful outcome. Delay in diagnosis has long been recognized as the only cause of failure of the treatment of ACS. Delay in diagnosis may be due to inexperience and lack of awareness of the

Table 6.2 Conditions causing acute compartment syndrome

Conditions increasing the volume of compartment contents
Fracture
Soft tissue injury
Crush syndrome (including use of the lithotomy position)
Revascularization
Exercise
Bleeding diathesis/anticoagulants
Fluid infusion (including arthroscopy)
Arterial puncture
Ruptured ganglia/cysts
Osteotomy
Snake bite
Nephrotic syndrome
Leukaemic infiltration
Viral myositis
Acute haematogenous osteomyelitis

Conditions reducing compartment volume
Burns
Repair of muscle hernia

Medical comorbidity
Diabetes
Hypothyroidism

possibility of ACS, an indefinite and confusing clinical presentation, or anaesthetic or analgesic techniques that mask the clinical signs.

Delay in treatment of ACS can be catastrophic, leading to serious complications such as permanent sensory and motor deficits, contractures, infection and, at times, amputation of the limb. In severe cases there may be systemic injury from the reperfusion syndrome. To avoid such complications it is essential for the treating surgeon to have a clear understanding of the clinical techniques necessary to make an early diagnosis. Early recognition and treatment of ACS also result in decreased indemnity risk in potential malpractice claims.[7]

CLINICAL DIAGNOSIS

Pain is considered to be the first symptom of ACS. The pain experienced is ischaemic and usually severe and out of proportion to the clinical situation. However, pain can be an unreliable indication of the presence of ACS because it can be variable in its intensity, may be absent in ACS associated with nerve injury or minimal in the deep posterior compartment syndrome. It cannot be elicited in the unconscious patient or where regional anaesthesia is used.[8] Elderly patients with dementia may not be able to express the severity of their pain, so restlessness, agitation and anxiety with increasing analgesic requirements should raise the suspicion of the presence of an ACS.

Pain has been shown to have a sensitivity of only 19% and a specificity of 97% in the diagnosis of ACS (i.e. a high proportion of false negative or missed cases but a low

Table 6.3 Risk factors for the development or delayed diagnosis of acute compartment syndrome

Demographic	Altered pain perception
Youth	Altered conscious level
Tibial fracture	Regional anaesthesia
High energy forearm fracture	Patient controlled analgesia
High energy femoral diaphyseal fracture	Children
Bleeding diathesis/anticoagulants	Associated nerve injury
Polytrauma with high base deficit, lactate levels and transfusion requirement	

proportion of false positive cases).[9] There is general agreement, however, that pain if present is a relatively early symptom of ACS in the awake alert patient.[9] Pain with passive stretch of the muscles involved is recognized as a symptom of ACS but is no more reliable than rest pain because the reasons for unreliability quoted above apply equally to pain on passive stretch. The sensitivity and specificity of pain on passive stretch are similar to those for rest pain.[9]

Paraesthesia and hypoesthesia in the territory of the nerves within the affected compartment are frequently the first signs of nerve ischaemia, although sensory abnormality may be the result of concomitant nerve injury. Ulmer reports a sensitivity of 13% and specificity of 98% for the clinical finding of paraesthesia in ACS, a false negative rate that precludes this symptom from being a useful diagnostic tool.[9] Paralysis of muscle groups affected by the ACS is recognized as being a late sign.[9] This sign has equally low sensitivity as others in predicting the presence of ACS, probably because of the difficulty of interpreting the underlying cause of the weakness, which could be inhibition by pain, direct injury to muscle or associated nerve injury. If a motor deficit develops, full recovery is unlikely[10,11] with full recovery in one series in only 13% of patients.[10]

Swelling is cited as a sign of ACS but the degree of swelling is difficult to assess accurately, making this sign very subjective. Casts or dressings often obscure compartments at risk[8] and some compartments such as the deep posterior compartment of the leg are difficult to access.

Peripheral pulses and capillary return are always intact in ACS unless there is major arterial injury or disease or in the very late stages of ACS when amputation is inevitable. If ACS is suspected and pulses are absent, then arteriography is indicated. Conversely, it is dangerous to exclude the diagnosis of ACS because distal pulses are present.

Using a combination of clinical symptoms and signs increases their sensitivity as diagnostic tools.[9] To achieve a probability of over 90% of ACS being present, however, three clinical findings must be noted. The third clinical finding is paresis, so to achieve an accurate clinical diagnosis of ACS the condition must be allowed to progress until a late stage. This is clearly unacceptable and has led to a search for earlier, more reliable methods of diagnosis.

COMPARTMENT PRESSURE MONITORING

Measurement of ICP was developed when it was established that ACS was caused by increased tissue pressure. Because raised tissue pressure is the primary event in ACS, changes in ICP precede the clinical symptoms and signs.[12] Most methods use a slit or wick catheter inserted into the relevant compartment connected to a pressure transducer through a column of saline. Patency can be confirmed by gentle pressure over the catheter tip; an immediate rise in the pressure should be seen. Care must be taken to avoid the presence of air bubbles in the system as this can result in falsely low readings. The slit and wick catheters are equally accurate.[13] ICP can also be measured by introducing a transducer into the compartment either by siting it in the lumen of the catheter or placing it at the tip. For continuous pressure measurement the latter requires an infusion of saline with a risk of increasing ICP; the former is expensive and difficult to resterilize. These methods all measure ICP which is an indirect measurement of muscle blood flow and oxygenation. Near infrared spectroscopy measures tissue oxygen saturation non-invasively by means of a probe placed on the skin and is a technique with promise but requires further validation in humans subjected to injury.

ICP is usually monitored in the anterior compartment in the tibia because this is most commonly involved in ACS and is easily accessible.[5] There is a risk of missing an ACS in the deep posterior compartments but measuring two compartments is much more cumbersome. If the anterior compartment alone is monitored, the ICP in the deep posterior compartment must be measured if there are unexplained symptoms in the presence of normal anterior compartment pressures. It is important to measure the peak pressure within the limb, which usually occurs within 5 cm of the level of the fracture.[14]

Threshold for decompression

Much debate has occurred about the critical pressure threshold, beyond which decompression of ACS is required. Historically tissue pressure measurements of between 30 and 50 mmHg were used as the threshold for decompression, but it is now recognized that apparent variation between individuals in their tolerance of raised ICP is because of variations in systemic blood pressure. Whitesides and his co-authors were the first to suggest the importance of the difference between the diastolic blood pressure and tissue pressure, or ΔP.[15] They stated that there is inadequate perfusion and relative ischaemia when the tissue pressure rises to within 10–30 mmHg of the diastolic pressure and this is supported by further evidence from experimental studies[16,17] or the similar concept that the difference between mean arterial pressure and tissue pressure should not be less than 30 mmHg in normal muscle or 40 mmHg in muscle subject to trauma[18] or antecedent ischaemia.[19] A clinical study of 116 patients with tibial diaphyseal fractures validated the experimental evidence. The authors concluded that a ΔP of 30 mmHg is a safe threshold for decompression in ACS.[5]

The use of ΔP as a threshold for fasciotomy has also been supported in other studies.[20,21]

The sensitivity and specificity of continuous compartment pressure monitoring has recently been reported.[6] Using a pressure threshold of a ΔP of 30 mmHg for more than 2 hours as an indication for fasciotomy in 850 patients, there were 11 false positives and 9 false negatives giving a sensitivity of 94% and a specificity of 98.4%. The positive predictive value was 92.8% and the negative predictive value was 98.7%. To achieve similar accuracy with clinical symptoms and signs, three signs need to be present with the third being paralysis.[9]

To derive the full benefit of monitoring for ACS, the diagnosis should be made on the basis of sequential differential pressure measurements rather than awaiting the development of clinical symptoms and signs. It has been demonstrated that this approach reduces both the delay to fasciotomy and the development of sequelae[22] and that the appearance of clinical symptoms and signs lags behind the pressure changes.[5] It has been assumed that these pressure thresholds apply equally to anatomic areas other than the leg, although this has not been formally examined.

Timing

Time factors are also important in making the decision to proceed to fasciotomy. It is well established experimentally and clinically that both the duration and severity of the pressure elevation influence the development of muscle necrosis and sequelae.[5,11,17,23] Continuous pressure monitoring allows a clear record of the trend of the tissue pressure measurements. In situations where the ΔP drops below 30 mmHg, if the ICP is dropping and the ΔP is rising, then it is safe to observe the patient in anticipation of the ΔP returning within a short time to safe levels. If the ICP is rising, the ΔP is dropping and less than 30 mmHg, and this trend has been consistent for a period of 2 hours, then fasciotomy should be performed. Fasciotomy should not be performed based on a single pressure reading except in extreme cases. Using this protocol, delay to fasciotomy and the sequelae of ACS are reduced without unnecessary fasciotomies being performed.[5] For ICP monitoring to be most effective in reducing delay, it must be used as the primary indication for fasciotomy.

Treatment

The single most effective treatment for ACS is fasciotomy, which if delayed can cause devastating complications. Nevertheless, other preliminary measures should be taken in cases of impending ACS. External limiting envelopes such as dressings or plaster casts, including the padding under the cast, should be split and spread. The limb should not be elevated above the height of the heart as this reduces the arteriovenous gradient.[24] Hypotension should be corrected, because this will reduce perfusion pressure. Oxygen therapy should be instituted to ensure maximum oxygen saturation.

FASCIOTOMY

The basic principle of fasciotomy of any compartment is full and adequate decompression. Skin incisions must be made along the full length of the affected compartment (Figure 6.2) and it is essential to visualize all contained muscles in their entirety. There is no place for limited or subcutaneous fasciotomy in ACS. Any muscle necrosis must be thoroughly debrided to avoid infection.

In the leg, all four compartments should be released using a double incision four-compartment fasciotomy. The anterior and lateral compartments are released through a lateral skin incision over the intermuscular septum between the compartments (Figure 6.2) and the two posterior compartments are accessed through a skin incision 2 cm from the medial edge of the tibia (Figure 6.3). It is important to allow a generous skin bridge between the two, especially in the elderly, when skin circulation may be compromised. Single incision fasciotomy of all four compartments has been described but double incision fasciotomy is faster and probably safer than single incision methods because the fascial incisions are all superficial. Using the single incision method, it can be difficult to visualize the full extent of the deep posterior compartment. Both methods seem to be equally effective at reducing ICP.

In other areas decompression is usually simple with incisions made directly over the affected compartments affording good exposure of the muscle groups. The exceptions are the foot and hand. In the foot there are a number of compartments to decompress, and a sound knowledge of the anatomy is essential. In most cases dorsal incisions are sufficient, but in hindfoot injury a separate medial incision may be required to decompress the calcaneal compartment. Decompression of the hand can usually be adequately achieved using two dorsal incisions that allow access to the interosseous compartments, but if there is clinical suspicion or raised ICP on measurement, then incisions may be made over the thenar and hypothenar eminences, allowing fasciotomy of these compartments.

Fasciotomy incisions must never be closed, primarily because this may result in persistent elevation of ICP. The wounds should be left open and dressed, and approximately 48 hours after fasciotomy a 'second look' procedure should be undertaken to ensure the viability of all muscle groups. Skin closure or cover should not be attempted unless all muscle groups are viable. Delayed primary closure should be used if possible but without tension on the skin edges. Commonly in the leg this technique is possible in the medial but not the lateral wound. Dermatotraction or gradual closure techniques should be used with caution as they may cause skin edge necrosis[25] and require a prolonged time to achieve closure. Split skin grafting is required less in the older patient, possibly because of reduced muscle bulk.[11] Although offering immediate skin

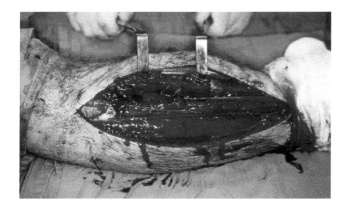

Figure 6.2 Fasciotomy of the anterior and lateral compartments of the leg using a lateral incision. Note the length of the incision which allows visualization of the full length of the compartments in order to ascertain the viability of the muscles.

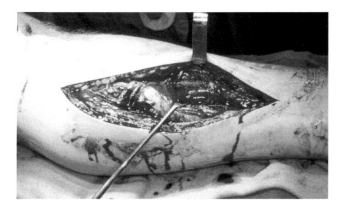

Figure 6.3 Fasciotomy of the superficial and deep posterior compartments of the leg through a medial incision. The superficial posterior compartment is being retracted to expose the deep posterior compartment. Care must be taken to ensure that there is a sufficiently wide skin bridge between the medial and lateral skin incisions.

cover this technique has the disadvantage of a high rate of long-term morbidity.[26] The recent introduction of vacuum assisted closure (VAC) systems is likely to be a significant advantage in this area and may reduce the need for split skin grafting.

MANAGEMENT OF ASSOCIATED FRACTURES

It is now generally accepted that fractures, especially of the long bones, should be stabilized in the presence of ACS treated by fasciotomy.[27-30] In reality the treatment of the fracture should not be altered by the presence of an ACS, although cast management of a tibial fracture is contraindicated in the presence of ACS. Fasciotomy should be performed prior to fracture stabilization in order to eliminate any unnecessary delay in decompression. Stabilization of the fracture allows easy access to the soft tissues and protects the soft tissues, allowing them to heal.

Complications of ACS

Complications of ACS are unusual if the condition has been treated expeditiously. Delay to fasciotomy of more than 6 hours is likely to cause significant sequelae,[31] including muscle contractures, muscle weakness, sensory loss, infection and non-union of fractures.[5,32-35] In severe cases amputation may be necessary because of infection or lack of function.[36]

REFERENCES

1. McQueen MM, Gaston P, Court-Brown CM. Acute compartment syndrome. Who is at risk? *J Bone Joint Surg Br*, 2000;82:200–3.
2. Court-Brown CM. The epidemiology of fractures and dislocations. In: Court-Brown CM, Heckman JD, McQueen MM, Ricci WM, Tornetta P, III, McKee MD, editors. *Rockwood and Green's Fractures in Adults*. 8th ed. Philadelphia, PA: Wolters Kluwer; 2015. pp. 59–108.
3. Buhr AJ, Cooke AM. Fracture patterns. *Lancet*, 1959;1:531–6.
4. Hope MJ, McQueen MM. Acute compartment syndrome in the absence of fracture. *J Orthop Trauma*, 2004;18:220–4.
5. McQueen MM, Court-Brown CM. Compartment monitoring in tibial fractures. The pressure threshold for decompression. *J Bone Joint Surg Br*, 1996;78:99–104.
6. McQueen MM, Duckworth AD, Aitken SA, et al. The estimated sensitivity and specificity of compartment pressure monitoring for acute compartment syndrome. *J Bone Joint Surg Am*, 2013;95:673–7.
7. Bhattacharyya T, Vrahas MS. The medical-legal aspects of compartment syndrome. *J Bone Joint Surg Am*, 2004;86-A:864–8.
8. Kosir R, Moore FA, Selby JH, et al. Acute lower extremity compartment syndrome (ALECS) screening protocol in critically ill trauma patients. *J Trauma*, 2007;63:268–75.
9. Ulmer T. The clinical diagnosis of compartment syndrome of the lower leg: Are clinical findings predictive of the disorder? *J Orthop Trauma*, 2002;16:572–7.
10. Bradley EL, III. The anterior tibial compartment syndrome. *Surg Gynecol Obstet*, 1973;136:289–97.
11. Duckworth AD, Mitchell SE, Molyneux SG, et al. Acute compartment syndrome of the forearm. *J Bone Joint Surg Am*, 2012;94:e63.
12. McQueen MM, Christie J, Court-Brown CM. Compartment pressures after intramedullary nailing of the tibia. *J Bone Joint Surg Br*, 1990;72:395–7.
13. Shakespeare DT, Henderson NJ, Clough G. The slit catheter: A comparison with the wick catheter in the measurement of compartment pressure. *Injury*, 1982;13:404–8.

14. Heckman MM, Whitesides TE, Jr., Grewe SR, et al. Compartment pressure in association with closed tibial fractures. The relationship between tissue pressure, compartment, and the distance from the site of the fracture. *J Bone Joint Surg Am*, 1994;76:1285–92.

15. Whitesides TE, Haney TC, Morimoto K, et al. Tissue pressure measurements as a determinant for the need of fasciotomy. *Clin Orthop Relat Res*, 1975;(113):43–51.

16. Heckman MM, Whitesides TE, Jr., Grewe SR, et al. Histologic determination of the ischemic threshold of muscle in the canine compartment syndrome model. *J Orthop Trauma*, 1993;7:199–210.

17. Matava MJ, Whitesides TE, Jr., Seiler JG, III, et al. Determination of the compartment pressure threshold of muscle ischemia in a canine model. *J Trauma*, 1994;37:50–8.

18. Heppenstall RB, Sapega AA, Scott R, et al. The compartment syndrome. An experimental and clinical study of muscular energy metabolism using phosphorus nuclear magnetic resonance spectroscopy. *Clin Orthop Relat Res*, 1988;(226):138–55.

19. Bernot M, Gupta R, Dobrasz J, et al. The effect of antecedent ischemia on the tolerance of skeletal muscle to increased interstitial pressure. *J Orthop Trauma*, 1996;10:555–9.

20. Ovre S, Hvaal K, Holm I, et al. Compartment pressure in nailed tibial fractures. A threshold of 30 mmHg for decompression gives 29% fasciotomies. *Arch Orthop Trauma Surg*, 1998;118:29–31.

21. White TO, Howell GE, Will EM, et al. Elevated intramuscular compartment pressures do not influence outcome after tibial fracture. *J Trauma*, 2003;55:1133–8.

22. McQueen MM, Christie J, Court-Brown CM. Acute compartment syndrome in tibial diaphyseal fractures. *J Bone Joint Surg Br*, 1996;78:95–8.

23. Petrasek PF, Homer-Vanniasinkam S, Walker PM. Determinants of ischemic injury to skeletal muscle. *J Vasc Surg*, 1994;19:623–31.

24. Matsen FA, III, Wyss CR, Krugmire RB, Jr., et al. The effects of limb elevation and dependency on local arteriovenous gradients in normal human limbs with particular reference to limbs with increased tissue pressure. *Clin Orthop Relat Res*, 1980;(150):187–95.

25. Janzing HM, Broos PL. Dermatotraction: An effective technique for the closure of fasciotomy wounds: A preliminary report of fifteen patients. *J Orthop Trauma*, 2001;15:438–41.

26. Fitzgerald AM, Gaston P, Wilson Y, et al. Long-term sequelae of fasciotomy wounds. *Br J Plast Surg*, 2000;53:690–3.

27. Gelberman RH. Upper extremity compartment syndromes. In: *Compartment Syndrome and Volkmann's Contracture*, Mubarak SJ, Hargens AR, editors. 1st ed. Philadelphia, PA: WB Saunders, 1981.

28. Gershuni DH, Mubarak SJ, Yaru NC, et al. Fracture of the tibia complicated by acute compartment syndrome. *Clin Orthop Relat Res*, 1987;(217):221–7.

29. Rorabeck CH. The treatment of compartment syndromes of the leg. *J Bone Joint Surg Br*, 1984;66:93–7.

30. Turen CH, Burgess AR, Vanco B. Skeletal stabilization for tibial fractures associated with acute compartment syndrome. *Clin Orthop Relat Res*, 1995;(315):163–8.

31. Rorabeck CH, Macnab L. Anterior tibial-compartment syndrome complicating fractures of the shaft of the tibia. *J Bone Joint Surg Am*, 1976;58:549–50.

32. Court-Brown, McQueen M. Compartment syndrome delays tibial union. *Acta Orthop Scand*, 1987;58:249–52.

33. Gelberman RH, Szabo RM, Williamson RV, et al. Tissue pressure threshold for peripheral nerve viability. *Clin Orthop Relat Res*, 1983;(178):285–91.

34. Hargens AR, Romine JS, Sipe JC, et al. Peripheral nerve-conduction block by high muscle-compartment pressure. *J Bone Joint Surg Am*, 1979;61:192–200.

35. Karlstrom G, Lonnerholm T, Olerud S. Cavus deformity of the foot after fracture of the tibial shaft. *J Bone Joint Surg Am*, 1975;57:893–900.

36. Finkelstein JA, Hunter GA, Hu RW. Lower limb compartment syndrome: Course after delayed fasciotomy. *J Trauma*, 1996;40:342–4.

COMPLEX REGIONAL PAIN SYNDROME IN THE ELDERLY

ROGER M. ATKINS

Introduction

Complex regional pain syndrome (CRPS) consists of abnormal pain, swelling, vasomotor and sudomotor dysfunction, contracture and osteoporosis. It used to be considered a rare complication of injury, caused by sympathetic nervous system abnormalities in psychologically abnormal patients. Modern research is altering this view radically. This review will examine CRPS within the context of orthopaedic trauma surgery in the elderly. Therefore, the emphasis, descriptions and concepts differ slightly from those found in publications from the International Association for the Study of Pain (IASP).

Some important definitions

A cardinal feature of CRPS is abnormalities of pain perception[1] which are unfamiliar to orthopaedic surgeons.

- *Allodynia:* painful perception of a stimulus which ought not to be painful, for example, gentle stroking of the affected part.
- *Hyperalgesia:* increased sensitivity to pain. Gentle touching with a pin is unbearably painful.
- *Hyperpathia:* temporal and spatial summation of an allodynia or hyperalgesia. Repetitive stimulus becomes increasingly unbearable. The pain continues and may be accentuated by stimuli such as sudden noise or a draft of cold air. These are genuine perceptions of pain. The patients are not malingering or mad.
- *Nociceptive pain* arises from direct stimulation of peripheral pain receptors, for example following fracture.
- *Neuropathic pain* arises from the nerves themselves without any precipitating stimulus. Spontaneous or burning pain, mechanical or thermal hyperalgesia, allodynia and hyperpathia are common.[1]
- *Sympathetically maintained pain* (SMP) consists of pain, hyperpathia and allodynia relieved by selective sympathetic blockade.

Taxonomy

Historically CRPS had many synonyms (Table 6.4) with differing diagnostic criteria. To overcome the resulting confusion, IASP reclassified the condition and proposed the name 'complex regional pain syndrome'' (CRPS)[2,3] with standardized diagnostic criteria.[1]

CRPS was divided into type 2 (CRPS 2) caused by nerve damage and type 1 (CRPS 1) without nerve damage. The clinical features differ.[4] From a surgeon's perspective,

Table 6.4 Synonyms for complex regional pain syndrome

Complex regional pain syndrome
Reflex sympathetic dystrophy
Sudeck's atrophy
Causalgia
Minor causalgia
Mimo-causalgia
Algodystrophy
Algoneurodystrophy
Post-traumatic pain syndrome
Painful post-traumatic dystrophy
Painful post-traumatic osteoporosis
Transient migratory osteoporosis

a diagnosis of CRPS 2 should indicate causative nerve damage susceptible to surgical intervention, for example, sural nerve entrapment following Achilles tendon surgery.

IASP's classification remains controversial, with suggestions that it medicalizes pain[5] and over diagnoses the condition.[6]

Clinical features

CRPS is a biphasic condition with early swelling and vasomotor instability (Figure 6.4) giving way over a variable timescale to late contracture and joint stiffness (Figures 6.5 and 6.6).[7] The hand and foot are the most frequent sites, although CRPS in the knee is increasingly recognized.[8,9] The elbow is rarely affected, whereas shoulder disease is common and some cases of frozen shoulder are probably CRPS.[10]

CRPS usually begins up to a month after a precipitating trauma but may be spontaneous.[7] As the direct effects of injury subside, a new diffuse, unpleasant, neuropathic pain arises.[11] Pain is unremitting (although sleep may be unaffected), worsening and radiating with time and may be increased by limb dependency, physical contact, emotional upset and by extraneous factors.

EARLY PHASE OF CRPS

Vasomotor instability (VMI) and oedema dominate the early phase, although this is less marked with more proximal CRPS. The classical description divides the early phase of CRPS into two stages depending on the type of VMI.[7,12-14] These stages are rarely seen except in severe cases.[7,14,15] Initially the limb is dry, hot and pink but after days or weeks, it becomes blue, cold and sweaty (Figure 6.4). Usually, however, VMI is accompanied by increased temperature sensitivity with variable abnormality of sweating.[4,14,15]

Oedema is marked, particularly where the distal part of the limb is affected and over time becomes more fixed and indurated with coalescence of tissue planes and structures.

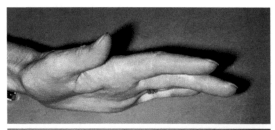

Figure 6.4 The hand in the early phase of CRPS. There is excessive sweating and the skin is bluish in colour.

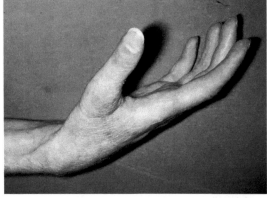

Figure 6.5 This patient's right hand is in the late phase of CRPS. There is atrophy of the hand with digital spindling, extension contractures and loss of joint creases and subcutaneous fat.

Loss of joint mobility is due to swelling and pain combined with an inability to initiate movement.[16–18] As the disease progresses, stiffness is increasingly due to contracture. Only if the disease can be halted before fixed contracture has occurred can complete resolution occur.

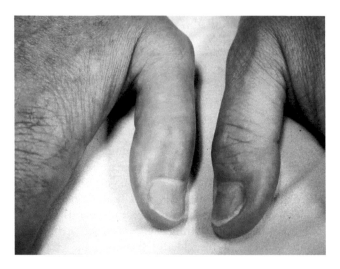

Figure 6.6 The thumbs of a patient with late CRPS 1 of the right hand. There is distal spindling of the affected thumb particularly distally with discolouration and ridging of the nail.

LATE PHASE OF CRPS

VMI recedes, oedema resolves and atrophy of the limb occurs affecting every tissue. The skin is thinned and joint creases and subcutaneous fat disappear (Figures 6.5 and 6.6). Hairs become fragile, thickened, uneven and curled, while nails are pitted, ridged, brittle and discoloured brown. Palmar and plantar fascias thicken, simulating Dupuytren's disease.[7,19] Tendon sheaths become constricted, causing triggering and increased resistance to movement which combined with muscle contracture and fibrosis leads to reduced tendon excursion. Joint capsules and collateral ligaments become shortened, thickened and adherent, causing joint contracture.

Within orthopaedic practice, the large majority of patients who demonstrate the features of early CRPS will not go on to develop severe contracture.

BONE CHANGES

Bone involvement is universal with increased uptake on the delayed bone scan in early CRPS throughout the affected region.[20] Later, this returns to normal and there are radiographic features of rapid bone loss: patchy, subchondral or sub-periosteal osteoporosis, metaphyseal banding and severe osteoporosis (Figure 6.7). Despite the osteoporosis, fracture is uncommon, presumably because the patients protect the painful limb very effectively.

INCIDENCE

Severe CRPS with major contracture is uncommon with a prevalence of less than 2% in retrospective series.[21,22] Population-based studies show 55 cases per 100,000 person-years in the United States[23] and 262 per 100,000 person-years in the Netherlands.[24]

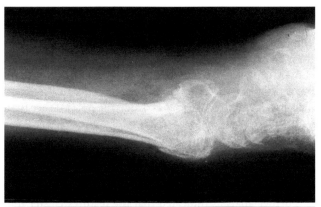

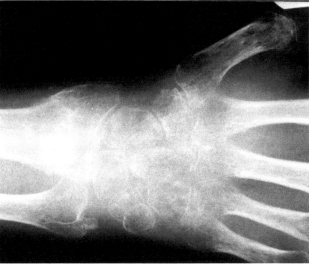

Figure 6.7 The radiographic appearance of a distal radius fracture complicated by the late phase of CRPS. There is profound osteoporosis.

Prospective studies specifically investigating the early features of CRPS show an incidence of up to 30% after every fracture and surgical trauma (for example total knee replacement).[15,25–32] The features occur together.[25,32] These common early cases of CRPS are usually not specifically diagnosed[30] and some would dispute the diagnosis.[33] They resolve substantially with standard treatment by physical therapy and analgesia within a year.[15,27,30,34] Stiffness may remain, suggesting that mild CRPS may be responsible for significant long-term morbidity.[15,35]

AETIOLOGY

CRPS occurs randomly uninfluenced by treatment method, and open anatomic reduction and rigid internal fixation do not abolish it.[28] Neither injury severity nor quality of fracture reduction are of major importance,[25,27] however it seems logical that some types of trauma (e.g. penetrating injury to a nerve) are more likely to be associated with its occurrence. There is an association with excessively tight casts[36] and there may be a genetic predilection.[37] The following aetiologies have been proposed.

PSYCHOLOGICAL ABNORMALITIES

Most orthopaedic clinicians immediately recognize a 'Sudecky' patient who appears to be likely to fare poorly after surgical intervention or trauma due to their inability to cooperate with mobilization, but CRPS is not primarily psychological[38] with no consistent pre-morbid personality abnormality.[39] Most patients are psychologically normal. There is an association with antecedent psychological stress[31,38,40–43] which probably exacerbates pain in CRPS, as in other diseases. It seems likely that the pain of CRPS causes depression and that a 'Sudecky' patient who develops early CRPS is at risk of a poor outcome because they cannot mobilize in the face of pain.

SOMATIC NERVOUS SYSTEM ABNORMALITIES

Pain is caused when a noxious stimulus activates nociceptors and it prevents tissue damage. Neuropathic pain in CRPS occurs without appropriate stimulus and has no protective function. Injured peripheral nerve fibres undergo cellular changes which cause usually innocuous tactile inputs to stimulate the dorsal horn cells via A-β fibres from low threshold mechanoreceptors, causing allodynia and causalgia in CRPS 2.[44] In CRPS 1, inflammatory mediators released by the initial trauma and retained sensitize nociceptors to respond to normally innocuous stimuli[11] causing allodynia. There is also evidence of small nerve fibre abnormality in amputated specimens from CRPS patients suggesting that a persisting injury to these nerves may be important.[45]

SYMPATHETIC NERVOUS SYSTEM ABNORMALITIES

Sympathetic nervous system (SNS) dysfunction in CRPS is suggested by abnormalities in skin blood flow, temperature regulation and sweating and oedema, and CRPS has long been treated by sympathetic manipulation. Recent studies however, cast doubt on whether sympathetic manipulation improves the long-term outcome.[34,46]

SNS activity is not usually painful. In CRPS, some pain[2] is SNS dependent, relieved by sympathetic blockade[47] and restored by noradrenalin.[48] The differential cutaneous sensory threshold between the limbs in CRPS may be reversed by sympathetic blockade,[49] while increasing sympathetic activity worsens pain.[50]

SMP is probably part of the body's reaction to injury. After partial nerve division, somatic axons express α-adrenergic receptors[51] and sympathetic axons surround sensory neuron cell bodies in dorsal root ganglia.[11,52] These temporary changes[48] make the somatic sensory nervous system sensitive to sympathetic mediators.

ABNORMAL INFLAMMATION

CRPS is associated with inflammatory changes including macromolecule extravasation[53] and reduced oxygen consumption.[54,55] Serum concentrations of substance P[56] and CGRP[57] are higher in CRPS patients than in controls, causing an augmented flare response[58] and excessive protein extravasation.[59] Cytokine levels are higher in CRPS affected limbs than in the contralateral limb or control patients.[60] This suggests that excess neuropeptide activity causes the extravasation, limb oedema and increased cytokine expression that characterize CRPS.

In animals, infusion of free radical donors causes a CRPS-like state[61] and amputated human specimens with CRPS show basement membrane thickening consistent with overexposure to free radicals.[62] These findings suggest that CRPS is an exaggerated local inflammatory response to injury[63,64] and that CRPS represents a local form of the systemic free radical disease after severe trauma. This concept is supported by preliminary evidence that vitamin C is effective prophylaxis against post-traumatic CRPS.[65]

The aberrant inflammatory response to tissue injury in CRPS is not caused by a cellular mediated immune response since systemic measures of inflammation are normal and histologically studies show minimal inflammatory cell infiltrate.[14,66]

AUTOIMMUNITY

Anti-neuronal autoantibodies occur in CRPS[67] and a randomized control study suggests that immunoglobulin administration reduces pain temporarily in chronic CRPS.[68] These findings suggest a possible autoimmune basis at least for the chronic disease. The barrier to the autoimmune theory is that CRPS is a local disease.

FAILURE TO USE THE AFFECTED LIMB

Abnormalities of motor function are found in the large majority of CRPS sufferers, varying from weakness to incoordination and tremor.[13,14,69,70] On objective testing, CRPS patients have impaired grip force coordination, target reaching and grasping.[71]

Interviews with CRPS patients demonstrate 'neglect' of the affected limb, similar to that seen after parietal lobe stroke. Statements are made such as 'my limb feels disconnected from my body' and 'I need to focus all my mental attention and look at the limb in order for it to move the way I want'.[16] Perceptions of the affected body part are bizarre[72] with central sensory confusion causing poverty of movement.[73,74]

CRPS patients ignore their affected limb and find it difficult to initiate or accurately direct movement and there is a mismatch between sensation, perception and movement.[18] Failure to use the limb appears to relate to this rather than the traditional view of learned pain avoidance behaviour in response to allodynia. Failure of mobilization may be central to the aetiology of CRPS since all the features of early CRPS, except pain, are produced by a period of cast immobilization possibly because normal tactile and proprioceptive input are necessary for correct central nerve signal processing.[58]

Treatment with mirror visual feedback (MVF) supports the central role of movement disorder.[75] MVF restores the congruence between sensory and motor information.[76] In early CRPS, MVF abolished or substantially improved pain and VMI.[75]

Making a diagnosis

The IASP work on CRPS has caused confusion. In 1994, the new diagnostic entity of CRPS was descriptive and consensus based.[1] It provided a set of standardized diagnostic criteria to improve clinical communication and facilitate research and to act as a starting point rather than a mature clinical diagnostic device.[77] The 1994 criteria were adequately sensitive *within the context of a pain clinic* (i.e. they rarely miss a case of actual CRPS), however, they had very poor specificity, over-diagnosing CRPS in up to 60% of cases.[78]

Further analysis indicated that the features cluster into four statistically distinct subgroups[79] which are similar to those suggested by others a decade earlier[14,25]:

1. Signs and symptoms indicating abnormalities in pain processing (allodynia, hyperalgesia, hyperpathia)
2. Skin colour and temperature changes, indicating vasomotor dysfunction
3. Oedema and abnormalities of sweating
4. Motor and trophic signs and symptoms.

A modified set of diagnostic criteria was proposed in 1999.[78–80] These are termed the Budapest, Bruehl or modified IASP criteria (Table 6.5) and they remain in widespread clinical use, but several points must be made. The statistics in Table 6.5 apply to the diagnosis of CRPS *within a pain clinic setting*. They do not therefore apply directly to the diagnosis of CRPS within the context of orthopaedic practice. The criteria are not pathologically based; they are a statistical association. Therefore if a patient fulfils the criteria, there remains a chance that they do not have the diagnosis. Finally, the criteria are consensus based and because the IASP wished to 'make a fresh start', much traditional knowledge of the subject has not been captured. Thus for example, algodystrophy is known to be associated with increased uptake on delayed bone scanning and to produce osteoporosis. These objective criteria do not form part of the IASP criteria. These are issues which need addressing in the future. At the moment, the 1999 modified IASP criteria remain the most widely employed diagnostic criteria.

Atkins et al. proposed a set of diagnostic criteria for CRPS specifically in an orthopaedic context (Table 6.6).[25,26,81] These were derived empirically in a manner similar to the IASP approach but critically in a fracture clinic rather than a pain clinic environment. The criteria were designed to be as objective as possible but the patient's veracity was assumed so no attempt was made to separate reports of vasomotor or sudomotor abnormalities from observation of them. A number of criteria are quantifiable,[25,26,82] which allows their powerful use to investigate treatment.[34,49,83] Diagnosis by these criteria, when used after Colles' fracture, maps almost exactly with the Bruehl criteria.[84]

Table 6.5 The modified IASP diagnostic criteria for complex regional pain syndrome

General definition of the syndrome

Complex regional pain syndrome (CRPS) describes an array of painful conditions that are characterized by a continuing (spontaneous and/or evoked) regional pain that is seemingly disproportionate in time or degree to the usual course of any known trauma or other lesion. The pain is regional (not in a specific nerve territory or dermatome) and usually has a distal predominance of abnormal sensory, motor, sudomotor vasomotor and/or trophic findings. The syndrome shows variable progression over time.

To make the *clinical* diagnosis, the following criteria must be met (sensitivity 0.85, specificity 0.69):

1. Continuing pain, which is disproportionate to any inciting event
2. Must report at least one symptom in *three of the four* following categories:

   Sensory: Reports of hyperesthesia and/or allodynia

   Vasomotor: Reports of temperature asymmetry and/or skin colour changes and/or skin colour asymmetry

   Sudomotor/oedema: Reports of oedema and/or sweating changes and/or sweating asymmetry

   Motor/trophic: Reports of decreased range of motion and/or motor dysfunction (weakness, tremor, dystonia) and/or trophic changes (hair, nail, skin)
3. Must display at least one sign **at time of evaluation** in *two or more* of the following categories:

   Sensory: Evidence of hyperalgesia (to pinprick) and/or allodynia (to light touch and/or temperature sensation and/or deep somatic pressure and/or joint movement)

   Vasomotor: Evidence of temperature asymmetry (>1°C) and/or skin colour changes and/or asymmetry

   Sudomotor/oedema: Evidence of oedema and/or sweating changes and/or sweating asymmetry

   Motor/trophic: Evidence of decreased range of motion and/or motor dysfunction (weakness, tremor, dystonia) and/or trophic changes (hair, nail, skin)
4. There is no other diagnosis that better explains the signs and symptoms.

   For *research* purposes, a diagnostic decision rule should be at least one symptom **in all four** symptom categories and at least one sign (observed at evaluation) in two or more sign categories (sensitivity 0.70, specificity 0.94).

Sources: From Bruehl, S., et al. *Pain*, 1999; 81(1–2): 147–54; Harden, R.N., et al. *Pain*, 1999; 83(2): 211–19.

Table 6.6 Suggested criteria for the diagnosis of complex regional pain syndrome (CRPS) within an orthopaedic setting

The diagnosis is made clinically by the finding of the following associated sets of abnormalities:

1. Neuropathic pain. Non-dermatomal, without cause, burning, with associated allodynia and hyperpathia.
2. VMI and abnormalities of sweating. Warm red and dry, cool blue and clammy or an increase in temperature sensitivity. Associated with an abnormal temperature difference between the limbs.
3. Swelling.
4. Loss of joint mobility with associated joint and soft tissue contracture, including skin thinning and hair and nail dystrophy.

These clinical findings are backed up by

1. Increased uptake on delayed bone scintigraphy early in CRPS.
2. Radiographic evidence of osteoporosis after 3 months.

The diagnosis is excluded by the existence of conditions that would otherwise account for the degree of dysfunction.

Sources: Modified from Atkins et al. *J Bone Joint Surg Br*, 1990; 72(1): 105–10; Atkins et al. *J Hand Surg Br*, 1989; 14(2): 161–4.

Clinical diagnosis in an orthopaedic setting

1. *Pain:* A history of excessive pain is elicited. Abnormalities of pain perception including allodynia and hyperpathia are sought. Excessive tenderness is found by squeezing digits between thumb and fingers.
2. *Vasomotor instability:* VMI is often transitory and so it may not be present at the time of examination. If the patient is reliable, history confirms its presence.

Visual inspection is the usual means of diagnosis. Thermography can be used but has not been validated within an orthopaedic context and must be employed with caution since inflammation from fracture would be expected to alter the result.

3. *Abnormal sweating:* This feature is also inconstant and it may be necessary to rely on history. Excessive sweating is usually obvious. In a doubtful case, the resistance to a biro gently stroked across the limb is useful.

4. *Oedema and swelling:* This is usually obvious on inspection. It may be quantified by hand volume, skinfold thickness and digital circumference measurement.[25,85]
5. *Loss of joint mobility and atrophy:* Loss of joint mobility is usually diagnosed by standard clinical examination. The range of finger joint movement may be accurately quantified.[25,82,85] As outlined above, atrophy will affect every tissue within the limb.
6. *Bone changes:* X-ray appearances and bone scans are discussed above. CRPS does not cause arthritis and joint space is preserved. Sudeck's technique of assessing bone density by radiographing two extremities on one plate remains useful but densitometry is not usually helpful. A normal bone scan without radiographic osteoporosis virtually excludes adult CRPS.

OTHER CLINICAL EXAMINATIONS

Sensory neglect can be elucidated by a difference in perceived sensory examination depending on whether or not the patient can see the affected limb being examined. Motor neglect is examined by asking the patient to undertake a simple task initially while looking away and then while watching the limb. If there is a significant improvement when the patient is watching the limb, motor neglect is present.[17]

General clinical examination is normal.

Investigations

There is no diagnostic test for CRPS. Biochemical markers and infection indices are negative.

The MRI shows early bone and soft tissue oedema with late atrophy and fibrosis but is not diagnostic. In CRPS 2 an MRI scan may demonstrate nerve involvement.

Electromyography and nerve conduction studies are normal in CRPS 1 but may demonstrate a nerve lesion in CRPS 2.

Differential diagnosis

Pain, swelling and VMI are common associations of trauma and orthopaedic surgery. The following are common differential diagnoses:

1. Soft tissue infection.
2. *'Mechanical' problems:* For example, incorrect sizing of a total knee replacement, overlong screws impinging on a joint or mal-reduction of an intra-articular fracture. All mechanical causes for the symptoms and signs must be excluded before making a diagnosis of CRPS (criterion 4).
3. *Conscious exaggeration of symptoms:* This is usually seen in the context of litigation but may also relate to pathological interpersonal relationships. This problem has been exacerbated by the IASP criteria for CRPS diagnosis which can readily provide a diagnosis of CRPS

in a deceitful patient. The rise of the internet means that any reasonably determined patient can be well informed about CRPS. The IASP criteria are designed to differentiate CRPS from other chronically painful conditions, not to deal with patient veracity. CRPS is a condition which inevitably leads to dystrophy[4,7,12,80] and in a patient who has suffered from significant CRPS for any significant length of time, objective features of dystrophy, such as nail or hair dystrophy, skin and subcutaneous tissue atrophy, fixed joint contracture and radiographic features of significant osteoporosis with abnormalities of bone scanning should be present.

4. *Psychiatric disease:* This may cause a patient unconsciously to exaggerate the impact of physical disease due to a somatoform or conversion disorder. These patients may have a history of an unusually severe reaction to multiple minor medical problems and they may show a tendency to 'catastrophize' life events. Patients with CRPS may also be depressed due to chronic pain and psychiatric disease may play an indirect part in the condition.[40]
5. *Neuropathic pain:* This is part of CRPS but a patient may have neuropathic pain without having CRPS. However, neuropathic pain may give rise to CRPS.

Management

A bewildering array of treatments have been proposed, but prospectively randomized blinded studies are few and uncontrolled investigations are particularly unreliable in CRPS. Modern treatment emphasizes functional limb rehabilitation to break the vicious cycle of disuse, rather than SNS manipulation. Initial orthopaedic treatment is by reassurance, excellent analgesia and intensive, careful physical therapy avoiding exacerbation of pain. Non-steroidal anti-inflammatory drugs may give better pain relief than opiates and a centrally acting analgesic such as amitriptyline is often useful at this early stage.

In achieving pain-free mobilization, epidural anaesthesia may be useful.[86] When the knee is affected this is combined with continuous passive motion.[8,9] Immobilization and splintage should generally be avoided but if used, joints must be placed in a safe position and splintage is a temporary adjunct to mobilization. Immobilization is most useful in cases where a relatively stiff but aligned joint is significantly more useful than a more mobile but contracted one, such as the ankle or wrist.

Abnormalities of pain sensation will often respond to desensitization. The patient strokes the allodynic area. They are reminded that simple stroking cannot be painful and they must stroke the affected part repetitively while looking at it and repeatedly saying 'this does not hurt, it is merely a gentle touch'. The earlier this is begun, the more effective it is. A similar attitude can be taken with early loss of joint mobility due to perceived pain rather than contracture. Mirror virtual therapy is an efficacious adjunct to desensitization.[75,76]

If the patient does not respond rapidly, a pain specialist should be involved and treatment continued on a shared basis. Psychological or psychiatric input may be important. Second line treatment is often unsuccessful and many patients are left with pain and disability. Further treatments include centrally acting analgesic medications such as amitriptyline, gabapentin or carbamazepine, regional anaesthesia, calcitonin, the use of membrane stabilizing drugs such as mexiletine, sympathetic blockade and manipulation, desensitization of peripheral nerve receptors with capsaicin and transcutaneous nerve stimulation or an implanted dorsal column stimulator.

It is important to ensure that a patient with CRPS within an orthopaedic context under the management of a pain clinic is reviewed by an orthopaedic surgeon with an interest in CRPS to ensure that there is no treatable orthopaedic condition which better explains the symptoms (Tables 6.4–6.6).[87]

The role of surgery is limited and hazardous. These patients are very fragile and difficult. They respond abnormally to pain and because of sensory and motor neglect, they rehabilitate poorly. Where the cause of CRPS is a surgically correctable nerve lesion, treatment should be cautiously directed at curing the nerve lesion. Occult nerve compression should be sought and dealt with. For example, decompression of a median nerve at the wrist may abort CRPS and should be undertaken cautiously in the presence of active disease.

Surgery is rarely indicated to treat fixed contractures which usually involve all of the soft tissues. Surgical release must therefore be radical and expectations limited. Surgery for contracture should be delayed until the active phase of CRPS has completely passed and ideally there should be a gap of at least a year since the patient last experienced pain and swelling.

Amputation of a limb affected by severe CRPS should be approached with great caution. Dielissen et al.[88] reported a series of 28 patients who underwent 34 amputations in 31 limbs. Surgery was usually performed for recurrent infection or to improve residual function. Pain relief was rare and unpredictable and neither was infection always cured or function universally improved. CRPS often recurred in the stump, especially if the amputation level was symptomatic at the time of surgery. For this reason only two patients wore prostheses. Similar poor functional outcomes were reported in a literature review of 111 cases.[89]

Generally, surgery represents a painful stimulus which may exacerbate CRPS or precipitate a new attack. This risk must be balanced carefully against the proposed benefit. The risk of surgically precipitated recurrence is greatest when the same site is operated upon in a patient with abnormal psychology in the presence of active disease and lowest when these conditions do not apply. Surgery must be performed carefully with minimal trauma with excellent and complete postoperative analgesia. The surgery may be covered by gabapentin. Ideally the anaesthetist will have a particular interest in the treatment of CRPS.

REFERENCES

1. Merskey, H. and N. Bogduk. *Classification of Chronic Pain: Descriptions of Chronic Pain Syndromes and Definitions of Pain Terms*. 2nd ed. Seattle, WA: IASP Press; 1994.
2. Stanton-Hicks, M., et al. Reflex sympathetic dystrophy: Changing concepts and taxonomy. *Pain*, 1995; 63(1): 127–33.
3. Boas, R. Complex regional pain syndromes: Symptoms, signs and differential diagnosis. In *Reflex Sympathetic Dystrophy: A Reappraisal*, W. Janig and M. Stanton-Hicks, Editors. Seattle, WA: IASP Press; 1996. pp. 79–92.
4. Bruehl, S., et al. Complex regional pain syndrome: Are there distinct subtypes and sequential stages of the syndrome? *Pain*, 2002; 95(1–2): 119–24.
5. Bass, C. Complex regional pain syndrome medicalises limb pain. *BMJ*, 2014; 348: g2631.
6. Del Pinal, F. Editorial. I have a dream … reflex sympathetic dystrophy (RSD or Complex Regional Pain Syndrome—CRPS I) does not exist. *J Hand Surg Eur Vol*, 2013; 38(6): 595–7.
7. Doury, P., Y. Dirheimer, and S. Pattin. *Algodystrophy: Diagnosis and Therapy of a Frequent Disease of the Locomotor Apparatus*. Berlin: Springer Verlag; 1981.
8. Cooper, D.E. and J.C. DeLee. Reflex sympathetic dystrophy of the knee. *J Am Acad Orthop Surg*, 1994; 2(2): 79–86.
9. Cooper, D.E., J.C. DeLee, and S. Ramamurthy. Reflex sympathetic dystrophy of the knee. Treatment using continuous epidural anesthesia. *J Bone Joint Surg Am*, 1989; 71(3): 365–9.
10. Steinbrocker, O. The shoulder-hand syndrome: Present perspective. *Arch Phys Med Rehabil*, 1968; 49(7): 388–95.
11. Woolf, C.J. and R.J. Mannion. Neuropathic pain: Aetiology, symptoms, mechanisms, and management. *Lancet*, 1999; 353: 1959–64.
12. Schwartzman, R.J. and T.L. McLellan. Reflex sympathetic dystrophy. A review. *Arch Neurol*, 1987; 44(5): 555–61.
13. Schwartzman, R.J. and J. Kerrigan. The movement disorder of reflex sympathetic dystrophy. *Neurology*, 1990; 40(1): 57–61.
14. Veldman, P.H., et al. Signs and symptoms of reflex sympathetic dystrophy: Prospective study of 829 patients. *Lancet*, 1993; 342(8878): 1012–16.
15. Bickerstaff, D.R. and J.A. Kanis. Algodystrophy: An under-recognized complication of minor trauma. *Br J Rheumatol*, 1994; 33(3): 240–8.
16. Galer, B.S., S. Butler, and M.P. Jensen. Case reports and hypothesis: A neglect-like syndrome may be responsible for the motor disturbance in reflex sympathetic dystrophy (Complex Regional Pain Syndrome-1). *J Pain Symptom Manage*, 1995; 10(5): 385–91.

17. Galer, B.S. and R.N. Harden. Motor abnormalities in CRPS: A neglected but key component. In *Complex Regional Pain Syndrome*, R.N. Harden, R. Baron, and W. Janig, Editors. Seattle, WA: IASP Press; 2001. pp. 135–40.

18. Butler, S.H. Disuse and CRPS. In *Complex Regional Pain Syndrome*, R.N. Harden, R. Baron, and W. Janig, Editors. Seattle, WA: IASP Press; 2001. pp. 141–50.

19. Livingstone, J.A. and J. Field. Algodystrophy and its association with Dupuytren's disease. *J Hand Surg Br*, 1999; 24(2): 199–202.

20. Atkins, R.M., et al. Quantitative bone scintigraphy in reflex sympathetic dystrophy. *Br J Rheumatol*, 1993; 32(1): 41–5.

21. Bacorn, R. and J. Kurtz. Colles' fracture: A study of 2000 cases from the New York State Workmen's Compensation Board. *J Bone Joint Surg Am*, 1953; 35A: 643–58.

22. Lidström, A. Fractures of the distal end of radius. A clinical and statistical study of end results. *Acta Orthop Scand Suppl*, 1959; 41: 1–118.

23. Sandroni, P., et al. Complex regional pain syndrome type I: Incidence and prevalence in Olmsted county, a population-based study. *Pain*, 2003; 103(1–2): 199–207.

24. de Mos, M., et al. The incidence of complex regional pain syndrome: A population-based study. *Pain*, 2007; 129(1–2): 12–20.

25. Atkins, R.M., T. Duckworth, and J.A. Kanis. Features of algodystrophy after Colles' fracture. *J Bone Joint Surg Br*, 1990; 72(1): 105–10.

26. Atkins, R.M., T. Duckworth, and J.A. Kanis. Algodystrophy following Colles' fracture. *J Hand Surg Br*, 1989; 14(2): 161–4.

27. Bickerstaff, D.R. *The Natural History of Post-Traumatic Algodystrophy.* MD thesis, Department of Human Metabolism and Clinical Biochemistry, University of Sheffield, 1990.

28. Sarangi, P.P., et al. Algodystrophy and osteoporosis after tibial fractures. *J Bone Joint Surg Br*, 1993; 75(3): 450–2.

29. Field, J. and R.M. Atkins. Algodystrophy is an early complication of Colles' fracture. What are the implications? *J Hand Surg Br*, 1997; 22(2): 178–82.

30. Stanos, S.P., et al. A prospective clinical model for investigating the development of CRPS. In *Complex Regional Pain Syndrome*, R.N. Harden, R. Baron, and W. Janig, Editors. Seattle, WA: IASP Press; 2001. pp. 151–64.

31. Harden, R.N., et al. Prospective examination of pain-related and psychological predictors of CRPS-like phenomena following total knee arthroplasty: A preliminary study. *Pain*, 2003; 106(3): 393–400.

32. Sandroni, P., et al. Complex regional pain syndrome I (CRPS I): Prospective study and laboratory evaluation. *Clin J Pain*, 1998; 14(4): 282–9.

33. Birklein, F., W. Kunzel, and N. Sieweke. Despite clinical similarities there are significant differences between acute limb trauma and complex regional pain syndrome I (CRPS I). *Pain*, 2001; 93(2): 165–71.

34. Livingstone, J.A. and R.M. Atkins. Intravenous regional guanethidine blockade in the treatment of post-traumatic complex regional pain syndrome type 1 (algodystrophy) of the hand. *J Bone Joint Surg Br*, 2002; 84(3): 380–6.

35. Field, J., D. Warwick, and G.C. Bannister. Features of algodystrophy ten years after Colles' fracture. *J Hand Surg Br*, 1992; 17(3): 318–20.

36. Field, J., D.L. Protheroe, and R.M. Atkins. Algodystrophy after Colles fractures is associated with secondary tightness of casts. *J Bone Joint Surg Br*, 1994; 76(6): 901–5.

37. Mailis, A. and J.A. Wade. Genetic considerations in CRPS. In *Complex Regional Pain Syndrome*, R.N. Harden, R. Baron, and W. Janig, Editors. Seattle, WA: IASP Press; 2001. pp. 227–38.

38. Bruehl, S. Do psychological factors play a role in the onset and maintenance of CRPS-1? In *Complex Regional Pain Syndrome*, R.N. Harden, R. Baron, and W. Janig, Editors. Seattle, WA: IASP Press; 2001.

39. Nelson, D.V. and D.M. Novy. Psychological characteristics of reflex sympathetic dystrophy versus myofascial pain syndromes. *Reg Anesth*, 1996; 21(3): 202–8.

40. Van Houdenhove, B. Neuro-algodystrophy: A psychiatrist's view. *Clin Rheumatol*, 1986; 5(3): 399–406.

41. Geertzen, J.H., et al. Reflex sympathetic dystrophy of the upper extremity—A 5.5-year follow-up. Part II. Social life events, general health and changes in occupation. *Acta Orthop Scand Suppl*, 1998; 279: 19–23.

42. Geertzen, J.H., et al. Reflex sympathetic dystrophy of the upper extremity—A 5.5-year follow-up. Part I. Impairments and perceived disability. *Acta Orthop Scand Suppl*, 1998; 279: 12–18.

43. Field, J. and F.V. Gardner. Psychological distress associated with algodystrophy. *J Hand Surg Br*, 1997; 22(1): 100–1.

44. Jensen, T.S. and R. Baron. Translation of symptoms and signs into mechanisms in neuropathic pain. *Pain*, 2003; 102(1): 1–8.

45. Oaklander, A.L. and H.L. Fields. Is reflex sympathetic dystrophy/complex regional pain syndrome type I a small-fiber neuropathy? *Ann Neurol*, 2009; 65(6): 629–38.

46. Jadad, A.R., et al. Intravenous regional sympathetic blockade for pain relief in reflex sympathetic dystrophy: A systematic review and a randomized, double-blind crossover study. *J Pain Symptom Manage*, 1995; 10(1): 13–20.

47. Price, D.D., et al. Analysis of peak magnitude and duration of analgesia produced by local anesthetics injected into sympathetic ganglia of complex regional pain syndrome patients. *Clin J Pain*, 1998; 14(3): 216–26.

48. Torebjork, E., et al. Noradrenaline-evoked pain in neuralgia. *Pain*, 1995; 63: 11–20.

49. Field, J., C. Monk, and R.M. Atkins. Objective improvements in algodystrophy following regional intravenous guanethidine. *J Hand Surg Br*, 1993; 18(3): 339–42.

50. Janig, W. CRPS 1 and CRPS 2: A strategic view. In *Complex Regional Pain Syndrome*, R.N. Harden, R. Baron, and W. Janig, Editors. Seattle, WA: IASP Press; 2001. pp. 3–15.

51. Campbell, J., S. Raga, and R. Meyer. Painful sequelae of nerve injury. In *Proceedings of the 5th World Congress on Pain*, R. Dubner, G. Gebhart, and M. Bond, Editors. Amsterdam: Elsevier Science; 1988. pp. 135–43.

52. McLachlan, E.M., et al. Peripheral nerve injury triggers noradrenergic sprouting within dorsal root ganglia. *Nature*, 1993; 363: 543–46.

53. Oyen, W.J., et al. Reflex sympathetic dystrophy of the hand: An excessive inflammatory response? *Pain*, 1993; 55(2): 151–7.

54. Goris, R.J. Conditions associated with impaired oxygen extraction. In *Tissue Oxygen Utilisation*, G. Gutierrez and J.L. Vincent, Editors. Berlin: Springer Verlag; 1991. pp. 350–69.

55. van der Laan, L. and R.J. Goris. Reflex sympathetic dystrophy. An exaggerated regional inflammatory response? *Hand Clin*, 1997; 13(3): 373–85.

56. Schinkel, C., et al. Inflammatory mediators are altered in the acute phase of posttraumatic complex regional pain syndrome. *Clin J Pain*, 2006; 22(3): 235–9.

57. Birklein, F., et al. The important role of neuropeptides in complex regional pain syndrome. *Neurology*, 2001; 57(12): 2179–84.

58. Marinus, J., et al. Clinical features and pathophysiology of complex regional pain syndrome. *Lancet Neurol*, 2011; 10(7): 637–48.

59. Leis, S., et al. Substance-P-induced protein extravasation is bilaterally increased in complex regional pain syndrome. *Exp Neurol*, 2003; 183(1): 197–204.

60. Uceyler, N., et al. Differential expression patterns of cytokines in complex regional pain syndrome. *Pain*, 2007; 132(1–2): 195–205.

61. van der Laan, L., et al. Clinical signs and symptoms of acute reflex sympathetic dystrophy in one hindlimb of the rat, induced by infusion of a free-radical donor. *Acta Orthop Belg*, 1998; 64(2): 210–17.

62. van der Laan, L., et al. Complex regional pain syndrome type I (RSD): Pathology of skeletal muscle and peripheral nerve. *Neurology*, 1998; 51(1): 20–5.

63. Goris, R.J. Treatment of reflex sympathetic dystrophy with hydroxyl radical scavengers. *Unfallchirurg*, 1985; 88(7): 330–2.

64. Goris, R.J., L.M. Dongen, and H.A. Winters. Are toxic oxygen radicals involved in the pathogenesis of reflex sympathetic dystrophy? *Free Radic Res Commun*, 1987; 3(1–5): 13–18.

65. Zollinger, P.E., et al. Can vitamin C prevent complex regional pain syndrome in patients with wrist fractures? A randomized, controlled, multicenter dose-response study. *J Bone Joint Surg Am*, 2007; 89(7): 1424–31.

66. Schinkel, C., et al. Systemic inflammatory mediators in post-traumatic complex regional pain syndrome (CRPS I)—Longitudinal investigations and differences to control groups. *Eur J Med Res*, 2009; 14(3): 130–5.

67. Kohr, D., et al. Autoantibodies in complex regional pain syndrome bind to a differentiation-dependent neuronal surface autoantigen. *Pain*, 2009; 143(3): 246–51.

68. Goebel, A., et al. Intravenous immunoglobulin treatment of the complex regional pain syndrome: A randomized trial. *Ann Intern Med*, 2010; 152(3): 152–8.

69. Bhatia, K.P. and C.D. Marsden. Reflex sympathetic dystrophy. May be accompanied by involuntary movements. *BMJ*, 1995; 311(7008): 811–12.

70. Marsden, C.D., et al. Muscle spasms associated with Sudeck's atrophy after injury. *Br Med J (Clin Res Ed)*, 1984; 288(6412): 173–6.

71. Schattschneider, J., et al. Kinematic analysis of the upper extremity in CRPS. In *Complex Regional Pain Syndrome*, R.N. Harden, R. Baron, and W. Janig, Editors. Seattle, WA: IASP Press; 2001. pp. 119–128.

72. Lewis, J.S., et al. Body perception disturbance: A contribution to pain in complex regional pain syndrome (CRPS). *Pain*, 2007; 133(1–3): 111–19.

73. Harris, A.J. Cortical origin of pathological pain. *Lancet*, 1999; 354: 1464–6.

74. McCabe, C.S., et al. Referred sensations in patients with complex regional pain syndrome type 1. *Rheumatology (Oxford)*, 2003; 42(9): 1067–73.

75. McCabe, C.S., et al. A controlled pilot study of the utility of mirror visual feedback in the treatment of complex regional pain syndrome (type 1). *Rheumatology (Oxford)*, 2003; 42(1): 97–101.

76. Ramachandran, V.S. and D. Roger-Ramachandran. Synaesthesia in phantom limbs induced with mirrors. *Proc R Soc Lond B Biol Sci*, 1996; 263: 377–86.

77. Harden, R.N., et al. Validation of proposed diagnostic criteria (the "Budapest Criteria") for Complex Regional Pain Syndrome. *Pain*, 2010; 150(2): 268–74.

78. Bruehl, S., et al. External validation of IASP diagnostic criteria for Complex Regional Pain Syndrome and proposed research diagnostic criteria. International Association for the Study of Pain. *Pain*, 1999; 81(1–2): 147–54.

79. Harden, R.N., et al. Complex regional pain syndrome: Are the IASP diagnostic criteria valid and sufficiently comprehensive? *Pain*, 1999; 83(2): 211–19.

80. Galer, B.S., S. Bruehl, and R.N. Harden. IASP diagnostic criteria for complex regional pain syndrome: A preliminary empirical validation study. International Association for the Study of Pain. *Clin J Pain*, 1998; 14(1): 48–54.

81. Atkins, R.M. and J.A. Kanis. The use of dolorimetry in the assessment of post-traumatic algodystrophy of the hand. *Br J Rheumatol*, 1989; 28(5): 404–9.
82. Field, J. Measurement of finger stiffness in algodystrophy. *Hand Clin*, 2003; 19(3): 511–15.
83. Field, J. and R.M. Atkins. Effect of guanethidine on the natural history of post-traumatic algodystrophy. *Ann Rheum Dis*, 1993; 52(6): 467–9.
84. Thomson McBride, A.R., et al. Complex regional pain syndrome (type 1): A comparison of 2 diagnostic criteria methods. *Clin J Pain*, 2008; 24(7): 637–40.
85. Atkins, R.M. Algodystrophy. In *Orthopaedic Surgery*. Oxford: University of Oxford; 1989.
86. Moufawad, S., O. Malak, and N.A. Mekhail. Epidural infusion of opiates and local anesthetics for Complex Regional Pain Syndrome. *Pain Pract*, 2002; 2(2): 81–6.
87. Goebel A, et al. *Complex Regional Pain Syndrome in Adults: UK Guidelines for Diagnosis, Referral and Management in Primary and Secondary Care*. London: Royal College of Physicians; 2012.
88. Dielissen, P.W., et al. Amputation for reflex sympathetic dystrophy. *J Bone Joint Surg Br*, 1995; 77(2): 270–3.
89. Bodde, M.I., et al. Therapy-resistant complex regional pain syndrome type I: To amputate or not? *J Bone Joint Surg Am*, 2011; 93(19): 1799–805.

ASEPTIC LONG BONE NON-UNIONS

PETER V. GIANNOUDIS

Introduction

Management of fractures and their associated complications has become a major health issue in the elderly population. One of the most frequent fracture complications is the development of an impaired fracture healing response expressed as delayed union or non-union. This complication could lead to loss of limb function, muscle atrophy, stiffness of the adjacent joints, diffuse limb osteopenia and eventually failure of fixation. Revision surgery can be challenging with dramatic consequences for the already frail elderly patient.

According to the United States Food and Drug Administration (FDA) fracture non-union is defined as the failure of a fracture to progress to osseous healing within 9 months following injury, alongside the absence of progressive signs of healing on serial radiographs over the course of three successive months.[1]

In the United States alone it has been estimated that over 100,000 fractures go on to develop non-union annually.[2] In a recent epidemiological study in Scotland, an overall incidence of 18.94 per 100,000 of the population per annum was reported with a peak incidence between 30 and 40 years of age.[3] The tibia and the femur are the most common long bones associated with the development of non-union.[4]

The incidence of fracture non-union is also known to be affected by the anatomical site of the injury, the type of fracture sustained as well as the method of fixation. For instance, the prevalence of humeral non-union is very low after conservative treatment of an upper arm fracture, estimated to be around 2.6%.[5,6]

After operative treatment, non-union is more common and the rate depends on the operative procedure, for example it is 4.2% after plate osteosynthesis, 11.6% after antegrade locking nailing and 4.5% after retrograde locking nailing.[5,7]

A multicentre prospective, randomized clinical trial carried out to evaluate the effectiveness of reamed and unreamed intramedullary (IM) nailing for the tibia provided some useful data about the prevalence of tibial non-union. The authors reported non-unions in 7.5% of cases treated without reaming compared with 1.7% of cases treated with reaming. They determined that the relative risk of non-union was 4.5 times greater without reaming and with the use of a relatively small diameter nail.[8]

Non-union after IM nailing of femoral shaft fractures is uncommon. Several authors have reported union rates of up to 99%.[4] In contrast to antegrade IM nailing, retrograde femoral nailing was found to have an overall non-union rate of 5.8%.[9] The prevalence of femoral non-union after other techniques of stabilization such as plating and external fixation has been reported to be approximately 12%.[10] However, recently the rate of non-union after these two methods of fixation has been reduced, which may be attributable to the

application of the concept of biological plating and the use of the newest generation of external fixator systems.[11]

The true incidence of long bone fracture non-union in the elderly is unknown and certainly underestimated. This can be attributed to loss to follow-up of patients and to the increased mortality rate seen in this patient population.

Non-unions can be classified as septic or aseptic according to the presence or absence of bacteria at the fracture site[1] and based on the radiographic appearance of hypertrophy (resulting from insufficient fracture stabilization; presence of extensive callus formation) or atrophy (fracture stabilization usually adequate but dysfunction of the local biological activity leading to little or no callous formation).[12] While the term atrophic non-union implies the absence of vascularity, this is actually not the case as it has been shown that blood vessels do exist at the non-union site. However, the mechanism which has led to the failure of bone repair remains unknown.

The focus of this section is on the management of aseptic long bone non-unions in the elderly.

Aetiology

Healing of fractures remains one of the most complex physiological processes of tissue repair. Molecular mediators, growth factors and cellular elements interact at different time points facilitating the formation of normal bone.[13] This process is unique when we take into account the fact that at completion there is no scar formation. Distinct types of healing have been described (primary and secondary) along with diverse molecular interactions of osteoprogenitor cells, signalling molecules and the extracellular matrix.[14] If any stage during these events is disturbed, it could lead to an impaired healing response.

A number of observations have been made over the years by clinicians managing these patients with regard to the aetiological factors leading to non-union. Although nowadays non-union is considered a multifactorial process (Table 6.7), potential risk factors have been documented and these have been grouped into four general categories: (i) patient related factors, (ii) environmental factors, (iii) injury related factors and (iv) treatment modality related factors.

Possible patient related factors are diabetes, rheumatoid arthritis, specific genotypes of important molecular mediators (i.e. Noggin, Smad-2), obesity, osteoporosis and advanced age.[15] In particular, elderly patients with osteoporosis could develop non-union due to mechanical instability after fixation of an osteoporotic bone, reduced availability of osteoprogenitor cells, and impaired influence and presence of signalling molecules.[16,17] Environmental factors comprise the intake of drugs or alcohol and smoking. Injury related factors include the topography of injury (some areas are more prone to the development of complications due to the peculiarity of distribution of blood supply compared to others), the type and magnitude of energy applied to produce the fracture, and whether the injury was an open or a

Table 6.7 Factors contributing to fracture non-union

Patient related
Age/Gender
Nutrition
Hormonal
Diabetes
Osteoporosis
Drugs
Smoking
Genetics

Fracture related
open fractures
fasciotomies
fasciotomies-actual loss of bone substance
interruption of the blood supply
extensive soft tissue damage

Iatrogenic
Poor reduction
Method of fixation
Lack of contact between the bone ends
Excessive soft tissue stripping
Reamed vs. Unreamed nailing

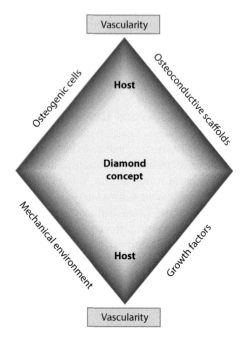

Figure 6.8 The diamond concept of bone healing interactions. (From Giannoudis PV, et al. *Injury* 2007;38(Suppl 4):S3–6.)

closed fracture.[18] Finally, treatment related causes embrace the degree of initial fracture displacement, the presence of periosteal stripping, distraction of fracture fragments, soft tissue interposition, the development of compartment syndrome and infection.[19]

Treatment principles

The management of aseptic long bone non-union in the elderly should follow the general principles of management of any other aseptic non-union. Initial assessment must include an accurate documentation of the natural history of the original injury and any subsequent interventions. Comorbidities and drug intake must be discussed with the patient, recorded and considered in the plan of treatment to be implemented. General haematological and biochemical investigations must include hormonal (i.e. thyroid function) and vitamin levels (i.e. vitamin D deficiency). A detailed clinical examination must be carried out to assess the state of the soft tissues, any leg length discrepancy, the presence of rotational or angular deformity, any muscular wasting and the range of motion of the joint above and below. Radiological examination in addition to the standard X-ray films should include long leg views and CT scanning. If there is uncertainty about whether low grade infection is present, then a bone scan, MRI and/or a bone biopsy can be considered and can assist in making the diagnosis.

Recently, a non–union scoring system was proposed in an attempt to assist the clinician to evaluate accurately the factors contributing to non-union and to guide treatment in terms of biological enhancement.[20] This non-union scoring system takes into account the state of the bone, the condition of the soft tissues as well as patient characteristics, comorbidities and drug use. According to this non-union scoring system, a score from 0 to 25 is a straightforward non-union which should respond well to standard treatments. Scores from 26 to 50 require more specialized care. For patients with scores from 51 to 75, specialized care and specialized treatments should be sought. Finally, patients with scores above 75 may be candidates for consideration of primary amputation.[21] Application of a biological based therapy should be considered in patients with a score of more than 26 points[20].

The so-called 'diamond concept' has recently been suggested for the successful management of fracture non-unions and bone defects (Figure 6.8).[22] It signifies a conceptual framework that takes into account all the essential biological prerequisites for a successful fracture healing outcome in the presence of an optimum mechanical environment. It stipulates the implantation of mesenchymal stem cells (MSCs), an osteoconductive scaffold and a growth factor in order to re-form the molecular milieu recognized to be essential for the initiation and effective completion of fracture repair.

Prior to the implantation of any of these biological based therapies, the non-union bed should be optimized, in terms of vascularity, containment and retention of sufficient mechanical support where molecular and physiological processes will evolve, facilitating successful osteogenesis in a timely fashion. While the diamond concept has been tested in the clinical environment with successful results,[23,24] it can be debated whether it is always necessary to apply the conceptual framework in terms of biological stimulation (signals, cells, scaffold and/or revision of the fixation) for a successful outcome.

Assessment of mechanical stability and the need for revision of fracture fixation can be evaluated by careful examination of the radiographs of the affected extremity. The following should be assessed:

- Is there evidence of loosening or osteolysis of the interface between the bone and the existing device?
- Is there breakdown of the metal work?
- Does the patient experience pain when walking?
- How long has the implant been in place?
- Following intervention, would the existing implant continue to provide adequate mechanical support for the succeeding 6–9 months or else until the anticipated amount of time for union to occur has been reached?

In the elderly population, with poor bone stock implant revision is frequently required and appropriate implant selection is essential. For stabilization of long bone nonunions, IM nailing remains the gold standard. Locking plates have also been used with variable success. Failure with locking plates has been attributed to the presence of large fracture gaps, mal-reduced fractures, short working length, monocortical screw fixation and inappropriate positioning of implants with an increased stiffness related profile (being too rigid).[25] Blade plates particularly for subtrochanteric non-unions have also been used with success.[23]

The decision of whether to apply only one of the biological constituents (monotherapy) of the 'diamond concept' or all of them simultaneously (cells, signals and a scaffold–polytherapy) remains more perplexing. The correct decision is critical in the elderly patient whose regeneration potential is known to be compromised[26] and it should not be forgotten that there may be only one chance to succeed. Ongoing failures in the elderly lead to increased morbidity and mortality.

It is important to document the history of the non-union by posing the following questions:

How many previous interventions have been done and failed?
Is the non-union recalcitrant?
What is the status of the surrounding soft tissues?
Is there localized muscular atrophy?
Is there a history of underlying host pathology (diabetes, peripheral vascular disease, smoking)?

In terms of biological stimulation, autologous bone graft is an excellent option for 'osteogenic' stimulation as it contains all the properties desirable in a bone graft material, those being osteoinduction, osteogenecity (availability of osteoprogenitor cells) and osteoconduction (properties of a matrix scaffold). Autologous bone is usually harvested from the iliac crest and is histocompatible and non-immunogenic,

thus diminishing the potential for the development of immunoreactions and transmission of infections as can occur with allograft materials. While iliac crest bone is one of the most commonly used autologous bone grafts (ABGs), one of its major limitations is the volume that can be harvested. This technique may be complicated by haematoma/seroma, fracture, nerve and vascular injuries, chronic donor site pain, hernias, unsightly scars and poor cosmesis.[27]

In the elderly patient the capacity to obtain bone graft is reduced. Due to reduced bone stock and medullary canal expansion secondary to osteoporosis, the red marrow is replaced by yellow marrow (fat) and the availability of pure cancellous bone is limited. Moreover, the risk of iatrogenic injury (i.e. fracture) is high (due to porotic bone) and pain from the donor site can be severe. Other forms of biological stimulation therefore must be sought, such as bone marrow aspirate (BMA; harvesting of MSCs, representing a form of cellular therapy), bovine cancellous chips and/or allograft and growth factors such as bone morphogenetic proteins (BMPs) and platelet-rich plasma (PRP) concentrations.

The reamer–irrigator–aspirator (RIA) system has been proven to be a useful tool to obtain autograph from the medullary canal of the femur.[28] It is of note that RIA initially was developed to simultaneously ream and aspirate the reaming debris to reduce the IM pressure, heat generation and systemic effects seen during the traditional reaming process. However, the application of a collection filter at the tip of the aspiration portal has allowed the collection of the reaming debris outside the medullary cavity. Such an approach led to the feasibility of collecting large volumes of corticocancellous graft (25–90 cm³). The safe use of RIA and how to minimise the risk of developing complications has been described previously in detail.[29] In the elderly, meticulous surgical technique is essential to minimize the risk of causing fractures due to the underlying osteoporotic bone.

Case examples

CASE 1

A 60-year-old woman sustained a right femoral fracture 10 months previously. It was stabilized with an IM nail. The patient was referred to our centre due to lack of progress in healing. Clinical examination revealed 1 cm of shortening of the right femur. Her biochemical profile was normal. Figure 6.9 shows the position 2 weeks and 10 months after stabilization. Bone graft was harvested from the contralateral femur using the RIA system and also from the iliac crest (Figure 6.10). After removal of the nail from the femoral non-union (Figure 6.11), the non-union gap could be seen (Figure 6.12). The non-union was mobilized with an osteotome and reduced following which bone morphogenetic protein 2 (BMP-2) was applied on a collagen sponge to minimize the effects of devascularisation with the subsequent application of cerclage wires (Figure 6.13). A cephalomedullary nail was inserted followed by the bone graft (Figure 6.14). Subsequent radiographs show progression to union (Figures 6.15 and 6.16).

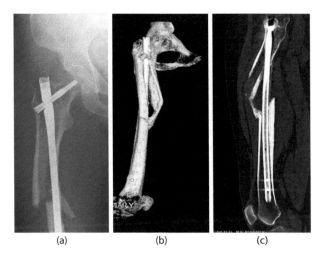

Figure 6.9 **(a)** Anteroposterior plain radiograph 2 weeks after initial stabilization. **(b)** 3D image and **(c)** CT scan at 10-month assessment.

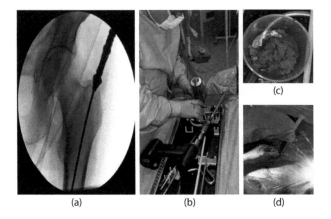

Figure 6.10 **(a)** Anteroposterior fluoroscopic image of the left hip demonstrating the insertion of a reamer–irrigator–aspirator (RIA) device for bone graft harvesting from the intramedullary canal. **(b)** Removal of the graft filter from the RIA device. **(c)** Demonstration of the volume of the RIA bone graft harvested with one passage of a 13 mm reamer head. **(d)** Harvesting of bone marrow aspirate from the left anterior iliac crest.

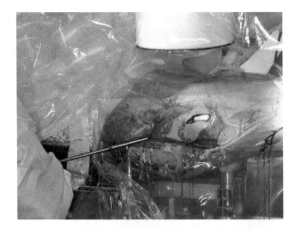

Figure 6.11 Removal of the nail from the right femoral non-union.

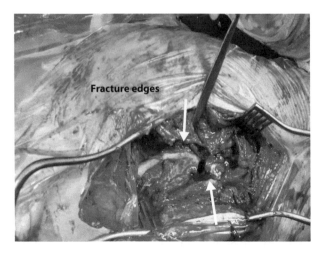

Figure 6.12 Intraoperative image demonstrating the gap between the fracture edges.

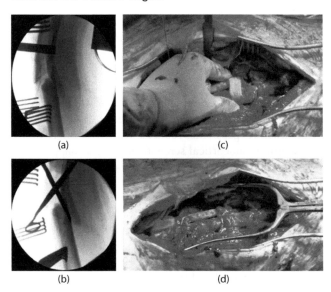

Figure 6.13 **(a, b)** Intraoperative fluoroscopic images showing mobilization of the non-union site with an osteotome. **(c)** After mobilization and reduction of the non-union fragments, pieces of collagen sponge loaded with BMP-2 are placed in the areas where cerclage wires are required to maintain reduction prior to nail insertion. **(d)** Application of the cerclage wiring over the pieces of the BMP-2 collagen sponge.

CASE 2

A 68-year-old man had sustained a subtrochanteric left femoral fracture 6 months previously. The fracture was stabilized with a cephalomedullary nail. The patient was referred to our centre with ongoing pain and a 1.5 cm shortening of the affected extremity. There were no conditions of note in his past medical history but the patient was a smoker. His biochemical profile was normal. Radiographs revealed a non-union which had been mal-reduced in varus (Figure 6.17) and a CT scan showed the non-union gap (Figure 6.18). The nail was removed and the non-union was mobilized (Figure 6.19). Reamings were harvested from

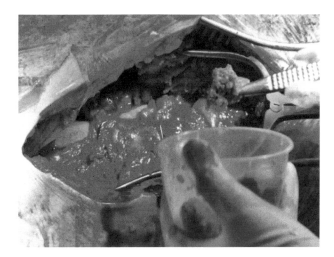

Figure 6.14 Intraoperative image showing the application of bone graft after stabilization of the right femoral non-union with a cephalomedullary nail.

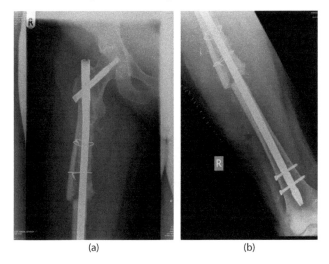

(a)   (b)

Figure 6.15 Postoperative (a) anteroposterior and (b) lateral radiographs of the right femur.

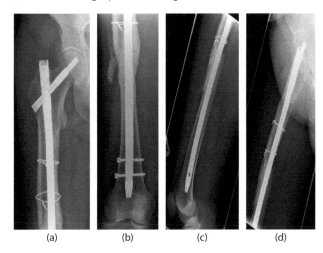

(a)   (b)   (c)   (d)

Figure 6.16 Radiographs taken at 6 months (a) AP proximal femur. (b) AP distal femur. (c) Lateral distal femur. (d) Lateral proximal femur demonstrating healing of the previous non-union.

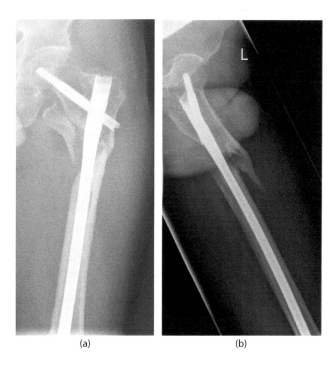

(a)   (b)

Figure 6.17 (a) Anteroposterior and (b) lateral radiographic views demonstrating a varus non-union.

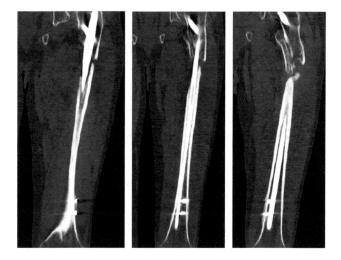

Figure 6.18 CT scan images showing the non-union gap.

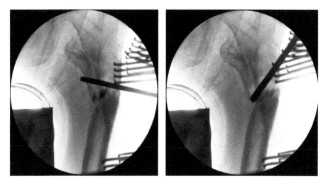

Figure 6.19 Intraoperative fluoroscopic images demonstrating mobilization of the non-union site after removal of the intramedullary nail.

the contralateral femur and the femur was stabilized with a blade plate and added anterior plate because of a deficient medial column (Figures 6.20 and 6.21). The RIA graft was placed at the non-union site before closure of the wound. Subsequent radiographs show progression to healing (Figures 6.22 and 6.23).

CASE 3

A 75-year-old woman sustained a distal femoral fracture following a fall while abroad. The fracture was stabilized with a locking plate and following repatriation she was followed up at her local hospital. At 7 months she was referred to our unit with a painful left distal femoral non-union when clinical examination revealed shortening of 1.6 cm and an external rotational deformity of 12 degrees. Her past medical history included hypertension and asthma. Her biochemical profile was normal. Radiographs at 3 months after injury showed mal-reduction of the fracture (Figure 6.24) and failure of the locking plate at 6 months (Figure 6.25). The plate was removed and the non-union debrided and mobilized (Figure 6.26). Microfractures were created at the non-union site using an osteotome. The femoral canal was reamed to induce osteogenesis (Figure 6.27) and the non-union was stabilized with an IM nail. Subsequent radiographs show progression to healing (Figures 6.28 and 6.29).

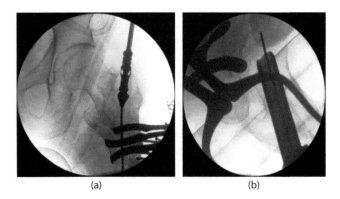

(a)　　　　　(b)

Figure 6.20 Intraoperative fluoroscopic images demonstrating (a) the use of a reamer–irrigator–aspirator in the left femur for harvesting autologous graft from the intramedullary canal. (b) Stabilization of the non-union with a blade plate.

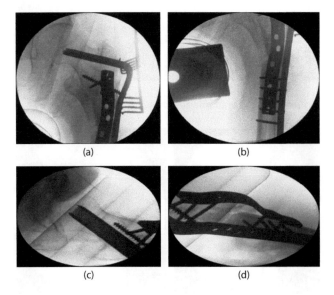

(a)　　　　　(b)

(c)　　　　　(d)

Figure 6.21 Intra-operative images of the left femur. (a,b) AP view proximal femur. (c,d) Lateral views of proximal femur showing stabilization with a blade plate and an anterior plate for optimum mechanical support.

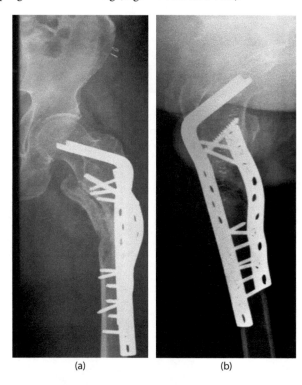

(a)　　　　　(b)

Figure 6.22 (a) Anteroposterior and (b) lateral radiographs at 3 months.

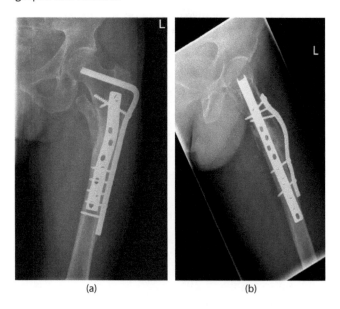

(a)　　　　　(b)

Figure 6.23 (a) Anteroposterior and (b) lateral radiographs at 6 months demonstrating healing of the left femoral non-union.

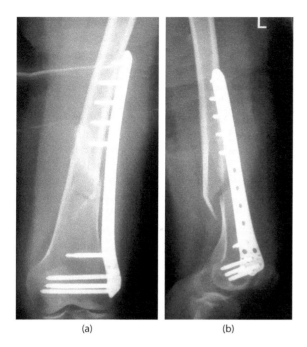

(a)   (b)

Figure 6.24 (a,b) Anteroposterior and lateral radiographs taken at 3 months illustrating fracture mal-reduction.

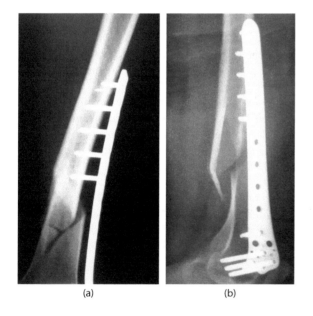

(a)   (b)

Figure 6.25 (a,b) Anteroposterior and lateral radiographs showing loosening of the locking plate at 6-month follow-up.

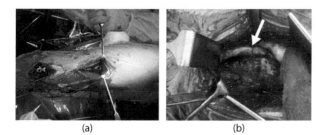

(a)   (b)

Figure 6.26 Intraoperative images showing (a) the incisions made for the removal of the locking plate and (b) the gap at the non-union site.

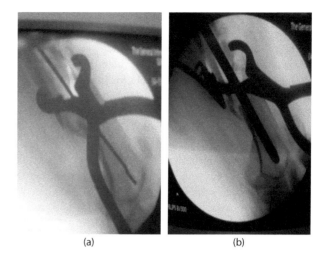

(a)   (b)

Figure 6.27 Intra-operative lateral view of the femur demonstrating. (a) The guide wire in the center of the femoral canal. (b) The insertion of the femoral nail for stabilisation.

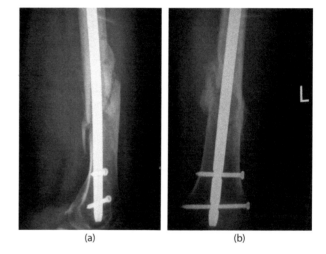

(a)   (b)

Figure 6.28 (a) Anteroposterior and (b) lateral radiographs at 3 months revealing the presence of a local osteogenic response.

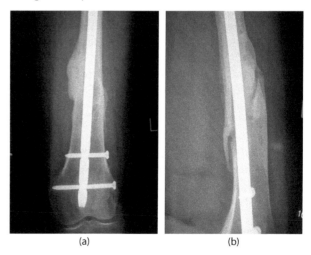

(a)   (b)

Figure 6.29 (a) Anteroposterior and (b) lateral radiographs at 5 months revealing osseous healing of the previous left distal femoral non-union.

Conclusion

Fracture healing represents a complex, well-orchestrated physiological process. It involves the blending of osteoconduction (the formation of a scaffold for ingrowth of bone), osteoinduction (promoted by cell migration, inflammatory cytokines and growth factors) and osteogenesis (the formation of new bone by osteoprogenitor cells). Inhibition of any of the above steps can lead to the development of non-union.

Due to the heterogeneity of long bone non-unions, their treatment is complex and challenging. Understanding the biological processes of fracture healing is essential and treatment should be tailored to each individual, addressing all the identified components of the problem. While there is no consensus with regard to the optimum treatment of aseptic long bone non-unions, mechanical stability and suitable biological enhancement should always be taken into consideration as per the diamond concept.

With regard to the type of biological enhancement used, a recent systematic review on this subject found that although the autologous bone graft (ABG) had a higher success rate compared to BMP-7 (95% vs 87%),[30] patients treated with BMP-7 had a higher number of previous failed interventions. The authors concluded that surgeon should decide the most appropriate treatment modality, depending on the nature and characteristics of the non-union and the patient.[30]

REFERENCES

1. Bishop JA, Palanca AA, Bellino MJ, et al. Assessment of compromised fracture healing. *J Am Acad Orthop Surg* 2012;20:273–82.
2. Miranda MA, Moon MS. Treatment strategy for nonunions and malunions. In Stannard JP, Schmidt AH, Kregor PJ, eds., *Surgical Treatment of Orthopaedic Trauma*. Vol. 1. New York: Thieme, 2007, pp. 77–100.
3. Mills LA, Simpson HRW. The relative incidence of fracture non-union in the Scottish population (5.17 million): A 5-year epidemiological study. *BMJ Open* 2013;3:e002276.
4. Tzioupis C, Giannoudis PV. Prevalence of long bone non-unions. *Injury* 2007;38(2):S3–9. Erratum in: *Injury* 2007;38(10):1224.
5. Koch PP, Gross DF, Gerber C. The results of functional (Sarmiento) bracing of humeral shaft fractures. *J Shoulder Elbow Surg* 2002;11:143–50.
6. Sarmiento A, Zaorski JB, Zych GA, et al. Functional bracing for the treatment of fractures of the humeral diaphysis. *J Bone Joint Surg Am* 2000;82:478–86.
7. McKee MD, Seiter JG, Jupiter JB. The application of the limited contact dynamic compression plate in the upper extremity: An analysis of 114 consecutive cases. *Injury* 1995;26:661–6.
8. Canadian Orthopaedic Trauma Society. Nonunion following intramedullary nailing of the femur with and without reaming. Results of a multicenter randomized clinical trial. *J Bone Joint Surg Am* 2003;85:2093–6.
9. Papadokostakis G, Papakostidis C, Dimitriou R, et al. The role and efficacy of retrograding nailing for the treatment of diaphyseal and distal femoral fractures: A systematic review of the literature. *Injury* 2005;36:813–22.
10. Alonso J, Geissler W, Hughes JL. External fixation of femoral fractures. Indications and limitations. *Clin Orthop Relat Res* 1989;241:83–8.
11. Papakostidis C, Grotz MR, Papadokostakis G, et al. Femoral biologic plate fixation. *Clin Orthop Relat Res* 2006;450:193–202.
12. Iwakura T, Miwa M, Sakai Y, et al. Human hypertrophic nonunion tissue contains mesenchymal progenitor cells with multilineage capacity in vitro. *J Orthop Res* 2009;27:208–15.
13. Giannoudis PV. Fracture healing and bone repair. *Injury* 2011;42:549–50.
14. Dimitriou R, Tsiridis E, Giannoudis PV. Current concepts of molecular aspects of bone healing. *Injury* 2005;36(12):1392–404.
15. Dimitriou R, Kanakaris N, Soucacos PN, et al. Genetic predisposition to non-union: Evidence today. *Injury* 2013;44(Suppl 1):S50–3.
16. Nikolaou VS, Efstathopoulos N, Kontakis G, et al. The influence of osteoporosis in femoral fracture healing time. *Injury* 2009;40:663–8.
17. Papanna MC, Al-Hadity N, Somanchi BV, et al. The use of bone morphogenic protein-7 (OP-1) in the management of resistant non-unions in the upper and lower limb. *Injury* 2012;43(7):1135–40.
18. Santolini E, Goumenos SD, Giannoudi M, et al. Femoral and tibial blood supply: A trigger for non-union? *Injury* 2014;45(11):1665–73.
19. Copuroglu C, Calori GM, Giannoudis PV. Fracture non-union: Who is at risk? *Injury* 2013;44(11):1379–82.
20. Calori GM, Phillips M, Jeetle S, et al. Classification of non-union: Need for a new scoring system? *Injury* 2008;39(Suppl 2):S59–63.
21. Abumunaser LA, AlSayyad MJ. Evaluation of the calori et al nonunion scoring system in a retrospective case series. *Orthopedics* 2011;34(5):356.
22. Giannoudis PV, Einhorn TA, Marsh D. Fracture healing: The diamond concept. *Injury* 2007;38(Suppl 4):S3–6.
23. Giannoudis PV, Ahmad MA, Mineo GV, et al. Subtrochanteric fracture non-unions with implant failure managed with the "Diamond" concept. *Injury* 2013;44(Suppl 1):S76–81.
24. Giannoudis PV, Kanakaris NK, Dimitriou R, et al. The synergistic effect of autograft and BMP-7 in the treatment of atrophic nonunions. *Clin Orthop Relat Res* 2009;467:3239–48.

25. Kanakaris NK, Giannoudis PV. Locking plate systems and their inherent hitches. *Injury* 2010;41(12):1213–19.

26. Goldhahn J, Jenet A, Schneider E, et al. Slow rebound of cancellous bone after mainly steroid-induced osteoporosis in ovariectomized sheep. *J Orthop Trauma* 2005;19(1):23–8.

27. Dimitriou R, Mataliotakis GI, Angoules AG, et al. Complications following autologous bone graft harvesting from the iliac crest and using the RIA: A systematic review. *Injury* 2011;42(Suppl 2):S3–15.

28. Kanakaris NK, Morell D, Gudipati S, et al. Reaming Irrigator Aspirator system: Early experience of its multipurpose use. *Injury* 2011;42(Suppl 4):S28–34.

29. Giannoudis PV, Tzioupis C, Green J. Surgical techniques: How I do it? The Reamer/Irrigator/Aspirator (RIA) system. *Injury* 2009;40(11):1231–6.

30. Pneumaticos SG, Panteli M, Triantafyllopoulos GK, et al. Management and outcome of diaphyseal aseptic non-unions of the lower limb: A systematic review. *Surgeon* 2014;12(3):166–75.

7

Systemic complications

HOUMAN JAVEDAN AND SAMIR TULEBAEV

IMPORTANT CONCEPTS AND INTRODUCTION

When looking at the topic of systemic complications it is important to view it through the lens of aging. As described in Chapter 2, the aging patient's complexity is defined not only by their comorbidities but also by the complex physiological changes associated with aging across all systems.

One way of summarizing the accumulative effect of aging is the loss of physiological reserve. In the context of homeostasis, this loss of physiological reserve represents decreasing capacity to maintain homeostasis in the setting of an insult or strain. For the purpose of this chapter we refer to this vulnerable state of maintaining homeostasis as 'homeostenosis'.[1] The homeostenotic baseline affects the response to strain placed on the organism at any given time.

As trauma and surgery will consume much of the already limited physiological reserve, it is important to evaluate these complications in each person and make the appropriate management changes to try and prevent them. Minimizing complications allows much of the physiological reserve to be dedicated to the acute trauma. This has implications for management before and after surgery. It demands astute clinical reasoning to decide whether an abnormality needs gentle homeostenotic support or aggressive intervention for a new disease process.

Cognitive reserve is also one of the homeostenotic physiological systems and has its own special demands throughout the clinical care pathway. Those with added neurodegenerative disorders may require even further input and thought for their care.

Adding further to the complexity is the fact that the field of orthopaedic trauma in the elderly is evolving as orthopaedic surgeons, geriatricians, anaesthesiologists, physical therapists, occupational therapists and others collaborate to better the care and understanding within the field. This means that there is not necessarily a consensus on how to define a complication. We have done our best to use consensus definitions and present complication incidences known at the time of writing. Interdisciplinary collaborations are increasing and may impact on the presented prevalence of complications in this chapter through prevention and early recognition.

Finally, it is impossible to cover all possible systemic complications in one chapter. The authors have chosen some of the most common and those they deem relevant to the clinician and student of musculoskeletal trauma in the elderly.

DELIRIUM

Definition

Delirium is a clinical syndrome consisting of distinct abnormalities in brain function due to a somatic illness. First codified in the *Diagnostic and Statistical Manual of Mental Disorders* (*DSM*),[2] in the first edition the syndrome was labelled 'acute brain syndrome' and finally crystallized as delirium with very specific diagnostic criteria in DSM-III-R.[3-5] To this day delirium remains a purely clinical diagnosis, and so the reference standard for delirium is a psychiatric evaluation in accordance with evolving DSM criteria. The current gold standard is DSM-V (Table 7.1).[6]

Table 7.1 DSM-V criteria for delirium

1. Disturbance in attention (i.e. reduced ability to direct, focus, sustain and shift attention) and awareness (reduced orientation to the environment).
2. The disturbance develops over a short period of time (usually hours to a few days), represents a change from baseline attention and awareness, and tends to fluctuate in severity during the course of a day.
3. An additional disturbance in cognition (e.g. memory deficit, disorientation, language, visuospatial ability or perception).
4. The disturbances in criteria 1 and 2 are not better explained by another pre-existing, established or evolving neurocognitive disorder and do not occur in the context of a severely reduced level of arousal, such as coma.
5. There is evidence from the history, physical examination or laboratory findings that the disturbance is a direct physiological consequence of another medical condition, substance intoxication or withdrawal (i.e. due to a drug of abuse or to a medication), or exposure to a toxin, or is due to multiple aetiologies.

Physiological risk factors/age related changes

Age itself is a risk factor for delirium. In addition to age, cognitive impairment such as dementia increases the risk for delirium. Individuals who are cognitively intact need a larger insult to cause delirium than those with underlying cognitive impairment.[7]

Incidence/epidemiology

Delirium is a common postoperative complication that increases both mortality and morbidity in elderly patients.[8] Delirium has been associated with higher in-hospital mortality (4–17%)[9–11] and postdischarge mortality (22.7-month mortality hazard ratio = 1.95).[8] In orthopaedic patients the prevalence and incidence are 17% and 12–51%, respectively.[7]

Prevention

In the context of delirium, it is hard to separate preventive measures from non-pharmacological treatment. Once delirium occurs, preventive measures become treatment modalities. This stems from the multifactorial nature of delirium and the incomplete understanding of the pathophysiology of delirium.[12] A non-pharmacological approach requires a multidisciplinary team which simultaneously attempts to address and manage multiple risk factors for delirium. It can only be implemented through education, reallocation of resources and reorganization of care for older adults by all those involved.

Identification/diagnosis

Unfortunately, a complete psychiatric evaluation is labour intensive and impractical to employ on a widespread basis. In one study, the psychiatric evaluation took a mean of 90 minutes.[13] Moreover psychiatric resources are scarce in comparison with the sheer number of patients

Table 7.2 Confusion Assessment Method (CAM) short form criteria

1. Acute onset and fluctuating course
2. Inattention
3. Disorganized thinking
4. Altered level of consciousness

Source: Confusion Assessment Method. © 1998, 2003. Hospital Elder Life Program. All rights reserved. Adapted from Inouye SK, van Dyck CH, Alessi CA, Balkin S, Siegal AP, Horwitz RI. Clarifying confusion: the confusion assessment method. A new method for detection of delirium. *Ann Intern Med* 1990, 113(12):941–948.

Note: Criteria 1 and 2 are required in addition to either criterion 3 or 4. Once there are at least three criteria, the diagnosis of delirium is established.

with delirium. As the medical community increasingly recognized the impact of delirium on morbidity, mortality, functional status and length of hospital stay, there was a need for more efficient instruments to diagnose delirium. This led to a proliferation of screening instruments with more than 24 of them described in published studies.[2] One of the most widely used clinical algorithms is the Confusion Assessment Method or CAM, which itself was developed from criteria based on the DSM-III-R.[13] It has been used in 4000 published studies, extensively validated and has a sensitivity of 94%, specificity of 89% and high reliability compared to expert psychiatric evaluation.[2]

CAM has been validated in surgical patients (Table 7.2).[2]

For the diagnosis of delirium, the presence of the first two criteria is required in addition to either criterion 3 or 4.[13] Once there are at least three criteria, the diagnosis of delirium is established.

Historical data on acute onset and fluctuating course are obtained from caregivers or healthcare professionals. Therefore knowledge of baseline cognitive status is essential. Sometimes a detailed history is not available during initial evaluation and a diagnosis of delirium is presumed. However, this underscores the fact that the clinician should make every effort to contact the primary caregiver or the patient's known health professionals. Fluctuating course is also assessed during daily clinical evaluations in the postoperative period.

Complex attention is one of the neurocognitive domains and describes ability to focus, sustain, divide and shift attention.[6] It also describes processing speed. Careful clinical observation during the interview is important to assess an individual's attention. Is the patient easily distractible, or do questions need to be repeated because the patient's attention wanders, or does the patient perseverate with an answer to a previous question rather than appropriately shift attention?[13] However, simple observation is not enough. Formal evaluation of attention must be done to decrease interobserver variability. A task such as naming days of the week backwards or months of the year backwards can serve as tests of attention.[2] Other commonly used methods are forward digit span (four or more random digits) or serially subtracting sevens from 100.[2] The test should be congruent to the person's cognitive ability. It is important to note that attention can be preserved in dementia.

Disorganized thinking is characterized by illogical flows of ideas, irrelevant or rambling conversation and frequent switches from one topic to another.[6] Disorganized thinking itself is likely driven in part by disturbances of complex attention and also perceptual abnormalities that might include misinterpretations, illusions and hallucinations in one or more sensory modalities.[6] There is no formal scale to quantify disorganized thinking and it is mostly based on the experience of the clinician.

Finally, identification of an altered level of consciousness depends on an observer's impression of whether a patient looked alert (normal), vigilant (hyperalert), lethargic (drowsy, easily aroused), stuporous (difficult to arouse) or comatose.[13] Altered level of consciousness may be formally assessed using the Richmond Agitation and Sedation Scale (RASS), which is a validated measure.[14] Additionally there are three variants of delirium based on psychomotor activity and level of consciousness.[6] Hyperactive delirium is fairly easily diagnosed and is what most clinicians think of when they mention delirium. It is characterized by psychomotor agitation and disturbed emotional state with patients calling out, screaming, cursing, muttering, moaning or making other sounds. Psychomotor agitation may significantly interfere with patient care, safety as well as the safety of healthcare personnel and is a frequent reason for indiscriminate administration of antipsychotic medications or sedatives. A less recognized form of delirium is the hypoactive variant with decreased level of consciousness and apathy. The hypoactive form has been shown to carry a poorer prognosis.[15] Finally, delirium may fluctuate between hyperactive and hypoactive forms, which is referred to a mixed delirium.

Management

The management goals of delirium start with preventing delirium, minimizing its duration and minimizing its severity (Table 7.3).[16]

Table 7.3 Management goals of delirium

- Prevent delirium
- Minimize length of delirium
- Minimize severity of delirium

Source: From Javedan H, Tulebaev S. *Clin Geriatr Med* 2014;30(2):271–8.

NON-PHARMACOLOGICAL STRATEGIES

Non-pharmacological measures have always been a foundation of delirium management. Pharmacological management consisting of antipsychotic medications is mostly directed towards agitation, which is a symptom of hyperactive delirium or mixed delirium. It is important to emphasize that antipsychotic medications and benzodiazepines do not treat the underlying causes of delirium and in the case of benzodiazepines may actually trigger delirium. Non-pharmacological management, on the other hand, attempts to address the multifactorial nature of delirium by early identification and elimination of risk factors.

One of the earliest landmark multicomponent intervention studies conducted on general medical wards by Inouye et al. focused on six components that were chosen because of known association with the risk of delirium and amenability to treatment.[17] The interventions were directed towards the management of:

- Cognitive impairment
- Sleep deprivation
- Immobility
- Visual impairment
- Hearing impairment
- Dehydration

This strategy was able to decrease delirium incidence by 40% and duration by 35%, but not the severity or recurrence rates.[17] It became known as the Hospital Elder Life Program (HELP) and was disseminated in the United States and abroad with some variations tailored to individual institutions. HELP required an interdisciplinary team and staff dedicated to implementation of the program.

Another landmark study by Marcantonio et al. used proactive geriatric consultation on hip fracture patients that also targeted multiple components.[20] Interventions included:

- Correcting fluid and electrolyte balance
- Providing adequate nutritional intake
- Actively eliminating medications that could potentially trigger delirium
- Early mobility
- Appropriate environmental stimuli

This study showed a reduction in delirium incidence of one third and in delirium severity of one half.[20]

Reorganization of medical care, appropriate resource allocation and education of staff with the focus on delirium prevention has also been shown to reduce duration of delirium and mortality in delirious patients.[18] The non-pharmacological measures are usually performed by trained medical staff; however, even intervention by family members who were briefly educated about some aspects of delirium has been shown to be effective.[19] Most studies in non-pharmacological management employed different variations and combinations of the strategies given in Table 7.4.

Controversies

Blood transfusion to a haemoglobin of 10 in a multicomponent intervention was helpful[20] but when looked at in isolation did not show any improvement.[21] Furthermore increased delirium was observed with intraoperative blood transfusions greater than 1000 ml red blood cells.[22] Please see the section on anaemia in this chapter for further discussion.

PHARMACOLOGICAL STRATEGIES

The multifactorial nature of delirium makes medications another tool to help address many of the driving and exacerbating factors. Antipsychotics are traditionally thought of

Table 7.4 Non-pharmacological interventions

- Removal of deliriogenic medications
  - Common deliriogenic medications
    - Antihistamines (e.g. diphenhydramine)
    - Antiemetics that effect dopamine (e.g. metoclopramide and prochlorperazine)
    - Benzodiazepines (e.g. lorazepam and clonazepam)
    - Antimuscarinics (e.g. oxybutynin)
    - Muscle relaxants (e.g. baclofen)
- Cognitive stimulation
  - Frequent reorientation
  - Provision of clocks, calendars, name of providers prominently displayed
  - Family present at bedside
- Improve sensory impairment
  - Provide glasses
  - Provide hearing aids
  - Provide dentures
- Mobility
  - Out of bed with meals
  - Reducing tethers (e.g. telemetry, catheters and feeding tubes)
  - Early physical therapy
- Correction of metabolic abnormalities
  - Maintain adequate hydration (encourage oral intake)
- Education of staff with focus on recognition of delirium and implementation of preventive measures
  - Evaluate for other acute issues (e.g. infection, hypoxia and urinary retention)

as the pharmaceutical approach to delirium. Antipsychotics in delirium do not treat the underlying cause but rather address the symptoms. Agitation for example is a symptom that can escalate to a level that is detrimental to the patient and dangerous to caregivers. At the same time treating pain and sleep deprivation with an appropriate medication addresses one of the underlying causes and can be far more effective than antipsychotics.

As a result, the medication and its timing and dosing need to be tailored to the specific patient with constant monitoring and adjustment as all such medications carry risk and side effects. The long-term risks of antipsychotics are well established, but smaller retrospective studies have shown likely safe use in short-term acute circumstances.[23,24] Table 7.5 outlines the pharmacological approaches to treating delirium and its symptoms.

Maximal effective dose

Haloperidol has been in use the longest and studies have shown that doses above 3.0 mg/24 hours increase medication side effects without significant added benefit to duration or severity of delirium.[33]

There is not enough evidence to definitively identify the maximal effective dose in other antipsychotic medications. However, based on geriatric pharmacokinetic principles it is best to use the lowest effective dose, which the authors recommend (Table 7.6).

Timing

The authors recommend evaluating the pattern of agitation throughout the day and giving a low dose of medication at the beginning of the agitation before it escalates. This will prevent escalation to a point where even maximum dosing will be ineffective and allows the overall 24-hour dosing to stay at a minimum.

Cholinesterase inhibitors

- Anticholinesterases have not been effective in treating delirium.[35]

Controversies

- There are no adequate controlled trials in non-alcohol withdrawal delirium to support the use of benzodiazepines.[36]
- Meta-analysis supports the possible prophylactic use of antipsychotics perioperatively.[37]

MYOCARDIAL INFARCTION

Definition

Acute myocardial infarction (MI) is defined as myocardial cell death due to inadequate blood supply according to the Third Universal Definition of Myocardial Infarction which was revised in 2012.[38] The definition distinguishes five types of MI. However in the context of the postoperative period,

Table 7.5 Pharmacological interventions.

- Treating causes
  - Pain
    - Standing acetaminophen addresses pain and reduces opiate requirement.[25,26]
    - Dosing of opiates is important as too much can cause delirium and yet poor pain control can also cause delirium.[27–29]
    - A retrospective study in hip fractures highlights the importance of 24-hour opiate dosing (0.15 mg/kg IV morphine in 24 hours was not associated with delirium).[30]
  - Sleep deprivation
    - Consider trazodone 25 mg PRN QHS.[31]
    - Consider quetiapine 12.5–25 mg QHS *if agitation of delirium* also needs to be treated.
    - Avoid use of diphenhydramine or benzodiazepines.
  - Constipation
    - Stimulant laxatives.
    - Osmotic laxatives if patient is taking sufficient oral hydration.
    - Suppository if above not effective.
- Treating symptoms[32]
  - Agitation/hallucinations
    - Haloperidol
      - Pros: Oldest and most accumulated historical evidence, IV/IM and PO availability.
      - Cons: QT prolongation, documented torsades de pointes with IV administration, extrapyramidal symptoms >4.5 mg daily.
    - Quetiapine
      - Pros: Most sedating – helpful for sleep, some evidence of safety in Lewy body dementia and Parkinson's dementia.
      - Cons: No IV/IM/SL form, QT prolongation.
    - Olanzapine
      - Pros: SL/IM form.
      - Cons: Most anticholinergic, QT prolongation.
    - Lorazepam – only for alcohol withdrawal
      - Pros: Not QT prolonging, benzodiazepine without active metabolites.
      - Cons: Can induce delirium itself, causes cognitive impairment, increases risk of falls, no good evidence to support its use in non-alcohol associated delirium.

Note: IM, intramuscular; IV, intravenous; PO, by mouth (per os); PRN, as needed (pro re nata); QHS, every night at bedtime (quaque hora somni); SL, sublingual.

Table 7.6 Dosing regimens for pharmacological interventions

Drug	Dosage
Haloperidol	0.25–1.0 mg PO/IM to be repeated every 30–60 minutes if needed. Maximum dose of 3.0 mg in 24 hours to minimize side effects.[33]
Risperidone	0.25–0.5 mg PO; repeat every 30–60 minutes if needed.
Quetiapine	12.5–50 mg PO; repeat every 30–60 minutes if needed. Consider maximum dose of 175 mg/day.[34]
Olanzapine	2.5–5.0 mg PO/SL/IM; repeat every 30–60 minutes if needed.
Lorazepam[a]	0.25 mg–1.0 mg PO/IM; repeat every 30–60 minutes if needed.

Source: From Javedan H, Tulebaev S. *Clin Geriatr Med* 2014;30(2):271–8.
Note: IM, intramuscular; PO, by mouth (per os); SL, sublingual.

[a] The authors recommend this as a choice of last resort as there is no good evidence to support its use except in alcohol withdrawal. If a benzodiazepine must be used, recommend shorter acting formulations with no active metabolites.

type I and II MI are the most relevant entities due to postoperative stress as well as increased prevalence of coronary atherosclerosis and diminished cardiac reserve in older adults. The distinction between type I and type II MI is important due to different approaches to management.

Type I is a spontaneous MI occurring as a result of the rupture of unstable atherosclerotic plaque in one or more coronary arteries with local formation of thrombus that interrupts blood flow to an area of myocardium. These patients usually have underlying coronary artery disease.

Type II MI occurs due to an imbalance between myocardial blood supply and oxygen demand. Examples include conditions that are fairly common in the postoperative period such as tachycardia, anaemia, respiratory failure, hypotension or severe hypertension.

Myocardial injury with non-cardiac surgery (MINS) is an emerging diagnostic entity and is defined as prognostically relevant myocardial injury due to ischaemia that occurs during or within 30 days after non-cardiac surgery.[39] It is characterized by isolated troponin elevation in the postoperative period without ischaemic symptoms or EKG changes. The definition of MINS does not apply to non-ischaemic elevation of troponin which may happen, for instance, with pulmonary embolism, sepsis or chronic kidney disease.

Physiological risk factors/age related changes

Aging of the cardiovascular system results in worsening of left ventricular diastolic dysfunction, increased cardiac afterload and increased arterial stiffness.[40] In addition, elderly patients have an increased prevalence of comorbidities such as hypertension, dyslipidemia, diabetes mellitus and chronic kidney disease that increase the risk of postoperative coronary events. Tachycardia due to pain or increased levels of catecholamines after surgery, hypotension or hypertension, and anaemia are common in the postoperative period and further increase the risk of either unstable plaque rupture in atherosclerotic coronary arteries or mismatch between oxygen supply and demand in aging myocardium.[41]

Incidence

There is a paucity of data regarding the incidence of postoperative MI in the setting of musculoskeletal injury in older adults. Most of the investigations report incidence of coronary events either after major non-cardiothoracic surgery or after hip fractures. The incidence of postoperative MI after hip fractures varies across studies and depends on the criteria used to establish the diagnosis. The incidence was reported as high as 10.4–13.8% within first 7 days after hip fracture surgery when the diagnosis relied on a combination of rise in cardiac troponin, ischaemic ECG changes and clinical symptoms.[42,43] It is worth noting that 92% of coronary events occurred in the first 48 hours.

Diagnosis

Currently the diagnosis of MI is based on the Third Universal Definition of Myocardial Infarction.

Cardiac biomarkers: The measurement of cardiac biomarkers became central to the diagnosis of MI. There should be a rise and/or fall of cardiac troponins (with at least one value above the 99th percentile of the upper reference limit).

ECG changes: Changes suggestive of ischaemia should be present such as either new ST segment elevation or new left bundle branch block or ST segment depression and T wave changes.

Clinical symptoms: Chest discomfort remains a common presentation of acute MI in older adults. However, elderly patients might also present primarily with atypical symptoms such as dyspnoea (49%), diaphoresis (46%), nausea and vomiting (24%) and syncope (19%).[44] New onset dysrhythmias or congestive heart failure (CHF) may also point to a possible coronary event.

In the postoperative period, the diagnosis of acute MI may be challenging. Patients may not be experiencing typical ischaemic pain due to the effects of anaesthesia, sedation or a postoperative pain regimen. Elderly patients with cognitive impairment may poorly communicate their symptoms or even manifest their pain with the development of delirium. One of the difficulties in making the diagnosis is that 75% of elderly patients with postoperative MI after hip fracture may be asymptomatic.[43] In this case, diagnosis may be established on the basis of cardiac troponin elevation and ischaemic ECG changes.

Another important distinction that should be made is between acute MI and MINS, myocardial injury which manifests itself with isolated troponin elevation without ischaemic symptoms or ECG changes. Elevated troponin may occur in up to 39% of elderly patients in the postoperative period.[45] The level of troponin is usually minimally elevated and does not have the rise and fall characteristic of acute MI. However even in the absence of MI, elevated troponin level independently predicted prolonged length of hospital stay, need for long-term care and all-cause mortality. Therefore cardiac troponin may serve as a prognostic factor. The question of whether cardiac troponins should be routinely measured in the postoperative period in the absence of clinical symptoms or EKG changes is controversial.

Management

The optimal management of postoperative MI in the elderly is unclear due to lack of relevant studies. In elderly patients a decision on the treatment modalities for acute myocardial ischaemia should be made in the context of general health, comorbidities and overall life expectancy.[46]

MYOCARDIAL INJURY WITH NON-CARDIAC SURGERY (MINS)

In patients with MINS, elevated troponin predicts an increase in 30-day and 1-year cardiovascular mortality.

Some authors suggest using aspirin and statins to treat MINS since these patients might have coronary artery disease with fixed obstruction.[47] However one randomized controlled study failed to show a difference in mortality between standard treatment and involvement of a cardiologist for postoperative troponin elevation after emergency orthopaedic geriatric surgery.[48]

NON-ST ELEVATION MYOCARDIAL INFARCTION (NSTEMI)

Non-ST segment elevation MI (NSTEMI) can occur as a result of unstable plaque rupture or a fissure (type I MI) or a mismatch between myocardial oxygen supply and demand (type II MI). The treatment decisions should be interdisciplinary and should involve an orthopaedic surgeon, a cardiologist and an internal medicine physician (ideally a geriatrician). The treatment decisions should be patient-centered and reflect his or her goals of care. Geriatric specific factors such as multimorbidity, cognitive impairment, frailty and functional impairment should be taken into account and will need to be discussed with the patient and/or a healthcare proxy. Other factors such as altered pharmacokinetics, presence of acute or chronic kidney failure and polypharmacy should be considered.

Aspirin and a statin should be started.

A P2Y12 receptor blocker is added (e.g. clopidogrel or prasugrel).[49]

If there are no contraindications, then anticoagulation with unfractionated or low molecular weight heparin should be initiated.

The decision to start a beta blocker should be individualized and will depend on postoperative blood pressure and the presence of dysrhythmias.

Early invasive versus early conservative management will depend on haemodynamic stability, the patient's risk and again on goals of care reflecting the patient's overall health.

ST SEGMENT ELEVATION MYOCARDIAL INFARCTION

These patients are at high risk of postoperative death without treatment and will require urgent primary percutaneous coronary intervention. Fibrinolytic treatment is generally not an option given recent surgery and risk of bleeding, but this again is best addressed with interdisciplinary input.

POSTOPERATIVE CONGESTIVE HEART FAILURE

Definition

CHF is defined as an inability of the heart to pump sufficient blood to meet the metabolic needs of the body. It combines both pump failure that leads to fatigue and poor exercise tolerance, and neurohormonal activation that leads to fluid retention and symptoms of congestion.

Physiological risk factors/age related changes

CHF is more complex in older adults due to the intersection of age related cardiovascular changes and non-cardiac comorbidities. Chronic kidney disease, anaemia, altered regulation of fluid volume, hypertension and other chronic conditions predispose to heart failure and stress in an already homeostenotic cardiovascular system. Heart failure is essentially a geriatric syndrome and needs to be viewed as a multifactorial condition.[50,51]

Incidence/epidemiology

The preoperative prevalence of CHF in hip fractures was reported to be 6–27%. The presence of CHF predisposes the elderly to musculoskeletal trauma. Osteopenia or osteoporosis is present in a significant number of CHF patients and there is an association between CHF severity, as expressed by lower left ventricular ejection fraction (LVEF) or higher New York Heart Association (NYHA) class, and bone mineral density (BMD) measurements.[52] In a population-based cohort of more than 16,000 elderly patients followed up for 1 year, heart failure was associated with a fourfold higher risk of sustaining any fracture requiring hospitalization compared with other cardiovascular diagnoses. This result remained significant after adjustment for age, sex, concurrent medications and other conditions associated with osteoporosis related fracture.[53]

Diagnosis

In the postoperative period, practitioners may encounter both typical and atypical presentations of CHF. One of the earliest indicators of CHF could be exercise intolerance that will manifest with fatigue and dyspnoea during physical therapy. The patient should be asked about their tolerance of physical therapy. Daily review of physical therapy notes and personal communication with a physical therapist is important for early detection of heart failure. However fatigue and dyspnoea on exertion are relatively non-specific signs and may be present in patients with lung problems, anaemia or general deconditioning. One should bear in mind that older adults frequently have multiple medical problems and a symptom can be a manifestation of several conditions at the same time. For instance dyspnoea on exertion might be caused by a combination of anaemia, chronic obstructive pulmonary disease (COPD) and worsening heart failure. The patient should be questioned about orthopnoea daily. Orthopnoea, which is shortness of breath in the recumbent position, may also manifest as a nocturnal cough. Orthopnoea is relieved by sitting upright or raising the head off the bed.

Nursing request for cough medication at night in orthogeriatric patients should prompt assessment of volume status and daily fluid balance. Paroxysmal nocturnal dyspnoea (PND) is shortness of breath, cough or wheezing that awakens the patient from sleep, usually 1–3 hours after the onset of sleep, and is one of the major Framingham criteria for CHF (Table 7.7).[54] Patients with cognitive impairment may have difficulties articulating their complaints and therefore nursing observation of poor sleep should alert a clinician to the possibility of orthopnoea or PND. Heart failure may also manifest with gastrointestinal symptoms such as anorexia, nausea and early satiety as a consequence of bowel oedema. Neurological symptoms such as confusion, disorientation and sleep disturbances may also occur due to underlying heart failure. Since the clinical manifestations in older adults may be diverse and atypical and there is a high prevalence in the elderly, clinicians should maintain a high index of suspicion with regard to the presence of heart failure.

Table 7.7 Framingham criteria for congestive heart failure

Major criteria

Complaints

    Paroxysmal nocturnal dyspnoea

Physical exam

    Neck vein distension

    Hepatojugular reflux

    Coarse crackles

    S3 gallop

Other

    Radiographic cardiomegaly (increasing heart size on chest radiography)

    Acute pulmonary oedema

    Increased central venous pressure (16 cm H_2O at right atrium)

    Weight loss of 4.5 kg in 5 days in response to treatment

Minor criteria

Complaints

    Dyspnoea on ordinary exertion

    Nocturnal cough

Physical examination

    Bilateral ankle oedema

Hepatomegaly

Tachycardia (heart rate of 120 beats per minute)

Other

    Pleural effusion

    Decrease in vital capacity by one third from maximum recorded

Source: Klein L. Heart failure with reduced ejection fraction. In: Crawford MH, ed. *Current Diagnosis & Treatment: Cardiology.* 4th ed. New York: McGraw-Hill Medical; 2014.

The common clinical signs of CHF are jugular venous distension and hepatojugular reflux, coarse crackles, S3 gallop and bilateral ankle oedema.

Management

NON-PHARMACOLOGICAL MANAGEMENT

Fluid restriction to <2000 mL/24 h, a sodium restricted diet of <1.5–2 g Na daily and monitoring of daily weight with strict input and output should be implemented. It is important to note however that these restrictions should not lead to actively impeding sufficient oral intake, especially during the early postoperative days when appetite may not be fully restored.

Pharmacological management

1. Diuretic therapy with the goal of a negative fluid balance of 300–500 mL/day. Diuretic therapy should be individualized and overdiuresis should be avoided because it can reduce systolic function and worsen azotemia.

2. In heart failure with preserved ejection fraction, tachycardia should be avoided. Use of beta blockers is important to achieve a heart rate of 65–70. This allows an increase in time for diastole. Tachycardia is triggered by pain, other discomfort such as urinary retention and constipation as well as hyperactive delirium. Therefore prevention of tachycardia whether it is sinus tachycardia or another dysrhythmia with a rapid ventricular rate is important to avoid precipitating heart failure. Pain management is important to this end as well.

POSTOPERATIVE CARDIAC DYSRHYTHMIA

Definition

Atrial fibrillation is the most common dysrhythmia and is characterized by disorganized electrical activation of the atria leading to uncoordinated atrial contractions and loss of 'atrial kick' which results in a decrease in cardiac output.

Physiological risk factors/age related changes

The increased prevalence of dysrhythmia in older adults occurs because of increased susceptibility of aging myocardium to abnormalities of electrical conduction due to fibrosis and loss of myocytes. Second, elderly patients have an increased prevalence of CHF, ischaemic heart disease and hypertension which are risk factors for the development of postoperative atrial fibrillation. Third, new dysrhythmias occur in susceptible myocardium due to perioperative triggers.

Systemic sympathetic flow can be increased because of a systemic inflammatory response due to trauma or surgery itself. There may be reflex catecholamine release due to hypovolemia and postoperative pain.

Hypotension and hypovolemia together with anaemia can also lead to ischaemia of atrial cells and conduction tissues altering the electrical properties of myocardium and triggering both atrial and ventricular dysrhythmias.

Hypervolemia due to excessive perioperative fluid administration may stretch myocardial cells and also trigger both atrial and ventricular dysrhythmias.

Metabolic abnormalities such as hyperglycemia, hypoglycemia, thyroid dysfunction and electrolyte disturbances, especially hypokalemia and hypomagnesemia, are seen commonly in older adults and may also trigger cardiac dysrhythmias.

Incidence/epidemiology

Atrial fibrillation is the most common dysrhythmia. The prevalence of atrial fibrillation increases with age and is approximately 2% at age 60–69 years, 4.6% at age 70–79 years and 8.8% at age 80–89 years. In patients undergoing non-cardiothoracic surgery the incidence of postoperative atrial fibrillation varies from 0.4% to 12%. There are sparse data on the incidence of postoperative atrial fibrillation specifically after orthogeriatric trauma surgery, but in one study the crude incidence of postoperative atrial fibrillation after orthopaedic surgery was 1.7%.[55] Atrial fibrillation is associated with higher postoperative mortality in patients undergoing non-cardiac surgery. In one study, a cohort of patients with atrial fibrillation who underwent emergent/urgent orthopaedic surgery had an unadjusted 30-day mortality of 10.2%.[56] Patients who develop atrial fibrillation also have longer hospital stay and increased hospitalization costs.

Diagnosis

Persistent atrial fibrillation may be asymptomatic, however, in the postoperative period patients frequently develop atrial fibrillation with rapid ventricular response. This may manifest with anxiety, palpitations, increased dyspnoea or chest discomfort. New atrial fibrillation may present with similar symptoms, however a sudden change in haemodynamics due to loss of atrial kick might also manifest with lightheadedness, dizziness or syncope. Cardiac auscultation reveals irregularly irregular rhythm. The diagnosis is established with ECG which shows an irregularly irregular rhythm with loss of p waves.

Treatment

The treatment of atrial fibrillation starts with the assessment of a patient's symptoms and haemodynamic stability. If a patient is unstable, that is, there is chest pain, dyspnoea or hypotension, then an immediate synchronized cardioversion may be required. If the patient is stable, then one should consider the three types of treatment for postoperative atrial fibrillation as detailed in Table 7.8.

A practitioner who encounters new atrial fibrillation or the worsening of previous atrial fibrillation with rapid

Table 7.8 Treatment of postoperative atrial fibrillation

Identification and correction of potential triggering factors
Rate or rhythm control
Prevention of stroke with systemic anticoagulation

ventricular response should consider cardiac ischaemia and the possibility of pulmonary embolism based on the clinical presentation. One of the most common postoperative triggering factors of atrial fibrillation is pain so this must be addressed first before moving on to other causes. One prospective study in thoracic patients showed a higher incidence of postoperative atrial fibrillation with poor pain control. Since the triggering mechanism of pain in atrial fibrillation is most likely common to all types of surgery, then control of pain becomes important in both the prophylaxis and treatment of atrial fibrillation. Maintenance of euvolemia by judicious administration of perioperative fluids may also reduce the incidence of postoperative atrial fibrillation. Correction of metabolic abnormalities such as hypoxemia, hypo- or hyperglycemia and electrolyte disturbances are part of both prophylaxis and treatment of atrial fibrillation. The next aspect of treatment is rate control. Immediate rate control can be achieved with intermittent boluses of IV beta blockers. This should be followed by oral beta blockers, which then can be titrated to heart rate and blood pressure. If beta blockers are not effective, then one can try calcium channel blockers. However, it is important that IV calcium channel blockers are not given immediately after IV beta blockers as complete nodal blockade may ensue. The target heart rate should be below 110. Rapid heart rate may cause tachycardia-induced cardiomyopathy and trigger heart failure. If a patient has a history of left ventricular dysfunction or if a patient becomes hypotensive with either beta blockers or calcium channel blockers, then an amiodarone bolus and drip can be considered. Of note, amiodarone is on the Beers Criteria list of medications to avoid in older adults and should be given for short periods only. The harm of prolonged use outweighs benefits in the elderly.

VENOUS THROMBOSIS AND THROMBOEMBOLISM

Definition

Venous thrombosis is the formation of an occluding blood clot in a vein. It is precipitated by blood stasis, vascular damage and disordered coagulation, which is referred to as Virchow's triad. Venous thrombosis commonly develops in the superficial or deep veins of the upper or lower extremities. Superficial venous thrombosis is a relatively benign condition. In deep venous thrombosis, a clot may form either in calf veins or in proximal veins, that is, the popliteal, femoral or iliac veins. Pulmonary thromboembolism occurs when a fragment of the blood clot breaks off and lodges in the pulmonary vascular bed. The consequences of pulmonary embolism range from an asymptomatic condition to significant hypoxemia, haemodynamic compromise and death. Most symptomatic pulmonary emboli originate from proximal vein thrombosis.

Physiological risk factors/age related changes

Advanced age is an independent risk factor for hypercoagulability. Aging is a prothrombotic state and is associated with markers of activated coagulation. Frail older adults have increased rates of venous thromboembolism compared with non-frail individuals due to an increase in procoagulant and inflammatory factors.[47] Additionally, older people have a higher prevalence of conditions that predispose them to venous thrombosis such as malignancy, heart failure, chronic kidney disease, atherosclerosis and immobility. In musculoskeletal trauma in older adults, there is a 'perfect storm' of conditions that precipitate venous thromboembolism. The prothrombotic state of aging is combined with immobility as well as vascular and tissue damage.

Prophylaxis

Thromboprophylaxis options include both mechanical and pharmacological approaches. Guidelines for the prevention of venous thromboembolism in orthopaedic surgery patients were recently revised. The American College of Chest Physicians recommends dual antithrombotic prophylaxis during the hospital stay for a major orthopaedic surgery with an antithrombotic agent and intermittent pneumatic compression device. In patients who undergo hip fracture surgery, low molecular weight heparins are the preferred agents. Recommended alternatives are low dose unfractionated heparin (LDUH), fondaparinux, adjusted dose warfarin or aspirin. Alternative medications have increased risk of bleeding such as fondaparinux or warfarin, or decreased efficacy such as aspirin, LDUH or mechanical prophylaxis alone. In patients undergoing hip fracture surgery thromboprophylaxis should continue for a minimum of 10–14 days and it is recommended the prophylaxis should be extended to 35 days postoperatively. For patients with isolated lower extremity injuries requiring leg immobilization, no thromboprophylaxis is recommended.[57]

Incidence/epidemiology

The reported risk of venous thromboembolism following hip fracture varies depending on how it is measured and when the study was completed. In the absence of thromboembolism prophylaxis the rates of venous thromboembolism in hip fractures can be as high as 46–75%, although many of these were determined through screening and were asymptomatic.[58,59] If only a physical prophylaxis was used, then the rate of venous thromboembolism ranged from 18% in pelvic fractures, 25.7% in distal fractures, 35% in multiple fractures to 50% in femoral shaft fractures.[60] The rate of fatal pulmonary embolism after hip fracture surgery was reported to be between 0.66% and 7.5% and is higher than with any other surgery.[61] In the thromboprophylaxis trials the thromboembolism rate ranges from 1.1% to 2.2%.[61,62]

Identification/diagnosis

The clinical features of deep vein thrombosis (DVT) are leg pain, increased swelling in the affected extremity, tenderness to palpation and palpable cords. The clinical findings are non-specific and should be combined with clinical prediction rules that include a risk factor profile and clinical signs and symptoms. Measurement of D-dimer is usually reserved for non-surgical patients; however, a small (n = 141) study in lower limb fracture patients demonstrated levels above 1000 ng/mL were 100% sensitive and 71% specific, so if access to ultrasonography is difficult and additional risk stratification is needed it may help.[63] Ultimately the diagnosis of venous thrombosis is established with either ultrasonography or, in selected patients, venography.

Pulmonary embolism is suspected in the presence of dyspnoea and tachypnoea, pleuritic chest pain and haemoptysis. Chest radiograph may show pulmonary infiltrates and pleural effusion. ECG may show non-specific dysrhythmias such as sinus tachycardia or atrial fibrillation. The patient may present with a wide range of symptoms or signs from anxiety and confusion to syncope and cardiovascular collapse. The symptoms are non-specific and therefore clinical prediction rules, similar to that used in DVT, is employed together with D-dimer measurements to guide further investigation and treatment. In both DVT and pulmonary embolism, assessment of clinical pretest probability is an important first step in establishing the diagnosis. Objective diagnosis of pulmonary embolism requires imaging studies. CT angiography (CTA) has a sensitivity of 83% and specificity of 96% for the diagnosis of pulmonary embolism. Combination of clinical assessment with CTA has a predictive value of 92–96%. Radionuclide scanning of the lungs is usually used when there is a high risk of contrast induced nephropathy, which is very relevant in elderly patients. A high probability scan has a positive predictive value of 85%. However, unfortunately most of the radionuclide scans are inconclusive, that is, have low or intermediate probability, especially in the presence of chronic lung disease. In these cases a combination of pretest probability, D-dimer and lower extremity ultrasonography is used to establish the diagnosis.

Management

Once the diagnosis of venous thromboembolism is established or strongly suspected, the treatment of choice is systemic anticoagulation. Absolute contraindications to anticoagulation are malignant hypertension, intracranial bleeding, severe active bleeding or recent brain, eye or spinal surgery. Clinical judgement is needed as to the timing, considering the bleeding risk with full anticoagulation and immediate orthopaedic surgery. Anticoagulation starts with either low molecular weight heparin, unfractionated heparin or fondaparinux. Warfarin should be initiated at the same time with parenteral anticoagulation. Heparin or fondaparinux should be continued for a minimum of 5 days and until the INR is between 2 and 3 for at least 24 hours. In the elderly a low initial starting dose of warfarin (we recommend a 2–5 mg starting dose) should be adjusted to maintain INR 2–3. The total duration of anticoagulation in the first episode of provoked venous thromboembolism should be at least 3 months. In the presence of absolute contraindications to anticoagulation, insertion of a retrievable inferior vena cava filter is indicated.

PULMONARY COMPLICATIONS

Definition

Postoperative pulmonary complications (PPCs) are defined as pulmonary abnormalities that result in identifiable disease or dysfunction and adversely impact the patient's clinical course.[64]

The most common of these are pneumonia, pneumonitis and COPD exacerbation.

Pneumonitis, also called chemical pneumonia, is due to irritant inflammation, commonly from gastric content aspiration.

Infectious pneumonia is due to pathogenic organisms causing pulmonary interstitial inflammation.

COPD exacerbation is a worsening obstruction of the airways due to an increase in bronchial inflammation.

Physiological risk factors/age related changes

The decrease in elastic recoil and increase in lung compliance leads to a greater predisposition to atelectasis in the recumbent position.[65] Older trauma patients who remain in a recumbent position due to immobilization easily become atelectatic, which coupled with poor ciliary clearance due to aging, creates a pulmonary environment suited for infection.

Although dysphagia is not a normal part of aging, the incidence of underlying swallowing difficulties is greater in older patients and may be worsened by stressors associated with hospitalization.[66]

Incidence/epidemiology

Pneumonia has been reported in 2% of inpatient rehabilitation hip fracture patients.[67] One study in hip fracture patients found PPCs during hospital stay to be 4%.[68]

Prevention

PNEUMONIA

Early mobility is an effective lung expansion manoeuvre which reduces pulmonary complications and decreases mortality, so having pathways in place to mobilize and get patients out of bed is essential.[69] Lung expansion manoeuvres (incentive spirometry, deep breathing exercises and continuous positive airway pressure) have shown to reduce PPCs and are worth implementing in patients who have the cognitive ability to do them.[64]

Previous swallowing difficulties should be assessed and precautions after surgery implemented if appropriate (e.g. elevating head of bed and modifying consistency of diet). The 'chin down' posture when swallowing can reduce the occurrence of aspiration.[66] Strict NPO may cause more harm than supervised hand feeding, especially in patients with dementia. Taste is an important reorienting modality in the context of delirium as well as in cognitively impaired patients.

COPD EXACERBATION

The intensity of preventive measures depends on the baseline severity of COPD.[64] If someone is oxygen dependent or has been hospitalized for their COPD, these are signs of severe COPD and must be communicated to the anaesthesiologist promptly. Bronchodilators and inhaled steroids must be continued and if a patient is expected to be too frail postoperatively to administer their inhalers, then regular nebulizers or assistance with spacers should be implemented.

Identification/diagnosis

PNEUMONIA

The clinical diagnosis of pneumonia is based on a combination of symptoms, signs and chest X-ray findings. The symptoms include cough, sputum, fever, chills and pleuritic chest pain. The signs include increased respiratory rate, dullness to percussion, bronchial breathing, aegophony, crackles, wheezes and pleural friction rub. The radiographic finding is a new opacity on chest radiograph that is not because of another condition.[70]

COPD EXACERBATION

The Winnipeg criteria are commonly used to diagnose COPD exacerbation, which is based on three symptoms: worsening of dyspnoea, an increase in sputum volume and an increase in sputum purulence. Patients with type I exacerbations have all of the above symptoms. Patients with type II exacerbations have two of the three symptoms, while those with type III exacerbations have at least one of these symptoms.[70]

Management

PNEUMONIA

Supplemental oxygen therapy is appropriate if the patient is hypoxic.

Antibiotic therapy is a central part of treating infectious pneumonia. The choice of antibiotic should be guided by the local microbiological surveillance of the institution. This will provide a much better empiric treatment based on local resistance and prevalence of pathogenic organisms.

Aspiration pneumonitis on its own does not justify antibiotics in frail older people especially because of the risk of antibiotic associated diarrhoea and *Clostridium difficile*. If a superimposed infectious pneumonia is present, antibiotics should be started; otherwise it is best to observe first.[71]

COPD EXACERBATION

A short course (2 weeks) of systemic steroids is an effective treatment modality for COPD exacerbations. In the elderly however it can be deliriogenic, particularly in cognitively impaired patients, and patients should be monitored for delirium when steroids are started.[70]

Inhaled bronchodilators should be intensified if they have not been maximized.

Antibiotics are indicated only in severe COPD exacerbations (type I).[70]

ACUTE HYPONATREMIA

Definition

An acute drop of serum sodium after surgery to less than 130 mmol/L.[71]

Physiological risk factors/age related changes

Water homeostasis in older adults is affected by changes in body composition, diminished renal function and alterations in hypothalamic–pituitary regulation of thirst and secretion of arginine vasopressin.[72] These changes diminish the ability to respond to mild volume shifts and other stressors such as pain and medications (diuretics and selective serotonin reuptake inhibitors). The fracture patient is subject to most of these stressors; therefore attempts at correcting hyponatremia should be focused on those stressors first before initiating aggressive osmotic interventions such as hypertonic saline which may cause an aging homeostenotic system to decompensate even further.[72]

Incidence/epidemiology

The incidence of acute postoperative hyponatremia (<130 mmol/L) in one retrospective study of 1131 orthopaedic trauma patients who underwent surgery was 2.8%. Up to 13% of fracture patients on admission present with a degree of hyponatremia (<135 mEq/L) but at the time of writing the cause and effect of this correlation is unclear.[73]

Prevention

Attention to volume status upon admission is important. Many patients have intravascular volume depletion on admission, which can be corrected with 250–500 mL volume increments. Maintenance fluids should be implemented when the patient is NPO prior to surgery. Excess use of free water via dextrose containing fluids should be avoided.[71]

Attention to medications is important. If a patient is on diuretics and/or selective serotonin reuptake inhibitors, the sodium should be monitored perioperatively. Diuretics may often be held while volume status is being optimized.

Attention to pain control is important. Pain is a common cause of syndrome of inappropriate antidiuretic hormone (SIADH) in the elderly.[72]

Identification/diagnosis

Serum sodium of <130 mmol/L.

Management

The patient's volume status should be assessed to decide whether they are euvolemic, hypovolemic or hypervolemic.

Hypovolemic patients require IV hydration, usually with normal saline. Dextrose should be avoided initially. Older adults may tolerate acute volume shifts poorly, so it is useful to hydrate with small increments of 250–500 mL at a time and reassess clinically for volume status before continuing.

Euvolemic patients normally have SIADH and need fluid restriction. Once again, adjust the severity of the restriction to the clinical situation of the patient.

Hypervolemic patients generally need to be diuresed. If overhydration is the cause, further overhydration can be limited by stopping or adjusting fluids. Patients who are overloaded are often in heart failure; please see section above on heart failure for management.

RENAL FAILURE OR KIDNEY DYSFUNCTION

Definition

A recent international consensus group for outcomes in hip fractures identified renal failure as a threefold increase of serum creatinine concentration, or serum creatinine ≥4 mg/dL with an acute rise of >0.5 mg/dL, or a urine output of <0.3 mL/kg/h×24 h, or anuria×12 h.[74]

Physiological risk factors/age related changes

Even though many studies in the aging kidney are based on rodents and do not necessarily translate to human beings, there are known changes that functionally result in a similar homeostenotic state as in other physiological systems.[75] These include loss of parenchymal mass, progressive glomerulosclerosis, tubulopathy, interstitial fibrosis and the development of afferent–efferent arteriolar shunts.[76] In addition medications like non-steroidal anti-inflammatory drugs (NSAIDs) can be particularly toxic to the prostaglandin dependent aging kidney. Prostaglandins play a bigger role in the aging kidney for free water excretion and vascular renal perfusion.[72,75] As a result hypotension and nephrotoxic medications can cause greater damage in an aging kidney.

Incidence

The incidence of kidney dysfunction in orthopaedic fracture patients varies from 8.9% to 16%.[77–79] In a large retrospective study 82.5% of these patients recovered their renal function to preoperative status.[77]

Prevention

Central to preventing kidney dysfunction perioperatively in older adults is avoiding hypotension and prolonged hypoperfusion of the kidney. Consider limiting the number of hypotensive medications given on the day of surgery or setting hold parameters based on blood pressure throughout the perioperative period. Once again the careful balance of fluid management is important perioperatively. Communicating with the anaesthesiology team is important to make sure this objective is followed throughout the entire care pathway.

After avoiding hypotension the next potential source of harm to the older kidney is nephrotoxic medications. Studies in orthopaedic patients have highlighted NSAIDs and nephrotoxic antibiotics as statistically significant, while a smaller study also questions the role of angiotensin converting enzyme inhibitors (ACEIs).[78,79]

Management

Once kidney dysfunction has occurred, then even greater scrutiny in maintaining intravascular volume should be implemented. Monitoring should be in accordance with the severity of the problem. Ideally this can be done without inducing delirium by excessive overnight disruptions and invasive procedures.

Medication dosages should be adjusted for renal dysfunction and non-critical potentially nephrotoxic medications should be stopped.

Finally if kidney dysfunction is severe it may be prudent to involve the care of a nephrologist. Careful dietary restrictions (sodium, potassium and protein) and medical management of electrolytes can be essential in preventing greater systemic complications.

URINARY TRACT INFECTION VERSUS ASYMPTOMATIC BACTERIURIA

Definition

Asymptomatic bacteriuria is defined as the isolation of bacteria from an adequately collected urine specimen in patients without signs or symptoms of urinary tract infection (UTI).

Symptoms of UTI include frequency, urgency, dysuria or suprapubic pain. Asymptomatic bacteriuria may be accompanied by pyuria.

Incidence/epidemiology

Asymptomatic bacteriuria is very common in the elderly population with the prevalence ranging from 3.6–19% in community-dwelling elderly to 25–50% in an institutionalized elderly population.[80] The presence of a chronic indwelling Foley catheter increases the prevalence of bacteriuria to 100%.[81]

Management

Asymptomatic bacteriuria or pyuria should not be treated in an elderly population. There are only two populations of patients that have been shown to benefit from antibiotic therapy in asymptomatic bacteriuria: pregnant women and patients undergoing invasive urological procedures.[81] Currently there is no strong evidence that asymptomatic bacteriuria increases the risk of prosthetic joint infections.[82] On the other hand, inappropriate treatment of asymptomatic bacteriuria with antibiotics may increase the risk of *C. difficile* infection, selection of resistant microbial pathogens and other adverse events.[83,84] Asymptomatic bacteriuria has become a major cause of antibiotic overuse. Studies have shown that 20–52% of hospitalized patients with asymptomatic bacteriuria were treated unnecessarily. Reducing *C. difficile* infection in hip fracture patients has decreased mortality.[85]

CONSTIPATION

Definition

Rome III criteria are used to define chronic constipation which address not only the frequency but also consistency and symptoms during defecation.[86] However, for postsurgical constipation, studies have taken the simple definition of failure of the bowel to open for 3 consecutive days.[87]

Physiological risk factors/age related changes

Susceptibility to dehydration, an aging myenteric nervous system and anorectal internal sphincter dysfunction predispose elderly patients to constipation.[88] Constipation in the elderly can be painful, deliriogenic and induce urinary retention, and so should be addressed quickly within the perioperative period.

Incidence/epidemiology

A small study of hip fracture patients found an incidence of 71.7% using the 3-day definition of constipation.[87] A proactive approach to start a bowel regimen routinely may reduce this rate.

Prevention

Most of the preventive studies using laxatives to address constipation in the setting of opiates come from palliative care and oncology studies; however, a small study in hip fracture patients also showed a trend but no statistical significance of laxatives given with opiates preventing constipation.[87] It is reasonable to use a stimulant laxative whenever prescribing opiates in the elderly, as the intake of fluids may not be sufficient for an osmotic laxative to be effective.

Identification/diagnosis

Nursing records should track bowel movements in patients so constipation can be easily identified. If not available, routine questioning in cognitively intact patients can be a good identifier.

Management

Non-pharmacological measures include early mobility, adequate oral intake and hydration.

If the stimulant laxatives are not effective by the third postoperative day a suppository is generally effective in addressing the anorectal sphincter dysfunction that tends to develop with aging. If a suppository is not effective then an enema can be tried. If an enema is not effective, rectal examination to look for faecal impaction should be considered.

POSTOPERATIVE FEVER

Definition

Fever is an increase in body temperature due to pyrogens commonly associated with inflammation, tissue injury and disease. Pyrogens include interleukin-1, interleukin-6 and tumour necrosis factor-α.[89,90]

Physiological risk factors/age related changes

Frail elderly individuals have lower mean baseline body temperatures than the generally accepted norm of 37°C (98.6°F). Animal models of aging demonstrate that temperature elevations in response to endogenous pyrogens are diminished with advanced age.[89]

Due to the diminished response to pryogens and possible lower baseline body temperatures, some have suggested that in the elderly fever be defined as (1) persistent elevation of body temperature of at least 1.1°C (2°F) over baseline values or (2) oral temperatures of 99°F (37.2°C) or greater on repeated measures or (3) rectal temperatures of 99.5°F (37.5°C) or greater on repeated measures.[89]

Incidence/epidemiology

The incidence of postoperative fever in elective arthroplasty ranges from 15% to 47%.[90,91] In elderly fracture patients a small study of 84 patients showed that blood cultures drawn within 4 days of surgery from patients whose temperature was >38°C in the setting of paracetamol (acetaminophen) produced <1% positive results and that test result was deemed to be a contaminant.[90]

Prevention

In elective arthroplasty patients it has been shown that adequate pain control can prevent unnecessary workup of postoperative fever without masking significant comorbidity.[92] Considering the benefits of adequate pain management for mobility, delirium and their relationship to improved mortality in hip fracture patients, masking fevers should not be a concern for adequate postoperative pain control with acetaminophen/paracetamol.

Identification/diagnosis

At the time of writing we still recommend oral and tympanic temperatures >38°C for diagnosing fever until better clinically relevant data in elderly hip fracture patients argue for a different definition.

It is very important to perform a good clinical assessment in the presence of fever to make sure there are no other signs or symptoms of sepsis. By the fifth postoperative day it is much less likely that the fever is simply due to postoperative inflammatory load and other sources should be considered.

Management

During the first 4 days following surgery without any other signs or symptoms of sepsis, postoperative fever requires simply clinical monitoring and supportive therapy with hydration, pain control and early mobilization.

New fever after the fourth day of surgery merits a closer look for new onset infection. Common sites of infection include catheter associated (urine or intravenous) infection, surgical site infection, pneumonia and C. difficile associated diarrhoea.[91] An infectious workup may include blood culture, urine culture, evaluation of stool and chest X-ray based on presentation.

ANAEMIA

Definition

Anaemia is defined as a decrease in the amount of red blood cells in the blood stream. The Word Health Organization definition includes a haemoglobin <12 g/dL in women and <13 g/dL in men.[93]

Physiological risk factors/age related changes

The aging bone marrow has a blunted haematopoietic response. The exact mechanism is still under study but an aging bone marrow cannot respond to a stressor including surgical blood loss in a timely manner.[94] This could explain the high prevalence of postsurgical anaemia in elderly hip fracture patients.

Age related stiffening of the left ventricle increases the incidence of heart failure with a normal ejection fraction so when transfusing blood the authors recommend transfusing 1 unit at a time and reassessing clinical symptoms and/or haemoglobin levels before further transfusion. This could avoid and explain why transfusion circulatory overload is the greatest risk in transfusion in hip fracture patients (1–4%).[95]

Incidence/epidemiology

More than 80% of hip fracture patients after surgery have a haemoglobin concentration <11 g/dL.[95]

Identification/diagnosis

Peripheral blood samples are generally used to perform blood counts and are done routinely before and after surgery.

Management

In a large trial, 2016 elderly hip fracture patients were randomized to receive blood transfusions after surgery to a goal of 8 g/dL versus 10 g/dL haemoglobin. There was no difference in 30-day mortality and 60-day ability to walk unassisted.[96] An ancillary study also found no difference in delirium between the two groups.[21]

Based on these results and in the context of no active ongoing bleeding, hypotension or tachycardia unresponsive to fluids or cardiac symptoms due to anaemia, we recommend a transfusion threshold of 8 g/dL haemoglobin and judicious consideration of transfusing 1 unit of packed red blood cells at a time for reasons explained under aging changes.

REFERENCES

1. Cowdry EV. *Problems of Ageing: Biological and Medical Aspects*. 2nd ed. Baltimore: Williams & Wilkins; 1942.
2. Lipowski ZJ. Delirium, clouding of consciousness and confusion. *J Nerv Ment Dis* 1967;145(3):227–55.
3. Committee on Nomenclature and Statistics, American Psychiatric Association. *Diagnostic and Statistical Manual of Mental Disorders*. Washington, DC: American Psychiatric Association; 1952.
4. Committee on Nomenclature and Statistics, American Psychiatric Association. *Diagnostic and Statistical Manual of Mental Disorders*. 2nd ed. Washington, DC: American Psychiatric Association; 1968.
5. American Psychiatric Association. *Work Group to Revise DSM-III. Diagnostic and Statistical Manual of Mental Disorders: DSM-III-R*. 3rd ed. Washington, DC: American Psychiatric Association; 1987.
6. American Psychiatric Association. *DSM-5 Task Force. Diagnostic and Statistical Manual of Mental Disorders: DSM-5*. 5th ed. Washington, DC: American Psychiatric Association; 2013.
7. Inouye SK, Westendorp RGJ, Saczynski JS. Delirium in elderly people. *Lancet* 2014;383(9920):911–22.
8. Witlox J, Eurelings LS, de Jonghe JF, et al. Delirium in elderly patients and the risk of postdischarge mortality, institutionalization, and dementia: A meta-analysis. *JAMA* 2010;304(4):443–51.
9. Rudolph JL, Jones RN, Rasmussen LS, Silverstein JH, Inouye SK, Marcantonio ER. Independent vascular and cognitive risk factors for postoperative delirium. *Am J Med* 2007;120:807–13.
10. Marcantonio ER, Goldman L, Mangione CM, et al. A clinical prediction rule for delirium after elective noncardiac surgery. *JAMA* 1994;271:134–9.
11. Norkiene I, Ringaitiene D, Misiuriene I, et al. Incidence and precipitating factors of delirium after coronary artery bypass grafting. *Scand Cardiovasc J* 2007;41:180–5.
12. Inouye SK. Delirium in older persons. *New Engl J Med* 2006;354(11):1157–65.
13. Inouye SK, van Dyck CH, Alessi CA, et al. Clarifying confusion: The confusion assessment method. A new method for detection of delirium. *Ann Intern Med* 1990;113(12):941–8.
14. Ely EW, Truman B, Shintani A, et al. Monitoring sedation status over time in ICU patients: Reliability and validity of the Richmond Agitation-Sedation Scale (RASS). *JAMA* 2003;289(22):2983–91.
15. Meagher DJ, Leonard M, Donnelly S, et al. A longitudinal study of motor subtypes in delirium: Relationship with other phenomenology, etiology, medication exposure and prognosis. *J Psychosom Res* 2011;71(6):395–403.
16. Javedan H, Tulebaev S. Management of common postoperative complications: Delirium. *Clin Geriatr Med* 2014;30(2):271–8.
17. Inouye SK, Bogardus ST, Jr., Charpentier PA, et al. A multicomponent intervention to prevent delirium in hospitalized older patients. *New Engl J Med* 1999;340(9):669–76.
18. Lundstrom M, Edlund A, Karlsson S, et al. A multifactorial intervention program reduces the duration of delirium, length of hospitalization, and mortality in delirious patients. *J Am Geriatr Soc* 2005;53(4):622–8.

19. Martinez FT, Tobar C, Beddings CI, et al. Preventing delirium in an acute hospital using a non-pharmacological intervention. *Age Ageing* 2012;41(5):629–34.

20. Marcantonio ER, Flacker JM, Wright RJ, et al. Reducing delirium after hip fracture: A randomized trial. *J Am Geriatr Soc* 2001;49(5):516–22.

21. Gruber-Baldini AL, Marcantonio E, Orwig D, et al. Delirium outcomes in a randomized trial of blood transfusion thresholds in hospitalized older adults with hip fracture. *J Am Geriatr Soc* 2013;61(8):1286–95.

22. Behrends M, DePalma G, Sands L, et al. Association between intraoperative blood transfusions and early postoperative delirium in older adults. *J Am Geriatr Soc* 2013;61(3):365–70.

23. Mittal V, Kurup L, Williamson D, Muralee S, Tampi RR. Risk of cerebrovascular adverse events and death in elderly patients with dementia when treated with antipsychotic medications: A literature review of evidence. *Am J Alzheimers Dis Other Dement* 2011;26(1):10–28.

24. Hatta K, Kishi Y, Wada K, et al. Antipsychotics for delirium in the general hospital setting in consecutive 2453 inpatients: A prospective observational study. *Int J Geriatr Psychiatry* 2014;29(3):253–62.

25. WHO. Cancer pain relief: with a guide to opioid availability. 2nd ed. 1996. http://apps.who. int/iris/bitstream/10665/37896/1/9241544821.pdf

26. Tsang KS, Page J, Mackenney P. Can intravenous paracetamol reduce opioid use in preoperative hip fracture patients? *Orthopedics* 2013;36(2 Suppl):20–4.

27. Morrison RS, Magaziner J, Gilbert M, et al. Relationship between pain and opioid analgesics on the development of delirium following hip fracture. *J Gerontol A Biol Sci Med Sci* 2003;58A:76–81.

28. Marcantonio ER, Juarez G, Goldman L, et al. The relationship of postoperative delirium with psychoactive medications. *JAMA* 1994;272:1518–22.

29. Marino J, Russo J, Kenny M, et al. Continuous lumbar plexus block for postoperative pain control after total hip arthroplasty. A randomized controlled trial. *J Bone Joint Surg Am* 2009;91:29–37.

30. Sieber FE, Mears S, Lee H, et al. Postoperative opioid consumption and its relationship to cognitive function in older adults with hip fracture. *J Am Geriatr Soc* 2011;59(12):2256–62.

31. Miura LN, DiPiero AR, Homer LD. Effects of a geriatrician-led hip fracture program: Improvements in clinical and economic outcomes. *J Am Geriatr Soc* 2009;57(1):159–67.

32. Mittal V, Muralee S, Williamson D, et al. Review: Delirium in the elderly: A comprehensive review. *Am J Alzheimers Disease Other Dement* 2011;26(2):97–109.

33. Lonergan E, Britton AM, Luxenberg J, et al. Antipsychotics for delirium. *Cochrane Database Syst Rev* 2007;(2):CD005594.

34. Tahir TA, Eeles E, Karapareddy V, et al. A randomized controlled trial of quetiapine versus placebo in the treatment of delirium. *J Psychosom Res* 2010;69(5):485–90.

35. Overshott R, Karim S, Burns A. Cholinesterase inhibitors for delirium. *Cochrane Database Syst Rev* 2008;(1):CD005317.

36. Lonergan E, Luxenberg J, Areosa Sastre A. Benzodiazepines for delirium. *Cochrane Database Syst Rev* 2009;(4):CD006379.

37. Teslyar P, Stock VM, Wilk CM, et al. Prophylaxis with antipsychotic medication reduces the risk of postoperative delirium in elderly patients: A meta-analysis. *Psychosomatics* 2013;54(2):124–31.

38. Thygesen K, Alpert JS, Jaffe AS, Simoons ML, Chaitman BR. ESC/ACCF/AHA/WHF Expert Consensus Document. *Circulation* 2012;126:2020–35.

39. Botto F, Alonso-Coello P, Chan MTV, et al. Myocardial injury after noncardiac surgery: A large, international, prospective cohort study establishing diagnostic criteria, characteristics, predictors, and 30-day outcomes. *Anesthesiology* 2014;120(3):564–78.

40. Kitzman DW, Taffet G. Effects of aging on cardiovascular structure and function. In: Halter JB, Ouslander JG, Tinettii, ME, Studenski S, High KP, Asthana S, eds. *Hazzard's Geriatric Medicine and Gerontology*. 6th ed. New York: McGraw-Hill, 2009.

41. Landesberg G, Beattie WS, Mosseri M, Jaffe AS, Alpert JS. Perioperative myocardial infarction. *Circulation* 2009;119(22):2936–44.

42. Huddleston JM, Gullerud RE, Smither F, et al. Myocardial infarction after hip fracture repair: A population-based study. *J Am Geriatr Soc* 2012;60:2020–6.

43. Gupta BP, Huddleston JM, Kirkland LL, et al. Clinical presentation and outcome of perioperative myocardial infarction in the very elderly following hip fracture surgery. *J Hosp Med* 2012;7(9):713–16.

44. Sandhu A, Sanders S, Geraci SA. Prognostic value of cardiac troponins in elderly patients with hip fracture—A systematic review. *Osteoporos Int* 2012;24(4):1145–9.

45. Brieger D, Eagle KA, Goodman SG, et al. Acute coronary syndromes without chest pain, an underdiagnosed and undertreated high-risk group: Insights from the Global Registry of Acute Coronary Events. *Chest* 2004;126(2):461–9.

46. Alexander KP, Newby LK, Cannon CP, et al. Acute coronary care in the elderly, Part I: Non-ST-segment-elevation acute coronary syndromes: A scientific statement for healthcare professionals from the American Heart Association Council on Clinical Cardiology: In collaboration with the Society of Geriatric Cardiology. *Circulation* 2007;115(19):2549–69.

47. Shammash JB, Kimmel SE. *Perioperative Myocardial Infarction after Noncardiac Surgery*. UpToDate. http://www.uptodate.com/contents/

perioperative-myocardial-infarction-after-noncardiac-surgery (accessed 7 Aug 2014).

48. Chong CP. Does cardiology intervention improve mortality for post-operative troponin elevations after emergency orthopaedic–geriatric surgery? A randomised controlled study. *Injury* 2012;43(7):1193–8.

49. Ershler WB, Longo DL. Hematology in older persons. In: Kaushansky K, Beutler E, Seligsohn U, et al., eds. *Williams Hematology*. 8th ed. New York: McGraw-Hill; 2010, pp. 115–28.

50. Forman DE, Ahmed A, Fleg JL. Heart failure in very old adults. *Curr Heart Fail Rep* 2013;10(4):387–400.

51. Chan M, Tsuyuki R. Heart failure in the elderly. *Curr Opin Cardiol* 2013;28(2):234–41.

52. Abou-Raya S, Abou-Raya A. Osteoporosis and congestive heart failure (CHF) in the elderly patient: Double disease burden. *Arch Gerontol Geriatr* 2009;49(2):250–4.

53. van Diepen S, Majumdar SR, Bakal JA, McAlister FA, Ezekowitz JA. Heart failure is a risk factor for orthopedic fracture: A population-based analysis of 16 294 patients. *Circulation* 2008;118(19):1946–52.

54. Klein L. Heart failure with reduced ejection fraction. In: Crawford MH, ed. *Current Diagnosis & Treatment: Cardiology*. 4th ed. New York: McGraw-Hill Medical; 2014.

55. Bhave PD, Goldman LE, Vittinghoff E, Maselli J, Auerbach A. Incidence, predictors, and outcomes associated with postoperative atrial fibrillation after major noncardiac surgery. *Am Heart J* 2012;164(6):918–24.

56. van Diepen S, Bakal JA, McAlister FA, Ezekowitz JA. Mortality and readmission of patients with heart failure, atrial fibrillation, or coronary artery disease undergoing noncardiac surgery: An analysis of 38 047 patients. *Circulation* 2011;124(3):289–96.

57. Falck-Ytter Y, Francis CW, Johanson MA, et al. Prevention of VTE in orthopedic surgery patients. *Chest* 2012;141(2 Suppl):e278S–325S.

58. Marsland D, Mears SC, Kates SL. Venous thromboembolic prophylaxis for hip fractures. *Osteoporos Int* 2010;21(Suppl 4):S593–604.

59. Friedman SM, Uy JD. Venous thromboembolism and postoperative management of anticoagulation. *Clinics Geriatr Med* 2014;30(2):285–91.

60. Niikura T, Lee SY, Oe K, et al. Venous thromboembolism in Japanese patients with fractures of the pelvis and/or lower extremities using physical prophylaxis alone. *J Orthop Surg (Hong Kong)* 2012;20(2):196–200.

61. Rosencher N, Vielpeau C, Emmerich J, Fagnani F, Samama CM. Venous thromboembolism and mortality after hip fracture surgery: The ESCORTE study. *J Thromb Haemost* 2005;3(9):2006–14.

62. McNamara I, Sharma A, Prevost T, Parker M. Symptomatic venous thromboembolism following a hip fracture. *Acta Orthop* 2009;80(6):687–92.

63. Bakhshi H, Alavi-Moghaddam M, Wu KC, Imami M, Banasiri M. D-dimer as an applicable test for detection of posttraumatic deep vein thrombosis in lower limb fracture. *Am J Orthop (Belle Mead NJ)* 2012;41(6):E78–80.

64. Lo IL, Siu CW, Tse HF, Lau TW, Leung F, Wong M. Pre-operative pulmonary assessment for patients with hip fracture. *Osteoporos Int* 2010;21(Suppl 4):S579–86.

65. Janssens JP, Pache JC, Nicod LP. Physiological changes in respiratory function associated with ageing. *Eur Resp J* 1999;13(1):197–205.

66. Love AL, Cornwell PL, Whitehouse SL. Oropharyngeal dysphagia in an elderly post-operative hip fracture population: A prospective cohort study. *Age Ageing* 2013;42(6):782–5.

67. Ahmed I, Graham JE, Karmarkar AM, Granger CV, Ottenbacher KJ. In-patient rehabilitation outcomes following lower extremity fracture in patients with pneumonia. *Respir Care* 2013;58(4):601–6.

68. Lawrence VA, Hilsenbeck SG, Noveck H, Poses RM, Carson JL. Medical complications and outcomes after hip fracture repair. *Arch Intern Med* 2002;162(18):2053–7.

69. Siu AL, Penrod JD, Boockvar KS, Koval K, Strauss E, Morrison RS. Early ambulation after hip fracture: Effects on function and mortality. *Arch Intern Med* 2006;166(7):766–71.

70. Yende S, Newman AB, Sin D. Chronic obstructive pulmonary disease. In: Hazzard WR, Halter JB, eds. *Hazzard's Geriatric Medicine and Gerontology*. 6th ed. New York: McGraw-Hill Medical; 2009.

71. Warner MA, Warner ME, Weber JG. Clinical significance of pulmonary aspiration during the perioperative period. *Anesthesiology* 1993;78(1):56–62.

72. Tambe AA, Hill R, Livesley PJ. Post-operative hyponatraemia in orthopaedic injury. *Injury* 2003;34(4):253–5.

73. Cowen LE, Hodak SP, Verbalis JG. Age-associated abnormalities of water homeostasis. *Endocrinol Metabol Clin North Am* 2013;42(2):349–70.

74. Gankam Kengne F, Andres C, Sattar L, Melot C, Decaux G. Mild hyponatremia and risk of fracture in the ambulatory elderly. *QJM* 2008;101(7):583–8.

75. Liem IS, Kammerlander C, Suhm N, et al. Identifying a standard set of outcome parameters for the evaluation of orthogeriatric co-management for hip fractures. *Injury* 2013;44(11):1403–12.

76. Wiggins J, Patel SR. Changes in kidney function. In: Hazzard WR, Halter JB, eds. *Hazzard's Geriatric Medicine and Gerontology*. 6th ed. New York: McGraw-Hill Medical; 2009.

77. Lamb EJ, O'Riordan SE, Delaney MP. Kidney function in older people: Pathology, assessment and management. *Clin Chim Acta* 2003;334(1–2):25–40.

78. Macheras GA, Kateros K, Koutsostathis SD, Papadakis SA, Tsiridis E. Which patients are at risk for kidney dysfunction after hip fracture surgery? *Clin Orthop Relat Res* 2013;471(12):3795–802.

79. Kateros K, Doulgerakis C, Galanakos SP, Sakellariou VI, Papadakis SA, Macheras GA. Analysis of kidney dysfunction in orthopaedic patients. *BMC Nephrol* 2012;13:101.

80. Bennet SJ, Berry OM, Goddard J, Keating JF. Acute renal dysfunction following hip fracture. *Injury* 2010;41(4):335–8.

81. Nicolle LE. Asymptomatic bacteriuria in the elderly. *Infect Dis Clin North Am* 1997;11:647–62.

82. Nicolle LE, Bradley S, Colgan R, et al. Infectious Diseases Society of America guidelines for the diagnosis and treatment of asymptomatic bacteriuria in adults. *Clin Infect Dis* 2005;40(5):643–54.

83. Cordero-Ampuero J, Gonzalez-Fernandez E, Martinez-Velez D, et al. Are antibiotics necessary in hip arthroplasty with asymptomatic bacteriuria? Seeding risk with/without treatment. *Clin Orthop Relat Res* 2013;471(12):3822–9.

84. Trautner BW. Asymptomatic bacteriuria: When the treatment is worse than the disease. *Nat Rev Urol* 2012;9(2):85–93.

85. Gulihar A, Nixon M, Jenkins D, et al. *Clostridium difficile* in hip fracture patients: Prevention, treatment and associated mortality. *Injury* 2009;40(7):746–51.

86. Fenton P, Singh K, Cooper M. *Clostridium difficile* infection following hip fracture. *J Hosp Infect* 2008;68(4):376–7.

87. Kurniawan I, Simadibrata M. Management of chronic constipation in the elderly. *Acta Med Indones* 2011;43(3):195–205.

88. Davies EC, Green CF, Mottram DR, Pirmohamed M. The use of opioids and laxatives, and incidence of constipation, in patients requiring neck-of-femur (NOF) surgery: A pilot study. *J Clin Pharm Ther* 2008;33(5):561–6.

89. Harari D. Constipation. In: Hazzard WR, Halter JB, eds. *Hazzard's Geriatric Medicine and Gerontology.* 6th ed. New York: McGraw-Hill Medical; 2009.

90. High KP. Infection in the elderly. In: Hazzard WR, Halter JB, eds. *Hazzard's Geriatric Medicine and Gerontology.* 6th ed. New York: McGraw-Hill Medical; 2009.

91. Sivakumar B, Vijaysegaran P, Ottley M, Crawford R, Coulter C. Blood cultures for evaluation of early postoperative fever after femoral neck fracture surgery. *J Orthop Surg (Hong Kong)* 2012;20(3):336–40.

92. Pile JC. Evaluating postoperative fever: A focused approach. *Cleve Clin J Med* 2006;73(Suppl 1):S62–6.

93. Karam JA, Zmistowski B, Restrepo C, Hozack WJ, Parvizi J. Fewer postoperative fevers: An unexpected benefit of multimodal pain management? *Clin Orthop Relat Res* 2014;472(5):1489–95.

94. Chaves PHM. Anemia. In: Hazzard WR, Halter JB, eds. *Hazzard's Geriatric Medicine and Gerontology.* 6th ed. New York: McGraw-Hill Medical; 2009.

95. Chatta GS, Lipschitz DA. Aging of the hematopoietic system. In: Hazzard WR, Halter JB. *Hazzard's Geriatric Medicine and Gerontology.* 6th ed. New York: McGraw-Hill Medical; 2009.

96. Willett LR, Carson JL. Management of postoperative complications: Anemia. *Clin Geriatr Med* 2014;30(2):279–84.

97. Carson JL, Terrin ML, Noveck H, et al. Liberal or restrictive transfusion in high-risk patients after hip surgery. *New Engl J Med* 2011;365(26):2453–62.

8

Rehabilitation after fracture

PATRICK KORTEBEIN

INTRODUCTION

Older adults are the fastest growing segment of the United States and global population, and so the prevalence of geriatric fracture and the associated healthcare and societal costs can be expected to increase in commensurate fashion.[1,2] As older adults in general have a more limited functional reserve, a fracture in this patient population can have significant adverse consequences, including loss of independence, institutionalization and even an increased risk of death. Hip fracture is the archetype of this phenomenon; in the year following hip fracture up to 50% of older adults may be institutionalized, while reported mortality rates range from 12% to 35%.[3,4] Other fragility fractures associated with increased morbidity and mortality include spine, proximal humerus and distal forearm fractures.[4] However, even a relatively minor fracture of an older adult's dominant hand may have a marked impact on an older individual's functional independence if they are, for instance, living alone with no family or social support. Rehabilitation is the process of restoring function, and the primary goal of a rehabilitation program in an older adult who has sustained a fracture is to optimize their functional recovery to at least, if not above, their pre-fracture level. For those living in the community, this goal would include returning to their previous living setting.

The purpose of this chapter is to present the key principles and components of a post-fracture rehabilitation program for geriatric patients. This includes a review of the main components of a rehabilitation assessment in an older adult patient, the key elements of a rehabilitation program including the healthcare practitioners involved in the rehabilitation process, the continuum of rehabilitation care post-fracture, including the rehabilitation facilities where post-fracture rehabilitation can occur, and other considerations during rehabilitation. It is beyond the scope of this chapter to discuss the rehabilitation program for all types of fractures, however the key principles and components of a post-fracture rehabilitation program are reviewed. A rehabilitation program should be tailored to each individual patient. It should also be recognized that a formal structured rehabilitation program is not necessary for all geriatric fracture patients merely because of their age. However, as older individuals tend to be at greater risk for functional compromise, even a minor fracture may offer an opportunity for a thorough geriatric assessment and initiation of preventive measures (e.g. osteoporosis evaluation and falls prevention).

REHABILITATION ASSESSMENT

While it has only relatively recently been reported that geriatric and orthopaedic co-management of hip fractures results in better outcomes with reduced healthcare costs, it is certainly reasonable to institute this type of management paradigm for other geriatric fracture patients.[5,6] However, as there are not enough geriatricians to manage all such patients, other physicians, including primary care specialists, will need to become familiar with these management programs. Fortunately, the standard rehabilitation assessment regimen typically encompasses many of the same elements as a comprehensive geriatric assessment.[7,8]

While this comprehensive assessment is perhaps more critical for individuals sustaining a major fracture (e.g. hip fracture), the key components of the rehabilitation assessment described below should be considered in all geriatric fracture patients, regardless of the particular type of fracture.

Pre-morbid function, cognition and family/social support

Compromised pre-fracture function and cognitive impairment have been identified as negatively impacting recovery from hip fracture and other geriatric fractures.[4,8,9] Similarly, having better social support, such as family or friends available to provide physical assistance, is associated with more positive outcomes in hip fracture patients. Consequently, it is important to determine an older individual's baseline physical function, cognitive status and available family/social support.

Physical function is assessed by inquiring as to an individual's ability to perform both basic and instrumental activities of daily living (ADL) before their fracture. Basic ADL include eating, grooming, bathing, toileting, transferring and walking, while instrumental ADL include more advanced activities such as shopping, driving/community transportation and managing personal finances. Basic ADL function may be assessed with either the Katz Index or the Barthel Index, while the Lawton instrument is often used to rate instrumental ADL function.[10–12] Assessment of ADL function should include ascertaining the amount of assistance, if any, required for each activity. This would include determining whether gait assistive devices (e.g. cane or walker) had been necessary, as post-fracture ambulatory function might be adversely impacted. For instance, in a patient who before the fracture utilized a walker for ambulation, a upper extremity fracture necessitating temporary non-weight bearing will require that an alternative means of mobilization will need to be identified (e.g. motorized scooter). As functional assessment is a standard part of physical or occupational therapy evaluation, this information may be obtained from or confirmed by these therapy specialists. Finally, the functional evaluation should also include inquiry as to the patient's status regarding driving (e.g. previous driver, plan to return to driving), as well as avocational (or vocational) activities. The ability to return to these activities can be particularly satisfying for many individuals; driving in particular affords freedom and thus many patients are eager to return to this activity.

Implicit in a functional evaluation is ascertainment of the individual's physical residence as it is vital to understand what obstacles may need to be overcome for them to return their prior living setting. This is particularly critical for individuals living in the community. For instance, for a patient living in a multi-level residence and unable to negotiate stairs after a fracture, it must be determined how the patient will access all essential living space (i.e. kitchen, bathroom and bedroom) for their basic ADL activities. All options should be considered, and may include, for instance, temporary home modification (e.g. bedside commode in the bedroom), assistance from family/friends (e.g. to mobilize the patient or provide meals) or temporary residence in a more accessible setting (e.g. a sibling's one-level home). Also, while it may be assumed that the patient will be returning to their previous living setting, this should be confirmed with the patient and their family (or other social support system). For instance, it may have been recognized that the patient's ability to remain living independently was rather tenuous and institutional settings (e.g. assisted living) had recently been considered.

Current and pre-fracture cognitive status are obtained as part of the rehabilitation assessment to determine if there is any baseline dysfunction, or any significant change since the fracture. Mild cognitive impairment may not have been overtly identified pre-fracture and may only become apparent on investigating the patient's cognitive status with family and/or friends. Delirium is quite common in older hospitalized patients and has significant adverse consequences. The symptoms of delirium (e.g. memory impairment and disorganized thinking) may persist for weeks and may adversely impact on an individual's ability to participate in rehabilitation activities. Thus, this syndrome should be proactively identified and managed.[13]

Current function and functional limitations secondary to fracture

In order to determine what functional elements require improvement, one must determine the post-fracture patient's current level of function, as well as any temporary functional restrictions and long-term prognosis. If temporary weight bearing or joint range of motion restrictions are in place, the timing for progression and/or discontinuation of the restrictions should be determined. The expected timing of follow-up evaluation with the orthopaedic surgeon should be clarified as well.

In a typical hospital setting, the current functional status of a patient is most commonly ascertained via a physical or occupational therapy consultation. Frequently, this is initiated immediately after surgery by the orthopaedic surgeon as the benefits of early mobilization are well recognized. The orthopaedic surgeon will include any relevant weight bearing restrictions; however, if there is any confusion the orthopaedist should be contacted directly for clarification. A recent review indicates that compliance with weight bearing restrictions is generally poor, but early weight bearing may be well tolerated and result in an earlier return to function for lower extremity periarticular fractures.[14]

If appropriate, wound care management plans including timing of suture/staple removal should be obtained from the orthopaedist. In concert with wound management, a pressure ulcer prevention program should also be considered, particularly for patients with limited mobility. As some orthopaedic surgeons have preferred post-operative care methodologies, additional patient management issues including the pain management regimen and venous thromboembolism (VTE) prophylaxis may be clarified with the orthopaedic service as well. Alternatively, if a geriatrician is co-managing or providing primary medical management, then this information can be obtained from him/her.

Medical comorbidities and medication review

This includes a review of current active medical problems and medications. For virtually all older fracture patients this affords an opportunity to make sure an osteoporosis evaluation is initiated as well as treatment if warranted (see Chapter 10).

As noted, it has been recognized that management of older adults sustaining a fracture is better when geriatricians co-manage these patients with an orthopaedist. Co-management of these older fracture patients has been reported to result in improved outcomes and reduced cost.[15] In the situation in which a hospitalized patient is transitioning to a post-acute care rehabilitation facility, continued primary medical management by the same geriatrician (or geriatric team) would be optimal. However, if the primary medical team will not be continuing to manage a patient, it is critical that the accepting rehabilitation service obtain a complete and accurate discharge summary including pertinent medical conditions managed during the acute care hospitalization, complications, current active medical conditions, past relevant medical conditions and a current list of medications including any planned modification (e.g. date/timing of VTE prophylaxis discontinuation). For facilities with a linked electronic medical record, review of this information may be more convenient, although the primary team may need to be contacted directly if there are any questions regarding the management plan.

REHABILITATION PROGRAM

As with any other fracture patient, post-fracture rehabilitation and recovery in an older adult should begin promptly after the fracture has been stabilized regardless of whether surgical repair was necessary. The post-fracture rehabilitation process is particularly important for older adults due to their greater risk for adverse consequences. However, it is also critical to recognize physiological age as opposed to chronological age. It should be readily apparent that, almost irrespective of the type of fracture, the functional reserve and prognosis, for example, of a 90-year-old community dwelling, functionally independent individual who is regularly engaged in vigorous exercise is most certainly greater than that of a frail 65-year-old with multiple medical comorbidities requiring assistance for bathing even before their injury. The development of an individualized rehabilitation program, including the requisite therapy resources, requires identifying each individual's functional deficit as obtained from their rehabilitation assessment, the likelihood of full functional recovery, and an assessment of their

living setting (e.g. home or apartment) and available social supports (e.g. family).

Each individual patient's functional deficit and resultant rehabilitation needs will depend in large part upon the extent and severity of their injury and their functional reserve. Fractures may range from relatively minor single bone injuries (e.g. metacarpal or phalanx fracture) to fractures associated with substantial morbidity and mortality (e.g. hip fracture) and multiple fractures associated with a major traumatic event (e.g. motor vehicle collision). Rehabilitation may be an informal process for minor fractures in a patient with substantial functional reserve and multiple family members available to provide assistance. Alternatively, individuals sustaining multiple or severe fractures related to a major traumatic event will often require ongoing direct medical care and a multidisciplinary rehabilitation program after discharge from the acute hospital setting (e.g. transfer to inpatient rehabilitation) with eventual transition to a community setting with continuation of therapy and medical management.

Determining the rehabilitation needs of a fracture patient requires a thorough functional history to ascertain the individual's pre-morbid function and an evaluation of their current functional capability. From this assessment, one can identify the patient's functional deficits and the rehabilitation provider(s) most well suited to address these deficits. Table 8.1 delineates the functional scope of physical, occupational and speech therapists. Physical therapists primarily focus on lower extremity function, including mobility and ambulation, while occupational therapists address basic ADL functional training; therapists with dedicated expertise in recovery of hand function are often occupational therapists, although some physical therapists may have expertise in this area as well.

For the patient in the acute hospital setting with an apparent functional deficit, it is recommended to obtain a therapist consultation to determine an individual's current functional ability, to provide training and/or equipment to improve their function and to assess their tolerance for therapy in case transfer to a post-acute rehabilitation facility is a consideration. Typically, physical therapy is initially consulted, as ambulation is the functional activity of greatest concern to patients and clinicians. However, for a patient with an upper extremity fracture and an evident basic ADL deficit, an occupational therapy evaluation may be more appropriate. In the acute hospital setting, therapists with orthopaedic expertise are typically readily available and therapist evaluations may be components of standard post-fracture order sets. For patients for whom discharge to a post-acute care rehabilitation facility is being considered, a physical medicine and rehabilitation (PM&R) physician (i.e. physiatrist) may be consulted to assist in identifying the optimal facility for a particular patient. As a PM&R physician consultation service may not always be available, alternative options may include recommendations from the patient's physical and/or occupational therapists, or from a nurse evaluating patients on behalf of a rehabilitation facility. In many outpatient

Table 8.1 Functional scope of physical, occupational and speech therapists

Physical therapy	Occupational therapy	Speech language pathology
Mobility training	Activities of daily living (ADL) training	Communication
Bed mobility	(+/– adaptive equipment)	Cognitive evaluation
Transfers (e.g. bed to chair)	Feeding	Feeding (including swallowing
Balance training (sitting/standing/	Grooming	evaluation)
gait)	Dressing	
Gait/stair training (+/– gait aid);	Toileting	
ambulatory endurance	Bathing	
Wheelchair seating/mobility	Instrumental ADL training	
	Hand fine motor skill training	
	Joint protection/energy conservation	
	Home safety evaluation	
	Cognitive assessment	
	Transfers	
Muscle strength/endurance training	Muscle strength/endurance training	
Joint range of motion/musculotendinous	Joint range of motion/musculotendinous	
stretching (focus on lower extremities)	stretching (focus upper extremities)	

orthopaedic practices, physical and occupational therapists are co-located on site and referral is also frequently part of a standardized care plan.

The specific components of a fracture rehabilitation program are mainly dependent upon the functional deficits of each individual patient. The overall goal of a fracture rehabilitation program is recovery to an individual's pre-morbid functional level or better. However, the rehabilitation program must also take into consideration any restrictions or limitations (e.g. joint range of motion, weight bearing) imposed by the treating orthopaedic surgeon; the specific duration of these limitations as well as any modification or progression should be confirmed with the orthopaedic surgeon to avoid any compromise of fracture healing. In addition, one needs to take into consideration the physical environment of a patient's living setting. Clearly, the functional training for an individual living in a handicap accessible single-level apartment is much less challenging than for a patient residing in a three-story home with the kitchen on the first floor and bathroom on the second floor.

A prescription for therapy should include several key elements including patient demographics (name, date of birth), the therapy discipline (e.g. physical therapy), diagnosis (i.e. specific fracture), goals of treatment (e.g. safe ambulation with progression to community mobility), restrictions/limitations (e.g. non-weight bearing right lower extremity for 4 weeks), relevant medical conditions or medications, the specific therapy orders (e.g. gait training with least restrictive gait aid), and the frequency and duration (e.g. two sessions/week for 3–4 weeks) of the requested therapy regimen. While a therapy prescription should delineate the specific requested therapeutic interventions, therapists should also have some discretion to modify the prescription based on their training and experience.

A therapy program often includes focused muscle strengthening and joint range of motion for the involved fracture region, however the primary emphasis is more typically on primary functional activities such as ambulation and performing basic ADL. Gait training focuses on recovery of a normal gait pattern, and an assistive device is recommended if the gait pattern is antalgic due to pain or may be a necessity for those patients with a lower extremity weight-bearing restriction. Formal resistance exercise programs have been evaluated in older adults after hip fracture. Binder et al. found that 6 months of additional rehabilitation, including resistance exercise training, after completion of standard rehabilitation resulted in improved strength, physical function and quality of life as compared to a home exercise program.[16] More recently, this paradigm was extended with the evaluation of a 6-month functional home exercise program compared to attention control in older hip fracture patients having completed a standard post-fracture rehabilitation program; modest functional benefits were demonstrated but additional studies were recommended to determine their clinical relevance.[17]

For individuals sustaining a fracture due to a fall, this affords an opportunity for initiation of a falls prevention program. This program may include lower extremity strengthening, balance training and other methods with demonstrated benefit (e.g. Tai Chi); this intervention may be deferred or delayed until the patient has mastered basic gait mobility and specific restrictions (e.g. weight bearing) have been removed. See Chapter 12 for more details on falls prevention.

For individuals unable to ambulate, either temporarily or chronically as a result of their fracture(s), a gait assistive device is typically warranted. There are a multitude of assistive devices available, ranging from canes, crutches and walkers to wheelchairs and scooters. The most appropriate gait aid for an individual patient is typically best determined by a skilled physical therapist. The key features of common ambulatory assistive devices are summarized in Table 8.2.[18]

Table 8.2 Ambulatory assistive devices for use after fracture

Assistive device	Positive characteristics	Negative characteristics	Typical weightbearing status
Single point cane	Assistance with balance and proprioception; decrease weight bearing on opposite side	Requires very good hand/upper extremity strength/function; mild decrease in weight bearing; only one upper extremity free to carry other objects	PWB/unilateral lower extremity
Quad (4-point) cane	Provides greater weight-bearing support than a single-point cane; stands unsupported	Requires very good hand/upper extremity function; heavier than a single point cane; trip/fall risk due to wider base of support	PWB/unilateral lower extremity
Crutches	Allows mobility if non-weight bearing one lower extremity; more rapid gait than with cane	Requires excellent bilateral hand/upper extremity strength/function and good coordination; neither upper extremity free to carry objects; trip/fall risk	PWB or NWB/ unilateral lower extremity
Standard walker (no wheels)	Very stable with wide base of support; allows mobility if non-weight-bearing one lower extremity	Requires good–very good upper extremity strength/function; must be lifted and advanced; slow gait pattern	PWB or NWB/ unilateral lower extremity
Two-wheel rolling walker	Stable with a wide base of support; roll to advance; allows faster, smoother gait pattern than standard walker	Requires good upper extremity strength/function; less stable than standard walker due to wheels	PWB/unilateral
Four-wheel rolling walker/ rollator	Stable with wide base of support; allows relatively normal gait speed; better for community mobility; if basket attachment, may carry objects; if seat available, allows intermittent rest	Requires very good bilateral grip strength/function to operate hand brakes; reduced forward/backward stability due to 4 wheels	PWB/unilateral
Knee scooter	Stable with moderately narrow base of support; more rapid mobility than cane/walker	Requires weight bearing on knee of injured lower extremity; requires good–very good strength/function of bilateral upper extremities and uninjured lower extremity	PWB/unilateral (distal lower extremity)
Manual wheelchair	Very good to excellent mobility (community settings)	Requires good–excellent upper extremity strength/function (or caregiver to provide mobility); very good–excellent cardiopulmonary function for longer distance/ community mobility	PWB or NWB/bilateral upper or lower extremities
Power wheelchair	Very good to excellent independent mobility (community settings); no significant upper extremity strength/function required; caregiver assistance not necessarily required	Requires adequate cognition and vision/hearing to operate; requires adequate manual dexterity to operate (or ability to operate alternate control system); very heavy; typically requires home/ vehicle modifications	PWB or NWB/bilateral lower extremities (typically requires at least one functionally intact upper extremity)
Scooter	Same as power wheelchair	Same as power wheelchair except adequate upper extremity function and manual dexterity required; lighter and easier to transport than power wheelchair	PWB or NWB/ unilateral

Source: From Brown CJ, Flood KL. JAMA 2013; 310(11): 1168–77.
Note: NWB, non-weight bearing; PWB, partial weight bearing.

Determining physical barriers to mobility in a patient's home environment is also critical. For example, if a patient has a two-story home with the bathroom on the second floor, then either learning to negotiate stairs will be necessary or an alternative plan identified (e.g. bedside commode on first floor).

Basic ADL training frequently includes adaptive techniques and/or adaptive equipment. An adaptive technique would include learning to button a shirt with the non-dominant hand when the dominant hand has been incapacitated due to fracture, while a device that allows one to button a shirt with one hand is an example of adaptive equipment. Implicit in ADL training is knowledge of the patient's home environment; this is one clear advantage of a home-based therapy program as functional training can be completed in the unique physical environment of the patient.

REHABILITATION FACILITIES

For patients in the United States admitted to an acute hospital after a fracture, there are basically three options regarding their discharge location: home, subacute rehabilitation in a skilled nursing facility (SNF) or acute rehabilitation in an inpatient rehabilitation facility (IRF). For patients discharged to home, therapy may be provided either in the patient's home or at an outpatient therapy facility. The specific characteristics of each of these potential post-acute rehabilitation settings are outlined in Table 8.3.[19]

There are many considerations in determining the optimal discharge location for a particular patient, however key variables are listed in Table 8.4. The discussion regarding discharge options should ideally be held together with the patient as well as his/her family. For patients previously living in a nursing home, transfer directly back to their

Table 8.3 Characteristics of post-acute care rehabilitation options

Setting	Care coordination requirements	Medical coverage	Therapy services	Nursing	Insurance
Inpatient rehabilitation facility	Multidisciplinary team patient care conferences (weekly)	Physician available 24 h/day, 7 days/week; physician evaluation typically ≥5 days/week	PT, OT and speech therapy available. Patients require ≥2 therapy services, and minimum of 15 hours per week	24-hour care	Medicare Part A: days 1–20: 100%; days 21–100: 80% plus co-payment; >100 days: no coverage
Skilled nursing facility		Physician supervised; physician evaluation within 2 weeks of admission and every 30 days; physician available in emergencies	PT and OT available; typically 3–5 sessions of each per week	24-hour care	Same as inpatient rehabilitation facility
Home health		Physician referral and recertification every 60 days	PT, OT and speech therapy available	Home health nursing	Typically 1–3 visits per week by PT/OT for 1–4 weeks
Outpatient (hospital or free standing clinic)		Physician referral and recertification every 30 days	PT, OT and speech therapy available	N/A	Typically 1–3 visits per week by PT/OT for 1–4 weeks Medicare Part B annual limits (2014): $1920 PT/speech therapy combined, $1920 OT

Note: PT, physical therapy; OT, occupational therapy.

Table 8.4 Considerations in determination of post-acute care discharge location

Pre-fracture functional status and living setting
Family/social support
Current active medical problems
Current physical and occupational therapy needs and theraphy tolerance
Potential for functional recovery
Cognition/ability to learn
Patient motivation
Patient/family preference
Financial resources/third party reimbursement

nursing home or to an affiliated SNF is most common. As inpatient rehabilitation facilities are specifically focused on returning patients to a community living setting, individuals from institutional settings are generally not considered appropriate for IRF admission.

OTHER ISSUES TO CONSIDER DURING REHABILITATION

While functional training is the key emphasis of a post-fracture rehabilitation program, often this process may be hampered by pain. While fracture related pain is common, geriatric patients may also have underlying painful conditions (e.g. osteoarthritis) that may compromise their functional training. The standard geriatric tenet of 'start low and go slow' is recommended for pharmacological pain management. An individualized pain management regimen is most appropriate as discussed in Chapter 9.

Many older adults are nutritionally compromised and thus a holistic post-fracture management program also affords an opportunity to address dietary deficiencies. This may be best accomplished by referral to a dietician to identify specific deficiencies and develop an individualized nutritional program. While it may appear self-evident that a nutritional intervention should be effective for this patient population, a recent Cochrane review noted only weak evidence for protein and calorie supplementation in older hip fracture patients.[20]

In addition to nutritional supplementation, some investigators have evaluated the use of anabolic agents to improve function after fracture. In older female hip fracture patients, Hedstrom et al. found that 12 months of treatment with the anabolic steroid nandrolone in concert with vitamin D and calcium resulted in maintenance of muscle mass, less bone loss and improved gait speed as compared to treatment with calcium alone.[21] A more recent trial in underweight women with hip fractures did not note any additional improvement in bone mineral density in subjects receiving nandrolone in addition to protein supplementation.[22] However, a recent Cochrane review noted methodological deficiencies with the few reported studies evaluating anabolic steroids in hip fracture patients and found insufficient data to make

any conclusions regarding this intervention.[23] While these interventions remain investigational, there is significant interest in hip fracture patients, in particular, as a target population for newer myoanabolics due to the substantial morbidity and mortality of this condition.[24]

As mentioned in the rehabilitation assessment section, the treating orthopaedic surgeon may address VTE prophylaxis. Regardless, VTE prophylaxis should be considered in virtually every geriatric fracture patient due to the high risk of morbidity and mortality; the American College of Chest Physicians publishes evidence based guidelines on this topic with regular updates.[25]

SUMMARY

Older adults are, in general, at greater risk of functional compromise, including potential loss of independence, after sustaining a bony fracture. The primary goal of a post-fracture rehabilitation program is to provide an individualized therapeutic program, in conjunction with continued orthopaedic and medical management, in order to optimize functional recovery. Ideally, a comprehensive individualized rehabilitation program will allow older adult fracture patients to recover at least their pre-morbid functional abilities, if not even greater functional independence.

REFERENCES

1. Ortmann JM, Velkoff VA, Hogan H. *An aging nation: The older population in the United States.* Current Population Reports, P25-1140. Washington, DC: US Census Bureau, 2014.
2. United Nations, Department of Economic and Social Affairs, Population Division. *World Population Ageing 2013.* ST/ESA/SER.A/348. New York: Department of Economic and Social Affairs, Population Division, 2013.
3. Sanders S, Geraci SA. Outpatient management of the elderly patient following fragility hip fracture. *Am J Med* 2011; 124(5): 408–10.
4. Roth T, Kammerlander C, Gosch M, Luger TJ, Blauth M. Outcome in geriatric fracture patients and how it can be improved. *Osteoporos Int* 2010; 21(Suppl 4): S615–19.
5. De Rui M, Veronese N, Manzato E, Sergi G. Role of comprehensive geriatric assessment in the management of osteoporotic hip fracture in the elderly: An overview. *Disabil Rehabil* 2013; 35(9): 758–65.
6. Kates SL, Mendelson DA, Friedman SM. Co-managed care for fragility hip fractures (Rochester model). *Osteoporos Int* 2010; 21(Suppl 4): S621–5.
7. Stuck AE, Siu AL, Wieland GD, Adams J, Rubenstein LZ. Comprehensive geriatric assessment: A meta-analysis of controlled trials. *Lancet* 1993; 342(8878): 1032–6.

8. Beaupre LA, Binder E, Cameron ID, Jones CA, Orwig D, Sherrington C, Magaziner J. Maximizing functional recovery following hip fracture in frail seniors. *Best Pract Res Clin Rheumatol* 2013; 27(6): 771–88.

9. Gill TM, Murphy TE, Gahbauer EA, Allore HG. Association of injurious falls with disability outcomes and nursing home admissions in community living older persons. *Am J Epidemiol* 2013; 178(3): 418–25.

10. Katz S, Ford AB, Moskowitz RW, Jackson BA, Jaffe MW. Studies of illness in the aged. The index of ADL: A standardized measure of biological and psychosocial function. *JAMA* 1963; 185: 914–19.

11. Mahoney FI, Barthel DW. Functional evaluation: The Barthel Index. *Md State Med J* 1965; 14: 61–5.

12. Lawton MP, Brody EM. Assessment of older people: Self-maintaining and instrumental activities of daily living. *Gerontologist* 1969; 9(3): 179–86.

13. Inouye SK, Wesendorp RG, Saczynski JS. Delirium in elderly people. *Lancet* 2014; 383(9920): 911–22.

14. Haller JM, Potter MQ, Kubiak EN. Weight bearing after a periarticular fracture: What is the evidence? *Orthop Clin North Am* 2013; 44(4): 509–19.

15. O'Malley NT, Kates SL. Co-managed care: The gold standard for geriatric fracture care. *Curr Osteoporos Rep* 2012; 10(4): 312–16.

16. Binder EF, Brown M, Sinacore DR, Steger-May K, Yarasheski KE, Schechtman KB. Effects of extended outpatient rehabilitation after hip fracture: A randomized controlled trial. *JAMA* 2004; 292(7): 837–46.

17. Latham NK, Harris BA, Bean JF, Heeren T, Goodyear C, Zawacki S, Heislein DM, et al. Effect of a home-based exercise program on functional recovery following rehabilitation after hip fracture: A randomized clinical trial. *JAMA* 2014; 311(7): 700–8.

18. Brown CJ, Flood KL. Mobility limitation in the older patient: A clinical review. *JAMA* 2013; 310(11): 1168–77.

19. UpToDate. *Overview of geriatric rehabilitation: Program components and settings for rehabilitation.* Available from: http://www.uptodate.com/contents/overview-of-geriatric-rehabilitation-program-components-and-settings-for-rehabilitation?source=machineLearning&search=geriatric+rehabilitation&selectedTitle=1%7E150&sectionRank=1&anchor=H4420023#H4420023 (accessed January 4, 2015).

20. Avenell A, Handoll HH. Nutritional supplementation for hip fracture aftercare in older people. *Cochrane Database Syst Rev* 2010; 1:CD001880.

21. Hedstrom M, Sjoberg K, Brosjo E, Astrom K, Sjoberg H, Dalen N. Positive effects of anabolic steroids, vitamin D and calcium on muscle mass, bone mineral density and clinical function after a hip fracture. A randomized study of 63 women. *J Bone Joint Surg Br* 2002; 84(4): 497–503.

22. Tengstrand B, Cederholm T, Soderqvist A, Tidermark J. Effects of protein-rich supplementation and nandrolone on bone tissue after a hip fracture. *Clin Nutr* 2007; 26(4): 460–5.

23. Farooqi V, van den Berg ME, Cameron ID, Crotty M. Anabolic steroids for rehabilitation after hip fracture in older people. *Cochrane Database Syst Rev* 2014; 10: CD008887.

24. Vellas B, Fielding R, Miller R, Rolland Y, Bhasin S, Magaziner J, Bischoff-Ferrari H. Designing drug trials for sarcopenia in older adults with hip fracture—A task force from the International Conference on Frailty and Sarcopenia Research (ICFSR). *J Frailty Aging* 2014; 3(4): 199–204.

25. Guyatt GH, Akl EA, Crowther M, Gutterman DD, Schuunemann HH, American College of Chest Physicians Antithrombotic Therapy and Prevention of Thrombosis Panel. Executive summary: Antithrombotic therapy and prevention of thrombosis, 9th ed: American College of Chest Physicians Evidence-Based Clinical Practice Guidelines. *Chest* 2012; 141(2): 7S–47S.

9

Outcome after fracture

SUSAN M. FRIEDMAN

INTRODUCTION

A fracture can be a sentinel event for an older adult, resulting in death or serious physical or psychological injury to the patient. Such injury can either trigger a decline or can be seen during the course of an ongoing decline and may require a significant amount of time for recovery. This chapter reviews different outcomes, their incidence and predictors, presenting both individual and situational risk factors, and approaches that may help to improve outcomes. This chapter addresses predominantly post-hospital outcomes; immediate outcomes and complications of fracture repair are discussed in Chapter 7. Because there are many types of fractures and a discussion of all outcomes for all fractures would be unwieldy, we focus on the fractures that are most common in older adults – proximal femur fractures, distal radial/ulnar fractures, proximal humerus fractures and vertebral fractures, which are all usually considered to be fragility fractures (see Chapter 1 for more on the incidence of these fractures). Discussion focuses on mortality, function and health-related quality of life for each of these fractures, and other outcomes of clinical concern are presented.

STAKEHOLDERS, GOALS AND PRIORITIZED OUTCOMES

There are multiple stakeholders whose goal is to optimize the outcome of a fracture. These include the patient, informal and formal caregivers, healthcare professionals, healthcare systems and payors. To this end, the goals in an optimal care setting have been noted to be those outlined in Table 9.1.[1] A recent consensus conference in the United Kingdom supported five domains as core outcomes to

measure for any trial related to hip fracture: mortality, pain, activities of daily living (ADL), mobility and health-related quality of life.[2]

PATIENT PREFERENCES

Understanding a patient's values and goals of care is important for providing optimal care for all patients, but particularly for older adults, where there may be trade-offs involved due to frailty and comorbidities. Although mortality is often viewed as the 'worst possible' outcome when assessing trade-offs, other outcomes, such as functional status, mobility, pain control and fear of being a burden, may take priority in an older or more frail individual's values.

It is therefore important to discuss goals of care with patients in order to weigh the risks and benefits of a procedure, and for care planning. This may be particularly challenging for patients with dementia or other conditions that limit their ability to weigh options or to state preferences, and in this situation, discussions with family members or others who are close to the individual can be invaluable in understanding meaningful outcomes.

INTER-RELATIONSHIP OF OUTCOMES

As thoroughly discussed in Chapter 7, frail patients, or those with limited physiological reserve, are at high risk for multiple adverse outcomes. These outcomes may be inter-related. As an example, hip fracture patients who develop neuropsychiatric symptoms, such as night-time behaviour disturbance, agitation or depression, are at higher risk for motor function decline.[3] Patients with functional or cognitive decline are at risk of needing an

Table 9.1 Goals for optimized care

1. Returning to pre-fracture status as soon as possible
2. Improving patient and family satisfaction
3. Reducing complications, readmission and mortality
4. Providing the best value of care to the healthcare system
5. Providing secondary fracture prevention

increased level of care. This has implications for prognosis as well as care. First, identifying individuals at high risk for adverse outcomes helps to frame discussions for care planning. Additionally, targeted care in the acute and rehabilitation setting may in turn lead to improvement in multiple outcomes and prevent a vicious spiral that may occur when one adverse outcome leads to another.

MORTALITY

Risk of mortality following a fracture depends primarily on the site of the fracture (Figure 9.1),[4] which is discussed under the subheadings below, but also on the characteristics of the patient. For many, fractures serve as a marker of frailty and comorbidity.

Osteoporotic fractures overall are associated with an increase in mortality risk.[5] For hip, vertebral and other major fractures, this is true for all older adults. In individuals aged 75 and over, even minor fractures are associated with increased mortality risk. Standardized mortality rates are higher for men than for women, and this is especially true for men over the age of 75. Age and quadriceps strength are predictive of mortality in both women and men with fractures, and sustaining a subsequent fracture is also a marker for increased mortality risk.

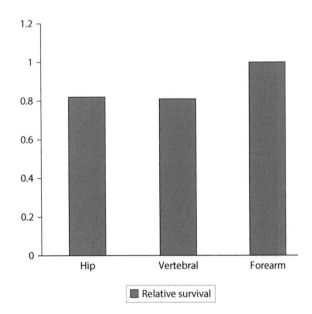

Figure 9.1 Relative survival at 5 years.

Hip fractures

Mortality following a hip fracture is increased. Mortality rates in the year following hip fracture vary substantially depending on the patient population, ranging from 12.7% in a community dwelling, cognitively intact patient population at baseline,[6] to 58.3% in male nursing home residents.[7] Although the demographics of hip fracture patients have changed in the past several decades, with increasing age at presentation, the overall mortality in the year following a hip fracture has not changed significantly.[8]

The excess mortality is highest immediately following a hip fracture. In the first 3 months, women are five times more likely to die, and men are eight times more likely to die than their counterparts who have not sustained a fracture. Excess mortality drops throughout the first year, but persists for at least 10 years for both women and men.[5,9] Viewed another way, hip fractures reduce life expectancy by 1.8 years or by about 25% relative to age- and sex-matched counterparts.[10]

It is estimated that fewer than a third of deaths following hip fracture are causally related, but that the predominance of mortality among hip fracture patients is due to their underlying frailty and comorbidity.[11,12] This has implications for clinical care. For those whose mortality is related to outcomes of caring for the fracture and its consequences, optimizing systems and the specifics of care to reduce adverse outcomes is the approach that will improve mortality. For those whose mortality is related to their underlying frailty, reducing comorbidity and improving function, treating osteoporosis and preventing falls is the approach that will ultimately reduce fracture mortality.

Predictors for mortality following a hip fracture are outlined in Table 9.2 and can be divided into baseline and incident predictors. Nursing home residents are at particularly high risk of mortality during the year following a hip fracture. At baseline, significant predictors include demographic characteristics, such as age, gender and residence. Poor baseline cognitive and physical function both predict higher mortality following a fracture. In terms of incident predictors, there is growing evidence that delay in surgery leads to higher mortality,[13] and this is particularly important in patients with functional impairment.[14] Development of postoperative delirium or pressure sores leads to a higher risk of 1-year mortality.[15] At the time of hospital discharge, function as measured by the motor Functional Independence Measure (FIM) score has been shown to be highly predictive of 1-year mortality.[16] Incident predictors are at least partially modifiable risk factors which, if reduced, may improve mortality outcomes.

Proximal humerus fractures

Although the proximal humerus is a common site for fragility fractures, there are less data on outcomes than for other sites, such as hip or vertebral fractures. Mortality has

Table 9.2 Predictors of mortality after a hip fracture

Baseline risk factors
Male gender
Older age
Admission from a nursing home
History of smoking
Low baseline activity level
ASA grade/significant comorbidity
Poor cognitive status
Poor baseline mobility
Quadriceps weakness
Incident risk factors
Delay in surgery
Incident delirium
Incident pressure sore
Function at hospital discharge

Note: ASA, American Society of Anesthesiologists.

been found to be high in patients with proximal humerus fracture, with a mortality rate that is approximately double that of individuals without fracture.[12] The impact on men appears to be greater than on women, with a median survival time of 6.5 and 11.8 years in male patients and their controls, respectively, and 9.0 and 11.5 years in female patients versus controls.[17]

As with other fracture sites, mortality appears to be driven by underlying frailty and comorbidity. In one case series of 100 patients with proximal humerus fracture,[18] patients with severe physical or mental disorders, such as dementia or severe cardiovascular disease, were much more likely to die in the year following their fracture. Forty percent of these patients died, compared with 2% of those with non-severe comorbidity and none of those without. In the case–control study above,[17] most patients died of cardiovascular disease or malignancy; in other words, they died of significant comorbidities.

Vertebral fractures

Vertebral fractures are associated with an increase in mortality in both women and men, with standardized mortality rates (the ratio of observed to expected deaths) of 1.8 and 2.1, respectively.[5] Similar to hip fractures, excess deaths appear to be a function of both the fracture itself and underlying comorbidity and frailty, with the predominance due to the latter.[19] The excess mortality at 5 years is similar to that seen in hip fractures (Figure 9.1), however the patterns are different. Patients with hip fractures see higher mortality immediately following the fracture, whereas among patients with vertebral fractures, the mortality curves relative to expected mortality continue to diverge over a 5-year period.[4]

Similar to hip fracture outcomes, men have higher mortality rates than women following a vertebral fracture.[4,20]

Older individuals are at higher risk of mortality as well.[4] Patients who sustain fractures as a result of mild to moderate trauma have an increased mortality risk, whereas those who fracture due to severe trauma do not. The most common cause for death in the former group is cardiovascular disease,[4] again supporting the idea that these are more frail patients with higher comorbidity.

Distal forearm fractures

The excess mortality does not appear to be elevated among patients with forearm fractures,[4,12] and, in fact, there is some evidence that women with distal fractures may have a lower mortality than the general population.[20] Similar to other types of fractures, this may reflect the patient population that sustains forearm fractures; this population tends to be younger and more vigorous than their counterparts with other osteoporotic fractures.[21] The mechanism for incurring a forearm fracture suggests both substantial forward momentum and preserved reflexes, consistent with a more active and robust individual.[22]

Other fractures

Rib fractures are also associated with an elevated mortality, particularly in women.[5] There is significant excess mortality in the months following rib fractures, but the mortality curves continue to diverge for several years, suggesting ongoing elevated risk.[12]

FUNCTION

Function involves multiple domains, including physical, cognitive, psychological and social. Physical functional status is often measured globally in older adults via ADL and instrumental activities of daily living (IADL). ADL cover activities related to self-care and the ability to live independently, namely, dressing, toileting, transferring, grooming, bathing and feeding oneself. IADL involve more complex tasks, such as using the telephone, managing medications, shopping, taking care of household finances, doing laundry, preparing meals, doing housework and managing transportation.

Other measures were developed to assess function related to the specific location affected. For example, the Michigan Hand Questionnaire measures outcomes in six domains via 37 questions: function, ADL, pain, work performance, aesthetics and patient satisfaction.[23] It is scored from 0 (poor) to 100 (excellent). A brief version that includes 12 items is also available, with a responsiveness that is similar to the original questionnaire.

The Disabilities of the Arm, Shoulder, and Hand (DASH) questionnaire is another self-reported score that is used to evaluate functional outcomes in the upper extremity.[24] It provides a score from 0 (no disability) to 100 (complete disability) based on 30 questions addressing activities, limitations and symptoms. A change of 10 points is considered to be clinically meaningful.

The Constant–Murley score is a 100-point score to evaluate shoulder function that encompasses both patient report and objective measurement. It evaluates pain, ADL, strength and range of motion. Higher scores denote better function.[25]

Osteoporotic fractures have a huge functional impact. It has been estimated that the 5.2 million fractures of the hip, spine and distal forearm that occur among postmenopausal white women in the United States in a 10-year period would lead to 2 million person-years of fracture-related disability.[26] A history of any osteoporotic fracture is associated with a two- to threefold increase in difficulty bending, lifting, reaching, walking, climbing stairs and descending stairs, and two- to almost seven times more difficulty in dressing, cooking, shopping and performing heavy housework.[27]

Hip fractures

The trajectory of functional recovery from a hip fracture depends on the area of function being assessed.[28] Most areas improve in the first year following the fracture, with earlier recovery for depressive symptoms, upper extremity function and cognition (4 months), and longer times to recovery of social, IADL and lower extremity functioning, which take about 11 months. Understandably, the IADL that are most likely to be impacted are those that depend on lower extremity functioning, such as housecleaning and shopping (62% and 42% dependent at 1 year, respectively, for those who were previously independent), whereas those that are not as dependent on lower extremity functioning, such as medication management and using the telephone, are less impacted (28% and 22%, respectively). Limitation in function 1 year

after a hip fracture is substantial (Figure 9.2)[28]; for those who were previously independent, new dependency in physical ADL at 1 year ranges from 20% for putting on pants to 90% for climbing five stairs. Two-thirds still have difficulty getting on and off the toilet. Most of these dependencies persist 2 years after the hip fracture.

There is considerable overlap between risk factors for mortality and those for functional impairment following a hip fracture (Table 9.3).[29–32] Older individuals, those with dementia, depression or other significant comorbidity, and those with poor baseline functioning are at higher risk for functional impairment after a hip fracture. Postoperative anaemia has been associated with decreased ambulation and reduced functional independence[31]; however, a liberal transfusion approach (transfusing for a haemoglobin level of 10 g/dL vs 8 g/dL) does not appear to improve functional outcomes.[33]

With respect to incident risk factors, longer length of stay and being rehospitalized are associated with worse postoperative function. Prolonged immobilization and delay in start of physical therapy can lead to loss of muscle function and higher risk of several medical complications (see Chapter 7), which in turn sets the stage for poor functional recovery. A surgical approach that allows for immediate weight bearing as tolerated will foster the start and progression of physical therapy; furthermore, patients with cognitive impairment may have difficulty following restrictions such as partial toe-touch weight bearing, and this may impede progress in therapy. The amount of contact with one's social support network following hospitalization is also predictive of functional recovery. The mechanism for this may be multifaceted. Those with more social support may have more opportunity to be physically active and may be less prone to depression that may impact progress.

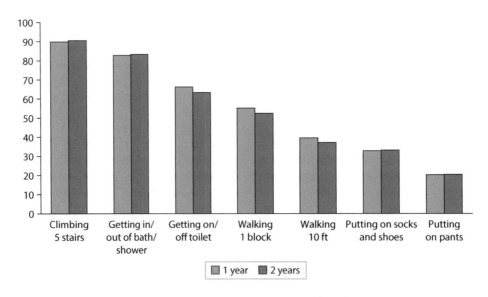

Figure 9.2 Percentage dependent among those who were independent before fracture.

Table 9.3 Predictors of poor recovery of function after a hip fracture

Baseline risk factors
Older age
Low pre-fracture physical function
Depression
Poor cognitive function, dementia
Poor nutritional status
Multiple comorbidities, ASA grade of 3 or 4 frailty
Incident risk factors
Length of stay
Less physical therapy in hospital
Rehospitalization
Low level of contact with social support network

Note: ASA, American Society of Anesthesiologists.

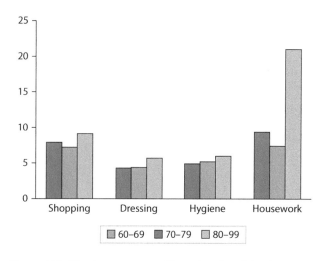

Figure 9.3 Weeks to return of functional activity, by age.

There is evidence that functional outcomes can be substantially impacted by the type of care that a patient receives. In an interdisciplinary program that incorporated geriatric consultation services, a continuous rehabilitation program and discharge planning services, patients were much more likely to have an excellent recovery than patients who received usual care.[29] Intensive and sustained rehabilitation is also useful; a 6-month program of supervised physical therapy in a rehabilitation centre and exercise training with home exercise led to significantly better physical performance, functional status, muscle strength, walking speed and balance than in controls who had a home based program three times a week.[34]

Proximal humerus fractures

Treatment and recovery from proximal humerus fractures depends in part on the degree of displacement of the fracture, as well as baseline function and comorbidities (see Chapter 20). For many proximal humerus fractures, the treatment that will lead to an optimal functional outcome is unclear.[35] Whether or not a patient has surgical intervention, they are often limited initially in their weight-bearing status and range of motion. Physical and occupational therapy are important care components for return of function.[36]

Overall, function as measured by the Constant score improves over the first year following a proximal humerus fracture.[37] Fracture-related complications, mainly shoulder impingement, are predictive of worse Constant scores. DASH scores were 10 points lower at 1 year than at baseline; however, this was felt to be below the threshold of detectable clinical change.

In a case series of 507 minimally displaced fractures, treated non-operatively with 2 weeks of immobilization via a sling followed by physical therapy,[38] return of function depended on both the realm being assessed, as well as the patient's age at the time of fracture (Figure 9.3). Outcomes were excellent or good in 87%, with progressive improvements over time from 6 weeks to a year. There was a positive correlation between duration of physical therapy and better outcome. The latter finding is consistent with a recent Cochrane report that found that immediate physical therapy was associated with better functional outcomes for patients with non-displaced or stable fracture.[35]

In one long-term follow-up study of patients with proximal humerus fractures, 61% had died by 13 years after the fracture, 21 of 47 patients (45%) examined after 13 years were pain free and had preserved function of their shoulder, and an additional two patients (4%) had preserved shoulder function with pain.[39] Most patients who had symptoms at 1 year still had symptoms after long-term follow-up, so functional result at a year is predictive of long-term outcome.

Vertebral fractures

Up to two-thirds of vertebral compression fractures may be undetected clinically,[20] and most do not require hospitalization,[40] yet the deformities that they cause can in turn lead to complications that result in disability. The interaction between these complications is complex and multifaceted (Figure 9.4), including bi-directional outcomes that reinforce each other and can lead to rapidly progressive disability. Adjacent fractures can lead to progressive thoracic kyphosis and/or lumbar lordosis, which may limit lung function, and lead to early satiety and weight loss. Kyphosis puts patients at risk for multiple medical complications, such as pressure sores, osteomyelitis and pneumonia. The disability resulting from vertebral fractures is also mediated through acute and chronic pain, which may limit activity, impair both appetite and sleep, and thereby lead to weakness, deconditioning and

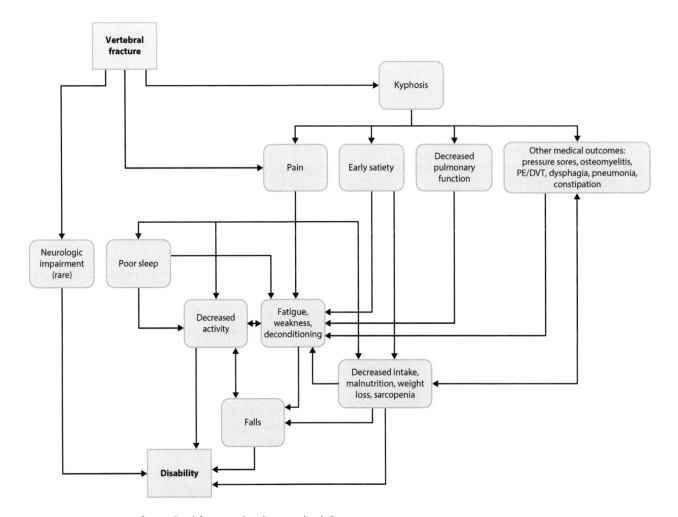

Figure 9.4 Outcomes of vertebral fracture leading to disability.

reduced activity. Rarely, vertebral fractures may cause neurological impairment, with damage to the spinal cord or cauda equina that may cause weakness or numbness or incontinence.[41]

Distal forearm fractures

Most people who sustain a distal forearm fracture have a good or acceptable clinical outcome eventually.[42] However, nearly half report unsatisfactory outcomes at 6 months, including hand pain, weakness and post-traumatic arthritis. Distal forearm fractures account for nearly 40% of physical therapy sessions due to osteoporotic fractures.[43] Functional tasks that depend on the upper extremities, such as meal preparation and grooming, are more heavily impacted by forearm fractures.[27] There is often poor correlation between radiological results, assessment of clinical variables such as grip strength and range of motion and patient self-reported outcomes.[44]

A discussion of specific treatments of distal radius and ulnar fractures and their outcomes is presented in Chapter 26. In one case series of distal radius fractures

with a mean age of 62 and follow-up period of 30 months, the DASH score on follow-up was excellent or good (0–15) in 75%, and poor (>35) in only 3%.[45] Age, gender (after adjustment for other characteristics), time to surgery, level of surgeon and duration of immobilization did not impact on functional outcome. A longitudinal evaluation of 49 women aged 50–75 with distal radius fractures showed a median DASH score of 14 at 1 year, decreasing to 8 at 2–4 years, suggesting that functional improvement continues to occur over several years. For those with moderate or severe malunion, the DASH score improved from 20 to 10 during that period.[46]

However, it appears that with advancing age, wrist fractures may have more functional implications. A study of 268 women aged 65 and above (mean age 71) with wrist fractures followed for over 7 years found that 15% developed clinically important functional decline. Even after adjusting for age, body mass index, health status, baseline functional status, lifestyle, comorbidities and neuromuscular function, the relative risk of clinically important decline increased by 48%. Other predictors of

Table 9.4 Predictors of functional decline among patient with wrist fractures

Age
Income
Hand dominance
Poor or fair health
Parkinson's disease
Stroke
Arthritis
Diabetes
Weight loss
Poor strength (hip, grip or triceps)
Using arms to step up or down
Incident hip fracture

function and functional decline in this population are listed in Table 9.4.[47-50]

HEALTH-RELATED QUALITY OF LIFE

Health-related quality of life is multidimensional and overlaps with concepts of function. It encompasses aspects of quality of life that can affect either physical or mental health and has been defined by the United States Centers for Disease Control and Prevention as 'an individual's or group's perceived physical and mental health over time'. It comprises multiple domains, including physical, mental, emotional and social well-being. With the increased aging population and growing prevalence of chronic disease, and greater focus on patient-centred outcomes, measuring and optimizing health-related quality of life has assumed a more prominent focus in health care. Measures of health-related quality of life incorporate such concepts as an overall self-assessment of health, fatigue, pain, emotional distress, social support and the ability to participate in work and social activities.

Several measures have been developed to assess health-related quality of life. One of the most commonly used is the Medical Outcomes Study Short Form, or SF-36. Others include the Sickness Impact Profile, the EuroQol-5D and the Quality of Well-Being Scale.

Hip fractures

Hip fractures adversely impact on both physical and mental health-related quality of life. Older adults understand the impact that a hip fracture can have, and when surveyed, 80% stated that they would rather be dead than sustain a hip fracture leading to admission to a nursing home.[51]

Patients with hip fracture have worse overall perception of health, physical role, physical functioning, pain, vitality, social function, emotional role and mental health a year after the hip fracture, when compared to matched controls who have not had a hip fracture.[52] Except for mental health, these differences persist 2 years after the fracture. Older individuals are at higher risk for worse physical health, and individuals with more comorbidity are at higher risk of worse mental health. In a longitudinal study that evaluated hip fracture patients after 7 years, there was no further deterioration in quality of life between 2 and 7 years.[53] Quality of life for those returning to the community has been found to be lower in all domains of the SF-36 compared to controls, suggesting that even among those who recover independence to the degree that they are able to return home are not able to fully regain baseline quality of life.[54]

There is evidence that the model of care can have an impact on the outcome of health-related quality of life. A home based physical therapy program that included exercises for muscle strengthening, range of motion, balance and functional training led to improvements in both psychological and physical domains of health-related quality of life.[55]

Proximal humerus fractures

Consistent with improvements in function over the year following a proximal humerus fracture, health-related quality of life appears to also improve.[56] Improvements occur progressively over the 12 months after the fracture, with most of the improvement in the first 6 months. Improvements occur more quickly in the mental than physical component of quality of life measures. Progress occurs more slowly for those aged 75 and over.

A longitudinal evaluation of quality of life of proximal humerus fractures showed that at 1 year, most measures were similar to those of patients who had not sustained a fracture. The only differences were among the physical functioning of patients who also had comorbidity; those without comorbidity did not have significant differences in health-related quality of life.[18]

Vertebral fractures

The impact of vertebral fractures on health-related quality of life crosses multiple domains. Vertebral fractures can cause acute or chronic pain. The deformities that result lead to kyphosis and height loss. In addition to the physical functional consequences, vertebral fractures may impact on body image, self-esteem and mood.

In a study comparing health-related quality of life over 7 years among patients with hip versus vertebral fractures, bodily pain increased among patients with vertebral fracture, who had also a high incidence of new fractures in the interim. Patients with vertebral fractures had reduced quality of life in physical functioning and role, bodily pain, vitality, social functioning and emotional role when compared to those without fracture.[53] This study suggests that the long-term impact of vertebral fractures on quality of life may be greater even than the impact of hip fractures, although this may in part be due to underlying frailty.

Distal forearm fractures

Compared to hip and vertebral fractures, wrist fractures are associated with less impact on quality of life, both immediately following and 1 year after the fracture.[57] The realms most impacted initially are usual activities, pain and self-care, with less of an effect on mobility or anxiety or depression. By 3 months, most expressed no problem with mobility, anxiety/depression, usual activities or self-care, but it took 6 months for most to have no problem with pain.

OTHER OUTCOMES OF IMPORTANCE

Increased level of care

The location of care following a fracture depends to a significant extent on the healthcare system and the type and intensity of care that can be provided in different settings. As described above, depending on the type of fracture, many patients have new care needs, either temporarily or long-term. Although there is some overlap in the types of care that can be provided in different settings, by and large, the greater the care needs, the more likely that an individual will need institutional, or skilled nursing facility, care. Other considerations that contribute to location of care include the patient's baseline living situation, cognition, and social and financial resources.

Overall, fractures and their outcomes are one of the leading causes of admission to a nursing home. It has been estimated that 7.8% of white women in the United States who are currently 50 years old will eventually require long-term nursing home admission due to an osteoporotic fracture.[58] Of all the osteoporotic fractures, hip fractures are most highly associated with risk of nursing home admission. Approximately 19% of patients require long-term nursing home care following a hip fracture. In the United States, 140,000 nursing home admissions every year are due to hip fracture.[43]

Recurrent or additional fracture

Although recurrent fracture may not be a direct consequence of a fracture, patients who present with fractures are at high risk for sustaining additional ones. Fractures of the clavicle, upper arm, forearm, vertebrae, ribs, hip, pelvis and upper and lower leg increase risk for future fractures, and patients who present with one fracture are at 50–100% higher risk of sustaining another one. This risk is highest in the first 5 years. Patients with vertebral fractures are at even higher risk, with a relative risk that is fourfold higher.[59]

This provides an important opportunity for secondary prevention. Unfortunately, for a variety of reasons, secondary prevention for fragility fractures remains suboptimal.

Less than half of patients with an osteoporotic fracture receive secondary evaluation and treatment. Identifying fragility fractures as osteoporotic fractures is a first step towards further preventive efforts.

Further discussion of the management of osteoporosis is discussed in Chapter 10. There is good evidence that a systems approach that involves dedicated personnel and bone mineral density testing optimizes management.[60]

Depression

Depression is common after a fragility fracture. There are many reasons for this. First, depression is a risk factor for osteoporosis and fracture. Patients with depression have an increased risk of falls, lower body mass index, higher rate of bone turnover, higher prevalence of smoking, lower use of calcium supplementation and higher risk for vitamin D deficiency than those without depression.[61]

In addition depression is often under-recognized in clinical practice and may be 'unmasked' by a hospital admission for fracture management that allows for longitudinal evaluation. Third, changes in function may increase the risk of depression and adjustment disorder.

Depression may complicate recovery from fracture in a variety of ways. First, it may limit participation in rehabilitation. It may lead to poor eating and drinking, which may impact nutritional status and wound healing. It may impair sleep. It may also alter the pain experience, so that patients either require more pain medication or under-report pain and thereby have undertreatment of pain. Conversely, undertreatment of pain is associated with increasing depressive symptoms.

Cognition

Cognitive decline can be seen following a fracture. There are several reasons for this. First, delirium is a common complication following surgery (see Chapter 7). Although delirium is typically a complication that lasts for hours to days, there is increasing evidence that some symptoms may persist. In one study, 32% of hip fracture patients who developed delirium had it at 1 month and 6% had it at 6 months.[62] Persistent delirium has the potential to impact on recovery through poor participation in rehabilitation, nutritional intake and mobility, as well as risk of rehospitalization.

There is also an increasing awareness of the overlap between delirium and dementia. Individuals with dementia are at higher risk of developing delirium, and that delirium may unmask a dementia that was unnoticed before its onset.

Finally, early dementia is often unrecognized or undiagnosed. Because of the often gradual progression, early cognitive changes may be attributed incorrectly to other things, including stress or age. Patients who develop coping strategies to compensate for cognitive changes may be unable to use these when they are out of their usual environment or challenged with new tasks, and this may also trigger recognition of the decline.

Falls and fear of falling

Falls and fear of falling are common after fractures. Among hip fracture patients, the risk of falls in the year following the fracture is over 50%.[63] The reason for this is twofold. First, fractures usually occur in the setting of a fall, and one fall with injury is a risk factor for future falls. Further discussion of falls, their predictors and ways to prevent them is presented in Chapter 12.

Second, the fracture and its complications may in turn put an individual at higher risk of falls. The '6 Ds' following a hip fracture increase risk, namely, deconditioning, dehydration, delirium, drugs, discrepancy in leg length and vitamin D deficiency.[64]

Fear of falling has increasingly been recognized as an important source of morbidity in older adults. Although it may occur in individuals who have not fallen, it is more common among those who have experienced a fall, and particularly among those who have sustained an injury due to fall. There is substantial overlap in risk factors for fear of falling and for fracture, including age, female gender, functional impairment, depression, cognition, and gait and balance.[65]

The approach to treatment following a fracture impacts on the future risk of falls. In a study by Bischoff-Ferrari et al., extended physical therapy lasting 60 minutes a day during the acute phase, followed by an unsupervised home program led to a 25% reduction in falls in the 12 months following a hip fracture.[66]

Pain

Postoperative pain can lead to multiple adverse consequences,[67] including delirium, decreased movement and poor sleeping and eating, which in turn may increase the risk of pneumonia, poor participation in therapy, poor wound healing, delay in return to ambulation and worse function 6 months after surgery (Table 9.5). Conversely, standardized and proactive treatment of pain should improve outcomes and facilitate the rehabilitation process.[68] Pain is often unrecognized and either untreated or undertreated.

As in the assessment of function, pain can be assessed globally or via scales targeted to the injured area. Assessment is predominantly via self-report and may be limited by a patient's cognitive status or by sensory impairment. Patients who are cognitively impaired may express pain in other ways, such as becoming agitated, moving less and eating less.

A common tool for global assessment of pain is the Numeric Rating Scale, which asks a patient to assign a number to their pain, with 0 indicating no pain at all and 10 representing the worst pain imaginable. A visual analog scale allows patients to mark where their pain is on a line that goes from 0 to 10. A similar scale that does not require numerical assessment, the Verbal Descriptor Scale, asks patients to describe pain ranging from 'no pain' to 'pain as bad as it could be'. For patients who have a difficult time

Table 9.5 Potential consequences of untreated or undertreated pain

Delirium
Decreased activity level
Poor sleep
Poor appetite
Slow improvement in rehabilitation
Functional decline
Depression

ranking by number or verbally, the Faces Pain Scale-Revised asks patients to match the severity of their pain to facial expressions. Finally, the FLACC (Face, Legs, Activity, Cry, Consolability) score is a physical assessment that provides a score from 0 (low) to 10 (high) to objectively assess evidence of pain for those who are unable to respond verbally.

A standardized approach that utilizes best practices ensures that all patients are assessed and treated for pain. Within a standardized framework, pain regimens may need to be individualized based on specific comorbidities, such as renal failure or delirium. Close monitoring of response includes assessment of pain control as well as monitoring for potential side effects of medications such as constipation, delirium or urinary retention.

SUMMARY

Fragility fractures occur in a patient population that is comprised primarily of older adults, with a high prevalence of comorbidity and functional impairment. The resulting risks of morbidity and mortality reflect, in part, this underlying vulnerability. Optimizing outcomes depends on, first, discussing goals of care with the patient and their caregiver(s), and, second, meticulous care that accounts for their comorbidities and lack of homeostatic reserve. Many of these outcomes are under-recognized, putting the onus on the clinician to screen patients for these different clinical entities. This is particularly important, because outcomes are often related and experiencing one adverse outcome can lead to another, thereby leading to increased risk of morbidity.

REFERENCES

1. Liem IS, Kammerlander C, Suhm N, Blauth M, Roth T, Gosch M, et al. Identifying a standard set of outcome parameters for the evaluation of orthogeriatric co-management for hip fractures. *Injury.* 2013;44(11):1403–12.
2. Haywood KL, Griffin XL, Achten J, Costa ML. Developing a core outcome set for hip fracture trials. *Bone Joint J.* 2014;96-B(8):1016–23.
3. Gialanella B, Ferlucci C, Monguzzi V, Prometti P. Determinants of functional outcome in hip fracture patients: The role of specific neuropsychiatric symptoms. *Disabil Rehabil.* 2015;37(6):517–22.

4. Cooper C, Atkinson EJ, Jacobsen SJ, O'Fallon WM, Melton LJ 3rd. Population-based study of survival after osteoporotic fractures. *Am J Epidemiol.* 1993;137(9):1001–5.

5. Bliuc D, Nguyen ND, Milch VE, Nguyen TV, Eisman JA, Center JR. Mortality risk associated with low-trauma osteoporotic fracture and subsequent fracture in men and women. *JAMA.* 2009;301(5):513–21.

6. Aharonoff GB, Koval KJ, Skovron ML, Zuckerman JD. Hip fractures in the elderly: Predictors of one year mortality. *J Orthop Trauma.* 1997;11(3):162–5.

7. Rapp K, Becker C, Lamb SE, Icks A, Klenk J. Hip fractures in institutionalized elderly people: Incidence rates and excess mortality. *J Bone Miner Res.* 2008;23(11):1825–31.

8. Haleem S, Lutchman L, Mayahi R, Grice JE, Parker MJ. Mortality following hip fracture: Trends and geographical variations over the last 40 years. *Injury.* 2008;39(10):1157–63.

9. Haentjens P, Magaziner J, Colon-Emeric CS, Vanderschueren D, Milisen K, Velkeniers B, et al. Meta-analysis: Excess mortality after hip fracture among older women and men. *Ann Intern Med.* 2010;152(6):380–90.

10. Braithwaite RS, Col NF, Wong JB. Estimating hip fracture morbidity, mortality and costs. *J Am Geriatr Soc.* 2003;51(3):364–70.

11. Kanis JA, Oden A, Johnell O, De Laet C, Jonsson B, Oglesby AK. The components of excess mortality after hip fracture. *Bone.* 2003;32(5):468–73.

12. Browner WS, Pressman AR, Nevitt MC, Cummings SR. Mortality following fractures in older women. The study of osteoporotic fractures. *Arch Intern Med.* 1996;156(14):1521–5.

13. Moja L, Piatti A, Pecoraro V, Ricci C, Virgili G, Salanti G, et al. Timing matters in hip fracture surgery: Patients operated within 48 hours have better outcomes. A meta-analysis and meta-regression of over 190,000 patients. *PLoS One.* 2012;7(10):e46175.

14. Pioli G, Lauretani F, Davoli ML, Martini E, Frondini C, Pellicciotti F, et al. Older people with hip fracture and IADL disability require earlier surgery. *J Gerontol A Biol Sci Med Sci.* 2012;67(11):1272–7.

15. Dubljanin-Raspopovic E, Markovic Denic L, Marinkovic J, Grajic M, Tomanovic Vujadinovic S, Bumbasirevic M. Use of early indicators in rehabilitation process to predict one-year mortality in elderly hip fracture patients. *Hip Int.* 2012;22(6):661–7.

16. Dubljanin-Raspopovic E, Markovic-Denic L, Marinkovic J, Nedeljkovic U, Bumbasirevic M. Does early functional outcome predict 1-year mortality in elderly patients with hip fracture? *Clin Orthop Relat Res.* 2013;471(8):2703–10.

17. Olsson C, Petersson C, Nordquist A. Increased mortality after fracture of the surgical neck of the humerus: A case-control study of 253 patients with a 12-year follow-up. *Acta Orthop Scand.* 2003;74(6):714–17.

18. Olsson C, Petersson CJ. Clinical importance of comorbidity in patients with a proximal humerus fracture. *Clin Orthop Relat Res.* 2006;442:93–9.

19. Kanis JA, Oden A, Johnell O, De Laet C, Jonsson B. Excess mortality after hospitalisation for vertebral fracture. *Osteoporos Int.* 2004;15(2):108–12.

20. Center JR, Nguyen TV, Schneider D, Sambrook PN, Eisman JA. Mortality after all major types of osteoporotic fracture in men and women: An observational study. *Lancet.* 1999;353(9156):878–82.

21. Kelsey JL, Browner WS, Seeley DG, Nevitt MC, Cummings SR. Risk factors for fractures of the distal forearm and proximal humerus. The Study of Osteoporotic Fractures Research Group. *Am J Epidemiol.* 1992;135(5):477–89.

22. Cummings SR, Nevitt MC. A hypothesis: The causes of hip fractures. *J Gerontol.* 1989;44(4):M107–11.

23. Chung KC, Pillsbury MS, Walters MR, Hayward RA. Reliability and validity testing of the Michigan Hand Outcomes Questionnaire. *J Hand Surg.* 1998;23(4):575–87.

24. Hudak PL, Amadio PC, Bombardier C. Development of an upper extremity outcome measure: The DASH (disabilities of the arm, shoulder and hand) [corrected]. The Upper Extremity Collaborative Group (UECG). *Am J Ind Med.* 1996;29(6):602–8.

25. Constant CR, Murley AH. A clinical method of functional assessment of the shoulder. *Clin Orthop Relat Res.* 1987;(214):160–4.

26. Chrischilles E, Shireman T, Wallace R. Costs and health effects of osteoporotic fractures. *Bone.* 1994;15(4):377–86.

27. Greendale GA, Barrett-Connor E, Ingles S, Haile R. Late physical and functional effects of osteoporotic fracture in women: The Rancho Bernardo Study. *J Am Geriatr Soc.* 1995;43(9):955–61.

28. Magaziner J, Hawkes W, Hebel JR, Zimmerman SI, Fox KM, Dolan M, et al. Recovery from hip fracture in eight areas of function. *J Gerontol A Biol Sci Med Sci.* 2000;55(9):M498–507.

29. Tseng MY, Shyu YI, Liang J. Functional recovery of older hip-fracture patients after interdisciplinary intervention follows three distinct trajectories. *Gerontologist.* 2012;52(6):833–42.

30. Magaziner J, Simonsick EM, Kashner TM, Hebel JR, Kenzora JE. Predictors of functional recovery one year following hospital discharge for hip fracture: A prospective study. *J Gerontol.* 1990;45(3):M101–7.

31. Kristensen MT. Factors affecting functional prognosis of patients with hip fracture. *Eur J Phys Rehabil Med.* 2011;47(2):257–64.

32. Beaupre LA, Binder EF, Cameron ID, Jones CA, Orwig D, Sherrington C, et al. Maximising functional recovery following hip fracture in frail seniors. *Best Pract Res Clin Rheumatol.* 2013;27(6):771–88.

33. Carson JL, Terrin ML, Noveck H, Sanders DW, Chaitman BR, Rhoads GG, et al. Liberal or restrictive transfusion in high-risk patients after hip surgery. *N Engl J Med.* 2011;365(26):2453–62.

34. Binder EF, Brown M, Sinacore DR, Steger-May K, Yarasheski KE, Schechtman KB. Effects of extended outpatient rehabilitation after hip fracture: A randomized controlled trial. *JAMA.* 2004;292(7):837–46.

35. Handoll HH, Ollivere BJ, Rollins KE. Interventions for treating proximal humeral fractures in adults. *Cochrane Database Syst Rev.* 2012;12:CD000434.

36. Price MC, Horn PL, Latshaw JC. Proximal humerus fractures. *Orthop Nurs.* 2013;32(5):251–8; quiz 259–60.

37. Hanson B, Neidenbach P, de Boer P, Stengel D. Functional outcomes after nonoperative management of fractures of the proximal humerus. *J Shoulder Elbow Surg.* 2009;18(4):612–21.

38. Gaebler C, McQueen MM, Court-Brown CM. Minimally displaced proximal humeral fractures: Epidemiology and outcome in 507 cases. *Acta Orthop Scand.* 2003;74(5):580–5.

39. Olsson C, Nordquist A, Petersson CJ. Long-term outcome of a proximal humerus fracture predicted after 1 year: A 13-year prospective population-based follow-up study of 47 patients. *Acta Orthop.* 2005;76(3):397–402.

40. Alexandru D, So W. Evaluation and management of vertebral compression fractures. *Perm J.* 2012;16(4):46–51.

41. Kammerlander C, Zegg M, Schmid R, Gosch M, Luger TJ, Blauth M. Fragility fractures requiring special consideration: Vertebral fractures. *Clin Geriatr Med.* 2014;30(2):361–72.

42. Wilcke MK, Abbaszadegan H, Adolphson PY. Patient-perceived outcome after displaced distal radius fractures. A comparison between radiological parameters, objective physical variables, and the DASH score. *J Hand Ther.* 2007;20(4):290–8; quiz 299.

43. Melton LJ 3rd. Adverse outcomes of osteoporotic fractures in the general population. *J Bone Miner Res.* 2003;18(6):1139–41.

44. Bentohami A, Bijlsma TS, Goslings JC, de Reuver P, Kaufmann L, Schep NW. Radiological criteria for acceptable reduction of extra-articular distal radial fractures are not predictive for patient-reported functional outcome. *J Hand Surg.* 2013;38(5):524–9.

45. Phadnis J, Trompeter A, Gallagher K, Bradshaw L, Elliott DS, Newman KJ. Mid-term functional outcome after the internal fixation of distal radius fractures. *J Orthop Surg Res.* 2012;7:4.

46. Brogren E, Hofer M, Petranek M, Dahlin LB, Atroshi I. Fractures of the distal radius in women aged 50 to 75 years: Natural course of patient-reported outcome, wrist motion and grip strength between 1 year and 2–4 years after fracture. *J Hand Surg.* 2011;36(7):568–76.

47. Edwards BJ, Song J, Dunlop DD, Fink HA, Cauley JA. Functional decline after incident wrist fractures— Study of Osteoporotic Fractures: Prospective cohort study. *BMJ.* 2010;341:c3324.

48. Morris NS. Distal radius fracture in adults: Self-reported physical functioning, role functioning, and meaning of injury. *Orthop Nurs.* 2000;19(4):37–48.

49. Chung KC, Kotsis SV, Kim HM. Predictors of functional outcomes after surgical treatment of distal radius fractures. *J Hand Surg.* 2007;32(1):76–83.

50. Beaule PE, Dervin GF, Giachino AA, Rody K, Grabowski J, Fazekas A. Self-reported disability following distal radius fractures: The influence of hand dominance. *J Hand Surg.* 2000;25(3):476–82.

51. Salkeld G, Cameron ID, Cumming RG, Easter S, Seymour J, Kurrle SE, et al. Quality of life related to fear of falling and hip fracture in older women: A time trade off study. *BMJ.* 2000;320(7231):341–6.

52. Rohde G, Haugeberg G, Mengshoel AM, Moum T, Wahl AK. Two-year changes in quality of life in elderly patients with low-energy hip fractures. A case-control study. *BMC Musculoskelet Disord.* 2010;11:226.

53. Hallberg I, Bachrach-Lindstrom M, Hammerby S, Toss G, Ek AC. Health-related quality of life after vertebral or hip fracture: A seven-year follow-up study. *BMC Musculoskelet Disord.* 2009;10:135.

54. Hall SE, Williams JA, Senior JA, Goldswain PR, Criddle RA. Hip fracture outcomes: Quality of life and functional status in older adults living in the community. *Aust N Z J Med.* 2000;30(3):327–32.

55. Tsauo JY, Leu WS, Chen YT, Yang RS. Effects on function and quality of life of postoperative home-based physical therapy for patients with hip fracture. *Arch Phys Med Rehabil.* 2005;86(10):1953–7.

56. Inauen C, Platz A, Meier C, Zingg U, Rufibach K, Spross C, et al. Quality of life after osteosynthesis of fractures of the proximal humerus. *J Orthop Trauma.* 2013;27(4):e74–80.

57. Hagino H, Nakamura T, Fujiwara S, Oeki M, Okano T, Teshima R. Sequential change in quality of life for patients with incident clinical fractures: A prospective study. *Osteoporos Int.* 2009;20(5):695–702.

58. Chrischilles EA, Butler CD, Davis CS, Wallace RB. A model of lifetime osteoporosis impact. *Arch Intern Med.* 1991;151(10):2026–32.

59. Klotzbuecher CM, Ross PD, Landsman PB, Abbott TA 3rd, Berger M. Patients with prior fractures have an increased risk of future fractures: A summary of the literature and statistical synthesis. *J Bone Miner Res.* 2000;15(4):721–39.

60. Sale JE, Beaton D, Bogoch E. Secondary prevention after an osteoporosis-related fracture: An overview. *Clin Geriatr Med.* 2014;30(2):317–32.

61. Friedman SM, Menzies IB, Bukata SV, Mendelson DA, Kates SL. Dementia and hip fractures: Development of a pathogenic framework for understanding and studying risk. *Geriatr Orthop Surg Rehabil*. 2010;1(2):52–62.

62. Marcantonio ER, Flacker JM, Michaels M, Resnick NM. Delirium is independently associated with poor functional recovery after hip fracture. *J Am Geriatr Soc*. 2000;48(6):618–24.

63. Lloyd BD, Williamson DA, Singh NA, Hansen RD, Diamond TH, Finnegan TP, et al. Recurrent and injurious falls in the year following hip fracture: A prospective study of incidence and risk factors from the Sarcopenia and Hip Fracture study. *J Gerontol A Biol Sci Med Sci*. 2009;64(5):599–609.

64. Friedman SM, Mendelson DA, Kates SL. Hip fractures. In: Hirth V, Wieland D, Dever-Bumba M, editors. *Case-Based Geriatrics*. New York: McGraw-Hill, 2011, pp. 529–43.

65. Scheffer AC, Schuurmans MJ, van Dijk N, van der Hooft T, de Rooij SE. Fear of falling: Measurement strategy, prevalence, risk factors and consequences among older persons. *Age Ageing*. 2008;37(1):19–24.

66. Bischoff-Ferrari HA, Dawson-Hughes B, Platz A, Orav EJ, Stahelin HB, Willett WC, et al. Effect of high-dosage cholecalciferol and extended physiotherapy on complications after hip fracture: A randomized controlled trial. *Arch Intern Med*. 2010;170(9):813–20.

67. Morrison RS, Magaziner J, McLaughlin MA, Orosz G, Silberzweig SB, Koval KJ, et al. The impact of postoperative pain on outcomes following hip fracture. *Pain*. 2003;103(3):303–11.

68. Friedman SM, Mendelson DA, Kates SL, McCann RM. Geriatric co-management of proximal femur fractures: Total quality management and protocol-driven care result in better outcomes for a frail patient population. *J Am Geriatr Soc*. 2008;56(7):1349–56.

10

Osteoporosis

ALEXANDRA STAVRAKIS, SUSAN V. BUKATA AND SUSAN M. FRIEDMAN

DEFINITION

Osteoporosis is a disease that is characterized by low bone mass, microarchitectural disruption, poor bone strength and an increase in the risk of fracture. The World Health Organization defines osteoporosis as a bone mineral density (BMD) at the hip or spine that is less than or equal to 2.5 standard deviations (SD) below the young normal mean reference population.

EPIDEMIOLOGY

Osteoporosis is the most common bone disease of humans. It is a major public health concern worldwide, impacting an estimated 200 million people[1] and contributing to approximately 9 million fractures in the year 2000.[2] It is estimated that more than 40% of postmenopausal women and 30% of men will eventually sustain osteoporosis related, or fragility, fractures. Fragility fractures lead to an increase in morbidity, mortality and cost.[3-8] Osteoporosis can be prevented, diagnosed and treated. It is typically silent until a patient sustains a fracture. Thus, early detection of osteoporosis is critical to prevent fragility fractures in the at-risk elderly population.

There are several risk factors for osteoporosis. These can be grouped into one of four categories: demographics and lifestyle, medical comorbidities, pharmacological agents and genetic polymorphisms (see Table 10.1). The risk of fragility fractures in both men and women is most closely related to low BMD, low body mass index, history of prior falls and prior fractures.[3]

PATHOPHYSIOLOGY

Fragility fractures result from a combination of decreased bone strength and an increase in fall risk. Several skeletal characteristics contribute to bone strength, including BMD, bone architecture, matrix and mineral composition, and rate of bone turnover. The most important of these is BMD. Patient BMD depends on the peak bone mass and the rate of bone mass loss. Peak bone mass is achieved in a patient's 20s and early 30s and, depending on genetic and environmental influences, generally decreases after this point. This bone loss occurs as a result of an age related, and in females, an estrogen related, imbalance in the activity of osteoblasts and osteoclasts. Additionally, several polymorphisms of genes coding for various receptors such as the vitamin D, estrogen and calcitonin receptors have also been linked to BMD and are thought to affect the rate of loss of BMD.[9]

Bone metabolism is a process of a balance between bone formation and bone resorption. Bone formation is primarily the result of active osteoblasts. Bone resorption occurs via active osteoclasts and is controlled by the RANK/RANKL pathway. RANKL (receptor activator of nuclear factor kappa-B ligand) is secreted by osteoblasts and binds to the RANK receptor on osteoclasts, stimulating osteoclast activation. This pathway can be controlled via several mechanisms, such as through osteoprotegerin (OPG) and parathyroid hormone (PTH). OPG is produced by osteoblasts and binds to and sequesters RANKL, thus inhibiting osteoclast activation. PTH is secreted by the parathyroid glands and binds to the adenylyl cyclase receptor on osteoblasts, stimulating RANKL secretion and thus osteoclast activation and bone resorption. Other factors that stimulate osteoclast activity and thus bone resorption include interleukin 1, 1,25-dihydroxy vitamin D and prostaglandin E2. Other factors, in addition to OPG, that inhibit osteoclast activity include calcitonin, estrogen, transforming growth factor β and interleukin-10.[9,10]

Estrogen plays a role in the normal remodelling of bone and its deficiency in postmenopausal women leads to an

Table 10.1 Osteoporosis risk factors

Demographics/ lifestyle	Comorbidities	Pharmacological agents	Genetic polymorphisms
Age	Liver disease	Furosemide	Vitamin D receptor
Female gender	Hyperthyroidism	Glucocorticoids	Estrogen receptor
Caucasian	Chronic renal failure	Phenytoin	Calcitonin receptor
Northern European	Chronic obstructive pulmonary disease	Selective serotonin reuptake inhibitors	
Alcohol (3 or more drinks per day)	Rheumatoid arthritis	Antineoplastic	
Family history	Malabsorption syndromes	Methotrexate	
Early menopause	Type 1 diabetes mellitus	Omeprazole	
Low body mass index	Gastric bypass	Anticoagulants (enoxaparin, heparin)	
Low dietary calcium intake	Vitamin D deficiency	Thiazolidinediones	
Smoking		Antiretroviral therapy	
Caffeine		Lithium	
Sedentary lifestyle			

increase in osteoclastogenesis secondary to interleukin-1 and tumour necrosis factors, which are normally inhibited by estrogen. Additionally estrogen normally directly promotes osteoclast apoptosis via production of transforming growth factor β, thus a decrease in estrogen levels would lead to an increase in osteoclast activity.[9]

DIAGNOSIS OF AND SCREENING FOR OSTEOPOROSIS

Imaging

Dual energy X-ray absorptiometry (DEXA) is considered the gold standard for the diagnosis of osteoporosis. DEXA is used to evaluate the bone mineral content of a region of interest, which is defined as the amount of mineral in the specific site scanned. The bone mineral content is then divided by the area measured, and this can be used to derive a value for the BMD.[11] The hip is generally the region analysed for diagnostic purposes since it has the highest predictive value for hip fractures as well as overall fracture risk. The L2–L4 region of the lumbar spine is another region commonly evaluated.[11,12] A patient's BMD is compared to the distribution of BMD from a sample of young adult females (aged 20–29 years old), who are used as a reference. The number of SD from this reference range is known as the T score.[13] A Z score is also available; this represents the number of SD of the patient's BMD in comparison to patients in the same age group; however, this value is not used in the diagnosis of osteoporosis.

The National Osteoporosis Foundation has four general diagnostic categories based on BMD: normal, osteopenia,

Table 10.2 Diagnostic categories of bone mineral density

Category	T score
Normal	≥–1
Osteopenia	Between –1 and –2.5
Osteoporosis	≤–2.5
Severe osteoporosis	≤–2.5, with fragility fracture

Source: National Osteoporosis Foundation. *Clinician's Guide to Prevention and Treatment of Osteoporosis.* http://nof. org/files/nof/public/content/file/917/upload/481.pdf (accessed 12 May 2015).

osteoporosis and severe osteoporosis (Table 10.2). Normal is defined as a hip BMD within 1 SD below the normal reference range (T score ≥–1). Osteopenia is defined as a T score between –2.5 and –1. Osteoporosis is diagnosed when the T score is ≤–2.5. Severe osteoporosis is defined as a T score ≤–2.5 with the presence of one or more fragility fractures.[11]

The United States Preventive Services Task Force recommends a screening DEXA in all women aged ≥65. The National Osteoporosis Foundation also recommends screening in men aged ≥70. It should be noted that, although lower BMD is associated with increased risk, there is no discrete value that clearly differentiates patients who will fracture from those who will not. In fact, although patients with BMD in the osteoporotic range are more likely to fracture than those who are osteopenic, more fragility fractures occur among patients who are in the osteopenic range, because of the higher prevalence of osteopenia.

Laboratory tests

Several serum and urine markers of bone turnover have been developed. The most commonly used markers include serum bone-specific alkaline phosphatase and amino-terminal propeptide of type 1 procollagen, which are markers of bone formation, and urine or serum telopeptides of collagen crosslinks, which are markers of bone resorption. Although these are generally not used for diagnostic purposes, they may be used to predict the risk of future fracture or to monitor the response to therapy. Additionally, levels of vitamin D can be evaluated to rule out vitamin D deficiency as related to the development of osteoporosis.[9]

FRAX score

The Fracture Risk Assessment Tool (FRAX) score is an algorithm developed by the World Health Organization based on several cohort studies to predict fracture risk. It has different calculators based on the patient's country of origin and race, and is validated for individuals aged 40–90. It provides the practitioner with the 10-year probability of fracture and of a major osteoporotic fracture (such as vertebral, wrist, hip or proximal humerus) in patients who are not already on antiresorptive treatment. This tool can be used to determine which patients are most at risk and likely to benefit from treatment. The FRAX calculator takes into account the following factors: patient race, age, sex, weight, height, history of prior fracture, family history of fracture, history of rheumatoid arthritis, current tobacco or alcohol use, current use of glucocorticoids, secondary osteoporosis and femoral neck BMD.[9] Although BMD can be used, it is not required to predict risk.

FRAGILITY FRACTURES

In general, a fracture is considered related to osteoporosis if it occurs with relatively low force such as a ground level fall, which would not be expected to cause a fracture in a young healthy patient. Although patients with osteoporosis are at increased risk of almost any type of fracture, those of most concern include fractures of the vertebral body, proximal femur, distal radius and proximal humerus.

Vertebral body fractures

Vertebral body compression fractures are the most common fragility fracture. In the year 2000, there were an estimated 1.4 million clinical vertebral fractures worldwide. Approximately 25% of patients over 70 years of age and 50% of patients over 80 years of age sustain vertebral fractures.[2] Only a quarter of these injuries result from falls and the majority are precipitated by routine everyday activities such as bending or lifting light objects. The occurrence of one vertebral fracture, even if asymptomatic, increases the likelihood of an additional fracture by at least fourfold.[14]

Vertebral body fractures can be diagnosed with plain radiographs. Radiographs should be taken of the entire spine in order to identify fractures at other levels given the high incidence of multiple simultaneous vertebral body fractures. Additional advanced imaging, such as CT or MRI, is generally not necessary unless the patient presents with neurological compromise in which case these imaging techniques should be used to evaluate for any spinal cord compression.

Although the majority of vertebral body compression fractures do not compromise the spinal canal, a thorough neurological examination is indicated in patients with these injuries to rule out any serious complications. Most patients can be treated non-operatively with pain control and bracing. The American Academy of Orthopaedic Surgeons strongly recommends administering a 4-week course of calcitonin, which has been shown to reduce pain significantly when started within 5 days of the fracture event. If patients continue to have severe pain for several weeks after a trial of non-operative treatment, they may benefit from kyphoplasty, which involves expanding the vertebral body height with a balloon followed by the injection of bone cement into the cavity created. Vertebroplasty is also available, where bone cement is injected directly into cancellous bone without cavity creation, however this procedure is not recommended given the much greater risk of cement extravasation into the spinal canal with vertebroplasty in comparison to kyphoplasty. If patients present with neurological compromise and imaging evidence of spinal canal compromise, surgical decompression and stabilization is urgently performed.[10,15] Further discussion of vertebral fractures can be found in Chapter 31.

Proximal femoral fractures

These fractures are considered the most devastating fragility fractures given that they are associated with a significant increase in patient morbidity and mortality.[16–20] A recent retrospective study evaluated 43,210 proximal femoral fracture patients with age matched controls and found that proximal femoral fractures were associated with more than a twofold increase in mortality risk and a fourfold increase in need of long-term nursing facility care.[20] Approximately 50% of patients who were ambulatory prior to sustaining a proximal femoral fracture could not do so independently after a proximal femoral fracture.[14] Early surgical intervention cannot be overemphasized as multiple studies have found that patients have significantly better outcomes if surgery is performed within 4 days of injury as this allows patients to be mobile quicker. Proximal femoral fractures are further defined based on the location of the fracture as this determines treatment. These include femoral neck fractures, intertrochanteric fractures and subtrochanteric fractures. The characteristics, treatment options and complications of each are summarized in Table 10.3.

Table 10.3 Proximal femoral fractures

Classification	Femoral neck	Intertrochanteric	Subtrochanteric
Physical exam	Short, externally rotated	Short, externally rotated	Short, varus
Patient population	Younger than intertrochanteric	Older than femoral neck	Bisphosphonate related
Treatment	Hemiarthroplasty (debilitated elderly) Total hip arthroplasty (active patients) Open reduction, internal fixation Cannulated screw fixation	Intramedullary nail Hip compression screw	Intramedullary nail Fixed angle plate
Complications	14–36% 1-year mortality Dislocation Osteonecrosis of femoral head	20–30% 1-year mortality Non-union Implant failure	Varus, procurvatum malunion Non-union Implant failure

In general, intertrochanteric femur fractures occur in an older age group than those who sustain femoral neck fractures.[20–22]

Although subtrochanteric femur fractures are generally considered high energy injuries, their incidence has increased recently in the osteoporotic population as it is associated with bisphosphonate use. Approximately 1% of patients on bisphosphonate therapy develop a subtrochanteric femur fracture. Many of these patients have prodromal symptoms of thigh pain with weight bearing and an associated lateral cortical thickening identified on radiographs.[23] In such a presentation, these patients should be followed closely for any sign of an increase in thigh pain and some may be candidates for prophylactic surgery to prevent fracture.[23] Subtrochanteric fractures are discussed further in Chapter 35.

In general, femoral neck fractures can be treated with cannulated screw fixation if non-displaced, versus hemiarthroplasty or total hip arthroplasty if displaced. In general, total hip arthroplasty is performed in healthy and active patients who are expected to continue to be active postoperatively. Hemiarthroplasty is performed in older and more debilitated patients and is chosen over total hip arthroplasty in this age group primarily because it involves less operative time and thus there is a potential decreased risk of complications. Additionally, postoperative dislocation following hip arthroplasty can be a devastating complication and the risk of dislocation is increased in patients who cannot follow postoperative hip precautions or who are at an increased risk of having subsequent falls. In general, hemiarthroplasty is associated with a lower dislocation risk and thus is considered a safer option in older patients. The downside of a hemiarthroplasty is primarily that it is less reliable for pain control postoperatively, especially if the patient has evidence of arthritis changes of the hip prior to femoral neck fracture. Intertrochanteric fractures can generally be treated with an intramedullary nail or hip compression screw, depending on fracture pattern, comminution and displacement. Subtrochanteric femur fractures can be treated with an intramedullary nail or fixed angle plate. Further discussion of hip fracture management can be found in Chapters 34 and 35.

Distal radial fractures

The incidence of distal radial fractures in females rises rapidly after menopause, likely secondarily to accelerated postmenopausal bone loss, but reaches a plateau after approximately age 75. This may be related to age related decreases in the speed with which an individual extends their arm to break a ground level fall, as well as the trajectory of the fall (forward vs down). In contrast, the incidence of distal radial fractures in males is low. As a result, the majority of distal radial fractures occur in women with a 4:1 female to male ratio, which is a much greater difference in comparison to other fragility fractures.[14] These injuries generally involve the distal aspect of the radius and/or ulnar styloid and can be diagnosed with plain radiographs. Treatment depends on the fracture pattern, displacement, comminution and whether the fracture extends into the wrist joint. Conservative treatment generally involves closed reduction and casting for several weeks. Surgical treatment involves open reduction and internal fixation with a plate and screws followed by casting. In older patients, presenting with low velocity injuries, there is little evidence that operative fixation results in better function, although an improved anatomical position is often achieved. Further studies of distal radial fractures in the elderly are required to examine the role of surgery in patients with reduced pre-fracture physical function. Distal radial fractures are discussed further in Chapter 26.

Proximal humeral fractures

Proximal humeral fractures are typical osteoporotic fractures with an increasing incidence in both males and females after middle age. Unlike distal radial fractures, the incidence of proximal humeral fractures continues to rise as patients age and in both males and females the incidence of these fractures is higher in the 90+ age group than in the 65–69 year group.[24] The majority of proximal humeral fractures are caused by a fall from standing height but the patients are relatively fit. Analysis of a group of 1027 proximal humeral fractures with an average age of 66 years showed that 91.6% were able to dress themselves, 90.6% lived at home and 79.5% did their own shopping.[25]

The treatment of proximal humeral fractures remains controversial. As with distal radial fractures, the introduction of proximal humeral locking plates has increased the rate of surgical treatment of these fractures. Previously most proximal humeral fractures were treated non-operatively with hemiarthroplasty and arthroplasty being reserved for more serious fractures. However recent studies have not shown improved results with operative management. Rangan et al.[26] undertook a randomized clinical trial of operative versus non-operative management in patients aged ≥16 years. They found no difference in outcome between the two groups. A retrospective study was undertaken by Okike et al.[27] who examined 207 patients aged ≥60 years who were treated operatively or non-operatively. There was no difference in clinical outcome scores despite the fact that 90.9% of non-operatively managed patients had a malunion compared with 31.8% of the operatively managed group. However, the complication rate in the operatively managed group was much higher. It is likely that some proximal humeral fractures will benefit from surgical treatment but further, more sophisticated, studies are needed to assess which fractures they are. Proximal humeral fractures are discussed further in Chapter 20.

Changing epidemiology of osteoporotic fractures

The epidemiology of the common osteoporotic fractures has changed considerably. It is difficult to assess the changing epidemiology of vertebral fractures as many do not present to doctors. However Table 10.4 gives information on the changing epidemiology of proximal femoral, proximal humeral and distal radial fractures in patients aged ≥65 years. The data come from the Royal Infirmary of Edinburgh, in Scotland, which is the only hospital treating orthopaedic trauma in a defined population. It shows the changing incidence of the three common osteoporotic fractures over a 20-year period.

Table 10.4 shows that the incidence of proximal femoral fractures is levelling off. The overall incidence increased in the 1990s but has begun to fall. This is particularly true of older females, but in older males the incidence of proximal femoral fractures has continued to rise. This presumably relates to improved male life expectancy. Analysis of the proximal humeral fractures shows that the incidence has continued to rise over a period of almost 20 years. This is true of both males and females. In distal radial fractures the situation would seem to be different. In females the incidence of distal radial fractures has continued to rise although it would seem to be levelling off. In males the incidence fell over the 10-year period between 2000 and 2010/11. It has already been pointed out that the incidence of distal radial fractures, unlike proximal humeral fractures, falls after about 75 years of age and the values in Table 10.4 probably represent this.

Table 10.4 Incidence of proximal femoral, proximal humeral and distal radial fractures over a 20-year period

	All patients	Males	Females
Proximal femur			
1991	674.1	286.5	901.8
2000	691.7	388.2	891.9
2010/11	679.2	425.9	862.7
Proximal humerus			
1993	155.6	90.1	196.1
2000	233.0	106.8	316.2
2010/11	265.5	139.6	356.8
Distal radius			
1991	376.6	93.8	546.5
2000	511.5	148.5	751.0
2010/11	507.1	127.8	782.1

Source: Data are taken from analysis of a 1-year period and are expressed as $\times/10^5/year$.

TREATMENT

Lifestyle approaches to treatment

The treatment of osteoporosis requires a multi-modal approach that includes diet, exercise and avoidance of smoking. Diet should include adequate calorie intake, as well as calcium and vitamin D. The optimal intake of calcium and vitamin D remains uncertain, and different organizations vary in their recommendations. Elemental calcium intake should approximate 1200 mg per day, and total vitamin D intake should be at least 800 international units daily. Heavy alcohol use should be avoided.

Exercise has been associated with a reduction in the risk of hip fractures, as well as the risk of fractures overall, with a relative risk reduction of 51%.[28,29] Prudent weight-bearing exercise for at least 30 minutes, three times a week, is recommended.[30] A sustained approach over time is important, as the benefits decline quickly after exercise is stopped. It is therefore important to choose an exercise regimen that is enjoyable and can be maintained long term. Furthermore, since a chief goal of the treatment of osteoporosis is prevention of fragility fractures, fall prevention is an important component of management. Balance exercise has been shown to be the most useful exercise approach to falls risk reduction.

Cigarette smoking accelerates bone loss. It is also associated with an increase in the risk of hip fracture in both women and men, with 19% of the risk of hip fracture attributable to smoking.[31]

Calcium and vitamin D

Calcium is necessary for adequate bone mineralization. With aging, serum calcium decreases, calcium absorption by the intestine decreases and urinary excretion of calcium increases. Vitamin D maintains serum calcium by increasing intestinal absorption and renal reabsorption of calcium, as well as increasing resorption of calcium from bone. Production of vitamin D in the skin declines with age, as does the renal conversion of 25-hydroxyvitamin D to 1,25-dihydroxyvitamin D, resulting in secondary hyperparathyroidism, with hypocalcemia and bone resorption.

Combined calcium and vitamin D supplementation has been shown to significantly reduce fracture risk in postmenopausal women in several studies, with rates of hip fracture decreasing anywhere by 26–43% and rates of total non-vertebral fractures by 23–32%.[9] Calcium supplementation (as distinct from dietary calcium) increases the risk of nephrolithiasis. The impact on cardiovascular disease remains unclear.

Pharmacological treatment

In addition to the interventions listed above, pharmacological treatment is indicated for high-risk individuals. In 2013, the National Osteoporosis Foundation released updated guidelines for pharmacological treatment of postmenopausal women and men aged 50 and over, as outlined in Table 10.5.[32] These guidelines should be individualized, following discussion between the clinician and patient (and, possibly, the patient's proxy), based on the patient's goals, life expectancy and specific comorbidities.

Pharmacological treatment of osteoporosis can be divided into two general categories: antiresorptive agents, which act primarily on bone resorption, or anabolic agents, which act on bone formation. Antiresorptive agents include bisphosphonates, hormone replacement therapy, denosumab, strontium ranelate and calcitonin. Teriparatide is the only anabolic agent currently approved for osteoporosis treatment.

ANTIRESORPTIVE AGENTS

Bisphosphonates are commonly used agents in both the prevention and treatment of osteoporosis. They are often used as first-line agents,[30] because of their efficacy, cost and availability of long-term data on safety. Bisphosphonates work primarily by inhibiting osteoclastic bone resorption, by reducing osteoclast effectiveness, as well as by decreasing osteoclast progenitor development promoting osteoclast apoptosis.

Table 10.5 Indications for pharmacological treatment of osteoporosis

History of hip or vertebral fracture
T score ≤2.5 by DEXA, at the femoral neck or spine
T score between −1 and −2.5 at the femoral neck or spine, with a 10-year probability of hip fracture ≥3% or any major fragility fracture ≥20%

Bisphosphonates are associated with significant reductions in fracture risk, with non-vertebral fractures decreasing by 20–40% and vertebral fractures by 40–50%.[5,9] Oral bisphosphonates are available in daily, weekly and monthly formulations. They are poorly absorbed from the gastrointestinal tract and must be taken alone on an empty stomach, with at least 8 ounces of water. They may also cause mucosal injury, so patients must not lie down for 30–60 minutes after taking them, to prevent reflux.

Patients who are unable to tolerate oral bisphosphonates may take intravenous formulations. Zoledronic acid is administered yearly and ibandronate is given every 3 months.

There is a theoretical concern that bisphosphonates could impair fracture healing, although there are not much data available to guide decision making. Because fracture healing involves the activation of both osteoclasts and osteoblasts in the remodelling of callus, a medication that inhibits osteoclast activity, such as a bisphosphonate, may impair this process. It is reasonable to wait 4–6 weeks after a fracture before initiating bisphosphonate therapy.

The optimal duration of treatment with bisphosphonates is not clear, given that the benefits of bisphosphonates on fracture endpoints have only been proven for the first 5 years after treatment initiation. Additionally, bisphosphonates have been associated with the rare but serious side effects of osteonecrosis of the jaw and subtrochanteric femur fractures.[9,10] These appear to increase with the duration of bisphosphonate use.

The role of long-term postmenopausal hormone therapy in the prevention of osteoporosis is currently controversial, primarily as the result of the publication of the Women's Health Initiative study, which evaluated the reduction in osteoporotic fractures in women on estrogen or estrogen and progesterone therapy. Combined hormone therapy patients had an increase in stroke, cardiovascular events and breast cancer. Following these findings, in general, hormone therapy should be avoided in favour of other antiresorptive agents such as bisphosphonates and should only be used in the short term in the perimenopausal period in symptomatic women with a high risk of fracture.[9]

Selective estrogen receptor modulators (SERMs), such as raloxifene, act as agonists on the estrogen receptor in bone, inhibiting bone resorption and resulting in an increase in BMD. This is in comparison to their antagonistic effects on the estrogen receptor in the breast and uterus. SERMs increase the risk of thromboembolic events and vasomotor symptoms. Raloxifene reduces the risk of vertebral fracture. This class of medication may be beneficial in a certain subgroup of postmenopausal women such as those with a history of hormone related malignancies and is usually chosen when there is also a need for breast cancer prophylaxis. Tamoxifen, which is also a SERM and is used mainly for the prevention and treatment of breast cancer, is not usually used for osteoporosis, but probably has some protective effect on bone.

The balance between bone formation and bone absorption is generally controlled by bone signalling via the RANKL pathway. Osteoblasts normally secrete RANKL, a ligand that binds to the RANK receptor on osteoclasts which activates osteoclast bone resorption. Denosumab is a monoclonal antibody against RANKL, thus its mechanism of action is to decrease RANKL induced osteoclast activation. It has been shown to increase BMD and reduce the incidence of hip, vertebral and non-vertebral fractures in postmenopausal women. Denosumab is administered via subcutaneous injection every 6 months. The most common side effects include hypocalcemia, rash, muscle and bone pain, and infection. Patients with hypocalcemia should have this corrected prior to starting denosumab.

Strontium ranelate is an oral medication available for use in Europe. It is theorized to enhance matrix mineralization. It appears to inhibit bone resorption with little impact on bone formation. It has been shown to reduce the risk of vertebral and, to a lesser extent, non-vertebral fractures in postmenopausal women, and to reduce hip fractures in a high-risk subgroup.

Calcitonin acts on osteoclasts to inhibit bone resorption. It is available as an intranasal spray and has been shown to reduce vertebral fracture incidence. It has a modest effect on BMD compared to bisphosphonates and PTH. It has not been shown to impact the risk of hip or non-vertebral fractures, and for this reason is not considered a first-line agent for the treatment of osteoporosis. It improves pain control in vertebral compression fractures.

ANABOLIC AGENTS

Teriparatide comprises the first 34 amino acids of the 84-amino acid sequence of PTH. Its mechanism of action is to reproduce the effects of PTH via the activation of adenylyl cyclase. When given intermittently it leads to a net anabolic effect on bone. It increases total body BMD, as well as vertebral and femoral BMD, reducing the risk of both vertebral and non-vertebral fractures.[33] The major contraindication to use of teriparatide is in patients with Paget's disease given its link with an increased risk of osteosarcoma in these patients.

Fluoride has been evaluated as a potential anabolic agent for osteoporosis treatment. Although it does increase BMD, it has not consistently been shown to reduce fracture incidence and is not recommended for treatment.

The increase in understanding of osteoporosis pathophysiology and bone metabolism has led to many new targets and approaches to osteoporosis treatment. Several new agents are in various phases of clinical trials and will likely increase the options available for treatment in the near future.

MONITORING OF PROGRESSION

There are few data to help guide rescreening individuals who do not have osteoporosis and are not receiving pharmacological intervention. In a recent study of almost 5000 postmenopausal women with either normal BMD or osteopenia and no history of fracture, osteoporosis developed in fewer than 10% of women with normal bone density or mild osteopenia during a 15-year interval, with a similar rate of progression in 5 years for women with moderate osteopenia (T score −1.5 to −1.99), and 1 year for women with advanced osteopenia (T score −2 to −2.49).[34]

There are several published guidelines for monitoring response to therapy for those who are already receiving treatment. The National Osteoporosis Foundation recommends repeat DEXA of the hip or spine 2 years after starting therapy, and then every 2 years thereafter, with more frequent testing for certain high-risk populations.[32] The American Association of Clinical Endocrinologists recommends DEXA of the hip and spine every 1–2 years until stability is attained, and then every 2 years or less frequently.[35]

SECONDARY PREVENTION

Unfortunately, despite its proven efficacy, the rates of treatment of osteoporosis among patients who have already sustained fractures remain low. Women with prior fractures are at twice the risk of subsequent fracture, making them an ideal population to target for treatment of osteoporosis and multifactorial fracture risk reduction. Absolute risk reduction with treatment ranges up to 6%, that is, a number needed to treat of 16. Although treatment rates have increased in the past two decades, many patients miss an opportunity for secondary prevention, and practice patterns vary considerably.[36] A recent meta-analysis showed that in patients who had had fractures, 1–45% carried a diagnosis of osteoporosis and 1–32% of patients had DEXA scans. In addition, 2–62% of patients received calcium/vitamin D and 1–65% of patients received pharmacological treatment. Men and older patients are less likely to receive treatment.[37] Several models have been initiated internationally to try to improve treatment rates, including the Fracture Liaison Services in Scotland, the Kaiser Permanente Healthy Bones Program in the US, the Osteoporosis Exemplary Care Program in Canada, the Minimal Trauma Fracture Liaison service in Australia and Osteoporosis Patient Targeted and Integrated Management for Active Living in Singapore.[36]

CONCLUSION

Osteoporosis is a major public health concern as it can lead to devastating complications when fragility fractures occur. Large strides have been made over the past two decades in screening at-risk populations and implementing treatment protocols for those patients with evidence of osteoporosis. These treatment protocols have resulted in a significant decrease in the incidence of fragility fractures. More research is needed to better understand the pathophysiology of osteoporosis which may aid in the development of new treatment options.

REFERENCES

1. Cooper C, Campion G, Melton LJ 3rd. Hip fractures in the elderly: A world-wide projection. *Osteoporos Int.* 1992;2(6):285–289.

2. Johnell O, Kanis JA. An estimate of the worldwide prevalence and disability associated with osteoporotic fractures. *Osteoporosis Int.* 2006;17:1726.

3. Office of Medical Applications Research, National Institutes of Health. Osteoporosis: Consensus conference. *JAMA.* 1984;252:799–802.

4. Berg RL, Cassells JS. Osteoporosis. *The Second Fifty Years: Promoting Health Preventing Disability.* National Academies Press, Washington, DC, 1990, pp. 76–100.

5. Abbott TA, Lawrence BJ, Wallach S. Osteoporosis: The need for comprehensive treatment guidelines. *Clin Ther.* 1996;18:127–149.

6. Ray NF, Chan JK, Thamer M, Melton LJ. Medical expenditures for the treatment of osteoporotic fractures in the United States in 1995: Report from the National Osteoporosis Foundation. *J Bone Miner Res.* 1997;12:24–35.

7. Ross PD. Osteoporosis: Frequency, consequences, and risk factors. *Arch Intern Med.* 1996;156:1399–1141.

8. Nguyen TV, Eisman JA, Kelly PJ, Sambrook PN. Risk factors for osteoporotic fractures in elderly men. *Am J Epidemiol.* 1996;144:255–263.

9. Sambrook P, Cooper C. Osteoporosis. *Lancet.* 2006;267:2010–2018.

10. Miller MD, Thompson SR, Hart J. *Review of Orthopaedics*, 6th Ed. Elsevier, Philadelphia, PA, 2012.

11. Kanis JA. Diagnosis of osteoporosis and assessment of fracture risk. *Lancet.* 2002;359(9321):1929–1936.

12. Marshall D, Johnell O, Wedel H. Meta-analysis of how well measures of bone mineral density predict occurrence of osteoporotic fractures. *BMJ.* 1996;312:1254–1259.

13. Kanis JA, Gluer CC, for the Committee of Scientific Advisors, International Osteoporosis Foundation. An update on the diagnosis and assessment of osteoporosis with densitometry. *Osteoporos Int.* 2000;11:192–202.

14. Cummings SR, Melton LJ. Epidemiology and outcomes of osteoporotic fractures. *Lancet.* 2002;359(9319):1761–1767.

15. Esses SI, McGuire R, Jenkins J, et al. The treatment of symptomatic osteoporotic spinal compression fractures. *J Am Acad Orthop Surg.* 2011;19(3):176–182.

16. Center JR, Nguyen TV, Schneider D, Sambrook PN, Eisman JA. Mortality after all major types of osteoporotic fracture in men and women: An observational study. *Lancet.* 1999;353:878–882.

17. Poór G, Atkinson EJ, O'Fallon WM, Melton LJ III. Determinants of reduced survival following hip fractures in men. *Clin Orthop.* 1995;319:260–265.

18. Browner WS, Pressman AR, Nevitt MC, Cummings SR. Mortality following fractures in older women: The Study of Osteoporotic Fractures. *Arch Intern Med.* 1996;156:1521–1525.

19. Cooper C, Atkinson EJ, Jacobsen SJ, O'Fallon WM, Melton LJ III. Population-based study of survival after osteoporotic fractures. *Am J Epidemiol.* 1993;137:1001–1005.

20. Tajeu GS, Delzell E, Smith W, Arora T, Curtis JR, Saag KG, Morrisey MA, Yun H, Kilgore ML. Death, debility, and destitution following hip fracture. *J Gerontol A Biol Sci Med Sci.* 2014;69(3):346–353.

21. Egol KA, Koval KJ, Zuckerman JD. Functional recovery following hip fracture in the elderly. *J Orthop Trauma.* 1997;11(8):594–599.

22. Moran CG, Wenn RT, Sikand M, Taylor AM. Early mortality after hip fracture: Is delay before surgery important? *J Bone Joint Surg Am.* 2005;87(3):483–489.

23. Puhaindran ME, Farooki A, Steensma MR, Hameed M, Healey JH, Boland PJ. Atypical subtrochanteric femoral fractures in patients with skeletal malignant involvement treated with intravenous bisphosphonates. *J Bone Joint Surg Am.* 2011;93(13):1235–1242.

24. Court-Brown CM, Clement ND, Duckworth AD, Aitken SA, Biant L, Mcqueen MM. The spectrum of fractures in the elderly. *Bone Joint J.* 2014;96-B(3):366–372.

25. Court-Brown CM, Garg A, McQueen MM. The epidemiology of proximal humeral fractures. *Acta Orthop Scand* 2001;72(4):365–371.

26. Rangan A, Handoll H, Brearley S, Jefferson L, Keding A, Martin BC, Goodchild L, Chuang LH, Hewitt C, Togerson D. Surgical vs nonsurgical treatment of adults with displaced fractures of the proximal humerus: The PROFHER randomized clinical trial. *JAMA.* 2015;313(10):1037–1047.

27. Okike K, Lee OC, Makanji H, Morgan JH, Harris MB, Vrahas MS. Comparison of locked plate fixation and nonoperative management for displaced proximal humerus fractures in elderly patients. *Am J Orthop.* 2015;44(4):E106–E112.

28. Feskanich D, Willett W, Colditz G. Walking and leisure-time activity and risk of hip fracture in postmenopausal women. *JAMA.* 2002;288:2300.

29. Kemmler W, Haberle L, von Stengel S. Effects of exercise on fracture reduction in older adults: A systematic review and meta-analysis. *Osteoporosis Int* 2013;24:1937.

30. Rosen HN, Drezner MK. *Overview of the Management of Osteoporosis in Postmenopausal Women.* UpToDate, 2014.

31. Hoidrup S, Prescott E, Sorensen TI, et al. Tobacco smoking and risk of hip fracture in men and women. *Int J Epidemiol.* 2000;29(2):253–259.

32. National Osteoporosis Foundation. *Clinician's Guide to Prevention and Treatment of Osteoporosis.* http://nof.org/files/nof/public/content/file/917/upload/481.pdf (accessed 12 May 2015).

33. Neer RM, Arnaud CD, Zanchetta JR, et al. Effect of parathyroid hormone (1–34) on fractures and bone mineral density in postmenopausal women with osteoporosis. *N Engl J Med.* 2001;344(19):1434–1441.

34. Gourlay ML, Fine JP, Preisser JS, et al. Bone-density testing interval and transition to osteoporosis in older women. *N Engl J Med.* 2012;366:225–233.

35. Watts NB, Bilezikian JP, Camacho PM, et al. American Association of Clinical Endocrinologists medical guidelines for clinical practice for the diagnosis and treatment of postmenopausal osteoporosis. *Endocr Pract* 2010;16(Suppl 3):1.

36. Sale EM, Beaton D, Bogoch E. Secondary prevention after an osteoporosis-related fracture. *Clin Geriatr Med* 2014;30:317–332.

37. Giangregorio L, Papaioannou A, Cranney A, et al. Fragility fractures and the osteoporosis care gap: An international phenomenon. *Semin Arthritis Rheum* 2006;35:293–305.

11

Other bone diseases in the elderly

STUART H. RALSTON

INTRODUCTION

Osteoporosis is by far the most important cause of fragility fractures in elderly people, but causes of musculoskeletal pain, deformity and fractures include metastatic bone disease, Paget's disease of bone (PDB) and osteomalacia. The reader is referred to Chapter 16 for a discussion of metastatic bone disease. Here the clinical presentation, differential diagnosis and treatment of PDB, osteomalacia, complex regional pain syndrome (CRPS), primary hyperparathyroidism (PHPT) and renal bone disease are discussed.

PAGET'S DISEASE OF BONE

PDB is a common metabolic bone disease in people of European descent. At a cellular level it is characterized by focal areas of increased and disorganized bone remodelling which can affect one or several bones in the skeleton.[1] Paget's disease preferentially affects the axial skeleton, and the bones that are most commonly affected include the pelvis, femur, tibia, lumbar spine, skull and scapula.[2] Paget's disease is often asymptomatic and reflecting this fact, it has been estimated that only 10–20% of patients come to medical attention.[3] Bone pain and other complications of the disease are common in those who do present clinically however, leading to significant morbidity in some patients.

Epidemiology

Paget's disease is rare before the age of 40, but gradually increases in incidence thereafter to affect up to 8% of the UK population by the age of 85. Paget's disease is common in Caucasians from north-west and southern Europe but is rare in Scandinavians, Asians, Chinese and Japanese. These ethnic differences persist after migration, supporting the importance of genetic factors in the aetiology. Nonetheless, the incidence of PDB has fallen in most countries over the past 25 years, suggesting that environmental factors also play a role. Suggested environmental triggers for PDB include paramyxovirus infections,[4] dietary calcium deficiency during childhood,[5] vitamin D deficiency,[6] repetitive mechanical loading or skeletal injury[7] and exposure to environmental toxins.[8] Paramyxovirus infection is the only factor that has been investigated experimentally, but the results of studies that have attempted to isolate viral proteins and nucleic acids from Pagetic tissue have been conflicting.[4,9]

Pathophysiology

The primary abnormality is increased osteoclastic bone resorption. The osteoclasts in PDB are larger than normal and some contain nuclear inclusion bodies (Figure 11.1). These were previously thought to represent paramyxovirus nucleocapsids,[10] but there is increasing evidence to suggest that they may be abnormal protein aggregates due to defects of the autophagy pathway.[10] Paget's disease is also associated with increased bone formation, marrow fibrosis and increased vascularity of bone. Although the density of affected bone is often increased due to osteosclerosis, the bone that is formed is structurally abnormal since the bone lamellae are laid down in a chaotic fashion (woven bone), reducing mechanical strength.

Over the past 10 years, it has become clear that genetic factors are important in the pathogenesis of PDB.[11] Many patients have a positive family history of the disease and the risk of PDB developing in a first degree relative of an affected patient is sevenfold increased as compared with an unrelated individual.[12] The disease can also be inherited in an autosomal dominant manner and this pattern is observed in between 15% and 40% of families.[13,14]

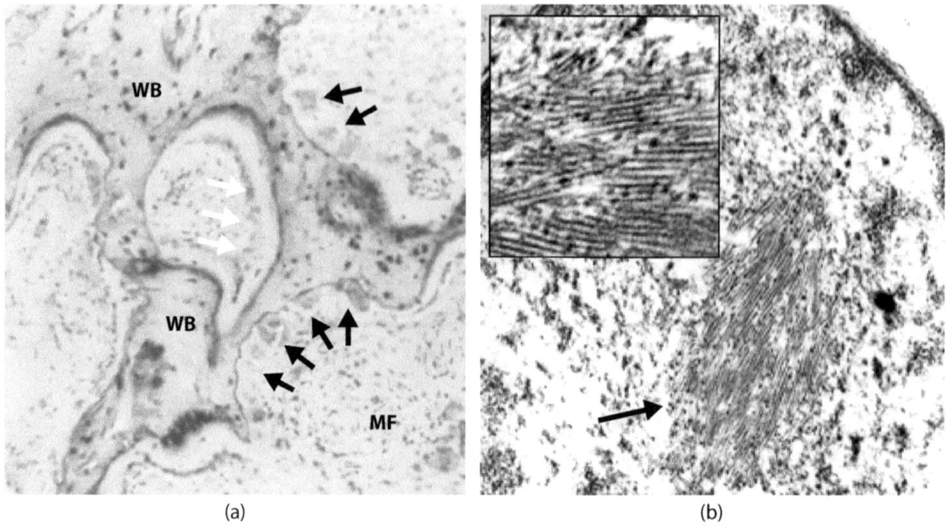

Figure 11.1 Histological features of PDB. **(a)** Toluidine blue stained transiliac bone biopsy in a patient with active Paget's disease. The calcified bone stains dark blue and the osteoid stains light blue. There are typical features of active PDB with a marked increase in osteoclast numbers and eroded surfaces (black arrows) juxtaposed with increased bone formation (white arrows). There is extensive marrow fibrosis (MF) and woven bone (WB). **(b)** Typical nuclear inclusion body in a Pagetic osteoclast visualized by transmission electron microscopy. The inset shows a higher power view of the same lesion.

Linkage analysis in families coupled with genome wide association studies (GWAS) have identified several genes and loci that predispose to PDB.[15–18] These are summarized in Table 11.1. Most implicated genes are known to play a role in osteoclast differentiation or function. The most important PDB-susceptibility gene is *SQSTM1* which lies on chromosome 5q35 and encodes the p62 protein. This protein acts as a scaffold in the receptor activator of the nuclear factor kappa B (RANK) signalling pathway which plays a key role in osteoclast differentiation and activity. The disease associated mutations in PDB cluster in the ubiquitin associated (UBA) domain of the protein and through various mechanisms cause activation of RANK signalling and stimulate osteoclastogenesis.[19,20] The *TNFRSF11A* gene which encodes the receptor activator of RANK is mutated in the rare PDB-like syndromes familial expansile osteolysis (FEO), expansile skeletal hyperphosphatasia (ESH) and early-onset familial Paget's disease (EoPDB). All of these conditions present with an early-onset severe PDB-like phenotype during adolescence. The mutations cluster in the signal peptide and cause osteoclast activation.[11] In addition, GWAS in classical PDB have identified an association between common variants at the *TNFRSF11A* locus and classical PDB. The molecular mechanisms responsible are incompletely understood. Loss of function mutations in the *TNFRSF11B* gene which encodes osteoprotegerin (OPG) cause juvenile PDB which presents with a severe phenotype during childhood. Mutations in the *VCP*, *hnRNPA2B1* and *hnRNPA1* genes cause the rare syndrome of inclusion body myopathy, Paget's disease and frontotemporal dementia. The causal mutations result in accumulation of abnormal protein aggregates in brain, muscle and bone.

The *OPTN* gene on chromosome 10p13 has been implicated as a cause of familial PDB in patients who do not have *SQSTM1* mutations by linkage analysis[21] and as a cause of non-familial PDB by genome wide association analysis.[18] The predisposing variant is associated with reduced mRNA expression of *OPTN*. This suggests that *OPTN* is an inhibitor of osteoclast differentiation and/or activity and that the reduced levels of expression predispose to PDB by causing osteoclast activation. At the present time the disease-causing mutations at the *OPTN* locus have not been identified. GWAS have identified other loci that predispose to PDB within or close to the *CSF1*, *RIN3*, *DCSTAMP*, *NUP205* and *PML* genes.[17,18] The *CSF1* gene encodes macrophage colony stimulating factor which plays an essential role in osteoclast differentiation[22]; the *DCSTAMP* gene encodes dendrocyte expressed seven transmembrane protein which plays an essential role in promoting the fusion of mononuclear osteoclast precursors to multinucleated osteoclasts.[23] At the present time the role of the *RIN3*, *NUP205* and *PML* genes in bone metabolism are unclear, but it seems likely that these genes (or genes nearby) will turn out to play a role in osteoclast differentiation or function.

Clinical features

Paget's disease can present in a variety of ways but the most common is with bone pain, which is the presenting feature in 50–70% of cases. Other modes of presentation include bone deformity, deafness and pathological fractures. In a recent case series from the United Kingdom, pain was a presenting feature in 50%, deformity in 18%, deafness in 6% and pathological fracture in 5%.[24] In the same series,

Table 11.1 Genes and loci that predispose to Paget's disease of bone

Gene	Locus	Mode of discovery	Phenotype	Protein	Function
SQSTM1	5q35	Linkage	PDB	p62	Scaffold protein downstream of RANK involved in NF-κB signalling and autophagy
TNFRSF11A	18q21	Linkage and GWAS	FEO, ESH, EoPDB, PDB	RANK	Essential receptor for osteoclast differentiation and activity
TNFRSF11B	8q24	Linkage, candidate gene	JPD	OPG	Decoy receptor which inhibits osteoclast differentiation and activity
VCP	9q21	Linkage	IBMPFD	VCP	Intracellular protein involved in NF-κB signalling, autophagy and various other functions
hnRNPA2B1	7p15	Linkage and exome sequencing	IBMPFD	Heterogeneous nuclear ribonucleoprotein A2/B1	RNA binding protein, mutations cause proteins to self-assemble into aggregates
hnRNPA1	12q13	Linkage and exome sequencing	IBMPFD	Heterogeneous nuclear ribonucleoprotein A1	RNA binding protein, mutations cause proteins to self-assemble into aggregates
OPTN	10p13	Linkage and GWAS	PDB	Optineurin	Signalling molecule
CSF1	1p13	GWAS	PDB	M-CSF	Essential cytokine for osteoclast and macrophage differentiation
TM7SF4	8q22	GWAS	PDB	DC-STAMP	Essential receptor for fusion of osteoclast precursors to form mature osteoclasts
RIN3	14q32	GWAS	PDB	Rab–Ras interactor protein-3	Involved in vesicular trafficking, role in bone as yet unclear
NUP205	7q33	GWAS	PDB	Nucleoporin 205 kDa	Plays a role in assembly of nuclear pore complex, role in bone unknown
PML	15q24	GWAS	PDB	Promyelocytic leukaemia protein	Plays a role in gene transcription, role in bone unknown

Note: EoPDB, early-onset familial Paget's disease; ESH, expansile skeletal hyperphosphatasia; FEO, familial expansile osteolysis; IBMPFD, inclusion body myopathy associated with Paget's disease of bone and/or frontotemporal dementia; JPD, juvenile Paget's disease; PDB, Paget's disease of bone.

about 20% of patients were truly asymptomatic and the disease was picked up as an incidental finding in patients who had blood tests or X-rays for other reasons.[24]

Clinical signs of PDB include bone deformity and expansion, increased warmth over affected bones, and pathological fracture. Bone deformity is most evident in weight-bearing bones such as the femur and tibia (Figure 11.2), but when the skull is affected the patient may complain that hats no longer fit properly due to cranial enlargement. Neurological problems, such as deafness, cranial nerve defects, nerve root pain, spinal cord compression and spinal stenosis, are recognized complications due to enlargement of affected bones and encroachment upon the spinal cord or cranial nerve foramina. Surprisingly, deafness seldom results from compression of the auditory nerve, but is instead conductive in nature due to osteosclerosis of the temporal bone.[25,26] The increased vascularity of Pagetic bone has been reported to precipitate high-output cardiac failure in elderly patients with limited cardiac reserve, but this is extremely rare. Hypercalcaemia may occur in patients who are immobilized. Osteosarcoma is a rare but serious complication affecting less than 0.01% of cases. The presentation is with worsening pain and/or swelling of an affected site.

Investigations

The diagnosis of PDB can usually be made by X-ray, which shows the typical features of bone expansion with an

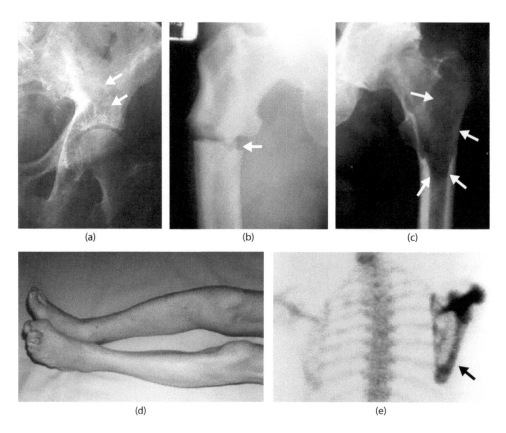

(a)   (b)   (c)

(d)   (e)

Figure 11.2 Clinical and radiographic features of PDB. (a) Radiograph of a patient with PDB of the left hemipelvis showing abnormal trabecular architecture with alternating areas of osteosclerosis and osteolysis (white arrows). (b) Pathological fracture (white arrow) in a patient with Paget's disease of the right femur. (c) Osteolytic lesion of the femoral shaft of a patient with Paget's disease of the left femur. The lytic area is highlighted by white arrows. There is also osteosclerosis of the femoral head and secondary osteoarthritis of the hip joint. (d) Tibial deformity in a patient with PDB. (e) Radionuclide bone scan of a patient with Paget's disease of the scapula showing intense homogeneous tracer uptake of the affected bone.

abnormal trabecular pattern, cortical thickening and alternating areas of radiolucency and osteosclerosis (Figure 11.2). The serum levels of alkaline phosphatase (ALP) are typically raised but may be normal, either because the disease is limited to a single bone, or because the disease is metabolically inactive. Routine biochemical tests in PDB are otherwise normal, resulting in a pattern of an 'isolated' elevation in ALP which is typical of the disease. Radionuclide bone scanning is a useful way of defining the presence and extent of PDB since tracer is avidly taken up by sites in which bone turnover is increased. This gives a picture of intense contiguous tracer uptake in an affected bone which is virtually diagnostic (Figure 11.2). Paget's disease can occasionally be confused with osteosclerotic metastases. Although the radiographic and bone scan appearances usually allow the correct diagnosis to be made, bone biopsy of an affected site can sometimes be required. In this regard it should be noted that PDB and bone metastases can co-exist.

Monitoring levels of metabolic activity in PDB is most easily and conveniently done by measurements of ALP which are raised in patients with high bone turnover and lowered by bisphosphonate therapy and other antiresorptive agents used in the treatment of PDB. Although ALP

levels give an indication of the levels of bone turnover in PDB, they do not correlate well with symptoms such as bone pain[1] and have not as yet been shown to act as a predictor of complications such as fracture or deformity.

Medical management

The main aim of medical management is to improve bone pain and this can be addressed by antiresorptive therapy or by the use of analgesics. There is no evidence as yet to show that medical treatment can prevent or reverse complications of PDB such as fracture, deformity, deafness and osteoarthritis.[2]

The increased bone turnover in PDB can be reduced by therapy with osteoclast inhibitors. Although various osteoclast inhibitors have been used in PDB, the current treatments of choice are bisphosphonates. Bisphosphonates are a class of compounds related to pyrophosphate in which phosphonate groups are linked by a carbon atom to which various side chains can be attached.[27] The phosphonate moiety binds calcium and causes the bisphosphonates to bind avidly to hydroxyapatite crystals in bone. Bisphosphonates particularly target to areas of increased bone turnover when they are taken up by osteoclasts that resorb bone. The bisphosphonate is then released within the osteoclast, impairing cellular function and causing cell death, making them ideal candidates for the treatment of PDB.[1]

The main indication for treatment with bisphosphonates in PDB is bone pain localized to an affected site which is thought to be due to increased metabolic activity.[1] Although bisphosphonates are effective at treating bone pain secondary to active PDB, it is sometimes difficult to differentiate this type of pain from that caused by a co-existing condition such as osteoarthritis or nerve compression. Therefore careful clinical evaluation is required to determine the likely cause of the pain in patients with PDB. This is not always easy; indeed in a recent case series from a specialist clinic, about one third of patients thought to have pain due to increased metabolic activity did not respond to bisphosphonate treatment, indicating that another cause may have been responsible.

Several bisphosphonates have been licensed for the treatment of PDB but the most widely used are the nitrogen containing bisphosphonates pamidronate, zoledronate and risedronate (Table 11.2). These are more effective than simple bisphosphonates such as etidronate and tiludronate at suppressing bone turnover in PDB. Zoledronic acid in particular is highly effective at restoring levels of bone turnover to normal in PDB with effects that last for several years after a single infusion.[33] It should be noted that the effectiveness with which bisphosphonates suppress bone turnover correlates poorly with the response of pain. This is most probably due to the fact that pain can arise from causes other than increased metabolic activity and that it may not be necessary to completely normalize bone turnover to get a positive response on pain.[2] Calcitonin is very occasionally used in the treatment of PDB where bisphosphonates are contraindicated. However this is less convenient to administer than bisphosphonates, is much more expensive and has a short duration of action. Repeated courses of antiresorptive drugs can be given if symptoms recur, particularly if this is accompanied by evidence of increased bone turnover.

Bone pain in PDB can also be treated with analgesics, non-steroidal anti-inflammatory drugs (NSAID) and anti-neuropathic agents. Although these agents have not specifically been studied in clinical trials of bone pain in PDB, clinical experience indicates that they are often effective. Indeed, in the Paget's Disease Randomized Trial of Intensive versus Symptomatic Management (PRISM) trial, therapy with analgesics and other painkillers coupled with intermittent bisphosphonate therapy in patients who did not respond adequately was found to be equivalent to intensive bisphosphonate therapy in the treatment of Pagetic bone pain.[2]

Surgical treatment

There are several indications for surgical treatment of PDB (Table 11.3), but the three most common are pathological fractures, osteoarthritis and spinal stenosis.

In general terms, surgical treatment of PDB can be challenging due to the increased vascularity of bone, bone deformity and osteosclerosis, but despite this the results of surgical treatment for PDB are generally good.[34] In particular, fracture healing in PDB seems to proceed normally with no real evidence to suggest an increased risk of non-union or delayed union.[35]

It has been traditionally considered that patients with PDB should be treated with osteoclast inhibitors to try and normalize bone turnover before surgery goes ahead, but there is no good evidence to suggest that this makes any difference. Indeed the only study to look at this, which was only published in abstract form, showed no evidence of a difference in blood loss in PDB patients treated with bisphosphonates as opposed to those who were untreated.

Orthopaedic surgery may also be required in patients who develop osteosarcoma, but the prognosis is poor even

Table 11.2 Bisphosphonates used in the treatment of Paget's disease

Drug	Regimen	Normalization of alkaline phosphatase	References
Etidronate	400 mg daily orally for 3–6 months	5–17%	Roux et al.,[28] Miller et al.,[29] Siris et al.[30]
Tiludronate	400 mg daily orally for 3–6 months	17%	Roux et al.[28]
Pamidronate[a]	60 mg i.v. on 3 days	56%	Walsh et al.[31]
Alendronate[b]	40 mg daily orally for 3 months	63–71%	Siris et al.,[30] Walsh et al.[31]
Risedronate	30 mg orally for 2 months	53–60%	Reid et al.,[32] Miller et al.[29]
Zoledronic acid	5 mg i.v. as a single infusion	88%	Reid et al.[32]

[a] Various other regimens have been used including 15, 30 and 45 mg i.v. on one or multiple occasions.
[b] Alendronate is not licensed in the United Kingdom or Europe for the treatment of PDB.

Table 11.3 Role of surgical treatment in Paget's disease of bone

Indication	Surgical technique
Osteoarthritis	Joint replacement surgery
Fracture	Fracture reduction with intramedullary nailing, pinning or plating
Long bone deformity	Osteotomy
Spinal stenosis	Spinal decompression
Impending fracture	Prophylactic intramedullary nailing, pinning or plating
Osteosarcoma	Tumour excision or amputation

with aggressive operative treatment with an overall 5-year survival of about 6%.[36]

OSTEOMALACIA

Osteomalacia is a syndrome characterized by defective mineralization of bone. By far the most common cause in elderly people is chronic vitamin D deficiency, but in the paediatric population and younger individuals it can be caused by genetic defects in the pathways involved in the activation and action of vitamin D and renal tubular phosphate absorption. A very rare cause is ectopic production of the hormone FGF23 by tumours. Osteomalacia is characterized clinically by bone and muscle pain, muscle weakness, fragility fractures and pseudofractures.

Epidemiology

Osteomalacia, once a common condition in the United Kingdom and other northern European countries, is now quite rare. It is difficult to estimate the incidence and prevalence of osteomalacia since the diagnosis is made clinically and/or histologically. Therefore information on the prevalence of osteomalacia principally comes from case series of patients who have presented to hospital with signs of symptoms of the disease or patients who have undergone bone biopsies. During the 1970s several studies from the United Kingdom indicated that osteomalacia predominantly affects Asian immigrants. For example in a series of 45 osteomalacia patients who presented to the Royal National Orthopaedic Hospital in London between 1975 and 1979, 44 (97%) were of Asian origin.[37] Similar findings were reported in studies from Glasgow in Scotland.[38] It is thought that the higher prevalence of osteomalacia in people of Asian origin is due to reduced synthesis of vitamin D in the skin and the practice of covering the skin in some Moslem women. Elderly housebound individuals are also at increased risk of osteomalacia and this may contribute in part to the pathogenesis of hip fractures in some patients. One study, based in Leeds during the 1970s, reported evidence of osteomalacia in 20–30% of hip fracture patients,[39] whereas another study, performed around the same time

in Cardiff, reported a prevalence of 5%,[40] The largest case series comes from the study of Priemel and colleagues who examined bone biopsies for evidence of osteomalacia in 675 subjects from the Hamburg area in Northern Germany who had died suddenly as the result of trauma, suicide and other causes. The cohort comprised 410 males of average age 58 years and 274 females of average age 68 years. In this study the investigators reported that about 1% of patients had osteomalacia as defined by an osteoid volume/bone volume of greater than 10%, which has previously been suggested as a threshold to make this diagnosis.[41]

Pathophysiology

The causes of osteomalacia are summarized in Table 11.4. Osteomalacia can be caused by deficiency of vitamin D (cholecalciferol) as the result of poor diet, malabsorption or lack of sunlight exposure, genetic defects in vitamin D metabolism and genetic defects in renal phosphate handling. Osteomalacia may also be caused by certain drugs and by over production of the hormone FGF23 by tumours. There are various causes of osteomalacia as will be discussed below and traditionally vitamin D deficient osteomalacia has been considered the most common. The relative frequency of these different causes has been little studied, but in a recently published series of 28 osteomalacia patients referred to a teaching hospital in Barcelona over a 20-year period, about half had osteomalacia related to vitamin D deficiency and half had osteomalacia due to hypophosphataemia.[42] Since the predominant cause of osteomalacia in the elderly is vitamin D deficiency, discussion of pathophysiology in this chapter will focus on mechanisms of vitamin D deficient rickets.

Table 11.4 Causes of osteomalacia

Cause	Mechanism
Vitamin D deficiency	Lack of sunlight exposure, poor diet or malabsorption
Chronic renal disease	Reduced production of $1,25(OH)_2D$ due to renal failure
Vitamin D resistant rickets	Loss of function mutations in the vitamin D receptor
Vitamin D dependent rickets	Loss of function mutations in CYPD17
Hereditary hypophosphataemic rickets	Renal phosphate wasting and hypophosphataemia
Aluminium	Physicochemical inhibition of mineralization
Bisphosphonates	Physicochemical inhibition of mineralization
Hypophosphatasia	Impaired mineralization due to accumulation of pyrophosphate caused by loss of function mutations in TNALP

The key steps in vitamin D metabolism are illustrated in Figure 11.3. Circulating vitamin D is derived from two sources. Endogenous synthesis occurs as the result of the action of ultraviolet light (UV) in the skin which converts 7-dehydrocholesterol to cholecalciferol. The remainder is absorbed from the diet. It has been estimated that about 70% of vitamin D is derived from the skin and 30% from the diet. Once in the circulation, vitamin D undergoes hydroxylation at the 25 position in the liver to give 25(OH)D and a second hydroxylation in the renal tubules to produce the active metabolite 1,25(OH)$_2$D. If production of vitamin D by the skin or absorption from the gut falls, there is a concomitant reduction in hepatic production of 25(OH)D. This in turn leads to a reduction in the amount of 1,25(OH)$_2$D produced by the kidney. Calcium absorption from the gut falls because of the low levels of 1,25(OH)$_2$D and this causes serum calcium levels to fall and parathyroid hormone (PTH) secretion to increase. The raised levels of PTH increase bone turnover and promote renal tubular phosphate excretion in an attempt to raise extracellular calcium levels. Initially these homeostatic responses are sufficient to maintain normocalcaemia, but if vitamin D deficiency persists in the longer term, there is progressive demineralization of bone with loss of both calcium and phosphate from the skeleton, resulting in accumulation of poorly mineralized bone.

Clinical features

During the early stages, osteomalacia may be asymptomatic or present with non-specific symptoms such as malaise and weakness. As the disease progresses, patients may experience muscle pain and weakness, bone pain, general malaise and fractures. The proximal limb muscles are particularly affected, causing the patient to walk with a waddling gait and struggle to climb stairs or get out of a chair. On clinical examination, bone pain and muscle tenderness may be detected and focal bone pain may occur due to fissure fractures of the ribs and pelvis.

Investigations

Typical findings on a routine biochemistry screen are raised levels of ALP, normal or low levels of serum calcium and low levels of serum phosphate. Serum levels of 25(OH)D are undetectable and PTH levels raised in untreated osteomalacia. Skeletal radiographs typically show osteopenia and with advanced disease pseudofractures may be observed in the ribs, pelvis or long bones (Figure 11.4). Vertebral fractures may be observed. Radionuclide bone scans may show multiple hot spots in the ribs and pelvis at the site of pseudofractures with appearances that can sometimes be confused with bone metastases. The diagnosis can be proven by transiliac bone biopsy, which shows the increased thickness and

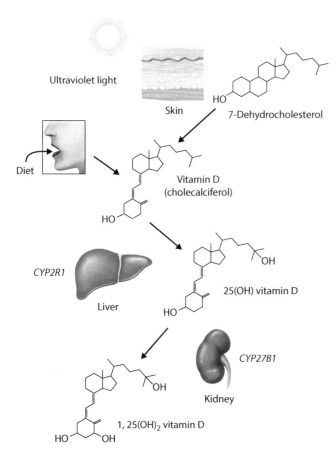

Figure 11.3 Vitamin D metabolism. Vitamin D is derived from the diet and conversion of 7-dehydrocholesterol in the skin. It then undergoes hydroxylation at the 25 position in the liver by the enzyme CYP2R1 and further hydroxylation in the kidney by the enzyme CYP2B1 to produce the active metabolite 1,25(OH)$_2$D. The 1,25(OH)$_2$D interacts with vitamin D receptors in the gut to increase calcium absorption and in the skeleton to regulate bone cell differentiation and function.

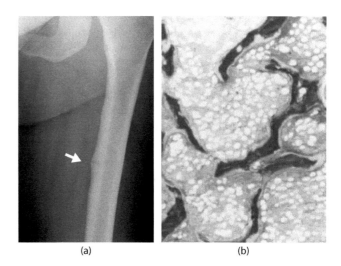

Figure 11.4 Radiographic and histological features of osteomalacia. **(a)** A pseudofracture in a patient with severe vitamin D deficiency. **(b)** Toluidine blue stained transiliac bone biopsy from a patient with osteomalacia. Calcified bone is stained dark blue and osteoid light blue. Virtually all of the bone surfaces are covered with thick osteoid consistent with severe osteomalacia.

extent of osteoid seams (Figure 11.4), although this is not necessary in patients with typical clinical and biochemical features of the disease.

Management

Vitamin D deficient osteomalacia responds promptly to treatment with vitamin D. Various dose regimens have been used with no evidence to suggest that one regimen is superior to another. One approach is to give 3200 units of vitamin D daily for up to 12–24 weeks, reducing thereafter to a maintenance dose of between 400 and 800 units daily depending on the response of ALP, serum calcium and serum phosphate. Another is to give a higher dose of vitamin D once or twice weekly (25,000–50,000 units) for up to 10 weeks and then to reduce to a maintenance dose of 400 or 800 units daily. There is often a rapid improvement in symptoms and general well-being following initiation of vitamin D therapy. Serum ALP levels may rise initially as the bone re-mineralizes but eventually ALP levels fall to within the normal range as the bone disease heals. Failure of the patient to respond clinically or biochemically suggests an alternative diagnosis such as hypophosphataemic osteomalacia.

Patients with hypophosphataemic osteomalacia and osteomalacia associated with chronic renal impairment require treatment with active vitamin D metabolites – either 1-alpha-hydroxyvitamin D or 1,25 dihydroxyvitamin D in doses of 1–3 micrograms daily. Patients with tumour induced osteomalacia may also require phosphate supplements.

METASTATIC BONE DISEASE

This may present in a variety of ways with localized or generalized progressive bone pain, generalized regional pain, symptoms of spinal cord compression or acute pain due to pathological fracture. Systemic features, such as weight loss and anorexia, and symptoms referable to the primary tumour are often present. Tumours which most commonly metastasize to bone are myeloma and tumours of the bronchus, breast, prostate, kidney and thyroid. More details are given in Chapter 16.

COMPLEX REGIONAL PAIN SYNDROME

CRPS, also known as reflex sympathetic dystrophy syndrome or algodystrophy, presents with gradual onset of local pain, swelling and tenderness, usually affecting a limb extremity. It can also affect the proximal femur when it is known as transient osteoporosis of the hip. It is characterized by localized osteoporosis of the affected bone and evidence of autonomic dysfunction, with abnormal sweating, colour and temperature change of the overlying skin. The cause is unknown but overactivity of the sympathetic nervous system is thought to be responsible for many of its features. Predisposing conditions are fracture, soft tissue

injury, pregnancy and intercurrent illnesses. It has been estimated that up to 25% of patients with Colles' fracture may develop CRPS to some degree.[43] It can also be associated with soft tissue injury, pregnancy and intercurrent illness or can develop spontaneously.

There are no abnormalities on biochemical or haematological testing, but radiographs show localized osteoporosis of the affected site. Radionuclide bone scans show a patchy localized increase in tracer uptake, whereas MRI scanning may show local bone marrow oedema. The differential diagnosis includes infection and malignancy. Usually the diagnosis of CRPS is clear on clinical grounds and by absence of an acute phase response or other systemic features of malignancy, but a biopsy of the affected site can be undertaken if necessary. In CRPS this typically shows local osteopenia only.

The aims of treatment are to control pain and encourage mobilization. Many treatments have been tried including analgesics, NSAID, anti-neuropathic agents, calcitonin, corticosteroids, β-adrenoceptor antagonists (β-blockers), sympathectomy and bisphosphonates, but none are particularly effective. In most cases the condition gradually improves spontaneously with time, although many patients have persistent symptoms and fail to regain normal function or mobility.

PRIMARY HYPERPARATHYROIDISM

PHPT affects about 0.15% of the population. Women are affected about three times more commonly than men and more than 90% of patients are over the age of 50 years. It is usually caused by an adenoma of one of the parathyroid glands. Many patients with PHPT are asymptomatic and the condition is discovered as an incidental finding on routine biochemical testing. The typical picture is hypercalcaemia with a low or low normal serum phosphate level and a normal or elevated serum PTH. Patients with PHPT are at an increased risk of developing osteoporosis since the raised levels of PTH stimulate bone resorption more than bone formation, resulting in bone loss, particularly in postmenopausal women. Accordingly the most common skeletal manifestation of PHPT is osteoporosis, which is discussed in more detail in Chapter 10.

Rarely PHPT can present with specific abnormalities in the skeleton, referred to as parathyroid bone disease. Patients with parathyroid bone disease tend to have large adenomas or parathyroid carcinomas, severe hypercalcaemia and elevated ALP levels. Serum phosphate levels are low and PTH levels are usually markedly elevated. Bone biopsies of these patients show markedly increased bone resorption and bone formation with marrow fibrosis – an appearance referred to as osteitis fibrosa cystica. The classical radiological feature of parathyroid bone disease is subperiosteal bone erosions which can be detected on hand radiographs although the condition can also present with focal osteolytic lesions that may be mistaken for bone metastases. Parathyroid bone disease can easily be differentiated from cancer associated bone disease by the fact that PTH levels are elevated in the former condition but low or undetectable in the latter.

Parathyroidectomy is advisable in patients with PHPT who have osteoporosis and those who have parathyroid bone disease. If surgery cannot be performed for any reason then osteoporosis can be treated with bisphosphonates or hormone replacement therapy.[44] Clinical experience indicates that osteoporosis often improves following parathyroidectomy in patients with mild PHPT.[45] Similarly, parathyroid bone disease also heals following parathyroidectomy although patients may experience hypocalcaemia postoperatively due to the 'hungry bone syndrome'. This is thought to be due to rapid mineralization of the skeleton as calcium from the extracellular compartment becomes deposited in osteoid. Anecdotal experience suggests that the risk of this can be minimized by giving calcium supplements and active metabolites of vitamin D preoperatively and for a few days postoperatively.

RENAL BONE DISEASE

Patients with chronic kidney disease (CKD) are at greatly increased risk of bone disease and this may take several forms, including osteoporosis, osteomalacia and secondary hyperparathyroidism. Osteoporosis is the most common problem and reflecting this fact, patients with CKD are at markedly increased risk of fracture as compared with the general population.[46] The sequence of events underlying these abnormalities is complex as depicted in Figure 11.5. There is reduced production of $1,25(OH)_2D$ due in part to an inhibitory effect of hyperphosphataemia on the CYP27B1 enzyme in the renal tubules. Production of the phosphaturic hormone FGF23 by osteocytes is increased in response to hyperphosphataemia and this also exerts an inhibitory effect on *CYP27B1*. Serum calcium levels fall as the result of the hyperphosphataemia which makes complexes with calcium causing soft tissue calcification and as the result of reduced intestinal calcium absorption because of the low $125(OH)_2D$ levels. This stimulates PTH secretion from the

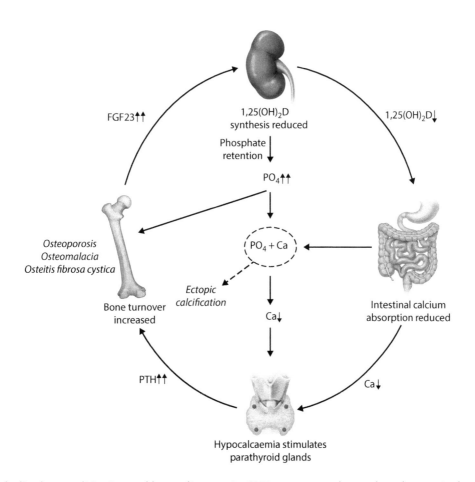

Figure 11.5 Metabolic abnormalities in renal bone disease. As CKD progresses, hyperphosphataemia develops, which causes hypocalcaemia by complexing with calcium and reducing $1,25(OH)_2D$ synthesis, thereby reducing intestinal calcium absorption. The hypocalcaemia stimulates PTH secretion by the parathyroid glands which increases bone turnover predisposing to osteoporosis, osteomalacia and osteitis fibrosa cystica (see text for details). Production of FGF23 by osteocytes in bone is increased in CKD as the result of hypophosphataemia. Although FGF23 normally causes phosphaturia, it is ineffective in CKD due to renal tubular damage and contributes to the pathogenesis of hypocalcaemia by inhibiting $1,25(OH)_2D$ production.

parathyroid glands, which increases bone turnover causing bone loss and in some cases, osteitis fibrosa cystica and osteomalacia.

The most common presentation is with fractures secondary to osteoporosis. Treatment of this is difficult since bisphosphonates – the most widely used drugs – are contraindicated in patients with a glomerular filtration rate (GFR) below 30. Denosumab is a potential option but experience in patients with advanced CKD is limited. Secondary hyperparathyroidism associated with CKD is usually treated with active metabolites of vitamin D (either alfacalcidiol or calcitriol) in combination with phosphate binders to prevent the development of hyperphosphataemia and ectopic calcification. In some patients it may be impossible to control hyperparathyroidism by medical means due to autonomous production of PTH by the parathyroid glands. This is referred to as tertiary hyperparathyroidism. This usually requires subtotal parathyroidectomy. Medical treatment with calcimimetic drugs such as cinacalcet which inhibit PTH production by the parathyroid gland are being explored as a medical treatment for hyperparathyroidism associated with CKD.[47]

REFERENCES

1. Ralston, S. H. Clinical practice. Paget's disease of bone. *N Engl J Med* 368 (2013): 644–50.
2. Langston, A. L., Campbell, M. K., Fraser, W. D., MacLennan, G. S., Selby, P. L., and Ralston, S. H. Randomised trial of intensive bisphosphonate treatment versus symptomatic management in Paget's disease of bone. *J Bone Miner Res* 25 (2010): 20–31.
3. van Staa, T. P., Selby, P., Leufkens, H. G., Lyles, K., Sprafka, J. M., and Cooper, C. Incidence and natural history of Paget's disease of bone in England and Wales. *J Bone Miner Res* 17 (2002): 465–71.
4. Rima, B. K., Gassen, U., Helfrich, M. H., and Ralston, S. H. The pro and con of measles virus in Paget's disease: Con. *J Bone Miner Res* 17 (2002): 2290–2.
5. Siris, E. S. Epidemiological aspects of Paget's disease: Family history and relationship to other medical conditions. *Semin Arthritis Rheum* 23 (1994): 222–5.
6. Barker, D. J., and Gardner, M. J. Distribution of Paget's disease in England, Wales and Scotland and a possible relationship with vitamin D deficiency in childhood. *Br J Prev Soc Med* 28 (1974): 226–32.
7. Solomon, L. R. Billiard-player's fingers: An unusual case of Paget's disease of bone. *Br Med J* 1 (1979): 931.
8. Lever, J. H. Paget's disease of bone in Lancashire and arsenic pesticide in cotton mill wastewater: A speculative hypothesis. *Bone* 31 (2002): 434–6.
9. Helfrich, M. H., Hobson, R. P., Grabowski, P. S., Zurbriggen, A., Cosby, S. L., Dickson, G. R., Fraser, W. D., et al. A negative search for a paramyxoviral etiology of Paget's disease of bone: Molecular, immunological, and ultrastructural studies in UK patients. *J Bone Miner Res* 15 (2000): 2315–29.
10. Rebel, A., Malkani, K., Basle, M., and Bregeon, Ch. Particularites ultrastructurales des osteoclasts de la maladie de Paget. *Rev Rhum Mal Osteoartic* 41 (1974): 767–71.
11. Ralston, S. H., and Layfield, R. Pathogenesis of Paget disease of bone. *Calcif Tissue Int* 91 (2012): 97–113.
12. Siris, E. S., Ottman, R., Flaster, E., and Kelsey, J. L. Familial aggregation of Paget's disease of bone. *J Bone Miner Res* 6 (1991): 495–500.
13. Hocking, L., Slee, F., Haslam, S. I., Cundy, T., Nicholson, G., Van Hul, W., and Ralston, S. H. Familial Paget's disease of bone: Patterns of inheritance and frequency of linkage to chromosome 18q. *Bone* 26 (2000): 577–80.
14. Morales-Piga, A. A., Rey-Rey, J. S., Corres-Gonzalez, J., Garcia-Sagredo, J. M., and Lopez-Abente, G. Frequency and characteristics of familial aggregation of Paget's disease of bone. *J Bone Miner Res* 10 (1995): 663–70.
15. Laurin, N., Brown, J. P., Lemainque, A., Duchesne, A., Huot, D., Lacourciere, Y., Drapeau, G., Verreault, J., Raymond, V., and Morissette, J. Paget disease of bone: Mapping of two loci at 5q35-qter and 5q31. *Am J Hum Genet* 69 (2001): 528–43.
16. Hocking, L. J., Herbert, C. A., Nicholls, R. K., Williams, F., Bennett, S. T., Cundy, T., Nicholson, G. C., Wuyts, W., Van Hul, W., and Ralston, S. H. Genomewide search in familial Paget disease of bone shows evidence of genetic heterogeneity with candidate loci on chromosomes 2q36, 10p13, and 5q35. *Am J Hum Genet* 69 (2001): 1055–61.
17. Albagha, O. M. E., Wani, S., Visconti, M. R., Alonso, N., Goodman, K., Cundy, T., Brandi, M. L., et al. Genome-wide association identifies three new susceptibility loci for Paget's disease of bone. *Nat Genet* 43 (2011): 685–9.
18. Albagha, O. M., Visconti, M. R., Alonso, N., Langston, A. L., Cundy, T., Dargie, R., Dunlop, M. G., et al. Genome-wide association study identifies variants at CSF1, OPTN and TNFRSF11A as genetic risk factors for Paget's disease of bone. *Nat Genet* 42 (2010): 520–24.
19. Jin, W., Chang, M., Paul, E. M., Babu, G., Lee, A. J., Reiley, W., Wright, A., Zhang, M., You, J., and Sun, S. C. Deubiquitinating enzyme CYLD negatively regulates RANK signaling and osteoclastogenesis in mice. *J Clin Invest* 118 (2008): 1858–66.
20. Chamoux, E., Couture, J., Bisson, M., Morissette, J., Brown, J. P., and Roux, S. The p62 P392L mutation linked to Paget's disease induces activation of human osteoclasts. *Mol Endocrinol* 23 (2009): 1668–80.
21. Lucas, G., Riches, P., Hocking, L., Cundy, T., Nicholson, G., Walsh, J., and Ralston, S. H. Identification of a major locus for Paget disease on chromosome 10p13 in families of British descent. *J Bone Miner Res* 23 (2008): 58–63.

22. Dobbins, D. E., Sood, R., Hashiramoto, A., Hansen, C. T., Wilder, R. L., and Remmers, E. F. Mutation of macrophage colony stimulating factor (Csf1) causes osteopetrosis in the tl rat. *Biochem Biophys Res Commun* 294 (2002): 1114–20.

23. Yagi, M., Miyamoto, T., Sawatani, Y., Iwamoto, K., Hosogane, N., Fujita, N., Morita, K., et al. DC-STAMP is essential for cell-cell fusion in osteoclasts and foreign body giant cells. *J Exp Med* 202 (2005): 345–51.

24. Tan, A., and Ralston, S. H. Clinical presentation of Paget's disease: Evaluation of a contemporary cohort and systematic review. *Calcif Tissue Int* 95 (2014): 385–92.

25. Monsell, E. M., Cody, D. D., Bone, H. G., Divine, G. W., Windham, J. P., Jacobson, G. P., Newman, C. W., and Patel, S. C. Hearing loss in Paget's disease of bone: The relationship between pure-tone thresholds and mineral density of the cochlear capsule. *Hear Res* 83 (1995): 114–20.

26. Monsell, E. M., Bone, H. G., Cody, D. D., Jacobson, G. P., Newman, C. W., Patel, S. C., and Divine, G. W. Hearing loss in Paget's disease of bone: Evidence of auditory nerve integrity. *Am J Otol* 16 (1995): 27–33.

27. Russell, R. G. Bisphosphonates: The first 40 years. *Bone* 49 (2011): 2–19.

28. Roux, C., Gennari, C., Farrerons, J., Devogelaer, J. P., Mulder, H., Kruse, H. P., Picot, C., Titeux, L., Reginster, J. Y., and Dougados, M. Comparative prospective, double-blind, multicenter study of the efficacy of tiludronate and etidronate in the treatment of Paget's disease of bone. *Arthritis Rheum* 38 (1995): 851–8.

29. Miller, P. D., Brown, J. P, Siris, E. S., Hoseyni, M. S., Axelrod, D. W., and Bekker, P. J. A randomized, double-blind comparison of risedronate and etidronate in the treatment of Paget's disease of bone. Paget's Risedronate/Etidronate Study Group. *Am J Med* 106 (1999): 513–20.

30. Siris, E. S., Weinstein, R. S., Altman, R., Conte, J. M., Favus, M., Lombardi, A., Lyles, K., et al. Comparative study of alendronate versus etidronate for the treatment of Paget's disease of bone. *J Clin Endocrinol Metab* 81 (1996): 961–7.

31. Walsh, J. P., Ward, L. C., Stewart, G. O., Will, R. K., Criddle, R. A., Prince, R. L., Stuckey, B. G., et al. A randomized clinical trial comparing oral alendronate and intravenous pamidronate for the treatment of Paget's disease of bone. *Bone* 34 (2004): 747–54.

32. Reid, I. R., Miller, P., Lyles, K., Fraser, W., Brown, J. P., Saidi, Y., Mesenbrink, P., et al. Comparison of a single infusion of zoledronic acid with risedronate for Paget's disease. *N Engl J Med* 353 (2005): 898–908.

33. Hosking, D., Lyles, K., Brown, J. P., Fraser, W. D., Miller, P., Curiel, M. D., Devogelaer, J. P., et al. Long-term control of bone turnover in Paget's disease with zoledronic acid and risedronate. *J Bone Miner Res* 22 (2007): 142–8.

34. Kaplan, F. S. Surgical management of Paget's disease. *J Bone Miner Res* 14(Suppl 2) (1999): 34–8.

35. Parvizi, J., Klein, G. R., and Sim, F. H. Surgical management of Paget's disease of bone. *J Bone Miner Res* 21(Suppl 2) (2006): 75–82.

36. Sharma, H., Jane, M. J., and Reid, R. Scapulohumeral Paget's sarcoma: Scottish Bone Tumour Registry experience. *Eur J Cancer Care (Engl)* 14 (2005): 367–72.

37. Stamp, T. C., Walker, P. G., Perry, W., and Jenkins, M. V. Nutritional osteomalacia and late rickets in Greater London, 1974–1979: Clinical and metabolic studies in 45 patients. *Clin Endocrinol Metab* 9 (1980): 81–105.

38. Ford, J. A., Colhoun, E. M., McIntosh, W. B., and Dunnigan, M. G. Rickets and osteomalacia in the Glasgow Pakistani community, 1961–71. *Br Med J* 2 (1972): 677–80.

39. Aaron, J. E., Gallagher, J. C., Anderson, J., Stasiak, L., Longton, E. B., Nordin, B. E., and Nicholson, M. Frequency of osteomalacia and osteoporosis in fractures of the proximal femur. *Lancet* 1 (1974): 229–33.

40. Compston, J. E., Vedi, S., and Croucher, P. I. Low prevalence of osteomalacia in elderly patients with hip fracture. *Age Ageing* 20 (1991): 132–4.

41. Priemel, M., von Domarus, C., Klatte, T. O., Kessler, S., Schlie, J., Meier, S., Proksch, N., et al. Bone mineralization defects and vitamin D deficiency: histomorphometric analysis of iliac crest bone biopsies and circulating 25-hydroxyvitamin D in 675 patients. *J Bone Miner Res* 25 (2010): 305–12.

42. Gifre, L., Peris, P., Monegal, A., Martinez de Osaba, M. J., Alvarez, L., and Guanabens, N. Osteomalacia revisited: A report on 28 cases. *Clin Rheumatol* 30 (2011): 639–45.

43. Atkins, R. M., Duckworth, T., and Kanis, J. A. Algodystrophy following Colles' fracture. *J Hand Surg Br* 14 (1989): 161–4.

44. Langdahl, B. L., and Ralston, S. H. Diagnosis and management of primary hyperparathyroidism in Europe. *QJM* 105 (2012): 519–25.

45. Silverberg, S. J., Shane, E., Jacobs, T. P., Siris, E., and Bilezikian, J. P. A 10-year prospective study of primary hyperparathyroidism with or without parathyroid surgery. *N Engl J Med* 341 (1999): 1249–55.

46. Nickolas, T. L., McMahon, D. J., and Shane, E. Relationship between moderate to severe kidney disease and hip fracture in the United States. *J Am Soc Nephrol* 17 (2006): 3223–32.

47. Nemeth, E. F., and Shoback, D. Calcimimetic and calcilytic drugs for treating bone and mineral-related disorders. *Best Pract Res Clin Endocrinol Metab* 27 (2013): 373–84.

12

Falls

ODDOM DEMONTIERO, DEREK BOERSMA AND GUSTAVO DUQUE

INTRODUCTION

The incidence of falls and related injuries will continue to pose significant challenges to healthcare systems globally as the world's population ages. This chapter describes the epidemiology, aetiologies, consequences and prevention of falls in the community, acute and long-term care settings.

DEFINITION OF FALLS

Earlier falls research employed inconsistent definitions of falls in the older age group, but one of the most accepted is that by Tinetti et al.[1] which defined a fall in the non-hospitalized geriatric patient as 'an event which results in a person coming to rest unintentionally on the ground or lower level, not as a result of a major intrinsic event (such as a stroke) or overwhelming hazard'. A similar definition is also used for the in-patient and long-term setting. The *International Classification of Diseases, Tenth Revision* defines several codes for falls, each with broad descriptions reflecting the place of occurrence and activity, such as a fall on the same level from slipping, tripping and stumbling (w01), to other fall on the same level including a fall from bumping against an object and from or off a toilet (w18).

EPIDEMIOLOGY OF FALLS

A myriad of studies on falls over the last three decades have reported different incidences. Varied definitions of falls used, marked heterogeneity of studied populations, differences in data collection methods, poor recall by participants particularly in retrospective studies and under-reporting of falls in cases without associated injuries are contributing factors.

Community setting

Approximately one in three adults above the age of 65 fall at least once in a year, increasing to more than one in two in the 85+ age group. Of those who fall in one year, half to two-thirds experience a repeat fall in the subsequent year. The majority of falls occur indoors and during the day, in a person's usual place of residence and in frequently used rooms such as bedrooms, kitchens and dining rooms. Those who fall indoors tend to be older, are female and have various indicators of poor health and frailty, while outdoor fallers are younger, male and are relatively physically active and healthy. US studies suggest similar rates of falls between different races, but a recent systematic review reported consistently lower fall prevalence rates for East Asians compared to Western populations.

Long-term care setting

Falls incidence in nursing care facilities are about three times those in the community, with more than half of residents experiencing at least one fall annually. Falls frequently occur in the residents' rooms or in bathrooms (75%), during transfers (41%) and when walking (36%). Most falls are observed between 10 am and midday and between 2 pm and 8 pm. Men fall more often than women and falls are less common in people requiring the least and highest levels of care.

Acute care setting

Although falls incidence varies with different wards and different healthcare systems, annual fall incidence rates in studies of hospitalized elderly patients reported double the rates of community dwelling populations. Nearly half of patients in stroke rehabilitation wards report at least one fall during an admission, and high rates of falls also occur in psychogeriatric and geriatric rehabilitation units.

The falls incidence of in-patients with any recent clinical fracture is also high. Within 3 months post-fracture, the falls rate is 15%, rising to 3.5 falls per patient-year. After hip fractures, up to one in two people fall again at least once within 2–12 months after subacute rehabilitation and 28% fall more than once, resulting in a new fracture in 12% of cases and a second hip fracture in 5% of cases.

EPIDEMIOLOGY OF INJURIOUS FALLS

In the community setting, 40–60% of falls lead to injuries: 30–50% result in minor injuries, 5–6% in major injuries other than fractures and 5% in fractures. In 2011, unintentional falls was the eighth leading cause of all deaths in the 65+ age group, but the most common cause of injury death and the most common cause of non-fatal injuries treated in US hospital emergency departments.

Numerous risk factors are associated with injurious falls, with the most important being lower-extremity muscle weakness, peripheral neuropathy, low pulmonary capacity, difficulties in gait, long acting benzodiazepines, cardiovascular medications and cognitive impairment (see Tables 12.1 and 12.2).

In the setting of long-term care, about 4% of falls (range, 1–10%) result in fractures, while other serious injuries such as head trauma, soft-tissue injuries and severe lacerations occur in about 11% of falls (range, 1–36%). Risk factors for these injurious falls are the same as those for falls in general, however, some risk factors show strong links, such as female sex, functional independence, the number of falls and use of mechanical restraints.

In the acute care setting, 30% of the hospitalized patients who fall suffer injuries, of which 4–6% are severe, including fractures, subdural haematomas, bleeding and even death.

CAUSES/RISK FACTORS

Community setting

A myriad of risk factors for falls have been identified and are classified broadly as intrinsic and extrinsic factors. Intrinsic factors generally include individuals' age related decline in systems involved in balance performance that may precipitate a fall, while extrinsic factors include medications, environmental hazards and hazardous activities. Risk factors have also been described in terms of possible causative categories, such as environment, medication, medical conditions, age related physiological changes, nutrition and lack of physical activity.

In the community setting early pivotal research of adults over 65 by Tinetti identified a number of risk factors: use of any sedative hypnotics or benzodiazepine, polypharmacy (four or more medications), postural hypotension, environmental hazards, muscular strength and range of motion impairments. Furthermore, half of the falls occurred in the presence of environmental hazards and only 5% and 10% during hazardous activity and acute illness, respectively. However more importantly, the risk of falling increased linearly with the number of risk factors, from 8% with none to 78% with four or more combination of risk factors.

Subsequent population studies since have identified a number of other risk factors (Table 12.1), however each risk factor on its own may not independently increase the risk of falling. The strongest associations were history of falls, gait problems, walking aids use, vertigo, Parkinson's disease and antiepileptic drug use. The others were less associated and some traditional factors such as orthostatic hypotension were not associated (Table 12.2).

Some of the more established risk factors are discussed in more detail below.

GAIT AND BALANCE

Gait disturbance is prevalent in older people. With age a decline in body-orienting reflexes, muscle strength and tone, step length and height produce a gait pattern that is stiffer and less coordinated with poorer posture control. The ability to shift weight or execute reach-to-grasp reactions rapidly or adopt an effective stepping reaction to maintain balance or recover equilibrium quickly after a perturbation is also impaired. Walking speed is slower with shorter stride length, greater propensity of landing flat-footed, less lateral sway, smaller ankle plantar flexion and hip extension during push-off and greater tendency to misstep.

Slower gait speed is the most significant gait parameter associated with increased risk of falls and is independent of other factors such as cognitive impairment and disability. Poorer performance on swing, double-support phase, swing time variability and stride length variability are also predictive of falls. Not surprisingly, both neurological gait pathologies (e.g. hemiparetic, frontal, Parkinsonian, unsteady, neuropathic and spastic) and 'higher-level gait disorder' are associated with increased risk of falls. Unsteady and neuropathic gait in particular are two gait subtypes that predict risk of falls independent of disability and cognitive status.

Overall, balance impairment alone confers only a moderate increase in falls risk in community dwelling older adults. However, differences in fall outcome, length of follow-up and balance measurement tools may underestimate the magnitude of association.

COGNITION

Global measures of cognition are linked with fall related injuries, and a diagnosis of dementia, in both community

Table 12.1 Risk factors for falls reported in epidemiological studies

Intrinsic risk factors	Demographic	Age
		Gender
		Race
	Systems	Gait and balance disturbance
		Reduced strength
		Poor vision
		Cognitive impairment
		ADL limitation
		Frailty
		Inability to comply with recommendation
		Falls history
	Symptoms/diseases	Fear of falling
		Dizziness/vertigo
		Cognitive impairment
		Anxiety/depression
		Syncope
		Diabetes/diabetic foot ulcer
		Stroke
		Anaemia
		Alzheimer's dementia
		Parkinson's disease
		Prostate hypertrophy
		Chronic lung disease/asthma
Extrinsic risk factors	Medications	Psychotropics
		Benzodiazepines
		Analgesics
		Digitalis
	Recent hospitalization	
	Home	Poor lighting and objects around the home, such as loose rugs
	Footwear	Inappropriate (slippers vs barefoot or with fastened shoes, barefoot or with socks vs athletic or canvas shoes)
		Shoes with heels greater than 2.5 cm high

Note: ADL, activities of daily living.

and institution dwelling older adults, confers a high risk for any fall and recurrent falls. However, even those with mild cognitive impairment are twice as likely to experience a fall as those with normal cognition.

Four cognitive domains are thought to influence fall prevalence: attention (especially dual tasking), executive function, information processing and reaction time. Among the subtypes of attention, divided attention, or dual tasking, has been found to be most related to balance, gait and fall risk. In situations which require both attention to a task and gait, subjects with limited attention capacity show a decline in one task or both. This deficit is evident in elderly fallers and patients with neurological disease, such as stroke, Alzheimer's disease or Parkinson's disease compared with healthy older adults.

In addition, systematic reviews have also demonstrated consistent evidence that executive function and dual-task performance are highly associated with falls or falls risk independently of their association with declines in gait speed.[2]

PHYSIOLOGICAL FACTORS

The maintenance of balance depends on the interaction of various sensory and motor inputs and integration by the central nervous system. With age there is a decline in the functioning of each sensori-motor component, and impairments in each function are associated with increased risk of falling. Impaired depth perception, reduced visual contrast sensitivity, reduced proprioception and poorer tactile sensitivity in the lower limbs, reduced quadriceps strength, slow reaction time, and impaired static and dynamic balance predict falls and multiple falls. Muscle strength, particularly of the lower extremities, decreases with age and is associated with falls. The falls incidence in frail older people is three times that of their more active and vigorous counterparts. Having a walking speed in the range stroll/very slow/

Table 12.2 Risk factors for falls in the community setting

Risk factors	Falls	Recurrent falls
History of falls	2.8	3.5
Walking aid use	2.2	3.1
Parkinson's disease	2.7	2.8
Gait problem	2.1	2.2
Use of antiepileptics	1.9	2.7
Dizziness and vertigo	1.8	2.3
Fear of falling	1.6	2.5
Physical disability	1.6	2.4
Instrumental disability	1.5	2
Self-perceived health status	1.5	1.8
Pain	1.4	1.6
Depression	1.6	1.9
History of stroke	1.6	1.8
Rheumatic disease	1.5	1.6
Urinary incontinence	1.4	1.7
Cognition impairment	1.4	1.6
Vision impairment	1.4	1.6
Use of sedatives	1.4	1.5
Comorbidity (increment of one condition)	1.2	1.5
Hearing impairment	1.2	1.5
Living alone	1.3	1.3
Gender (female)	1.3	1.3
Use of antihypertensives	1.3	1.2
Diabetes	1.2	1.3
No. medications (for one-drug increase)	1.1	1.1
Age (5-year increase)	1.1	1.1
Physical activity (limitation)	1.2	ND

Note: Odds ratio for falls (at least once in 6 months) and recurrent falls (at least twice in 6 months). ND, no data.

Table 12.3 Drug class and risk of falls

Medication class	Odds or RR for falls
Any psychotropic drug	1.8
Antipsychotics	1.5–1.7
Antidepressants	1.7
Benzodiazepines	1.4–1.6
Type 1a anti-arrhythmics	1.6
Sedatives and hypnotics	1.3–1.5
Opioids	1.4
Antihypertensive agents	1.3
Tranquilizers	1.3
Non-steroidal anti-inflammatory drugs	1.2
Digoxin	1.2
Diuretics	1.1

its use in the previous 30 days for alprazolam, 2 previous weeks' exposure for flurazepam and temazepam use has a statistically significant association with the risk of fall related injuries only when the effects of both the cumulative use and current dose are jointly taken into account. The risk of fall related injuries associated with cumulative use of temazepam may be driven mostly by a withdrawal effect, especially among the elderly who have been using it over a prolonged period.

Falls are associated with other medications as well, such as antihypertensive agents. They are associated with a 24% increased odds of falling but the relationship between initiating different antihypertensive medications and the occurrence of falls and fractures is variable. Insulin treated patients are at increased risk compared to non-insulin treated patients and non-diabetics. Metformin and secretagogues are not linked to falls but patients on thiazolidinediones are more prone to having fractures after a fall. Surprisingly, β-blockers and opiates are not independently associated with increased risk of falls unless orthostatic hypotension is present. Other cardiovascular medications, however, are implicated in fall risk, including digoxin, type 1a anti-arrhythmics and diuretics. With diuretics there is an increased risk in falling the day following a change in diuretics medication or an increase in the dose.

In addition to the effects of individual drugs or drug class, the interactions between multiple drugs, that is, polypharmacy, and in particular multiple drugs that have associations with falls, that is, falls risk increasing drugs (FRIDs), are important factors to consider. The prevalence of falls increases with overall number of drugs prescribed, certain drug combinations (e.g. a TCA plus any hypotension producing drug) and multiple FRIDs. Polypharmacy and in particular in the context of its association with falls has been defined as four or more medications. However the optimal discriminating number of concomitant medications associated with not only falls but also frailty, disability and mortality is five or more. The number of medications on hospital discharge and FRIDs on discharge in one study

non-ambulant compared with normal/brisk/fast doubles the risk of falls. In fact, slow gait velocity (<0.7 m/s) at baseline is associated with future adverse events, hospitalizations, new falls and requirement for a caregiver.

MEDICATIONS

Several commonly used medications have shown association with falls, but each class confers different levels of risk (Table 12.3).[3] Benzodiazepines, antipsychotics (both atypical and typical) and antidepressants, in particular selective serotonin reuptake inhibitors (SSRIs) and tricyclic antidepressants (TCAs), significantly increase the risk of falls. Psychotropic medications, which include those used in dementia, increase the risk of falling by 47% in older adults living in the community. This risk is further increased when two or more psychotropic drugs are combined. Benzodiazepine use in the older population is prevalent and adverse outcomes often involve prolonged exposure, but the mechanisms affecting the risk of falls may differ across benzodiazepines. For example, the cumulative duration of also was significantly associated with recurrent falls. More importantly, recurrent falls were most likely to occur with only 1.5 FRIDs in the frail and 2.5 FRIDs in the robust. In this study antidepressants and anxiolytics were the most frequently dispensed FRIDs.

VERTIGO AND DIZZINESS

Vestibular dysfunction is common in older people and often results in impairments in posture and gait, characterized by postural instability and a broad-based, staggering gait pattern with unsteady turns placing the older adult at an increased risk of recurrent falls. However, there is no clear causal relationship between age-associated changes in vestibular function and falls when visual and peripheral sensations are intact.

VISION IMPAIRMENT

Intact vision is integral to enable planning and coordination of movements in response to environmental hazards as well as assisting with the maintenance of balance. Inputs from the visual, vestibular and somatosensory systems are integrated centrally and instructions are sent to the motor system to maintain balance. Optical flow provides information about anteroposterior body sway and information from eye movements provides information about lateral body sway. Both the central and peripheral visual system assesses optical flow and thus postural control. It is not surprising that standing postural control is poorer in individuals with cataract, age related macular degeneration or glaucoma.

Vision is also used to scan the travel pathway for obstacles and changes in terrain, typically one to two steps ahead to enable safe ambulation through the environment and when negotiating steps and stairs. The lower peripheral visual fields in particular provide exteroception (position of the lower limbs relative to the environment) information, which is used to fine tune the gait. In this respect vision plays a major role in successful stair negotiation.

Visual impairment increases with age affecting 3.1% of 65–74 year olds, 11.6% of 75–84 year olds and 35.5% of 85+ year old individuals. The most prevalent age related causes are cataract, macular degeneration, glaucoma and presbyopia. Glaucoma sufferers have limited perception due to restricted visual fields and loss of peripheral vision. Individuals with age related macular degeneration have poorer vision, slower visual reaction times, and visuomotor and balance deficits, and are prone to clumsiness and increased risk of falls.

Aside from a poor level of visual acuity, visual field deficits, impaired depth perception, low contrast sensitivity, stereoacuity and changes in visual acuity demonstrate even stronger links with falls. Surprisingly, the effect of vision improvement through cataract surgery may in fact increase falls rate. This effect on falls rate is similar to that seen in patients with new spectacles. New spectacles may be associated with changes in magnification, optical centres, lens type (e.g. progressive addition lens [PAL] rather than single vision lens) and position of bifocals/PALs, which could adversely affect falls risk. A change from a distance single vision lens to PALs or bifocals distorts the peripheral visual field in PALs and provides a blurred and magnified view of the lower visual field beyond near working distance in both PALs and bifocals. This affects the peripheral optic flow information used for postural control and makes it difficult to judge the position of obstacles in the lower visual field, including obstacles, step and stair edges and/or foot placements relative to such environmental obstacles. Thus the recommendation is that changes to refractive corrections in older people should be conservative, and PALs or bifocals should never be prescribed to patients who are used to wearing single vision glasses and who could be categorized as at high risk for falls.

COMORBIDITIES

A number of chronic diseases are independently associated with falls (Table 12.1) and both number and type of chronic conditions play a role in falls. Fall prevalence increases linearly with the number of chronic conditions, suggesting an additive effect of chronic disease on fall risk, irrespective of the specific condition. However not all clusters of chronic conditions are associated with falls. Patients with a number of chronic conditions, which include hypertension or chronic obstructive pulmonary disease (COPD), tend to be at higher risk of falls. With hypertension both the condition itself and treatment side effects known to induce orthostatic hypotension may be the underlying mechanisms. People with uncontrolled hypertension and orthostatic hypotension are 2.5 times more likely to have recurrent falls than those with uncontrolled hypertension and no orthostatic hypotension.

Similarly, people with COPD have both increased prevalence of falls as well as dysfunction in physiological risk factors for falls, such as impaired postural control. Skeletal muscle dysfunction and cerebral hypoxemia have been postulated as contributing factors.

Acute and subacute care setting

Risk factors for falls in these settings include advanced age, agitation, confusion or disorientation, generalized muscle and/or leg weakness, unstable gait, urinary incontinence, a history of previous falls, visual deficit or the use of certain medications (hypnotics, sedatives, etc). The hospital environment itself, such as the presence/absence of bed rails, the height and stability of any type of seat (including the toilet) or furniture and equipment may present as new obstacles. Also hospitalization itself may make older people become more disoriented or agitated, or suffer a decline in function and thus be at increased risk of falls.

Status at discharge such as a decline in mobility, use of assistive device, cognitive impairment and self-report of confusion after hospital discharge are also major risk factors for falls. More significantly, patients who were functionally dependent and needed professional help after discharge had the highest rate of falls (20.2%).

A recent meta-analysis by Deandrea et al.[4] showed a number of risk factors resembling those in the community setting (Table 12.4). Age was less associated and gender did not confer increased risk compared to community setting.

Patients with recent hip fractures present a higher risk group. Recurrent falls affect those who are less mobile and less active, have a higher number of chronic diseases and medications, have higher pre-fracture disability, have chronic heart failure, have lower vitamin D levels, have lower handgrip strength and have reduced quality of life.

Similar to patients without hip fracture in the community, the use of a rollator frame (rolling walker) and nocturnal urinary incontinence are also associated with falls. The measures of impairment before hip fracture (disability, poor vitamin D status and a more sedentary lifestyle), combined with strength and balance impairments persistent after surgery, identified the most vulnerable individuals who would go on to suffer injurious falls again. Among these risk factors, hip abductor weakness postoperatively had the strongest relationship with fall related injuries risk.

Notably, the other risk factors associated with falls after hip fractures resemble those in the population without hip fracture: age, female sex, difficulties in activities of daily living (ADL), orthostatic hypotension and polypharmacy, more handicap, lower Activities-specific Balance Confidence (ABC) Scale and falls efficacy score, worry over further falls, previous falls and poor performance with the 5-metre Timed Up and Go (TUG) test, timed 10-metre walk and the Turn180 test.

Long-term care setting

Prospective studies have shown hip weakness, poor balance and number of prescribed medications to be factors most strongly associated with falling among institutionalized subjects. Other factors reported in the literature include

Table 12.4 Risk factors for falls in in-patient settings

Intrinsic risk factors	Demographic systems	Age
		Gait instability
		Agitated confusion
		Need for transfer assistance
		Previous falls/falls history
		Cognitive impairment
	Symptoms/ diseases	Vertigo
		Urinary incontinence
		Sleep disturbance
		Stroke
Extrinsic factors	Hospital environment	Carpet flooring
	Medications	Psychotropic medications
		Sedatives
		Antidepressants
		Anticonvulsants
		Tranquillizers
		Antihypertensives

increased age, male sex, higher care classification, incontinence, psychoactive medication use, previous falls and slow reaction times. Use of walking aids, presence of moderate disability, wandering tendencies, Parkinson's disease and dizziness were other independent risk factors reported in an earlier meta-analysis.[4] However in contrast to the community dwelling setting, age, gender, vision impairment, depression, stroke and incontinence were not associated with an increased risk of falls.

Dementia is another significant independent risk factor for falls. Residents with dementia were twice as likely to fall and more likely to suffer injurious falls compared to residents without dementia.

CONSEQUENCES OF FALLS

Older individuals have an increased susceptibility for injury due to the higher prevalence of comorbidities. Falls and associated injuries cause substantial physical, social and psychological morbidity in the individual and cost for the health system.

Fractures and other injuries

Although the probability of sustaining a hip fracture from a fall is estimated to be 1.0% and that of some other fracture is 4–10%, falls precede nearly 90% of non-hip non-vertebral, more than 90% of hip, and nearly half of vertebral fractures among women aged 64–85 years. The proportion increases with age and up to 92% of all fractures are osteoporotic. In fact having both a fall and osteoporosis or osteopenia puts such women at 7–9 times higher odds of a fracture compared with community dwelling postmenopausal women having a fall or osteoporosis/osteopenia only.

Significant mortality and morbidity is associated with fractures. Both hip fracture and other fall related injuries are associated with significantly greater disability during the first 6 months and patients are more than three times more likely to require nursing home admission after hospitalization than for non-fall related admissions. In the first year following a hip fracture, 25% of older patients die, 76% have a decline in their mobility, 50% have a decline in their ability to perform ADL and 22% move into a nursing home.

The consequences for patients with proximal femoral fractures (PFFs) sustained in a hospital setting are even worse. Compared with PFFs sustained in the community, similar fractures sustained in hospital were associated with a threefold higher death rate, a threefold higher institutionalization rate and such patients are three times less likely to reach premorbid baseline ambulation and six times less likely to regain premorbid ADL status.

Medical/psychological

Approximately one-half of elderly individuals who fall are unable to get up and remain on the ground. These 'long-lies' can lead to dehydration, rhabdomyolysis, pressures sores and pneumonia. Up to 73% of recent fallers can develop a marked fear of falling which can impair ADL and instrumental activities of daily living (IADL), and physical and social functioning. Even in the absence of falls, fear of falling affects 46% of the older age group and 40% of affected people self-impose restrictions on their ADL. Fear of falling can also negate gains made through rehabilitation, leading to a vicious cycle with further declines in physical fitness, social isolation and depression, in turn causing further increases in the risk of falls, reduced ADL, increased dependence, lower quality of life and increased institutionalization.

Costs

Falls consume a disproportionate share of hospital resources and the healthcare budget worldwide. Hospital stays are almost twice as long in elderly patients who are hospitalized after a fall than in elderly patients who are admitted for another reason.

Fall related costs ranged between 0.85% and 1.5% of the total healthcare expenditures within the United States, Australia, the EU15 and the United Kingdom.[5] A systematic review[6] comparing the costs of falls internationally reported a range of the falls cost. The total direct medical cost for fall related injuries among older adults in the United States was US$23.3 billion and US$1.6 billion in the United Kingdom. Comparing global data, the mean cost of falls ranged from US$3476 per faller to US$10,749 per injurious fall and US$26,483 per fall requiring hospitalization.

In the United States, a substantial fraction of direct medical costs resulting from falls is attributable to fractures followed by superficial injuries and contusions. A recent systematic review[7] estimated the cost of fall related osteoporotic fractures to range from US$12.9 to US$16.6 billion in 2010 dollars. This estimate did not include nursing home stays attributable to fractures, which are an important contributor to costs, or the costs of non-fatal falls in the institutionalized population. Other costs not accounted for include costs on the health system due to nursing home placement or additional, often prolonged, rehabilitation resulting from fear of falling.

Functional/social

Falls, particularly those resulting in injury, are independently associated with a decline in the ability to carry out important functional activities, such as bathing, dressing, shopping and housekeeping, and with an increased risk of a long-term nursing home admission. Among the strongest predictors of nursing home admission are three or more ADL dependencies. Up to 40% of nursing home admissions are precipitated by falling or instability.

Mortality related to falls

One in four elderly persons who sustain a hip fracture die within 6 months of the injury. More than 50% of older patients who survive hip fractures are discharged to a nursing home, and nearly one-half of these patients are still in a nursing home 1 year later. Hip fracture survivors experience a 10–15% decrease in life expectancy and a meaningful decline in overall quality of life.

Among long-term care residents, fall related injuries account for an in-hospital death rate of 15% and a survival rate of only 66%. Older people who sustain a hip fracture while in hospital have been shown to have poor outcomes compared with age matched controls sustaining similar fractures in the community.

EVALUATION OF THE ELDERLY INDIVIDUAL WHO FALLS

A single fall may simply be an isolated event and is not always indicative of increased risk for subsequent falls. However, elderly patients with known risk factors for falling should be screened about falls periodically and patients with recurrent falls, defined as more than two falls in a 6-month period, should be assessed. A number of guidelines currently exist for screening and assessment. One such guideline from The American Geriatrics Society and British Geriatrics Society recommends a panel of questions followed by focused history, physical examination, functional and environmental assessment (Table 12.5). The components of this guideline and others are derived from risk assessment tools which have been validated in community, in-patient and nursing home settings. These tools however are not applicable to all patients even in similar settings. These instruments are described below.

Community setting

Risk assessment of community dwelling, elderly individuals are either purely functional mobility assessments (FMAs) of gait, strength and balance (e.g. Tinetti Performance Oriented Mobility Assessment [POMA], Berg Balance Scale, Functional Reach, TUG or Dynamic Gait Index) or combined with clinical risk factors to generate a multifactorial assessment tool for falls. A number of FMAs have been tested and validated in the community setting (Table 12.6).[8]

Given that falls are usually multifactorial and a complex interaction between factors determines whether a person falls, multifactorial assessment tools are the recommended strategy. One of the earliest and most widely accepted is that proposed by Tinetti et al.[9] This risk assessment index used nine risk factors: mobility, morale, mental status, distance vision, hearing, postural blood pressure, back examination, medications and ability to perform ADL. The risk of falling ranges from 0% with 0–3 risk factors, to 31% with 4–6 risk factors, to 100% with ≥7 risk factors. A specificity of 74% and sensitivity of 80% has been reported. Graafmans et al. [10] showed that a combination of impaired mobility, dizziness upon standing, history of stroke, reduced mental state (Mini Mental State Examination [MMSE] ≤24 and Global

Deterioration Scale [GDS] ≥10/30) and orthostatic hypotension yielded an 84% probability of having another fall over a period of 28 weeks.

Tromp et al.[11] showed that any combination of two independent risk factors such as previous falls, urinary incontinence, visual impairment, use of benzodiazepines or functional limitations would yield a greater than 25% risk of recurrent falls. Similarly in a model proposed by Stalenhoef and colleagues,[12] having two or more of the following predictors: depression, previous falls, reduced hand grip strength and an abnormal postural sway, is associated with a 60–90% risk of recurrent falls.

Table 12.5 AGS/BGS Clinical Practice Guideline: prevention of falls in older persons: summary of recommendations

Screening and assessment

1. All older individuals should be asked whether they have fallen (in the past year).
2. An older person who reports a fall should be asked about the frequency and circumstances of the fall(s).
3. Older individuals should be asked if they experience difficulties with walking or balance.
4. Older persons who present for medical attention because of a fall, report recurrent falls in the past year, or report difficulties in walking or balance (with or without activity curtailment) should have a multifactorial fall risk assessment.
5. Older persons presenting with a single fall should be evaluated for gait and balance.
6. Older persons who have fallen should have an assessment of gait and balance using one of the available evaluations.
7. Older persons who cannot perform or perform poorly on a standardized gait and balance test should be given a multifactorial fall risk assessment.
8. Older persons who have difficulty or demonstrate unsteadiness during the evaluation of gait and balance require a multifactorial fall risk assessment.
9. Older persons reporting only a single fall and reporting or demonstrating no difficulty or unsteadiness during the evaluation of gait and balance do not require a fall risk assessment.
10. The multifactorial fall risk assessment should be performed by a clinician (or clinicians) with appropriate skills and training.

Multifactorial fall risk assessment

Focused history	• History of falls: Detailed description of the circumstances of the fall(s), frequency, symptoms at time of fall, injuries, other consequences
	• Medication review: All prescribed and over-the-counter medications with dosages
	• History of relevant risk factors: Acute or chronic medical problems (e.g. osteoporosis, urinary incontinence, cardiovascular disease)
Physical examinations	• Detailed assessment of gait, balance, and mobility levels and lower-extremity joint function
	• Neurological function: Cognitive evaluation, lower-extremity peripheral nerves, proprioception, reflexes, tests of cortical, extrapyramidal and cerebellar function
	• Muscle strength (lower extremities)
	• Cardiovascular status: Heart rate and rhythm, postural pulse, blood pressure, and, if appropriate, heart rate and blood pressure responses to carotid sinus stimulation
	• Assessment of visual acuity
	• Examination of the feet and footwear
Functional assessment	• Assessment of activities of daily living (ADL) skills including use of adaptive equipment and mobility aids, as appropriate
	• Assessment of the individual's perceived functional ability and fear related to falling (assessment of current activity levels with attention to the extent to which concerns about falling are protective [i.e. appropriate given abilities] or contributing to deconditioning and/or compromised quality of life [i.e. individual is curtailing involvement in activities he or she is safely able to perform due to fear of falling])
Environmental assessment	• Environmental assessment including home safety

Note: AGS, American Geriatrics Society; BGS, British Geriatrics Society.

Table 12.6 Falls risk assessment tools in community settings

Tool	Components	Sensitivity	Specificity
Berg Balance Scale (cut-off 45/56)	1. Sitting to standing 2. Standing unsupported 3. Sitting unsupported 4. Standing to sitting 5. Transfers 6. Standing with eyes closed 7. Standing with feet together 8. Reaching forward with an outstretched arm 9. Retrieving object from floor 10. Turning to look behind 11. Turning 360° 12. Placing alternate foot on stool 13. Standing with one foot in front of the other foot 14. Standing on one foot	77%	86%
Elderly Fall Screening Test (cut-off 3/5)	1. One fall or more reported in previous year 2. An injurious fall in the last year 3. Reporting 'near falls' 4. Slow walking speed (>10 s over 5 m) 5. Unsteady or uneven gait	93%	78%
Dynamic Gait Index (cut-off 19/24)	1. Gait on even surfaces 2. Gait when changing speeds 3. Gait and head turns in a vertical direction 4. Gait and head turns in a horizontal direction 5. Gait when stepping over 6. Gait around obstacles 7. Gait with pivot turns 8. Gait with steps	85%	38%
Timed Get Up and Go (cut-off 14 s)	Rise up from standard armchair Walk to line on floor 10 feet away Turn and return to chair Sit in chair again	87%	87%

(Continued)

Table 12.6 (*Continued*) Falls risk assessment tools in community settings

Tool	Components	Sensitivity	Specificity
Tinetti Performance Oriented Mobility Assessment (POMA) (cut-off 18/28)	1. Balance section Sitting balance, Rises from chair, Attempts to rise, Immediate standing balance, Standing balance, Nudged, Eyes closed, Turning 360°, Sitting down (score: /16) 2. Gait section Indication of gait, Step length and height, Foot clearance, Step symmetry, Step continuity, Path, Trunk, Walking time (score: /12)	70–80%	52–74%
Functional gait assessment (cut-off score ≤22/30)	Walk at normal speeds, at fast and slow speeds, with vertical and horizontal head turns, with eyes closed, over obstacles, in tandem, backwards, and while ascending and descending stairs	100	83
FRAT (≥3 risk factors)	1. History of any fall in previous year 2. ≥ 2 prescribed medications 3. Stroke or Parkinson's disease 4. Reported problems with balance 5. Inability to rise from a chair without using arms	42% (NPV 86%)	92% (PPV 57%)
Fall risk assessment tool for predicting repeat fallers	Alternate step test Sit-to-stand test Tandem stand test	70 66 55	55 55 62
FROP-Com screen (cut-off 4/9)	1. Falls in previous 12 months (0–3) 2. Function: ADL status (0–3) 3. Balance (0–3)	67	67
Modified Gait Abnormality Rating scale	1. Variability – a measure of inconsistency and arrhythmicity of stepping and/or arm movement 2. Guardedness – hesitancy, slowness, diminished propulsion, and lack of commitment in stepping and arm swing 3. Staggering – sudden and unexpected laterally directed partial losses of balance 4. Foot contact – the degree to which the heel strikes the ground before the forefoot 5. Hip ROM – the degree of loss of hip range of motion seen during a gait cycle 6. Shoulder extension – a measure of the decrease of shoulder range of motion 7. Arm-heel-strike synchrony – the extent to which the contralateral movements of an arm and leg are out of phase		

Note: ADL, activities of daily living; FRAT, falls risk assessment tool; NPV, negative predictive value; PPV, positive predictive value; ROM, range of motion.

In the primary care setting, a simple and quick tool such as the falls risk assessment tool (FRAT)[13] may be very useful for initial screening. The tool uses five risk factors: history of any fall in the previous year, four or more prescribed medications, diagnosis of stroke or Parkinson's disease, reported problems with balance and inability to rise from a chair without using arms. The presence of three or more risk factors had a positive predictive value for a fall in the next 6 months of 57%. Less than three risk factors had a negative predictive value of 86% and a specificity of 92%.

Another risk profile that was derived from a 3-year prospective study can also be used to identify community dwelling elderly at a high risk of recurrent falling.[14] A number of risk factors were predictive of recurrent falls over a 1- and 3-year period, and the probability of having two or more falls in the next year and in the next 3 years as predicted by this profile is up to 90% and 97%, respectively, with all nine predictors present.

To identify young relatively healthy older adults living in the community who are at risk of falls, a tool that incorporates FMA with risk factors and which has a simple clinical score that reflects the cumulative effect of risk factors may be needed. Such a model proposed by Bongue et al.[15] showed gender, living alone, psychoactive drug use, osteoarthritis, previous falls and a change in the position of the arms during the one-leg balance (OLB) test to be strong predictors of falls.

In the setting of patients presenting to the emergency department after a fall, the FROP-Com screen[16] was shown to have reasonable capacity to predict falls and may be useful in time-limited situations to classify those at high risk of falls who require more detailed assessment and management. The items in the screen are falls in the previous 12 months, observation of the person's balance and the need for assistance to perform domestic ADL.

Slightly different to the FROP-Com screen, the LASA (Longitudinal Aging Study Amsterdam) fall risk profile predicts the risk of recurrent falling in older persons who present to the emergency department after a fall. This profile consists of nine items including fall history, dizziness, functional limitations, grip strength, body weight, having a dog or cat in the household, fear of falling, alcohol intake and level of education. Its predictive validity was moderate.[17]

A 'physiological' rather than 'disease-oriented' assessment[18] consisting of a series of simple tests of vision, peripheral sensation, muscle force, reaction time and postural sway may also be useful. The Physiological Profile Assessment (PPA) measurements correctly classify subjects into a multiple falls group or a non-multiple falls group with an accuracy of 75%.

Lastly, despite good evidence of an association between gait and balance abnormalities in older adults with dementia and impaired executive function and gait changes suggesting that executive function and gait impairments may underpin the increased risk of falls in dementia, tests of executive function are not part of routine fall risk assessment.

Long-term care settings

Similar to the community population, a number of risk assessment tools have been studied in long-term care settings (Table 12.7). Of these the Morse Fall Scale (MFS) demonstrated high predictive values and can be completed in less than a minute making it probably the most useful nursing assessment tool for falls risk in long-term care facilities.

The Peninsula Health-Falls Risk Assessment Tool (PH-FRAT) is a moderately predictive, reliable and brief method of screening fall risk in subacute and residential aged care. It incorporates the four strongest falls predictors (Table 12.7) derived from a panel of known risk factors. It showed good reliability and achieved high compliance rate of application due to its ease of use with little training requirement.

Similarly, Robbins and colleagues[19] proposed a fall prediction model consisting of three of the most strongly associated risk factors (hip weakness, poor balance and number of prescribed medications). The predicted 1-year risk of falling ranges from 12% with none of these risk factors to 100% for long-term care residents having all three risk factors.

Physiological factors have also shown correlation with falls. A battery of 13 sensorimotor, vestibular and visual tests was able to correctly classify subjects into a multiple falls group (two or more falls) or a non-multiple falls group (no falls or one fall) with an accuracy of 79%.[20]

Recently there has been greater interest in more objective measurement of short-term risk of falls. A modified Berg Balance Scale (mod-Berg), the Short Physical Performance Battery (SPPB) and spatiotemporal gait measures using the GaitRITE Walkway system have shown potential as predictors of falls in older adults living in dementia-specific assisted living in a short-term study. Reduced velocity and reduced mean stride length measured with an electronic walkway system were the best gait predictors of a fall among nursing home residents with moderate to severe dementia.[21]

Acute care setting

A number of falls risk assessment instruments have been developed such as the Downton scale, the Morse Fall Scale (MFS), the St. Thomas Risk Assessment Tool in Falling Elderly Inpatients (STRATIFY), the Tinetti test, the Conley scale, the Hendrich Fall Risk Model (HFRM) and its later version HFRM II. The elements of these scales are described in Table 12.8. However, only the MFS, STRATIFY and HFRM have been validated in multiple studies across different populations.

Several systematic reviews have compared these three tools, and while some confirmed the usefulness of the MFS, STRATIFY and HFRM, others found them to show relatively low-pooled specificity and sensitivity and even lower

Table 12.7 Falls screening tools in long-term care setting

Tools	Components	Sensitivity	Specificity
Elderly Fall Screening Test (cut-off 3/5)	1. More than one fall reported in the previous year	93%	78%
	2. A fall that resulted in injury in the last year		
	3. Reporting 'near falls' occasionally or often		
	4. Slow walking speed (>10 s over 5 m)		
	5. Unsteady or uneven gait		
Reassessment Is Safe Kare tool	Unsteady gait/dizziness/imbalance	ND	ND
	Weakness		
	Impaired memory or judgement		
	History of falls		
	Use of a wheelchair		
Resident Assessment Instrument		ND	ND
High Risk for Falls Assessment		ND	ND
Tinetti Balance Subscale		ND	ND
Care Dependency Scale (≤54/75) (item scores: '1=completely dependent' to '5=almost independent')	1. Eating and drinking	60–74%	60–74%
	2. Continence		
	3. Body posture		
	4. Mobility		
	5. Day/night pattern		
	6. Getting dressed and undressed		
	7. Body temperature		
	8. Hygiene		
	9. Avoidance of danger		
	10. Communications		
	11. Contact with others		
	12. Sense of rules and values		
	13. Daily activities		
	14. Recreational activities		
	15. Learning activities		
Downton Index (score 3/11=high risk of fall)	1. Known previous falls	91%	39%
	2. Medications (tranquillizers/sedatives, diuretics, antihypertensives, antiparkinsonian drugs, antidepressants)		
	3. Sensory deficits (visual impairment, hearing impairment, limb impairment)		
	4. Mental state (confused or cognitively impaired)		
	5. Gait (unsafe, with/without walking aids)		

(Continued)

Table 12.7 (Continued) Falls screening tools in long-term care setting

Tools	Components	Sensitivity	Specificity
Mobility Fall Chart	1. Test of the ability to walk and simultaneously interact with a person or an object 2. A vision test 3. A concentration rating	43%	69%
Morse Fall Scale (cut-off 45–55/125)	1. History of falls [25] 2. Medical diagnoses [15] 3. Ambulatory aid (15 or 30) 4. Intravenous access [20] 5. Gait [20] 6. Mental status [15]	78–83%	83%
Spartanburg Fall Risk Assessment	1. Previous falls 2. Medications 3. Gait 4. Age 5. Altered mental status 6. Cognitive impairment 7. Environment 8. Impaired mobility 9. Incontinence 10. Hypertension 11. Get Up and Go Test	100%	28%
PH-FRAT (cut-off score 14/20)	1. Recent falls (last 3–12 months)/8 2. Medications (sedatives, antidepressants, antiparkinsonian drugs diuretics, antihypertensives)/4 3. Psychological (anxiety, depression, cooperation, ↓insight especially concerning mobility)/4 4. Cognitive status (Hodkinson AMTS)/4	69%	70%

Note: AMTS, Abbreviated Mental Test Score; ND, no data; PH-FRAT, Peninsula Health-Falls Risk Assessment Tool.

Table 12.8 Falls screening tools in in-patient settings

Tools	Components	Sensitivity	Specificity
Morse Fall Scale (cut-off 45–55/125)	1. History of falls [25] 2. Medical diagnoses [15] 3. Ambulatory aid (15 or 30) 4. Intravenous access [20] 5. Gait [20] 6. Mental status [15]	78–83	68–83
STRATIFY (cut-off 2/5)	1. History of falls 2. Agitation 3. Visual impairment 4. Frequent visits to the toilet 5. Impaired ability to transfer and walk	93	88
Hendrich Fall Risk Model (cut-off 6/25)	Recent history of falls, depression, altered elimination patterns, dizziness or vertigo, primary cancer diagnosis, confusion and altered mobility	77	72
Hendrich Fall Risk Model II (cut-off 5/16)	1. Confusion, disorientation, impulsivity 2. Symptomatic depression 3. Altered elimination 4. Dizziness or vertigo 5. Male gender 6. Prescribed antiepileptics 7. Prescribed benzodiazepines 8. Timed up and go Test	86	43
Fall Prediction Index (cut-off 5/11)		100	44
Fall Assessment Questionnaire (cut-off 3/10)	1. Age, mental status, elimination, history of falling, sensory impairment, activity and medications	73	88
Fall Risk Assessment Tool (cut-off 3/5)	2. Mobility, mental status, elimination, history of falling and medications	93	78
Tinetti Performance Oriented Mobility (cut-off 10/28)	1. Balance section Sitting balance, rises from chair, attempts to rise, immediate standing, balance, standing balance, nudged, eyes closed, turning 360°, sitting down (score: /16) 2. Gait section Indication of gait, step length and height, foot clearance, step symmetry, step continuity, path, trunk, walking time (score: /12)	80	74

(Continued)

Table 12.8 (*Continued*) Falls screening tools in in-patient settings

Tools	Components	Sensitivity	Specificity
Downton Index (cut-off 3/11)	1. Known previous falls 2. Medications (tranquillizers/sedatives, diuretics, antihypertensives, antiparkinsonian drugs, antidepressants) 3. Sensory deficits (visual impairment, hearing impairment, limb impairment) 4. Mental state (confused or cognitively impaired) 5. Gait (unsafe, with/without walking aids)	92	34
Care Dependency Scale (≤54/75) (item scores: '1=completely dependent' to '5=almost independent')	1. Eating and drinking 2. Continence 3. Body posture 4. Mobility 5. Day/night pattern 6. Getting dressed and undressed 7. Body temperature 8. Hygiene 9. Avoidance of danger 10. Communications 11. Contact with others 12. Sense of rules and values 13. Daily activities 14. Recreational activities 15. Learning activities	75	46
Conley Scale (cut-off 3/8)	1. History of falling /2 2. Impaired judgement or lack of safety awareness /3 3. Agitation /2 4. Impaired mobility /1 5. Dizziness or vertigo /1 6. Incontinence on way to bathroom /1	69	61

Note: STRATIFY, St. Thomas Risk Assessment Tool in Falling Elderly Inpatients.

positive predictive value. One meta-analysis concluded that the MFS and STRATIFY were comparable with nurses' clinical judgement, while another showed that the MFS has the highest sensitivity, the STRATIFY the highest specificity and the HFRM is the tool of choice when a more comprehensive assessment is required. However in a more recent meta-analysis,[22] the STRATIFY tool was shown to be the best tool for assessing the risk of falls among hospitalized acutely ill adult patients, followed by the MFS and HFRM II. STRATIFY produced the best values for sensitivity and had a specificity similar to that of the MFS, and obtained the best values for the diagnostic odds ratio.

By and large reviews of falls risk assessment tools in the acute care setting have shown them not to work and even when they do, they may not provide any greater clinical benefit than identifying the risk factors for falls and doing something to modify them. For example, Wong Shee et al.[23] recently compared a new modified STRATIFY to another version of STRATIFY which had been previously validated in a different acute hospital. Both tools showed only fair predictive accuracy but showed that the locally modified STRATIFY tool combined with associated nursing care plan falls documentation, improved the targeting of prevention strategies for key risk factors such as cognitive impairment, incontinence and mobility impairment. Indeed, a recent analytical review by Lee et al.[24] of fall screening tools across all care settings recommended specific tools for specific settings combined with overall clinical evaluation of falls risk. They recommended the TUG test with a cut-off of >12.34 seconds and functional gait assessment among community dwelling elderly; the St. Thomas Risk Assessment Tool in medical in-patients <65 years old and surgical in-patients; the HFRM II in medical in-patients; the 10-Metre Walk Test in patients in post-stroke rehabilitation; and the Berg Balance Scale or the Step Test in patients in post-stroke rehabilitation who had fallen during their in-patient stay.

Thus it is clear that it is difficult to accurately predict the risk of falls among hospitalized adult patients with any single instrument because they all generally fail to adequately take into account extrinsic factors specific to the hospital environment and intrinsic factors which may be modified by the acute hospitalization process. Selecting the instrument is further complicated by the lack of agreement of sensitivity and specificity thresholds because these risk assessment instruments' behaviours vary considerably depending on the population and the environment in which they are administered. Consequently, no single instrument can be recommended for implementation in all hospital settings without its prior testing in the healthcare setting of the intended implementation.

FALL PREVENTION

Falls are not an inevitable result of aging and available best evidence suggests that prevention interventions can reduce falls. The relative reduction in fall related injuries range from 6% to 75% in studies conducted in Australia, Denmark, Norway, Taiwan and Sweden over up to 8 years. Cost savings can also be achieved with some interventions such as home based exercise in over 80-year-olds and home safety assessment and modification in those with a previous fall, and a multifactorial programme targeting specific risk factors.

Community

EXERCISE BASED INTERVENTIONS

As a single intervention, exercise is the most effective way to reduce falls risk in older fallers, and is comparable with other multifaceted interventions. A meta-analysis by Sherrington et al.[25] showed that a balance training (of moderate or high challenge intensity) combined with higher dose exercise (2 hours a week for a 6-month period) regime without a walking component resulted in a 38% reduction in falls. It is however important that the correct type of exercise is implemented, as not all types of exercise improve balance to an extent that actually prevents falls. Furthermore, although some exercise interventions with balance and muscle strengthening components have been shown to reduce falls, there have also been many unsuccessful exercise interventions. The types of exercise are described in Table 12.9.

A recent Cochrane review[26] found different modalities of exercise achieved different falls outcomes. Group and individual exercise classes that included just gait, balance or functional training reduced the rate of falls but not the risk of falling, whereas strength/resistance training delivered in a group setting did not seem to reduce rate of falls or number of people falling and may in fact cause some injuries. There was insufficient evidence for other single interventions such as general physical activity (walking or cycling), exercise involving computerized balance programmes and vibration plates.

However the same Cochrane systematic review concluded that overall, exercise classes containing multiple components (i.e. a combination of two or more categories of exercise) reduce rate of falls and risk of falling. The intervention was effective in participants at higher risk of falling (history of falling or one or more risk factors for falls at enrolment) and lower risk of falling (not selected on falls risk at enrolment). Similarly, home based exercises containing multiple components were found to reduce rate of falls and risk of falling. However the components vary (Table 12.10) and not all are effective. Tai Chi reduces risk of falling but the effect on rate of falls was not conclusive. The effect on falls rate was greater and the intervention appears to be more effective in people who are not at high risk of falling at baseline.

Although small in number, exercise studies that assess fracture outcomes showed that exercise interventions reduced the risk of sustaining a fall related fracture by 66%.

Table 12.9 Exercises with positive effect on balance

Exercise	Timed up and go test	Single leg stance on the floor with eyes open	Single leg stance on the floor with eyes closed	Gait speed	Berg Balance Scale
Gait, balance coordination and functional tasks	↓	–	–	↑	↑
Strengthening exercise	↓	↑	–	↑	–
3D exercise (Tai Chi, Gi Gong, dance, yoga)	↓	↑	↑	–	↑
General physical activity (walking)	–	–	–	–	ND
General physical activity (cycling)	ND	ND	ND	–	ND
Computerized balance	ND	ND	ND	ND	ND
Vibration	–	ND	ND	ND	ND
Multiple exercise	↓	↑	↑	–	↑

Note: '–' indicates no difference between exercise and control group outcomes. ND, no data.

Table 12.10 Single interventions in the community

Interventions and components	Effect	
	Rate of falls	Risk of falling
Group exercise: multiple categories of exercise versus control	↓	↓
Individual exercise at home: multiple categories of exercise versus control	↓	↓
Group exercise: Tai Chi versus control	↓	↓
Group and individual exercise: balance training versus control	↓	–
Group and individual exercise: strength/resistance training versus control	–	–
Individual exercise: general physical activity (walking) versus control	–	–
Exercise versus exercise: higher intensity multiple component exercise vs lower intensity exercise	↓	↓
Vitamin D (with or without calcium) versus control/placebo/calcium	–	–

Note: '–' indicates no difference between exercise and control group outcomes.

OTHER SINGLE INTERVENTIONS

Home safety assessment and modification interventions are effective in reducing rate of falls and risk of falling, particularly when delivered by an occupational therapist. These interventions are more effective in people at higher risk of falling, including those with severe visual impairment. However a recent systematic review was unable to reach any conclusion about the effectiveness of environmental or behavioural interventions for increasing physical activity in community dwelling visually impaired older people, as no eligible studies were found. In addition, although behavioural interventions delivered by occupational therapists have been shown to reduce the rate of falls, it is not clear whether this is due to reduced activity restriction (increased mobility) or reduced activity (lessening exposure to risk). There are also inconclusive and conflicting results from trials evaluating the effectiveness of behavioural and environmental interventions aimed at improving quality of life.

Interventions to treat vision problems have shown conflicting results on the rate of falls and risk of falling. Contributing factors may include: patients who regularly seek optometric care may be over-represented in randomized controlled trials (RCTs), control group participants in optometric intervention RCTs cannot be told to avoid optometric services and are typically asked to keep to their 'usual care', and some participants in control groups could be tempted to obtain additional ophthalmic care beyond 'the usual', having been alerted to their potential benefits by study participation. More likely, these interventions cause major changes in refractive correction and lens form inducing magnification changes which in turn change the vestibulo-ocular reflex gain affecting everyday actions such as stepping over curbs or obstacles or walking upstairs. The vestibulo-ocular reflex links the vestibular system with the extraocular muscles and produces the rapid compensatory eye movements needed to maintain stable vision of an object of interest as the head moves. However when regular wearers of multifocal glasses were given single lens glasses, all falls and outside falls were significantly reduced in the patients who regularly took part in outside activities. This is because multifocals produce a blurred and magnified view of the lower visual field beyond the near working distance, thus affecting the peripheral optic flow information used for postural control and making it difficult to judge the position of obstacles in the lower visual field, including obstacles and step and stair edges and/or foot placements relative to such environmental obstacles. Similar conflicting results occur with RCTs and observational studies with cataract surgery.

Gradual withdrawal of psychotropic medication reduced rate of falls, but not risk of falling. Medication review carried out by a pharmacist (or nurse or geriatrician) and recommendations regarding modification sent to the participant's family physician for implementation and modification were not effective in reducing rate of falls or risk of falling. However a comprehensive prescribing modification programme for primary care physicians that included face-to-face education by a clinical pharmacist, feedback on prescribing practices, and financial rewards combined with self-assessment of medication use by their patients and subsequent medication review and modification, significantly reduced risk of falling.[27]

Practical recommendations in the literature also include making a list of FRIDs, establishing a computerized alert system for when to de-prescribe FRIDs, seeking an alternative drug with lower fall risk, withdrawing FRIDs if clinically indicated, taking pertinent cautions when the use of FRIDs cannot be avoided, paying attention to prescribing appropriateness, simplifying the medication regimen, strengthening pharmacist-conducted clinical medication review, ensuring the label of each FRID dispensed contains a corresponding warning sign, being careful when medication change occurs, enhancing medication adherence and mandating for periodic reassessment of potential risk associated with the patient's medication regimen.[28]

Multifaceted podiatry including foot and ankle exercises compared with standard podiatry in people with disabling foot pain significantly reduced the rate of falls but not the risk of falling. Overall, supplementation with vitamin D, either alone or with calcium co-supplementation did not reduce rate of falls or risk of falling irrespective of falls risk status at baseline. However, there was a reduction in rate of falls and risk of falling in people with lower vitamin D levels before treatment. Higher dose of vitamin D (2000 IU/day) as opposed to lower dose (800 IU/day) did not have a preventative effect on falls but however showed a trend towards reducing risk of fracture. There is no evidence of effect for cognitive behavioural interventions or interventions to increase knowledge/educate about fall prevention alone on rate of falls or risk of falling.

Whole body vibration (WBV) has a significant treatment effect on the Tinetti Body Balance Score and the TUG test but the effect on other balance/mobility outcomes and fall rate remains inconclusive. In WBV, exercises are performed on a platform that generates vertical sinusoidal vibrations to produce a stimulation of the muscle spindles and induce muscles contractions.

MULTICOMPONENT AND MULTIFACTORIAL INTERVENTIONS

Combinations of some interventions were effective in reducing rate of falls but have inconsistent effect on risk of falling, while some combinations were not effective at all

(Table 12.11). Most of the effective combinations contain exercises that provide a moderate or high challenge to balance and of sufficient dose and duration.

Similarly, multifactorial interventions, which include individual risk assessment, reduce rate of falls but not risk of falling. Some of the components of intervention in these trials are described in Table 12.11. Managing falls in people with dementia however has proven difficult, and multifactorial interventions fail to demonstrate the same reduction. However, studies aiming to improve executive function through exercise, dual-task training or cognitive enhancing medications have shown promising results.

Long-term care

Exercise as a single intervention does not reduce the rate of falls or risk of falling. However, there appeared to be a trend towards an increase in rate of falls in facilities providing high level nursing care and a trend towards a decrease in intermediate level care facilities. This possibly is associated with the levels of dependency of cohorts where exercise reduces falls in people who are less frail in intermediate level facilities, and increase falls in frail people in high level nursing homes.

Some types of exercise may have beneficial outcomes (Table 12.12).[29] Of the various exercise components tested, only balance training using a mechanical apparatus in intermediate level care facilities reduced rate of falls. Nevertheless through physical rehabilitation interventions compared with usual care, ADL independence and performance are enhanced, or decline less, and there are possibly some positive effects on mood, cognition and fear of falling. However, the size, duration of the effects, the specific type(s) with most benefit and how these relate to resident characteristics is unclear. Among other single interventions, vitamin D supplementation reduced the rate of falls but not risk of falling. Medication review, education and other interventions did not affect falls rate or falls risk.

For multifactorial interventions in care facilities, the rate of falls and risk of falling suggested possible benefits (Table 12.13), but this evidence was not conclusive. Individually, some studies demonstrated a significant reduction in rate of falls and risk of falling. The study design of these multifactorial trials did not allow evaluation of their individual components however.

Interpretation of the multifactorial interventions is complex because of the variation in components, frailty of the population, duration and intensity of the intervention and how the interventions were implemented. In practice care provided in care facilities differs between countries and even when interventions seem effective careful consideration of the context is needed. Considerations of cultural and organizational contexts need to be taken into account when generalizing the results from these studies.

Table 12.11 Multiple components and multifactorial interventions in the community

Interventions and components	Rate of falls (RaR)	Risk of falling (RR)
Exercise + home safety intervention	↓ (0.77)	↓ (0.76)
Exercise + vision assessment	↓ (0.72)	↓ (0.73)
Exercise + home safety + vision assessment	↓ (0.71)	↓ (0.67)
Exercise + education + home safety intervention vs control	↓ (0.69)	–
Exercise + education + home safety intervention vs education	–	–
Exercise + education + home safety intervention + clinical assessment vs education	–	–
Exercise + education vs education	–	–
Exercise + education + risk assessment vs control	–	–
Exercise + home safety + multifactorial assessment and referral vs multifactorial assessment and referral	↓ (0.19)	ND
Exercise + nutritional supplementation + vitamin D and calcium vs calcium and vitamin D	–	ND
Exercise + vitamin D vs no exercise/no vitamin D	–	–
Exercise + cognitive behavioural therapy vs control	–	–
Exercise + 'individualized fall prevention advice' vs control	–	ND
Physical training + education vs control	–	–
Home safety + vision assessment	–	ND
Home safety + medication review vs control	ND	–
Education + free access to geriatric clinic vs control	ND	↓ (0.77)
Centre based rehabilitation programme (exercise + education) vs comparable home based programme	↓ (0.46)	↓ (0.57)
Multifunctional training + whole body vibration vs light physical exercise	↓ (0.46)	ND
'Multifaceted podiatry' (customized orthoses, footwear review, foot and ankle exercises, fall prevention education and 'usual podiatry care') vs 'usual podiatry care' alone	↓ (0.64)	–
Multidisciplinary rehabilitation + home safety visit vs multidisciplinary rehabilitation (no home visit)	↓ (0.46)	–

Note: ND, no data; RaR, rate ratio; RR, risk ratio. '–' indicates no difference between exercise and control group outcomes.

Acute care setting

For patients who are in hospital for more than a few weeks, interventions targeting multiple risk factors, and some single interventions, are effective. Additional physiotherapy (supervised exercises) in subacute wards reduced the risk of falling and an educational session by a trained research nurse targeting individual fall risk factors in patients at high risk of falling in acute medical wards reduces the risk of falls in these patients. Wards in which 85% of beds are visible from nursing staff stations have lower falls rate compared to wards where 15% of beds are visible from nursing stations. Carpet flooring increased the rate of falls and potentially increased the risk of falling while the effectiveness of other single interventions is limited (Table 12.14).

On the other hand, multifactorial interventions in hospitals reduce rate of falls as well as risk of falling and multidisciplinary care in a geriatric ward after hip fracture surgery compared with usual care in an orthopaedic ward

significantly reduce rate of falls and risk of falling. The different components are shown in Table 12.15. However, similar to long-term care settings, interpretation of the effectiveness of multifactorial interventions in this setting is complex because of the variation in components, case mix of the samples, duration and intensity of the interventions, and how the interventions were implemented. Care provided in healthcare systems differs between countries and even when interventions seem effective careful consideration of the context is needed. Considerations of cultural and organizational contexts need to be taken into account when applying the results of these studies in practice.

Falls prevention after a fracture

The strategies to prevent falls in patients with recent fractures should be implemented as a continuum beginning with assessments and interventions in the in-patient setting and continuing to the community or out-patient setting.[30]

Table 12.12 Single interventions in care facilities

Interventions	Effect	
	Rate of falls	Risk of falls
Exercise: overall	–	–
Supervised exercises vs usual care	–	–
Balance training using mechanical apparatus: perturbed walking exercise using a bilateral separated treadmill	↓	–
Balance training on a force platform with a visual feedback screen: standing balance exercises on one leg	–	–
'Functional Walking' programme, consisting mainly of functional balance training	↑	–
'Goal setting and individualized activities of daily living activity programme' by a gerontology nurse	–	–
Tai Chi intervention	ND	–
Combination of exercises	–	–
Medication review		–
Single clinical medication review	–	–
Pharmacist transition coordinator for patients discharged from a hospital to a long-term care facility for the first time	–	–
Pharmacist led outreach programme of audit and feedback, and education of staff regarding medications and falls risk	–	–
GRAM software for decision support for prescribing practices	–	–
Vitamin D + calcium vs calcium	↓	–
Staff training/education		
Half-day education programme on fall and fracture prevention for managers, nurses and healthcare assistants, given by specialist osteoporosis nurses	–	–
Education to implement a patient-safety programme directed at falls, urinary tract infection and pressure ulcers based on available guidelines	–	–
Care model change		
Fall risk assessment tool vs nurses' judgement alone	–	–
Lavender olfactory stimulation	↓	–
Increased sunlight exposure	–	–
Multisensory stimulation in a Snoezelen room	–	ND

Note: ND, no data. '–' indicates no difference between exercise and control group outcomes.

Table 12.13 Multifaceted interventions in care facilities

Interventions and components	Effect
Overall	Possible benefit for rate of falls and risk of falling
Supervised exercises + fluids + regular toileting	Possibly some reduction in risk of falls, no effect on fracture and rate of falls
Increased sunlight exposure + calcium supplementation	No significant reduction in rate of falls, risk of falling or risk of fracture
Fall prevention programme for staff and residents: 1. Staff training on risk factors and preventive measures (60 min), audit and monthly feedback concerning falls and injuries 2. Check list of 76 environmental hazards (lighting, chair and bed height, floor surfaces, etc). Feedback to staff and administrators	Reduction in rate of falls and reductions in risk of falling

(Continued)

Table 12.13 *(Continued)* Multifaceted interventions in care facilities

Interventions and components	Effect
3. Resident education: all received written information, offered personal consultation by study nurse or exercise instructor	
4. Group exercise programme (progressive balance and resistance training) for 75 min, twice a week	
5. Hip protectors	
Multifactorial, multidisciplinary intervention: Baseline assessments by physiotherapist, nurse and OT and interventions based on these	Reduction in rate of falls
1. Exercise: supervised gait, balance, coordination and functional + strength/resistance + flexibility + general physical exercises, 3×40 min sessions per week for 3 months Progressive exercises individually tailored and delivered by exercise assistants supported by physiotherapists. Carried out in groups or individually if residents unable to participate in groups because of frailty or cognitive impairment	
2. Staff education	
3. Medical review: baseline assessments screened by geriatrician. Recommendations concerning medication review, orthostatic hypotension and osteoporosis prevention sent to participant's GP for GP to implement	
4. Environmental modification: OT assistant visited facilities to assess and report on falls hazards, with facilities being alerted of major hazards	
5. Optician and podiatry referrals based on baseline assessment	
Multidisciplinary programme including general and resident-specific tailored interventions for 11 weeks: supervised exercises, medication review, modifying environmental hazards, supplying and repairing aids, hip protectors, education of staff, post-fall problem-solving conferences and staff guidance. Individually tailored supervised exercises (gait, balance, coordination and functional + strength/resistance) 2–3 times a week. Intervention delivered by registered nurses, physician and physiotherapists	Reduction in risk of falling
Falls risk management programme of 12 months duration	Increase in rate of falls
1. Falls coordinator in each home (carried out fall risk assessment of all residents using tool, developed specific recommendations and care plans, coordinated with other healthcare professionals, and ensured that recommendations were followed)	
2. Evidence based risk assessment tool + detailed management strategies relating to mobility impairments, mental impairments, medications, continence, sensory impairments	
3. Tailored care plan based on assessment + OT, PT, medical and specialist referrals	
4. Logo on high-risk residents walls + colour coded dots showing fall prevention strategies	
5. Manual containing the risk assessment form, information for strategies, high-risk fall logos, all forms and educational information for nurses, doctors, physiotherapists and OTs	
Consultation service with individual assessment and recommendations targeting environmental and personal safety, wheelchair use, psychotropic medication use, transferring and ambulation. Falls coordinator at each site. Intervention delivered by study team	Significant difference in the proportion of recurrent fallers

Note: GP, general practitioner; OT, occupational therapist; PT, physical therapist.

Table 12.14 Single interventions in hospital settings

Interventions	Effect
Exercises – additional physiotherapy in rehabilitation wards	Reduction in risk of falling No reduction in rate of falls
Vitamin D supplementation and calcium: 800 IU oral cholecalciferol (vitamin D3) plus 1,200 mg calcium daily until separation from the facility vs control: 1,200 mg calcium daily until discharge or death	No difference in risk of falling or fractures
Carpeted floors compared with vinyl floors	Increased rate of falls and potentially increased risk of falling
One low-low bed per 12 existing beds in acute and subacute wards	No effect on rate of falls
Blue identification bracelet on high-risk patients in a subacute hospital setting	No reduction in rate of falls or risk of falling
Bed exit alarms	No difference in the number of bed falls
Staff training	
Multifaceted fall prevention guideline implementation vs routine dissemination in acute care hospitals	No significant difference in rate of falls
Implementation of three guidelines (falls, urinary tract infection, pressure ulcers) targeted nursing staff in acute care hospital wards	No difference in rate of falls
Service model change	
Computer based fall prevention tool kit	No difference in rate of falls or risk of falling
Acute care for the elderly service vs usual care in general medical wards	No reduction in rate of falls
Behavioural advisory service for people with confusion	No change in number of people falling
Knowledge interventions	Reduction in risk of falling
Education + usual care: participants received one educational session (no more than 30 min) based on identified risk factors	
Designed to increase awareness of risk of falling during hospitalization and teach risk-reduction strategies. Relatives of confused participants received the educational session vs control: usual care and including usual fall prevention interventions	
Two forms of multimedia patient education (written and video based materials plus one-on-one bedside follow-up from a trained health professional (complete programme) or educational materials only compared with usual care in a mixture of acute and subacute wards	Falls were less frequent in people who were cognitively intact receiving the complete programme

Table 12.15 Multifaceted interventions in hospital settings

Interventions and components	Effect

Targeted falls risk prevention programme based on identified falls risk (Peter James Centre Falls Risk Assessment Tool). Potential interventions were:
1. Supervised exercise programme: 45 min sessions three times a week from commencement of intervention until discharge. Exercises comprised gait, balance and coordination + strengthening/resistance + 3D (Tai Chi)
    Exercises were individually tailored
    Exercises were delivered by a physiotherapist
2. Falls risk alert card
3. Up to four educational sessions from OT at bedside to individual participants of up to 30 min duration
4. Hip protectors
	Rate of falls was reduced (most obvious after 45 days of observation) but not risk of falling

(Continued)

Table 12.15 *(Continued)* Multifaceted interventions in hospital settings

Interventions and components	Effect
Targeted risk factor reduction care plan for patients with a history of falls or a near fall during admission. Based on assessment (and subsequent referral/ action) relating to: eyesight (referral to ophthalmologist); medications check for sedatives, antidepressants, diuretics, polypharmacy, etc (medical review of benefit vs harm); lying and standing blood pressure (advice to participant and referral to medical staff); ward urine test (midstream urine if positive for nitrites, blood or protein); difficulty with mobility (referral to physiotherapist); review of bed rail use; footwear safety (advice on replacement); bed height (kept at lowest height); position in ward (placing high risk patients near nurses' station); environmental causes (act to correct); nurse call bell (explained and in reach)	Reduced risk of falling
Multidisciplinary team providing comprehensive geriatric assessment, management and rehabilitation	Reduction in the rate of falls and in the risk of falling at discharge, even in patients with dementia
Targeted multifactorial intervention: a nurse and a physiotherapist each worked for 25 hours per week for 3 months in all intervention wards. Provided risk assessment of falls, staff and patient education, drug review, modification of bedside and ward environments, an exercise programme, and sock alarms for selected patients (maximum of two per ward)	No effect on falls rate

Note: OT, occupational therapist.

The baseline falls risk and any risk factors for delirium and functional decline should be evaluated on admission. The subsequent assessment and care plan should involve a multidisciplinary team responsible for preventing new in-hospital episodes. This team should also identify all potential risk factors for subsequent falls, integrating a fracture risk assessment tool within the equation. Once the patient is out of hospital, multifaceted evaluation should continue, with a view to implementing targeted multicomponent interventions as part of an effective falls prevention programme.

CONCLUSION

Falls prevention in the older population is a major health priority in all healthcare settings, which will continue to pose significant challenges given the aging population. There is good evidence that falls prevention works and is cost-effective with appropriately designed intervention programmes. These programmes should be guided by the best available evidence in each care setting.

REFERENCES

1. Tinetti M, Speechley M, Ginter S. Risk factors for falls among elderly persons living in the community. *N Engl J Med*. 1988;319(26):1701–7.
2. Kearney F, Harwood R, Gladman J, Lincoln N, Masud T. The relationship between executive function and falls and gait abnormalities in older adults: A systematic review. *Dement Geriatr Cogn Disord*. 2013;36(1–2):20–35.
3. Woolcott J, Richardson K, Wiens M, Patel B, Marin J, Khan K, et al. Meta-analysis of the impact of 9 medication classes on falls in elderly persons. *Arch Intern Med*. 2009;169(21):1952–60.
4. Deandrea S, Bravi F, Turati F, Lucenteforte E, Vecchia CL, Negri E. Risk factors for falls in older people in nursing homes and hospitals. A systematic review and meta-analysis. *Arch Gerontol Geriatr*. 2013;56(3):407–15.
5. Heinrich S, Rapp K, Rissmann U, Becker C, König H. Cost of falls in old age: A systematic review. *Osteoporos Int*. 2010;21(6):891–902.
6. Davis J, Robertson M, Ashe M, Liu-Ambrose T, Khan K, Marra C. International comparison of cost of falls in older adults living in the community: A systematic review. *Osteoporos Int*. 2010;21(8):1295–306.
7. Morrison A, Fan T, Sen S, Weisenfluh L. Epidemiology of falls and osteoporotic fractures: A systematic review. *Clinicoecon Outcomes Res*. 2013;5:9–18.
8. Perell K, Nelson A, Goldman R, Luther S, Prieto-Lewis N, Rubenstein L. Fall risk assessment measures: An analytic review. *J Gerontol A Biol Sci Med Sci*. 2001;56(12):M761–6.
9. Tinetti M, Williams T, Mayewski R. Fall risk index for elderly patients based on number of chronic disabilities. *Am J Med*. 1986;80(3):429–34.
10. Graafmans W, Ooms M, Hofstee H, Bezemer P, Bouter L, Lips P. Falls in the elderly: A prospective study of risk factors and risk profiles. *Am J Epidemiol*. 1996;143(11):1129–36.

11. Tromp A, Pluijm S, Smit J, Deeg D, Bouter L, Lips P. Fall-risk screening test: A prospective study on predictors for falls in community-dwelling elderly. *J Clin Epidemiol.* 2001;54(8):837–44.

12. Stalenhoef P, Diederiks J, Knottnerus J, Kester A, Crebolder H. A risk model for the prediction of recurrent falls in community-dwelling elderly: A prospective cohort study. *J Clin Epidemiol.* 2002;55(11):1088–94.

13. Nandy S, Parsons S, Cryer C, Underwood M, Rashbrook E, Carter Y, et al. Development and preliminary examination of the predictive validity of the Falls Risk Assessment Tool (FRAT) for use in primary care. *J Public Health (Oxf).* 2004;26(2):138–43.

14. Pluijm S, Smit J, Tromp E, Stel V, Deeg D, Bouter L, et al. A risk profile for identifying community-dwelling elderly with a high risk of recurrent falling: Results of a 3-year prospective study. *Osteoporos Int.* 2006;17(3):417–25.

15. Bongue B, Dupré C, Beauchet O, Rossat A, Fantino B, Colvez A. A screening tool with five risk factors was developed for fall-risk prediction in community-dwelling elderly. *J Clin Epidemiol.* 2011;64(10):1152–60.

16. Russell M, Hill K, Day L, Blackberry I, Gurrin L, Dharmage S. Development of the Falls Risk for Older People in the Community (FROP-Com) screening tool. *Age Ageing.* 2009;38(1):40–6.

17. Peeters G, Pluijm S, van Schoor NM, Elders P, Bouter L, Lips P. Validation of the LASA fall risk profile for recurrent falling in older recent fallers. *J Clin Epidemiol.* 2010;63(11):1242–8.

18. Lord S, Menz H, Tiedemann A. A physiological profile approach to falls risk assessment and prevention. *Phys Ther.* 2003;83(3):237–52.

19. Robbins A, Rubenstein L, Josephson K, Schulman B, Osterweil D, Fine G. Predictors of falls among elderly people. Results of two population-based studies. *Arch Intern Med.* 1989;149(7):1628–33.

20. Lord S, Clark R, Webster I. Physiological factors associated with falls in an elderly population. *J Am Geriatr Soc.* 1991;39(12):1194–2000.

21. Sterke C, van Beeck EF, Looman C, Kressig R, van der Cammen TJ. An electronic walkway can predict short-term fall risk in nursing home residents with dementia. *Gait Posture.* 2012;36(1):95–101.

22. Aranda-Gallardo M, Morales-Asencio J, Canca-Sanchez J, Barrero-Sojo S, Perez-Jimenez C, Morales-Fernandez A, et al. Instruments for assessing the risk of falls in acute hospitalized patients: A systematic review and meta-analysis. *BMC Health Serv Res.* 2013;13:122.

23. Wong Shee A, Phillips B, Hill K. Comparison of two fall risk assessment tools (FRATs) targeting falls prevention in sub-acute care. *Arch Gerontol Geriatr.* 2012;55(3):653–9.

24. Lee J, Geller A, Strasser D. Analytical review: Focus on fall screening assessments. *PM R.* 2013;5(7):609–21.

25. Sherrington C, Tiedemann A, Fairhall N, Close J, Lord SR. Exercise to prevent falls in older adults: An updated meta-analysis and best practice recommendations. *N S W Public Health Bull.* 2011;22(3–4):78–83.

26. Gillespie L, Robertson M, Gillespie W, Sherrington C, Gates S, Clemson L, et al. Interventions for preventing falls in older people living in the community. *Cochrane Database Syst Rev* 2012;(9):CD007146.

27. Pit S, Byles J, Henry D, Holt L, Hansen V, Bowman D. A quality use of medicines program for general practitioners and older people: A cluster randomised controlled trial. *Med J Aust* 2007;187(1):23–30.

28. Chen Y, Zhu L, Zhou Q. Effects of drug pharmacokinetic/pharmacodynamic properties, characteristics of medication use, and relevant pharmacological interventions on fall risk in elderly patients. *Ther Clin Risk Manag.* 2014;10:437–48.

29. Cameron I, Gillespie L, Robertson M, Murray G, Hill K, Cumming R, et al. Interventions for preventing falls in older people in care facilities and hospitals. *Cochrane Database Syst Rev.* 2012;12:CD005465.

30. Demontiero O, Gunawardene P, Duque G. Postoperative prevention of falls in older adults with fragility fractures. *Clin Geriatr Med.* 2014;30(2):333–47.

13

Open fractures

LISA K. CANNADA AND TINA K. DREGER

INTRODUCTION

Our population is aging with the number of people in the United States older than 65 expected to double to 60 million or 17% of the population by 2030.[1] Compared to the past, this is a more active population with an increased lifespan and has been working and maintaining their independence for longer. In addition, in 2010 the United States census found that the population aged between 45 and 64 had a growth rate of 32%, primarily due to the baby boomers.[2] This population growth will be reflected in the years to come in North America.

The increasingly elderly population can be expected to lead to an increased number of trauma patients over 65. Trauma is currently the fifth leading cause of death in those above 65 and accounts for 23% of hospital admissions and 28% of all hospital charges.[1] This will have significant implications for future healthcare cost as the population grows. The elderly generally have more medical comorbidities, and so longer lengths of stay can be anticipated after trauma.

The geriatric population has been well studied in terms of certain types of fractures including distal radius and hip fractures. However, geriatric open fractures are not a well-researched subset of injuries. In the past, it has been hard to record large enough numbers to evaluate these injuries although the current literature is increasing studying geriatric traumatic fractures. With the growing elderly population, these fractures will affect many healthcare disciplines, including the subspecialty of orthopaedic trauma.

EPIDEMIOLOGY

Despite the aging population and frequency of fractures among the elderly, the literature on open fractures in this group of patients is limited. We do know that unlike open fractures in the young, 60% of open fractures in the elderly occur due to low energy mechanisms such as a fall. The most common open fractures are sustained in the distal radius, ankle, fingers and the tibial diaphysis. Much of the information we have on epidemiology comes from the Royal Infirmary of Edinburgh and the work of Court-Brown et al.[3] Prospective data on fractures occurring in 4,786 consecutive outpatients and inpatients ≥65 years of age were collected over a 2-year period. The majority of fractures in the elderly population were in women (77%), and only 1.2% were open fractures, 13.6% of which were Gustilo type III. This trend towards a higher incidence of Gustilo type III open fractures would typically be expected as the energy mechanism increases, although in the elderly they can occur after ground level falls.

Court-Brown et al.[4] reviewed 484 open fractures in patients ≥65 years of age over a 15-year period and compared them to open fractures in patients below 65. The incidence of open fractures was noted to increase with age. Interestingly, males aged 15–19 and females ≥90 showed a similar incidence of open fractures. These results are from the United Kingdom and may be different elsewhere. However, females were noted to have an increase in open fractures throughout their life, but with a sharp increase starting in the seventh decade. This could be due to a physical decline with decreased bone mineral density, and decreased physical activity leading to balance issues perpetuating a vicious cycle. The main mechanism of injury was a fall in 60% of patients, representing a low energy mechanism, yet there was a high incidence of type III fractures. This was true especially in women. There is a definitive increase in open fractures in post-menopausal women. The decline in bone quality in post-menopausal women is also accompanied by changes in the skin.

Animal studies show that the male dermis is 190% thicker than in the female, while the epidermis is thicker in female mice.[5] This is similar to the situation in humans.[6] Applying this to the results of a simple ground level fall, the higher grade of open fracture can possibly be attributed to the skin quality in elderly patients and may not be reflective of the energy of the injury. The skin is thinner and may tear more easily, resulting in a higher grade of open fracture due to the size of the wound (Figure 13.1).

Cox et al.[7] specifically compared the comorbidities and mechanism of injury for tibial shaft fractures sustained in the elderly. Comorbidities were found to be similar between patients sustaining closed or open fractures. The mechanism of injury was also similar, with ground level falls and pedestrian versus motor vehicle accidents predominating. Patients with Gustilo type III open fractures had more complications, and increased length of stay and need for additional surgery compared to those with lower Gustilo types.

Keller et al.[1] retrospectively reviewed all high energy trauma in patients ≥65 over a 5.5-year period at their academic trauma centre. Clavicle, midfoot, proximal humerus, sacroiliac joint and distal ulna fractures were predictors of mortality in geriatric patients. It was also highlighted that the elderly present with worse injuries, remain in hospital longer, require greater resources after discharge and die at a rate three times higher than the younger population after high energy trauma. The impact or frequency of open fractures in this study population of 597 was not studied.

In a similar study, Abdelfattah et al. reviewed 154 geriatric patients, admitted over a 6-year period, who sustained high energy trauma (Injury Severity Score [ISS] >16).[2] Clavicle, scapula and femur fractures were found to predispose this population to worse outcomes. Increased mortality was found in those with pelvic or acetabular fractures requiring operative fixation and spine fractures that were treated non-operatively. Again no assessment of those patients with open fractures was delineated.

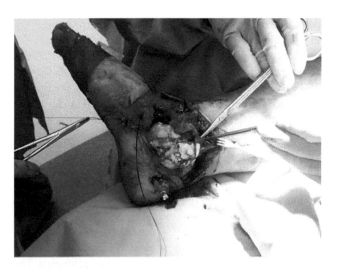

Figure 13.1 Geriatric open fracture with large open wound due to skin tearing.

In this chapter we hope to draw attention to the important issue of geriatric open fractures as there is very little literature to guide care. Several articles do discuss geriatric trauma, both low and high energy, but open fractures are frequently not mentioned or evaluated.

CLASSIFICATION

The Gustilo classification of open fractures has been commonly utilized to grade all open fractures. In this system, a type I is an open fracture with a clean wound less than 1 cm long, a type II has a laceration over 1 cm long without extensive soft tissue damage and type III fractures have more extensive soft tissue damage. Type III fractures are subdivided into IIIA, IIIB and IIIC fractures. Type IIIA fractures are those which can be closed primarily. Type IIIB fractures require the soft tissue injury to be closed secondarily by skin grafting, flaps or other techniques. Type IIIC fractures are those with a vascular injury requiring repair.[8]

The Gustilo classification has been used extensively. However, in the elderly population even the mechanism leading to the open fracture is not the same as in younger patients. Often the geriatric patient has very thin skin, which may contribute to larger wounds. As one ages, there is an increase in soft tissue fragility. In addition to the changes which we know occur with aging of the elderly bone and the decrease in bone mineral density, elderly skin has decreased organization of collagen making it more susceptible to injury.[4] The skin loses elasticity and often feels 'loose' without significant connection to the underlying soft tissue. In addition, the skin turgor is not the same as in the younger patient. Thus, the older patient may have propagation of skin trauma from a small bony insult yielding a much larger skin tear. As the skin tears, it causes a much higher grade injury due to the larger size of the soft tissue injury.

A common example is an open ankle fracture dislocation. An eversion type of mechanism is common. The medial malleolus fracture may be quite small but the wound presents as a transverse laceration 10 cm or more in length. This is because the skin is quite fragile and tears more easily. The open fracture classification of Gustilo and Anderson is useful in the younger and high energy trauma patient, but in the geriatric fracture patient, its applicability may be more limited. Surgeons should perhaps consider an alternative classification which evaluates multiple factors.

The value of classification systems for mangled extremities was evaluated in the Lower Extremity Assessment Project (LEAP) study.[9] There are several classifications for mangled extremities taking into consideration the injury to the skin, muscle and nerves; ischaemia; chronological age; energy of injury; and other factors. Those scoring systems were used to predict amputation versus limb salvage. The various scoring systems proved unreliable in predicting outcome.[10] In the elderly open fracture we have already established that there often is a higher grade of open fracture due to the size of the wound. The literature is limited but suggests that outcomes in higher fracture grades are worse.[7]

Table 13.1 Geriatric open fracture considerations to further assess severity of the fracture

Pre-existing venous stasis	Yes/No
Pitting oedema	Yes/No
CHF/CVD	Yes/No
Fracture comminution	Yes/No
Fracture contamination	Yes/No
Length of skin tear	<1 cm, 1–5 cm, >5 cm
Proximal based flap	Yes/No

Note: CHF, congestive heart failure; CVD, cardiovascular disease.

Table 13.1 shows a number of additional factors which, we believe, should be taken into consideration when classifying elderly open fractures. These are all questions relating to the injury, which should be answered to assist in planning the treatment of the elderly open fracture. We suggest evaluation of these additional factors when considering the severity of open fractures in the geriatric population.

TREATMENT

As with any open fracture there are several considerations before operative fixation. The first involves a thorough clinical evaluation consisting of the basic principles of Airway-Breathing-Circulation (ABC) management. Early resuscitation is essential for decreasing mortality in this often fragile population. Once the patient is stabilized, exposure of all injured extremities will allow complete assessment of the viability of the limb, degree of soft tissue damage and amount of contamination present. Compartment syndrome cannot be excluded despite the open nature of the fracture or because of the age of the patient. If vascular injury is suspected, ankle brachial indices (ABIs) should be used as a screening tool. Complete radiographic evaluation of the fractured limb to include the adjacent joints is essential. In periarticular fractures, CT scans can be very useful after spanning external fixation has been applied as they may reveal fracture morphology better than X-rays. This can be indispensable for preoperative planning.

Once the general assessment is complete, specific emergency room management should be tailored to the fracture and soft tissue injury. Wound haemorrhage must be controlled. If the bleeding is from one of the extremities, direct pressure is preferable with application of a tourniquet if the former is insufficient. If there is an open pelvic fracture, intra-pelvic packing may be necessary. If the pelvic fracture is an open book fracture, a binder or sheet may be required, applied over the greater trochanters to decrease blood loss.

Antibiotic administration is also important in the emergency room. The antibiotics will depend on the initial classification of the open fracture. This has been historically based on the Gustilo and Anderson classification (Table 13.2). However, in the elderly, with an increased risk of renal dysfunction and potential for decreased creatinine clearance, the choice and dose of antibiotic regimens may need to be altered.

Table 13.2 Antibiotics recommended for different fracture grades as defined by the Gustilo–Anderson Classification

Open fracture type	Antibiotic recommendations
Type I	First generation cephalosporin
Type II	First generation cephalosporin
Type III	First generation cephalosporin + aminoglycoside + penicillin for farm injuries

Fractures will then need provisional irrigation and reduction followed by placement in a properly padded splint before transfer to the operating room. Formal irrigation and debridement (I&D) in the operating room should be initiated as soon as deemed safe by all care teams, and haemodynamic stability achieved. Meticulous assessment of the zone of injury is important, with a systematic debridement being undertaken. This should start with the most superficial structures and proceed down to the bone. Any non-viable structures or foreign bodies should be excised. Extension of the wound is usually necessary for complete assessment.

Irrigation with normal saline should follow debridement. No advantage has been shown with the addition of antibiotic solution to normal saline irrigation. Debate continues as to whether there is an advantage to pulsatile lavage versus low flow irrigation. Some surgeons feel that tissue is traumatized with pulsatile lavage and foreign material is driven further into the wound than with gentle high volume irrigation. In the elderly, the skin is thinner and more friable making it less tolerant of even minimal tissue trauma. This favours low flow irrigation.

Based on the amount of contamination and extent of injury at initial I&D, a decision regarding wound closure or repeat debridement must be made. The level of soft tissue viability following a high energy mechanism of injury may not be apparent on initial debridement and a second look is likely to be beneficial. The fragility of the soft tissues and potential vascular compromise by pre-morbid conditions in the elderly may make even a low energy injury best managed with a second look. Other situations where this may apply is in a moderate to severely contaminated wound, when there has been a delay in transfer to the operating room due to polytrauma or comorbidities, or in a damage control situation where the time required for wound closure places the patient at greater risk. In these situations negative pressure wound therapy (NPWT) allows for control of drainage at the site of injury, provides a sterile environment and allows ease of exposure on return to the operating room (Figure 13.2). Closure may follow when the wound is felt to be clean and there is no concern about further progression. The use of vessel loops sequentially crossing the wound and secured with staples tends to ensure better approximation of the wound edges as opposed to the sponge alone which tends to push the skin edges further apart. The negative pressure device has adaptations that may protect fragile

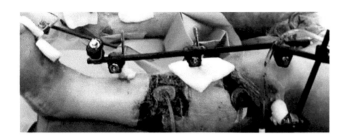

Figure 13.2 Use of negative pressure wound therapy for an open fracture.

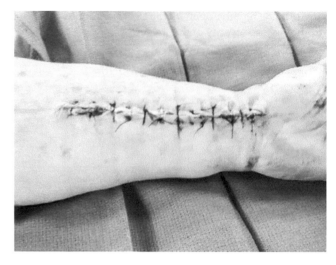

Figure 13.3 Multiple suture techniques used to close an open both-bones forearm fracture.

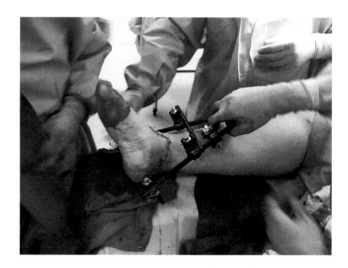

Figure 13.4 Use of a mattress suture technique to reapproximate an open fracture (from Figure 13.1). This figure also demonstrates the use of a delta frame external fixator to stabilize an open fracture.

elderly tissue. The pressure can be lower than the typically used 125 mmHg especially if placed over nerves or vessels, or traumatized muscle tissue. Different sponge types or dressings beneath the sponge provide added protection. Intermittent suction has the same benefits of tissue protection as the continuous mode.

Some debate exists in the literature as to whether post-irrigation wound cultures should be obtained. Post-irrigation wound cultures have been used to guide antibiotic therapy should a deep infection develop after treatment of an open fracture. These have proven to be more accurate than pre-irrigation cultures. Lenarz et al.[11] retrospectively reviewed 346 open fractures at a single level 1 trauma centre. A standard protocol was utilized to determine timing of closure for open fractures. Type II and III fractures were included as the majority of type I fractures were closed primarily after initial I&D. Post-irrigation cultures were taken and an NPWT device applied. If the cultures remained negative at 48 hours, the wound underwent repeat I&D and closure. If the cultures were positive at this point in time, the wound underwent a further I&D and the NPWT was replaced. This process was repeated until the cultures remained negative, at which time the wound was closed. The authors found a decrease in deep infection across all open fracture grades when compared to historic controls.

If the injury is amenable to primary closure, many factors must be considered. As soft tissue in the elderly is prone to swelling, early meticulous closure can avoid future complications and decrease the need for plastic surgery coverage. The basic principles of suturing are even more important in the elderly. One must avoid strangulation and prevent necrosis of the tissue edges. Many aspects should be thoughtfully evaluated for the best outcomes. The use of a reverse cutting needle can prevent tearing of the suture through the skin towards the wound edge once tension is placed. Also, entering the skin at a 90 degree angle minimizes the tissue trauma of needle placement and allows proper eversion of the skin edges. The use of non-toothed rather than toothed forceps can prevent crushing the tissue as sutures are placed. Various suture techniques can also be used to aid closure. At times multiple closure techniques will need to be combined for the best closure (Figure 13.3). Use of far-near near-far retention sutures spaced along the incision is useful when wound approximation is difficult and can decrease the tension on any one suture, preventing them from tearing fragile skin. These can

be left in for a period of time until the tension has decreased, or on initial closure once the remaining sutures are placed. Horizontal mattress sutures perform the same function of distributing skin and suture tension while everting the skin edges for improved healing (Figure 13.4).

Once the open fracture is thoroughly debrided, the fracture requires stabilization. The type of stabilization will be guided by the extent of soft tissue damage, the severity and location of the fracture as well as the medical status of the patient and any ancillary interventions that are required. For example, the patient may require an exploratory laparotomy or vascular repair due to concomitant injuries allowing inadequate time for definitive fixation of one or all fractures.

An external fixator can be applied to stabilize the fracture which not only protects the soft tissues from further trauma but can also decrease bleeding and patient discomfort and facilitate bedside care for the nursing staff. In the setting of pelvic ring or femur fractures it eliminates the need for skeletal traction facilitating offloading of bony prominences and preventing pressure ulcers. In certain circumstances the fixator may serve as definitive fixation. There are several 'tricks' that can improve the use of external fixators. First the surgeon should consider the approach that will be necessary for definitive fixation. The pins should be placed outside of the area where plates will be applied. This can decrease the risk of infection as the pin tracts are open to bacterial contamination. When possible the pins should also be placed outside the zone of injury to prevent further trauma as well as decreasing the risk of bacteria tracking to bone. Using a C-arm is invaluable to prevent misplacement and multiple unnecessary screw holes thereby placing the patient at risk of fracture by further decreasing the strength of osteoporotic bone. Next a strong construct should be built to prevent malreduction once the frame is placed. Basic principles such as the use of multiple bars, increasing the working length, and decreasing the distance between the bars and skin should be employed. For unstable open ankle fractures adding a first metatarsal pin to the standard delta frame can aid in positioning and maintaining reduction (Figure 13.4).

Intramedullary nailing is an excellent option when long bone fractures are present together with soft tissue injury. Closed reduction techniques can be utilized and minimal incisions applied out of the affected area. The open wound can frequently be utilized to assist with reduction of the fracture as well. This technique allows for less periosteal stripping that accompanies standard open reduction and internal fixation and may maintain a greater amount of blood flow and osteogenic cells at the fracture site.

When open reduction and internal fixation is chosen for stabilizing a fracture, the treating surgeon must decide what type of plating will best balance stability yet allow healing of the fracture. If the fracture is transverse it may be stabilized in such a way to allow primary bone healing. Bridge plating techniques can be utilized for comminuted fractures. With osteoporotic bone, one might consider locked plating techniques. Very rigid fixation can be achieved with these locked techniques. However the surgeon must carefully balance stability and micromotion to allow secondary bone healing and prevent non-union.

Crucial issues to consider include the timing of surgery which must be balanced with the condition of the patient and the insult to the system. Careful evaluation of the polytrauma patient and teamwork with general surgery, trauma and critical care teams is essential for a good outcome. Serum markers of particular value are base deficit and lactic acid. A base deficit of ≤ -6 was associated with a significantly higher mortality rate in individuals older than 55.[12] This has been supported in more recent articles even in elderly blunt trauma patients who were normotensive.[13]

Early surgery with the goal of stabilization of the fracture with minimal soft tissue trauma should be the goal.

This goes a long way to allowing mobilization and decreasing the complications from prolonged recumbency and multiple trips to the operating room.

SPECIFIC OPEN FRACTURE TYPES IN THE ELDERLY

Distal radial fractures

Just like open fractures in the elderly, there are few studies to guide treatment of open distal radius fractures in the elderly. In a recently published article, Kaufman et al.[14] reported good results with immediate open reduction and internal fixation of these fractures. The numbers were quite small with only 21 geriatric open distal radius fractures in one of the largest trauma centres in the United States over an 8-year period with adequate follow-up. There was only one deep infection and one non-union noted in this group. There were four operative complications requiring repeat surgery. The authors also completed functional outcome measures. The conclusion was that there was an acceptable risk/benefit ratio with immediate fixation of open distal radius fractures and immediate closure.

Ankle fractures

There are multiple questions with geriatric ankle fractures, including optimum plate fixation. It was thought that locked plates provided a stronger fixation construct less prone to failure in osteoporotic bone. However, the use of locking plates has not proven superior in biomechanical or clinical studies. Locking plates can be thicker, increasing the incidence of symptomatic hardware in the elderly patient with thin, compromised soft tissue.[15,16]

Foot fractures

It is hard to find specific literature related to the elderly with open foot fractures. Court-Brown et al. specifically examined open foot fractures in adults.[17] Over a 23-year period, there were 348 open fractures of the foot. There were only 41 fractures in patients who were aged 65 years or older (11.8%). The numbers were quite interesting with 68% of the fractures being open phalangeal fractures, 19.5% metatarsal fractures and 9.8% calcaneal fractures. There were no open talus fractures. These fractures may have been considered minor in terms of fracture grade with only 26.8% being Gustilo type III. There was a 17.1% amputation rate with 71.4% of the amputations being for open fractures of the phalanges. This underscores the importance of prompt attention to open fractures with a timely debridement being undertaken. One must consider the pre-existing morbidities which can definitely affect the treatment and outcome. That is why evaluation of all aspects of the soft tissue injury and open fracture, as suggested in Table 13.1, is important.

Tibial fractures

Although there are no specific treatment recommendations for open tibial fractures in the elderly, or any comparison of different techniques, in the literature, there are two studies that look at outcomes. Cox et al. reviewed the trauma database from Leeds Teaching Hospitals in the United Kingdom for all patients over 65 years of age with closed and open tibial diaphyseal fractures.[7] Over a 2-year period they had 28 open fractures and 26 closed fractures. These patients were followed for 16–23 months. There were no significant differences in comorbidities between the groups. The mean ISS was greater in the open fracture group, at 18.9 versus 10, although mean age was the same. Each open fracture received antibiotic prophylaxis immediately and this was continued for 5 days postoperatively. If any soft tissue procedures were required to close the wound, they were undertaken within 5 days of injury. In the open fracture group several stabilization methods were used. Intramedullary nailing was used in 17, plating in 8 and an Ilizarov frame in 3 patients. No open fractures were treated in a cast compared to three in the closed group. Additional surgical procedures were required in 54%, which was significantly higher than in the closed fracture group. This had a direct impact on hospitalization time as the mean length of stay increased from 17 to 44 days. Mortality on the other hand was not significantly different between the two groups. This study also highlights the importance of the team approach to elderly open fractures. Of the open fractures, 10 were classified as type IIIB and required soft tissue coverage. This same subset also had a significantly higher complication rate, a greater rate of ICU admission and a longer mean length of stay when compared to all lower grade open fractures.

Clement et al. also sought to evaluate the outcome of tibial diaphyseal fractures in the elderly.[18] Over a 10-year period the Royal Infirmary of Edinburgh had 238 fractures of the tibial shaft in patients ≥65 years of age, 69 (30%) of which were open. There was a high rate of morbidity and mortality with two patients requiring primary amputation and eight dying within 3 days of injury. They followed this group of patients for 1 year and found an increased mortality rate at 120 days and at 1 year in the open fracture group compared to the group with closed fractures.

COMPLICATIONS

The open fractures in the elderly most commonly studied are those of the ankle, tibia and distal radius. Obviously there are other fractures which have a high prevalence of open injuries including phalangeal fractures and both-bone forearm fractures (see Chapter 1). The complications of open fractures in the elderly should be looked at in two main categories, these being complications of the bone, which would include non-union, malunion and deep infection, and complications of the soft tissues, which would include postoperative wound dehiscence, prominent hardware and need for soft tissue coverage. In addition, there is a risk of systemic complications when open fractures become infected.

Non-union

Open fractures in any patient are more prone to developing non-union because of the increased periosteal stripping, contamination and bone damage. In patients with osteopenia or osteoporosis union can be difficult to achieve even with minimal periosteal stripping. However there are aspects of treatment which can decrease the incidence of non-union in the elderly. We will use the tibia as an example.

In elderly patients the intramedullary canal can be wide and may require a larger diameter nail. With the decreased blood supply which can occur with open fractures and the extensive reaming which may be necessary for larger diameter nails, it is important that one considers the soft tissues carefully and plans definitive fixation appropriately. The rate of non-union in tibial fractures is higher in open fractures, no matter what the age,[18–21] mainly due to surgical and patient factors. Multiple publications have demonstrated that a transverse fracture can be at an increased risk of non-union. The reason is that there may be a lack of cortical continuity in these fractures. If an intramedullary nail is used to treat an open tibial fracture, one may use intra-operative techniques to minimize this risk. These include the use of a two-pin external fixator to reduce the fracture before nailing (Figure 13.5), placing an interlocking screw distally and back slapping, the use of a temporary plate for fixation before nailing and meticulous attention to detail. In some instances, plate fixation may be an alternative fixation for a distal open tibia fracture (Figure 13.6).[19] These are some hints to minimize surgical factors contributing to non-union.

The patient factors that may contribute to non-union of geriatric open fractures are numerous (Table 13.3). We will address each of these factors separately. In the

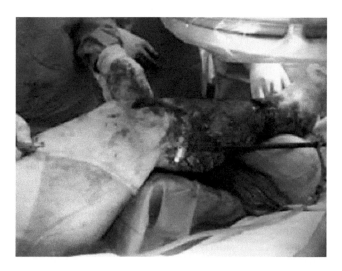

Figure 13.5 Two-pin external fixator for temporary stabilization.

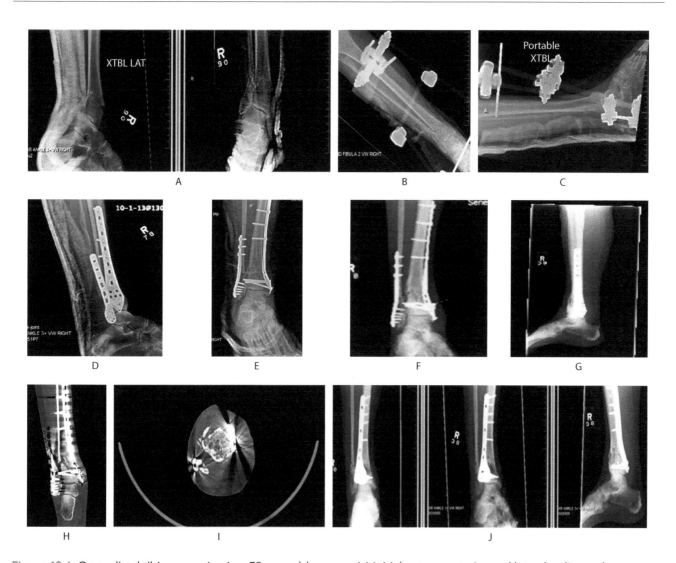

Figure 13.6 Open distal tibia non-union in a 73 year old woman. **(a)** Initial anteroposterior and lateral radiographs. **(b,c)** Temporary external fixation with an external fixator after wound debridement. **(d,e)** Definitive fixation using open reduction and internal fixation (ORIF). **(f,g)** fracture non-union at 9 months. **(h,i)** CT demonstrating non-union. **(j)** Revision of ORIF with bone graft substitute.

geriatric patient bone quality may dictate fixation type. It is important to question the patient or family before definitive fixation of open fractures regarding these important risk factors for healing.

Bone quality is often compromised in the elderly. A history of osteoporosis or osteopenia should be looked for. It should be determined how it was diagnosed and whether a DEXA scan was used. The World Health Organization defines osteopenia as a bone density that is not normal, but also not as low as osteoporosis. Osteopenia is defined by bone densitometry as a T-score of −1 to −2.5. Osteoporosis is defined as a T-score of less than −2.5 compared to norms. It is important to realize the osteoporosis may be a cause of the fracture as it is known to cause more than 8.9 million fractures worldwide annually. It is not just geriatric hip fractures that fall into this category. Distal radius fractures are common osteoporotic fractures and may be open in the elderly population.

Table 13.3 Factors to evaluate in non-union of geriatric open fractures

Bone quality
Metabolic disease
Nutrition
Medication
Medical morbidity
Personal habits
Infection

A consideration in the patient with pre-existing osteoporosis is whether they are being treated with medications which may affect fracture healing. Bisphosphonate therapy is used in the treatment of osteoporosis. A recent meta-analysis reviewed eight eligible trials with 2508 patients.[22] The authors found no detectable delay to fracture healing via external callous following bisphosphonate treatment. However, this result must be interpreted with caution. These were not high energy or open fractures that were studied. In addition, depending on the type of fracture stabilization, there may be primary bone healing without callous.

Ng et al.[23] completed a review of upper extremity fractures in patients having bisphosphonate therapy. This review included only six studies. They found post-fracture bisphosphonate use was associated with a doubling of the risk of non-union. Overall, they felt that the benefits of the therapy were not worth changing practice patterns.

It is important to consider the bone quality in the patient when considering treatment options for open fractures and tailor the fixation appropriately.

We know that decreased bone quality can affect fracture healing and essentially represents metabolic bone disease. However additional metabolic bone disease may exist in the geriatric patient with an open fracture that may affect fracture healing. This 'umbrella' term can refer to a broad range of disorders affecting bone. In the geriatric patient, there may be Paget's disease of bone. This condition is more common in the elderly and may even be a contributing factor to the fracture. In Paget's disease there is disorganized bone remodelling due to excessive breakdown of bone. This leads to weakening of the bone. If there is characteristic Pagetoid bone on radiographs, this should be taken into account when treating the fracture.

One of the most common metabolic deficiencies affecting bone is calcium and vitamin D deficiency. Other mineral deficiencies include phosphorus and magnesium. Brinker et al. suggested evaluating patients with non-union for underlying metabolic abnormalities and felt that certain fracture non-unions might heal without surgical intervention if these are corrected.[24] In his study, Brinker et al. found that 84% of patients with non-union had undiagnosed metabolic or endocrine abnormalities and 70% were vitamin D deficient or insufficient. The interesting fact from these data is that this was a younger, supposedly healthier male population. The incidence therefore may be greater in the geriatric population.

Complications can also occur due to the nutritional status of the patient. An article by Dwyer et al.[25] evaluated 43 patients with an average age of 28, although the range went up to 74. These patients were studied prospectively for 40 weeks to ascertain the relationship of anthropometric, biomechanical and haematological parameters with wound healing following injury. Interestingly, nearly half of the patients were malnourished at the time of admission. With proper dietary advice and better food intake, there was improved nutritional status with only 13 patients out of 43 malnourished at the end of the study period.

It is important to recognize what happens to the nutritional state in the trauma patient. The stress of the trauma produces a catabolic state. There is loss of total body protein and excessive nitrogen secretion proportional to the magnitude of the injury.[26] An open fracture alone is a significant insult to the system and this is increased because the patients may be kept 'nil per os' (NPO, nothing by mouth) on numerous occasions waiting for the operating room. The caloric requirements for bone and wound healing place additional strain on the patient's nutritional status. In addition to the physiological changes patients experience with an injury, pain and narcotics can lead to decreased appetite and nausea.

Laboratory values which can be assessed to determine nutritional status include pre-albumin, albumin, total protein and total lymphocyte count. A nutrition consult can be helpful. In the geriatric patient, we recommend evaluation of the nutritional state and metabolic state after the initial injury. That is one instance in which prevention is prudent in treating those factors affecting healing before initial hospital discharge.

Medications and medical comorbidities are factors which definitely affect fracture healing, but are difficult to control by the treating surgeon. The medications for chronic medical conditions typically cannot be altered but may require dose adjustment due to the tremendous strain of the trauma on a geriatric patient. Medical comorbidities are, again, diagnoses which cannot be altered to affect fracture healing. However, optimizing medical management of comorbid conditions can be very helpful for patient readiness for the operating room especially in those requiring multiple operative procedures.

The American Society of Anesthesiologists (ASA) score is a measure of physical status. Often elderly patients have higher ASA scores of 3 or more. There are several articles on ASA score and hip fracture mortality,[27-30] but they are not particularly useful in the geriatric open fracture population. However, there have been a few recent articles on ASA score and orthopaedic injuries. Kay et al.[31] evaluated ASA and length of stay and cost due to length of stay after common, isolated orthopaedic fractures. The authors found that ASA score was a strong predictor of length of stay and also a significant predictor of inpatient costs. A larger study by Sathiyakumar et al.[32] used the ASA score to predict 30-day readmission rates using the National Surgical Quality Improvement Program (NSQIP) database. The ASA score was found to be the strongest predictor for readmission following surgery for orthopaedic trauma. Those patients with an ASA score of 3 were 3.77 times as likely to have a hospital readmission, while those with an ASA score of 4 were 13.7 times as likely to have a readmission! Since the ASA score is collected in all patients undergoing surgery, it can be used no matter what hospital or service is involved in patient care. The ASA score can be a useful tool in geriatric open fracture patients to help predict the risk of complications and increased costs following fracture care.

The geriatric trauma patient may be thought not to have significant personal habits that affect fracture healing. However, the patients all need to be questioned and counselled appropriately. Regular use of tobacco, alcohol or illicit drugs can impact outcomes making screening in the geriatric population imperative. One aspect of their lifestyle to ask about is exercise. Those geriatric trauma patients who exercise, whether it be walking, tennis, water aerobics or other activities, should all be commended as the exercise can help with bone quality, balance and recovery following geriatric open fractures. This is one personal habit to encourage! Knowing your patient's lifestyle can aid in goal setting and expectation management.

The treatment of non-union in the geriatric open fracture patient must be tailored to the aetiology. The evaluation of patient factors has been discussed. Any fracture that does not heal must be evaluated for infection. The white blood cell (WBC) count and differential should be obtained, along with infectious indices such as erythrocyte sedimentation rate (ESR) and C-reactive protein (CRP). With a known infection, without systemic illness, the literature supports the maintenance of the hardware until the fracture has healed.[33] There are several issues regarding the infected geriatric open fracture. The length of time to fracture healing can be delayed in the geriatric trauma patient. In addition, the patient may have less physiological reserve and may not tolerate the stress of an infection. The antibiotic treatment of the infection may lead to systemic complications including adverse reactions from *Clostridium difficile* colitis, gastrointestinal symptoms and impaired renal function. This is where multidisciplinary teamwork is essential.

If infection has been ruled out as a cause of non-union, treatment planning may commence. As mentioned, there are patient and surgical factors to consider. There is considerable debate regarding the time when a non-union can be stated to have occurred. Previously non-union was defined as failure to heal by 9 months.[34] The geriatric fracture patient may be slower to heal, especially with open fracture. Thus the physician must allow adequate time to heal. Close radiographic evaluation can be helpful. One cannot draw a definite healing curve with two consecutive radiographs, but the curve can begin to be appreciated with three or more consecutive radiographs. Computed tomography scans are also an effective tool in the diagnosis of non-union (Figure 13.6).

Once the diagnosis of non-union is established, treatment planning can begin. The surgeon should closely evaluate the aetiology of the non-union. Is the biology adequate to permit healing? If not, what can be done to improve the biology? Is the construct too stiff to promote healing? Is the construct of adequate size or working length to promote healing? Was there bone–on-bone contact for those fractures healing by primary bone healing? What type of implant is appropriate for the non-union? (Figure 13.6). Preoperative planning is essential. One cannot forget that the removal of existing hardware may not be easy and there could be complications. It is always crucial to have a back-up plan. The need for biological augmentation to promote healing is another consideration. The management of non-unions in the elderly is discussed further in Chapter 6.

Soft tissue complications

The thin skin of the elderly requires special attention to minimize complications. We discussed specialized soft tissue handling in the treatment section. Complications affecting the soft tissues can range from hardware prominence (Figure 13.7) to wound dehiscence and infection. Wound dehiscence is not reported in many studies as a complication, but when you consider that the fracture was open in an already compromised soft tissue environment it is definitely an issue. We recommend close observation of any geriatric open fracture wound, including delayed discharge, if there is persistent drainage. Often, the geriatric patient is sent to a rehabilitation facility and a draining wound at hospital discharge can turn into a much bigger problem. Draining wounds should be taken seriously, and the aetiology should be carefully considered. Is the compromised skin and drainage due to an underlying haematoma? If there is concern about a possible haematoma, irrigation and drainage should be considered. Sometimes the wound 'spreads' over time leaving gaping sutures. This wound may be optimally treated with a wet-to-dry dressing. Alternatively, NPWT could be applied. NPWT settings are often at 125 mmHg. In the geriatric population with their sensitive skin, a lesser setting can be used while still providing the same benefit.

Prominent plates can also be an issue due to thin skin and decreased subcutaneous fat necessitating hardware removal. We encourage consideration of the plates and implants chosen for fixation in areas where prominence can be an issue. While locking plates are often used in osteoporotic

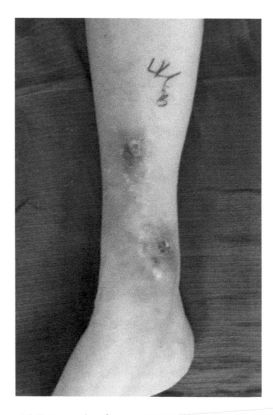

Figure 13.7 Example of a prominent plate with skin lesions.

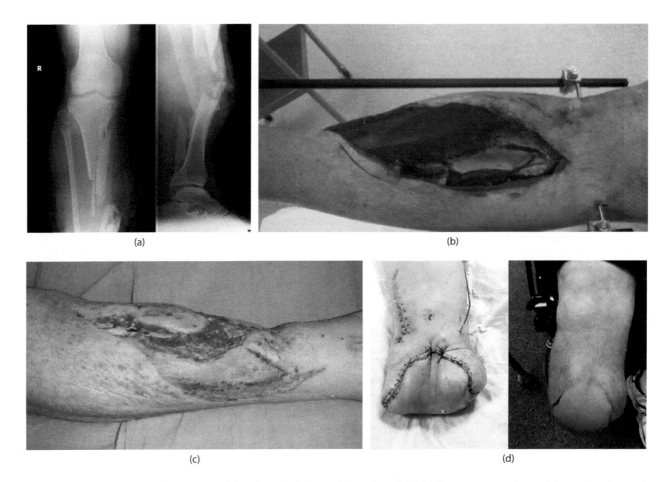

(a)

(b)

(c)

(d)

Figure 13.8 Case example of a 65-year-old male with failure of free flap. **(a)** Initial anteroposterior and lateral radiographs of a Gustilo type IIIB fracture. **(b)** Soft tissue before free flap. **(c)** Failed free flap at 2 months after injury. **(d)** Residual limb after amputation and when ready for prosthesis.

bone, they are thicker than their non-locking counterparts. Consideration of stability of fixation and plate thickness is a factor in preoperative planning to try to minimize postoperative complications. The percentage of patients requiring plate removal especially around the ankle or elbow region from an open fracture may not be avoidable as adequate fixation and stability take priority in fracture treatment. Plate or prominent hardware removal should not occur until the fracture has healed.

Some open fractures in the geriatric population may require a free tissue transfer. The question that should be considered in severe lower extremity injuries is: Should limb salvage proceed? The outcomes of limb salvage versus amputation indicate no difference in outcome at 7 years.[35] However in the LEAP, patients over 55 years of age were prone to a worse outcome. Geriatric fracture patients with severe soft tissue injury should be counselled appropriately. Even if limb salvage is attempted, it can ultimately fail (Figure 13.8).

Systemic complications

A number of systemic complications can occur in geriatric fracture cases. These are discussed in Chapter 7.

CONCLUSIONS

Geriatric open fractures represent serious injuries to the patient. There is limited information available on this topic. The purpose of this chapter was to discuss the epidemiology, classification, treatment and outcomes. It is important to realize that the soft tissue is the most important factor affecting outcome. Often geriatric open fractures are 'up classified' in the Gustilo system as the geriatric patient has fragile skin due to changes as one ages. This chapter has provided information to assist the practitioner to treat geriatric open fracture patients and expand knowledge on this topic.

REFERENCES

1. Keller JM, Sciadini MF, Sinclair E, O'Toole RV. Geriatric trauma: Demographics, injuries, and mortality. *J Orthop Trauma*, 2012; 26(9): e161–5.
2. Abdelfattah A, Del Core M, Cannada LK, Watson JT. Geriatric high-energy polytrauma with orthopedic injuries: Clinical predictors of mortality. *Geriatr Orthop Surg Rehabil*, 2014; 5(4): 173–7.

3. Court-Brown CM, Clement ND, Duckworth AD, Aitken S, Biant LC, McQueen MM. The spectrum of fractures in the elderly. *Bone Joint J*, 2014; 96-B(3): 366–72.

4. Court-Brown CM, Biant LC, Clement ND, Bugler KE, Duckworth AD, McQueen MM. Open fractures in the elderly. The importance of skin ageing. *Injury*, 2015; 46(2): 189–94.

5. Azzi, L, El-Alfy M, Martel C, Labrie F. Gender differences in mouse skin morphology and specific effects of sex steroids and dehydroepiandrosterone. *J Invest Dermatol*, 2005; 124(1): 22–7.

6. Makrantonaki E, Brink TC, Zampeli V, Elewa RM, Mlody B, Hossini AM, Hermes B, et al. Identification of biomarkers of human skin ageing in both genders. Wnt signalling—A label of skin ageing? *PLoS One*, 2012; 7(11): e50393.

7. Cox G, Jones S, Nikolaou VS, Kontakis G, Giannoudis PV. Elderly tibial shaft fractures: Open fractures are not associated with increased mortality rates. *Injury*, 2010; 41(6): 620–3.

8. Gustilo RB, Anderson JT. Prevention of infection in the treatment of one thousand and twenty-five open fractures of long bones: Retrospective and prospective analyses. *J Bone Joint Surg Am*, 1976; 58(4): 453–8.

9. Bosse MJ, MacKenzie EJ, Kellam JF, Burgess AR, Webb LX, Swiontkowski MF, Sanders RW, et al. A prospective evaluation of the clinical utility of the lower-extremity injury-severity scores. *J Bone Joint Surg Am*, 2001; 83-A(1): 3–14.

10. Cannada LK, Cooper C. The mangled extremity: Limb salvage versus amputation. *Curr Surg*, 2005; 62(6): 563–76.

11. Lenarz CJ, Watson JT, Moed BR, Israel H, Mullen JD, MacDonald JB. Timing of wound closure in open fractures based on cultures obtained after debridement. *J Bone Joint Surg Am*, 2010; 92(10): 1921–6.

12. Davis JW, Kaups KL. Base deficit in the elderly: A marker of severe injury and death. *J Trauma*, 1998; 45(5): 873–7.

13. Callaway DW, Shapiro NI, Donnino MW, Baker C, Rosen CL. Serum lactate and base deficit as predictors of mortality in normotensive elderly blunt trauma patients. *J Trauma*, 2009; 66(4): 1040–4.

14. Kaufman AM, Pensy RA, O'Toole RV, Egiseder WA. Safety of immediate open reduction and internal fixation of geriatric open fractures of the distal radius. *Injury*, 2014; 45(3): 534–9.

15. Lynde MJ, Sautter T, Hamilton GA, Schuberth JM. Complications after open reduction and internal fixation of ankle fractures in the elderly. *Foot Ankle Surg*, 2012; 18(2): 103–7.

16. Davis AT, Israel H, Cannada LK, Bledsoe JG. A biomechanical comparison of one-third tubular plates versus periarticular plates for fixation of osteoporotic distal fibula fractures. *J Orthop Trauma*, 2013; 27(9): e201–7.

17. Court-Brown C, Honeyman C, Bugler K, McQueen M. The spectrum of open fractures of the foot in adults. *Foot Ankle Int*, 2013; 34(3): 323–8.

18. Clement ND, Beauchamp NJ, Duckworth AD, McQueen MM, Court-Brown CM. The outcome of tibial diaphyseal fractures in the elderly. *Bone Joint J*, 2013; 95-B(9): 1255–62.

19. Vallier HA, Cureton BA, Patterson BM. Randomized, prospective comparison of plate versus intramedullary nail fixation for distal tibia shaft fractures. *J Orthop Trauma*, 2011; 25(12): 736–41.

20. Schemitsch EH, Bhandari M, Guyatt G, Sanders DW, Swiontkowski M, Tornetta P, Walter SD, et al. Prognostic factors for predicting outcomes after intramedullary nailing of the tibia. *J Bone Joint Surg Am*, 2012; 94(19): 1786–93.

21. Fong K, Truong V, Foote CJ, Petrisor B, Williams D, Ristevski B, Sprague S, Bhandari M. Predictors of nonunion and reoperation in patients with fractures of the tibia: An observational study. *BMC Musculoskelet Disord*, 2013; 14: 103.

22. Xue D, Li F, Chen G, Yan S, Pan Z. Do bisphosphonates affect bone healing? A meta-analysis of randomized controlled trials. *J Orthop Surg Res*, 2014; 9: 45.

23. Ng AJ, Yue B, Joseph S, Richardson M. Delayed/non-union of upper limb fractures with bisphosphonates: Systematic review and recommendations. *ANZ J Surg*, 2014; 84(4): 218–24.

24. Brinker MR, O'Connor DP, Monla YT, Earthman TP. Metabolic and endocrine abnormalities in patients with nonunions. *J Orthop Trauma*, 2007; 21(8): 557–70.

25. Dwyer AJ, John B, Mam MK, Anthony P, Abraham R, Joshi M. Nutritional status and wound healing in open fractures of the lower limb. *Int Orthop*, 2005; 29(4): 251–4.

26. Switzer JA, Gammon SR. High-energy skeletal trauma in the elderly. *J Bone Joint Surg Am*, 2012; 94(23): 2195–204.

27. Hu F, Jiang C, Shen J, Tang P, Wang Y. Preoperative predictors for mortality following hip fracture surgery: A systematic review and meta-analysis. *Injury*, 2012; 43(6): 676–85.

28. Bjorgul K, Novicoff WM, Saleh KJ. American Society of Anesthesiologist Physical Status score may be used as a comorbidity index in hip fracture surgery. *J Arthroplasty*, 2010; 25(6 Suppl): 134–7.

29. Garcia AE, Bonnaig JV, Yoneda ZT, Richards JE, Ehrenfeld JM, Obremskey WT, Jahangir AA, Sethi MK. Patient variables which may predict length of stay and hospital costs in elderly patients with hip fracture. *J Orthop Trauma*, 2012; 26(11): 620–3.

30. Ricci WM, Brandt A, McAndrew C, Gardner MJ. Factors effecting delay to surgery and length of stay for hip fracture patients. *J Orthop Trauma*, 2015; 29(3): e109–14.

31. Kay HF, Sathiyakumar V, Yoneda ZT, Lee YM, Jahangir AA, Ehrenfeld JM, Obremskey WT, Apfeld JC, Sethi MK. The effects of American Society of Anesthesiologists physical status on length of stay and inpatient cost in the surgical treatment of isolated orthopaedic fractures. *J Orthop Trauma*, 2014; 28(7): e153–9.

32. Sathiyakumar V, Molina CS, Thakore RV, Obremskey WT, Sethi MK. ASA score as a predictor of 30-day perioperative readmission in patients with orthopaedic trauma injuries: A NSQIP analysis. *J Orthop Trauma*, 2015; 29(3): e127–32.

33. Berkes M, Obremskey WT, Scannell B, Ellington JK, Hymes RA, Bosse MJ. Maintenance of hardware after early postoperative infection following fracture internal fixation. *J Bone Joint Surg Am*, 2010; 92(4): 823–8.

34. Cannada LK, Anglen JO, Archdeacon MT, Herscovici D, Ostrum RF. Avoiding complications in the care of fractures of the tibia. *Instr Course Lect*, 2009; 58: 27–36.

35. MacKenzie EJ, Bosse MJ, Pollak AN, Webb LX, Swiontkowski MF, Kellam JK, Smith DG, et al. Long-term persistence of disability following severe lower-limb trauma. Results of a seven-year follow-up. *J Bone Joint Surg Am*, 2005; 87(8): 1801–9.

14

Polytrauma in the elderly

JULIE A. SWITZER AND LISA K. SCHRODER

INTRODUCTION

Trauma, in general, and polytrauma, in particular, are widely recognized as conditions afflicting the young. Consequently, the study of polytraumatized or multiply injured patients has focused historically on young, male adults, commonly considered the population most affected by trauma. More recently, however, there has been recognition that high-energy trauma affects all populations. In fact, approximately 35% of all trauma occurs in individuals over 65 years of age.[1,2]

The elderly make up the population demographic whose numbers are increasing at the greatest rate. Prior to 2007, at no time in human history did the number of individuals over the age of 65 exceed the number of individuals under the age of 5. Since 2007, however, the number of the elderly in the world's population has begun to exceed the number of young children. In fact, the global population of elderly individuals (generally considered to be 60+ years of age) is expected to increase from 287 million in 2013 to 417 million by 2050.[1]

Additionally, older individuals are participating in activities that put them at high risk for sustaining severe injuries that may involve multiple organ systems. The number of older individuals who drive or are passengers in motor vehicles, who ride motorcycles or who engage in other high speed or high-energy activities is increasing. It stands to reason that, given the demographic and behavioural trends, the prevalence of polytrauma in the elderly will increase (Figure 14.1).

When older individuals sustain polytrauma, their outcomes, when compared to a younger population, are generally poorer and result in higher complication and mortality rates. This poses unique challenges to medical, trauma and orthopaedic providers.

EPIDEMIOLOGY

The elderly constitute an increasing proportion of polytraumatized patients. Although recent census reports estimate that people aged 65 and older make up 13–14% of the US population, the 2014 report of the US National Trauma Data Bank indicates that patients aged 65 and older comprise 28% of all reported trauma patients.[3] An analysis of the same data reveals that 30% of all polytrauma incidents were in this older age group.[4]

In 1986, a Swiss study focused attention on polytraumatized elderly patients. In a cohort of 300 patients who sustained polytrauma, defined as either a visceral injury associated with significant fractures or a minimum of two major fractures, 27 (9%) were aged 70 and older.[5] Similarly, in 1988, Broos et al. described 416 multiply injured Belgian patients, of whom 49 (12%) were aged 65 and over.[6] Before these reports, only a small number of authors in the English literature had written on the topic of polytrauma in the elderly and even fewer had reported on the orthopaedic implications of polytrauma in the elderly.

In the nearly three decades since these initial reports, only a limited number of studies have expanded our epidemiological knowledge about these patients. As illustrated in the summary of the literature in Table 14.1, few authors have specifically described older trauma victims as a unique patient cohort that might require specific protocols of care and that could benefit from specific study.[4–16] As this summary

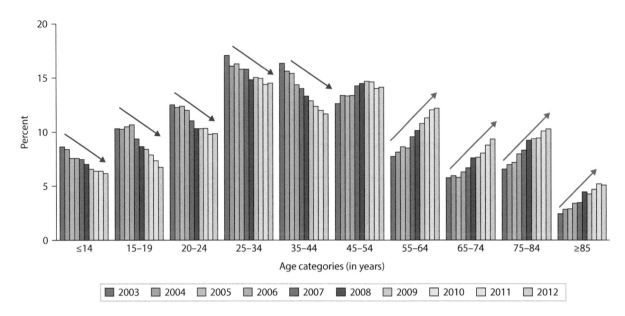

Figure 14.1 A 10-year history of weighted estimates of the incidents of trauma admissions from the US National Trauma Databank illustrate a clear declining trend in trauma admissions in patients aged 44 years and younger, but an increasing trend for all age categories in patients aged 55 and older. (Reprinted from the Committee on Trauma, American College of Surgeons. NTDB Annual Report 2014. Chicago, IL. With permission. The content reproduced from the NTDB remains the full and exclusive copyrighted property of the American College of Surgeons. The American College of Surgeons is not responsible for any claims arising from works based on the original data, text, tables or figures.)

elucidates, most authors have defined 'elderly' or 'geriatric' as patients aged 65 and older. Only a few reports have used an older[5,8,10] or younger[7] definition for the elderly patient.

Most reports on trauma in the elderly have employed an inclusion criterion of a minimum Injury Severity Score (ISS) of 10–17 to indicate 'polytrauma' or 'severely' injured (Table 14.1). One study found that 5% of all trauma patients admitted to a level 1 trauma centre were elderly patients (≥65 years old) with multisystem trauma.[16] From these reports, we can see that 'elderly' patients comprise 8–30% of reported polytrauma cohorts, with one study from Australia reporting an incidence of 41% of trauma patients with an ISS >12 at 55 years of age or over.[7]

In a review of the changing characteristics of all trauma patients across the decades, a study of 501 polytraumatized patients found an age increase of 0.75 years for each subsequent year.[17] In other words, older age is becoming an increasingly important characteristic of polytrauma patients. A report from the national hospital registries in Spain found similar trends in the decade from 2000 to 2010, when the incidence of all trauma patients under the age of 75 remained stable, but the incidence of trauma patients over the age of 75 increased significantly.[18] This trend has also been noted across Europe; in an analysis of a large prospective single centre database from Switzerland from 1996 to 2009, the percentage of patients over 75 years of age increased from 6.5% in years one and two to 11.8% in the final 3 years of the study data.[10] Similarly, a US based study from Texas noted a nearly 3% increase in annual elderly admissions to a level 1 trauma centre between 2005 and

2008 (P<0.001),[9] further indicating the global phenomena of the increasing elderly polytrauma patient population.

The sexual dimorphism of polytrauma in the elderly occurs at a rate that is neither consistent with the rate of low-energy injury in the elderly nor the rate of high-energy injury in the young. The proportion of male to female elderly polytrauma patients is nearly 50/50, while the proportion of male to female low-energy trauma patients is approximately 25/75. Most reports in younger trauma populations show an approximately 75/25 male to female proportion.[9]

RISK FACTORS AND MECHANISMS OF INJURY IN OLDER POLYTRAUMA

As in all orthopaedic trauma related events, the greatest predictor of injury is participation in risky activities. Increased independence, increased life expectancy and an expectation of a more active lifestyle are the primary characteristics of elder individuals that predispose them to polytrauma.

Although there has been an increase in the number of elderly polytrauma patients, focused reports indicate that, across the past quarter of a century, mechanisms of injury in this patient population have not changed significantly. Blunt trauma, as opposed to penetrating trauma, is reported as the cause of injury in nearly 99% of all polytrauma in the older adult population.[12] However, the elderly are participating in higher energy activities such as motor vehicle usage, motorcycling, climbing or working at heights.

Data from the National Hospital Ambulatory Medical Care Survey show that between 2003 and 2007 there were

Table 14.1 Global reporting of the incidence of elderly polytrauma

Author	Publication year	Country	Date	N	Inclusion ISS	Inclusion age	Mean age of Elderly	M:F ratio in 'Elderly'	% Polytrauma	% 'Elderly'	% of Mortality in 'Elderly'	% of Mortality in 'Non-Elderly'
Cox	2014	Australia	2007–2011	7,461	>12	>55	NR	39%:61%	2	41	25	6%
NTDB	2014	USA	2013	174,351	≥16	≥65	NR	41%:59%	21	30	18	NR
Pfortmueller	2014	Switzerland	2006–2010	780	NR	≥75	83	44%:56%	12	16	10	3%
Adams	2012	Texas, USA	2005–2008	6,013	≥16	≥65	NR	50%:50%	39	14	NR	NR
Schonenberger	2012	Switzerland	1996–2009	2,090	≥16	>75	NR	49%:51%	NR	8	64	37%
Grzalja	2011	Croatia	2006–2010	381	≥17	≥65	74	58%:42%	NR	14	31	11%
Labib	2011	Canada	2004–2006	283	≥16	≥65	82	59%:41%	NR	NR	27	NR
Giannoudis	2009	UK	1996–2001	2,667	≥16	≥65	75	48%:42%	13	16	42	20%
Aldrian	2005	Austria	1992–2001	466	NR	≥65	75	44%:46%	NR	10	53	27%
Grant	2000	Scotland	1996–1998	1,436	≥16	≥65	NR	NR	12	20	42	20%
Zietlow	1994	Minnesota, USA	1991	94	≥10	≥65	79	45%:55%	NR	5	23	NR
Broos	1988	Belgium	1978–1986	416	Multi-injured	≥65	72	NR	NR	12	18	8%
Marx	1986	Switzerland	1974–1980	300	Multi-injured	≥70	75	59%:41%	NR	9	41	11%

Note: ISS, Injury Severity Score; NR, not reported.

an average of approximately 240,000 annual visits by elderly individuals (>65 years of age) to US emergency departments for motor vehicle related injuries.[19] In fact, motor vehicle collisions are the second most common cause of non-fatal injury in elderly individuals, the most common being falls. Broos et al., when first drawing attention to elderly polytrauma patients in 1993, found that motor vehicle accidents (MVA) and falls were the leading cause of injury, with 57% and 30% of the 126 cases reporting these mechanisms, respectively.[20] Interestingly, these authors also determined that, in 44% of these cases, the patient was a pedestrian hit by a motor vehicle. Similarly, in a 1994 study by Zietlow et al., 59% of the multiply injured elderly patients included in the study were injured due to a fall and 36% were due to MVA[16] (Figure 14.2).

These same commonalities in mechanism of injury (MOI) hold true globally as well. In a large study from the United Kingdom's Trauma Audit and Research Network (TARN) database of 438 polytrauma patients aged 65 and older, road traffic accidents were determined to be the MOI in 42%. Falls from a low height were the cause of injury in 31% of older patients but in only 8% of the younger adult trauma population.[13] In registry reports from both Scotland (Scottish Trauma Audit Group)[15] and Australia,[7] MVA were determined to be the predominant cause of injury in older adults, although falls from a low height were found to have a significantly older mean age than other mechanisms.[15]

Falls are the leading cause of death due to injury in the elderly. Multiple studies have shown that as a result of falls, the elderly sustain injuries of a similar severity to those in younger patients resulting from higher energy mechanisms.[21,22] Not surprisingly, in studies that stratify polytrauma patients by age, increasing age correlates with falls as an increasingly more prevalent injury mechanism. One such study found that falls from a low height were the MOI in only 9.7% of adult trauma patients aged 25–49, 19.7% in patients aged 50–75 and 37.3% in patients over the age of 75.[10]

COMORBIDITIES IN OLDER POLYTRAUMA

Older patients have blunted physiological responses to trauma. Secondary to changes associated with aging and diminished physiological reserve, older patients cannot mount the same type of haemodynamic and metabolic response to trauma as younger patients. Additionally, other factors such as the use of medications that complicate resuscitation of elderly polytrauma patients also challenge their care.

Specific physiological changes that may lead to challenges in the treatment of polytraumatized individuals are listed in Table 14.2. These include decreased renal, hepatic and pulmonary function, impaired cardiovascular reserve, an inability to launch an appropriate physiological response to stress and shock, frailty and dementia. In a study of abstracted data from over 33,000 medical records of trauma patients over the age of 65, hepatic disease, renal disease and cancer, in particular, were shown to contribute to poorer outcome in polytraumatized older patients.[23]

The elderly may also have deceptively normal vital signs, even when they are hypovolemic and close to shock. A normal adult haemodynamic response to hypovolemic shock, as a result of trauma, is increased heart rate and blood pressure. When elderly trauma patients present with normal

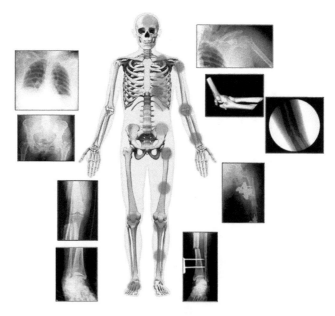

Figure 14.2 A 64-year-old female patient was involved in a head-on motor vehicle collision. The patient sustained subarachnoid haemorrhage, splenic laceration, L rib fractures with pneumothorax, R subtalar fracture dislocation, R patella fracture, L tibia and fibula fracture, L tibial plateau fracture, L femur fracture, L inter-trochanteric hip fracture, L both-bone forearm fracture, open L transolecranon fracture dislocation and L clavicle fracture with L four-part proximal humerus fracture.

Table 14.2 Physiological considerations and comorbidities in older polytrauma patients

Considerations

Heart disease and hypertension

Diabetes

Chronic obstructive pulmonary disease
  (steroid treatment: reduced wound healing, clinical
    adrenal insufficiency)

Dementia
  (antipsychotics: effect neurological exam)

Cancer

Chronic renal failure

Hepatic disease

Medications
  (beta blockers: masking normal vital signs, under-
    recognition of tachycardia) (anticoagulation/
    antiplatelet agents, warfarin, blood thinners, cardiac
    medications) (polypharmacy)

Pacemaker

heart rate and/or a normal or low blood pressure, they can be misdiagnosed as being either less injured or better resuscitated than they actually are; hypertension is common in the elderly, therefore normal vital signs might indicate hypovolemia. Low volume and hypoperfusion, as a result of trauma in the elderly, are often further complicated by a decreased ability to generate responses to stress, the effect of medications commonly prescribed in the elderly (i.e. beta blockers, ACE inhibitors, steroids) and/or the fact that, when compared to body weight, the elderly have a lower gross blood volume and cardiac output.

Also complicating evaluation and management in the setting of trauma in the elderly is the decreased reporting of pain by the elderly, as well as mental status change that can occur as a result of age. These patients may have a history of Alzheimer's disease, cognitive decline, Parkinson's disease or a history of cerebrovascular insults that can contribute to difficulty in communication that, in turn, lead to difficulties in diagnosis and treatment. Even mild dementia can be precipitously worsened by trauma, and the delirium that often accompanies stress and trauma in the elderly can make challenging the interpretation of information available in the setting of polytrauma in the elderly.

PATTERNS OF INJURY AND SPECIFIC ASSOCIATED INJURIES

Given the lack of robust investigative focus on elderly polytrauma patients, it is difficult to well characterize common patterns of injury in this patient population. There are, however, important injury types and injury constellations that may guide future study in this area.

In the 1984 report by Oreskovich et al.,[24] a review of 100 patients over the age of 70 who were admitted to a metropolitan trauma centre, 80% of the patients were classified as 'multi-trauma', having at least two body regions injured. In this cohort, the authors reported that the extremities and pelvis were the most common body regions to be injured and that one-third of the patients had an injury to the thorax or abdomen that required surgery. In 1994, in a similar single centre cohort of 94 subjects, Zietlow et al. found that 57% experienced thorax injury, 56% experienced an extremity fracture and 13% experienced combined abdominal and pelvic injuries. The mean ISS in this cohort was 18. Closed head injury and fractures were cited as the most frequent injuries.[16]

Two studies that focused specifically on elderly pedestrian trauma reported the increasing occurrence of specific fracture patterns in the elderly when compared to younger victims.[1,25,26] Both reports found that the elderly had significantly higher rates of fractures of the pelvis, upper extremities and lower extremities. The elderly patients also had a higher rate of intracranial injuries, but sustained lower rates of hepatic injuries when compared to younger age groups (Figure 14.3). These reports contrast with a 2009 database analysis that compared young and old, severe and multiply injured trauma patients, and found similar anatomic injury distribution regardless of age. These authors reported 63% had serious head injury, 18% serious thoracic or lower limb injury and 9% serious abdominal injury.[13] A 2011 report of 283 elderly trauma patients with ISS ≥16 and a mean age of 81.5 years found that rates of injury in this population included: 88.4% traumatic brain injury, 22.8% thoracic injuries (with rib fractures and flail chest the most common), 17% spine injuries and 8%, 7.6% and 6.5% long bone, pelvic and hip fractures, respectively.[12] Most recently, a single centre report that included 154 older polytrauma patients with orthopaedic injuries found that spine fractures followed by pelvic/acetabulum injuries were most common. These authors excluded all low-energy mechanisms and the most severely injured patients with an Abbreviated Injury Scale (AIS) ≥4, which could have skewed the results.[27]

Pelvic and acetabular fractures that occur as a result of trauma in elderly patients demonstrate characteristics that differ from those in younger patients. Lateral compression pelvic factures are the most common pelvic ring injury in the elderly and, when they occur, result in greater blood loss and need for transfusion, longer length of stay and higher mortality than those in younger patients.[28] Anterior column, both-column, and anterior column with posterior hemitransverse acetabular fractures are also more common in the elderly.[1]

Clavicle and/or rib fractures that occur in the elderly as a result of blunt trauma also demonstrate increased morbidity and mortality when compared with the same injuries in younger patients. In an analysis of 277 patients >65 years of age, the morbidity and mortality of blunt chest trauma was such that, for each additional rib fracture, mortality increased by 19% and the risk of pneumonia increased by 27%.[29] A study by Keller et al. of high-energy skeletal trauma in the elderly, found, in addition to a high association

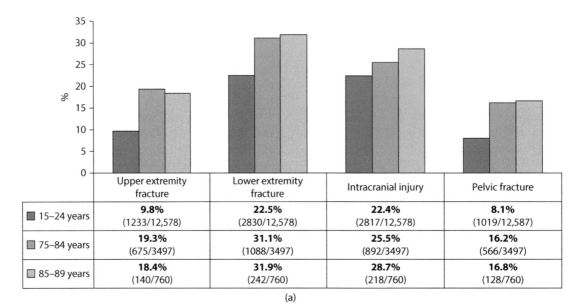

	Upper extremity fracture	Lower extremity fracture	Intracranial injury	Pelvic fracture
■ 15–24 years	**9.8%** (1233/12,578)	**22.5%** (2830/12,578)	**22.4%** (2817/12,578)	**8.1%** (1019/12,587)
■ 75–84 years	**19.3%** (675/3497)	**31.1%** (1088/3497)	**25.5%** (892/3497)	**16.2%** (566/3497)
□ 85–89 years	**18.4%** (140/760)	**31.9%** (242/760)	**28.7%** (218/760)	**16.8%** (128/760)

(a)

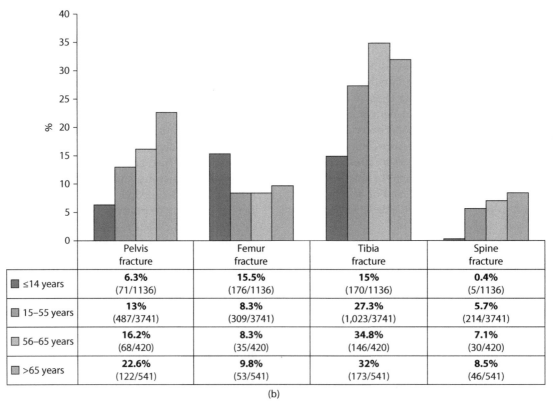

	Pelvis fracture	Femur fracture	Tibia fracture	Spine fracture
■ ≤14 years	**6.3%** (71/1136)	**15.5%** (176/1136)	**15%** (170/1136)	**0.4%** (5/1136)
■ 15–55 years	**13%** (487/3741)	**8.3%** (309/3741)	**27.3%** (1,023/3741)	**5.7%** (214/3741)
□ 56–65 years	**16.2%** (68/420)	**8.3%** (35/420)	**34.8%** (146/420)	**7.1%** (30/420)
□ >65 years	**22.6%** (122/541)	**9.8%** (53/541)	**32%** (173/541)	**8.5%** (46/541)

(b)

Figure 14.3 **(a)** Chart showing data from the study by Siram et al.[25] which illustrates the rate of pedestrian trauma by age group and location of injury. **(b)** Chart showing data from the study by Demetriades et al.[26] which illustrates the rate of pedestrian trauma by age group and location of injury. (Reprinted from Switzer JA, Gammon SR. *J Bone Joint Surg Am.* 2012;94(23):2195–2204. With permission.)

between pelvic, spine injuries with increased mortality, an increase in mortality associated with clavicle fracture.[30]

SCORING SYSTEMS

In the trauma literature, the ISS has been utilized as the standard determinant for predicting outcome. Understanding the impact, morbidity and survivability of trauma in the elderly poses a more nuanced problem. Several investigators have found in the elderly that the ISS score, when coupled with cardiac and pulmonary disease, is a more reliable predictor of prognosis than the ISS alone. The Shock Index (ratio of heart rate divided by systolic blood pressure) has also been determined to be a reasonable predictor of outcome following trauma in the elderly. In 1987, investigators combined age, ISS, sepsis and cardiac complications to create a Geriatric Trauma Scoring System (GTSS) that, in their elderly cohort of polytraumatized patients, predicted survivability better than other single variables.[31] Some work has also been done to determine the usefulness of scoring systems that incorporate injury severity but also comorbidities (reported in ICD-9 or ICD-10 coding systems). Finally, more recently, frailty as a determinant of outcome in polytraumatized elderly has gained greater attention. In a recently published study of elderly trauma patients, frailty was highly correlated with mortality, in-hospital complications and adverse discharge disposition.[32]

TRIAGE OF THE ELDERLY POLYTRAUMA PATIENT

Unfortunately, the little data available on polytrauma in the elderly suggest that we are slow to recognize it, slow to triage it and slow to manage it aggressively. Multiple studies from the USA and Canada have reported that, even when physiological or injury mechanism criteria for transfer to a trauma centre are met, older individuals are less likely to be transported to those trauma centres.[33,34] In one study of the trauma system in Maryland, under-triage of trauma patients (the missed transfer of a trauma patient to a state-designated trauma centre) was observed starting at age 50. Another decrease in the probability of transfer began at age 70.[35] When, in another report, emergency medical providers were asked for reasons for undertriage of elderly patients, they mentioned possible age bias, perceived lack of negative reaction from trauma staff and lack of training in elderly trauma.

Regardless of the reasons for its occurrence, the under-triage of elderly trauma patients has been recognized as one of three current crucial issues in elder polytrauma.[36] It has been shown that their survivability improves when elderly individuals are triaged to trauma centres. In one well-designed trial in which the age of 70 was used as a cut-off for triage to a trauma centre, there was a substantial risk-adjusted improvement in survival.[37] Several other reports have shown that when older patients are transported to trauma centres, they have a better chance of survival.[38]

EVALUATION AND CARE OF ELDERLY POLYTRAUMA PATIENTS

The principles of the acute management of the poly-traumatized older patient are similar to the principles of the management and resuscitation of younger trauma patients. A focus on the basics of Advanced Trauma Life Support (ATLS), with the achievement of adequate access and monitoring, as well as aggressive resuscitation, has been shown to improve outcomes in elderly trauma patients. The principles best employed in the goal directed care of older polytrauma patients are shown in Table 14.3.

Table 14.3 Goal directed care of the older polytrauma patient

Treatment goals
Aggressive early resuscitation
Invasive monitoring, if necessary
Monitoring and treatment of comorbidities
Laboratory tests every 4 hours as necessary
Monitoring and responding to lactate and/or base deficit levels
Avoidance of drugs that predispose to delirium
Focused secondary and tertiary surveys
Appropriate pain management
Special consideration of treatment involving common medications
• Beta blockers
• Anticoagulation therapies
On-going consideration of the patient's goals of care

Invasive monitoring and aggressive resuscitation

Just as older trauma patients are more likely to be under-triaged to trauma centres, they are also less likely to be transferred to units where invasive monitoring and intervention may be carried out, despite studies which have shown that early invasive haemodynamic monitoring and directed interventions, such as reversal of coagulopathies, improve outcomes in elderly trauma patients.[37,39] A study by Scalea et al., published in 1990, underscored the benefit of invasive monitoring in elderly trauma patients. The adoption of a protocol focused on invasive monitoring and aggressive resuscitation in elderly trauma patients improved survival from 7% to 53%.[40]

Additionally, aggressive treatment and care following trauma in the elderly may include other interventions. Avoidance of hypothermia, acidosis and coagulopathy; emergent surgery to control haemorrhage or to repair vital structures; nutritional supplementation as soon as possible and at least provisional skeletal stabilization are all indicated in the polytraumatized elderly individual. There is no evidence to show that the elderly do not benefit from early damage control of trauma and orthopaedic intervention in the same manner as younger patients. In fact, with their more 'fragile' physiology, a more interventional approach may be beneficial. In a recent cross-sectional retrospective analysis of trauma registry patients in Pennsylvania, in which a specific protocol was adopted for identifying elderly trauma patients at risk for poor outcomes, a protocol that included moderately aggressive monitoring and intervention was enacted (Tables 14.4 and 14.5).

Whether this approach is warranted can be determined through monitoring a patient's base deficit, which is a fairly reliable guide to resuscitation and injury survivability.

Table 14.4 High-risk geriatric patient indicators

High-risk injuries	Medical history indicators	Assessment indicators
Traumatic brain injury	Anticoagulation: Coumadin/Plavix	Admission Glasgow Coma Scale score ≤14
≥2 Rib fractures	Cardiac history: CHF/HTN/arrhythmias	Need for blood products
Pulmonary contusion	Chronic liver failure: cirrhosis	PRBC/FFP
Pneumothorax	Chronic renal failure: Cr ≥1.8 and/or GFR ≤60	Surgical intervention
Haemothorax	Pulmonary disease: COPD	Base deficit >–6 mmol/L
Blunt cardiac injury		Systolic block pressure <90 mmHg
Haemoperitoneum		Lactic acid ≥2.4 mmol/L
Pelvic fracture		
Long bone fractures		
Open fractures		

Source: Bradburn E et al. *J Trauma Acute Care Surg.* 2012;73(2):1035.
Patients were enrolled in the 'geriatric protocol' when they were >65 and had one high-risk injury, one or more medical history indicators and one or more assessment indicator.
CHF, congestive heart failure; COPD, chronic obstructive pulmonary disease; Cr, creatinine; FFP, fresh frozen plasma; GFR, glomerular filtration rate; HTN, hypertension; PRBC, packed red blood cells.

Table 14.5 High-risk geriatric protocol

STAT ABG

If base deficit ≥–6 mmol/L, ABG every 4 h until base deficit ≤–2 mmol/L

STAT EKG

Basic metabolic profile, magnesium and phosphorus in AM

PT/PTT INR in AM

ICU admission and neuro checks every hour for 24 h

For unexplained haemodynamic instability, obtain STAT echocardiogram

Consult geriatrics

Source: Bradburn E et al. *J Trauma Acute Care Surg.* 2012;73(2):1035.
Note: ABG, arterial blood gases; EKG, electrocardiogram; INR, international normalized ratio; PT, prothrombin time; PTT, partial thromboplastin time.

A base deficit of –6 mmol/L has been found to correspond with severe injury and increased mortality. In a study by Davis and Kaups, individuals over the age of 55 had a mortality rate of 60% with a base deficit of –6 mmol/L or lower, while those with a base deficit of –5 mmol/L or higher had an overall mortality rate of 23%.[41]

Geriatric comanagement

Although the outcomes of elderly polytrauma patients treated at trauma centres are better than those treated at non-trauma designated hospitals, trauma designation alone does not directly translate into excellent outcomes.

In a recent analysis of regional US trauma centres, those with a greater volume of trauma patients did not demonstrate an improvement in the outcomes of elder trauma patients commensurate with the improvement seen in the younger population.[42]

Involvement of a geriatrician in the care of the elderly trauma patient has been shown to reduce hospital-acquired complications and to improve outcomes in this patient population.[43] The impact of frailty and comorbid conditions on an elderly trauma patient's recovery is such that multiple, collaborative care partnerships that take into account both the impact of the trauma and also the effect of the patient's age and comorbidities on the patient's course provide benefit. Fallon et al. analysed data from a prospective descriptive study of the impact on elderly trauma patient outcomes of consultation by a specialist in geriatrics. A positive impact, in terms of appropriate management of comorbidities, medication selection and administration, and facilitation of disposition was seen in the majority of patients.[43] Other researchers have found that ICU management of polytraumatized elderly patients that includes geriatric consultation decreases morbidity and mortality.

Multiple studies have shown that comanagement of patients, with collaboration between orthopaedists and other appropriate providers, such as geriatricians or hospitalists, anaesthesiologists, nurses and care managers, decreases morbidity and mortality in hip fracture patients.[44,45] In a multivariate analysis of data collected over time, elderly trauma patients in one US study who were cared for under a protocol that emphasized geriatric comanagement, demonstrated a decrease in mortality.[46] There is every reason to believe that comanagement of polytraumatized elderly patients will result in the same positive outcomes as seen in patients who have sustained hip fractures.

OUTCOMES

Mortality

Elderly polytrauma patients have worse outcomes and more complications than younger polytrauma patients and sustain more serious injuries with lower energy mechanisms. Age, pre-existing disease, decreased physiological reserve and more challenging management may predispose to these worse outcomes. However, due to a lack of prospective trials and evidence-based research, determining the individual influence of these factors is difficult.

Nevertheless, there are several published studies on mortality, complications and outcomes in elderly polytrauma patients, most of which have been summarized by Jacobs et al.[47] and by Switzer and Gammon.[1]

Age, increased ISS, frailty, comorbidities, and head and cervical spine injuries in elderly polytrauma patients correlate with mortality. Shock—diagnosed on admission—and a sustained Glasgow Coma Scale (GCS) ≤8 in elderly trauma patients have been shown to independently predict mortality. Several studies have also shown increased mortality in the elderly following trauma, specifically head injury, and especially in the first 24 hours following admission.[17]

Complications

Although one recent study found similar types of complications, but increased complication rates with increasing age, beginning at age 45, specific negative outcomes and complications are clearly associated with polytrauma in the elderly.[9] Aldrian et al. found in a cohort of Austrian patients that polytrauma in an older population resulted in a significantly higher incidence of multi-organ failure (P=0.02).[14] In another published series, a trauma patient cohort demonstrated a complication rate of 14% while older trauma patients (≥65) had a 34% complication rate. In this study of data from the National Trauma Data Bank, many of the reported complications were infectious in nature.[48] Perhaps secondary to impaired immune response in the elderly, infectious complications are not uncommon in elderly trauma patients. In a study published in 2001, Bochicchio et al. found a nosocomial infection rate of 34% in elderly trauma patients compared to 17.4% in younger patients. Patients in this study who contracted an infection also had longer hospital and ICU lengths of stay.[49]

Not surprisingly, older trauma patients are more likely to be discharged from hospital to a care facility as opposed to their own home. This transfer, known as an 'adverse discharge disposition', increases in likelihood with increasing age.[50] In spite of this, it is important to note that several authors have followed elderly trauma patients over time and have reported that, when they survive, many of these patients have fairly high levels of independence.[16,51]

Withdrawal of care

Early recognition of unsurvivable injuries in the elderly is preferred. 'Unsurvivable' generally has been accepted to mean a persistent GCS ≤8 for 72 hours and a base deficit of −6 mEq/L or greater in a patient >65 years of age, despite aggressive resuscitation and treatment. The discussion with families of limiting extremely aggressive care in these patients should be thought of as compassionate individual care and thoughtful stewardship (Figure 14.4). Appropriate withdrawal of care was one of the three emphasized foci in the recent practice management guidelines for trauma in the elderly published by The Eastern Association for the Surgery of Trauma.[36]

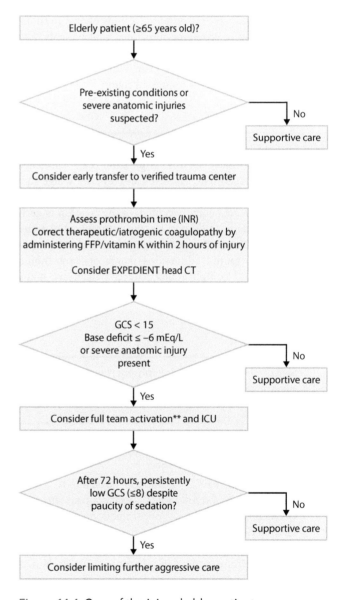

Figure 14.4 Care of the injured older patient: an evidence-based flow diagram. (Reprinted from Calland JF, et al. *J Trauma Acute Care Surg.* 2012;73(5):S345–S350. With permission.)

PREVENTION

With increasing awareness of the prevalence and the individual and societal impact of polytrauma in the elderly, comes the realization that injury prevention in this population is paramount. Programmes that focus on fall prevention and on safe motor vehicle operation in the elderly should be supported. Older motor vehicle collision victims are more likely to be female, to wear safety restraints, to be travelling at <60 mph and to be struck at urban intersections.[52] A recognition that motor vehicle trauma in the elderly affects a different population than motor vehicle trauma in the young should be used to inform prevention strategies. It is also important to overcome biases about the elderly that could result in a lost opportunity to address substance abuse or trauma recidivism. In a study from Illinois, just under 50% of older trauma patients tested positive for alcohol and 12% tested positive for other illicit substances.[53] In addition, a study of data from the Longitudinal Study on Aging illustrated that patients who had been hospitalized for traumatic injury were over three times more likely to have a subsequent injury related hospitalization than those from the uninjured cohort.[54]

CONCLUSION

Polytrauma in elderly individuals is becoming more common. Comorbidities in this population can challenge diagnosis and treatment. However, appropriate triage to a trauma centre and aggressive resuscitation can improve outcomes. Dedicated comanagement or the creation of geriatric trauma teams could help decrease complications and improve mortality in this patient population. As the number of elderly trauma admissions increases, care should be improved and complications reduced. There are many opportunities to improve care in this growing population of trauma patients.

REFERENCES

1. Switzer JA, Gammon SR. High-energy skeletal trauma in the elderly. *J Bone Joint Surg Am*. 2012;94(23):2195–2204. doi: 10.2106/JBJS.K.01166.
2. Davidson GH, Hamlat CA, Rivara FP, Koepsell TD, Jurkovich GJ, Arbabi S. Long-term survival of adult trauma patients. *JAMA*. 2011;305(10):1001–1007. doi: 10.1001/jama.2011.259.
3. US Census Bureau. *2012 National Population Projections: Summary Tables*. Available from: http://www.census.gov/population/projections/data/national/2012/summarytables.html
4. Stewart RM. *National Trauma Data Bank 2014*. 2014. Available from: https://www.facs.org/~/media/files/quality programs/trauma/ntdb/ntdb annual report 2014.ashx
5. Marx AB, Campbell R, Harder F. Polytrauma in the elderly. *World J Surg*. 1986;10(2):330–334. doi: 10.1007/BF01658158.
6. Broos PL, Stappaerts KH, Rommens PM, Louette LK, Gruwez JA. Polytrauma in patients of 65 and over. Injury patterns and outcome. *Int Surg*. 1988;73(2):119–122.
7. Cox S, Morrison C, Cameron P, Smith K. Advancing age and trauma: Triage destination compliance and mortality in Victoria, Australia. *Injury*. 2014;45(9):1312–1319. doi: 10.1016/j.injury.2014.02.028.
8. Pfortmueller CA, Kunz M, Lindner G, Zisakis A, Puig S, Exadaktylos AK. Fall-related emergency department admission: Fall environment and settings and related injury patterns in 6357 patients with special emphasis on the elderly. *ScientificWorldJournal*. 2014;2014:256519. doi: 10.1155/2014/256519.
9. Adams SD, Cotton BA, McGuire MF, et al. Unique pattern of complications in elderly trauma patients at a Level I trauma center. *J Trauma Acute Care Surg*. 2012;72(1):112–118. doi: 10.1097/TA.0b013e318241f073 [doi].
10. Schönenberger A, Billeter ATA, Seifert B, Neuhaus V, Trentz O, Turina M. Opportunities for improved trauma care of the elderly—A single center analysis of 2090 severely injured patients. *Arch Gerontol Geriatr*. 2012;55(3):660–666. doi: 10.1016/j.archger.2012.02.013.
11. Grzalja N, Saftić I, Marinović M, Stiglić D, Cicvarić T. Polytrauma in elderly. *Coll Antropol*. 2011;35(Suppl 2):231–234.
12. Labib N, Nouh T, Winocour S, et al. Severely injured geriatric population: Morbidity, mortality, and risk factors. *J Trauma*. 2011;71(6):1908–1914. doi: 10.1097/TA.0b013e31820989ed.
13. Giannoudis PV, Harwood PJ, Court-Brown C, Pape HC. Severe and multiple trauma in older patients; incidence and mortality. *Injury*. 2009;40(4):362–367. doi: 10.1016/j.injury.2008.10.016.
14. Aldrian S, Nau T, Koenig F, Vécsei V. Geriatric polytrauma. *Wien Klin Wochenschr*. 2005;117(4):145–149. doi: 10.1007/s00508-004-0290-y.
15. Grant PT, Henry JM, McNaughton GW. The management of elderly blunt trauma victims in Scotland: Evidence of ageism? *Injury*. 2000;31(7):519–528.
16. Zietlow SP, Capizzi PJ, Bannon MP, Farnell MB. Multisystem geriatric trauma. *J Trauma* 1994;37(6):985–988.
17. Aldrian S, Koenig F, Weninger P, Vécsei V, Nau T. Characteristics of polytrauma patients between 1992 and 2002: What is changing? *Injury*. 2007;38(9):1059–1064. doi: S0020-1383(07)00174-X [pii].
18. Cirera E, Pérez K, Santamariña-Rubio E, Novoa AM, Olabarria M. Incidence trends of injury among the elderly in Spain, 2000–2010. *Inj Prev*. 2014;20(6):401–407. doi: 10.1136/injuryprev-2014-041199.

19. Vogel JAJ, Ginde AAA, Lowenstein SR, Betz ME. Emergency department visits by older adults for motor vehicle collisions. *West J Emerg Med*. 2013;14(6):576–581. doi: 10.5811/westjem.2013.2.12230.

20. Broos PLO, D'Hoore A, Vanderschot P, Rommens PM, Stappaerts KH. Multiple trauma in elderly patients. Factors influencing outcome: Importance of aggressive care. *Injury*. 1993;24(6):365–368.

21. Sterling DA, O'Connor JA, Bonadies J. Geriatric falls: Injury severity is high and disproportionate to mechanism. *J Trauma*. 2001;50(1):116–119.

22. Spaniolas K, Cheng JD, Gestring ML, Sangosanya A, Stassen NA, Bankey PE. Ground level falls are associated with significant mortality in elderly patients. *J Trauma*. 2010;69(4):821–825. doi: 10.1097/TA.0b013e3181efc6c6; 10.1097/TA.0b013e3181efc6c6.

23. Grossman MD, Miller D, Scaff DW, Arcona S. When is an elder old? Effect of preexisting conditions on mortality in geriatric trauma. *J Trauma*. 2002;52(2):242–246.

24. Oreskovich MR, Howard JD, Copass MK, Carrico CJ. Geriatric trauma: Injury patterns and outcome. *J Trauma Acute Care Surg*. 1984;24(7):565–572.

25. Siram SM, Sonaike V, Bolorunduro OB, et al. Does the pattern of injury in elderly pedestrian trauma mirror that of the younger pedestrian? *J Surg Res*. 2011;167(1):14–18. doi: 10.1016/j.jss.2010.10.007.

26. Demetriades D, Murray J, Martin M, et al. Pedestrians injured by automobiles: Relationship of age to injury type and severity. *J Am Coll Surg*. 2004;199(3):382–387. doi: 10.1016/j.jamcollsurg.2004.03.027.

27. Abdelfattah A, Core MD, Cannada LK, Watson JT. Geriatric high-energy polytrauma with orthopedic injuries: Clinical predictors of mortality. *Geriatr Orthop Surg Rehabil*. 2014;5(4):173–177. doi: 10.1177/2151458514548578.

28. Dechert TA, Duane TM, Frykberg BP, Aboutanos MB, Malhotra AK, Ivatury RR. Elderly patients with pelvic fracture: Interventions and outcomes. *Am Surg*. 2009;75(4):291–295.

29. Bulger EM, Arneson MA, Mock CN, Jurkovich GJ. Rib fractures in the elderly. *J Trauma*. 2000;48(6):1040–1047.

30. Keller JM, Sciadini MF, Sinclair E, O'Toole RV. Geriatric trauma: Demographics, injuries, and mortality. *J Orthop Trauma*. 2012;26(9):e161–e165. doi: 10.1097/BOT.0b013e3182324460

31. DeMaria EJ, Kenney PR, Merriam MA, Casanova LA, Gann DS. Survival after trauma in geriatric patients. *Ann Surg*. 1987;206(6):738–743.

32. Joseph B, Pandit V, Zangbar B, et al. Superiority of frailty over age in predicting outcomes among geriatric trauma patients: A prospective analysis. *JAMA Surg*. 2014;149(8):766–772. doi: 10.1001/jamasurg.2014.296.

33. Lane P, Sorondo B, Kelly JJ. Geriatric trauma patients—Are they receiving trauma center care? *Acad Emerg Med*. 2003;10(3):244–250.

34. Ma MH, MacKenzie EJ, Alcorta R, Kelen GD. Compliance with prehospital triage protocols for major trauma patients. *J Trauma*. 1999;46(1):168–175.

35. Lehmann R, Beekley A, Casey L, Salim A, Martin M. The impact of advanced age on trauma triage decisions and outcomes: A statewide analysis. *Am J Surg*. 2009;197(5):571–574; discussion 574–575. doi: 10.1016/j.amjsurg.2008.12.037.

36. Calland JF, Ingraham AM, Martin N, et al. Evaluation and management of geriatric trauma. *J Trauma Acute Care Surg*. 2012;73(5):S345–S350. doi: 10.1097/TA.0b013e318270191f.

37. Demetriades D, Karaiskakis M, Velmahos G, et al. Effect on outcome of early intensive management of geriatric trauma patients. *Br J Surg*. 2002;89(10):1319–1322. doi: 10.1046/j.1365-2168.2002.02210.x.

38. Mann NC, Cahn RM, Mullins RJ, Brand DM, Jurkovich GJ. Survival among injured geriatric patients during construction of a statewide trauma system. *J Trauma*. 2001;50(6):1111–1116.

39. McKinley BBA, Marvin RGR, Cocanour CS, Marquez A, Ware DN, Moore FA. Blunt trauma resuscitation. *Arch Surg*. 2000;135(6):688. doi: 10.1001/archsurg.135.6.688.

40. Scalea TM, Simon HM, Duncan AO, et al. Geriatric blunt multiple trauma: Improved survival with early invasive monitoring. *J Trauma*. 1990;30(2):129–136.

41. Davis JW, Kaups KL. Base deficit in the elderly: A marker of severe injury and death. *J Trauma*. 1998;45(5):873–877.

42. Matsushima K, Schaefer EW, Won EJ, Armen SB, Indeck MC, Soybel DI. Positive and negative volume-outcome relationships in the geriatric trauma population. *JAMA Surg*. 2014;149(4):319–326. doi: 10.1001/jamasurg.2013.4834.

43. Fallon WF, Rader E, Zyzanski S, et al. Geriatric outcomes are improved by a geriatric trauma consultation service. *J Trauma*. 2006;61(5):1040–1046. doi: 10.1097/01.ta.0000238652.48008.59.

44. Friedman SM, Mendelson DA, Bingham KW, Kates SL. Impact of a comanaged Geriatric Fracture Center on short-term hip fracture outcomes. *Arch Intern Med*. 2009;169(18):1712–1717. doi: 10.1001/archinternmed.2009.321.

45. Kates SL, Mendelson DA, Friedman SM. The value of an organized fracture program for the elderly: Early results. *J Orthop Trauma*. 2011;25(4):233–237. doi: 10.1097/BOT.0b013e3181e5e901.

46. Bradburn E, Rogers FB, Krasne M, et al. High-risk geriatric protocol. *J Trauma Acute Care Surg*. 2012;73(2):1035. doi: 10.1097/TA.0b013e318274e87a.

47. Jacobs DG, Plaisier BR, Barie PS, et al. Practice management guidelines for geriatric trauma: The EAST Practice Management Guidelines Work Group. *J Trauma Acute Care Surg.* 2003;54(2):391–416. doi: 10.1097/01.TA.0000042015.54022.BE.

48. Min L, Burruss S, Morley E, et al. A simple clinical risk nomogram to predict mortality-associated geriatric complications in severely injured geriatric patients. *J Trauma Acute Care Surg.* 2013;74(4):1125–1132. doi: 10.1097/TA.0b013e31828273a0.

49. Bochicchio GV, Joshi M, Knorr KM, Scalea TM. Impact of nosocomial infections in trauma: Does age make a difference? *J Trauma.* 2001;50(4):612–619.

50. Bennett KM, Scarborough JE, Vaslef S. Outcomes and health care resource utilization in super-elderly trauma patients. *J Surg Res.* 2010;163(1):127–131. doi: 10.1016/j.jss.2010.04.031 [doi].

51. Battistella F, Din A, Perez L. Trauma patients 75 years and older long terms followup results justify aggressive management. *J Trauma* 1998;44(4):618–623; discussion 623.

52. Clark DE. Motor vehicle crash fatalities in the elderly: Rural versus urban. *J Trauma.* 2001;51:896–900. doi: 10.1097/00005373-200111000-00011.

53. Zautcke JL, Coker SB, Morris RW, Stein-Spencer L. Geriatric trauma in the State of Illinois: Substance use and injury patterns. *Am J Emerg Med.* 2002;20(1):14–17. doi: 10.1053/ajem.2002.30107.

54. McGwin G, May AK, Melton SM, Reiff DA, Rue LW. Recurrent trauma in elderly patients. *Arch Surg.* 2001;136:197–203. doi: 10.1001/archsurg.136.2.197.

15

Multiple fractures

NICHOLAS D. CLEMENT

INTRODUCTION

The incidence of fractures in the elderly population is increasing and most occur as the result of low energy falls, usually in their place of domicile.[1,2] Most of the literature concerning fractures in the elderly has focused on isolated fractures, particularly those of the proximal femur,[3] proximal humerus[4] and distal radius.[5] Although elderly patients frequently present with more than one fracture,[6] there has been little published regarding the epidemiology and outcome of multiple fractures in the elderly.[7,8] Potentially, these polytraumatized elderly patients should be managed differently compared to those with isolated fractures, as early intervention and rehabilitation may improve outcome.[9] Early medical assessment, with the aim of optimizing physiological status and early rehabilitation, is now an accepted part of the management of the multiply injured elderly patient.[10]

Despite the relative paucity of multiple fractures in the elderly, which occur in approximately 5% of patients presenting with a fracture, the burden upon the trauma workload in the future will likely increase with the growing elderly population and with increasing longevity. This will result in major repercussions on medical resources, both acutely and for the ongoing care of these frail patients.[11,12]

Patients with multiple fractures are more likely to be admitted to hospital, have a longer length of stay, and are less likely to return to their original place of domicile.[7,8] Hence, the optimal management of these patients is essential to minimize the impact of their injuries and optimize outcome. In order to do this it is essential to have an understanding of the epidemiology and the current outcome of multiple fractures in the elderly.

This chapter presents the prevalence of multiple fractures in the elderly and describes the mechanisms of injury, common injury patterns and the effect of socioeconomic status. The evidence surrounding admission rates, operative intervention, length of stay, rehabilitation and mortality will be discussed.

EPIDEMIOLOGY

The Centers for Disease Control and Protection in the United States has suggested that the cost of falls in 2020 may reach $54.9 billion in the USA alone.[13] The main reason for this increased cost is a growing elderly population in the Western world, as it is estimated that the population aged 65 years or more will almost double by 2030.[14] A third of all fractures occur in patients above 65 years of age, and a quarter occur in patients above 75 years of age.[6] The majority of these patients suffer fragility fractures following low energy mechanisms, which account for 30% of male fractures and 66% of female fractures.[6]

PATIENT POPULATION

There is relatively little literature describing the epidemiology and outcome of multiple fractures other than that published from Edinburgh.[7] Much of the data presented in this chapter will be from this work, with supportive data presented when available.

The study population discussed in this chapter is based on all patients presenting to the Royal Infirmary of Edinburgh with fractures during a 1-year period between July 2007 and June 2008, which were prospectively documented. The Royal Infirmary of Edinburgh is the only hospital receiving adult trauma for a predominately urban population of 780,000, of which 15.4% are 65 years of age or above.[15] Patients with multiple fractures are divided into three groups for the purposes of this chapter: upper limb multiple fractures only, lower limb multiple fractures only and combined, involving both the upper and lower limbs. Pelvic fractures are included with lower limb fractures.

DEMOGRAPHIC AND INJURY PATTERNS

It has been estimated that about one-third of adults aged 65 years or more who live at home will fall each year, which increases to two-thirds for adults who live in residential homes.[16] Approximately 10% of falls result in a serious injury[17] and a recent Swedish study has suggested that 7% of falls in the elderly result in fracture.[18] It is likely that the incidence of fall related fractures will increase in the future, resulting in considerable expense for healthcare systems.

There is no significant difference in the average age or gender ratios in elderly patients who present with single or multiple fractures. From the Edinburgh data, 2,335 patients aged at least 65 presented with 2,465 fractures over a 1-year period, 119 (5.1%) of whom had multiple fractures. Of these, 109 (91.6%) patients presented with two fractures, 9 (7.6%) presented with three fractures and 1 (0.8%) presented with four fractures. Multiple fractures were found to be common in females (78%) and the mean age is 79 years. As would be expected, females are significantly older than males. A comparison of the demographic characteristics of elderly patients presenting to Edinburgh with single and multiple fractures

is found in Table 15.1. Distal radial, proximal humeral and pelvic fractures are associated with an increased risk of sustaining associated fractures (Table 15.1).

The incidence of multiple fractures is influenced by socioeconomic deprivation (Figure 15.1), with a significant increase in the incidence of multiple fractures in the fifth quintile (least deprived) compared to quintiles one to four. This pattern is also seen with isolated fractures in the elderly. There is also evidence that demonstrates an increased incidence of fractures in socially deprived patients after falls.[19] From this one might hypothesize that there is an association with multiple fractures and deprivation.

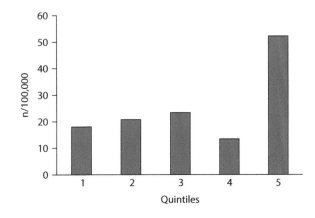

Figure 15.1 A histogram showing the relationship between social deprivation and the incidence of fractures. (Reproduced with permission and copyright © of the British Editorial Society of Bone and Joint Surgery from: Clement ND, et al. *J Bone Joint Surg Br* 2012;94(2):231–6.)

Table 15.1 Demographic characteristics of elderly patients who present with single or multiple fractures from all modes of injury

	Single fractures	Multiple fractures	Odds ratio	P value
Patients (%)	2,216 (94.9)	119 (5.1)	–	–
Average age (years)				
All	78.9	78.7	–	0.78[a]
Male	77.7	76.5	–	0.61[a]
Female	79.2	79.4	–	0.54[a]
Male/female	23/77	22/78	1.0	0.9[b]
Fracture prevalence (%)				
Proximal femur	30.6	32.8	1.1	0.34[b]
Distal radius	21.1	37.0	2.2	<0.0001[b]
Proximal humerus	9.9	35.3	5.1	<0.0001[b]
Ankle	6.7	9.2	1.4	0.19[b]
Finger phalanx	3.8	7.6	2.1	0.05[b]
Pelvis	3.1	12.6	4.9	<0.0001[b]

Source: Reproduced with permission and copyright © of the British Editorial Society of Bone and Joint Surgery from: Clement ND, et al. *J Bone Joint Surg Br* 2012;94(2):231–6.
Note: The prevalence and risk of sustaining one of the most common six fractures are shown.
[a] Mann–Whitney U test.
[b] Chi-square test.

Mechanism of injury

Multiple fractures in the elderly may occur as a result of high energy or low energy injuries. However, it is not correct to assume that the primary causes are motor vehicle accidents or falls from a height.[7] Certainly some combinations of fractures indicate the high energy mechanism through which they were sustained, such as the association of calcaneal and spinal fractures. Conversely, the proximal humeral fracture associated with a hip fracture is a relatively common presentation, occurring in approximately one in 50 patients presenting with a hip fracture, and is more likely to be sustained through a simple fall.[7]

The mechanism of injury is noted to influence the prevalence and number of elderly patients presenting with multiple fractures (Table 15.2). The highest prevalence is observed for road traffic accidents and falls from a height, but in the elderly population these modes of injury are uncommon. Although only 5% of patients have multiple fractures after a simple fall, because of the frequency of falls in the elderly population, this mechanism results in 81% of all multiple fractures. Female gender is a risk factor for multiple fractures after a simple fall when compared to other modes of injury. Combined upper and lower limb fractures and proximal femoral fractures are more likely to occur after a simple fall (Table 15.3).

Table 15.2 Numbers and percentages of multiple fractures caused by different modes of injury

	Patients (n)	Multiple fractures	%	Average age (year)	Male/ female (%)
Simple fall	2,111	96	4.5	79.0	16/84
Fall from height	11	3	27.3	72.0	67/33
Fall downstairs	80	10	12.5	77.0	30/70
Motor vehicle accident	22	8	36.4	80.2	75/25
Direct blow/assault	45	2	4.4	77.5	0/100
Sport	17	0	–	–	–
Spontaneous	24	0	–	–	–
Others	25	0	–	–	–
Total	2,335	119	5.1	78.7	22/78

Source: Reproduced with permission and copyright © of the British Editorial Society of Bone and Joint Surgery from: Clement ND, et al. J Bone Joint Surg Br 2012;94(2):231–6.
Note: The average ages and gender ratios are also shown.

Table 15.3 Comparison of the demographic characteristics of double fractures caused by a fall with those caused by other modes of injury

	Falls	Other modes of injury	Odds ratio	P value
Number of patients	90	19	–	–
Fractures	180	38	–	–
Average age (years)	79.1	77.9	–	0.4[a]
Male/female (%)	16/84	42/58	3.8	0.03[b]
Fracture combinations				
Upper limb fractures (%)	32.2	47.4	1.8	0.29[b]
Lower limb fractures (%)	12.2	31.6	3.4	0.04[b]
Combined fractures (%)	55.5	21.0	4.6	0.007[b]
Fracture types				
Proximal femur (%)	21.7	5.3	5.0	0.01[b]
Distal radius (%)	21.1	18.4	1.0	0.59[b]
Proximal humerus (%)	18.8	10.5	2.0	0.16[b]
Pelvis (%)	8.9	10.5	1.2	0.47[b]

Source: Reproduced with permission and copyright © of the British Editorial Society of Bone and Joint Surgery from: Clement ND, et al. J Bone Joint Surg Br 2012;94(2):231–6.
[a] Mann–Whitney U test.
[b] Fisher's exact test.

SIMPLE FALLS

The commonest fractures involved in fall related double fractures are those involving the proximal femur, distal radius, proximal humerus or pelvis (Table 15.4). Elderly patients with upper limb fracture combinations are significantly younger than those in the lower limb and combined fracture groups. The distal radius is involved in 66% of fracture combinations and the proximal humerus in 38%. The combination of a proximal femoral fracture, with either a proximal humeral or distal radial fracture, accounts for 31% of all fall related double fracture combinations. Only 10% of upper limb fracture combinations do not involve a distal radial or proximal humeral fracture. Only 12% of patients sustain lower limb fracture combinations (Table 15.5).

Over 50% of elderly patients have combined upper and lower limb fractures of which proximal femoral fractures with proximal humeral or distal radial fractures are the most common (Table 15.5). The Edinburgh data showed 16 different combinations, but only seven occurred more than once during the year. The proximal femur was involved in over two-thirds of the fracture combinations.

These patterns of fall related injuries probably reflect the natural epidemiological history of fragility fractures, as the mean age of isolated distal radial, proximal humeral and proximal femoral fractures is 56, 65 and 81 years, respectively.[6] Hence, fragility fractures of the upper limb occur at a younger age, which may explain the observed age difference between the upper limb multiple fracture group and the lower limb and combined fracture groups.

FALLS DOWNSTAIRS

Overall, 13% of patients sustain multiple fractures after a fall down stairs (Table 15.2). There were 70% with double fractures and 30% had three fractures. Analysis of the patients with double fractures demonstrated that 43% presented with upper limb fracture combinations and the remaining patients having combined upper and lower limb fracture combinations.

Table 15.4 Epidemiology of fractures that occurred most commonly in fall-related double fracture combinations

Fracture	Number (%)	Average age (years)	Male/ female (%)
Proximal femur	39 (21.7)	81.4	21/79
Distal radius	38 (21.1)	77.6	13/87
Proximal humerus	34 (18.8)	79.7	15/85
Pelvis	11 (6.1)	88.4	9/91

Source: Reproduced with permission and copyright © of the British Editorial Society of Bone and Joint Surgery from: Clement ND, et al. *J Bone Joint Surg Br* 2012;94(2):231–6.

Table 15.5 Double fracture combinations according to fracture combination group

Fracture combinations	Number (%)	Average age (years)	Male/female (%)
Upper limb			
Distal radius/distal radius	8 (27.6)	74.7	25/25
Distal radius/proximal humerus	4 (13.8)	79.5	0/100
Distal radius/finger phalanx	3 (10.3)	74.6	0/100
Distal radius/proximal radius	2 (6.9)	73.0	50/50
Proximal humerus/scapula	2 (6.9)	80.5	0/100
Proximal humerus/finger phalanx	2 (6.9)	74.5	0/100
All combinations	29 (100)	75.1	17/83
Lower limb			
Ankle/metatarsal	3 (27.3)	75.3	0/100
Pelvis/proximal femur	3 (27.3)	92.3	0/100
All combinations	11 (100)	83.4	18/82
Combined			
Proximal femur/proximal humerus	17 (34.0)	80.9	18/82
Proximal femur/distal radius	11 (22.0)	80.1	18/82
Pelvis/proximal humerus	4 (8.0)	87.5	25/75
Pelvis/distal radius	3 (6.0)	85.0	0/100
Distal radius/patella	2 (4.0)	76.5	0/100
Distal radius/metatarsal	2 (4.0)	74.5	0/100
Patella/proximal forearm	2 (4.0)	74.5	0/100
All combinations	50 (100)	80.5	14/86

Source: Reproduced with permission and copyright © of the British Editorial Society of Bone and Joint Surgery from: Clement ND, et al. *J Bone Joint Surg Br* 2012;94(2):231–6.

Note: The numbers, percentages, average age and gender ratio of each combination are shown.

REHABILITATION

The majority of elderly patients sustaining multiple fractures require admission, despite a large proportion not needing surgical fixation, and more than half require an increased level of care before discharge. Looking at data from Edinburgh, the rate of admission is above 80% for all types of management in elderly patients with multiple fractures (Table 15.6). This high admission rate is not solely due to the need for operative fixation of the fracture, with only 24% of upper limb combinations undergoing surgery in contrast to 80% of upper and lower limb combinations. The length of stay is significantly less for upper limb fractures, as to be expected (Table 15.6). There is no reported difference in length of stay or rate of discharge to original domicile for patients who undergo surgical fixation. The rate of return to original place of domicile is low, with less than 50% of the combined upper and lower limb fracture group and 20% of the lower limb fracture group returning to their original home (Table 15.6).

Literature regarding the effect of multiple fractures upon rehabilitation after injury is limited.[8,20,21] Weatherall[8] described the outcome of nine patients (6%) admitted to an orthopaedic trauma rehabilitation unit for elderly people who had multiple fractures secondary to falls. All of their patients were female with a mean age of 83 years. The mean length of stay in hospital was 37 days, being 7 days longer than that observed in Edinburgh.[7] In contrast to the Edinburgh cohort, the majority of patients were able to return to their own homes. In addition, it was claimed that 30% of patients admitted from their own homes were discharged 'considerably more dependent'. Fractures of the hip and humerus were the most common, as observed in Edinburgh.[7] Cardiovascular and neurological systemic diseases were most prevalent, with neurological systemic disease the cause of the fall in a third of the patients. Weatherall[8] concludes by stating 'rehabilitation of these patients is more difficult than for those with single fractures, and a multidisciplinary approach is needed'. This would seem to be a conclusion that would not only optimize the patient's functional outcome, but also potentially improve survival.

In contrast to Weatherall,[8] a study from Italy by Di Monaco et al.[20] found no difference in length of stay if patients sustained a concomitant fracture of an upper limb with a hip fracture.

Di Monaco et al.[20] assessed 586 consecutive inpatient hip fractures, of which 24 (4%) presented with a concomitant fracture of the upper limb. They assessed functional recovery using the Barthel Index score, which is an ordinal scale to assess activities of daily living. After adjustment for confounding variables, a significant reduction in the Barthel Index score was found on admission, but not on discharge, for patients with multiple fractures compared to those with single fractures. The length of stay was not significantly associated with the presence of a concomitant upper limb fracture. These data may be skewed as the majority of patients in this cohort had a concomitant distal radial fracture, which the Edinburgh data suggest are a more physiologically robust group relative to other fracture combinations, which is supported by a lower standardized mortality ratio (SMR).

The equivocal effect of a concomitant fracture of the distal radius with a hip fracture is supported by Shabat et al.,[21] who actually demonstrated a better pre-injury morbidity. They identified 46 patients over a 10-year period presenting with a combination of distal radial and hip fractures who were older than 65 years. They assessed age, gender, pre-fall function, use of medication, chronic and acute comorbidities, circumstance of the fall, length of hospital stay, management, complications and rehabilitation. Eighteen (39%) patients were totally independent, while the remaining patients needed some assistance with the activities of daily living. Twenty-six (57%) patients returned to pre-injury activity levels after an average of 60 days. Among the remaining 18 patients, 11 gained full recovery and seven patients had a slight reduction. The authors concluded that 'the double trauma represents a better pre-morbid condition relative to patients in the same age group, and thus it may serve as a prognostic indicator for success in rehabilitation'. This is supported by the short hospital stay, which ranged from 5 to 23 days, compared to 30 days in Edinburgh for all double fracture combinations.

MORTALITY

Data from Edinburgh has demonstrated that the SMR at 1 year is significantly greater after sustaining both single and multiple fractures involving the pelvis, proximal femur and proximal humerus (Table 15.7). However, the mortality

Table 15.6 Rate of admission, operative intervention, fixation of both fractures, length of stay and rate of discharge to original domicile (for those patients admitted to hospital) for each double fracture group

Outcome	Upper limb	Lower limb	Combined	P value
Admission (%)	24/29 (82.8)	11/11 (100)	46/50 (92.0)	0.14[a]
Operative intervention (%)	7/29 (24.1)	5/11 (45.5)	40/50 (80.0)	<0.001[a]
Both fractures fixed (%)	2/29 (6.9)	1/11 (9.1)	6/50 (12.0)	0.75[a]
Length of stay (days)	8.3	32.8	29.3	0.002[b]
Return to original place of domicile (%)	21/24 (87.5)	2/11 (18.2)	21/46 (45.6)	<0.001[a]

Source: Reproduced with permission and copyright © of the British Editorial Society of Bone and Joint Surgery from: Clement ND, et al. *J Bone Joint Surg Br* 2012;94(2):231–6.

[a] Chi square test.
[b] ANOVA.

Table 15.7 One-year standardized mortality ratios and P values for single and multiple fractures of the ankle, distal radius, pubic rami, proximal femur and proximal humerus for patients 65 years and older.

Fractures	Single fracture (95% CI)	P value[a]	Multiple fractures (95% CI)					
			All ages	P value[a]	65–79 years	P value[a]	≥80 years	P value[a]
Ankle	1.85 (1.03 to 3.10)	0.02	1.95 (0.34 to 6.61)	0.32	2.66 (0.33 to 6.61)	0.31	No deaths	–
Distal radius	0.75 (0.50 to 1.08)	0.13	1.43 (0.64 to 4.82)	0.15	2.18 (0.33 to 6.61)	0.31	1.07 (0.16 to 3.30)	1.0
Pelvis	2.28 (1.35 to 3.63)	<0.001	10.50 (2.43 to 13.05)	<0.001	11.64 (5.38 to 19.22)	0.03	3.45 (1.27 to 9.65)	0.003
Proximal femur	3.41 (2.99 to 3.87)	<0.001	4.66 (2.66 to 7.64)	<0.001	8.39 (1.83 to 11.08)	<0.001	3.53 (1.46 to 5.51)	<0.001
Proximal humerus	2.06 (1.47 to 2.80)	<0.001	4.95 (2.66 to 7.64)	<0.001	6.64 (1.83 to 11.08)	<0.001	4.34 (2.19 to 8.25)	<0.001

Source: Reproduced with permission and copyright © of the British Editorial Society of Bone and Joint Surgery from: Clement ND, et al. J Bone Joint Surg Br 2012;94(2):231–6.

[a] Chi square test.

rate is only significantly increased, relative to patients sustaining single fractures, for pelvic fractures ($p=0.04$) and proximal humeral fractures ($p=0.008$). A subgroup analysis found a lower SMR for very-elderly patients (aged 80 years or older) after sustaining multiple fractures relative to the SMR for elderly patients between 65 and 79 years of age (Table 15.7). Proximal femoral fractures in this younger elderly subgroup have a significantly increased mortality risk compared to patients with a fractured proximal femur in isolation. In addition, a proximal femoral fracture sustained in combination with a proximal humeral fracture is associated with a significantly increased mortality risk at 1 year relative to an isolated proximal femoral fracture (47%). In contrast, the mortality of patients with a proximal femoral fracture is reduced if associated with a distal radial fracture (18%).

The reason that a higher 1-year mortality rate is associated with the most common double fracture combination of a proximal femoral and proximal humeral fracture (47%) compared to that of a proximal femoral fracture and a distal radial fracture (18%) is not clear. Allum et al.[22] studied age-dependent balance correction and arm movements for falls in different age groups and found that compensatory movements to facilitate protection from falls were less effective with increasing age. Frailer patients were more likely to incur proximal limb girdle fractures due to diminished protective reflexes, and hence sustain proximal humeral and femoral fractures.[22,23] Patients who retain protective reflexes are more likely to sustain a distal radial fracture, which may reflect a superior physiological status. This may account for the observed improved survival rate of proximal femoral fractures associated with distal radial fracture.

A previous study assessing polytrauma in elderly patients with mild to moderate injuries (injury severity score [ISS] <16), such as multiple extremity fractures, demonstrated

that those patients with pre-existing comorbidity were at an increased risk of late death from medical complications that were not directly related to their original injury.[9] Those elderly patients with a high ISS are more likely to die early during their admission (<48 h), in contrast to those with a low ISS who are more likely to die later in their admission (>13 days).[9] The cause of death in the early group is the trauma insult that is reflected by a high ISS, but those dying later do so because of medical complications.[9] It is already known that mortality is predicted by ISS and medical complications in older patients,[24] of which infections and chest complications are twice as common and dysrhythmias five times more frequent.[25] Age alone has been shown to be an independent risk factor for mortality.[26] Also, the presence of pre-existing comorbidity increases the odds of experiencing a complication by over threefold.[27] The combination of age and pre-existing comorbidity is additive, with increasing mortality risk.[28]

Hollis et al.[28] demonstrated that pre-existing comorbidity and increasing age are independent risk factors for mortality after trauma. However, this increased risk diminishes with increasing ISS and is no longer statistically significant with scores of >24, which may suggest the trauma insult causes death before medical complications ensue. This trend could be due to these risk factors predisposing patients to medical complications which are not directly related to their trauma insult, after sustaining minor to moderate injuries.

A study by Clement et al.[9] supports this theory. They reported that irrespective of age after sustaining a severe trauma insult, the majority who die do so within 48 hours, but elderly patients with pre-existing comorbidity die of medical complications not directly related to the initial trauma insult late in their admission after suffering injuries that they may be expected to survive with low ISS (Figure 15.2) and high predicted survival scores. This pattern of increased mortality risk later during admission

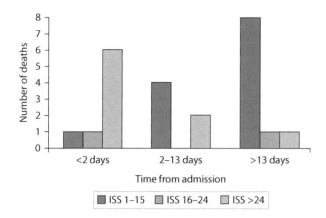

Figure 15.2 Deaths of patients ≥65 years of age in relation to time from admission and injury severity score. (From Clement ND, et al. *Scand J Trauma Resusc Emerg Med* 2010;18:26.)

has also been observed in more severely injured elderly patients (ISS >15).[29] It may be that early medical/physician intervention may avert these late deaths due to medical complications, and patients older than 65 years with pre-existing comorbidity could be targeted with early multidisciplinary input.

Early intensive monitoring, evaluation and resuscitation of elderly patients does improve survival after trauma.[30] This support can be justified by the fact that few require nursing home care on discharge and the majority return to their original domicile.[31] It was first suggested by Richmond et al.[27] that a care of the elderly consultation service could be an important addition to the trauma team, optimizing pre-existing comorbidity and managing medical complications that arise. This was confirmed by Fallon et al.[32] who demonstrated improved medical care in elderly patients after review by a physician, addressing new and existing medical issues and reducing hospital acquired complications, such as functional decline, falls, delirium and death.

A study comparing the differences between severely (ISS >15) injured patients 65 years or older with those less than 65 years of age found that the older age group were at an increased risk of inpatient mortality despite normal physiological parameters on admission.[29] Due to this phenomenon, the authors suggest it may be difficult to predict which older patients would benefit from aggressive monitoring and management using physiological parameters only. The authors hypothesize the observed discrepancy may relate to pre-existing comorbidities, which were not analysed in their study. A smaller retrospective study supports this theory identifying those patients with pre-existing comorbidity as being at an increased risk of inpatient mortality, which was independent of age and so would need to be accounted for in a statistical analysis of physiological parameters.[9]

The question remains as to how those patients with an increased risk of mortality late in admission after sustaining multiple fractures can be identified early. Skaga et al.[33] described using the American Society of Anesthesiologists (ASA) Physical Status classification to predict mortality, finding it to be an independent predictor. Clement et al.[9] retrospectively assigned a pre-injury ASA score to the 12 individuals who died beyond 13 days after injury with an ISS of <16. All except one had an ASA score of III, which is associated with an increased risk of mortality (adjusted OR 2.25).[33] For patients with an ISS of <16, mortality increases from <1% in those with an ASA grade of I to approximately 8% in those with an ASA grade of III or IV. In conjunction with other risk factors of morality, the ASA grade could be used to identify those individuals most at risk, and early medical intervention and physiological optimization could potentially avert late mortality.

From the evidence it would seem that the frailty of patients who present with double fractures is affirmed by the associated increased SMR at 1 year. This is supported by the fact that elderly patients, relative to very-elderly patients, have an increased mortality risk that may reflect the frailty of this younger age group after sustaining low energy multiple fractures. The mortality risk is significantly increased for multiple fractures that includ pelvic or proximal humeral fractures in all elderly patients, or proximal femoral fractures in those 65–79 years old, relative to factures sustained in isolation. However, this increased mortality risk diminishes with increasing age, with very-elderly patients having a lower risk. Combined fractures of the proximal humerus and femur are associated with the highest mortality risk at 1 year. Patients sustaining these multiple fracture combinations should be recognized, and both the medical and surgical management should be prioritized in an effort to improve their outcome.

CONCLUSIONS

The literature suggests that a majority of multiple fractures in the elderly happen after low energy trauma and occur predominantly in females. Distal radius, proximal humerus and pelvic fractures are associated with an increased risk of sustaining multiple fractures. The commonest multiple fracture group is that of combined fractures involving the upper and lower limbs.

It seems likely that, with increasing longevity, multiple fractures secondary to low energy injuries will become more prevalent and form a greater proportion of the trauma workload in the future. There will be financial repercussions associated with the management and ongoing care of these frail elderly patients sustaining multiple fractures, with high admission rates, prolonged length of stay and increased level of care needed upon discharge.

A large proportion of these patients undergo conservative management and rehabilitation. Hence, these frail patients with an increased mortality risk and prolonged rehabilitation may benefit from early identification and medical optimization. A multidisciplinary approach should be adopted to facilitate rehabilitation and to potentially provide increased care needs, in an effort to improve functional outcome, survival and shorten admission stay.

REFERENCES

1. Court-Brown CM, Aitken SA, Forward D, O'Toole RV. The epidemiology of fractures. In: Bucholz RW, Heckman JD, Court-Brown CM, Tornetta P, editors. *Rockwood and Green's Fractures in Adults*. 7th ed. Philadelphia, PA: Lippincott Williams & Wilkins; 2010. pp. 53–77.

2. Kannus P, Parkkari J, Koskinen S, Niemi S, Palvanen M, Jarvinen M, et al. Fall-induced injuries and deaths among older adults. *JAMA* 1999;281(20):1895–9.

3. Clement ND, Green K, Murray N, Duckworth AD, McQueen MM, Court-Brown CM. Undisplaced intracapsular hip fractures in the elderly: Predicting fixation failure and mortality. A prospective study of 162 patients. *J Orthop Sci* 2013;18(4):578–85.

4. Clement ND, Duckworth AD, McQueen MM, Court-Brown CM. The outcome of proximal humeral fractures in the elderly: Predictors of mortality and function. *Bone Joint J* 2014;96(7):970–7.

5. Clement ND, Duckworth AD, Court-Brown CM, McQueen MM. Manipulation of displaced distal radial fractures in the superelderly: Prediction of malunion and the degree of radiographic improvement. *Adv Orthop* 2014;2014:785473.

6. Court-Brown CM, Caesar B. Epidemiology of adult fractures: A review. *Injury* 2006;37(8):691–7.

7. Clement ND, Aitken S, Duckworth AD, McQueen MM, Court-Brown CM. Multiple fractures in the elderly. *J Bone Joint Surg Br* 2012;94(2):231–6.

8. Weatherall M. Rehabilitation of elderly patients with multiple fractures secondary to falls. *Disabil Rehabil* 1993;15(1):38–40.

9. Clement ND, Tennant C, Muwanga C. Polytrauma in the elderly: Predictors of the cause and time of death. *Scand J Trauma Resusc Emerg Med* 2010;18:26.

10. Switzer JA, Gammon SR. High-energy skeletal trauma in the elderly. *J Bone Joint Surg Am* 2012;94(23):2195–204.

11. Ray NF, Chan JK, Thamer M. Medical expenditures for the treatment of osteoporotic fractures in the United States in 1995: Report from the National Osteoporosis Foundation. *J Bone Miner Res* 1997;12:24–35.

12. Johnell O. The socioeconomic burden of fractures: Today and in the 21st century. *Am J Med* 1997;103(2A):20S–25S.

13. Centers for Disease Control and Prevention. Cost of falls among older adults. 2010. http://www.cdc.gov/homeandrecreationalsafety/falls/fallcost.html (accessed 10 October 2010).

14. Office of National Statistics. http://www.dft.gov.uk/pgr/statistics (accessed 10 October 2010).

15. National Records of Scotland. http://www.nrscotland.gov.uk/

16. Masud T, Morris RO. Epidemiology of falls. *Age Ageing* 2001;30(Suppl 4):3–7.

17. Tinetti ME, Speechley M, Ginter SF. Risk factors for falls among elderly persons living in the community. *N Engl J Med* 1988;319(26):1701–7.

18. Von Heideken P, Gustafson Y, Kallin K, Jensen J, Lundin-Olsson L. Falls in the very old people: The population based Umea study in Sweden. *Arch Gerontol Geriatr* 2009;49:390–396.

19. Court-Brown CM, Aitken SA, Ralston SH, McQueen MM. The relationship of fall-related fractures to social deprivation. *Osteoporos Int* 2011;22(4):1211–18.

20. Di Monaco M, Vallero F, Di MR, Mautino F, Cavanna A. Functional recovery after concomitant fractures of both hip and upper limb in elderly people. *J Rehabil Med* 2003;35(4):195–7.

21. Shabat S, Gepstein R, Mann G, Stern A, Nyska M. Simultaneous distal radius and hip fractures in elderly patients – Implications to rehabilitation. *Disabil Rehabil* 2003;25(15):823–6.

22. Allum JHJ, Carpenter MG, Honegger F. Age-dependant variations in the directional sensitivity of balance corrections and compensatory arm movements in man. *J Physiol* 2002;542:643–663.

23. Rankin JK, Woollacott MH, Shumway-Cook A. Cognitive influence on postural stability: A neuromuscular analysis in young and older adults. *J Gerontology A Biol Sci Med Sci* 2000;55:M112–19.

24. Tornetta P III, Mostafavi H, Riina J, Turen C, Reimer B, Levine R, et al. Morbidity and mortality in elderly trauma patients. *J Trauma* 1999;46(4):702–6.

25. Schiller WR, Knox R, Chleborad W. A five-year experience with severe injuries in elderly patients. *Accid Anal Prev* 1995;27(2):167–74.

26. Taylor MD, Tracy JK, Meyer W, Pasquale M, Napolitano LM. Trauma in the elderly: Intensive care unit resource use and outcome. *J Trauma* 2002;53(3):407–14.

27. Richmond TS, Kauder D, Strumpf N, Meredith T. Characteristics and outcomes of serious traumatic injury in older adults. *J Am Geriatr Soc* 2002;50(2):215–22.

28. Hollis S, Lecky F, Yates DW, Woodford M. The effect of pre-existing medical conditions and age on mortality after injury. *J Trauma* 2006;61(5):1255–60.

29. Giannoudis PV, Harwood PJ, Court-Brown, Pape HC. Severe and multiple trauma in older patients; incidence and mortality. *Injury* 2009;40(4):362–7.

30. Demetriades D, Karaiskakis M, Velmahos G, Alo K, Newton E, Murray J, et al. Effect on outcome of early intensive management of geriatric trauma patients. *Br J Surg* 2002;89(10):1319–22.

31. DeMaria EJ, Kenney PR, Merriam MA, Casanova LA, Gann DS. Aggressive trauma care benefits the elderly. *J Trauma* 1987;27(11):1200–6.

32. Fallon WF Jr., Rader E, Zyzanski S, Mancuso C, Martin B, Breedlove L, et al. Geriatric outcomes are improved by a geriatric trauma consultation service. *J Trauma* 2006;61(5):1040–6.

33. Skaga NO, Eken T, Sovik S, Jones JM, Steen PA. Pre-injury ASA physical status classification is an independent predictor of mortality after trauma. *J Trauma* 2007;63(5):972–8.

16

Metastatic fractures

WAKENDA K. TYLER

INTRODUCTION

As we age, the incidence of cancer increases exponentially, making the elderly population most susceptible to the development of cancer and unfortunately many of the sequelae associated with it. Two-thirds of all cancer deaths occur above the age of 65 in the United States.[1] The most commonly seen forms of cancer in the elderly, which are lung, breast, prostate and the haematopoietic cancers, all have a high propensity to involve bone. Overall, 70–80% of patients with metastatic prostate or breast cancer and 40% of patients with metastatic lung cancer will have bone involvement from their cancers.[2,3] Unfortunately, in the case of older patients with metastatic disease, the bone involvement occurs in the setting of age related osteopenia or osteoporosis. To further complicate the picture, many patients with metastatic cancer are receiving systemic therapies that can further compromise the quality of the bone. These therapies include the hormone blocking agents and frequently steroids.

Skeletal related events, such as compression fractures or long bone fractures, occur in more than half of patients with metastatic breast, prostate or lung cancer.[4] A pathological fracture is often a devastating event for a patient with cancer as it not only dramatically impacts their functional status but can also greatly interfere with treatment. Patients who do not meet certain criteria for functional status often cannot participate in many of the available chemotherapy protocols. Without systemic treatment, cancer progression in vital organs and in bone is often greatly accelerated. Once a pathological fracture occurs, length of survival greatly diminishes.[5] This phenomenon of decreased survival after a metastatic cancer related fracture is partly due to disruption of treatment and decreased mobility, but also often indicates a disease process that has reached a more terminal state and may no longer be responding to systemic and available local therapies.

Certain solid organ cancers have a higher predilection for bone than others. This is due to a complex interaction between the tumour cells and their host environment. There is some evidence to suggest that the tumour cells, either at the primary site or circulating in the blood stream, can induce the bone environment to be more prepared for the tumour cells' adherence and growth in that environment.[6] The tumour cells are capable of secreting a myriad of proteins that enhance their ability to adhere and invade into the bone microenvironment. Once in that environment, they can then replicate and further induce the local cells to increase or decrease bone formation and activate a series of events that leads to an appropriate condition for the tumour to propagate. The solid organ cancers most likely to induce this series of events are lung, breast, prostate, renal and thyroid. Although these are often reported as the most common cancers to spread to bone, it should be noted that other solid organ cancers, such as liver, colon, rectal, pancreatic and uterine, can all spread to bone and lead to pathological fracture (Figure 16.1). The haematopoietic cancers frequently involve bone and in some cases, like multiple myeloma, bone involvement is an essential component of the cancer's pathogenesis. Any patient with a haematopoietic cancer should have close monitoring of their bone disease to detect early risk of pathological fracture.

Once cancer cells have entered into the bone environment, they frequently will induce osteoclast and/or osteoblast activation depending on the gene expression within the cell. The vast majority of lung, thyroid and renal cancers in bone are lytic (Figure 16.2), meaning that they have induced bone resorption, while 98% of prostate cancers in bone are blastic (Figure 16.3), with the cells inducing abnormal bone formation. Breast cancer can lie on

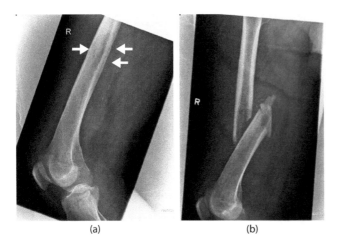

Figure 16.1 **(a)** Patient with metastatic colon cancer who presented with right leg pain. X-rays were obtained, but films were not closely scrutinized for a pathological process because of a perceived low incidence of metastatic bone disease in this patient population. Black arrows show area of concern. **(b)** Three months later the patient presented to the emergency room with this fracture.

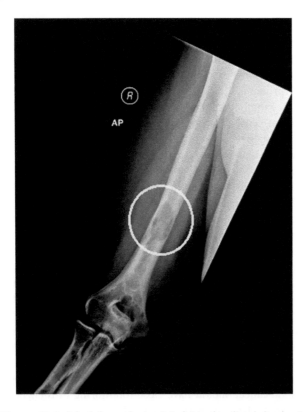

Figure 16.2 A lytic bone lesion (circle) in the distal diaphysis of the humerus in a patient with multiple myeloma. Note the thinning of the cortex and loss of bone density around the lesion in comparison to the rest of the uninvolved bone.

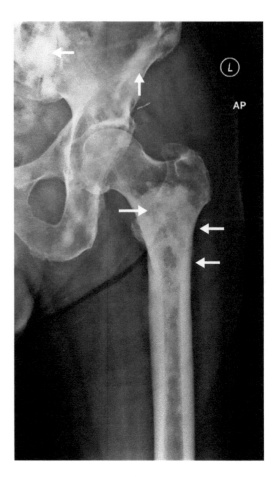

Figure 16.3 Blastic bone lesions throughout the femoral shaft and pelvis (white arrows) in a patient with metastatic prostate cancer. Note the increased density on the plain film illustrating the abnormal bone formation that is induced by the prostate cancer cells.

a spectrum anywhere from purely blastic to purely lytic, but most breast cancers in bone are a mix of lytic and blastic. The significance of the type of lesion created by the tumour in bone is relevant to the risk of fracture in that a greater degree of bone lysis results in an increased risk

of fracture. Blastic lesions also have an increased risk of fracture because the bone that is induced to form in this setting is abnormal both in structure and strength.

The more recent trends have suggested that patients with advanced cancer are living longer and as a result there is a trend towards an increased prevalence of older patients with metastatic disease of bone.[1] Although cancer metastasizing to bone is generally considered a terminal diagnosis for patients with cancer, patients with metastatic bone cancer can and often do live for many years after diagnosis of bone involvement. Not every patient with metastatic bone disease is at risk for a pathological fracture. Therefore it is important to determine who is at risk, so that we do not over- or undertreat this patient population. The goals of any treatment for this cohort are (1) to improve or maintain function, (2) to reduce pain and (3) to prolong survival if possible. Determining the best treatment for each individual patient can be a daunting task. Preventing pathological fracture from occurring in a patient who will regain function after treatment is the ideal approach. The development of a pathological fracture is not an imminent terminal event as once believed and these patients need equal consideration with a treatment plan that will best improve their quality of life.

Several recent analyses have looked at the cost of skeletal events in patients with metastatic cancer and have found that the burden to healthcare systems is very high.[7–9] Spinal cord compression and the need for surgical intervention rank highest among cost, with US$20,000 per patient being spent on spinal cord compression treatment and approximately US$18,000 on surgical intervention for pathological fracture.[10] Not surprisingly, spinal cord compression is also associated with the shortest life expectancy.[10] Reducing the likelihood of these two catastrophic events would greatly reduce healthcare costs, but more importantly improve quality of life.

Metastatic fractures are a serious threat to the well-being of the elderly population. Identifying patients at risk for fracture and treating them before the event occurs is ideal. However, despite our best efforts, fractures can still occur. Patients with metastatic fractures need prompt identification of the fracture and appropriate treatment that takes into account both quality and quantity of life remaining.

DIAGNOSIS AND CLINICAL PRESENTATION

Patients at risk for metastatic fracture will often present as one of three scenarios: (1) known metastatic disease and usually known bone involvement, (2) a remote history of cancer and a new finding of a bone lesion or (3) no known history of cancer and a new bone lesion. Each of these scenarios requires a different protocol for workup and management of the bone lesion. The first priority in all of these scenarios is determining what the bone lesion is, followed by a determination of the risk of fracture. If the risk of fracture is determined to be high, the next important step is to identify if fracture in a particular part of the skeleton will lead to major loss of function or not, as this will ultimately influence treatment.

For the patient with a known history of metastatic disease, it is not uncommon to have multiple sites of bone involvement. In this situation it is appropriate to assume that a bone lesion is due to metastatic cancer and therefore a major workup to identify the aetiology of the lesion is not necessary. If a particular site is causing pain, this should raise the concern of possible fracture risk. Bone pain often manifests as pain associated with weight bearing and can also present as deep aching pain at rest, usually at the site of concern within the skeleton.

Bone pain is the most common presenting symptom of a patient with an impending metastatic fracture. In some instances, patients will report no pain prior to fracture, but an extremely low energy event, such as opening a door or standing up from a sitting position, results in fracture. Pain is not always an indication of impending fracture as back pain with nerve root compression may present with leg pain but without risk of femoral or tibial fracture. Radicular pain such as this will often originate in the buttock region and

radiate down the entire length of the leg, lacking localization to a discrete area.

Two classification systems are frequently used to help determine risk of fracture in a patient with known metastatic disease to bone. These systems are good tools to help guide decision making, but should not be used as absolute rules. Tables 16.1 and 16.2 contain the Mire and Harrington classification systems for determining impending fracture risk. In the case of the Mirel classification, a score equal or greater than 9 is high risk of fracture and likely warrants fixation. In the case of the Harrington classification, any one of these criteria should warrant strong consideration for prophylactic fixation. Both use clinical presentation as well as findings on plain X-ray. Plain X-rays are considered the gold standard for assessing the structural integrity of bone and therefore the true risk of fracture. CAT scans can also be used to assess the structural integrity of bone, but are not necessary for determining fracture. Magnetic resonance imaging (MRI) is useful for looking at soft tissue involvement and extent of tumour involvement within the marrow space, but lacks the ability to assess the cortical structure of bone and is therefore not a good tool for determining fracture risk (Figure 16.4). Technitium-99 bone and positron emission tomography (PET) scans are useful in locating the site of bone involvement, but give no information about the structural integrity of bone and therefore should not be used as the sole method for assessing risk of fracture. PET scans and bone scans help determine the metabolic activity and cellular activity at a particular site and this may be a surrogate for the virulence of the tumour cells, but does not provide details on what the tumour cells are actually doing to the bone at that site. When obtaining plain films, full length anterior–posterior and lateral films of the entire limb should be ordered. It is common for patients with metastatic disease with bone involvement at the upper end of the bone to also have a significant lesion at the lower end

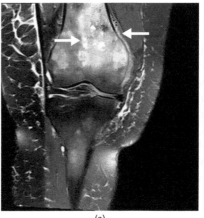
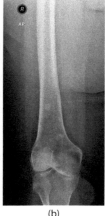

(a)   (b)

Figure 16.4 (a) T2 weighted MRI of the knee in a patient with metastatic breast cancer. White arrows indicate significant oedema seen on MRI within the bone, but without plain film (b), one cannot accurately determine the degree of loss of bone architecture. In this case bone architecture is intact.

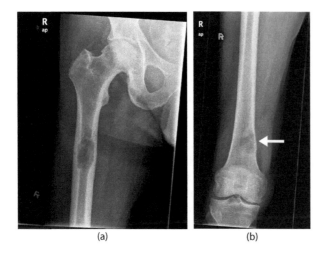

Figure 16.5 Anterior–posterior (AP) view of the femur of a patient with metastatic renal cancer. (a) A lesion was first identified at the proximal end of the femur. (b) Full length femur films revealed a lesion at the distal end of the bone (white arrow). An intramedullary implant should not end at the location of this distal lesion or a stress riser will be created.

of the same bone. Missing this could be quite serious with regard to treatment planning (Figure 16.5).

Harrington first described a fairly simplistic method for assessing risk of fracture in the early 1980s. His system has stood the test of time and is one that is easy to remember for those who may not treat or see patients with impending fractures on a daily basis (Table 16.1 and Figure 16.6). The other classification system that is commonly used is the Mirels classification system (Table 16.2). Unlike the Harrington system, it takes into account type of metastatic lesion (lytic or blastic) and location. For the Harrington system, if any one of the criteria is met, the patient is considered at high risk of fracture.[11] For the Mirels system (Table 16.2), the patient is assigned a number from 1 to 3 for each of the four criteria assessed: site, pain with activity (functional pain), type of lesion and size of lesion in relation to the diameter of the bone region being assessed for fracture risk. The numbers are then added together. A score of <7 has a very low risk of fracture (<4%), while a score of >9 is considered to have a fairly high risk of fracture (33% or more likely to fracture in the next 6 months).[12]

Using the images in Figure 16.6 as an example, the patient has a lesion in the peritrochanteric region of the femur. It is lytic and greater than 2.5 cm in size as well as about two-thirds the diameter of the entire bone in that location of the femur. If you are also told that the patient has significant pain with both taking a step and straight leg raise when supine on a bed, then you also know that the patient has significant functional pain. Based on this clinical scenario and image presentation, the Mirels score would be 12, the highest possible score indicating a very high risk of fracture over the next 6 months. By Harrington's criteria (>2.5 cm and persistent functional pain), the patient also would be considered at high risk for fracture. Treatment to

Table 16.1 Harrington system for determining risk of fracture

| Cortical bone destruction of 50% or more |
| Lesion of 2.5 cm or more in the proximal femur |
| Pathological avulsion fracture of lesser trochanter |
| Persistent stress pain (functional pain) |

Source: Harrington KD. *Instr Course Lect* 1986;35:357–381.

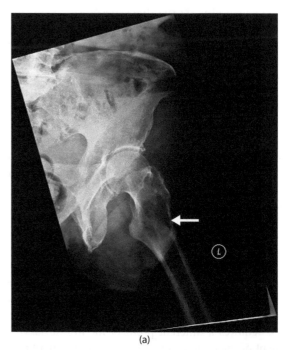

(a)

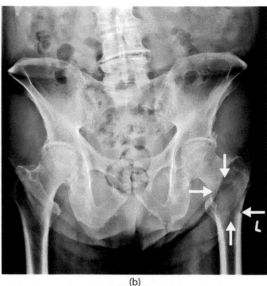

(b)

Figure 16.6 Lateral hip (a) and anterior–posterior (AP) view of the pelvis (b) of a patient with metastatic lung cancer in the left proximal femur. Note the cortical erosion on both the lateral and AP views (white arrows). Compare the contralateral hip on the AP pelvis to see the more medially located erosion. This patient has a very high risk of metastatic fracture using both Harrington's and Mirels' criteria.

Table 16.2 Mirels algorithm for determining risk of pathological fracture

	1	2	3
Site	Upper extremity	Lower extremity	Peritrochanteric
Pain	Mild	Moderate	Functional
Lesion	Blastic	Mixed	Lytic
Size	<1/3	1/3–2/3	>2/3

Source: Mirels H. Clin Orthop Relat Res 1989;(249):256–264.
Note: <1/3, 1/3-2/3 and >2/3 is in reference to diameter of bone on the AP or lateral plain radiographs.

prevent fracture would likely be recommended assuming no other mitigating factors.

For a patient with a remote history of cancer who presents with a new bone lesion and the patient who presents with no known history of cancer and a bone lesion, it is imperative that the aetiology of the lesion in question be determined before proceeding with treatment. Primary bone sarcomas tend to present in two patient populations. The first is in patients under the age of 21, who will present with tumours such as rhabdomyosarcoma, Ewing's sarcoma and osteosarcoma. The second is in patients over the age of 65, who will present with chondrosarcoma, high-grade pleomorphic sarcoma and osteosarcoma. Wrongfully treating or missing a primary sarcoma of bone can result in loss of limb (amputation) or more significantly, loss of life. This occurs most commonly in patients over the age of 65 in part because of the misconception that primary sarcomas of bone are only a paediatric condition. Therefore any patient presenting with a new bone lesion and no known history of metastatic bone disease should be investigated appropriately to exclude primary sarcoma of bone. The workup should include a CT scan of the chest, abdomen and pelvis (to look for a primary site of cancer origin), a bone scan (to look for other bony sites of involvement), serum protein electrophoresis and urine protein electrophoresis (to look for multiple myeloma) and often a biopsy. If the CT scan, bone scan and laboratory results do not reveal obvious metastatic disease or an obvious primary lesion, then a biopsy is warranted. In most cases, biopsies can be done through an image guided technique that does not require general anaesthesia. These biopsies are usually coordinated through the interventional or musculoskeletal radiology team. Rarely, an open biopsy is indicated if a needle biopsy fails to determine the diagnosis or if the lesion has features that would suggest a higher quantity of tissue may be necessary to determine the diagnosis.

Once a metastatic lesion is identified and confirmed, a decision regarding appropriate treatment can be made. The most common sites of bone involvement from metastatic disease are the spine (lumbar>thoracic>cervical), ribs, pelvis, skull and proximal long bones. In any patient with metastatic cancer, these sites should be monitored.[13] It is also worth noting that patients with metastatic cancer have a multitude of conditions that can arise as a result of their cancer. In the case of patients with bone involvement, the treating physician should be aware of the possibility of hypercalcemia which is estimated to occur in 5–10% of all patients with metastatic bone disease.[14] Hypercalcemia is a potentially fatal complication of metastatic bone disease and one that can be treated if identified early. It is recommended that any patient being evaluated for metastatic fracture or metastatic bone disease also be evaluated for hypercalcemia either through basic laboratory work or monitoring of symptoms for hypercalcemia (confusion, lethargy, excessive thirst and urination, nausea, vomiting and diffuse bone pain). Unfortunately the symptoms of hypercalcemia are also symptoms one finds in conjunction with chemotherapy, so good clinical judgment is required. First line treatment of hypercalcemia is hydration, followed by use of intravenous (IV) bisphosphonates if oral or IV hydration is not enough to bring calcium levels close to normal.

TREATMENT

Treatment of metastatic and impending metastatic fractures is determined by a multitude of factors. Type of malignancy, location of lesion and life expectancy are important factors to take into account. The vast majority of metastatic bone lesions do not require any direct intervention and even among those at increased risk of fracture, intervention is not necessarily surgical in nature. The top four most common sites of metastatic bone involvement (spine, ribs, pelvis and skull) rarely require surgical intervention for treatment of metastatic fractures. The majority of patients with metastatic bone disease do not wish to spend most of their remaining life recovering from an extensive surgical procedure and it is unfair to both the patient and their family not to take this into consideration when determining a treatment plan. Both surgical and non-surgical interventions should be considered together when deciding on an appropriate treatment plan for patients with metastatic or impending metastatic fractures (Box 16.1).

Radiation and radionucleotide therapy

Radiation therapy has several important roles in the treatment of patients with metastatic bone disease. It can be a very effective modality for reducing cancer related bone pain. It can also reduce the likelihood of metastatic fracture or progression of disease after surgical treatment of a metastatic fracture. It is also a useful tool in the prevention

---

BOX 16.1: Treatments for metastatic fractures

- Surgery
- Radiation and radionucleotide therapy
- Chemotherapy
- Cryoablation, radiofrequency ablation, embolization
- Assistive devices (canes, walkers, slings)

and treatment of spinal cord compression. Approximately 50–80% of patients will experience some level of pain relief following radiation therapy for painful metastatic bone lesions and up to 35% will report complete pain relief at the site of treatment.[15] It is the treatment of choice at sites of bone involvement that are not amenable to surgical intervention and it can be used to avoid surgery in areas where surgery might be considered but radiographic or clinical presentation do not yet warrant that degree of intervention. Radiation therapy should be reserved for patients at risk for fracture or with significant pain, since there is a limit to the amount of radiation a given area of the body can receive. If that limit is reached early in the disease process, then radiation can no longer be used as a treatment modality later on when the patient may have greater need for it.

The skull, ribs, sternum, scapula, clavicle and pelvis (the flat bones of the body) are sites where surgery is not considered particularly helpful for improving function or reducing pain. These are areas of the body where there is no direct load bearing through the bone or the distribution of load bearing is such that a fracture in one area does not dramatically alter the biomechanics of weight distribution (as in the pelvis). Painful lesions and even full fractures in these bones should be treated with radiation therapy as a first line approach. A major exception to this is the peri-acetabular area of the pelvis, through which, unfortunately, the body's full weight is transferred with standard activities, such as walking. Small fractures and small lesions in this area are usually tolerable because there is some sharing of the load by the surrounding pelvic ilium, ischium and pubic rami. However, if bone lesions in this area reach a critical size and level of bone destruction, they can have a significant impact on the ability to ambulate.

External beam radiation therapy for metastatic bone lesions is usually given by one of two methods. The traditional method is to deliver smaller doses of radiation over a 2–3-week period totalling around 30 Gy. A newer method that has gained in popularity over the past few years is to give one large dose (between 4 and 10 Gy) in 1 day. Several studies have suggested equivocal pain relief for patients between the two methods.[16–18] The benefits to patients with one-time dosing in terms of convenience is obvious. The one-time dosing also significantly reduces cost to the healthcare system. The disadvantage is that a greater percentage of patients have been shown to require a second treatment with the one-time dosing modality.[15]

Another method of controlling metastatic bone related pain in patients is the use of radionucleotide agents, such as strontium-89, samarium-153 and radium-223. These radionucleotides will aggregate at sights of rapid bone formation and cause tumour cell death. These agents are given as a single infusion and can be repeated with bone marrow toxicity being the limiting factor for number of times this approach can be used.[15] Patients will often experience pain relief for more than 6 months, usually starting 2–4 weeks after treatment. They will also have a nadir in their blood counts at around 6 weeks after treatment and this requires close monitoring. These agents work best for blastic lesions, where rapid bone formation is occurring. This method is therefore most useful in prostate cancer and more blastic forms of breast cancer. It is often most beneficial in a patient with multiple painful boney sites that would be more challenging to treat with external beam radiation. It is *not* useful as a tool to prevent fracture in a bone whose structural integrity has been compromised by tumour. In those circumstances, appropriate treatment for the impending fracture should be given first before radionucleotide therapy.

It is important for both providers and patients to understand that although many patients will report pain relief within a few days of the initiation of radiation therapy, the full benefit may not be felt for up to 2 months after treatment. It is therefore important in some cases to have patience with this treatment modality.[15] There can also be the unfortunate event of a transient radiation induced increase in bone pain after the initiation of radiation therapy.[15] This is usually short-lived and can be treated with appropriate acute pain management modalities. The other major concern that is important to be aware of in radiation treatment of patients with metastatic bone cancer is that during treatment and for a few months following treatment, there can be an increased risk of pathological fracture. Unfortunately the doses of radiation that generally kill tumour cells can also inhibit or lead to the death of the cells within the bone that are responsible for restoring the bone architecture (the osteoblasts). The bone itself can also develop changes in its mechanical properties as a direct result of radiation. For this reason, the radiation oncology team will often want an evaluation by the orthopaedic surgeon of any long bone sites that they are considering for radiation. If there is any question about the integrity of the bone then prophylactic fixation prior to radiation should be considered. Although radiation therapy is a key modality in the treatment of metastatic fractures, there are cancers that can be quite radio-resistant and yield little or no improvement in pain or function after radiation therapy.

Chemotherapy

Chemotherapy, including the newer targeted molecular therapies and hormone receptor antagonists, is a critical component in the management of patients with metastatic bone disease and pathological fractures. In many instances, the main goal of treatment for metastatic fractures is to return the patient to a state where they can continue to receive chemotherapy. Although the skeleton is an important organ, metastatic cancer to the lungs, liver and brain are usually best treated with chemotherapy. Chemotherapy can also greatly reduce the likelihood of a metastatic fracture and can reduce disease progression in the bone after treatment of a metastatic fracture. In several cancers that are thought to be very chemo-sensitive, chemotherapy alone can result in complete healing of a pathological fracture. This is a common phenomenon in many forms of lymphoma and has also been seen in hormone responsive forms of breast cancer. It is important to make sure that a patient being treated for a metastatic fracture is being appropriately reviewed by a medical oncologist. It is also essential that communication between the treating surgeon, radiation oncologist, general practitioner and medical oncologist be frequent and clear. The surgeon and radiation oncologist should give a clear point at which chemotherapy can be restarted after treatment of a metastatic fracture. They should also consider the importance of returning to systemic treatment in their decisions for types of interventions.

Surgical intervention

Surgical intervention for metastatic and impending metastatic fractures is an extremely valuable tool in the care of patients with metastatic bone disease. As outlined above, it should be reserved for those patients who are most likely to benefit from such an intervention. Recovery from orthopaedic surgery can be challenging under the most ideal circumstances. In an elderly patient who is compromised both by factors related to age and by factors related to cancer, this is an even more arduous task. Most patients with metastatic bone disease do not require surgery because the risk of fracture is low or the fracture is at a site where it will not greatly impede function.

The long bones are the sites that are most likely to require surgical intervention because fractures in these locations will greatly compromise mobility and function. The peri-acetabular region compromised by tumour may also require surgery, but the surgical intervention is usually extensive and requires 3–6 months of recovery. When surgery is indicated, it should be followed by radiation therapy to the involved bone to prevent disease progression and hardware failure.

Life expectancy must be taken into consideration when determining if surgical intervention is appropriate. If a patient is not going to live long enough to recover from the surgery, then surgery is contraindicated. A careful discussion between the medical treatment teams and surgeon should be undertaken before surgical planning to make sure that all caregivers are clear on the estimated length of survival. This information is also important for determining the type of implant used for surgery in some instances. Table 16.3 provides an overview of the types of surgery performed and the general requirements for life expectancy. These criteria are to be used as guidelines only. There are certainly circumstances where surgery is indicated when life expectancy is

thought to be short if it is deemed that the pain relief benefits from surgery outweigh the risks, even if the patient will not fully recover from the surgery by the end of their life. In these situations, the aim is to minimize the time spent in hospital. For example, a femoral intramedullary nailing for a metastatic fracture may reduce the need for analgesia and allow easier transfer thereby allowing care at home. In these circumstances the procedure should be considered even if life expectancy is only a few weeks.

There are several different ways in which metastatic fractures can be surgically treated. The surgical intervention chosen for the patient should generally try to adhere to the orthopaedic principle of one bone-one surgery, which will reduce the re-hospitalization rate and re-operation rate. To comply with this rule, an implant should protect the entire length of the bone and it should be durable enough to support the patient's entire body weight for several months and possibly the rest of their life since pathological fractures rarely heal.[19] For these reasons, intramedullary nail fixation is preferred over plate fixation in patients with metastatic fractures (Figure 16.7). Intramedullary nails are weight sharing devices and biomechanically less likely to break if loaded with normal body weight over several months. They can also protect the entire bone with a percutaneous surgical approach. They are less technically demanding and can be performed by non-specialist orthopaedic surgeons with relative ease. There are occasions when plate fixation is the only option available,

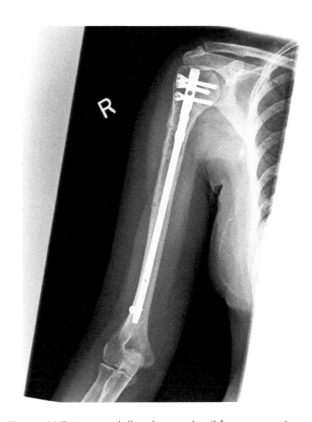

Figure 16.7 Intramedullary humeral nail for metastatic breast cancer. The implant extends the entire length of the bone and can be placed through small incisions at the shoulder and elbow.

Table 16.3 Guidelines for surgical intervention and life expectancy

Site of fracture	Life expectancy
Lower extremity long bone fracture	>6 weeks
Upper extremity long bone fracture	>3 months
Spine stabilization (excluding cord compression)	>6 months
Peri-acetabular fractures	>3 months

such as in radius and ulna fractures, in which case a plate can be used, frequently supplemented with methylmethacrylate (bone cement) (Figure 16.8).

Another important principle of the surgical treatment of metastatic fractures is that the surgical intervention chosen should be one that will allow for immediate weight bearing following surgery. There are rare occasions when this principle cannot be met, but all attempts should be made to meet this goal. Limited ability to weight-bear can greatly impede function and make it very difficult for a patient to live independently at home.

When fractures or impending fractures occur close to the joint surfaces, joint replacement surgery should be considered (Figure 16.9). It is often quite difficult to get adequate fixation in the metaphyseal bone adjacent to the joint surface when cancer has eroded the normal bone architecture. It is also likely that even despite good radiation and chemotherapy, there will be progression of the tumour in these regions resulting in failure of fixation. Joint replacement in these regions has the added benefit of removing gross tumour from the area, which improves the effects of chemotherapy and radiation therapy.[11,20] Pain relief is often more substantial and immediate following joint replacement for metastatic fractures. When performing joint replacement surgery it is still important to protect the entire length of the bone and therefore long stemmed implants are often used (Figure 16.10). The major downside and reason that surgeons will sometimes avoid joint replacement surgery in the setting of metastatic fractures is because surgery is more extensive, more technically demanding, often with longer anaesthesia time, greater blood loss and a higher risk of intraoperative and postoperative complications. Preoperative embolization can sometimes reduce blood loss.

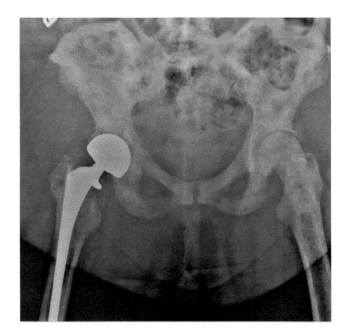

Figure 16.9 Long stem, cemented hemiarthroplasty for right femoral neck and head metastatic breast cancer.

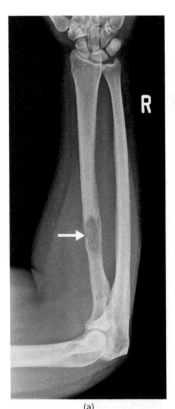 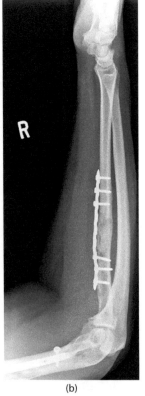

(a)　　　　　　(b)

Figure 16.8 Preoperative (a) and postoperative (b) X-rays of plate stabilization of the radius in a patient with multiple myeloma. Bone cement has been used to fill in the bone void after tumour curettage.

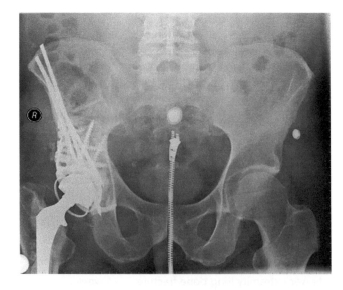

Figure 16.10 Anterior–posterior (AP) view of the pelvis of Harrington's procedure done in a patient with isolated metastatic lung cancer to bone. Pins and bone cement are used to recreate the lost pelvic bone. The patient is still alive 12 years after this initial procedure.

On rare occasions, a peri-acetabular lesion that involves the weight-bearing dome of the acetabulum can be amenable to surgical intervention. Patients often present when the tumour involvement is extending into or adjacent to the joint surface leading to pain with weight bearing. Tumours that are small and not directly adjacent to the joint surface are generally best treated with radiation therapy or if isolated, percutaneous ablation can sometimes be helpful. For surgical intervention to be appropriate in this region, the patient needs to have adequate bone within the ilium that is not extensively involved with tumour. This is important because the surgical procedure that has been described for extensive tumours in this area requires adequate fixation within the ilium.[21] The patient also should have a life expectancy of greater than 3 months, to allow the benefit of recovery from the surgery. Surgery in this region usually requires removal of the tumour, which often includes removal of most of the acetabulum, followed by creating a new scaffold with large diameter pins and bone cement replacing the lost bone (Figure 16.10). The reconstruction is then completed with a total joint arthroplasty.

The vertebral body is the most common boney location for metastatic carcinoma. As a result, vertebral compression fractures, spinal instability and spinal cord compromise by tumour are frequent among patients with metastatic bone disease. Vertebral compression fractures are the most common consequence of metastatic spine disease. These compression fractures can be painful and occasionally lead to neurological compromise. In general, if there is no major neurological compromise and no evidence of significant nerve root or cord impairment from a bone fragment or tumour, open spine surgery is not indicated. External beam radiation therapy is often the best way to reduce pain from a metastatic compression fracture without neurological deficit. Recent randomized trials have shown that the clinical difference between placebo procedure and vertebroplasty is minimal in non-oncology related compression fractures.[22] Because of these findings, many clinicians are moving away from the use of vertebroplasty or kyphoplasty in the acute fracture setting and in particular for patients with cancer, since risk of cement extrusion is higher in cancer involved vertebrae.

An indication for the use of vertebroplasty in cancer patients still exists in the setting of a patient who has not yet developed a compression fracture but is at high risk of doing so. This scenario is often seen in myeloma patients with extensive vertebral body marrow involvement. In this circumstance, percutaneous vertebroplasty can be used to augment the strength of the bone before radiation treatment.

Spinal instability as a result of tumour involvement within the posterior and anterior elements of the spine is rare, but when it occurs, it can present as excruciating and unrelenting pain with almost any type of movement of the spine. There is a gradual onset of symptoms that progress with time. Pain is less when lying supine and immobile and exacerbated by weight bearing or rotational motion of the spine. Flexion and extension views of the spine can often detect this level of instability. If a patient cannot tolerate flexion and extension spine X-rays, then MRI of the area in question can be very helpful. Surgical stabilization of significant spinal instability is warranted for patients with a life expectancy of greater than 6 months and whose functional status would be close to normal were it not for their spinal instability. Spinal stabilization involves extensive surgery and is fraught with complications, particularly in elderly cancer patients whose bone quality may not allow for adequate fixation. Therefore careful consideration by the spine surgeon, oncology team and patient should be undertaken prior to surgery. If bracing or radiation alone can address the problem, then this should be considered.

Spinal cord compression is a devastating complication of metastatic bone disease. It usually presents with a gradual onset of increasing lower extremity weakness and numbness, with associated loss of bowel or bladder function. Often patients will report increasing difficulty emptying their bladder or sudden episodes of uncontrolled urination, which usually represents overflow incontinence. They will also report onsets of diarrhoea or severe constipation. The key to the treatment of spinal cord compression is early detection. Unfortunately, symptoms such as bladder and bowel dysfunction are common complaints among the elderly population. As a result, the complaints are frequently not recognized as early spinal cord compromise. Early identification allows for initiation of steroid treatment, which can greatly diminish ultimate neurological deficit. In many cases if detected early, emergent spinal cord decompressive surgery can be performed to prevent further neurological loss. However, if the process is allowed to continue until complete motor and sensory nerve loss has occurred, often surgery will not allow neurological recovery. Many of these patients will have permanent neurological compromise, which is one of many reasons why this event is associated with a greatly shortened life expectancy.

Assistive devices

A discussion of the treatment of patients with metastatic fractures would not be complete without mentioning use of assistive devices, braces and slings as part of the treatment considerations. In patients with lower extremity and pelvic fracture pain that has been deemed inappropriate for surgery, supplying the patient with a cane or walker to off-load the forces on the bone can be very beneficial. This approach can be used in patients deemed too medically unstable for surgery who may have areas of the lower extremity long bones at risk for fracture. A sling on the upper extremity can similarly serve to protect the limb, reduce motion that may be leading to pain and remind the patient to limit heavy lifting with that arm. These simple approaches can be extremely beneficial to patients at the end of their life.

Cryoablation, radiofrequency ablation and embolization

Other modalities that should be considered as alternatives to surgery or radiation or as augmentation of these treatments are some of the less invasive procedures such as radiofrequency ablation (RFA) or cryoablation. These techniques are useful in painful lesions that are generally small (<5 cm), well contained and in locations where surgery is less useful (like the pelvis or scapula). They can obliterate tumour cells and allow for bone healing in an area without major surgical intervention.

PREVENTION

The ideal method to treat metastatic fractures is to prevent them from occurring. Patients who sustain a complete fracture often do not return to baseline functional status, have significant delays in treatment for their cancer and have a reduced life expectancy compared to patients treated prior to completion of fracture.[5] Detecting an impending metastatic fracture before it occurs and treating it with either radiation or surgical stabilization before fracture is likely to provide the best outcome for a patient. Any patient with known metastatic cancer should be monitored by their medical team for the onset of symptoms that might suggest an impending fracture. Pain with activity and weight bearing is the most frequent indicator of an impending metastatic fracture. An initial X-ray of the area of concern can facilitate identifying a bone at risk for fracture.

The other major way to prevent fracture in patients with metastatic bone disease is the use of bisphosphonates or denosumab.[23,24] Both agents work to inhibit osteoclast activity, which leads to slowing of tumour cell induced bone turnover and bone destruction by the osteoclasts. Amino containing bisphosphonates, such as zoledronic acid, are pyrophosphate analogues that inhibit protein prenylation ultimately leading to reduced osteoclast activity and apoptosis. They are usually given as an IV infusion over 30 minutes monthly. Denosumab is an antibody directed at RANK-ligand, which inhibits the binding of endogenous RANK-ligand to its receptor (RANK) on osteoclasts. This critical step is needed for osteoclast activation and without it, osteoclast activity is greatly hindered. Denosumab is given as a monthly subcutaneous injection. Both agents are effective at reducing skeletal related events in patients with metastatic bone cancer. Data are emerging to suggest that denosumab in the elderly population may be more clinically and cost effective than zoledronic acid.[23,25,26] In the case of IV bisphosphonates, renal insufficiency with a glomerular filtration rate (GFR) of less than 30 mL/min/1.73 m^2 is considered a relative contraindication for use of these agents. Elderly patients frequently have marginal renal function that is already placed under significant stress from the chemotherapy they are receiving. The trends in clinical practice are moving towards the use of denosumab in elderly patients with metastatic bone disease.

CONCLUSION

Early detection and prophylactic treatment of impending metastatic fractures is the key to improved function, reduced pain and prolonged survival for elderly patients with metastatic cancer to bone. The elderly population is at greatly increased risk of developing metastatic bone cancer and at highest risk of a major complication related to it. All patients with metastatic disease should be considered for treatment with bone anti-resorptive medications (IV bisphosphonates or denosumab) to reduce the likelihood of a skeletal event. Radiation therapy, chemotherapy, bracing, assistive devices and surgery are all tools that should be considered to prevent metastatic fracture. Often these should be used in combination. If fractures do occur, it is important to note that patients often can live a very long and high quality life after such an event. Good coordination between medical, surgical and radiation oncology teams is extremely important in the care of this patient population.

Key points

- Individuals with cancer are living longer with advanced disease.
- Bone involvement from metastatic cancer is common.
- Identifying those patients with bone involvement that would benefit from interventions to prevent fracture is paramount to appropriate care of these patients.
- Not all interventions are surgical in nature and surgery should be reserved for those who will have significant benefit from it.
- Goals of care are to prevent fractures and thereby maintain function.
- Secondary goals are to improve pain and prolong survival.
- Denosumab and zoledronic acid are important medications in the prevention of metastatic fractures.

REFERENCES

1. Howlader N, Noone A, Krapcho M, Neyman N, Aminou R, Altekruse S, et al. *SEER Cancer Statistics Review, 1975–2009 (Vintage 2009 Populations)*. National Cancer Institute, Bethesda, MD, 2011. http://seer.cancer.gov/csr/1975_2009_pops09/, based on November 2011 SEER data submission, posted to the SEER web site, 2012.
2. Coleman RE. Clinical features of metastatic bone disease and risk of skeletal morbidity. *Clin Cancer Res* 2006;12(20 Pt 2):6243s–6249s.
3. Weilbaecher KN, Guise TA, McCauley LK. Cancer to bone: A fatal attraction. *Nat Rev Cancer* 2011;11(6):411–425.

4. Oster G, Lamerato L, Glass AG, Richert-Boe KE, Lopez A, Chung K, et al. Natural history of skeletal-related events in patients with breast, lung, or prostate cancer and metastases to bone: A 15-year study in two large US health systems. *Support Care Cancer* 2013;21(12):3279–3286.

5. Ratasvuori M, Wedin R, Keller J, Nottrott M, Zaikova O, Bergh P, et al. Insight opinion to surgically treated metastatic bone disease: Scandinavian Sarcoma Group Skeletal Metastasis Registry report of 1195 operated skeletal metastasis. *Surg Oncol* 2013;22(2):132–138.

6. Kaplan RN, Riba RD, Zacharoulis S, Bramley AH, Vincent L, Costa C, et al. VEGFR1-positive haematopoietic bone marrow progenitors initiate the premetastatic niche. *Nature* 2005;438(7069):820–827.

7. Habib MJ, Merali T, Mills A, Uon V. Canadian health care institution resource utilization resulting from skeletal-related events. *Hosp Pract (1995)* 2014;42(1):15–22.

8. Luftner D, Lorusso V, Duran I, Hechmati G, Garzon-Rodriguez C, Ashcroft J, et al. Health resource utilization associated with skeletal-related events in patients with advanced breast cancer: Results from a prospective, multinational observational study. *Springerplus* 2014;3:328. eCollection 2014.

9. Lorusso V, Duran I, Garzon-Rodriguez C, Luftner D, Bahl A, Ashcroft J, et al. Health resource utilisation associated with skeletal-related events in European patients with lung cancer: Alpha subgroup analysis from a prospective multinational study. *Mol Clin Oncol* 2014;2(5):701–708.

10. Carter JA, Ji X, Botteman MF. Clinical, economic and humanistic burdens of skeletal-related events associated with bone metastases. *Expert Rev Pharmacoecon Outcomes Res* 2013;13(4):483–496.

11. Harrington KD. Impending pathologic fractures from metastatic malignancy: Evaluation and management. *Instr Course Lect* 1986;35:357–381.

12. Mirels H. Metastatic disease in long bones: A proposed scoring system for diagnosing impending pathologic fractures. *Clin Orthop Relat Res* 1989;(249):256–264.

13. Coleman RE. Skeletal complications of malignancy. *Cancer* 1997;80(8 Suppl):1588–1594.

14. Lazaretti-Castro M, Kayath M, Jamnik S, Santoro IL, Tadokoru H, Vieira JG. Prevalence of hypercalcemia in patients with lung cancer. *Rev Assoc Med Bras* 1993;39(2):83–87.

15. Lutz S, Lo SS, Chow E, Sahgal A, Hoskin P. Radiotherapy for metastatic bone disease: Current standards and future prospectus. *Expert Rev Anticancer Ther* 2010;10(5):683–695.

16. Chow E, Harris K, Fan G, Tsao M, Sze WM. Palliative radiotherapy trials for bone metastases: A systematic review. *J Clin Oncol* 2007;25(11):1423–1436.

17. Lutz ST, Chow EL, Hartsell WF, Konski AA. A review of hypofractionated palliative radiotherapy. *Cancer* 2007;109(8):1462–1470.

18. Price P, Hoskin PJ, Easton D, Austin D, Palmer SG, Yarnold JR. Prospective randomised trial of single and multifraction radiotherapy schedules in the treatment of painful bony metastases. *Radiother Oncol* 1986;6(4):247–255.

19. Gainor BJ, Buchert P. Fracture healing in metastatic bone disease. *Clin Orthop Relat Res* 1983;(178):297–302.

20. Harrington KD. Orthopedic surgical management of skeletal complications of malignancy. *Cancer* 1997;80(8 Suppl):1614–1627.

21. Rock MG, Harrington K. Pathologic fractures of the acetabulum and the pelvis. *Orthopedics* 1992;15(5):569–576.

22. Kallmes DF, Comstock BA, Heagerty PJ, Turner JA, Wilson DJ, Diamond TH, et al. A randomized trial of vertebroplasty for osteoporotic spinal fractures. *N Engl J Med* 2009;361(6):569–579.

23. Henry D, Vadhan-Raj S, Hirsh V, von Moos R, Hungria V, Costa L, et al. Delaying skeletal-related events in a randomized phase 3 study of denosumab versus zoledronic acid in patients with advanced cancer: An analysis of data from patients with solid tumors. *Support Care Cancer* 2014;22(3):679–687.

24. Mathew A, Brufsky A. Bisphosphonates in breast cancer. *Int J Cancer* 2015;137(4):753–764.

25. Lothgren M, Ribnicsek E, Schmidt L, Habacher W, Lundkvist J, Pfeil AM, et al. Cost per patient and potential budget implications of denosumab compared with zoledronic acid in adults with bone metastases from solid tumours who are at risk of skeletal-related events: An analysis for Austria, Sweden and Switzerland. *Eur J Hosp Pharm Sci Pract* 2013;20(4):227–231.

26. Balla J. The issue of renal safety of zoledronic acid from a nephrologist's point of view. *Oncologist* 2005;10(5):306–308; author reply 311–312.

17

Periprosthetic fractures

ADAM SASSOON AND GEORGE HAIDUKEWYCH

INTRODUCTION

Periprosthetic fractures about the hip and knee are a cause of significant morbidity in the geriatric population. These fractures often occur in the setting of poor bone stock secondary to osteoporosis, osteolysis or both, thereby adding a further level of complexity to already challenging reconstructions. The incidence of these fractures is increasing in parallel with the continued rise in demand for primary and revision total joint arthroplasty.[1] This chapter discusses the presentation, work-up and classification of periprosthetic fractures about the hip and knee. Technical considerations and principles in the treatment of these injuries are highlighted and a review of the reported results and complications following surgical treatment of periprosthetic fractures is presented.

CLINICAL PRESENTATION AND INITIAL EVALUATION OF PERIPROSTHETIC FRACTURES ABOUT THE HIP AND KNEE

Periprosthetic fractures occurring about a total hip or knee arthroplasty can occur intraoperatively during component placement or remotely from surgery in the setting of either low or high energy trauma. This section focuses on those occurring remotely from surgery, but the technical principles applied to the surgical treatment of these fractures are universally applicable.

Evaluation of the patient with a periprosthetic fracture in the setting of high energy trauma must initially follow the guidelines of appropriate resuscitation with emphasis being placed on the airway, breathing and circulation of the patient. A thorough secondary survey is important in ruling out associated injuries. Fractures resulting from low energy injuries such as ground level falls should initiate an appropriate

work-up in a geriatric patient including adequate head and neck imaging when warranted. Additionally, other organic reasons for a non-mechanical fall such as a myocardial infarction or stroke must be ruled out. Patients may benefit from a provisional reduction and splint/brace application or traction during this period of medical stabilization.

Once the appropriate initial medical work-up and resuscitation has been completed and the patient is clinically stable, important details regarding the history of the affected implant must be collected. Sometimes these details need to be gathered from family members or previous medical providers if the patient is unable to provide them. Key components of this history include antecedent pain in the affected joint, a history of infection or wound healing complications and previous operative reports that include implant types and sizes. If details in the history raise concern for the possibility of a coexistent periprosthetic infection, the joint should be aspirated to obtain a synovial fluid nucleated cell count, differential and cultures prior to reconstructive efforts.[2] Intraoperative issue biopsy in conjunction with aspiration results may also improve sensitivity and specificity for the diagnosis of a concurrent periprosthetic infection.[3] Serum markers for inflammation in the setting of fracture may be falsely elevated and should not be relied upon solely in dictating treatment.[4]

Appropriate imaging is paramount in accurately classifying periprosthetic fractures to determine the appropriate treatment strategy. Radiographs of the hip and entire femur should be obtained for all periprosthetic hip fractures around a femoral component. The presence of a long-stemmed total knee below such a fracture will greatly affect the reconstruction options available to the treating surgeon and should be anticipated. Conversely, femur views are also important in detecting a total hip arthroplasty (THA) above a periprosthetic fracture occurring around the femoral component of a total knee arthroplasty. All radiographs should be scrutinized for evidence of prosthetic loosening indicated by either a shift in prosthetic position, concentric radiolucent lines, fractured cement mantles or prosthetic subsidence. Judet views should be obtained for periprosthetic acetabular fractures to determine the columnar integrity and rule out a pelvic discontinuity. Computed tomography with three-dimensional reformatting is also useful in these instances and plays an important role in evaluating the extent of pre-existing osteolysis in the pelvis when present.

The status of the unaffected components must also be scrutinized radiographically. For the hip this is usually the acetabular component and liner. Surgical intervention to treat a periprosthetic fracture around a femoral component often affords a surgeon with a valuable opportunity to bone-graft areas of osteolysis behind an otherwise stable acetabular component, change an eccentrically worn liner or increase the head size of the reconstructed femur and potentially enhance postoperative stability. For periprosthetic fractures about the knee, the fate of two components are more closely linked, as revision of one component will often dictate the revision of the other so that the articulation and level of constraint match.

The majority of periprosthetic fractures occur in geriatric patients with osteoporosis. As such, the comprehensive care of these elderly patients should include an evaluation of their bone health. This usually involves obtaining vitamin D levels, referring the patient for bone densitometry, and potentially evaluation by a metabolic bone specialist. Often, developing a standing partnership between surgeons, endocrinologists or other primary care physicians is critical in reliably establishing a bisphosphonate treatment program for these patients to prevent future fragility fractures.

INCIDENCE, CLASSIFICATION AND TREATMENT ALGORITHMS

Hip

Periprosthetic fractures of the hip can occur in both the femur and acetabulum. Fractures of the femur occur more commonly in a revision setting and when uncemented stems are used. The risk of intraoperative fractures reported from the Mayo Clinic was 0.3% for cemented and 5.4% for uncemented stems.[5] This study and others have estimated the cumulative incidence of postoperative periprosthetic femoral fractures to be 1% and 4% for primary and revision THAs, respectively.[5,6] Intraoperative fractures of press-fit acetabular components have been reported with an incidence of 0.4%, and have been noted more commonly in ellipsoidal cup designs.[7] Periprosthetic acetabular fractures can also occur as late sequelae of osteolysis behind acetabular components, or ground level falls in osteoporotic bone.[8] Recent studies have indicated that the number of periprosthetic fractures is increasing, which places a significant burden on the healthcare system secondary to the high cost associated with the care of these complex injuries.

Multiple classification schemes exist for periprosthetic fractures about a THA; however, the most widely used and accepted is the Vancouver classification system.[9,10] This system focuses on fractures occurring around the femoral component and is particularly useful in that it guides treatment strategies. It divides fractures based on location, with Vancouver A fractures occurring at a trochanteric level, Vancouver B fractures occurring about the indwelling prosthesis (usually involving the tip of the stem) and Vancouver C stems occurring distal to the stem. There is further subclassification of Vancouver A fractures depending on whether the greater trochanter (AG) or lesser trochanter is involved (AL). Vancouver B fractures are also subclassified according to the stability of the indwelling femoral component and surrounding bone quality. Vancouver B1 fractures occur around a stable femoral component, while Vancouver B2 fractures have either directly resulted from component loosening or have occurred around an already loose component. Vancouver B3 fractures involve a loose component in the setting of poor bone stock (osteoporosis, extensive osteolysis, etc).

The treatment of Vancouver A fractures (both AG and AL) usually involves a period of protected weight bearing with an assistive device. If significant displacement of an AG fracture exists, resulting in compromise of abductor function, a symptomatic limp or instability, then open reduction internal fixation (ORIF) may be indicated. Isolated periprosthetic fractures of the lesser trochanter are rare, and careful evaluation of imaging is required to ensure that other osseous involvement is not present. The majority of Vancouver A fractures occur through areas of advanced osteolysis, prompting evaluation of the bearing couple and revision when indicated to eliminate the potential particulate debris generator.

Vancouver B fracture treatment depends primarily on the status of femoral component fixation. Fractures around stable femoral implants (B1s) can be treated with open reduction and internal fixation. The use of locking plates to create balanced fixation proximal and distal to the femoral component is particularly important when performing these fracture repairs. Unicortical locking screws and judicial use of cables around the proximal segment are often required to achieve fixation. Some plates with offset screw trajectories allow for bicortical screw placement around the stem proximally which is biomechanically favourable and should be sought.[11] This is more easily achieved if the indwelling implant has a dual taper design (Figure 17.1a through e).

Fractures occurring around loose stems or resulting in stem dislodgement (B2s and B3s) require advanced reconstructive efforts, combining ORIF of the femur and revision THA. Revision to long-stemmed components which bypass the fracture by two cortical diameters is recommended. Fracture patterns that involve the trochanter or fractures with significant comminution may also benefit from

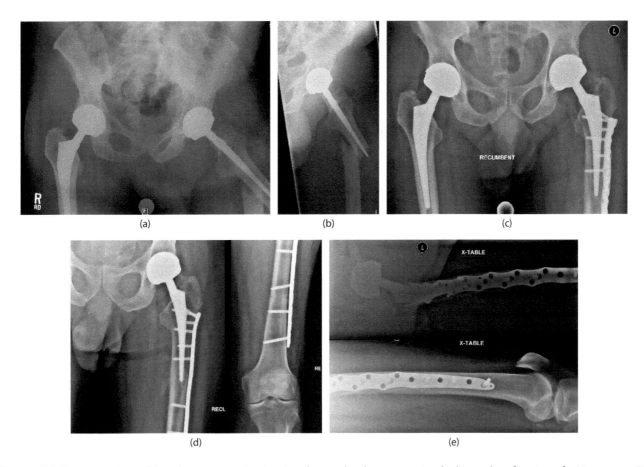

Figure 17.1 Preoperative (a,b) and postoperative (c–e) radiographs demonstrating locking plate fixation of a Vancouver B1 periprosthetic fracture. Note the screw trajectory allows for bicortical fixation proximal and distal to the tip of the stem, facilitating balanced fixation and improvement of mechanical strength.

augmentation with a cable plate or locking plate around the revision stem. If fracture length precludes bypassing it with a stem, then plating around the revision stem with a distal femoral locking plate is also recommended.

The choice of revision stem type is dependent on the available bone stock (Figure 17.2a through d). Diaphyseal fixation should be relied on in all instances; however, if 4 cm of press fit distal to the fracture cannot be reliably achieved or the bone stock is otherwise compromised (B3), a tapered-fluted stem might be preferred.[12,13] (Figure 17.3a through e). In cases where proximal bone stock is completely unsupportive of prosthetic revision, proximal femoral replacement may be indicated (Figure 17.4a through e).

As treatment of Vancouver B fractures is dictated by component stability, accurate determination of component fixation status is of paramount importance when treating these injuries.[14] Preoperative imaging needs to be carefully scrutinized for signs of loosening. For cemented stems this includes fractures of the cement mantle, concentric radiolucent lines around the component or cement mantle or a shift in component position noted on serial films. For uncemented stems this includes concentric radiolucent lines, component migration or subsidence and a pedestal sign. Even in the absence of these radiographic signs, intraoperative assessment and testing of the stem should be performed,

as failure to recognize a loose stem can lead to early failure of internal fixation and reconstructive efforts.

Vancouver C fractures should be treated with open reduction and internal fixation. The indwelling stem proximal to the fracture limits the role of intramedullary fixation. Good results with fixation constructs employing locking plates with balanced fixation between distal and proximal fracture segments have been observed.[15] Mechanical stability is optimized with long constructs that bypass the end of the proximal stem.[16] One potential caveat arises in a patient who sustains a Vancouver C fracture below a symptomatic loose stem. In this instance a revision arthroplasty with a long-stemmed component can be considered in conjunction with ORIF of the fracture, especially if the fracture is proximal enough to allow bypassing with the revision stem.

Knee

Periprosthetic fractures occurring around a TKA can occur in the femur, tibia or patella, with the femur being most commonly affected. These fractures occur intraoperatively and postoperatively, and are more commonly encountered during or following revision TKA. The reported incidence of periprosthetic fractures about a TKA is between 0.3%

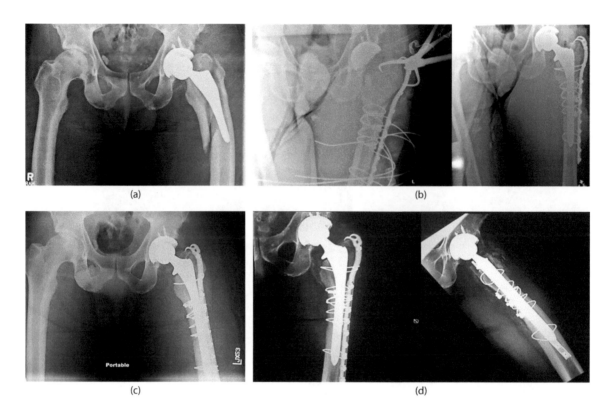

Figure 17.2 Preoperative **(a)**, intraoperative **(b)** and postoperative **(c,d)** radiographs of a Vancouver B2 fracture treated with open reduction internal fixation (ORIF) of the femoral fracture and revision total hip arthroplasty (THA) to a monolithic, fully-porous, cylindrical stem. Note the intraoperative films which demonstrate anatomic reconstruction of the femur prior to revision stem preparation.

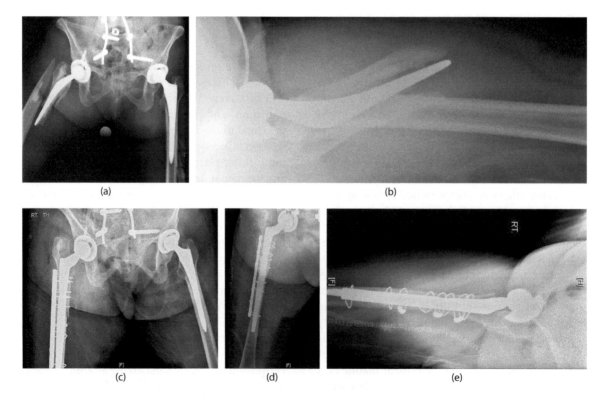

Figure 17.3 Preoperative **(a,b)** and postoperative **(c–e)** radiographs of a Vancouver B3 periprosthetic fracture which occurred around a cemented stem that was revised to a fluted, tapered, modular stem. The distal segment was prepared, the stem potted, the proximal stem assembled and the proximal fragments then cabled around the proximal body of the stem to facilitate their reduction. The acetabular liner was also changed so that a 36 mm head could be utilized to maximize stability.

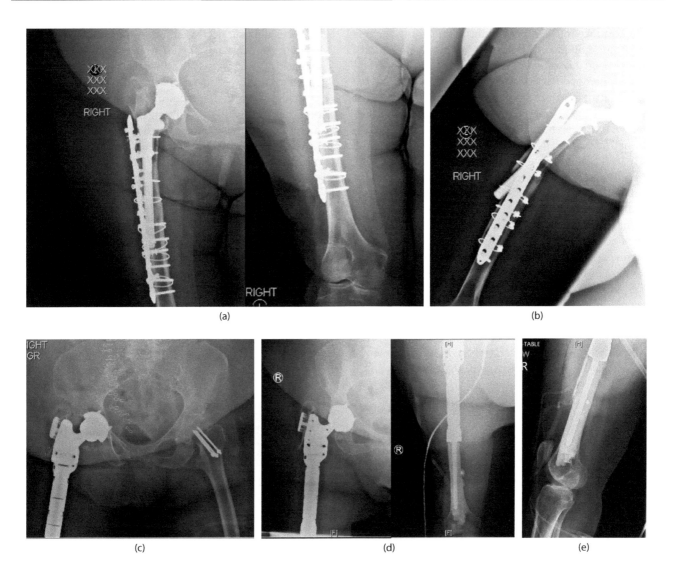

Figure 17.4 Preoperative **(a,b)** and postoperative **(c–e)** radiographs of a patient who had failed ORIF of a periprosthetic B3 fracture twice at outside institutions. The proximal segment had malunited with subsequent stem subsidence and anterior cortex perforation. The patient was subsequently revised to a proximal femoral replacement.

and 2.5%[17] and they have been reported to account for 4.7% of revision TKA volume.[18]

Various classification systems exist for periprosthetic fractures involving a TKA, and can be broadly divided based on whether the fracture occurs in the femur, tibia or patella. The majority of these fractures occur in an elderly population and involve the femur secondary to the stress mismatch zone occurring between the osteopenic metaphyseal bone and the components. The most commonly used classification system for these supracondylar periprosthetic fractures is that of Rorabeck et al. which divides fractures into non-displaced around a stable component (type 1), displaced around a stable component (type 2, and most common) and fractures around a loose component (type 3).[17]

While occurring from similar mechanisms, tibial periprosthetic fractures are less common than those observed in the femur, and have been classified by Felix et al.[19] The classification system is based on fracture location, with type I fractures occurring in the tibial plateau,

type II fractures occurring around the stem of the tibial component, type III fractures occurring distal to the prosthesis and type IV fractures involving the tibial tubercle. The system also subclassifies fractures based on whether the prosthesis is well-fixed (type A), loose (type B) or if the fracture occurred intraoperatively (type C).

Periprosthetic fractures occurring about the patella are rare events. Despite their relative infrequency, several classification schemes have been developed. Subtle differences exist between these systems but the main distinctions between fracture types, which dictate treatment, are the integrity of the extensor mechanism and the stability of the indwelling patellar component. The classification system of Berry and Ortiguera categorizes fractures as occurring around a stable implant with an intact extensor mechanism (type 1), a stable implant with a disrupted extensor mechanism (type 2) or a loose implant (type 3).[20] Type 3 fractures are subclassified based on whether the remaining patellar bone stock is good (3A) or poor (3B).

The treatment of TKA periprosthetic fractures occurring in the femur around a stable implant can mostly be achieved with non-operative measures or ORIF. If the fracture is non-displaced, non-operative treatment in the form of protected weight bearing and bracing can be attempted with close follow-up. In the setting of fracture displacement ORIF is preferred. ORIF can be performed with either plate or retrograde nail fixation. Nails are load-sharing devices, leave blood supply to the fracture site undisturbed and allow for early mobilization. The presence of a proximal THA will limit the role of nail fixation, as the authors do not recommend fixation with short intramedullary (IM) nails. Restrictions on nail fixation may occur if the box design of the indwelling component will not accommodate nail passage. Additionally, if the box forces an IM nail starting point too far posterior relative to the anatomic axis of the femur, a malunion will result from flexion of the distal segment. A compatibility guide has recently been published to help guide patient selection for the use of IM nail fixation for periprosthetic fractures about the knee.[21] Plates offer the advantage of being applicable regardless of prosthesis and maximize distal fixation. Minimally invasive plate osteosynthesis (MIPO) techniques have been developed

that also allow for decreased soft tissue stripping around the fracture site. Initial postoperative reduction may be more reliably achieved than observed with nail fixation; however, varus drift can occur over time during fracture healing.

Fractures occurring around a loose femoral component, non-unions, and those occurring in the setting of very short highly comminuted, or osteoporotic distal segments should receive further consideration. In these situations the patient may benefit from revision to a distal femoral replacement (DFR) (Figure 17.5a through d). This allows for immediate weight bearing and may decrease the risk of bedsores, clots, pneumonia and other perioperative complications that come from immobilization. Revision to a DFR also removes non-union as a potential postoperative complication.

Periprosthetic TKA fractures occurring in the tibia should be closely scrutinized for any evidence of implant loosening. Fractures around stable implants can be treated with ORIF using either medial or lateral based locking plates. MIPO techniques can also be employed in these instances to limit the amount of soft tissue stripping at the fracture site (Figure 17.6). In the setting of a loose implant revision TKA with a long-stemmed component to bypass

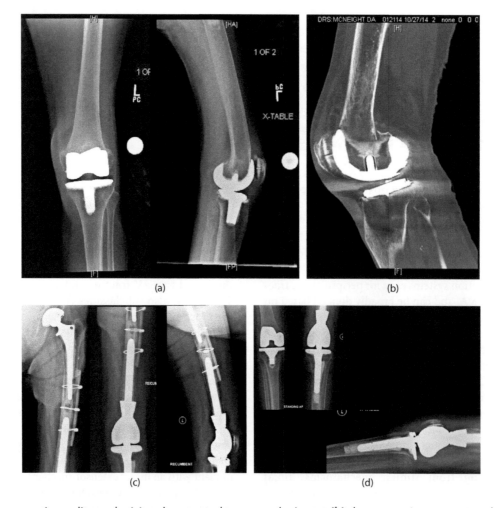

(a)

(b)

(c)

(d)

Figure 17.5 Preoperative radiographs (a) and computed tomography image (b) demonstrating an extremely distal interprosthetic fracture in osteoporotic bone. The patient was revised to a distal femoral replacement (c,d) with placement of an allograft strut to help mitigate the stress riser created between the femoral stems.

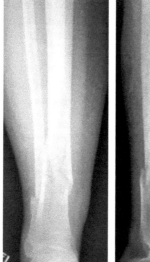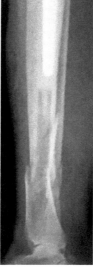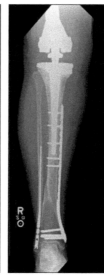

Figure 17.6 Pre- and postoperative radiographs of a tibial periprosthetic fracture with an associated fibular fracture demonstrate successful treatment with minimally invasive plate osteosynthesis (MIPO) tibial plating techniques and an intramedullary (IM) fibular nail.

the fracture site should be performed. If fracture comminution compromises metaphyseal bone stock, sleeves or cones may be required for base plate support. In extreme cases of metaphyseal bone loss, proximal tibial replacement can also be performed.

Non-surgical management of periprosthetic patellar fractures is preferred in cases with an intact extensor mechanism and a stable implant. In instances where patellar component stability is questionable (i.e. in the presence of radiographic lucencies) and the extensor mechanism remains intact, the decision for surgical treatment should be made based on whether the treating surgeon believes there is a risk for patellar component displacement.[22] In these instances, the implant should be removed, and in the setting of an intact extensor mechanism, the surgical treatment should be limited to implant retrieval. Fracture treatment should be subsequently continued via closed means through postoperative bracing or casting. Patellar revision should be avoided, as the results following revision are not encouraging and patellar resection arthroplasty has been shown to be affective in cases of compromised bone stock.

In patients with a disrupted extensor mechanism and good bone stock, ORIF of the patella can be performed with component retention if stable, or following a resection if loose. Fixation is usually performed with cannulated screws and a figure-of-eight wire passed through the screws, as a modified tension-band technique. If screw purchase cannot be achieved secondary to poor bone stock, or the patellar fragment is too small to accommodate screw fixation, then a partial patellectomy is preferred. Suture repair of the tendon to the remaining patella can then be performed through drill holes.

When periprosthetic patellar fractures result in extensor mechanism disruption and are treated in a subacute fashion or have failed a previous attempt of ORIF,

a patellectomy with allograft reconstruction of the extensor mechanism may be indicated, employing either an Achilles allograft on a bone block or a complete extensor mechanism allograft.[23] Alternatively, use of synthetic polymer mesh materials has been reported and shown to provide encouraging results.[24]

TECHNICAL PRINCIPLES AND CONSIDERATIONS

Discussion of all techniques used to treat these injuries is beyond the scope of this chapter. As such we have elected to focus on the techniques that require knowledge of both fracture reduction techniques and arthroplasty. For more in depth discussion of MIPO plating and endoprosthetic replacement, please refer to other texts and articles on these techniques.

Open reduction and internal fixation of periprosthetic hip fractures

The keys to successful plate fixation for periprosthetic hip fracture treatment include ensuring component stability and balanced fixation which does not compromise the biology at the fracture site. If there is any question regarding the stability of the indwelling component, the authors favour formal testing of the femoral stem intra-operatively. This can be performed in a bottom-up fashion with mechanical testing directed at the tip of the stem if it is accessible through the fracture site. Alternatively it can be performed in a more traditional fashion following an arthrotomy and dislocation of the proximal fragment. Plate selection should favour long constructs, generally spanning the entire femur. The fracture zone is usually avoided to preserve blood supply; bridging constructs are used to span areas of comminution. A balance must be struck between adequate fixation and creating a construct that is too stiff leading to increased strain at the fracture site. Additionally, attention must be paid to having an equal amount of fixation points on both sides of the fracture as having dense fixation below the stem and sparse fixation around the stem may increase failure rates.

Variable angle locking plates or plates with offset screw options help target screws around the stem proximally and increase the chances of obtaining bicortical fixation in the proximal segment (Figure 17.1). If bicortical fixation cannot be achieved, then a balance of unicortical locking screws and cables should be employed. Overuse of cerclage cables should be avoided as this may compromise blood supply to the fracture site. Fixation augmentation with femoral struts has become less commonly performed as locking plates have generally shown successful results and strut application and fixation can compromise blood supply to the zone of fracture healing.

Revision THA in the setting of periprosthetic femur fractures

Revision THA can be accomplished, either following reduction and provisional fixation of the fracture or via preparation of the distal segment with reduction of the proximal segment(s) to a potted prosthesis. If a monolithic stem is selected for the reconstruction (good bone stock, young patient), the fracture is typically reduced and provisionally fixed with two to three cerclage cables. The femur is then reamed and broached to accept the desired stem (Figure 17.2). Following stem placement additional fixation in the form of a cable plate can be performed. If 4 cm of diaphyseal press fit cannot be achieved with a monolithic stem, or extensive proximal comminution exists, a tapered modular stem should be selected for the reconstruction. In these instances where proximal comminution exists and the proximal fragments do not form an intact tube, it is often easier to prepare the distal femoral segment, seat the implant, construct the proximal body and then reduce the proximal fragments around the femoral component (Figure 17.3). Prior to preparation of the distal fragment a prophylactic cable is placed around the femur to prevent fracture propagation. Maximizing osseous coverage over the stem–body junction in these implants is important in supporting the junction mechanically and preventing failure over time.

IM nail fixation of supracondylar periprosthetic fractures

Retrograde nail fixation is performed through a formal arthrotomy, as this allows for complete visualization of the starting point and helps prevent iatrogenic damage to the components with reamers. An arthrotomy in conjunction with fluoroscopy also allows for confirmation that the starting point is in line with the axis of the femur and not excessively posterior. The authors prefer maximizing fixation in the distal fragment. Some nail designs have mechanisms with a setscrew that allow for static locking of multiple distal interlocking bolts. Additionally, nail fixation is augmented with two proximal locking screws at a level close to the lesser trochanter. Short nails are not used, as reliance on metaphyseal fixation is unreliable in these patients.

RESULTS AND REPORTED COMPLICATIONS

Reduction and internal fixation of periprosthetic hip fractures occurring in the femur

The reported literature regarding internal fixation of periprosthetic hip fractures around stable femoral stems has provided encouraging results. Ricci et al.[25] reported on 41 Vancouver B1 fractures that were treated with indirect reduction and locked plating techniques, which all went on to heal at 3 months postoperatively. This contrasts with data from the Swedish registry, which reported a 34% failure rate of operative fixation of B1 fractures and cited a missed diagnosis of a loose stem for their high rate of failure.[26] Further support for isolated locked plating of B1 fractures was reported by Bryant et al., who noted a union rate of 100% in 10 subjects at a mean of 17 weeks, without any complications.[27] Complications of ORIF include, but are not limited to, infection, progressive loosening of components, non-union and malunion. The use of longer constructs, which span the entire length of the involved femur, has been shown to decrease the incidence of hardware failure, non-unions and fractures distal to fixation hardware.[28]

Revision THA in the setting of periprosthetic fractures

The results of revision THA in the setting of a periprosthetic fracture around a loose stem (B2/B3) have been encouraging as well. The Swedish registry reported a revision rate of approximately 18% following this treatment, compared to a 34% revision rate noted following ORIF of periprosthetic hip fractures.[26,29] Additionally, mortality rates following revision THA (12%) are better than those observed after ORIF (33%), which may be related to a potential for earlier weight bearing.[30] Clinical results following revision THA with monolithic stems for B2 and B3 fractures have been reported by Garcia-Rey et al.,[31] who noted a 100% union rate in 35 fractures treated with fully porous stems. Complications in this series included >1 cm subsidence of stems in 48% of patients between 6 and 12 weeks. Moreover, 15% had a clinically significant limb length discrepancy related to this subsidence. Other reported complications included postoperative haematoma, intraoperative trochanteric fractures and missed fracture extension distal to the tip of the stem. Another study of 21 patients treated in a similar fashion for B2 and B3 fractures yielded a 33% complication rate, indicating the technical difficulties encountered when treating these injuries.[32]

Revision THA with modular stems is gaining momentum given the ease of adjusting for length, offset and version. Additionally, these stems are preferred in situations where 4 cm of press fit cannot be achieved with a cylindrical stem in the revision setting. While there have been a few reports of junctional failures for some stem designs and modular junctions can be a source of corrosion, these stems are rapidly becoming popular because of their ease of use. A recent study by Abdel et al. demonstrated 98% fracture union in 44 patients, at a mean of 4.5-year follow-up, with an average Harris Hip Score of 83.[33] A slightly larger series by Munro et al. also demonstrated a 98% fracture union rate in 54 fractures; of these, only two stems required revisions.[34] Noted complications in both series were stem subsidence, infection and instability.[33,34]

Open reduction and internal fixation of femoral and tibial periprosthetic fractures around a TKA

Supracondylar periprosthetic fractures above a stable TKA component treated with locked plating techniques have shown mixed results in the literature. Ricci et al. reported on 22 fractures treated in this fashion with a union rate of 86%.[35] All non-unions in this series were noted in obese diabetic patients. Furthermore, they noted satisfactory postoperative alignment in 20 of 22 fractures and the 17 patients who healed returned to baseline ambulatory status. Despite satisfactory union rates, other studies have noted a high complication rate in these patients. Ebraheim et al. reported a series of 27 patients with a complication rate of 37% including non-unions, delayed unions and hardware failure.[36] Another mixed series including both nail and plate fixation of periprosthetic fractures demonstrated successful fracture healing in only 75%. This series noted that the most common reason for treatment failure was patient death, occurring in 17%. Additionally, the authors noted a 9% non-union rate, 9% malunion rate and 6% infection rate in patients treated with locked plates.[37]

Uniform series of IM nail fixation for periprosthetic supracondylar fractures exist and support good clinical outcomes with this technique. Lee et al. reported on 25 patients treated with long IM nails and noted a 100% union rate. At final follow-up the average knee flexion was 111° with a mean Knee Society Score of 81.5.[38] Overall, 16% of patients treated in this series demonstrated malalignment postoperatively but still achieved knee flexion greater than 90°. Other studies comparing IM nail fixation to plate fixation exist. A recent retrospective review of 95 consecutive fractures treated with either nail (n=29) or plate fixation (n=66) demonstrated a failure rate in plated fractures that was twice as high as in fractures treated with nails.[39] The retrospective nature of this study introduces selection bias such that one possible interpretation of the data is that patients with fracture patterns and implants that permit IM nail fixation are predisposed to better results. Conflicting data from another comparison study reported by Horneff et al. reported that in a review of 63 patients treated with either nails (n=35) or plates (n=28), a higher union rate at 36 weeks was observed in plated fractures. Additionally, patients who underwent plate fixation had a lower re-operation rate.[40]

Periprosthetic fractures occurring in the tibia are much less frequent than those occurring in the supracondylar femur, and the reported literature is, accordingly, less frequent. Felix et al. classified and reported on 102 tibial periprosthetic fractures treated with a variety of techniques including protected weight bearing, ORIF and revision TKA.[19] The authors concluded that fractures about stable prostheses could be treated with adherence to general principles of orthopaedic trauma. Subanalysis of results of patients undergoing ORIF was not performed and this series was published before locked fixation became popular, making it difficult to apply to current methods of treatment. A large uniform series of tibial periprosthetic fractures treated with locked plating has yet to be published due to the relative infrequency of this injury pattern.

Revision TKA for periprosthetic fractures

The results of revision TKA for periprosthetic fractures are scattered within multiple revision series throughout the literature, the analysis of which are beyond the scope of this chapter. One study highlighting revision TKA in the setting of failed ORIF of periprosthetic fracture has been reported by Abbas and Morgan-Jones.[41] This series of six patients, with a mean follow-up of 4.5 years, noted a union of 100% and an 84° average arc of motion. Another series looking at revision to a DFR for the initial treatment of periprosthetic femur fractures in patients with poor bone stock demonstrated 100% implant survivorship free from revision at an average follow-up of 33 months, and an average Oxford Knee Score of 22.5.[42]

Periprosthetic patellar fractures

The results of treatment following periprosthetic fractures of the patella indicate that surgery should be avoided whenever possible as there is a high risk of complications in these patients.[20,43,44] Berry and Ortiguera reviewed 85 periprosthetic patellar fractures, 38 of which were associated with stable components and intact extensor mechanisms.[20] Of these, 37 were treated non-operatively with good results in 97%. Eleven fractures with associated extensor mechanism disruption were treated operatively with ORIF (n=6) or partial patellectomy with tendon repair (n=5). A complication rate of 55% was observed in these patients undergoing surgical intervention. Twelve additional fractures in this series were associated with loose patellar components in good bone stock, of which four were treated non-operatively, while eight underwent surgery. Two of the five knees treated with resection of patellar component and internal fixation required a re-operation. Sixteen fractures were associated with a loose patellar component in poor bone stock. Twelve of these patients were treated operatively, the majority of whom experienced persistent pain, patellar or extensor instability or weakness.

CLOSING REMARKS

Periprosthetic fractures require an understanding of both the principles of orthopaedic trauma and hip and knee arthroplasty. They almost exclusively occur in a geriatric patient population with compromised bone stock and medical comorbidities, factors that play a pivotal role in choice of fixation and the need to tailor treatments promoting ambulation as soon as possible. The development of locked plating techniques has enabled many of these fractures to be treated without revision arthroplasty, but great care needs to be exercised with respect to patient selection for ORIF, as undiagnosed component loosening can lead to early failure of appropriately performed fixation.

REFERENCES

1. Kurtz, S.M., et al. Impact of the economic downturn on total joint replacement demand in the United States: Updated projections to 2021. *J Bone Joint Surg Am*, 2014; 96(8): 624–30.
2. Preston, S., et al. Are nucleated cell counts useful in the diagnosis of infection in periprosthetic fracture? *Clin Orthop Relat Res*, 2015; 473(7): 2238–43.
3. Meermans, G. and F.S. Haddad. Is there a role for tissue biopsy in the diagnosis of periprosthetic infection? *Clin Orthop Relat Res*, 2010; 468(5): 1410–17.
4. Chevillotte, C.J., et al. Inflammatory laboratory markers in periprosthetic hip fractures. *J Arthroplasty*, 2009; 24(5): 722–7.
5. Berry, D.J. Epidemiology: Hip and knee. *Orthop Clin North Am*, 1999; 30(2): 183–90.
6. Kavanagh, B.F. Femoral fractures associated with total hip arthroplasty. *Orthop Clin North Am*, 1992; 23(2): 249–57.
7. Haidukewych, G.J., et al. Intraoperative fractures of the acetabulum during primary total hip arthroplasty. *J Bone Joint Surg Am*, 2006; 88(9): 1952–6.
8. Berry, D.J. Periprosthetic fractures associated with osteolysis: A problem on the rise. *J Arthroplasty*, 2003; 18(3 Suppl 1): 107–11.
9. Duncan, C.P. and B.A. Masri. Fractures of the femur after hip replacement. *Instr Course Lect*, 1995; 44: 293–304.
10. Brady, O.H., et al. The reliability and validity of the Vancouver classification of femoral fractures after hip replacement. *J Arthroplasty*, 2000; 15(1): 59–62.
11. Hoffmann, M.F., et al. Biomechanical evaluation of fracture fixation constructs using a variable-angle locked periprosthetic femur plate system. *Injury*, 2014; 45(7): 1035–41.
12. Berry, D.J. Treatment of Vancouver B3 periprosthetic femur fractures with a fluted tapered stem. *Clin Orthop Relat Res*, 2003; (417): 224–31.
13. Sporer, S.M. and W.G. Paprosky. Revision total hip arthroplasty: The limits of fully coated stems. *Clin Orthop Relat Res*, 2003; (417): 203–9.
14. Yasen, A.T. and F.S. Haddad. The management of type B1 periprosthetic femoral fractures: When to fix and when to revise. *Int Orthop*, 2015; 39(9): 1873–9.
15. Froberg, L., et al. Periprosthetic Vancouver type B1 and C fractures treated by locking-plate osteosynthesis: Fracture union and reoperations in 60 consecutive fractures. *Acta Orthop*, 2012; 83(6): 648–52.
16. Kubiak, E.N., et al. Does the lateral plate need to overlap the stem to mitigate stress concentration when treating Vancouver C periprosthetic supracondylar femur fracture? *J Arthroplasty*, 2015; 30(1): 104–8.
17. Rorabeck, C.H. and J.W. Taylor. Periprosthetic fractures of the femur complicating total knee arthroplasty. *Orthop Clin North Am*, 1999; 30(2): 265–77.
18. Sharkey, P.F., et al. Why are total knee arthroplasties failing today—Has anything changed after 10 years? *J Arthroplasty*, 2014; 29(9): 1774–8.
19. Felix, N.A., et al. Periprosthetic fractures of the tibia associated with total knee arthroplasty. *Clin Orthop Relat Res*, 1997; (345): 113–24.
20. Ortiguera, C.J. and D.J. Berry. Patellar fracture after total knee arthroplasty. *J Bone Joint Surg Am*, 2002; 84-A(4): 532–40.
21. Thompson, S.M., et al. Periprosthetic supracondylar femoral fractures above a total knee replacement: Compatibility guide for fixation with a retrograde intramedullary nail. *J Arthroplasty*, 2014; 29(8): 1639–41.
22. Adigweme, O.O., et al. Periprosthetic patellar fractures. *J Knee Surg*, 2013; 26(5): 313–17.
23. Rosenberg, A.G. Management of extensor mechanism rupture after TKA. *J Bone Joint Surg Br*, 2012; 94(11 Suppl A): 116–19.
24. Browne, J.A. and A.D. Hanssen. Reconstruction of patellar tendon disruption after total knee arthroplasty: Results of a new technique utilizing synthetic mesh. *J Bone Joint Surg Am*, 2011; 93(12): 1137–43.
25. Ricci, W.M., et al. Indirect reduction and plate fixation, without grafting, for periprosthetic femoral shaft fractures about a stable intramedullary implant. *J Bone Joint Surg Am*, 2005; 87(10): 2240–5.
26. Lindahl, H., et al. Risk factors for failure after treatment of a periprosthetic fracture of the femur. *J Bone Joint Surg Br*, 2006; 88(1): 26–30.
27. Bryant, G.K., et al. Isolated locked compression plating for Vancouver Type B1 periprosthetic femoral fractures. *Injury*, 2009; 40(11): 1180–6.
28. Moloney, G.B., et al. Treatment of periprosthetic femur fractures around a well-fixed hip arthroplasty implant: Span the whole bone. *Arch Orthop Trauma Surg*, 2014; 134(1): 9–14.

29. Lindahl, H., et al. Three hundred and twenty-one periprosthetic femoral fractures. *J Bone Joint Surg Am*, 2006; 88(6): 1215–22.

30. Bhattacharyya, T., et al. Mortality after periprosthetic fracture of the femur. *J Bone Joint Surg Am*, 2007; 89(12): 2658–62.

31. Garcia-Rey, E., et al. Increase of cortical bone after a cementless long stem in periprosthetic fractures. *Clin Orthop Relat Res*, 2013; 471(12): 3912–21.

32. Sheth, N.P., et al. Operative treatment of early periprosthetic femur fractures following primary total hip arthroplasty. *J Arthroplasty*, 2013; 28(2): 286–91.

33. Abdel, M.P., et al. Periprosthetic femur fractures treated with modular fluted, tapered stems. *Clin Orthop Relat Res*, 2014; 472(2): 599–603.

34. Munro, J.T., et al. Tapered fluted titanium stems in the management of Vancouver B2 and B3 periprosthetic femoral fractures. *Clin Orthop Relat Res*, 2014; 472(2): 590–8.

35. Ricci, W.M., et al. Locked plates combined with minimally invasive insertion technique for the treatment of periprosthetic supracondylar femur fractures above a total knee arthroplasty. *J Orthop Trauma*, 2006; 20(3): 190–6.

36. Ebraheim, N.A., et al. High complication rate in locking plate fixation of lower periprosthetic distal femur fractures in patients with total knee arthroplasties. *J Arthroplasty*, 2012; 27(5): 809–13.

37. Herrera, D.A., et al. Treatment of acute distal femur fractures above a total knee arthroplasty: systematic review of 415 cases (1981–2006). *Acta Orthop*, 2008; 79(1): 22–7.

38. Lee, S.S., et al. Outcomes of long retrograde intramedullary nailing for periprosthetic supracondylar femoral fractures following total knee arthroplasty. *Arch Orthop Trauma Surg*, 2014; 134(1): 47–52.

39. Meneghini, R.M., et al. Modern retrograde intramedullary nails versus periarticular locked plates for supracondylar femur fractures after total knee arthroplasty. *J Arthroplasty*, 2014; 29(7): 1478–81.

40. Horneff, J.G., 3rd, et al. Intramedullary nailing versus locked plate for treating supracondylar periprosthetic femur fractures. *Orthopedics*, 2013; 36(5): e561–6.

41. Abbas, A.M. and R.L. Morgan-Jones. Revision total knee arthroplasty for failure of primary treatment of periprosthetic knee fractures. *J Arthroplasty*, 2014; 29(10): 1996–2001.

42. Jassim, S.S., et al. Distal femoral replacement in periprosthetic fracture around total knee arthroplasty. *Injury*, 2014; 45(3): 550–3.

43. Keating, E.M., et al. Patella fracture after post total knee replacements. *Clin Orthop Relat Res*, 2003; (416): 93–7.

44. Parvizi, J., et al. Periprosthetic patellar fractures. *Clin Orthop Relat Res*, 2006; 446: 161–6.

18

Scapular fractures

JAN BARTONÍČEK

INTRODUCTION

Unlike most other fractures in the elderly, scapular fractures are not typically associated with osteoporosis. According to the reported data, scapular fractures account for only 3–5% of all injuries to the shoulder girdle and for about 1% of all fractures.[1] The reason is that the scapula is well protected by a thick muscular envelope, is highly mobile and is located on the elastic chest wall. Scapular fractures result mostly from high-energy trauma and therefore are often found in younger patients.

EPIDEMIOLOGY

There are no detailed epidemiological studies of scapular fractures and the data indicating their proportion of the total number of fractures are almost 80 years out of date.[1,2] Until now, most authors have used data on patient age, the male–female ratio and the distribution of types of fractures from older studies. However, a detailed analysis of those studies shows that they cannot be considered representative. Their main drawbacks are small numbers of patients and a questionable diagnosis of individual fracture patterns, based on radiographs without CT data.[3] Therefore, the epidemiological data presented here are based on an analysis of our own group of 250 patients with scapular fractures.

The group comprised 199 men (80%) and 51 women (20%). The average age of the whole group was 45 years (range: 15–92 years), with the average age of men 43.5 years and that of women 52.4 years. CT examination was used in 204 patients and 100 patients underwent surgical fixation. When the whole cohort was subdivided into two subgroups of patients under and over the age of 60 years based on our experience in previous epidemiological studies, particularly of proximal femoral fractures,[4] the basic characteristics of each subgroup changed. In the group of patients under 60 years of age, the male–female ratio was 84:16, while in the group of patients older than 60 years, it was 64:36 (Table 18.1).

Patients older than 60 years accounted for 17% of the whole group. They constituted 12% of the men and up to 38% of the women in the whole group. The peak incidence of fractures in men was between the fourth and sixth decades, while in women it was between fifth and seventh decades (Table 18.2 and Figure 18.1).

Overall, 52% were fractures of the scapular body, 29% were fractures of the glenoid, 11% were fractures of the processes and 8% were fractures of the scapular neck. In patients older than 60 years, a slight increase was noted in the proportions of fractures of the glenoid and the processes, but no fracture of the scapular neck was recorded (Table 18.3). At the same time, the number of associated fractures of the proximal humerus was significantly higher, probably due to progressing osteoporosis.

Comparison of our groups of patients with a fracture of the scapula, the ankle, the distal radius, the proximal humerus or the proximal femur shows that the group with a scapular fracture had the lowest average age and the highest proportion of men versus women (Table 18.4). With advancing age, the proportion of women rose and, ultimately, in the eighth decade, exceeded that of men. For these reasons scapular fractures cannot logically be considered as osteoporotic injuries.

Table 18.1 Group of patients

Group of patients	All patients	Male (N)	Female (N)	Male:Female ratio
Under 60 years	204	171	33	84:16
Over 60 years	46	28	18	64:36
All patients	250	199	51	80:20

Table 18.2 Age distribution of scapular fractures

Decade	N	Male	Female	%	% Male	% Female
2	11	8	3	4.4	3.2	1.2
3	32	27	5	12.8	10.8	2.0
4	60	55	5	24.0	22.0	2.0
5	53	45	8	21.2	18.0	3.2
6	51	40	11	20.4	16.0	4.4
7	32	20	12	12.8	8.0	4.8
8	8	3	5	3.2	1.2	2.0
9	2	1	1	0.8	0.4	0.4
10	1	0	1	0.4	0.0	0.4

ANATOMY

The scapula is part of the shoulder girdle. It is attached to the axial skeleton by the clavicle via the acromioclavicular (AC) and sternoclavicular (SC) joints. This articulation chain maintains a constant distance between the scapula and the sternum. The scapula is located on the posterior chest wall between the second and seventh ribs and is held in this position by the tone of the attached muscles, mainly the upper part of the trapezius and the levator scapulae. The angle between the scapula and the frontal plane is approximately 30 degrees. The scapula is primarily responsible for providing efficient support to the humeral head in all positions of the arm. Smooth motion of the scapula over the chest wall is possible thanks to the gliding fibro-fatty tissue that fills the space between the muscles covering the anterior surface of the scapula and those of the chest wall.

Bone anatomy

The scapula is a flat triangular bone, defined by the superior, medial and lateral borders and three angles, including two flat angles: the *superior* and *inferior angles*, and the *lateral angle*, a three-dimensional structure formed by the *scapular neck* and the *glenoid*. On the posterior surface of the scapula, the division between the scapular body and neck is marked by the spinoglenoid notch. The anterosuperior surface of the scapular neck bears the origin of the coracoid process. The glenoid has a pear-shaped articular surface with a prominent ring of fibrocartilage at its wider

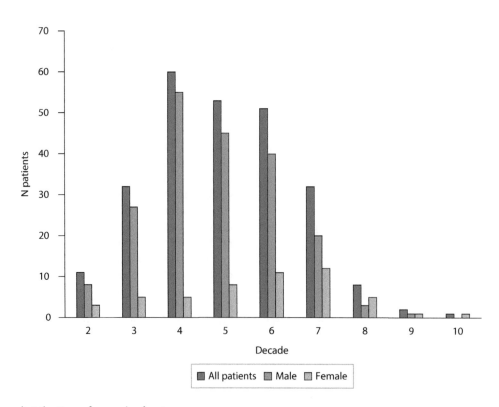

Figure 18.1 Age distribution of scapular fractures.

Table 18.3 Types of scapular fractures

Type of fractures	All patients (N)	%	<60 years (N)	<60 years (%)	>60 years (N)	>60 years (%)
All fractures	250	100	204	100	46	100
Body	131	52	107	52	24	52
Glenoid	73	29	58	28	15	33
Processes	27	11	20	10	7	15
Neck	19	8	19	10	0	0
Sca+PH	8	3	4	2	4	9

Note: PH, proximal humerus; Sca, scapula.

Table 18.4 Comparison of our groups of patients with a fracture of the scapula, the ankle, the distal radius, the proximal humerus or the proximal femur

Fracture type	N	Male (N)	Female (N)	Male:Female ratio	Average age, all (years)	Average age, male (years)	Average age, female (years)	Male–female age difference (years)
Scapula	250	199	51	80:20	45	44	52	8
Ankle	1,195	665	660	50:50	49	43	55	12
DR	2,514	723	1,791	29:71	59	46	65	19
PH	1,464	441	1,023	30:70	67	59	71	12
PF	3,340	911	2,429	27:73	78	72	80	9

Note: DR, distal radius; PF, proximal femur; PH, proximal humerus.

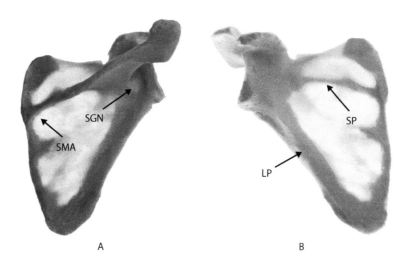

A   B

Figure 18.2 Anatomy of the scapula. (a) Anterior view, (b) posterior view. LP, lateral pillar; SGN, spino-glenoidal notch; SMA, spino-medial angle; SP, spinous pillar.

end – the *glenoid labrum*. The anterior surface of the scapula is concave. The posterior surface of the scapula is divided by a bony ridge – the *scapular spine* – into the supra- and infraspinous fossae. In its lateral extent, the scapular spine becomes more elevated and ends in a robust bony process – the *acromion* – which is flattened and curves forward.

The distribution of the bony mass of the scapula is very uneven. When held up to the light, the scapula shows the highest concentration of bony mass in the glenoid, the scapular neck, including the base of the coracoid process, and the lateral border of the scapular spine. Cancellous bone is to be found only in the region of the lateral angle of the scapula.

Two bony pillars, which pass from the glenoid to the scapular body, transmit compression forces from the glenoid fossa. The *lateral pillar* is identical with the lateral border of the scapular body and connects the inferior border of the glenoid with the inferior angle. The *spinal pillar* arises from the central part of the glenoid and continues medially to become part of the base of the scapular spine. Its course can be seen better by viewing the scapula from the front against the light (Figure 18.2). The spinal pillar and the medial border of the scapular body form an open *spino-medial angle*. From the posterior view, it is evident that the two pillars and their connection via the markedly thinner

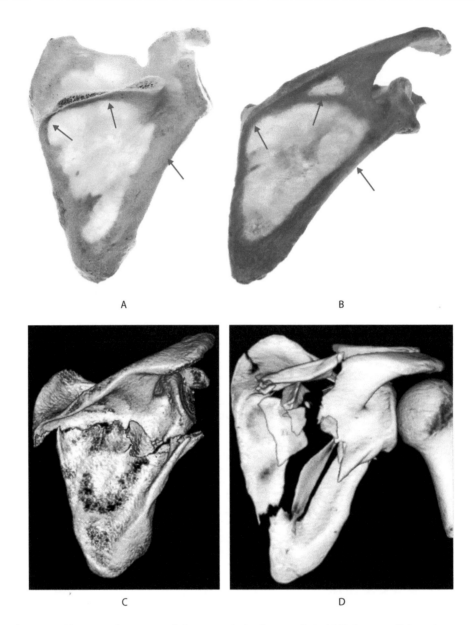

Figure 18.3 Critical zones of bony architecture of the scapula (red arrows). **(a,b)** Spino-medial angle, central scapular spine, lateral border, **(c)** two part fractures of the scapular (biomechanical) body, the fracture line passes from the lateral border into the spino-medial angle, **(d)** comminuted fracture of the scapular (anatomical) body, fracture lines pass through the lateral body, spino-medial angle and central scapular spine.

medial border of the scapular body constitute the basic, triangular load-bearing structure of the scapular body. This triangle is effectively the *biomechanical body of the scapula*, as the superior angle and the adjacent part of the supraspinous fossa form merely an appendage, which serves as a surface for the insertion, or origin, of muscles, but does not transmit compressive forces from the glenoid. For this reason, it is necessary to distinguish between the *anatomical and biomechanical bodies* of the scapula.

The weak areas of the scapula are mainly the central parts of the supra- and infraspinous fossae, where the bone is only a few millimetres thick. The weakest area of the circumference of the biomechanical body of the scapula is the spino-medial angle which is demonstrated by the fact that in the majority of scapular body fractures one of the main fracture lines passes through this region. Another area of weak bone is in the central part of the scapular spine where, quite often, fracture lines can also be seen, as shown by analysis of the course of fracture lines[5] (Figure 18.3).

Muscles

The muscles of the scapula may be divided into two systems. The first, the *scapulo-axial* system connects the scapula with the axial skeleton, the spine and the chest wall in particular. This system is responsible for movement of the scapula over the chest wall. The other, the *scapulo-brachial* system, is formed by the muscles arising from the scapula and attaching to the bones of the free part of the upper limb, more specifically to the humerus, the proximal radius and the proximal ulna. Its role is to control movement between the scapula and the free part of the upper limb, that is, control of the motion in the glenohumeral joint and, to a small extent, the elbow.

In total, 18 muscles are attached to the scapula. Only three of them, namely the subscapularis, supraspinatus and infraspinatus, originate from the broad surface of the scapula in their respective fossae; the rest of them are attached to the borders of the scapula or its processes. Other muscles reinforce individual borders, angles and processes by their attachments, namely the levator scapulae at the superior angle, the rhomboid minor at the medial border at the level of the scapular spine posteriorly, the rhomboid major located directly inferior to it, and the latissimus dorsi at the inferior angle. From the same angle and partially from the lateral border of the scapula there originates the teres major and in the upper half of the lateral border, the teres minor. The serratus anterior inserts along the entire anterior length of the medial border of the scapula; the trapezius is attached to the scapular spine and the anterior rim of the acromion; the deltoid muscle arises from the distal border of the scapular spine and subsequently from the posterior rim of the acromion. The long head of biceps originates above the superior rim and the long head of triceps from below the inferior rim of the glenoid. Attached to the central part of the coracoid process is the pectoralis minor and from the apex of the coracoid there arise the coracobrachialis and the short head of biceps.

Nerves and blood vessels

The suprascapular nerve passes under the superior transverse scapular ligament, and travels together with the suprascapular artery and vein along the supraspinous fossa. This neurovascular bundle runs under the inferior transverse scapular ligament and enters the spinoglenoid notch on the posterior surface of the scapular neck. The suprascapular nerve gives off motor branches to the supraspinatus and infraspinatus muscles. The suprascapular artery anastomoses with the scapular circumflex artery on the lateral border of the scapula, about 2–3 cm distal to the glenoid.

INJURY MECHANISM AND ASSOCIATED INJURIES

By virtue of its thick muscular envelope, its considerable mobility and its location on the elastic chest wall, the scapula is well protected against injury. A majority of scapular fractures are reported to be caused by a high-energy mechanism, but this is not entirely true.[6] From the viewpoint of the energy of the injury mechanism, the patients may be divided into three groups.

The first group comprises those with high-energy injuries, sustained mostly during a traffic accident, by a fall from height or by a heavy object falling onto the patient. They are found mostly in polytrauma patients with a range of injuries to individual organ systems, particularly to the chest (ribs, lungs), head, spine and abdomen. Injuries to the scapula are often discovered coincidentally, towards the end of the diagnostic and therapeutic process.

The second group comprises patients with medium-energy trauma caused usually by a fall from a bicycle or a slowly travelling motorcycle. The injury to the scapula and the shoulder girdle usually dominates, associated sometimes with cerebral contusion or another injury (e.g. tibial fracture).

The third group comprises mostly elderly patients who sustained a scapular fracture in a simple fall from standing height, down stairs or even as a result of a smaller object falling onto the scapula. In the majority of these patients it is an isolated injury to the shoulder girdle.

Scapular fractures are caused by exogenous and endogenous mechanisms. With the exogenous (external) mechanism, the impact acts directly on individual parts of the scapula, or is transmitted through the humeral head. In cases of direct impact, the scapula hits surrounding objects (e.g. when the chest hits the car body) or vice versa, when for instance a heavy object hits the scapula. The result is most often a fracture of the scapular body or scapular processes. In cases of transmitted forces, the impactor is the humeral head. The fracture pattern depends on the position of the arm at the time of injury. With the arm in abduction, the humeral head is driven against the inferior glenoid, which separates off, often together with a part of the lateral border of the scapula. With the arm in adduction, a blow on the elbow along the axis of the humeral shaft proximally dislocates the humeral head, which hits the acromion or the coracoid. Anterior or posterior dislocation of the humeral head may result in a fracture of the respective rim of the glenoid. The endogenous cause of scapular fractures is most frequently a violent muscle contracture as the result of an electrical injury or an epileptic seizure.

Pathological scapular fractures (e.g. bone cyst, osteodystrophy and tumour metastasis) are rare.[6,7] Fatigue fractures of the scapular spine and the acromion have been reported in cases of insufficiency of the rotator cuff.[8] A specific group are periprosthetic scapular fractures in patients following shoulder arthroplasty.

Our patients older than 60 years most often sustained a scapular fracture in a fall from standing height, on stairs or from a bicycle. We have recorded one fracture in a tumour metastasis. None of our patients older than 60 years was classified as a polytrauma patient.

DIAGNOSTICS

The diagnostic procedure in patients with scapular injuries depends on their general condition. In polytrauma patients, the priority is to save life. The treatment of a scapular fracture, even if detected during primary examination, may be postponed to a later time, except for an open scapular fracture. In a number of polytrauma patients, scapular fractures are often found coincidentally, for example, on a radiograph of lungs or a CT scan of chest.

Clinical examination

Patients in a less severe general condition, who are able to communicate, may undergo standard clinical examination. Scapular fractures are often associated with other injuries and, therefore, it is essential first to conduct a thorough and comprehensive examination of the patient before focusing on the shoulder. If one fracture of a shoulder girdle is found (e.g. of the clavicle), it is necessary to exclude other potential injuries.

PATIENT'S MEDICAL HISTORY

Knowledge of the exact mechanism of the injury and the patient's subjective complaints are essential to a proper diagnosis. Elderly patients are asked about any past problems with the shoulder (rotator cuff lesion, osteoarthritis) or other systemic diseases (tumours, metabolic disease).

VISUAL ASSESSMENT

Careful examination of the shoulder and the entire chest, including the axilla, is performed. The shoulder may be deformed by a clavicular fracture, acromioclavicular dislocation, humeral head dislocation, by a markedly displaced scapular fracture or significant swelling. Examination of the integrity of the skin cover is important as a skin abrasion may indicate a site of impact.

PALPATION

A large part of the skeleton of the shoulder girdle may be examined by palpation, that is, the clavicle, sternoclavicular joint, acromioclavicular joint, the scapular spine and acromion, the tip of the coracoid and the humeral head; in the elderly who tend to be less muscular, the inferior angle and medial border of the scapula are also accessible. Palpation may reveal crepitus or pathological mobility. It is also important to palpate the axilla and the adjacent chest wall, and to identify the pulse of the axillary artery. As the fracture may be combined with a lesion of the brachial plexus, sensation in the upper limb should be examined to exclude an injury to the brachial plexus.

RANGE OF MOTION

Examination of the range of motion, mainly active motion, in scapular fractures is significantly limited by pain. If possible, passive motion in the glenohumeral joint is carefully examined.

PERIPHERY

It is also important to thoroughly assess other parts of the ipsilateral extremity including its peripheral innervation and vascularity in order to exclude associated injuries.

Imaging methods

Radiological examination is essential to the diagnosis of scapular fractures, the determination of the fracture patterns and the treatment procedure. Other imaging methods may include MRI and ultrasound scanning, although they are indicated only exceptionally and their contribution is limited.[6,7,9] When scapular fractures occur in polytrauma patients or in the elderly, the radiodiagnostic algorithm described below has to be adjusted to the patient's general condition.

RADIOLOGY

Part of the basic examination is a general radiograph of the entire shoulder girdle covering the whole scapula, the proximal humerus and the whole clavicle, including acromioclavicular and sternoclavicular joints. Scapular fractures are often associated with a clavicular fracture or acromioclavicular dislocation and, in the elderly, with a proximal humeral fracture. In cases with a suspected or detected scapula fracture, it should be combined with both Neer projections, if allowed by the patient's general condition (Figure 18.4).

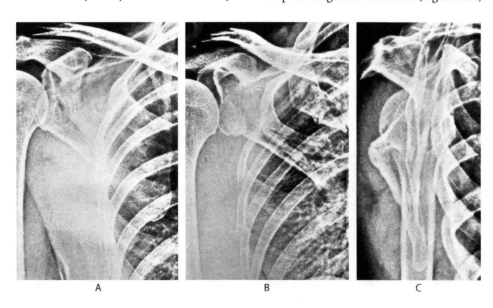

A B C

Figure 18.4 Radiological examination of scapular fractures. (a) Anteroposterior (AP) shoulder view, (b) Neer I view, (c) Neer II view.

Neer I projection, or the true anteroposterior radiograph of the scapula, is used to assess the glenohumeral joint space, displacement of the glenoid in relation to the lateral border of the scapula and to measure the glenopolar angle (GPA). In this projection, the scapular plane is parallel to the X-ray cassette. This may be achieved by rotating the patient with his/her back to the X-ray cassette by 30 degrees towards the affected side.

Neer II projection, also called Y-view, is a true lateral scapular projection. In this projection the scapular plane is perpendicular to the X-ray cassette. This may be achieved by rotating the patient, facing the X-ray cassette, by 60 degrees towards the affected side. The Y-view projection allows assessment of scapular body fractures in terms of translation, angulation and overlap of fragments, particularly of the lateral border. In addition, it displays clearly the relationships between the coracoid, the acromion and the lateral clavicle, as well as the acromioclavicular joint. It can be used to identify any avulsion of the anterior rim of the glenoid.

General radiograph of the chest, indicated to examine the lungs, heart and chest wall, in polytrauma patients often provides the first clue leading to a diagnosis of a scapular fracture. It is important mostly for assessment of the position of both scapulae in relation to the spine (scapulothoracic dissociation).

Other special projections, axillary in particular, are recommended by some authors as complementary views, to diagnose fractures of the glenoid, acromion and coracoid. However, axillary projection is, for most patients with a scapular or rib fracture, highly unpleasant and should not be used as a substitute for CT examination.

The complicated shape of the scapula and its position on the chest makes an unambiguous interpretation of findings and determination of the fracture pattern with the use of radiographic projections alone often very difficult or even impossible, For this reason, CT examination is very important.[7,9]

CT EXAMINATION

CT examination has fundamentally changed the radiodiagnostics of scapular fractures. It is always indicated when radiographic examination cannot reveal the exact fracture pattern, involvement of the articular surface or displacement of fragments.

CT transverse sections are valuable in the assessment of the condition of the glenoid fossa. They also help to detect undisplaced fractures of the scapular processes, especially those of the coracoid and the acromion. However, they do not provide a three-dimensional image of the fracture anatomy.

Two-dimensional CT reconstructions (2D CT), mainly in the sagittal plane, are used to assess the articular surface, especially in fractures of the base of the coracoid process involving the glenoid fossa.

Three-dimensional CT reconstructions (3D CT) are the only way to determine reliably the exact fracture pattern, particularly in fractures of the scapular body and neck, although they do not show fine fracture lines, especially in minimally displaced fragments. Reconstructions should be made in three basic views (Figure 18.5), with subtraction of ribs, clavicle and proximal humerus.[10]

The posterior view allows assessment of the course of fracture lines with regard to the scapular spine. It is important that it covers the entire infraspinous and also part of the supraspinous fossa.

The anterior view is essential in fractures of the scapular neck. This view helps to identify different courses of fracture lines in fractures of the anatomical and surgical necks of the scapula.

Glenoid fractures require a lateral view, always with subtraction of the humeral head. This is the only way to get exact information about the number of fragments and the course of fracture lines involving the glenoid. In fractures of the lateral border of the scapular body, this lateral view helps to assess its shortening, angulation and translation, or the shape and displacement of small intermediate fragments.

In certain fracture patterns it may be useful to obtain other views in order to assess the course of the fracture line, for example, a view of the supraspinous fossa, the spino-glenoid notch or a medial view.

CLASSIFICATION OF SCAPULAR FRACTURES

All classification systems published in the literature have one common drawback: they have been developed only on the basis of radiographs, often taken in a non-standard way.[3,11,12] A number of fracture patterns previously proposed do not, in fact, correspond to the reality. In spite of this, they may persist in the newly developed classifications.[13]

Based on the analysis of our own group of 250 scapulae, with 3D CT reconstruction in 204 of them and 100 of them treated surgically, we have divided scapular fractures into five basic groups.[7,14,15]

Fractures of scapular processes

Fractures of scapular processes account for 11% of all scapular fractures in our group and for 15% of those in patients over 60 years of age (Table 18.3). They include fractures of the superior angle and the upper border of the scapula, fractures of and in the acromion and the scapular spine, and coracoid fractures. These fractures result from a direct blow to the upper part of the scapula, the pull of muscles and ligaments or impact by the displaced humeral head (Figure 18.6).

Fractures of the scapular body

Fractures of the scapular body account approximately for 52% of all scapular fractures in both the older and younger groups. We divide them into two basic groups, namely fractures of the

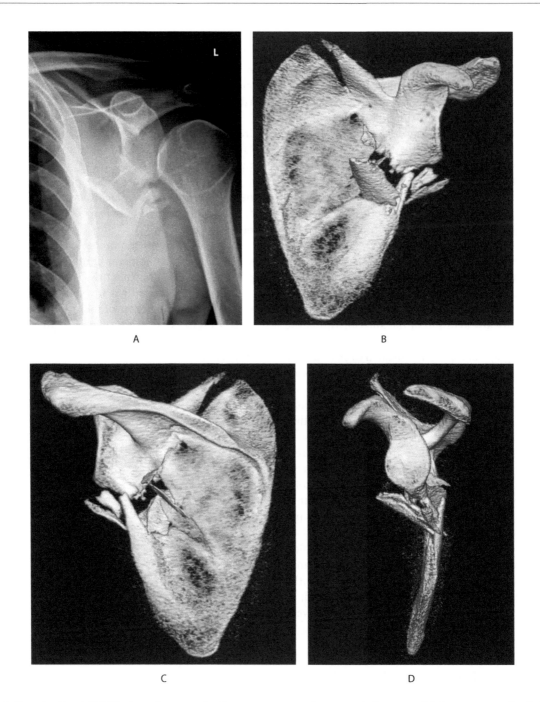

A   B

C   D

Figure 18.5 Standardized CT 3D views for scapular fractures: transspinous neck fracture. **(a)** Anteroposterior (AP) shoulder radiograph, **(b)** anterior 3D CT view, **(c)** posterior 3D CT view, **(d)** lateral 3D CT view.

biomechanical and of the anatomical bodies (Figure 18.7). The decisive criterion is the course of fracture lines in relation to the scapular spine.[5,14]

Fractures of the biomechanical body affect only the infraspinous fossa, always with damage to the lateral border of the scapula. Based on the number of fragments, we distinguish two-, three- and multi-part (comminuted) fractures.

Fractures of the anatomical body involve the entire scapular body and fracture lines pass across the scapular spine. They mostly result from direct high-energy impacts and are often comminuted.

Fractures of the scapular neck

Fractures of the scapular neck are defined as extra-articular fractures of the lateral scapular angle, separating the glenoid from the scapular body. In our group they comprise 8% of all scapular fractures although none occurred in the older patients. According to the course of the fracture line and the shape of the glenoid fragment, we distinguish between three basic types.[15]

Fractures of the anatomical neck separate only the glenoid from the scapular body. The fracture line passes proximally

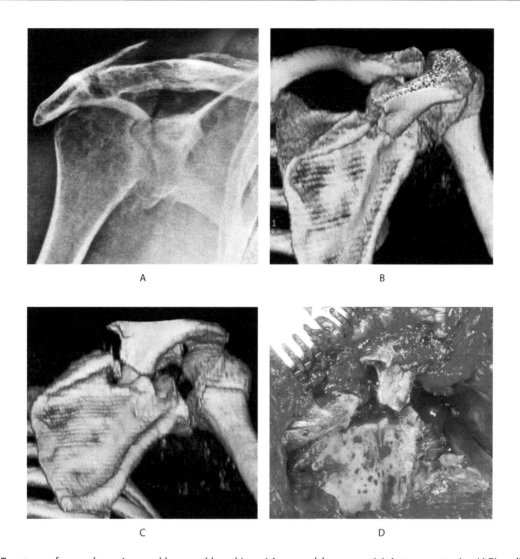

Figure 18.6 Fracture of scapular spine and humeral head in a 64-year-old woman. (a) Anteroposterior (AP) radiograph of the shoulder, (b) posterior 3D CT view, (c) postero-inferior 3D CT view, (d) intraoperative view.

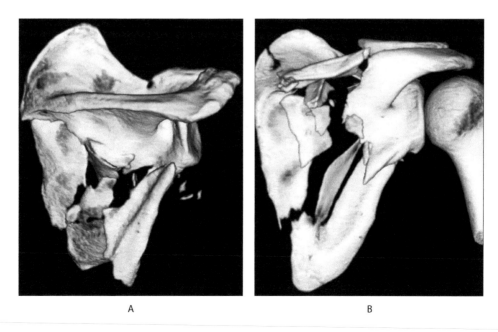

Figure 18.7 Fractures of the scapular body. (a) Fracture of the biomechanical body, (b) fracture of the anatomical body.

between the upper rim of the glenoid and the coracoid base. This rare fracture is unstable and usually displaces into valgus.

Fractures of the surgical neck of the scapula are the most frequent of the three types of surgical neck fractures. Part of the glenoid fragment is the coracoid. The pull of muscles attached to this process (the short head of biceps, the coracobrachialis and the pectoralis minor) may displace the glenoid fragment inferomedially. The decisive factor in this respect is the integrity of the coracoacromial and coracoclavicular ligaments. If they are intact, the fracture is stable in relation to the acromion and the clavicle. A rupture of the coracoacromial ligament affects the relationship between the glenoid fragment and the acromion, but not the clavicle; the fracture is unstable rotationally. In cases of a rupture of the coracoclavicular ligament, the fracture is fully unstable, which is shown by a larger separation between the coracoid and the clavicle.

Transspinous fractures of the scapular neck are rare and little is known about them. The lateral fragment is formed by the glenoid, the coracoid and the acromion and the adjacent lateral part of the scapular spine.

Intra-articular fractures of the glenoid

Intra-articular fractures of the glenoid account in our group for 29% of all scapular fractures and are roughly equally distributed in the older and younger groups (Table 18.3). They may be divided into four basic groups with varying anatomy of the fragment, depending on the involvement of the glenoid fossa.

Fractures of the superior pole of the glenoid fossa are in fact intra-articular fractures of the coracoid base, where the fragment also carries a portion of the superior border of the scapula. They are probably caused by the impact of the humeral head on the coracoid, with the arm in adduction.

Avulsion of the anteroinferior rim of the glenoid fossa is caused by a glenohumeral dislocation mechanism, and is often associated with an impaction fracture of the humeral head. A fracture of the anterior rim of the glenoid results from anterior glenohumeral dislocation and is much more common than fracture of the posterior rim. The extent of involvement of the anteroinferior rim of the glenoid fossa varies. With a larger fragment, the shoulder is unstable after reduction (Figure 18.8). A similar fracture of the posterior rim of the glenoid caused by posterior glenohumeral dislocation is quite rare and takes the form, as a rule, of several small fragments.

Fractures of the inferior glenoid fossa are the most severe injury to the glenoid fossa. They are caused by direct impact of the humeral head onto the glenoid fossa, with the arm in abduction. The impact is directed at the inferior half of the glenoid fossa and, consequently, also at the lateral border of the scapular body. The size of the avulsed part of the glenoid fossa varies, involving usually one to two thirds of the articular surface. The fracture line extends into the lateral border of the scapula for a variable distance. Most fractures of the inferior glenoid are combined with a fracture of the scapular body that may be involved to a varying extent.

Fractures of the entire glenoid fossa are very rare. The glenoid fossa is completely separated from the scapular neck and broken into several fragments.

Combined fractures

Combined fractures are divided into two groups. The first group includes combinations of two, and more basic, fractures of the scapula, for example, a fracture of the scapular body combined with a fracture of the surgical neck of the scapula. The second group comprises scapular fractures in combination with injuries to the proximal humerus (Figure 18.9), the clavicle or acromioclavicular joint. The most frequent pattern is a combined fracture of the scapular body and the clavicular shaft.

TREATMENT

Treatment of scapular fractures depends on the fracture pattern, its displacement, local conditions and the patient's general condition.[7,9,16–21]

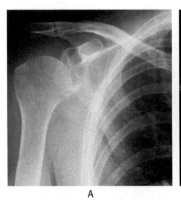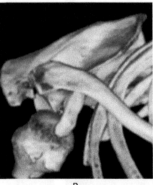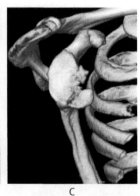

A B C

Figure 18.8 Fracture of the antero-inferior rim of the glenoid fossa in a 77-year-old woman. **(a)** Anteroposterior (AP) radiograph of the shoulder, **(b)** superior 3D CT view demonstrates anterior subluxation of the humeral head, **(c)** lateral 3D CT view into the glenoid fossa.

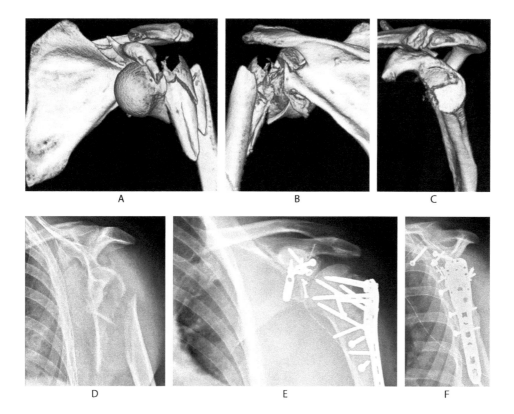

Figure 18.9 Fracture of the superior glenoid and anterior glenoid rim, combined with a proximal humeral fracture in a 70-year-old woman. (a) Anterior 3D CT view, (b) posterior 3D CT view, (c) lateral 3D CT view, (d) anteroposterior (AP) shoulder radiograph after injury, (e) Neer I view after surgery, (f) Neer II view after surgery.

Indication

Undisplaced intra- and extra-articular fractures of the scapula are treated non-operatively; similarly displaced intra- or extra-articular fractures when the patient's general or local condition does not allow operative treatment.

Displaced intra-articular fractures involving more than 20–30% of the articular surface, together with a step-off of more than 3 mm, require operative treatment to restore congruity and stability of the glenohumeral joint.

The treatment of displaced extra-articular fractures is currently the subject of intense debate.[7,8,16–21] In general, operative stabilization is preferred in severely displaced fractures of the scapular body and neck in active individuals, if allowed by their local and general condition. Indications for operative treatment are fractures of the scapular body and neck with the following types of displacement: 100% translation of fragments of the lateral border of the scapular body, angulation of main fragments of the lateral border exceeding 30–40 degrees, medio-lateral displacement of the fragments of the lateral border of the scapular body of more than 1–2 cm and a GPA of less than 20 degrees.[7,9,19]

In displaced fractures of the processes, particularly the coracoid, acromion and scapular spine, which give attachments to prominent muscles and ligaments, the aim is to achieve healing in an anatomical position, as malunion may compromise the rotator cuff.[19] Non-union of these processes is often painful, due to muscle pull.

The indications for operative treatment of fractures in elderly patients must be carefully considered. Sometimes osteosynthesis of a scapular fractures may take 2 or more hours with the patient resting in a semi-prone position on the intact shoulder. As these fractures are often associated with rib fractures and the elderly patient may have compromised lung function, this position is suboptimal.

In our group, 46 patients were older than 60 years, and 12 (26%) of them had indications for operation. Only one of the operated patients was older than 70 years (a fracture of the anterior glenoid rim associated with an unstable anterior dislocation of the humeral head). We have always carefully taken into consideration not only the fracture pattern but also the patient's general condition and physical activities. Eight cases were intra-articular fractures, that is, a fracture of the glenoid fossa, three cases involved severely displaced fracture of the scapular body and one case a fracture of the scapular spine. By comparison, of 204 patients under 60 years of age, 88 (43%) were treated operatively (Table 18.1).

Non-operative treatment

Non-operative care consists of pain relief and about 2 weeks of sling immobilization. It is then possible to start a passive range of motion exercises. A full passive range of motion should be achieved within 1 month of the injury[7,9] and the restoration of a full range of active motion could reasonably be expected during the second month after injury. Beginning from the third month, strengthening of the rotator cuff muscles and parascapular muscles may be started, and during the fourth month all restrictions can be lifted.

Operative treatment

The aim of operative treatment depends on the fracture pattern.[7,8,13,18–21] In displaced intra-articular fractures, the aim of the operation is to restore both congruity and stability of the glenohumeral joint. In displaced extra-articular fractures of the processes, particularly the coracoid, acromion and scapular spine, which give attachments to prominent muscles and ligaments, the aim is to achieve healing in an anatomical position, to avoid compromise of the rotator cuff. Non-union of these processes is often painful, due to muscle pull. Displaced extra-articular fractures of the scapular body and neck require restoration of the original alignment of the glenoid with the scapular body (GPA), primarily by reconstruction of the length and integrity of the lateral border (Figure 18.10). This will restore the normal course of muscles, particularly those of the rotator cuff. From the standpoint of physiological mobility of the scapula, it is also important to restore the congruity between its anterior surface and the chest wall and, if necessary, to remove fragments of the scapula impacted into the chest wall.

Operative treatment of a closed fractured scapula is never an acute intervention and it should be postponed until the patient's general and local condition allow, especially in the elderly patient. Therefore most patients undergo surgery several days to weeks after their injury.

SURGICAL APPROACHES

In operating on scapular fractures, one of the following surgical approaches may be used.[7,9]

A *deltopectoral approach* is indicated for isolated fractures of the anteroinferior rim of the glenoid and of the coracoid process.

A *Judet posterior approach* provides excellent exposure of the entire infraspinous fossa, the lateral and medial borders of the scapula, the anatomical and surgical scapular necks and the posterior and inferior rims of the glenoid. The Judet posterior approach is indicated as a universal exposure in fractures of the scapular body, scapular neck and the inferior glenoid. In some cases it is possible to make only medial and lateral para-muscular windows without mobilizing the infraspinatus. On the lateral side, it is sufficient to detach the infraspinatus from the lateral border of the scapula only in the required field; on the medial side it is typically released in the spino-medial angle. The exposure depends on the fracture pattern and the surgeon's experience. Patients without mobilization of the infraspinatus

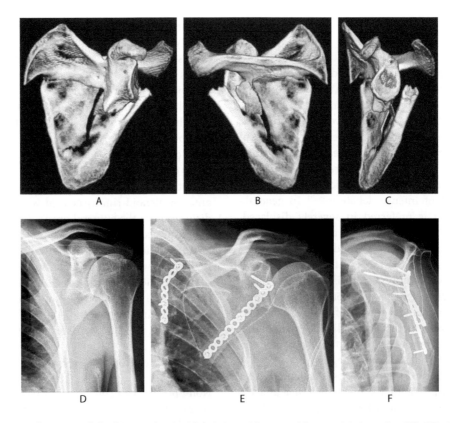

Figure 18.10 Three-part fracture of the biomechanical body in a 68-year-old man. (a) Anterior 3D CT view, (b) posterior 3D CT view, (c) lateral 3D CT view, (d) anteroposterior (AP) shoulder radiograph after injury, (e) Neer I view after surgery, (f) Neer II view after surgery.

muscle experience less postoperative pain and restoration of the range of motion is much faster.

A *posterosuperior approach* is indicated in fractures of the acromion and the scapular spine, sometimes also in fractures of the posterior rim of the glenoid fossa. It uses the horizontal part of the Judet incision and passes along the posterior border of the acromion and the lateral part of the scapular spine. When necessary, this approach may be extended to a full Judet approach.

IMPLANTS

No special implants are required for the operative treatment of scapular fractures in elderly patients. In most cases, adequate stabilization may be achieved using 3.5 mm DCP reconstruction plates, 1/3 semitubular plates or the 3.5 mm T-plate designed for the distal radius. Currently, we prefer reconstruction, with straight, T- or L-shaped 2.7 mm plates with standard 2.7 mm cortical screws, and only exceptionally do we use locking plates and screws.

INTERNAL FIXATION OF INDIVIDUAL FRACTURE TYPES

Sufficient anchorage of implants is offered primarily by the lateral border of the scapular body, the scapular spine, the scapular neck and the glenoid. Additional fixation purchase may be gained in the spino-medial or inferior angles of the scapula.

Glenoid fossa fractures are, in terms of operative treatment, a heterogeneous group of injuries.[6,7,18,22,23] Fractures of the anteroinferior rim of the glenoid, resulting from glenohumeral dislocation, usually do not pose any particular problems. The deltopectoral approach is used to reduce and fix the avulsed fragment by lag screws and, if necessary, supported by a buttress plate. The adjacent part of the labrum is examined and treated if necessary. In suitable cases, an alternative may be arthroscopically assisted reduction and internal fixation with a lag screw.

More difficult, in terms of reduction and stabilization, are fractures of the superior glenoid, which also need a deltopectoral approach. Reduction is not always easy, due to the pull of muscles attached to the coracoid. These fractures may be fixed by cannulated lag screws fitted with washers, inserted through the coracoid into the glenoid or the scapular neck.

Fractures of the inferior glenoid that almost always involve the scapular body are the most severe scapular injuries. Reduction and stabilization are performed via the Judet approach. Fractures of the inferior glenoid are usually associated with fractures of the scapular body. If the posterior joint capsule and labrum are not ruptured, incision of the capsule should run parallel to the posterior rim of the glenoid and labrum. This allows both a visual check and palpation of the glenoid fossa reduction. Reduction and fixation depend on the shape of the inferior joint fragment. This fragment may be small and carry only a small part of the lateral border or it may include a large part of the lateral border. Reduction and fixation of a short fragment is usually easier. Reduction of a long fragment must be accurate along the whole length of the fracture line. This is the only guarantee of an anatomical reduction of the joint surface (Figures 18.11 and 18.12). If another, usually smaller, fragment has separated from the articular surface, it has to be anatomically reduced and fixed by lag screws, as a rule 2.0 mm or 2.4 mm. The main two fragments may be fixed using a variety of techniques, most often by a combination of different plates, that is, 3.5-mm T-plate; 2.7 mm L- shaped, T-shaped or straight plates; and lag screws. Reconstruction of the articular surface of the glenoid will also often ensure the repositioning of the lateral border of the scapula. If not, the lateral border of the scapula is reconstructed in the next step and, where necessary, reduction and internal fixation of the scapular body in the spino-medial and inferior angles of the scapula are performed.

Fractures of the scapular neck are rare in elderly patients but if encountered are always accessed via the Judet approach; mobilization of the infraspinatus is usually not necessary. In fractures of the surgical neck, potential entrapment of the suprascapular nerve in the fracture line at the spino-glenoid notch must be taken into account. Special attention should be paid to the insertion of screws into the glenoid fragment, in order to prevent their penetration into the joint cavity. Therefore, it is necessary to identify accurately the posterior rim of the glenoid and respect the inclination of its articular surface. Stabilization of fractures of the anatomical neck may sometimes be difficult due to the size and instability of the glenoid fragment. For this reason it is beneficial to use a T-shaped or L-shaped plate. In fractures of the surgical neck, it is recommended to use additional fixation using 3.5 mm cortical screws inserted through the scapular spine.[15]

Fractures of the scapular body require restoration of the so-called biomechanical triangle, that is, the circumference of the infraspinous fossa.[5,14] A key structure from the viewpoint of internal fixation of a fracture of the scapular body is the lateral border which must be reduced and fixed as the first step. Prior to internal fixation, all main fragments of the scapular body must be identified and carefully cleaned. If a fracture is operated on with a delay of a week or more after the injury, callus formation makes identification of fracture lines more difficult. In most cases translation occurs with overlap of the main fragments of the lateral border resulting in considerable shortening. The lateral border may be reduced using different techniques.[7,9,14,24] The simplest method has proved to be careful reduction using a small rasp inserted between the two fragments of the lateral border. Another option is to drill a 3.5 mm cortical screw into the distal fragment as a support for a bone hook. In a more robust skeleton, it is sufficient to drill a hole through both cortices for insertion of the tip of the bone hook but this may not be advisable in the elderly patient with poor bone stock. Cole et al.[9,24] recommend reduction by a small external fixator but this may impair visualization and manipulation in the surgical wound.

Final stabilization may be performed with a 2.7 DCP or reconstruction plate fixed to each of the main fragments of the lateral border by two or, where necessary, three screws.

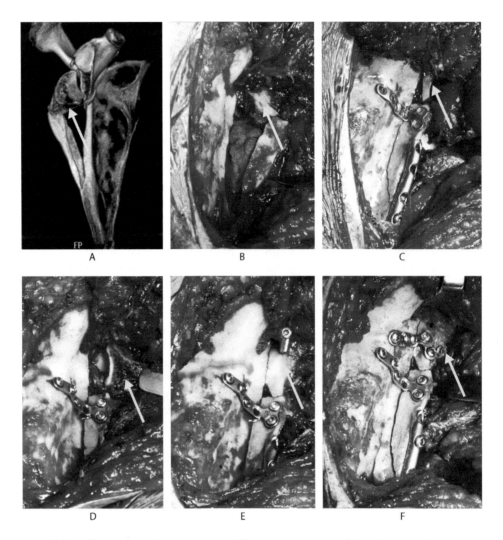

Figure 18.11 Fracture of the inferior glenoid in a 68–year-old woman. **(a)** Lateral 3D CT view, **(b)** intraoperative view before reconstruction, **(c–f)** step-by-step reconstruction in the infero-superior direction. The yellow arrow indicates an articular fragment of the inferior glenoid.

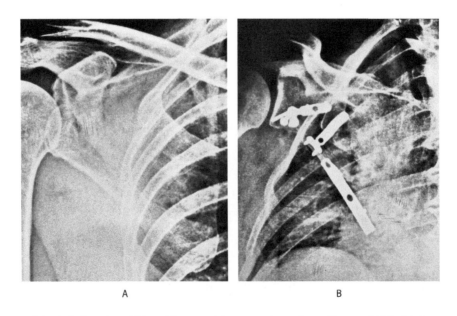

Figure 18.12 Fracture of the inferior glenoid in a 68-year-old woman (case from Figure 18.11). **(a)** Anteroposterior (AP) shoulder radiograph after injury, **(b)** AP shoulder radiograph after surgery.

In muscular individuals, or in case it is necessary to eliminate shear and bending forces, it is better to use a 3.5 mm plate. Stabilization of a fracture of the medial border of the scapular body in the region of the spino-medial angle is of secondary importance, compared with the internal fixation of the lateral border and is only required if the fracture is insufficiently stabilized after completion of internal fixation of the lateral border.

Fractures of processes may be fixed by cerclage wiring, lag screws, or 2.7 L-shaped or T-shaped plates. Displaced small fragments of the rim of the acromion or tip of the coracoid should preferably be excised and the muscle reinserted. Fractures of the finger-like projection of the coracoid may be well stabilized by a cannulated lag screw fitted with a washer.[18]

POSTOPERATIVE TREATMENT

Postoperatively, the arm is immobilized in a sling. Drainage is removed by 48 hours after operation. Radiographs of the shoulder are obtained using the Neer I and II views. The patient is checked as an outpatient for the first time 2 weeks after operation to ensure wound healing and remove sutures. Radiographs are taken at 6 weeks (Neer I and II views), 3 months (Neer I view) and 1 year after operation (Neer I and II views). As a rule scapular fractures heal in 6–12 weeks.

Of great importance for the final outcome is proper rehabilitation. Passive range of motion exercises of the shoulder begin on the first postoperative day and continue for about 6 weeks. A continuous passive motion (CPM) machine can be very helpful in the early stages. Active range of motion exercises start at approximately 4–5 weeks postoperatively, depending on the extent of the surgical approach and presence of other injuries (clavicular fracture, acromioclavicular dislocation). The range of motion is assessed at 6 weeks and, if unsatisfactory, motion is examined under general anaesthesia and gentle manipulation performed, as necessary. Active resistance exercises may be started approximately 8 weeks after operation. All restrictions of the shoulder range of motion are lifted, as a rule, 3 months postoperatively (Figures 18.13 and 18.14). The final subjective, objective and radiological outcomes of the operation cannot be assessed before 1 year after the operation at the earliest.

COMPLICATIONS

Both conservative and operative treatment of scapular fractures can result in a number of early and late complications, leading to pain and limitation of the range of motion.[7,14–30]

Complications of non-operative treatment

These complications manifest themselves usually some time after the injury.

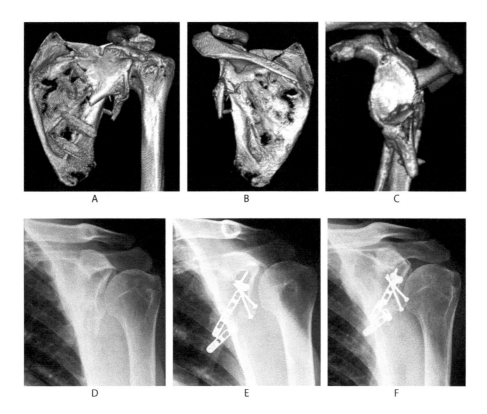

Figure 18.13 Fracture of the inferior glenoid and anatomical body fracture in a 70–year-old man. (a) Anterior 3D CT view, (b) posterior 3D CT view, (c) lateral 3D CT view, (d) anteroposterior (AP) shoulder radiograph after injury, (e) Neer I view after surgery, (f) Neer I view 3 months after surgery; the fracture has healed, but the plate broke due to the patient's failure to respect the postoperative programme as he started intensive body building 3 weeks after operation!

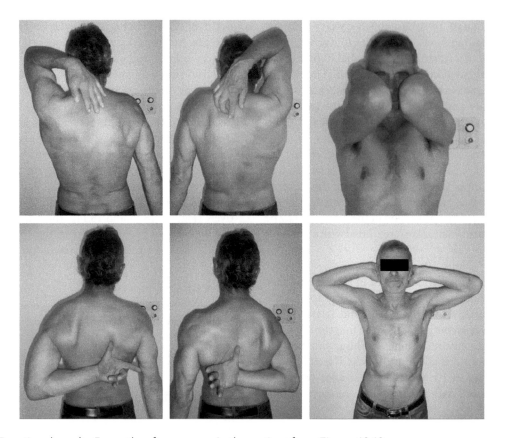

Figure 18.14 Functional results 5 months after surgery in the patient from Figure 18.13.

MALUNION

Malunion is the most frequent complication of non-operative treatment of scapular fractures. Healing of extra-articular fractures in a non-anatomical position has several consequences. It changes the relationship between the glenoid and the scapular body, and, as a result, the course of muscles of the rotator cuff, which affects their function. Subjectively, it is manifested by feelings of weakness, pain and limitation of the range of motion. Pace et al.[26] described secondary degenerative changes of the rotator cuff in these cases. Malunion may also result in impingement syndrome. Fractures of the glenoid that have healed in displacement result in incongruity, instability of the joint, or both, and subsequently lead to osteoarthrosis.

The prominence of a bony fragment healed in displacement may be painful. Irregularity of the surface of the scapular body limits smooth motion of the scapula over the chest wall. The solution is excision of the projecting part of the bone.[25]

DELAYED UNION

Delayed union is rare in the elderly but was described by Curtis et al.[27] in a 15-year-old sportsman with an undisplaced fracture of the scapular neck. CT examination at 6 months after the injury, undertaken because of persisting pain of the shoulder, revealed non-union of the undisplaced fracture of the scapular neck that healed after transcutaneous electrical stimulation.

NON-UNION

Non-unions of the scapular body are rare. In 2009, Marek et al.[28] found only 15 in the English literature, all of them after non-operative treatment. Non-unions of the acromion were also reported.[6] The solution is internal fixation or excision of the ununited fragment.

INJURY TO THE SUPRASCAPULAR NERVE

In fractures of the scapular neck, the suprascapular nerve may become entrapped in the fracture line. This injury is manifested by atrophy of the infraspinatus.

RIB NON-UNION

Rib non-union may be a rare cause of chronic pain after a scapular fracture. In the four reported cases,[29] the situation was successfully treated by internal fixation.

Complications of operative treatment

These complications may be divided into intraoperative, early postoperative and late postoperative complications. Their numbers reported by individual authors vary.

INTRAOPERATIVE COMPLICATIONS

Intraoperative complications include injuries to the suprascapular nerve, malreduction and intra-articular perforation by screws. In an analysis of 212 cases, Lantry et al.[18] found injury to the suprascapular nerve in 2.4%, with atrophy of the infraspinatus developing postoperatively. It is difficult to distinguish whether the injury was caused by the original trauma or during operation. Reduction of the fragments may be hard to achieve in comminuted fractures of the scapular body or in significantly displaced fractures of the scapular neck, particularly if operation is performed late after the injury. Insertion of screws into the joint cavity is a rare complication that may occur particularly during internal fixation of the scapular neck or of the lateral border of the scapula.

EARLY POSTOPERATIVE COMPLICATIONS

Early postoperative complications include first of all haematoma, and superficial and deep infection.[20,22,23] Haematoma has to be evacuated and washed out surgically. Most cases of superficial infection may be treated with antibiotics and local care. Deep infection requires debridement of the surgical wound and, where necessary, removal of any unstable implant. A relatively common complication is a limited range of motion of the shoulder, requiring manipulation if it persists for more than 6 weeks after surgery.[20,23]

LATE COMPLICATIONS

Late complications are reported quite frequently. Failure of internal fixation required re-operation in several cases,[18,20,23] as did non-union after internal fixation.[26]

Malreduction of the glenoid fossa fragment results in residual incongruity. Hardegger et al.[20] had to reoperate for joint instability. Malunion of the inferior scapular angle was recorded by Bartoníček et al.[14] Several cases of heterotopic ossification have been described, in one of which there occurred entrapment of the axillary nerve requiring surgical decompression.[18] Acromial impingement after internal fixation of the glenoid has had to be treated by acromioplasty.[23] Prominence of implants, requiring their removal, is a problem mainly in fractures of the acromion, scapular spine, or associated clavicular fractures.[18,30] One report also describes a late infection, 11 months after operation, requiring hardware removal.[23] In addition, one breakage of a plate was recorded after several years in a healed scapular fracture.[23]

Post-traumatic osteoarthrosis after scapular fractures occurs in 1.9% of cases. In two cases it had to be managed by arthrodesis.[18,20,22] Currently, the method of choice in such cases is shoulder arthroplasty.

CONCLUSION

Scapular fractures are not typical osteoporotic injuries; nevertheless, in patients older than 60 years they show certain differences as compared to younger patients. Most injuries in older patients are caused by a medium- or low-energy mechanism, usually a fall. The number of fractures of the glenoid and processes, and of associated injuries to the proximal humerus, is slightly higher, while fractures of the scapular neck are almost absent. In addition, it is also necessary to take into account insufficiency of the rotator cuff. The treatment of older patients is predominantly conservative. Indications for surgery are primarily displaced intra-articular fractures with an unstable glenohumeral joint. Surgery for extra-articular fractures is only indicated in physically active patients, particularly in cases of marked displacement. Fractures can be fixed with standard implants; locking plates are usually not necessary. Older patients usually require more postoperative physiotherapy and the functional outcome is as a rule worse as compared to younger patients.

ACKNOWLEDGEMENT

Preparation of this chapter was supported by a grant from the IGA, Ministry of Health, Czech Republic NT/14092: Diagnostics and operative treatment of displaced intra-articular fractures of the scapula.

REFERENCES

1. Bartoníček J, Cronier P. History of the treatment of scapular fractures. *Arch Orthop Trauma Surg* 2010;130:83–92.
2. Court-Brown C, McQueen MM, Tornetta P. *Trauma*. Philadelphia, PA: Lippincott Williams & Wilkins, 2006, pp. 68–88.
3. Ideberg R, Grevsten S, Larsson S. Epidemiology of scapular fractures. *Acta Orthop Scand* 1995;66:395–397.
4. Bartoníček J, Džupa V, Frič V, Pacovský V, Skála-Rosenbaum J, Svatoš F. Epidemiology and economic implications of fractures of proximal femur, proximal humerus, distal radius and fracture-dislocation of ankle. *Rozhl Chir* 2008;87:213–219.
5. Tuček M, Bartoníček J, Frič V. Osseous anatomy of scapula: Its importance for classification of scapular body fractures. *Ortopedie (Czech Orthopaedics)* 2011;5:104–109.
6. Goss TP. Fractures of the scapula. In: Rockwood CA, Matsen FA, Wirth MA, Lippitt SB (eds.). *The Shoulder*. 3rd ed. Philadelphia, PA: Saunders, 2004, pp. 413–454.
7. Shindle MK, Wanich T, Pearle AD, Warren RF. Atraumatic scapular fractures in the setting of chronic rotator cuff tear arthropathy: A report of two cases. *J Shoulder Elbow Surg* 2008;17:e4–e8.
8. Bartoníček J. Scapular fractures. In: Court-Brown CM, Heckman JD, McQueen MM, Ricci WM, Tornetta P III (eds.). *Rockwood and Green's Fractures in Adults*. 8th ed. Philadelphia, PA: Wolters Kluwer, 2015, pp. 1475–1501.
9. Cole PA, Marek DJ. Shoulder girdle injuries. In: Standard JP, Schmidt AH, Gregor PJ (eds.). *Surgical Treatment of Orthopaedic Trauma*. New York: Thieme, 2007, pp. 207–237.
10. Chochola A, Tuček M, Bartoníček J, Klika D. CT diagnostics of scapular fractures. *Rozhl Chir* 2013;92:385–388.

11. Ada JR, Miller ME. Scapular fractures. Analysis of 113 cases. *Clin Orthop Rel Res* 1991;269:174–180.

12. Euler E, Habermeyer P, Kohler W, Schweiberer L. Skapulafrakturen—Klassifikation und Differentialtherapie. *Orthopäde* 1992;21:158–162.

13. Orthopaedic Trauma Association. Fracture and dislocation compendium. Scapular fractures. *J Orthop Trauma* 2007;(Suppl 1): S68–71.

14. Bartoníček J, Frič V. Scapular body fractures: Results of the operative treatment. *Int Orthop* 2011;35:747–753.

15. Bartoníček J, Tuček M, Frič V, Obruba P. Fractures of the scapular neck: Diagnosis, classifications and treatment. *Int Orthop* 2014;38(10):2163–2173.

16. Hersovici D, Roberts CS. Scapular fractures: To fix or not to fix? *J Orthop Trauma* 2006;20:227–229.

17. Zlowodski M, Bhandari M, Zelle BA, Kregor PJ, Cole PA. Treatment of scapular fractures: Systematic review of 520 fractures in 22 case series. *J Orthop Trauma* 2006;20:230–233.

18. Lantry JM, Roberts CS, Giannoudis PV. Operative treatment of scapular fractures: A systematic review. *Injury* 2008;39:271–283.

19. Cole PA, Gauger EM, Schroder LK. Management of scapular fractures. *J Am Acad Orthop Surg* 2012;20:130–141.

20. Hardegger F, Simpson LA, Weber BG. The operative treatment of scapular fractures. *J Bone Joint Surg Br* 1984;66-B:725–731.

21. Bauer G, Fleischmann W, Dussler E. Displaced scapular fractures: Indication and long-term results of open reduction and internal fixation. *Arch Orthop Trauma Surg* 1995;114:215–219.

22. Adam FF. Surgical treatment of displaced fractures of the glenoid cavity. *Int Orthop* 2002;26:150–153.

23. Schandelmaier P, Blauth M, Schneider C, Krettek C. Fractures of the glenoid treated by operation. *J Bone Joint Surg Br* 2002;84-B:173–177.

24. Cole PA, Gauger EM, Herrera DA, Anavian J, Tarkin IS. Radiographic follow-up of 84 operatively treated scapular neck and body fractures. *Injury* 2012;43:327–333.

25. Martin SD, Weiland AJ. Missed scapular fracture after trauma. A case report and a 23-year follow-up report. *Clin Orthop Rel Res* 1994;299:259–262.

26. Pace AM, Stuart R, Brownlow H. Outcome of glenoid neck fractures. *J Shoulder Elbow Surg* 2005;14:585–590.

27. Curtis C, Sharma V, Micheli L. Delayed union of a scapular fracture—An unusual cause of persistent shoulder pain. *Med Sci Sport Exerc* 2007;12:2095–2098.

28. Marek DJ, Sechriest VF, Swiontkowski MF, Cole PA. Case report: Reconstruction of a recalcitrant scapular neck nonunion and literature review. *Clin Orthop Relat Res* 2009;467:1370–1376.

29. Anavian J, Guthrie T, Cole PA. Surgical management of multiple painful rib nonunions in a patient with a history of severe shoulder girdle trauma: A case report and literature review. *J Orthop Trauma* 2009;23:600–604.

30. Cole PA, Talbot M, Schroder LK, Anavian J. Extra-articular malunions of the scapula: A comparison of functional outcome before and after reconstruction. *J Orthop Trauma* 2011;25:649–656.

19

Clavicle fractures

PATRICK D.G. HENRY AND MICHAEL D. McKEE

INTRODUCTION

Non-operative management is the mainstay of treatment for most fractures of the clavicle in elderly patients. The decision to pursue surgery in the elderly patient is influenced by medical and social factors. Biological and technical factors related to fracture patterns unique to osteoporotic bone are also a consideration. The goals of orthopaedic surgery, which are typically to achieve a united fracture with good alignment, must be balanced with a thorough appreciation of the risks, needs and expectations of the elderly patient with a clavicle fracture.

EPIDEMIOLOGY AND FRACTURE TYPES

Fractures of the clavicle account for approximately 2.6–4% of all fractures, and 35–44% of all fractures involving the shoulder girdle, making it one of the most commonly fractured bones in the human body.[1-3] In 1967, Allman published an anatomic classification system of clavicle fractures, dividing the clavicle into medial third, middle third and lateral third types.[4] Several variations of this system have been proposed which account for more specific morphological patterns such as comminution and degree of displacement including the AO/OTA system,[5] but none have taken into account the factors of patient age (paediatric vs elderly) or bone quality (i.e. osteoporosis).

Bone quality declines slowly after 30 years of age and osteoporosis most commonly develops after the age of 50.[6,7] Osteoporotic bone is known to have a greater propensity to fracture, and elderly patients have a greater propensity to fall.[8,9] Taken together, it would seem that clavicle fractures would be most likely to occur in elderly individuals.

Surprisingly, this is not observed in practice, as clavicle fractures are most commonly observed young males.[1,3,10] However, there is a second, smaller peak in elderly patients, and this peak has nearly equal male and female preponderance (Figure 19.1). In the young male population, the mechanism of injury is most commonly a sporting injury or motor vehicle crash, whereas simple falls are the most frequent mechanism in older patients.[3,10,11]

Between the ages of 18 and 30, medial third fractures account for 2% of all fractures, middle third 80% and lateral third 18%.[3] Among patients aged 61 and over, 10% of clavicle fractures involve the medial third, 67% the middle third and 23% the lateral third.[3] Therefore, while middle third fractures remain the most common subgroup, there is a higher proportion of both lateral and medial third clavicle fractures in the elderly compared to the younger population.[10]

For midshaft fractures, patients over 50 have a higher incidence of comminuted and displaced fractures than patients below 50.[11] Since the fracture mechanism is more commonly low energy in older patients, the increased complexity of fracture morphology in elderly patients can likely be attributed to poor bone quality.

ASSOCIATED INJURIES AND COMORBIDITIES

Comorbidities and associated injuries frequently complicate both the management and outcome of trauma in the elderly. Clavicle fractures, particularly those associated with higher energy trauma, are commonly associated with other injuries.[12] Elderly patients have less ability to tolerate these injuries, which is reflected by the finding in the

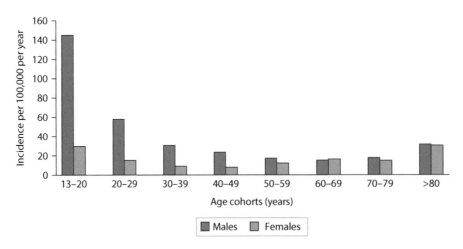

Figure 19.1 Epidemiology of clavicle fractures according to gender and age (From Robinson CM. *J Bone Joint Surg Br.* 1998;80:476–84. Reprinted with permission and copyright of the British Editorial Society of Bone and Joint Surgery.)

orthopaedic literature that the elderly are 4–4.6 times more likely to die than younger patients as a result of a traumatic event of similar severity, and age older than 65 years is an independent predictor of death after trauma.[13]

The presence of a clavicle fracture may be a particular sign of associated injuries and subsequent poor outcomes in higher energy geriatric trauma patients. Of all long bone fractures, the presence of a clavicle fracture is the strongest predictor of mortality in the geriatric trauma population, with a mortality rate of 23% in those patients (compared to a mortality rate of 13% in geriatric trauma patients without clavicle fractures).[12] In contrast, young major trauma patients with clavicle fractures have a mortality rate of only 7%.

Interestingly, while associated injuries are found in greater prevalence in the population of elderly high-energy trauma patients,[14,15] this may not be the case with high-energy clavicle fracture patients. In a recent study by Keller et al., geriatric patients with clavicular fractures had an average admission Injury Severity Score, Glasgow Coma Scale score, and Brain, Thorax, and Lower Extremity Abbreviated Injury Scores that were worse compared with the average scores of elderly or younger patients without clavicle fractures, but were similar to the average scores of younger patients with clavicle fractures.[12] The authors concluded that the increased mortality rate in elderly clavicle fracture patients is due to the associated injuries being less well tolerated by the elderly, rather than the associated injuries being more severe in the elderly.

CLINICAL EVALUATION OF THE ELDERLY PATIENT WITH A CLAVICLE FRACTURE

History

The same principles apply to history taking for the elderly patient as for younger patients, and some may argue that the history is even more important in the elderly patient.

The history is important both for determining the diagnosis and for deciding on treatment. One must bear in mind that due to the prevalence of osteoporosis, lower energy injuries may lead to significant fractures in the older patient, and therefore descriptions of a relatively benign fall should not diminish the surgeon's suspicion for fracture. Similarly, geriatric patients are often better able to tolerate clavicle fractures and their sequelae and are frequently far less symptomatic (and in some cases asymptomatic) compared with younger patients[1]; therefore in elderly patients, the absence of pain should not lead the surgeon to rule out a fracture without carrying out a thorough work-up.

In addition, it should be remembered that a fall in an elderly person might have resulted from a cardiac or neurological event that may require further investigation and treatment, especially if surgical intervention is contemplated.

Despite the importance of history, unfortunately, history taking can be challenging if dementia or delirium is present. In these cases, witnesses or family members may be able to describe the injury in order to indicate to the physician the injured body part. As important as identifying the injured body part is determining the patient's baseline functional level and daily physical demands, which are crucial in order to decide on the best treatment plan.

Physical examination

The physical examination of the clavicle is no different for elderly patients than it is for the rest of the population and includes observation of skin abnormalities (swelling, bruising, ecchymosis and deformity), palpation for pain, an upper extremity neurological examination and a thorough shoulder evaluation (within the patient's limitations) in order to rule out concomitant injury to the shoulder girdle.

What is different is that greater attention should be paid to the general physical examination of the other body systems. This is important for two reasons. First, it can rule out injury to other body systems that, if missed, may lead to worse consequences than in the younger patient. Second, it may identify underlying comorbidities, which are more common in elderly patients and play a large role in determining the appropriate treatment. If surgery is being considered, an underlying comorbidity may be identified which may alter the risk–benefit ratio of surgical intervention and affect the decision to proceed.

Imaging

Anteroposterior (AP) radiographs of the clavicle are sufficient to diagnose clavicle fractures and should be performed in all elderly patients complaining of shoulder pain after trauma. A chest radiograph may also suffice, and in some cases provides additional information by including the contralateral clavicle for comparison, and will likely be needed as part of the preoperative evaluation if surgery is being considered. Surgical decision-making is aided by assessing displacement on the AP view; however, this can be misleading as the deformity may occur in the AP plane and thus the true displacement will be masked by bony overlap. Dedicated views such as the Zanca view (cephalic tilt of 15 degrees) can be particularly helpful in this regard and are also used for lateral clavicle fractures (as well as direct views of the acromioclavicular joint) in order to avoid overlap from the upper ribs.[16] This is a standard part of our evaluation of these injuries.

As is the case with younger patients, advanced imaging of the clavicle such as CT scanning is rarely required, except in cases of medial clavicle fracture or dislocation, or to evaluate for associated fractures in the shoulder girdle. However, in elderly trauma patients who often receive a chest CT in the emergency department, the scan should be carefully scrutinized for a clavicle fracture, as these are a prognostic marker for increased mortality in the geriatric population.[12]

CLAVICLE FRACTURE MANAGEMENT OPTIONS: SPECIAL CONSIDERATIONS IN THE ELDERLY PATIENT

Non-operative management

Non-operative management remains the mainstay of treatment for all non-displaced or minimally displaced fractures of both the midshaft and distal clavicle in elderly patients. The decision of when to consider surgery is complex and discussed below, although even displaced fractures may be successfully managed non-surgically in the elderly. Several points should be considered that are unique to the elderly patient with a clavicle fracture being treated non-operatively.

A standard protocol for non-operative management of both midshaft and distal clavicle fractures is the use of a conventional sling for 4–8 weeks, with active self-assisted stretching exercises initiated when fracture healing is established.[8,17] The sling must be worn with adequate padding, as elderly patients lose collagen and fat within the subcutaneous layer of the skin, making the skin vulnerable to frictional or pressure-related injury from the shoulder strap, which has been reported.[18] In addition, the effect of the sling on the independent function of an elderly patient must be considered.

Operative indications

The role of surgery for displaced midshaft clavicle fractures is still debated. Numerous prospective and randomized studies demonstrate improved functional outcomes for certain subsets of patients treated with surgical management of displaced midshaft clavicle fractures, as well as a reduced incidence of non-union and malunion.[16,19–22] As observed in a recent large-scale population study, the dissemination of this information led to an increase in the number of clavicle fractures treated operatively in the past decade.[23] This study excluded patients over the age of 60, therefore it is not known if this trend has occurred in elderly patients as well.

Similarly, there is ongoing debate regarding the appropriate indications for operative treatment of distal clavicle fractures in patients of all ages. Non-operative management is the mainstay for non-displaced fractures, but displaced fractures have a high rate of non-union.[24,25] Surgery reduces the risk of non-union for displaced fractures,[26] but several studies have shown similar outcomes in patients treated with surgery or non-operatively (Figure 19.2).[27–29]

The issue of choosing surgery over non-operative treatment for clavicle fractures (both midshaft and distal) is considerably more complex in the elderly patient. Osteoporotic bone might be more prone to delayed and non-union.[17,30] Elderly patients have more comorbidities and anaesthesia poses a greater risk. Older patients are also more prone to postoperative delirium and confusion. The soft tissues are thinner and more prone to dehiscence and wound complications, which in turn can lead to colonization or infection. The bone is weaker, and thus more prone to failure of fixation. Physical demands are usually much less, making the problem of non-union (or malunion) less of a functional deficit compared to a younger person who engages in manual work or sport. Finally, non-union of the clavicle seems to be more readily tolerated in elderly individuals compared to younger patients (Figure 19.3).

In 2004, a study by Robinson et al. followed a cohort of 101 patients who had sustained displaced distal clavicle fractures and were treated non-operatively.[28] At 7–24 months after injury, 14 patients had severe persistent symptoms and underwent delayed surgical treatment. The remaining 87 patients never progressed to surgery, and the non-union rate in those patients was 21%. Surprisingly, there was no difference in the Constant or SF-36 scores between those who had delayed surgery, those who developed non-union with non-operative management and those who healed with non-operative management. These results suggest that an

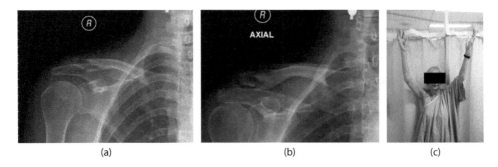

(a)   (b)   (c)

Figure 19.2 **(a)** A displaced distal clavicle fracture. The 75-year-old low demand patient was treated non-operatively with a sling for 4 weeks followed by progressive passive, then active range of motion exercises and return to full activity by 3 months. **(b)** The same fracture at 6 months after injury, demonstrating non-union. **(c)** Despite the non-union, the patient is asymptomatic with no pain and has an excellent range of motion.

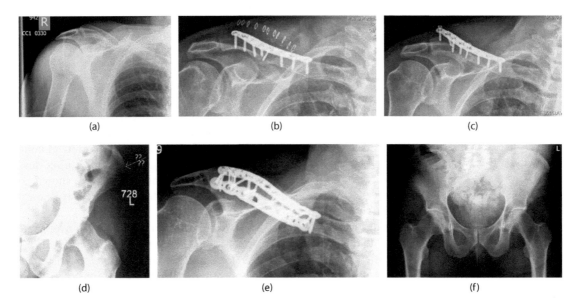

(a)   (b)   (c)

(d)   (e)   (f)

Figure 19.3 **(a)** A 68-year-old man with a painful clavicle non-union 9 months after injury. **(b)** The patient was treated with open reduction and internal fixation using a pre-contoured non-locking plate and iliac crest bone graft. **(c,d)** The patient presented 5 weeks after surgery with sudden onset of hip pain that occurred when rising from a chair. In addition, he complained of persistent shoulder discomfort. He admitted to using his arm for light activities and removing his sling after 2 weeks, but had not engaged in any heavy lifting. Radiographs revealed his plate had loosened and failed, and he had sustained a minimally displaced fracture of the iliac crest at the bone harvest site. The loosening of the distal part of a superior plate via axial pull out of the screws is typical. **(e)** Revision surgery was carried out using two plates for added stability, and strict instructions for sling use for 6 weeks followed by passive range of motion exercises for another 4 weeks. The fracture had appeared to fully heal by 3 months postoperatively. **(f)** The pelvic fracture was treated symptomatically and healed by 3 months after injury.

initial trial of non-operative management seems prudent in the large majority of displaced clavicle fractures, and that the indication for surgery should be unacceptable symptoms that can be addressed with surgery, and it might be wise to wait a year.

In summary, for elderly patients, the surgical indications for clavicle fractures should be largely based on the physical requirements and goals for the individual patients, comorbidities, associated soft-tissue injuries and the specific fracture morphology. For example, open (Figure 19.4) and impending open (Figure 19.5) fractures are indications for surgical intervention even in the elderly patient.

Operative techniques

If surgery is chosen, several devices are available for the management of midshaft clavicle fractures, including non-locking plates, locking plates, pre-contoured plates and intramedullary devices (modified large calibre pins, modern 'locking' clavicle nails and titanium elastic nails). While osteoporosis predisposes elderly patients to clavicle fracture, it is also a problem in osteosynthesis of these fractures. The major technical problem that surgeons face is the difficulty in obtaining stable fixation of the implant due to osteoporotic bone, which experiences significant forces, even at

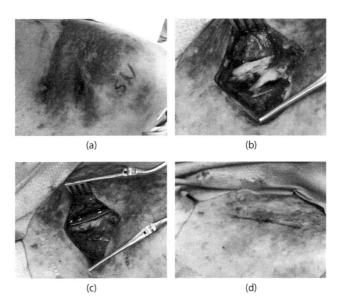

Figure 19.4 (a) An open clavicle fracture in an elderly patient after a fall downstairs. There is extensive bruising, a small puncture wound and tethering of the adjacent soft tissues in the fracture site (case courtesy of Dr. Sarah Ward). (b) Intraoperative photograph of the fracture site following extrication of the entrapped soft tissue, debridement and thorough irrigation. (c) Anatomic reduction and fixation with a pre-contoured clavicular plate. (d) A two-layered closure with mattress sutures for the skin resulted in a much improved clinical picture. The underlying stability provided by the plate fixation enhanced rapid soft-tissue healing and resulted in infection-free bony union.

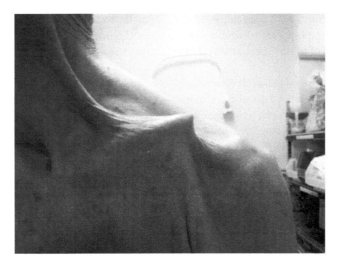

Figure 19.5 An impending open fracture of the midshaft clavicle in a 90-year-old patient. As with an open fracture, this degree of soft-tissue tenting is an indication for operative fixation, even in an elderly patient.

rest. The load transmitted at the bone–implant interface can often exceed the reduced strain tolerance of osteoporotic bone, and pullout strength is reduced.[31,32] These features result in compression-plate fixation being less reliable in osteopenic or osteoporotic bone,[33] and therefore alternatives to standard non-locked plating should be considered when fixing clavicle fractures in geriatric patients, such as the utilization of locked plates, longer plates, multiple plates (superior and anterior) or intramedullary fixation.[31]

A study comparing non-locked to locked plating of displaced midshaft clavicle fractures in patients over the age of 60 found an 11% rate of hardware failure in the non-locked group, with zero failures in the locked plating group.[34] An additional study compared non-locking plates to intramedullary fixation with a Knowles pin, finding that the plated group had longer surgical incisions, longer operative time, a higher infection rate, more complaints of symptomatic hardware and a hardware failure rate of 7% compared to 0% in the Knowles pin group.[35] These studies reinforce the notion that clavicular bone in the elderly is biologically and mechanically weaker than in the younger population. Locking plates and intramedullary devices have biomechanical advantages over simple plates when treating osteopenic fractures,[36,37] and alternative techniques should be considered when fixing clavicle fractures in such patients.

Our treatment of choice for displaced midshaft fractures of the clavicle is a pre-contoured clavicular plate with locking capability, typically in the superior position. A minimum of four screws proximal and distal to the fracture site are typically used. Anteriorly placed plates are used in very thin patients where hardware prominence is a concern or can be used to supplement a superior plate when fixation is poor (Figure 19.3).

Operative treatment of distal clavicle fractures can be a challenge in patients of all ages because of the small and usually comminuted distal metaphyseal fragment and the proximity to the acromioclavicular joint.[38] These issues are compounded in the elderly patient as the poor quality bone leads to additional challenges with fixation. Options for fixation include hook plates, distal locking plates and variations on techniques that indirectly reduce the fracture through coracoclavicular fixation (either rigid or flexible).[39-42] Transacromial K-wire fixation leads to high complication rates, is largely historical and not recommended.[43] To date, no studies have compared these techniques in the elderly patient. In osteoporotic bone the hook plate has several biomechanical advantages over other methods in that the fixation can be spread over a large area of the clavicle, locking plates are available and the acromion is also used as part of a lever mechanism that provides additional bony support.

Our treatment of choice for displaced distal clavicle fractures in the elderly is to use a pre-contoured distal clavicular plate with a distal 'flare' to allow for the insertion of multiple (locked) screws into the metaphyseal fragment. We also have a hook plate available for use if the distal fixation is suboptimal.

OUTCOMES AND COMPLICATIONS

There is a general belief that outcomes following management of displaced clavicle fractures in adults and elderly patients are in general much less satisfactory than in the young.[44] As discussed above, mortality is significantly greater in elderly patients who sustain clavicle fractures due to high-energy injury, with a mortality rate of 23% in those patients compared to only 7% in young patients. This is typically related to a reduced capacity to tolerate associated injuries.[12] In lower energy fractures, there is also evidence that outcomes tend to be worse in elderly patients.

Simple fracture patterns with minimal displacement have been shown to have excellent healing rates and outcomes with non-operative management. In the elderly population, even with low-energy injury mechanisms, comminution and displacement of clavicle fractures is greater than in young patients (11), which is likely a reflection of the reduced bone quantity and quality in patients with osteoporosis. Several high-quality studies have demonstrated that comminution

and displacement are important factors that portend a greater risk of non-union and malunion in non-operatively treated midshaft clavicle fractures.[19,28] In addition to this, elderly patients have reduced bone healing capacity due to both local and systemic factors,[30,45] and age has been shown to be an independent risk factor for non-union in the clavicle.[46,47] Taken together, these features suggest treatment of midshaft clavicle fractures through operative or non-operative means has a greater likelihood of failure and subsequent non-union than in young patients.

The corollary to this observation is the finding that elderly patients have a much better tolerance of non-union and malunion in the clavicle than younger patients.[1,27,28] The phenomenon of elderly patients adapting well to fracture non-union and malunion has been observed in other upper extremity fractures as well, including the distal radius[48] and the proximal humerus.[49,50] This is likely related in part to decreased activity levels, but there may be other factors at play as well.

Despite lower activity levels in the elderly, and an observed ability to tolerate non-union better than the younger population, elderly patients are at a disadvantage in recovering from clavicle fractures, and this effect is multifactorial. First, the fracture patterns tend to be worse, as described above. Second, the effect of comorbidities (such as cardiac disease or diabetes) indirectly complicates the management plan and can have acute and unexpected negative affects during recovery (Figure 19.3). Third, whether or not surgery is planned, sling use and minimal resisted activity through the shoulder is almost universally prescribed for a certain period of time with any clavicle fracture. This would preclude the use of a cane or walker for ambulatory support, which many elderly people utilize. This may be particularly disruptive as the sling use combined with narcotic pain medication may affect the patient's equilibrium. Even if ambulatory aids are not used, older patients have less ability to compensate by using only one hand for their daily activities. If their independence is compromised, these problems may result in the patient being unable to continue independently and requiring inpatient care at a care facility.

CONCLUSION

In the last decade our understanding and management of clavicle fractures has undergone a major transition.[23] Once considered benign and universally treated conservatively with presumed excellent results, the clavicle is now identified as a complex bone with important functions in the shoulder girdle that is prone to complications if injured and managed incorrectly. Non-operative management remains the mainstay of treatment; however, operative treatment is now indicated for displaced fractures in active young (<60 years of age) individuals. The threshold for operative intervention is higher in older patients, given the higher operative complication rate and the lower physical demands of elderly patients. Special challenges in the elderly include osteoporotic bone with a higher intrinsic non-union rate, the greater likelihood of fixation failure and need for revision surgery, associated comorbidities which can complicate decision-making, increased mortality in high-energy injuries and greater difficulties in the recovery period. A case-by-case decision-making process can tailor both the management plan and surgical techniques (if necessary) to the individual. Measures to achieve union should be tempered by evaluation of the surgical risks and the patient's needs.

REFERENCES

1. Khan LA, Bradnock TJ, Scott C, Robinson CM. Fractures of the clavicle. *J Bone Joint Surg Am.* 2009;91(2):447–60.

2. Nordqvist A, Petersson C. The incidence of fractures of the clavicle. *Clin Orthop Relat Res.* 1994;(300):127–32.

3. Postacchini F, Gumina S, De Santis P, Albo F. Epidemiology of clavicle fractures. *J Shoulder Elbow Surg.* 2002;11(5):452–6.

4. Allman FL Jr. Fractures and ligamentous injuries of the clavicle and its articulation. *J Bone Joint Surg Am.* 1967;49(4):774–84.

5. Marsh JL, Slongo TF, Agel J, Broderick JS, Creevey W, DeCoster TA, et al. Fracture and dislocation classification compendium—2007: Orthopaedic Trauma Association classification, database and outcomes committee. *J Orthop Trauma.* 2007;21(10 Suppl):S1–133.

6. Dennison E, Cole Z, Cooper C. Diagnosis and epidemiology of osteoporosis. *Curr Opin Rheumatol.* 2005;17(4):456–61.

7. Mosekilde L. Age-related changes in bone mass, structure, and strength—Effects of loading. *Z Rheumatol.* 2000;59(Suppl 1):1–9.

8. Sambrook P, Cooper C. Osteoporosis. *Lancet.* 2006;367(9527):2010–18.

9. van Helden S, van Geel AC, Geusens PP, Kessels A, Nieuwenhuijzen Kruseman AC, Brink PR. Bone and fall-related fracture risks in women and men with a recent clinical fracture. *J Bone Joint Surg Am.* 2008;90(2):241–8.

10. Robinson CM. Fractures of the clavicle in the adult. Epidemiology and classification. *J Bone Joint Surg Br.* 1998;80(3):476–84.

11. Stegeman SA, Nacak H, Huvenaars KH, Stijnen T, Krijnen P, Schipper IB. Surgical treatment of Neer type-II fractures of the distal clavicle: A meta-analysis. *Acta Orthop.* 2013;84(2):184–90.

12. Keller JM, Sciadini MF, Sinclair E, O'Toole RV. Geriatric trauma: Demographics, injuries, and mortality. *J Orthop Trauma.* 2012;26(9):e161–5.

13. Tornetta P 3rd, Mostafavi H, Riina J, Turen C, Reimer B, Levine R, et al. Morbidity and mortality in elderly trauma patients. *J Trauma.* 1999;46(4):702–6.

14. Lehmann R, Beekley A, Casey L, Salim A, Martin M. The impact of advanced age on trauma triage decisions and outcomes: A statewide analysis. *Am J Surg.* 2009;197(5):571–4; discussion 4–5.

15. Perdue PW, Watts DD, Kaufmann CR, Trask AL. Differences in mortality between elderly and younger adult trauma patients: Geriatric status increases risk of delayed death. *J Trauma.* 1998;45(4):805–10.

16. McKee MD. Clavicle fractures. In: Court-Brown CM, Heckman JD, McQueen MM, et al., editors. *Rockwood & Green's Fractures in Adults.* Part 2. Philadelphia, PA: Lippincott Williams & Wilkins; 2010. pp. 1427–74.

17. Lopez MJ, Edwards RB III, Markel MD. Healing of normal and osteoporotic bone. In: An YH, editor. *Orthopaedic Issues in Osteoporosis.* Boca Raton, FL: CRC Press; 2003, pp. 55–70.

18. Radha S, Vaghela KR, Konan S, Radford W. Polysling skin pressure necrosis—A complication of shoulder immobilisation. *BMJ Case Rep.* 2012;2012. doi: 10.1136/bcr-2012-006671.

19. Canadian Orthopaedic Trauma Society. Nonoperative treatment compared with plate fixation of displaced midshaft clavicular fractures. A multicenter, randomized clinical trial. *J Bone Joint Surg Am.* 2007;89(1):1–10.

20. Kulshrestha V, Roy T, Audige L. Operative versus nonoperative management of displaced midshaft clavicle fractures: A prospective cohort study. *J Orthop Trauma.* 2011;25(1):31–8.

21. Zlowodzki M, Zelle BA, Cole PA, Jeray K, McKee MD, Evidence-Based Orthopaedic Trauma Working Group. Treatment of acute midshaft clavicle fractures: Systematic review of 2144 fractures: On behalf of the Evidence-Based Orthopaedic Trauma Working Group. *J Orthop Trauma.* 2005;19(7):504–7.

22. Evaniew N, Simunovic N, McKee MD, Schemitsch E. Cochrane in CORR®: Surgical versus conservative interventions for treating fractures of the middle third of the clavicle. *Clin Orthop Relat Res.* 2014;472(9):2579–85.

23. Leroux T, Wasserstein D, Henry P, Khoshbin A, Dwyer T, Ogilvie-Harris D, et al. Rate of and risk factors for reoperations after open reduction and internal fixation of midshaft clavicle fractures: A population-based study in Ontario, Canada. *J Bone Joint Surg Am.* 2014;96(13):1119–25.

24. Edwards DJ, Kavanagh TG, Flannery MC. Fractures of the distal clavicle: A case for fixation. *Injury.* 1992;23(1):44–6.

25. Neer CS 2nd. Fractures of the distal third of the clavicle. *Clin Orthop Relat Res.* 1968;58:43–50.

26. Flinkkila T, Ristiniemi J, Hyvonen P, Hamalainen M. Surgical treatment of unstable fractures of the distal clavicle: A comparative study of Kirschner wire and clavicular hook plate fixation. *Acta Orthop Scand.* 2002;73(1):50–3.

27. Nordqvist A, Petersson C, Redlund-Johnell I. The natural course of lateral clavicle fracture. 15 (11–21) year follow-up of 110 cases. *Acta Orthop Scand.* 1993;64(1):87–91.

28. Robinson CM, Cairns DA. Primary nonoperative treatment of displaced lateral fractures of the clavicle. *J Bone Joint Surg Am.* 2004;86-A(4):778–82.

29. Rokito AS, Zuckerman JD, Shaari JM, Eisenberg DP, Cuomo F, Gallagher MA. A comparison of nonoperative and operative treatment of type II distal clavicle fractures. *Bull Hosp Jt Dis.* 2002;61(1–2):32–9.

30. Giannoudis P, Tzioupis C, Almalki T, Buckley R. Fracture healing in osteoporotic fractures: Is it really different? A basic science perspective. *Injury.* 2007;38(Suppl 1):S90–9.

31. Giannoudis PV, Schneider E. Principles of fixation of osteoporotic fractures. *J Bone Joint Surg Br.* 2006;88(10):1272–8.

32. Stromsoe K. Fracture fixation problems in osteoporosis. *Injury.* 2004;35(2):107–13.

33. Gardner MJ, Demetrakopoulos D, Shindle MK, Griffith MH, Lane JM. Osteoporosis and skeletal fractures. *HSS J.* 2006;2(1):62–9.

34. Pai HT, Lee YS, Cheng CY. Surgical treatment of midclavicular fractures in the elderly: A comparison of locking and nonlocking plates. *Orthopedics.* 2009;32(4).

35. Lee YS, Lin CC, Huang CR, Chen CN, Liao WY. Operative treatment of midclavicular fractures in 62 elderly patients: Knowles pin versus plate. *Orthopedics.* 2007;30(11):959–64.

36. Cornell CN, Ayalon O. Evidence for success with locking plates for fragility fractures. *HSS J.* 2011;7(2):164–9.

37. Johanson NA, Litrenta J, Zampini JM, Kleinbart F, Goldman HM. Surgical treatment options in patients with impaired bone quality. *Clin Orthop Relat Res.* 2011;469(8):2237–47.

38. Tiren D, van Bemmel AJ, Swank DJ, van der Linden FM. Hook plate fixation of acute displaced lateral clavicle fractures: Mid-term results and a brief literature overview. *J Orthop Surg Res.* 2012;7:2.

39. Ballmer FT, Gerber C. Coracoclavicular screw fixation for unstable fractures of the distal clavicle. A report of five cases. *J Bone Joint Surg Br.* 1991;73(2):291–4.

40. Jackson WF, Bayne G, Gregg-Smith SJ. Fractures of the lateral third of the clavicle: An anatomic approach to treatment. *J Trauma.* 2006;61(1):222–5.

41. Mall JW, Jacobi CA, Philipp AW, Peter FJ. Surgical treatment of fractures of the distal clavicle with polydioxanone suture tension band wiring: An alternative osteosynthesis. *J Orthop Sci.* 2002;7(5):535–7.

42. Yamaguchi H, Arakawa H, Kobayashi M. Results of the Bosworth method for unstable fractures of the distal clavicle. *Int Orthop.* 1998;22(6):366–8.

43. Kona J, Bosse MJ, Staeheli JW, Rosseau RL. Type II distal clavicle fractures: A retrospective review of surgical treatment. *J Orthop Trauma.* 1990;4(2):115–20.

44. Van Houwelingen A, McKee M, Schemitsch E. Clavicular fractures: Open reduction internal fixation. In: Wiss D, editor. *Master Techniques in Orthopaedic Surgery: Fractures.* 2nd ed. Philadelphia, PA: Lippincott Williams & Wilkins; 2006.

45. Nikolaou VS, Efstathopoulos N, Kontakis G, Kanakaris NK, Giannoudis PV. The influence of osteoporosis in femoral fracture healing time. *Injury.* 2009;40(6):663–8.

46. Robinson CM, Court-Brown CM, McQueen MM, Wakefield AE. Estimating the risk of nonunion following nonoperative treatment of a clavicular fracture. *J Bone Joint Surg Am.* 2004;86-A(7):1359–65.

47. Wu CL, Chang HC, Lu KH. Risk factors for nonunion in 337 displaced midshaft clavicular fractures treated with Knowles pin fixation. *Arch Orthop Trauma Surg.* 2013;133(1):15–22.

48. Arora R, Lutz M, Deml C, Krappinger D, Haug L, Gabl M. A prospective randomized trial comparing nonoperative treatment with volar locking plate fixation for displaced and unstable distal radial fractures in patients sixty-five years of age and older. *J Bone Joint Surg Am.* 2011;93(23):2146–53.

49. Court-Brown CM, Garg A, McQueen MM. The translated two-part fracture of the proximal humerus. Epidemiology and outcome in the older patient. *J Bone Joint Surg Br.* 2001;83(6):799–804.

50. Zyto K. Non-operative treatment of comminuted fractures of the proximal humerus in elderly patients. *Injury.* 1998;29(5):349–52.

20

Proximal humeral fractures

STIG BRORSON

INTRODUCTION

Recent data indicate that many elderly patients with displaced proximal humeral fractures do not benefit from surgical treatment even for complex fracture patterns. In most elderly there is some degree of physical impairment after fracture regardless of the fracture anatomy and treatment modality. The degree of impairment does not always correlate with the complexity of the injury, and some patients with minimally displaced fractures end up with pain and poor function. Pre-injury infirmity and medical comorbidity may strongly influence outcome after surgery. Poor bone quality and degenerative changes in the rotator cuff may further compromise outcome after surgery. Studies of outcome in the average patient or younger patients with proximal humeral fractures may not apply to older patients, and observer administrated measures of shoulder function (e.g. the Constant score) used to evaluate patients in clinical studies may overemphasize the importance of range of motion and strength. Some elderly patients have lower functional demands and may accept restricted strength and range of motion if pain is limited.

Evidence based recommendations for management according to age are sparse and the optimal treatment for proximal humeral fractures in the elderly has yet to be determined. The methodological quality of clinical studies has generally been low and recommendations are inconsistent. Current best evidence consists largely of uncontrolled case series with a high risk of bias. Systematic reviews have been unable to demonstrate statistically and clinically significant benefits from surgical treatment of displaced fractures.[1-12] However, within the last 5 years new data from randomized trials have appeared in the literature[13-21] and protocols for planned randomized studies have been published.[22-26] It is likely that the next updated Cochrane review will contain some evidence based treatment recommendations.

This chapter is based on data from current randomized clinical trials, systematic reviews and large epidemiological studies. Whenever possible, data on elderly (65–79 years) and very elderly (80 and above) patients are reported separately.

EPIDEMIOLOGY

Proximal humeral fractures account for 4–6% of all fractures.[27-29] They are associated with advanced age and osteoporosis. Falls from standing height account for about 94% of proximal humeral fractures in patients older than 65.[30] The incidence of proximal humerus fractures is third only to fractures of the distal radius and the proximal femur. The lifetime risk of a fracture of the proximal humerus in women aged 50 or more is 13%.[31] An increase in incidence from 32 to 105/100,000 per year between 1970 and 2002 has been reported.[32] In women older than 80 years the incidence increased from 90 to 294/100,000 per year. Kannus et al. reported an incidence of 298/100,000 per year in women older than 60,[33] and Court-Brown et al. recently reported an incidence of 392/100,000 per year in women older than 65, and 520/100,000 per year in women older than 80, compared to 147 and 261/100,000 per year in men.[34] At least one previous fracture was found in 47% of patients. Together with low bone mineral density and diminished stature, a previous fracture is an independent risk factor for fracture of the proximal humerus.[30] The odds ratio for sustaining concomitant fractures in patients with a proximal humeral fracture is 2.2.[35] In a Swedish population the median survival time after a proximal humeral fracture was 9 years compared to 12 years in controls.[36] In women aged 60–79 years with a proximal humeral fracture, the lifetime risk for a hip fracture is about 2.4.[37] In an unselected population of 629 elderly patients a poor functional outcome (Constant score <55) after a proximal humeral fracture was reported in 27% of the patients after 1 year.[38] The functional outcome was unrelated to fracture severity.

Distribution of fracture types

In Neer's classic article from 1970,[39] minimally displaced fractures accounted for 85% of all proximal humeral fractures in a population of patients with a mean age of 56 years (Figure 20.3). More recent studies in elderly populations have reported less than 50% minimally displaced fractures (Table 20.1).[28,40,41] Three fracture patterns within the Neer classification (minimally displaced, two-part surgical neck and three-part [surgical neck and greater tuberosity]) account for 86% of all proximal humerus fractures.[28] Fracture complexity is age and sex specific. Overall, 70% of three- and four-part displaced fractures occur in patients older than 60 years with a 1.72 times higher rate of three- and four-part fractures in women compared to men.[42]

Rotator cuff integrity

Fjalestad et al.[43] obtained MRI scans of 76 non-operatively treated fractures of the proximal humerus at the time of injury and 1 year after injury and reported 22 full thickness defects presented at the time of injury and 10 more 1 year after fracture. Function measured with the Constant score 1 year after fracture corresponded with the presence of a rotator cuff defect at the time of injury. Given that rotator cuff degeneration is a normal part of human aging, it is not clear if this rate is greater than expected for age.

Bahrs et al.[44] sonographically examined 302 patients with proximal humeral fractures 4 years after the injury. In 17% a full thickness rotator cuff defect was found on the fractured side, compared to 4% on the contralateral side. There was a significant correlation between four-part fractures and full thickness rotator cuff defects.

Table 20.1 The reported 'prevalence' of minimally displaced fractures in four populations

Study	Fractures (n)	Minimally displaced fractures (%)	Age (mean and range)
Neer[39]	300	85	56 (22–89)
Court-Brown et al.[28]	1,027	49	66 (13–98)
Tamai et al.[41]	509	36	65 (18–95)
Roux[40]	329	43	70 (16–97)

IMAGING

Preoperative assessment of proximal humeral fractures is usually limited to radiographs. A series including an anterior-posterior view, a perpendicular lateral/scapular view and an axillary view is most useful. In some institutions the axillary view is omitted because it can be painful. This may be unwise because the axillary view is the best view for ensuring the glenohumeral joint is not dislocated, it can add important information on tuberosity displacement, and it improved observer agreement on classification in one study.[45] Most institutions have access to computed tomography (CT) and three dimensional (3D) CT scans (Figures 20.1 and 20.2). CT may be useful in preoperative planning and might improve reliability of classification but no study has reported a beneficial effect on patient outcome. There is generally limited correspondence between imaging appearance and functional outcome in proximal humeral fractures.

CLASSIFICATION

Agreement on classification

The most frequently used classification systems for proximal humeral fractures are the Neer classification (Figure 20.3) and the AO classification (Figure 20.4). They are based on assessment of two or three perpendicular preoperative radiographs.

Within the last two decades, more than 20 observer studies and systematic reviews have reported that orthopaedic surgeons greatly disagree when classifying according to the Neer and the AO classification. They have consistently reported low kappa values for interobserver agreement ranging from 0.17 to 0.52.[46,47] A review on agreement on four commonly used classification systems between experienced shoulder surgeons only, reported kappa values of between 0.15 and 0.44.[48] Lack of consistency in classification may explain some of the discrepancies in treatment recommendations and outcome found in the scientific literature.

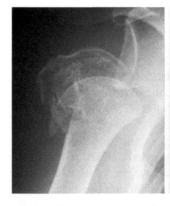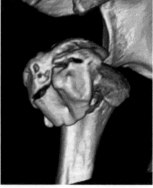

Figure 20.1 Radiograph (anterior-posterior view) and 3D CT reconstruction of a proximal humeral fracture.

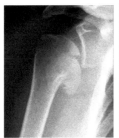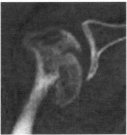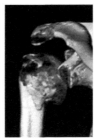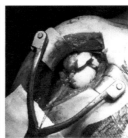

Figure 20.2 Imaging modalities in an articular surface fracture (AO C3.3). Radiograph, CT-scan, 3D CT reconstruction and intraoperative view.

Figure 20.3 The 16 categories of the Neer classification. A fracture is considered displaced if one or more of the four anatomical segments (greater tuberosity, lesser tuberosity, humeral head and humeral shaft) are displaced more than 1 cm or angulated more than 45°. (Modified from Neer CS. *J Bone Joint Surg Am* 1970;52(6):1077–89. With permission from Rockwater, Inc.)

The low agreement does not improve through selection of experienced observers, by using high quality radiographs only, by reducing the number of classification categories, or by adding advanced pictorial modalities like CT scans or 3D CT reconstructions.[46] However, systematical training of observers seems to improve agreement especially among shoulder specialists.[49] There seems to be less agreement on complex fracture patterns.[50]

Agreement on treatment

One study found significantly higher agreement on treatment recommendations than on classification in a consecutive series of 193 radiographs from emergency units or orthopaedic wards.[50] Only one third of changes in classification were followed by changes in treatment recommendation. The highest agreement was found on non-surgical treatment. It was concluded that the low observer agreement on the Neer classification may have less clinical importance than previously assumed.

Translation between classification systems

A common 'fracture language' is lacking in the scientific literature on proximal humeral fractures and the two most common classification systems are partly incompatible.[51] The result is difficulty comparing outcome from clinical studies and 'translation' of treatment recommendations into other populations. For example, minimally displaced fractures can correspond to 15 different AO subgroups, 'classic' four-part fractures (Neer category 12) can be classified into at least eight different AO subgroups and AO type C fractures can appear as one-, two-, three- or four-part fractures in the Neer classification.[51]

Important clinical information is lost within both classification systems. Most importantly, a distinction between varus and valgus displacement is not found in the Neer classification, and a concise definition of displacement is lacking in the AO classification. Researchers and surgeons are encouraged to report data from both classification systems and cross-check their coding.[51] Classification of proximal humeral fractures remains a challenge in clinical and scientific orthopaedics.

TREATMENT

Non-surgical treatment includes sling immobilization with immediate pendulum exercises or delayed active and passive exercises. Some advocate attempted manipulative reduction (usually impaction of the humeral shaft into the head of the humerus) followed by non-operative treatment. Surgical treatments include manipulative reduction and percutaneous pinning, and open reduction and internal fixation with

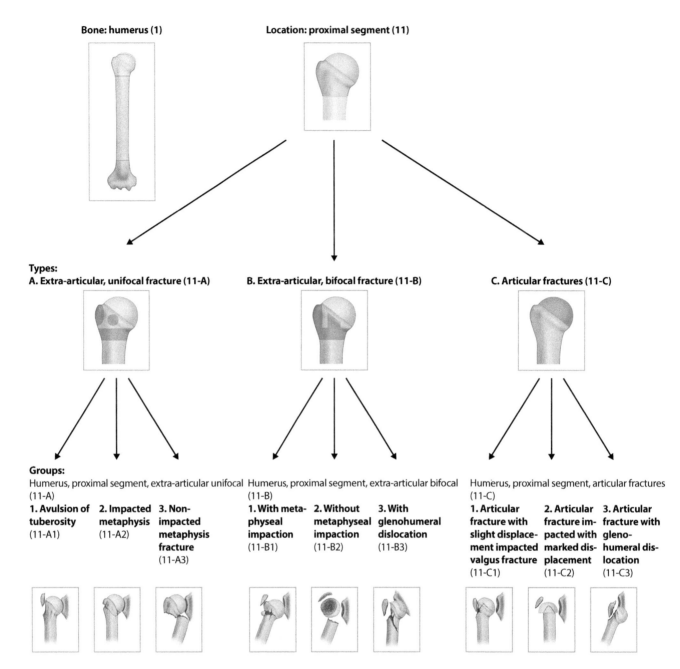

Bone: humerus (1)

Location: proximal segment (11)

Types:
A. Extra-articular, unifocal fracture (11-A)

B. Extra-articular, bifocal fracture (11-B)

C. Articular fractures (11-C)

Groups:

Humerus, proximal segment, extra-articular unifocal (11-A)

1. Avulsion of tuberosity (11-A1)	**2. Impacted metaphysis (11-A2)**	**3. Non-impacted metaphysis fracture (11-A3)**

Humerus, proximal segment, extra-articular bifocal (11-B)

1. With metaphyseal impaction (11-B1)	**2. Without metaphyseal impaction (11-B2)**	**3. With glenohumeral dislocation (11-B3)**

Humerus, proximal segment, articular fractures (11-C)

1. Articular fracture with slight displacement impacted valgus fracture (11-C1)	**2. Articular fracture impacted with marked displacement (11-C2)**	**3. Articular fracture with glenohumeral dislocation (11-C3)**

Figure 20.4 The three types and nine groups of the AO classification. The 27 subgroups are not shown. (Reprinted from Marsh JL et al. *J Orthop Trauma* 2007;21(10 Suppl):S1–133. With permission from RightsLink.)

a plate and screws, tension-band wiring, suture anchors, Kirschner wires, helix wiring, transosseous suture or intramedullary fixation. Arthroplasty options include proximal humerus hemiarthroplasty and reverse total shoulder arthroplasty.

The proportion of surgically treated patients has increased within the last two decades. Khatib et al.[52] reviewed 50,100 patients aged 65 years or older in New York State between 1990 and 2010 with a proximal humeral fracture. The incidence of proximal humeral fractures increased by 28% in the period, but the number of operatively treated fractures increased by more than 40%. The use of locking plates increased from 2001 to 2010 and the

use of reverse arthroplasty increased from 2006 to 2010. The use of hemiarthroplasty decreased correspondingly from 2000 to 2010.

Treatment decision

An offer of operative treatment is based on patient age, comorbidity, pre-injury function, fracture anatomy, bone quality, soft tissue injury, the surgeon's experience and the expectations of the patient.

In a retrospective review of 229 proximal humeral fractures (mean age 77), Okike et al.[53] reported factors associated with the decision for operative treatment in patients older than 60. Factors associated with operative treatment included younger age, other orthopaedic injury requiring surgery, AO type C fractures, associated dislocation, translation displacement and management by shoulder or upper extremity specialists compared to trauma specialists.

Medical comorbidity merits careful consideration. Each additional medical comorbidity increases the risk of readmission after surgery by 20%.[54] A 90-day readmission rate of 14% was reported among 27,017 surgically treated proximal humeral fractures. Three out of four readmissions were associated with medical diagnoses. Among surgical causes, locking plate osteosynthesis had a significant higher readmission rate (29%) compared to hemiarthroplasty (16%) and reverse prostheses (20%). Mechanical complications after locking plate use accounted for 11% of all readmissions. Infections were also more common in locking plates.[55]

Surgical or non-surgical treatment in the elderly?

There is limited high level evidence to inform decision making for displaced fractures in elderly patients. A Cochrane review[5] included 23 small and heterogeneous randomized trials with a total of 1,238 included patients. Six studies with 270 patients compared surgical and non-surgical treatments. It was concluded that the current evidence is weak, and shows no benefit with surgery. One out of nine surgically treated patients needed additional surgery.

Den Hartog et al.[4] included 1096 patients from 33 randomized and non-randomized trials comparing hemiarthroplasty and non-surgical treatment for three- or four-part fractures and found no advantage with surgery.

Kontakis et al.[7] included 810 hemiarthroplasties, mainly for four-part fractures, from 16 randomized and non-randomized studies and concluded that there is inadequate evidence to support the effectiveness of primary hemiarthroplasty in the treatment of complex proximal humerus fractures.

Jia et al.[6] included 286 three- and four-part fractures from seven randomized trials. They found no clinically important differences between surgical treatment (hemiarthroplasty or internal fixation with tension band or locking plate) and non-surgical treatment.

Nanidis et al.[56] included 486 patients from two randomized trials and eight observational studies comparing surgical and non-surgical treatment modalities. They concluded that there was no demonstrable difference in outcomes between fractures managed surgically or non-surgically.

A large randomized clinical trial comparing non-surgical and surgical management of displaced fractures involving the surgical neck has recently been published.[57] A total of 250 patients referred for surgical treatment were randomized into non-surgical treatment or surgical treatment. The surgical group was managed according to the surgeon's preference. Patients were recruited from 33 British orthopaedic departments and all patients followed the same

rehabilitation protocol. After 24 months, 215 patients were evaluated with the Oxford Shoulder Score. No difference in outcome between the two groups was found. The rates of complications and secondary surgery were not significantly different, but the cost of surgery was significantly higher.

Timing of surgery

There is no consensus on the optimal time for surgery. Both patient related and potentially modifiable factors influence the time to surgery.

Menendez and Ring[58] reported data on 70,000 surgically managed proximal humeral fractures from a national database. Of these, 87% were operated on within 2 days and 13% had surgery after 3 days or more. Increased inpatient morbidity was found after delayed surgery, even when comorbidities and fracture complexity were controlled for. Late surgery was associated with inpatient adverse events (odds ratio 2.1) and prolonged postoperative stay (odds ratio 1.7). In the late surgery group, 57% were discharged to rehabilitation or skilled nursing facility compared to 28% in the early surgery group. Weekend admission was the most common reason for delay in surgery caused by unavailability of the surgeon or operating room facilities.

Outcome assessment with the Constant score in the elderly

The most commonly used outcome assessment instrument in studies of proximal humeral fractures is the Constant–Murley Shoulder score.[59-61] It is an observer administrated shoulder specific outcome instrument consisting of four parts: pain (15 points), activities of daily living (20 points), range of motion (40 points) and strength (25 points). The maximum score is 100 points indicating a shoulder with no disability.

Several problems in the use of the Constant score in the elderly should be mentioned. First, the Constant score can be non-adjusted, age- and sex-adjusted or compared to the opposite shoulder. In several studies it is not clear which version is used. Comparison across studies is therefore problematic. Second, the Constant score decreases with age. Better strength and range of motion is expected in younger patients and the non-adjusted Constant score will therefore underestimate outcome in the elderly. Third, strength cannot be assessed in patients with less than 90 degrees of abduction. This means a subtraction of 25 points from the total Constant score plus the points withdrawn due to the impaired mobility. A satisfied elderly patient with a pain-free shoulder but less than 90 degrees of abduction may therefore have a misleading poor Constant score.

NON-SURGICAL TREATMENT

Only few studies have systematically collected data on outcome after non-surgical treatment of different fracture patterns.

In a systematic review Iyengar et al.[62] reported data from 12 studies covering 650 non-surgically treated fractures. There were 49% minimally displaced, 25% two-part, 21% three-part and 5% four-part displaced fractures. Mean age was 65 years and the mean follow-up time was 46 months. Radiographically, healing was obtained in 98% but 13% had complications. Only 2% developed avascular necrosis of the humeral head. The mean Constant score was 74.

Court-Brown et al.[63] reported outcome after non-surgical treatment of 125 AO B1.1 fractures followed for 1 year. This fracture pattern represents about 15% of all proximal humeral fractures and appears as minimally displaced fractures, two-part greater tuberosity fractures, two-part surgical neck fractures or three-part fracture fractures (Figure 20.5) within the Neer classification (Figure 20.3). Mean age was 71 years and 81% of the patients reported a good to excellent result after non-surgical treatment with a mean Constant score of 72 overall and 67 in patients aged 80–89. The outcome depended on age and displacement of the fractures, but generally B1.1 fractures can be managed non-surgically.

Hanson et al.[64] prospectively followed 160 non-surgically treated fractures. There were 75 minimally displaced, 60 two-part, 23 three-part and 2 four-part fractures according to the Neer classification, and 85 type A, 71 type B and 4 type C according to the AO classification. Four underwent surgical fixation with locking plates or screws, and five had arthroscopic subacromial decompression because of impingement. After 1 year, the difference in mean Constant score between the injured and the contralateral shoulder was 8%. The risk for delayed union and non-union was 7%.

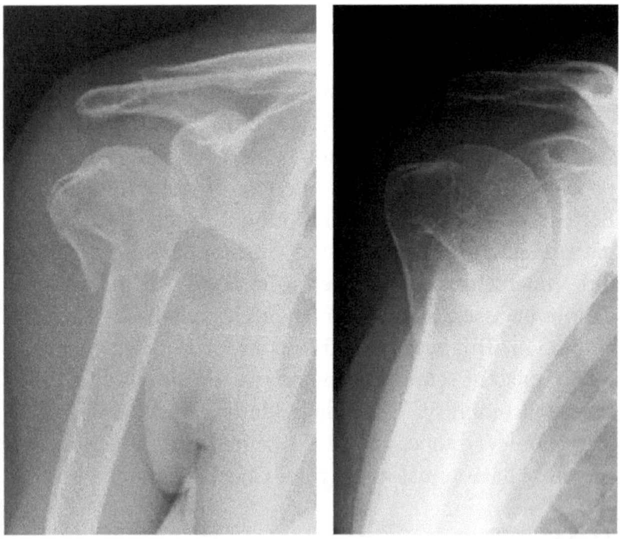

Gaebler et al.[65] followed 376 minimally displaced fractures for 1 year after non-surgical treatment. According to the AO classification, there were 76% type A, 23% type B and 2% type C fractures. Good or excellent results were seen in 88%. A strong association between age and outcome was reported. Accounting for the influence of age, there was no difference in outcome between fracture types. They found no association between displacement of the greater tuberosity and outcome.

Olsson et al.[36] reported 253 non-surgically treated patients followed for 12 years. The median survival time was 9 years compared to 12 years in controls with no proximal humeral fractures. Cardiovascular disease and malignancy were the most common causes of death in both groups. A 16% cumulative survival difference compared to matched controls was reported.

Minimally displaced fractures

The AO classification (Figure 20.4)[66] has enabled a more detailed analysis of fracture patterns classified as minimally displaced within the Neer classification (Figure 20.3). Fractures classified as minimally displaced according to Neer can appear as 15 different subtypes within the AO classification.[51]

Calvo et al.[67] reported epidemiological data from 912 postmenopausal women aged 50 years or older with minimally displaced fractures treated non-surgically on an outpatient basis. A subpopulation of proximal humeral fractures was evaluated by phone after 6 months with the Disabilities of the Arm, Shoulder and Hand (DASH) (n = 25) and EuroQol 5D (EQ-5D) questionnaires (n = 46). Overall, 67% reported pain and discomfort and a significant reduction in functional capacity especially in self-care (45%), activities of daily living (57%) and anxiety or depression (33%).

Rehabilitation in non-surgically treated patients

Non-surgically treated patients are usually referred to training. Few randomized trials have studied the effect and optimal timing of training in non-surgically treated patients with proximal humeral fractures.

Lefevre-Colau et al.[68] randomized 74 patients with impacted proximal humeral fractures to mobilization after 3 days or 3 weeks. Early mobilization was safer and more effective. The difference was statistically significant after 3-month follow-up, but not after 6 and 12 months.

Hodgson et al.[69] randomized 86 minimally displaced two-part fractures to training within 1 week or training after 3 weeks of immobilization. Slow recovery continued for 2 years after injury. Better recovery after 1 year with immediate physiotherapy was found. The Constant score was significantly higher after 8 and 16 weeks in the early mobilization group but the difference at 1 year was not statistically significant.

Admission   16 months

Figure 20.5 A 62-year-old woman with a valgus-impacted fracture (AO B1.1) treated with a sling and early exercises pre-injury function was obtained despite healing with slight angulation.

Kristiansen et al.[70] randomized 85 mainly non-displaced fractures to training after 1 or 3 weeks. They reported significantly less pain after early mobilization at 3 months but the effect could not be found after 6 months. No further recovery was found after 1 or 2 years.

SURGICAL TREATMENT

Locking plate osteosynthesis

Within the last two decades, the advent of locking plate technology has changed the possibilities for operative management of proximal humeral fractures. However, an increase in operatively treated patients has been followed by a proportional increase in revision surgery.[71] Bell et al.[72] reported a 26% increase in surgically managed proximal humeral fractures between 2000 and 2005. The absolute rate of surgically managed proximal humeral fractures increased from 13% to 16%. Osteosynthesis increased by 29% compared to 20% for hemiarthroplasty.

Primary hemiarthroplasty

Hemiarthroplasty was introduced half a century ago to treat unrepairable fractures of the proximal humerus. Functional outcome can be satisfactory in the elderly if the tuberosities heal without resorption and with an intact rotator cuff. Pain is usually satisfactory, but the average motion is poor, especially when there is rotator cuff insufficiency. Olerud et al.[18] randomized 55 elderly (mean age 77) with acute displaced four-part fractures to hemiarthroplasty or non-surgical treatment. There was a significant difference in EQ-5D favouring hemiarthroplasty, but no difference in the Constant score. Additional surgery was performed for three hemiarthroplasties and one non-surgically treated fracture. The authors suggested that the difference between the EQ-5D and Constant score could be ascribed to the subjectivity of self-reported outcome measurement.

Intramedullary locking nails

Zhu et al.[73] compared intramedullary nailing and locked plating in a randomized trial of 51 two-part fractures (mean age 55 years). A slightly better American Shoulder and Elbow Surgeons (ASES) score in locked plating, but no difference in Constant score, was found after 1 year. No difference in function was found after 3 years. The complication rate was 31% in locking plates compared to 4% in nails. In a review of eight observational studies with 215 patients treated with intramedullary nails for two-, three- and four-part fractures, Giannoudis et al.[74] reported good functional outcome, even in four-part fractures. Mean union rate was 96% and the mean complication rate was 25%. However, the mean age was younger than 70 years in all included studies. The use of intramedullary nails in the elderly has not been addressed in randomized trials and no recommendations can be given based on the current literature.

Primary reverse prosthesis

In elderly patients with poor bone stock it may be impossible to obtain satisfactory fixation of the tuberosities to an anatomical hemiarthroplasty, and in some elderly patients the rotator cuff is deficient. In such cases the primary insertion of a reverse shoulder arthroplasty can be an option. By moving the centre of rotation laterally and distally, the deltoid muscle can be mobilized and some forward elevation and abduction can be obtained, but at the cost of poor rotation. Pain relief and early mobilization have been reported, but randomized trials comparing reverse shoulder arthroplasty with hemiarthroplasty or non-surgical treatment are sparse. Nevertheless, reverse shoulder arthroplasty is increasingly used to treat acute proximal humeral fractures.

Sebastia-Forcada et al.[20] randomized 61 patients older than 70 years with four-part fractures, three-part fracture dislocations or head splitting fractures to reverse prosthesis or hemiarthroplasty. After 2 years of follow-up reverse arthroplasty had a better functional outcome measured with the Constant score, University of California-Los Angeles (UCLA) score and DASH score, less pain and a lower revision rate compared to hemiarthroplasty. In the hemiarthroplasty group the functional result was dependent on tuberosity healing.

One systematic review of observational studies on reverse shoulder arthroplasty[3] identified 18 observational studies with 430 reverse shoulder arthroplasties in acute fractures. Four studies compared outcome in reverse shoulder arthroplasty with a historical group of hemiarthroplasties. The mean Constant score was 58 which is comparable with outcome after hemiarthroplasty in four-part fractures.[4] Another systematic review[75] identified nine studies with 247 patients with a mean age of 78 (range 57–94) followed for an average of 44 months. The mean Constant score was 56. A third systematic review[76] analysed 15 studies with 377 patients. Outcome was compared to 504 matched patients treated with hemiarthroplasty. The authors reported improved forward elevation but less external rotation in 430 reverse shoulder arthroplasties. The complication rates were comparable. A fourth systematic review[11] included seven studies with 232 patients with reverse shoulder arthroplasty compared to hemiarthroplasty a mean of 44 months after surgery. The authors found no difference in the Constant score and ASES score, or range of motion between reverse shoulder arthroplasty and hemiarthroplasty, but the odds ratio for complications was 4.0 in the reverse shoulder arthroplasty group compared to the hemiarthroplasty group. The cost of reverse shoulder arthroplasty was twice the cost of hemiarthroplasty.

Other surgical options

Recently, several randomized clinical trials have compared the effect of different surgical techniques. Voigt et al.[77] randomized 56 three- and four-part fractures in patients older than 60 to locking plate osteosynthesis with fixed head screws or polyaxially locked screws positioned according to the surgeons' preference. They found no difference in functional outcome or reoperation rate. Smejkal et al.[78] randomized 55 A2, A3, B1 and C1 fractures in patients aged 18–80 years to K-wire fixation or locking plates. They found no difference in functional outcome or complication rates. Liao et al.[17] randomized 70 three- and four-part fractures (mean age 62) to K-wire tension band or screw fixation, locking plate or hemiarthroplasty. They reported more complications in K-wire fixation. The average Constant score was better in the locking plate group.

Exercises after surgery

Wirbel et al.[79] randomized 77 patients to 1 or 3 weeks of immobilization after closed reduction and percutaneous fixation. They found no statistically significant difference in Neer score after a mean follow-up of 14 months. Agorastides et al.[80] compared early mobilization (after 2 weeks) and late mobilization (after 6 weeks) after hemiarthroplasty in 49 three- and four-part fractures. They found no significant difference between groups in the Constant score or Oxford Shoulder Score after 12 months.

TREATMENT OF TWO-PART FRACTURES

Two-part surgical neck fractures comprise about 28% of all proximal humeral fractures.[28] Displaced fractures show medialization of the humeral shaft due to the pull of the pectoralis major muscle and varus or valgus angulation. Court-Brown et al.[81] analysed 126 translated two-part fractures of the surgical neck classified according to the Neer classification (mean age 72). The highest incidence was found in women older than 80. They found no difference in 1-year functional outcome between surgical and non-surgical management.

Court-Brown and McQueen[82] further reported outcome after non-surgical treatment (except for closed reduction of fracture dislocations) of 287 two-part fractures classified as AO subtype A1.2, A1.3, A2.1, A2.2, A2.3, A3.1, A3.2 or A3.3, accounting for 28% of all proximal humeral fractures. Overall, 30% of fractures occurred in patients older than 80 years. AO A3.2 (Figure 20.6) was the most common two-part fracture, and 40% of these occurred in patients older than 80. The final radiographic alignment did not correlate with outcome measured with the Constant score and Neer score. Inferior outcome was found in metaphyseal comminution (AO A3.3).

In a randomized trial with 68 displaced fractures, Zhang et al.[55] found no benefits from adding medial support screws in two-part fractures. They found, however, a significantly increased loss of reduction in three- and four-part fractures without medial support screws.

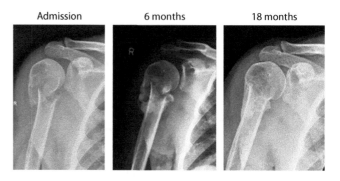

Figure 20.6 A displaced two-part surgical neck fracture (AO A3.2) in a 62-year-old woman. The radiographic appearance shows abundant callus and a persistent fracture line 6 months after injury. After 18 months of healing, full function was obtained. The patient was pain-free and has obtained pre-injury function.

TREATMENT OF THREE- AND FOUR-PART FRACTURES

Boons et al.[13] randomized 50 elderly patients with four-part fractures to hemiarthroplasty (mean age 80 years) or non-surgical treatment (mean age 76 years). They found no significant differences in function, strength or pain and concluded that no clear benefits could be detected in the patients treated with a hemiarthroplasty compared with the patients treated non-surgically, at a follow-up of 12 months.

Olerud et al.[19] randomized 60 elderly patients (mean age 74) with three-part fractures to locked plating or non-surgical treatment. At 2-year follow-up there were no significant differences in the Constant score, DASH or EQ-D5, but 30% of the locked plates had revision surgery (2 deep infections, 1 non-union, 2 avascular necroses, 3 stiffness and 2 impingement). Most fractures in the non-surgical group healed with malunion but the range of motion was surprisingly good. It was concluded that conservative treatment is sufficient in elderly patients with low functional demands.

Fjalestad et al.[15] randomized 50 patients aged 60 or more with three- or four-part fractures (AO B2 or C2) to non-surgical treatment or locking plate osteosynthesis. They found no statistically significant difference in the Constant score and functional outcome at 1-year follow-up. A functional improvement was found between 6 and 12 months, but not between 1 and 2 years.[16]

Cai et al.[14] reported a better functional outcome, pain and quality of life after hemiarthroplasty compared to locking plate osteosynthesis after 2 years of follow-up in a randomized trial of 32 four-part fractures in the elderly (mean age 72), but the difference was not statistically significant.

COMPLICATIONS

Complications can be patient-, injury- or surgeon-related.

Inpatient adverse events

Neuhaus et al.[83] reported registry data from 867,282 admissions for proximal humeral fractures. Inpatient adverse events occurred in 20%, and 2.3% died in hospital. Risk factors for adverse events were alcoholism (odds ratio 3.2), surgical treatment of other fractures (odds ratio 2.5) and concomitant fracture of the femur (odds ratio 2.5). Risk factors for discharge to a short- or long-term facility included femur fracture (odds ratio 2.9), pneumonia (odds ratio 2.5), obesity (odds ratio 2.3), congestive heart failure (odds ratio 1.8) and dementia (odds ratio 1.6).

Neuhaus et al.[84] further reported outcome after surgical and non-surgical treatment of proximal humeral fractures in 132,005 patients older than 65 years (mean age 79). Overall, 61% were non-surgically treated, 22% had osteosynthesis and 17% had hemiarthroplasty; 21% had adverse events. The risk for adverse events compared to non-surgical treatment had an odds ratio of 4.4 for hemiarthroplasty and an odds ratio of 2.7 after osteosynthesis. After accounting for comorbidities, surgical treatment was an independent risk factor for inpatient adverse events and death in elderly patients with an isolated proximal humeral fracture. It was concluded that operation carries short-term medical risks, which should be considered in decision making.

Non-surgical treatment

Data on complications after non-surgical treatment are sparse. Malunion, joint stiffness, avascular necrosis, secondary displacement and non-union should be considered. Malunion is inevitable in non-surgical treatment of displaced fractures (Figures 20.5, 20.8 and 20.10) and can be symptomatic or non-symptomatic. Capsular contracture and stiffness can result from prolonged immobilization or from non-compliance in rehabilitation. Some non-surgically treated patients develop symptomatic avascular necrosis of the humeral head. Avascular necrosis is the result of loss of perfusion of the humeral head. It can

occur after minimal displaced or displaced fractures managed non-surgically (Figure 20.9) or it can follow operative management with manipulation or soft tissue stripping. Some patients develop cephalic collapse but some heal without blood supply. Foruria et al.[85] reported 8.5% avascular necrosis in a prospective cohort of 93 non-surgically treated fractures. Secondary displacement may appear within the first weeks after trauma especially if the greater tuberosity is involved in the fracture. The initial radiographs can show a degree of inferior displacement. It usually resolves within 2 weeks after injury after pain control and early exercises. The risk of non-union in non-surgical management seems to be overestimated. Court-Brown and McQueen[86] found non-union in only 1.1% of 1,027 proximal humeral fractures. Metaphyseal comminution was followed by non-union in 8%. Translation displacement in 33–100% was followed by non-union in 10%. Hanson et al.[64] reported non-union in 7% of 160 non-surgically treated proximal humeral fractures.

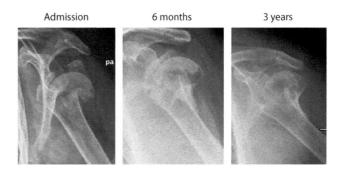

Admission   6 months   3 years

Figure 20.8 A 77-year-old infirm woman with a displaced four-part fracture treated non-surgically. Comorbidities included diabetes, hypertension and chronic obstructive lung disease. Malunion occurred and mobility was restricted to abduction and flexion of 40° and no internal or external rotation. The patient was satisfied with the functional result and reported only slight pain.

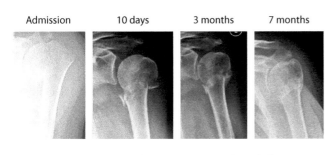

Admission   10 days   3 months   7 months

Figure 20.7 A displaced two-part surgical neck fracture (AO A3.1) in a 71-year-old woman. Spontaneous reduction of the varus displacement occurred after use of a sling and non-opioid pain management. A good functional result was obtained.

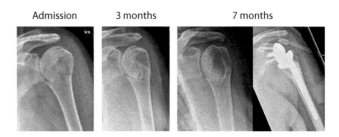

Admission   3 months   7 months

Figure 20.9 A varus impacted two-part fracture (AO C1.2) in a 67-year-old woman treated with sling immobilization. Avascular necrosis appeared and the fracture healed in varus position. The patient requested reverse total shoulder arthroplasty for severe pain and lack of motion related in part to advanced rotator cuff tendinopathy.

Admission	6 months	12 months	14 months

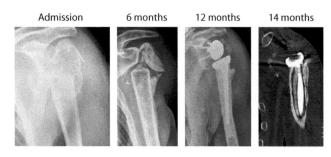

Figure 20.10 A displaced four-part fracture was treated non-operatively in a 62-year-old man with severe alcohol abuse. The fracture healed with substantial malunion with pain and limited motion. A reverse prosthesis was inserted but became infected and the stem loosened. After one-stage revision with debridement, insertion of a new reverse prosthesis and antibiotic suppression, the patient obtained abduction and flexion of 70° but no internal or external rotation. The patient had a slightly painful shoulder in activity but remained self-reliant.

Hemiarthroplasty

Insertion of a hemiarthroplasty is usually followed by good pain relief but also some degree of impaired mobility and functional loss. Most complications after hemiarthroplasty are associated with poor tuberosity fixation, but tuberosity necrosis or retraction can appear in several fracture types. Tuberosity fixation is a precondition for a good functional result. Retraction of the tuberosities will eventually lead to impaired rotation leaving the only surgical option a reverse arthroplasty. Registry data have reported a lower revision rate after fracture hemiarthroplasties compared to shoulder replacements on other indications.[87]

The importance of biceps tenodesis in hemiarthroplasty is disputed. Soliman and Koptan[21] randomized 37 four-part fractures, fracture dislocations and head-split fractures to biceps tenodesis or no tenodesis. Significantly less pain after tenodesis was reported.

Intramedullary nails

Primary insertion of an intramedullary nail enables rigid fixation in displaced fractures with minimal tuberosity displacement, especially in displaced two-part metaphyseal fractures. Complications include iatrogenic rotator cuff injury, rotator cuff dysfunction, loss of reduction, implant failure and malunion. Hardware removal is often needed.

Locking plates

The advent of locking plate technology has been considered a breakthrough in the treatment of osteoporotic fractures. However, a new generation of implant specific complications have appeared including primary and secondary screw cut-out eventually leading to glenoid destruction

Admission	Postoperative	6 months postoperative

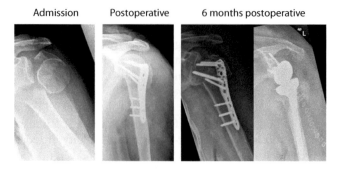

Figure 20.11 A 68-year-old woman with a displaced three-part fracture (AO B2.2) treated with a locking plate. The fracture healed, but osteonecrosis of the head resulted in screw penetration and severe glenoid destruction treated with a reverse total shoulder arthroplasty.

(Figure 20.11). Other complications commonly seen after locking plate osteosynthesis are loss of fixation, varus fracture collapse, tuberosity displacement and resorption, plate impingement and plate or screw breakage. Varus collapse is a sign of failure of the osteosynthesis and will eventually lead to screw cut-out. Predictors of poor outcome after osteosynthesis include disruption of the medial hinge, short or comminuted metaphyseal head extension and varus malreduction.

In a systematic review of observational studies Brorson et al.[88] included 12 studies with 282 AO type C fractures treated with locking plates. The mean Constant score ranged from 53 to 75. Complications included humeral neck necrosis (4–33%), screw perforations (5–20%), loss of fixation (3–16%), impingement (7–11%) and infections (4–19%). Reoperation rates varied from 6% to 44%. In another systematic review Brorson et al.[2] included 14 observational studies with 374 displaced four-part fractures treated with locking plates. Complication rates of between 16% and 64% and reoperation rates of 11–27% were reported.

Jost et al.[89] reported outcome in 121 patients (mean age 59 years) revised for a failed locking plate osteosynthesis in a tertiary referral centre. In this negatively selected cohort, a mean of three complications occurred per patient including malreduction (55%), primary screw cut-out (12%), malunion (63%), non-union (13%), avascular necrosis (68%), infection (4%), secondary screw cut-out (57%) and glenoid destruction (33%). More than 50% had four-part fractures and 20% had fracture dislocations. Anatomical reduction was obtained in less than half of the patients. Secondary arthroplasty was needed in more than half of the revisions. The mean Constant score increased from 24 to 55 after 2 years.

Shoulder mobility is often substantially restricted after revision surgery. However, not all revisions should be considered failures. Early removal of screws penetrating into the joint can save the glenoid and should be done without hesitation. Removal of the locking plate is often successful in case of impingement.[90]

Reverse prosthesis

The biomechanics of reverse shoulder arthroplasty have led to a new group of complications. Scapular notching is unique to this implant and has been reported in 0–94% of patients.[3] The long-term consequences of scapular notching remain to be evaluated. A prospective cohort study[91] with 1–17 years of follow-up concluded that the results after reverse shoulder arthroplasty in acute fractures were clinically disappointing and radiographically worrying and associated with a substantial rate of complications and reoperations. Randomized trials with long-term follow-up comparing reverse shoulder arthroplasty to hemiarthroplasty or non-surgical treatment are needed. The complication rate is high and revision surgery is challenging. Treatment options in failure of reverse shoulder arthroplasty are limited and this surgical option should be followed carefully within clinical protocols.

AUTHOR'S PREFERRED TREATMENT

Non-surgical treatment is always considered. Minimally displaced fractures are treated with sling and analgesics. Passive exercises are started within a week for faster recovery and less pain.[68-70] The patients are reassessed clinically within 2 weeks and active exercises and self-training supervised by a physiotherapist are initiated in stable fractures. Minimally displaced greater tuberosity fractures are reassessed radiographically after 10 days. Operative treatment is considered in the active elderly if the greater tuberosity displaces into the subacromial space or posteriorly.

Displaced two-part greater tuberosity fractures (Neer category 4) are often associated with glenohumeral dislocation (Neer category 6). If the greater tuberosity is in place after closed reduction the patients are managed non-surgically. In case of severe displacement of the greater tuberosity in the active elderly, operative fixation with screws, sutures through bone holes or suture anchors is done within 2 weeks.

Two-part surgical neck fractures (Neer category 3), even those with substantial displacement, are treated non-operatively. In elderly patients treated with a simple sling and analgesics the alignment sometimes improves during the first 2 weeks (Figure 20.7). Osteosynthesis with a locking plate or intramedullary nail is considered in active elderly patients if there is no contact between the fracture fragments.

I prefer non-operative treatment of three-part surgical neck and greater tuberosity fractures (Neer category 8); however, in severely displaced fractures in the active elderly hemiarthroplasty is considered. Because of the limited evidence for the benefits of using reverse arthroplasty in acute fractures, we do not use these implants in acute fractures outside clinical protocols. The result of surgical treatment depends on good tuberosity fixation. Locking plate osteosynthesis or nailing is not used in displaced three-part fractures because of the risk of primary screw penetration or secondary screw penetration due to humeral head collapse. Four-part fractures are treated non-surgically or with hemiarthroplasty. The result after surgery depends on good tuberosity fixation. Valgus-impacted four-part fractures are usually treated non-operatively. Locking plate osteosynthesis is not used in displaced four-part fractures because of high rates of severe complications in intra-articular fracture patterns.[2,88,89]

A deltopectoral approach is used in internal fixation and hemiarthroplasty except in greater tuberosity fractures where a deltoid split is preferred. Reverse prosthesis is not used in acute fractures outside clinical protocols.

CONCLUSIONS

- Non-surgical treatment should always be considered in elderly patients with fracture of the proximal humerus.
- Some elderly patients have lower functional demands and may accept a restricted range of motion if pain is limited.
- The data on treatment of proximal humeral fractures in the elderly consist largely of uncontrolled case series with a high risk of bias. A growing number of randomized trials are appearing, and they are having trouble demonstrating an advantage of operative over non-operative treatment.
- Observer agreement is low for preoperative fracture assessment.
- There is a poor correlation between radiographical alignment and symptom intensity and magnitude of disability.
- Observer administered measures of shoulder function tend to overemphasize the importance of range of motion and strength in the elderly.
- Intraoperatively conversion to a primary hemiarthroplasty should be considered if anatomical reduction and fixation is not possible with a locking plate. Failed locking plates can severely damage the glenohumeral joint in cases of screw penetration.
- Tuberosity healing in good alignment is important for a good outcome after surgical reconstruction.
- High complication rates for locking plates have been reported.
- Until higher quality evidence is available, the use of locking plates or primary reverse prostheses in complex fractures is not recommended outside clinical protocols.

REFERENCES

1. Bhandari M, Matthys G, McKee MD. Four part fractures of the proximal humerus. *J Orthop Trauma* 2004;18(2):126–7.
2. Brorson S, Frich LH, Winther A, Hrobjartsson A. Locking plate osteosynthesis in displaced 4-part fractures of the proximal humerus. *Acta Orthop* 2011;82(4):475–81.

3. Brorson S, Rasmussen JV, Olsen BS, Frich LH, Jensen SL, Hrobjartsson A. Reverse shoulder arthroplasty in acute fractures of the proximal humerus: A systematic review. *Int J Shoulder Surg* 2013;7(2):70–8.

4. Den Hartog D, de Haan J, Schep NW, Tuinebreijer WE. Primary shoulder arthroplasty versus conservative treatment for comminuted proximal humeral fractures: A systematic literature review. *Open Orthop J* 2010;4:87–92.

5. Handoll HH, Ollivere BJ, Rollins KE. Interventions for treating proximal humeral fractures in adults. *Cochrane Database Syst Rev* 2012;12:CD000434.

6. Jia Z, Li W, Qin Y, Li H, Wang D, Zhang C, et al. Operative versus nonoperative treatment for complex proximal humeral fractures: A meta-analysis of randomized controlled trials. *Orthopedics* 2014;37(6):e543–51.

7. Kontakis G, Koutras C, Tosounidis T, Giannoudis P. Early management of proximal humeral fractures with hemiarthroplasty: A systematic review. *J Bone Joint Surg Br* 2008;90(11):1407–13.

8. Lanting B, MacDermid J, Drosdowech D, Faber KJ. Proximal humeral fractures: A systematic review of treatment modalities. *J Shoulder Elbow Surg* 2008;17(1):42–54.

9. Mao Z, Zhang L, Zhang L, Zeng X, Chen S, Liu D, et al. Operative versus nonoperative treatment in complex proximal humeral fractures. *Orthopedics* 2014;37(5):e410–19.

10. Misra A, Kapur R, Maffulli N. Complex proximal humeral fractures in adults—A systematic review of management. *Injury* 2001;32(5):363–72.

11. Namdari S, Horneff JG, Baldwin K. Comparison of hemiarthroplasty and reverse arthroplasty for treatment of proximal humeral fractures: A systematic review. *J Bone Joint Surg Am* 2013;95(18):1701–8.

12. Sproul RC, Iyengar JJ, Devcic Z, Feeley BT. A systematic review of locking plate fixation of proximal humerus fractures. *Injury* 2011;42(4):408–13.

13. Boons HW, Goosen JH, van Grinsven S, van Susante JL, van Loon CJ. Hemiarthroplasty for humeral four-part fractures for patients 65 years and older: A randomized controlled trial. *Clin Orthop Relat Res* 2012;470(12):3483–91.

14. Cai M, Tao K, Yang C, Li S. Internal fixation versus shoulder hemiarthroplasty for displaced 4-part proximal humeral fractures in elderly patients. *Orthopedics* 2012;35(9):e1340–6.

15. Fjalestad T, Hole MO, Hovden IA, Blucher J, Stromsoe K. Surgical treatment with an angular stable plate for complex displaced proximal humeral fractures in elderly patients: A randomized controlled trial. *J Orthop Trauma* 2012;26(2):98–106.

16. Fjalestad T, Hole MO. Displaced proximal humeral fractures: Operative versus non-operative treatment–A 2-year extension of a randomized controlled trial. *Eur J Orthop Surg Traumatol* 2014;24(7):1067–73.

17. Liao C, Wang P, Xie Y, Fan T, Li P, Liang W. Different surgical methods for treatment of senile osteoporotic comminuted proximal humerus fracture. *Zhongguo Xiu Fu Chong Jian Wai Ke Za Zhi* 2009;23(12):1443–6.

18. Olerud P, Ahrengart L, Ponzer S, Saving J, Tidermark J. Hemiarthroplasty versus nonoperative treatment of displaced 4-part proximal humeral fractures in elderly patients: A randomized controlled trial. *J Shoulder Elbow Surg* 2011;20(7):1025–33.

19. Olerud P, Ahrengart L, Ponzer S, Saving J, Tidermark J. Internal fixation versus nonoperative treatment of displaced 3-part proximal humeral fractures in elderly patients: A randomized controlled trial. *J Shoulder Elbow Surg* 2011;20(5):747–55.

20. Sebastia-Forcada E, Cebrian-Gomez R, Lizaur-Utrilla A, Gil-Guillen V. Reverse shoulder arthroplasty versus hemiarthroplasty for acute proximal humeral fractures. A blinded, randomized, controlled, prospective study. *J Shoulder Elbow Surg* 2014;23(10):1419–26.

21. Soliman OA, Koptan WM. Proximal humeral fractures treated with hemiarthroplasty: Does tenodesis of the long head of the biceps improve results? *Injury* 2013;44(4):461–4.

22. Brorson S, Olsen BS, Frich LH, Jensen SL, Johannsen HV, Sorensen AK, et al. Effect of osteosynthesis, primary hemiarthroplasty, and non-surgical management for displaced four-part fractures of the proximal humerus in elderly: A multi-centre, randomised clinical trial. *Trials* 2009;10:51.

23. den Hartog D, Van Lieshout EM, Tuinebreijer WE, Polinder S, Van Beeck EF, Breederveld RS, et al. Primary hemiarthroplasty versus conservative treatment for comminuted fractures of the proximal humerus in the elderly (ProCon): A multicenter randomized controlled trial. *BMC Musculoskelet Disord* 2010;11:97.

24. Handoll H, Brealey S, Rangan A, Torgerson D, Dennis L, Armstrong A, et al. Protocol for the ProFHER (PROximal Fracture of the Humerus: Evaluation by Randomisation) trial: A pragmatic multi-centre randomised controlled trial of surgical versus non-surgical treatment for proximal fracture of the humerus in adults. *BMC Musculoskelet Disord* 2009;10:140.

25. Launonen AP, Lepola V, Flinkkila T, Strandberg N, Ojanpera J, Rissanen P, et al. Conservative treatment, plate fixation, or prosthesis for proximal humeral fracture. A prospective randomized study. *BMC Musculoskelet Disord* 2012;13:167.

26. Verbeek PA, van den Akker-Scheek I, Wendt KW, Diercks RL. Hemiarthroplasty versus angle-stable locking compression plate osteosynthesis in the treatment of three- and four-part fractures of

the proximal humerus in the elderly: Design of a randomized controlled trial. *BMC Musculoskelet Disord* 2012;13:16.

27. Buhr AJ, Cooke AM. Fracture patterns. *Lancet* 1959;1(7072):531–6.

28. Court-Brown CM, Garg A, McQueen MM. The epidemiology of proximal humeral fractures. *Acta Orthop Scand* 2001;72(4):365–71.

29. Knowelden J, Buhr AJ, Dunbar O. Incidence of fractures in persons over 35 years of age. *Br J Prev Soc Med* 1964;18:130–41.

30. Olsson C, Nordqvist A, Petersson CJ. Increased fragility in patients with fracture of the proximal humerus: A case control study. *Bone* 2004;34(6):1072–7.

31. Johnell O, Kanis J. Epidemiology of osteoporotic fractures. *Osteoporos Int* 2005;16(Suppl 2):S3–7.

32. Palvanen M, Kannus P, Niemi S, Parkkari J. Update in the epidemiology of proximal humeral fractures. *Clin Orthop Relat Res* 2006;442:87–92.

33. Kannus P, Palvanen M, Niemi S, Parkkari J, Jarvinen M, Vuori I. Increasing number and incidence of osteoporotic fractures of the proximal humerus in elderly people. *BMJ* 1996;313(7064):1051–2.

34. Court-Brown CM, Clement ND, Duckworth AD, Aitken S, Biant LC, McQueen MM. The spectrum of fractures in the elderly. *Bone Joint J* 2014;96-B(3):366–72.

35. Clement ND, Aitken S, Duckworth AD, McQueen MM, Court-Brown CM. Multiple fractures in the elderly. *J Bone Joint Surg Br* 2012;94(2):231–6.

36. Olsson C, Petersson C, Nordquist A. Increased mortality after fracture of the surgical neck of the humerus: A case-control study of 253 patients with a 12-year follow-up. *Acta Orthop Scand* 2003;74(6):714–17.

37. Nguyen TV, Center JR, Sambrook PN, Eisman JA. Risk factors for proximal humerus, forearm, and wrist fractures in elderly men and women: The Dubbo Osteoporosis Epidemiology Study. *Am J Epidemiol* 2001;153(6):587–95.

38. Clement ND, Duckworth AD, McQueen MM, Court-Brown CM. The outcome of proximal humeral fractures in the elderly: Predictors of mortality and function. *Bone Joint J* 2014;96-B(7):970–7.

39. Neer CS. Displaced proximal humeral fractures. I. Classification and evaluation. *J Bone Joint Surg Am* 1970;52(6):1077–89.

40. Roux A, Decroocq L, El Batti S, Bonnevialle N, Moineau G, Trojani C, et al. Epidemiology of proximal humerus fractures managed in a trauma center. *Orthop Traumatol Surg Res* 2012;98(6):715–19.

41. Tamai K, Ishige N, Kuroda S, Ohno W, Itoh H, Hashiguchi H, et al. Four-segment classification of proximal humeral fractures revisited: A multicenter study on 509 cases. *J Shoulder Elbow Surg* 2009;18(6):845–50.

42. Bahrs C, Bauer M, Blumenstock G, Eingartner C, Bahrs SD, Tepass A, et al. The complexity of proximal humeral fractures is age and gender specific. *J Orthop Sci* 2013;18(3):465–70.

43. Fjalestad T, Hole MO, Blucher J, Hovden IA, Stiris MG, Stromsoe K. Rotator cuff tears in proximal humeral fractures: An MRI cohort study in 76 patients. *Arch Orthop Trauma Surg* 2010;130(5):575–81.

44. Bahrs C, Rolauffs B, Stuby F, Dietz K, Weise K, Helwig P. Effect of proximal humeral fractures on the age-specific prevalence of rotator cuff tears. *J Trauma* 2010;69(4):901–6.

45. Sidor ML, Zuckerman JD, Lyon T, Koval K, Schoenberg N. Classification of proximal humerus fractures: The contribution of the scapular lateral and axillary radiographs. *J Shoulder Elbow Surg* 1994;3(1):24–7.

46. Brorson S, Hrobjartsson A. Training improves agreement among doctors using the Neer system for proximal humeral fractures in a systematic review. *J Clin Epidemiol* 2008;61(1):7–16.

47. Brorson S, Frich LH, Hrobjartsson A. The Neer classification for fractures of the proximal humerus: A narrative review. *Minerva Ortop Traumatol* 2009;60:447–60.

48. Majed A, Macleod I, Bull AM, Zyto K, Resch H, Hertel R, et al. Proximal humeral fracture classification systems revisited. *J Shoulder Elbow Surg* 2011;20(7):1125–32.

49. Brorson S, Bagger J, Sylvest A, Hrobjartsson A. Improved interobserver variation after training of doctors in the Neer system. A randomised trial. *J Bone Joint Surg Br* 2002;84(7):950–4.

50. Brorson S, Olsen BS, Frich LH, Jensen SL, Sorensen AK, Krogsgaard M, et al. Surgeons agree more on treatment recommendations than on classification of proximal humeral fractures. *BMC Musculoskelet Disord* 2012;13:114.

51. Brorson S, Eckardt H, Audige L, Rolauffs B, Bahrs C. Translation between the Neer- and the AO/OTA-classification for proximal humeral fractures: Do we need to be bilingual to interpret the scientific literature? *BMC Res Notes* 2013;6:69.

52. Khatib O, Onyekwelu I, Zuckerman JD. The incidence of proximal humeral fractures in New York State from 1990 through 2010 with an emphasis on operative management in patients aged 65 years or older. *J Shoulder Elbow Surg* 2014;23(9):1356–62.

53. Okike K, Lee OC, Makanji H, Harris MB, Vrahas MS. Factors associated with the decision for operative versus non-operative treatment of displaced proximal humerus fractures in the elderly. *Injury* 2013;44(4):448–55.

54. Zhang AL, Schairer WW, Feeley BT. Hospital readmissions after surgical treatment of proximal humerus fractures: Is arthroplasty safer than open reduction internal fixation? *Clin Orthop Relat Res* 2014;472(8):2317–24.

55. Zhang L, Zheng J, Wang W, Lin G, Huang Y, Zheng J, et al. The clinical benefit of medial support screws in locking plating of proximal humerus fractures: A prospective randomized study. *Int Orthop* 2011;35(11):1655–61.

56. Nanidis TG, Majed A, Liddle AD, Constantinides VA, Sivagnanam P, Tekkis PT, et al. Conservative versus operative management of complex proximal humeral fractures: A meta-analysis. *Shoulder Elbow* 2010;2:166–74.

57. Rangan A, Handoll H, Brealey S, Jefferson L, Keding A, Martin BC, et al. Surgical vs nonsurgical treatment of adults with displaced fractures of the proximal humerus: The PROFHER randomized clinical trial. *JAMA* 2015;313(10):1037–47.

58. Menendez ME, Ring D. Does the timing of surgery for proximal humeral fracture affect inpatient outcomes? *J Shoulder Elbow Surg* 2014;23(9):1257–62.

59. Constant CR. *Age related recovery of shoulder function after injury.* Master thesis, University College, Cork, Ireland, 1986.

60. Constant CR, Murley AH. A clinical method of functional assessment of the shoulder. *Clin Orthop Relat Res* 1987;(214):160–4.

61. Constant CR, Gerber C, Emery RJ, Sojbjerg JO, Gohlke F, Boileau P. A review of the Constant score: Modifications and guidelines for its use. *J Shoulder Elbow Surg* 2008;17(2):355–61.

62. Iyengar JJ, Devcic Z, Sproul RC, Feeley BT. Nonoperative treatment of proximal humerus fractures: A systematic review. *J Orthop Trauma* 2011;25(10):612–17.

63. Court-Brown CM, Cattermole H, McQueen MM. Impacted valgus fractures (B1.1) of the proximal humerus. The results of non-operative treatment. *J Bone Joint Surg Br* 2002;84(4):504–8.

64. Hanson B, Neidenbach P, de Boer P, Stengel D. Functional outcomes after nonoperative management of fractures of the proximal humerus. *J Shoulder Elbow Surg* 2009;18(4):612–21.

65. Gaebler C, McQueen MM, Court-Brown CM. Minimally displaced proximal humeral fractures: Epidemiology and outcome in 507 cases. *Acta Orthop Scand* 2003;74(5):580–5.

66. Marsh JL, Slongo TF, Agel J, Broderick JS, Creevey W, DeCoster TA, et al. Fracture and dislocation classification compendium–2007: Orthopaedic Trauma Association classification, database and outcomes committee. *J Orthop Trauma* 2007;21(10 Suppl):S1–133.

67. Calvo E, Morcillo D, Foruria AM, Redondo-Santamaria E, Osorio-Picorne F, Caeiro JR. Nondisplaced proximal humeral fractures: High incidence among outpatient-treated osteoporotic fractures and severe impact on upper extremity function and patient subjective health perception. *J Shoulder Elbow Surg* 2011;20(5):795–801.

68. Lefevre-Colau MM, Babinet A, Fayad F, Fermanian J, Anract P, Roren A, et al. Immediate mobilization compared with conventional immobilization for the impacted nonoperatively treated proximal humeral fracture. A randomized controlled trial. *J Bone Joint Surg Am* 2007;89(12):2582–90.

69. Hodgson SA, Mawson SJ, Saxton JM, Stanley D. Rehabilitation of two-part fractures of the neck of the humerus (two-year follow-up). *J Shoulder Elbow Surg* 2007;16(2):143–5.

70. Kristiansen B, Angermann P, Larsen TK. Functional results following fractures of the proximal humerus. A controlled clinical study comparing two periods of immobilization. *Arch Orthop Trauma Surg* 1989;108(6):339–41.

71. Maier D, Jaeger M, Izadpanah K, Strohm PC, Suedkamp NP. Proximal humeral fracture treatment in adults. *J Bone Joint Surg Am* 2014;96(3):251–61.

72. Bell JE, Leung BC, Spratt KF, Koval KJ, Weinstein JD, Goodman DC, et al. Trends and variation in incidence, surgical treatment, and repeat surgery of proximal humeral fractures in the elderly. *J Bone Joint Surg Am* 2011;93(2):121–31.

73. Zhu Y, Lu Y, Shen J, Zhang J, Jiang C. Locking intramedullary nails and locking plates in the treatment of two-part proximal humeral surgical neck fractures: A prospective randomized trial with a minimum of three years of follow-up. *J Bone Joint Surg Am* 2011;93(2):159–68.

74. Giannoudis PV, Xypnitos FN, Dimitriou R, Manidakis N, Hackney R. Internal fixation of proximal humeral fractures using the Polarus intramedullary nail: Our institutional experience and review of the literature. *J Orthop Surg Res* 2012;7:39.

75. Anakwenze OA, Zoller S, Ahmad CS, Levine WN. Reverse shoulder arthroplasty for acute proximal humerus fractures: A systematic review. *J Shoulder Elbow Surg* 2014;23(4):e73–80.

76. Mata-Fink A, Meinke M, Jones C, Kim B, Bell JE. Reverse shoulder arthroplasty for treatment of proximal humeral fractures in older adults: A systematic review. *J Shoulder Elbow Surg* 2013;22(12):1737–48.

77. Voigt C, Geisler A, Hepp P, Schulz AP, Lill H. Are polyaxially locked screws advantageous in the plate osteosynthesis of proximal humeral fractures in the elderly? A prospective randomized clinical observational study. *J Orthop Trauma* 2011;25(10):596–602.

78. Smejkal K, Lochman P, Dedek T, Trlica J, Koci J, Zvak I. Surgical treatment for proximal humerus fracture. *Acta Chir Orthop Traumatol Cech* 2011;78(4):321–7.

79. Wirbel R, Knorr V, Saur B, Dühr B, Mutschler W. Minimalinvasive osteosynthese dizlozierter proximaler Humerusfrakturen. *Oper Orthop Traumatol* 1999;11(1):44–53.

80. Agorastides I, Sinopidis C, El Meligny M, Yin Q, Brownson P, Frostick SP. Early versus late mobilization after hemiarthroplasty for proximal humeral fractures. *J Shoulder Elbow Surg* 2007;16(3 Suppl):S33–8.

81. Court-Brown CM, Garg A, McQueen MM. The translated two-part fracture of the proximal humerus. Epidemiology and outcome in the older patient. *J Bone Joint Surg Br* 2001;83(6):799–804.

82. Court-Brown CM, McQueen MM. Two-part fractures and fracture dislocations. *Hand Clin* 2007;23(4): 397–414, v.

83. Neuhaus V, Swellengrebel CH, Bossen JK, Ring D. What are the factors influencing outcome among patients admitted to a hospital with a proximal humeral fracture? *Clin Orthop Relat Res* 2013;471(5):1698–706.

84. Neuhaus V, Bot AG, Swellengrebel CH, Jain NB, Warner JJ, Ring DC. Treatment choice affects inpatient adverse events and mortality in older aged inpatients with an isolated fracture of the proximal humerus. *J Shoulder Elbow Surg* 2014;23(6):800–6.

85. Foruria AM, de Gracia MM, Larson DR, Munuera L, Sanchez-Sotelo J. The pattern of the fracture and displacement of the fragments predict the outcome in proximal humeral fractures. *J Bone Joint Surg Br* 2011;93(3):378–86.

86. Court-Brown CM, McQueen MM. Nonunions of the proximal humerus: Their prevalence and functional outcome. *J Trauma* 2008;64(6):1517–21.

87. Annual Report 2013. Competence Centre for Clinical Quality and Health Informatics. The Danish Shoulder Arthroplasty Registry 2013.

88. Brorson S, Rasmussen JV, Frich LH, Olsen BS, Hrobjartsson A. Benefits and harms of locking plate osteosynthesis in intraarticular (OTA Type C) fractures of the proximal humerus: A systematic review. *Injury* 2012;43(7):999–1005.

89. Jost B, Spross C, Grehn H, Gerber C. Locking plate fixation of fractures of the proximal humerus: Analysis of complications, revision strategies and outcome. *J Shoulder Elbow Surg* 2013;22(4):542–9.

90. Kirchhoff C, Braunstein V, Kirchhoff S, Sprecher CM, Ockert B, Fischer F, et al. Outcome analysis following removal of locking plate fixation of the proximal humerus. *BMC Musculoskelet Disord* 2008;9:138.

91. Cazeneuve JF, Cristofari DJ. Long term functional outcome following reverse shoulder arthroplasty in the elderly. *Orthop Traumatol Surg Res* 2011;97(6):583–9.

21

Dislocations around the shoulder

SANG-JIN SHIN

INTRODUCTION

The prevalence of traumatic dislocations of the shoulder in the elderly is increasing due to lifestyle changes and prolonged life expectancy. However, injury mechanisms, clinical manifestations and treatment modalities are routinely determined from data on younger patients.

The literature has demonstrated differences between the clinical manifestations and prognosis of elderly and young patients who sustain a dislocation of the shoulder. A dislocation of the shoulder is usually due to a low energy fall onto the outstretched hand in the elderly, unlike younger patients where it is commonly due to higher energy injuries, for example during sports.[1] Recurrence is less commonly seen in the elderly, although higher morbidity can be expected due to associated rotator cuff tears, greater tuberosity fractures and/or nerve injuries.[2]

EPIDEMIOLOGY

Rowe reported an equivocal incidence for shoulder dislocations in patients below and above the age of 45 years.[3] Recent studies have reported that 20–44% of patients with an anterior shoulder dislocation are over the age of 60 years.[3–5] Rotator cuff tears are common sequelae of traumatic shoulder dislocations in the elderly, with the incidence ranging from 34% to 100%.[4,6–9]

McLaughlin[10] suggested that a dislocation of the shoulder may occur due to failure of either the anterior structures that include the antero-inferior glenoid and labrum (anterior mechanism), or the posterior structures that include the postero-superior rotator cuff (posterior mechanism) (Figure 21.1).

In elderly patients, since the rotator cuff is the weakest structure due to normal age related degenerative changes, it is the first structure to give way and hence the anterior capsulolabral structures are relatively well preserved.[10] Labral lesions are less commonly found in patients over 40 years compared to young patients following a traumatic dislocation.[11] However, Gumina and Postacchini found anterior labral tears in all their patients and concluded that the anterior capsulolabral structures may be damaged and may contribute to recurrent dislocation in the elderly patient.[4] Patients with recurrent dislocation over 55 years are routinely found to have either a Bankart lesion or glenoid rim fracture, along with a concomitant large or massive tear of the rotator cuff.[12]

The spectrum of injury mechanism may vary. At one end are patients with pre-existing degeneration of the rotator cuff that is disrupted as a consequence of the dislocation and results in a tear. The other end of the spectrum is where the rotator cuff is relatively intact and the anterior capsulolabral structures give way. In some patients both rotator cuff tear and Bankart lesion may coexist (Figure 21.2). Clinicians must be aware of the common associated pathologies and evaluate for these injuries as part of a thorough clinical assessment.

CLINICAL PRESENTATION

Patients can present with an acute dislocation in the emergency room or subacutely with a history of dislocation which has been reduced with persistent pain, weakness of the shoulder, neurological deficit, stiffness due to prolonged immobilization or recurrent dislocation. In an acutely dislocated shoulder, after reduction is achieved, the affected shoulder and upper limb are carefully examined. The first priority is to rule out neurovascular injury. The radial and brachial arteries are assessed and if the pulse is absent, further evaluation and treatment is the priority. Neurological assessment focuses on a thorough assessment of the brachial plexus and specifically the axillary nerve. The axillary

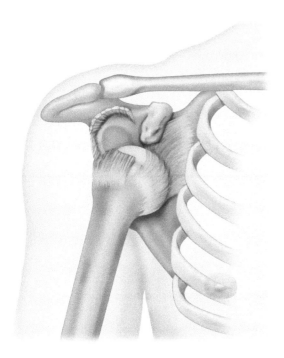

Figure 21.1 Posterior injury mechanism. Elderly patients with shoulder dislocation are prone to a tear of the rotator cuff. (Please note the direction of the dislocation is still anterior)

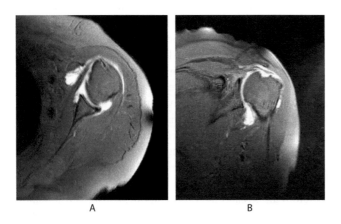

A   B

Figure 21.2 MRI of a 65-year-old patient following a primary anterior shoulder dislocation. The axial image shows a Bankart lesion (a) and the coronal image shows a medium sized full-thickness rotator cuff tear (b).

nerve may be difficult to examine in the acute setting as a diminished or absent sensation in the military badge area may not be a reliable way of detecting a deficit.[13]

Diagnostic imaging

In a patient with an acute dislocation, detailed plain radiographs include a true anteroposterior, modified axial and scapular lateral views prior to reduction. Associated injuries around the shoulder (e.g. greater tuberosity fracture) and other injuries in the upper limb should be excluded. After reduction of the dislocation the views have to be repeated to confirm congruency of the joint and to rule out other injuries. If there is any suspicion of associated fractures, a 3D CT scan should be performed.

FURTHER IMAGING

Ultrasound can aid in the diagnosis of rotator cuff tears. A recent Cochrane review concluded that ultrasound has a sensitivity and specificity similar to MRI for diagnosing a full-thickness rotator cuff tear and slightly inferior for diagnosing a partial-thickness tear.[14] While it may allow for evaluation of tuberosity fractures or a Hill–Sachs lesion, ultrasound is not the ideal imaging modality for evaluating the labrum.[15]

An MRI or a MR arthrogram may help in determining the size of an associated rotator cuff tear, Bankart lesion and/or another anterior bony or capsulolabral lesion such as an anterior capsular tear (Figure 21.3). MRI is recommended when patients present with persistent weakness, pain or instability despite appropriate following dislocation. If an MRI is contraindicated e.g. due to metallic implants, a CT arthrogram may be useful for evaluation of the rotator cuff and has demonstrated comparable accuracy to MRI. The timing of MRI is a matter of controversy. One study recommended evaluating patients at 7–10 days post injury,[16] while other authors have recommended an MRI can be done at 4 weeks without any increased incidence of stiffness.[9,17]

If a neurological deficit is suspected, an electromyography-nerve conduction velocity test (EMG-NCV) may be done at 4 weeks and repeated at 3 months if no improvement is seen. Although findings on EMG-NCV may be delayed, it may act as a baseline for further evaluation.

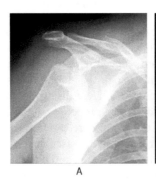
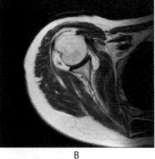
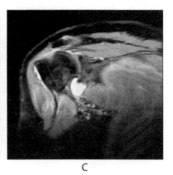

A   B   C

Figure 21.3 A 64-year-old patient following primary anterior shoulder dislocation (a). MRI axial image shows an anterior capsular tear with intact anterior labrum (b) and the coronal image shows a medium sized full-thickness rotator cuff tear (c).

Associated injuries

PERIPHERAL NERVE INJURIES

A prospective study reported that the prevalence of associated nerve injuries in patients over the age of 65 years was 54%, which was more than the 26% seen in younger patients.[13] The increased prevalence may be due to lower muscle tone, which allows the humeral head to displace more and therefore lead to greater disruption of the surrounding soft tissues. Another reason for the high prevalence of nerve injuries could be due to age related neural degeneration making injury following a simple dislocation more likely.

The most commonly involved nerve is the axillary nerve. The prevalence quoted in a large prospective study was 9.3%, compared to 4.6% in younger patients.[4] However, the prevalence is increased when all patients are tested with electromyography.[13] The proportion of nerve injuries as confirmed on NCV studies is found in Table 21.1.

AXILLARY ARTERY INJURIES

Although uncommon, an injury to the axillary artery can lead to devastating complications, particularly if there is a delay in diagnosis. A review of the literature demonstrates that of the axillary artery injuries reported following a dislocation of the shoulder, 86% are found in patients over 50 years of age[18]. Most injuries occur in the third part of the artery distal to the pectoralis minor, with 68% presenting with an axillary mass. Distal pulses may rarely be present due to collateral vessel flow and should not rule out an arterial injury. Any patient presenting with an axillary mass and diminished pulses after a shoulder dislocation should be investigated with an arteriogram for possible axillary artery injury and early vascular input is required. Atherosclerotic changes in the artery associated with tenting of the artery over the pectoralis minor may be responsible for the increased incidence of this injury in the elderly patient.[18]

ASSOCIATED FRACTURES

Approximately 15–30% of anterior shoulder dislocations are associated with a greater tuberosity fracture.[3,19] Fracture occurs either due to a shearing mechanism or as a result of avulsion. Shearing injuries are due to the greater tuberosity abutting against the glenoid and eccentric contraction of the rotator cuff during dislocation. In a retrospective review of 103 patients, 57% of the fractures were due to an anterior shoulder dislocation.[20]

The standard anteroposterior radiographs may underestimate the displacement of the greater tuberosity, with axillary and scapular Y views more indicative. These fractures usually are displaced superiorly and posteriorly due to the pull of the intact attachment of the posterosuperior cuff. A CT scan can better delineate such fractures (Figure 21.4). Glenoid rim fractures are less common in elderly patients, with one study reporting two cases among the 52 patients studied.[16]

ROTATOR CUFF TEARS

Rotator cuff tears are frequently reported following a traumatic shoulder dislocation in the elderly with the incidence ranging from 34% to 100%.[4,6–9] Neviaser et al. reported that all 31 patients in their series, all of whom were more than 35 years of age and were unable to abduct their arm after a dislocation of the shoulder and adequate immobilization, had a rotator cuff tear, with the rate of axillary nerve injury of 7.8%.[8]

While some authors have found the incidence of cuff tears in patients with shoulder dislocation increases with age,[6,21] others have found no such association.[4,7,17] A prospective study comparing the incidence of rotator cuff tears found a significant increase in the rate of rotator cuff tears after shoulder dislocation in elderly patients. However, the increase was only of statistical significance among patients below the age of 60 years when compared to patients above 60 years of age.[6] There is considerable debate as to whether a rotator cuff tear leads to a dislocation or a dislocation leads to rotator cuff tear. Many biomechanical studies have shown that the cuff is an important dynamic stabilizer of the shoulder and large to massive tears have been demonstrated to cause shoulder instability (Figure 21.5).[22]

Table 21.1 Incidence of nerve injuries following a dislocation of the shoulder

Nerve	Percentage injury
Axillary	37
Suprascapular	29
Radial	22
Musculocutaneous	19
Ulnar	8

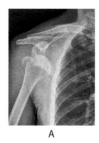 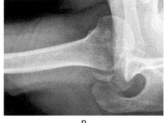 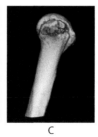 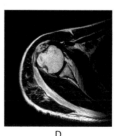

A   B   C   D

Figure 21.4 A 67-year-old patient with anterior shoulder dislocation with greater tuberosity fracture confirmed on radiographs (a,b), 3D-CT (c) and MRI (d).

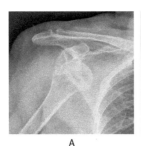 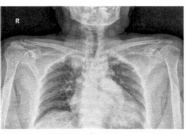 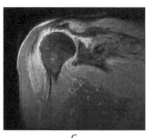

A   B   C

Figure 21.5 An 81-year-old patient who sustained an anterior shoulder dislocation following a fall from standing height (a). The patient was found to have a rotator cuff arthropathy after reduction of the shoulder (b). Coronal MRI shows a massive rotator cuff tear with arthropathy (c). This implies that in essentially asymptomatic patients, a massive cuff tear may predispose the patient to primary dislocation following minimal injury.

A cadaveric study has found that less capsular disruption is needed in the presence of cuff defects to result in a shoulder dislocation.[23] Similarly, a large rotator cuff tear is a significant risk factor for redislocation within the first week following reduction of a primary dislocation.[24] A study utilizing ultrasound found 15.1% of patients presenting with a shoulder dislocation have chronic tears that were large to massive in size.[6] Similarly a population based study of the prevalence of rotator cuff tears found 20.7% of patients had a rotator cuff tear and 16.9% of asymptomatic patients had a cuff tear.[25] One study reported no difference in the incidence of cuff tears in patients with pre-existing shoulder symptoms and those with no symptoms prior to dislocation in a study of 95 patients over 60 years of age.[4]

It might be inferred that large to massive tears predispose to instability, which can lead to shoulder dislocation after a provocative trivial traumatic event. In these patients the degree of trauma required to dislocate the shoulder might be less than required when the cuff is intact. In patients with a degenerate cuff, the shoulder dislocation may be a causative factor in a subsequent tear. It is important to appreciate that rotator cuff tears may be asymptomatic prior to dislocation, with subsequent trauma and dislocation precipitating symptoms in such patients.

TREATMENT

Acute dislocation

After a thorough examination, the shoulder joint should be reduced (Figure 21.6). This can be done under sedation or general anesthesia depending on patient comorbidities and the degree of anticipated difficulty in reduction. Gentle manoeuvring is needed and excessive traction should be avoided. The arm is held close to the shoulder to prevent concomitant fractures of the humerus. A study reported five cases of iatrogenic fracture of the humeral neck after closed reduction of shoulder dislocation under sedation, but with all patients having a greater tuberosity fracture prior to reduction.[26]

The duration of subsequent immobilization is controversial. Some authors suggest shorter periods of 7–10 days,[16] while some suggest 3–4 weeks.[4] Longer periods of immobilization may lead to stiffness and difficult rehabilitation, whereas shorter periods may lead to persistent pain that may not allow the patient to follow a rehabilitation protocol. A prudent approach is to immobilize the shoulder for 2 weeks. At the end of 2 weeks, if pain is tolerable, a detailed clinical and neurological examination can be performed, with or without ultrasound as indicated to detect the presence of an associated rotator cuff tear.[17,21] In the absence of pain, rehabilitation progressing from passive to active movements and strengthening exercises can be commenced once shoulder motion is restored. If the patient continues to experience pain after 2 weeks, a further 2 weeks of immobilization can be used with rehabilitation initiated after a further thorough evaluation has been performed. If patients are comfortable at the end of 4 weeks then rehabilitation is initiated.

Rotator cuff tears

NON-OPERATIVE

In patients who do not have a rotator cuff tear and respond well to rehabilitation,[6,17] conservative treatment has been reported to give good to excellent results in 79% of patients with a shoulder dislocation 2 years following injury (Figure 21.6). The patients without associated rotator cuff tears who were treated conservatively had a better outcome than patients who had surgical repair of a cuff tear.[17] Patients with a dislocation of the shoulder who improve with physiotherapy and have no significant rotator cuff tear are ideal candidates for conservative treatment.

Conservative treatment may also be indicated in some patients with shoulder instability and large rotator cuff tears. These include patients with multiple comorbidities and low functional demands where the risk of surgery outweighs the benefit, moribund patients, those who would not be expected to co-operate with a rehabilitation protocol after surgery and those who refuse surgery. Such patients should be counseled to accept the functional disability and avoid provocative activities. Treatment in such patients is aimed at pain relief and achieving a functional range of motion for activities of daily living.

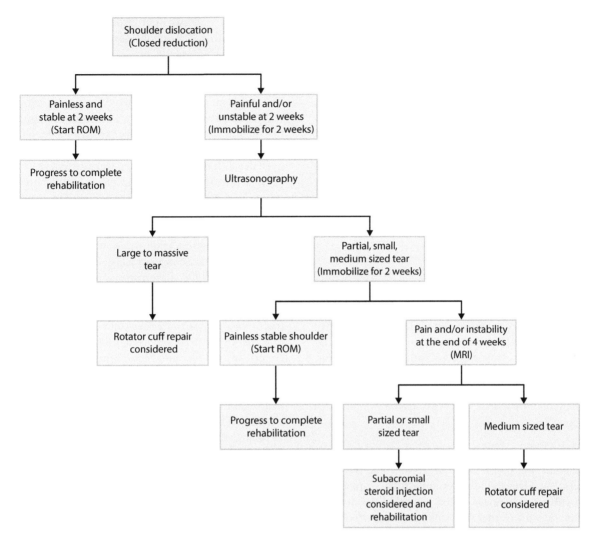

Figure 21.6 Treatment algorithm following a dislocation of the shoulder in elderly patients, with and without rotator cuff tears.

OPERATIVE

Indications

Various studies have documented that a majority of patients who are symptomatic 3–4 weeks post shoulder dislocation will have some form of a rotator cuff tear.[6,8,17,27] Pain and some amount of stiffness may be present following a period of immobilization. Local corticosteroid injections into the glenohumeral joint and a supervised exercise program can be effective in such situations. However, persistent pain, stiffness, instability or weakness may necessitate investigation (e.g. with MRI) and possibly surgical intervention (Figure 21.6). The rotator cuff may be repaired if a concomitant tear is found in such patients. Persistent symptoms and clinical signs of instability even in the presence of small tears can also be an indication for surgery. In patients where the rotator cuff tear is too small to cause instability, the MRI should be studied carefully for an anterior capsulolabral lesion.

Patients with a rotator cuff tear may present with weakness or pseudoparalysis. A brachial plexus injury should be ruled out in such patients. The indications, prognosis and techniques for repair remain the same as in patient otherwise presenting with a degenerate rotator cuff tear. If a rotator cuff tear is recognized, then patients should be counseled regarding the risk and benefits of surgical repair. Excellent results have been documented with this protocol.[6,17]

Outcome

Inferior results have been documented for conservative treatment in patients with a rotator cuff tear following an anterior dislocation.[7,9,16] In patients with shoulder instability and a rotator cuff tear, cuff repair has been found to produce an excellent or good result in 84% of patients as compared to 50% with conservative treatment.[16] Surgical repair gives superior results as compared to conservative treatment even in patients with a single primary dislocation and associated cuff tear.[4] Surgical stabilization has been found to decrease the rate of recurrence in the elderly patient. However, the improvement in clinical outcome scores and function is not as impressive as in younger patients with shoulder instability undergoing surgical stabilization.[11]

Neviaser et al. reported on 31 patients with weakness of arm abduction following a primary anterior dislocation of the shoulder.[8] The mean age was 58 years and the mean followup was 5 years. Of the 19 patients with an associated rotator cuff tear alone, all had a reduction in pain (none had pain at night) and 16 patients regained full abduction following intervention. Itoi et al. reported on 12 patients over the age of 40 years with a rotator cuff tear associated with a traumatic anterior dislocation of the shoulder.[28] Open repair was performed in 11 patients, with eight (73%) reporting a good or excellent outcome at a mean of 32 months following surgery. No repair of the Bankart lesion was performed in these patients and no effect on the outcome was reported by the authors.

Associated fractures

Treatment of greater tuberosity fractures following a shoulder dislocation depends on patient specific and fracture specific factors. Patient specific factors include age, activity level and associated comorbidities. Fracture specific factors include displacement, comminution and size of the fragment. Neer[29] advocated intervention for fractures displaced more than 1 cm. However, some have suggested that displacement of more than 0.5 cm is associated with an inferior outcome.[30]

NON-OPERATIVE

The indications for conservative treatment are fractures that are displaced less than 0.5 cm and displaced fractures in elderly patients where associated comorbidities and the level of function mean that the benefits of surgery do not outweigh the risks. For many patients, non-operative management will likely be the mainstay of treatment.

The shoulder is immobilized for 2 weeks and as the pain subsides, active and passive ranges of motion exercises are initiated. Abduction and external rotation are not allowed for 4–6 weeks. The patient should be monitored both clinically and radiologically to check for any displacement during the first 6–8 weeks following injury.[30]

Conservative treatment in undisplaced fractures yields good results. Platzer et al. reported that 97% of 135 patients with greater tuberosity fractures displaced less than 5 mm treated conservatively had good to excellent results at a mean followup of 3.7 years following injury.[31] Rath et al. reported retrospectively on 69 patients with an isolated greater tuberosity fracture managed non-operatively, all of which were displaced <3 mm.[32] At a mean of 31 months following injury the mean Constant score was 95 points and the mean satisfaction score was 9.5 out of 10. On average, patients had 8 months of pain and decreased range of motion.

OPERATIVE

Fractures displaced more than 0.5 cm, in active adults more than 0.3 cm, and a displaced fragment preventing closed reduction of the dislocation are relative indications for surgery. There are two approaches: deltopectoral and lateral deltoid splitting. The deltopectoral approach gives extensive exposure and is usually employed if there is a concurrent proximal humerus fracture. The lateral deltoid splitting approach provides excellent visualization of the posterolateral fragment and can be utilized for simultaneous rotator cuff repairs and acromioplasty. The various fixation modalities include screw fixation, suture fixation over a screw and suture anchor fixation. Arthroscopic techniques have also been developed but have a steep learning curve.

In a retrospective comparative study of non-operative (n = 9) and operative (n = 52) treatment for displaced fractures, patients treated surgically (open reduction internal fixation [ORIF] or closed reduction with percutaneous fixation) had significantly better function and union rates than those treated conservatively at a mean of 5.5 years following injury.[33] Ji et al. retrospectively analyzed 16 patients who underwent arthroscopic fixation with a double row suture anchor technique for displaced greater tuberosity fractures at a mean of 2 years following surgery.[34] Good or excellent results were reported in 14 patients, with the mean American Shoulder and Elbow Surgeons (ASES) score 88.

In a study of 17 patients managed with ORIF (n = 15) and arthroscopic fixation (n = 2), 16 had a satisfactory or excellent outcome at a mean of 5 years following surgery, with a mean ASES score of 82.9% and 87% achieving evidence of radiographic union.[35] Factors such as the presence of a concomitant rotator cuff tear requiring repair, history of dislocation, age 60 years or older and delayed time to surgery over 10 days did not significantly affect the final active forward elevation or ASES scores.

COMPLICATIONS

Neurovascular injuries

PERIPHERAL NERVE INJURIES

The axillary nerve is the most common nerve injury following a dislocation of the shoulder. Increasing age, bruising about the shoulder and an associated fracture of the proximal humerus are risk factors.[36] Axillary nerve palsy is usually transient, with recovery occurring between 6 weeks to 1 year following dislocation.[7,13] A persistent disabling neurological deficit is uncommon, with one study reporting that although three of four patients with an axillary nerve palsy following dislocation did not completely recover, all patients had at least grade 4 muscle power at final followup.[8,28]

If a patient is noted to have a persistent motor deficit, a rotator cuff tear should be first ruled out through further imaging. In such patients, an EMG is warranted at approximately 4 weeks to document the type of injury, which helps to provide a prognosis for recovery and outcome. Injury can range from neuropraxia to denervation due to an axonal injury. Absence of F-waves and positive sharp waves with normal recruitment is correlated with neuropraxia and excellent prognosis. These patients can be observed for up to 6 months for spontaneous recovery. If there is no recovery after 6 months, nerve exploration with or without repair or nerve grafting may be required depending on the functional demands of the patient. However, even complete EMG recovery does not guarantee normal shoulder function as patients with recovery on EMG have been found to have persistent poor shoulder function.[36]

AXILLARY ARTERY INJURIES

In addition to absent distal pulses axillary artery injury should be suspected in the presence of an expanding local axillary swelling and/or bruising, delayed onset neurological deficit after reduction or worsening neurological deficit and pain despite successful reduction of the shoulder. Doppler ultrasound aids in making the diagnosis, with CT arteriography or MR arteriography definitive for diagnosis and planning management. Early referral to the local vascular team is recommended. Treatment options include endarterectomy, vein patch repair or resection of the lacerated segment.

Recurrent dislocation

Recurrent dislocation of the shoulder in the elderly patient has been reported in very few studies and is known to be less common when compared to younger counterparts.[10] The incidence varies, with one study reporting a recurrent dislocation rate of 22.1% in the 95 patients reviewed.[4] Levy et al. reported an incidence of 11% recurrence in patients more than 60 years of age,[12] while Rowe et al. found a recurrence rate of 16% in 60–70 years and 14% in age group of 51–60 years.[19]

Most episodes of redislocation appear to occur within the first 2 weeks following the primary injury. Risk factors identified for early dislocation include high energy injuries, associated neurological deficit, large rotator cuff tear, fracture of the glenoid rim or a fracture of both the glenoid rim and greater tuberosity (highest risk).[24] Patients with an isolated fracture of the greater tuberosity have been found not to have an increased incidence of recurrent dislocation, with some studies reporting that a concomitant greater tuberosity fracture reduces the incidence of redislocation.[3,19]

The mechanism of recurrent shoulder dislocation in the elderly is controversial. Levy et al. reported that all 16 patients older than 55 years with recurrent shoulder dislocation had a large to massive tear, with an anterior capsulolabral injury in the form of a Bankart lesion or a bony Bankart lesion.[12] One study has reported large to massive tears in 96% of patients with recurrent instability,[37] while other studies have concluded that anterior capsulolabral avulsions are the major cause of recurrence.[7,38,39] Kinnett et al. reported on six patients with a mean age of 64 years with multiple recurrent dislocation of the shoulder, with four treated with an anterior capsulolabral repair (Bankart).[40] However, another study did not find any capsulolabral lesions in 11 older patients with

a recurrent dislocation and instead consistently found an isolated subscapularis tear with capsular avulsion from the greater tuberosity.[8,27]

TREATMENT

A careful evaluation of the capsulolabral structures, the rotator cuff and ligamentous laxity is necessary for all patients. Poor results have been reported in this subgroup if rotator cuff repair is neglected.[37] A study on six active patients over the age of 50 years with multiple recurrent shoulder dislocations found that all the patients had significant general ligamentous laxity and the dislocation was precipitated by minimal trauma. During surgery in all six patients, the authors found a small Bankart lesion, a redundant and capacious capsule, and the rotator cuff was intact in all patients. A subsequent Bankart repair was done with good results and the authors concluded that the outcome was comparable to that of younger patients.[39]

There is a wide variety of opinion regarding the need to repair a torn rotator cuff and the avulsed anterior capsulolabral structures. Levy et al. reported the results in 10 patients over 55 years of age with recurrent shoulder dislocation, a large to massive tear and an anterior capsulolabral injury in the form of a Bankart lesion or a bony Bankart lesion.[12] The technique described involves the anterior capsule being shifted posterosuperiorly and sutured to the infraspinatus stump through a combined deltopectoral and lateral approach, with no attempt made to repair the supraspinatus or the infraspinatus tendon. This achieves a capsulodesis effect and active centring of the humeral head. However, an intact subscapularis tendon is a prerequisite for this procedure. At a mean followup of 52 months there were seven excellent results, two good and one fair according to the Rowe criteria. The average Constant score was 83% and there were no episodes of recurrent instability.

In a study of 11 patients over 40 years of age with a recurrent anterior shoulder dislocation, an anterior capsular and subscapularis tear from the lesser tuberosity was found.[27] In all these patients the capsule and subscapularis tear were repaired and all were reported to have pain relief, shoulder function restoration and no recurrence after a mean followup of 5 years. Anterior capsular disruption and subscapularis tears from the lesser tuberosity have not been reported in subsequent studies. One study reported that a third of patients (n = 12) with a dislocation of the shoulder had a Bankart lesion and rotator cuff tear,[28] with two of four of these patients having a recurrent dislocation. Satisfactory results were obtained following an isolated rotator cuff repair and no repair of the Bankart lesion. However, in the same study the authors did recommend Bankart repair when the shoulder remained unstable following cuff repair.

Jouve et al. reported on 28 cases (mean age 47 years) of recurrent anterior shoulder instability with an associated full-thickness rotator cuff tear, with 19 patients (mean age 59 years) undergoing open anterior stabilization alone either when the rotator cuff was not repairable or when the patient was not willing to undergo a rotator cuff repair.[37] The remaining nine cases underwent a Latarjet procedure with cuff repair (mean age 40 years). The authors found that 92.5% of patients had a Bankart or a bony Bankart lesion. At a mean of 74 months following surgery three patients (16%) in the stabilization alone group had a recurrence, with no recurrences in the combined repair group. Subjective satisfaction overall was 96%.

In a retrospective study of 11 patients with recurrent anterior instability with onset after the age of 40 years, the authors found two patients with large rotator cuff tears and nine patients with a Bankart lesion and small cuff tear.[39] In the two patients with a large cuff tear only the cuff was repaired while in the remaining nine patients a Bankart repair with cuff repair was done. All patients were reported to have an excellent outcome with no recurrence and a functional range of motion. In a study on patients with an early redislocation after closed reduction, the authors reported good results with no recurrent instability and equivocal functional scores at 1 year after repair of the rotator cuff and anterior capsulolabral structures with closure of the rotator interval.[24] The authors advised repair of the disrupted anterior capsulolabral structures in addition to rotator cuff repair for good results.

A prudent approach would seem to be to repair the rotator cuff when a large to massive tear is present because such tears by themselves have a destabilizing effect. However, in the presence of small to medium sized tears (Figure 21.6), an anterior capsulolabral repair may be required.[17]

ACROMIOCLAVICULAR JOINT DISLOCATIONS

Acromioclavicular joint (ACJ) dislocations in the elderly should be approached by considering the symptoms and functional demands of the patients. ACJ dislocations are classified according to the Rockwood classification (Table 21.2).

The aim of management of an ACJ dislocation is a painless and functional range of shoulder movement, recovery of strength and resumption of pre-trauma activities of daily living. Types 1, 2 and 3 are routinely managed non-operatively, the management of type 4 is controversial, and types 5 and 6 routinely require operative intervention in the active patient.[40] The majority of elderly patients can likely be managed with non-operative intervention.

Non-operative management consists of rest in an arm sling and physical therapy.[40] Operative treatment routinely involves one of the following procedures:

1. Intra-articular fixation: K-wires, Steinmann pins, hook plates
2. Extra-articular fixation:
   a. Coraco-clavicular screw fixation
   b. Dacron or mersilene tape fixation using encirclage or tunnels through the coracoid and clavicle
   c. Suture anchors in the coracoid
3. Anatomical reconstruction:
   a. Numerous procedures have been described using autograft and allograft tendons.
   b. It is necessary to reconstruct both the coraco-clavicular and acromio-clavicular ligaments.

CONCLUSIONS

Rotator cuff tears are the predominant pathological lesion associated with a dislocation of the shoulder in elderly patients. Following reduction of the shoulder, patients should undergo supervised rehabilitation following 2–4 weeks of immobilization. Ultrasound and MRI are indicated when the patient has persistent pain, weakness or instability.

In the absence of a symptomatic rotator cuff tear, patients can be managed with conservative treatment and a supervised rehabilitation program. Symptomatic and disabling tears should be repaired with the aim to improve clinical outcome and prevent recurrence. Associated injuries such as significant labral tears, displaced greater tuberosity fractures and proximal humerus fractures should be addressed on an individual patient basis.

Table 21.2 Rockwood classification of acromio-clavicular joint dislocation

Type	AC ligament	CC ligament	DT fascia	Displacement
1	Sprained	Intact	Intact	None
2	Rupture	Sprained	Intact	AC displacement <100%
				CC displacement <20%
3	Ruptured	Ruptured	Intact	AC displacement >100%
				CC displacement 20–100%
4	Ruptured	Ruptured	Ruptured	Posterior displacement of distal end clavicle
5	Ruptured	Ruptured	Ruptured	AC displacement >100%
				CC displacement 100–300%
6	Ruptured	Ruptured	Ruptured	Inferior displacement of the distal end clavicle

Note: AC, acromioclavicular; CC, coracoclavicular; DT, deltotrapezial.

REFERENCES

1. Robinson CM, Shur N, Sharpe T, Ray A, Murray IR. Injuries associated with traumatic anterior glenohumeral dislocations. *J Bone Joint Surg Am.* 2012;94(1):18–26.

2. McLaughlin HL, Cavallaro WU. Primary anterior dislocation of the shoulder. *Am J Surg.* 1950;80(6):615–21.

3. Rowe CR. Prognosis in dislocations of the shoulder. *J Bone Joint Surg Am.* 1956;38-A(5):957–77.

4. Gumina S, Postacchini F. Anterior dislocation of the shoulder in elderly patients. *J Bone Joint Surgery Br.* 1997;79(4):540–3.

5. Kazar B, Relovszky E. Prognosis of primary dislocation of the shoulder. *Acta Orthop Scand.* 1969;40(2):216–24.

6. Berbig R, Weishaupt D, Prim J, Shahin O. Primary anterior shoulder dislocation and rotator cuff tears. *J Shoulder Elbow Surg.* 1999;8(3):220–5.

7. Hawkins RJ, Bell RH, Hawkins RH, Koppert GJ. Anterior dislocation of the shoulder in the older patient. *Clin Orthop Relat Res.* 1986;(206):192–5.

8. Neviaser RJ, Neviaser TJ, Neviaser JS. Concurrent rupture of the rotator cuff and anterior dislocation of the shoulder in the older patient. *J Bone Joint Surg Am.* 1988;70(9):1308–11.

9. Sonnabend DH. Treatment of primary anterior shoulder dislocation in patients older than 40 years of age. Conservative versus operative. *Clin Orthop Relat Res.* 1994;(304):74–7.

10. McLaughlin HL, MacLellan DI. Recurrent anterior dislocation of the shoulder. II. A comparative study. *J Trauma.* 1967;7(2):191–201.

11. Maier M, Geiger EV, Ilius C, Frank J, Marzi I. Midterm results after operatively stabilised shoulder dislocations in elderly patients. *Int Orthop.* 2009;33(3):719–23.

12. Levy O, Pritsch M, Rath E. An operative technique for recurrent shoulder dislocations in older patients. *J Shoulder Elbow Surg.* 1999;8(5):452–7.

13. de Laat EA, Visser CP, Coene LN, Pahlplatz PV, Tavy DL. Nerve lesions in primary shoulder dislocations and humeral neck fractures. A prospective clinical and EMG study. *J Bone Joint Surg Br.* 1994;76(3):381–3.

14. Lenza M, Buchbinder R, Takwoingi Y, Johnston RV, Hanchard NC, Faloppa F. Magnetic resonance imaging, magnetic resonance arthrography and ultrasonography for assessing rotator cuff tears in people with shoulder pain for whom surgery is being considered. *Cochrane Database Syst Rev.* 2013;9:CD009020.

15. Daenen B, Houben G, Bauduin E, Lu KV, Meulemans JL. Ultrasound of the shoulder. *JBR-BTR* 2007;90(5):325–37.

16. Pevny T, Hunter RE, Freeman JR. Primary traumatic anterior shoulder dislocation in patients 40 years of age and older. *Arthroscopy.* 1998;14(3):289–94.

17. Shin SJ, Yun YH, Kim DJ, Yoo JD. Treatment of traumatic anterior shoulder dislocation in patients older than 60 years. *Am J Sports Med.* 2012;40(4):822–7.

18. Gates JD, Knox JB. Axillary artery injuries secondary to anterior dislocation of the shoulder. *J Trauma.* 1995;39(3):581–3.

19. Rowe CR, Sakellarides HT. Factors related to recurrences of anterior dislocations of the shoulder. *Clin Orthop.* 1961;20:40–8.

20. Bahrs C, Lingenfelter E, Fischer F, Walters EM, Schnabel M. Mechanism of injury and morphology of the greater tuberosity fracture. *J Shoulder Elbow Surg.* 2006;15(2):140–7.

21. Simank HG, Dauer G, Schneider S, Loew M. Incidence of rotator cuff tears in shoulder dislocations and results of therapy in older patients. *Arch Orthop Trauma Surg.* 2006;126(4):235–40.

22. Shin SJ, Yoo JC, McGarry MH, Jun BJ, Lee TQ. Anterior capsulolabral lesions combined with supraspinatus tendon tears: Biomechanical effects of the pathologic condition and repair in human cadaveric shoulders. *Arthroscopy.* 2013;29(9):1492–7.

23. Pouliart N, Gagey O. Concomitant rotator cuff and capsuloligamentous lesions of the shoulder: A cadaver study. *Arthroscopy.* 2006;22(7):728–35.

24. Robinson CM, Kelly M, Wakefield AE. Redislocation of the shoulder during the first six weeks after a primary anterior dislocation: Risk factors and results of treatment. *J Bone Joint Surg Am.* 2002;84-A(9):1552–9.

25. Yamamoto A, Takagishi K, Osawa T, Yanagawa T, Nakajima D, Shitara H, et al. Prevalence and risk factors of a rotator cuff tear in the general population. *J Shoulder Elbow Surg.* 2010;19(1):116–20.

26. Atoun E, Narvani A, Even T, Dabasia H, Van Tongel A, Sforza G, et al. Management of first-time dislocations of the shoulder in patients older than 40 years: The prevalence of iatrogenic fracture. *J Orthop Trauma.* 2013;27(4):190–3.

27. Neviaser RJ, Neviaser TJ, Neviaser JS. Anterior dislocation of the shoulder and rotator cuff rupture. *Clin Orthop Relat Res.* 1993;(291):103–6.

28. Itoi E, Tabata S. Rotator cuff tears in anterior dislocation of the shoulder. *Int Orthop.* 1992;16(3):240–4.

29. Neer CS. Displaced proximal humerus fractures. Part I. Classification and evaluation. *J Bone Joint Surg Am.* 1970;52(6):1077–89.

30. McLaughlin HL. Dislocation of the shoulder with tuberosity fracture. *Surg Clin North Am.* 1963;43:1615–20.

31. DeBottis D, Anavian J, Green A. Surgical management of isolated greater tuberosity fractures of the proximal humerus. *Orthop Clin North Am.* 2014;45(2):207–18.

32. Platzer P, Kutscha-Lissberg F, Lehr S, Vecsei V, Gaebler C. The influence of displacement on shoulder function in patients with minimally displaced fractures of the greater tuberosity. *Injury.* 2005;36(10):1185–9.

33. Rath E, Alkrinawi N, Levy O, Debbi R, Amar E, Atoun E. Minimally displaced fractures of the greater tuberosity: Outcome of non-operative treatment. *J Shoulder Elbow Surg.* 2013;22(10):e8–11.

34. Platzer P, Thalhammer G, Oberleitner G, Kutscha-Lissberg F, Wieland T, Vecsei V, et al. Displaced fractures of the greater tuberosity: A comparison of operative and nonoperative treatment. *J Trauma.* 2008;65(4):843–8.

35. Ji JH, Shafi M, Song IS, Kim YY, McFarland EG, Moon CY. Arthroscopic fixation technique for comminuted, displaced greater tuberosity fracture. *Arthroscopy.* 2010;26(5):600–9.

36. Yin B, Moen TC, Thompson SA, Bigliani LU, Ahmad CS, Levine WN. Operative treatment of isolated greater tuberosity fractures: Retrospective review of clinical and functional outcomes. *Orthopedics.* 2012;35(6):e807–14.

37. Visser CP, Coene LN, Brand R, Tavy DL. The incidence of nerve injury in anterior dislocation of the shoulder and its influence on functional recovery. A prospective clinical and EMG study. *J Bone Joint Surg Br.* 1999;81(4):679–85.

38. Jouve F, Graveleau N, Nove-Josserand L, Walch G. [Recurrent anterior instability of the shoulder associated with full thickness rotator cuff tear: Results of surgical treatment]. *Rev Chir Orthop Reparatrice Appar Mot.* 2008;94(7):659–69.

39. Araghi A, Prasarn M, St Clair S, Zuckerman JD. Recurrent anterior glenohumeral instability with onset after forty years of age: The role of the anterior mechanism. *Bull Hosp Jt Dis.* 2005;62(3–4):99–101.

40. Kinnett JG, Warren RF, Jacobs B. Recurrent dislocation of the shoulder after age fifty. *Clin Orthop Relat Res.* 1980;(149):164–8.

41. Epstein D, Day M, Rokito A. Current concepts in the surgical management of acromioclavicular joint injuries. *Bull NYU Hosp Jt Dis.* 2012;70(1):11–24.

22

Humeral diaphyseal fractures

AMY S. WASTERLAIN AND KENNETH A. EGOL

INTRODUCTION

The incidence of diaphyseal humerus fractures nearly doubles with every decade of life after age 60.[1] The management of diaphyseal humerus fractures in elderly patients merits specific considerations. On the one hand, elderly patients may be less able to adapt to restricted use of the affected extremity during non-operative treatment. They may not be able to live independently. On the other hand, operative fixation must account for challenges in achieving adequate fixation in osteoporotic bone and the potential for increased medical risks.

ANATOMY

The AO classification system defines the proximal and the distal segments of long bones by a square whose sides have the same length as the widest part of the epiphysis; the diaphysis is the remaining middle portion of the bone (Figure 22.1). The humeral diaphysis is covered by muscle on all sides, contributing to a good blood supply and high union rates. The extensive range of motion at the shoulder helps patients compensate for relatively substantial angular deformity of the humeral shaft.

EPIDEMIOLOGY

The majority of diaphyseal humerus fractures occur in elderly patients after a simple fall.[1] The annual incidence of diaphyseal humerus fractures among the elderly in the United States was estimated as 12.0 or 23.5 per 100,000.[2,3] In a study of 361 humeral shaft fractures in Europe, Ekholm et al. reported a bimodal age distribution with a minor peak in the third decade represented by young men sustaining high-energy trauma, and a second major peak in the eighth decade attributed to low-energy falls in elderly women (Figure 22.2).[1] Whereas most fractures occurring in patients up to age 50 are attributed to high-energy mechanisms, among patients older than 50 years, over 75% occurred in women and were due to a fall from standing height.[4]

EVALUATION AND CLASSIFICATION

A fracture caused by relatively minimal trauma should raise suspicion for pathological fracture through a tumour. Loss of consciousness may point to syncope or an underlying cardiac condition.

The reported mechanism should be consistent with the fracture pattern. For example, a spiral fracture is typically caused by a rotational force rather than by a direct lateral blow. Discordance between the history and objective findings is a hallmark of domestic or elder abuse.[5,6] The PRAISE study recently revealed that 1 in 6 women presenting to an orthopaedic clinic has a history of abuse within the past year, and 1 in 50 women present as a direct consequence of intimate partner violence.[6] Although no specific fracture pattern is considered pathognomonic of elder abuse, suspicion may be raised by implausible or vague explanations provided by the patient or caregiver, delays in seeking medical treatment, frequent emergency room visits and partially healed fractures.[5]

When associated with high-energy polytrauma, Advanced Trauma Life Support (ATLS) guidelines should be followed to resuscitate and stabilize a trauma patient prior to addressing the humerus fracture. In the setting of a high-energy injury, humeral shaft fractures may be associated with intra-abdominal injuries.[7]

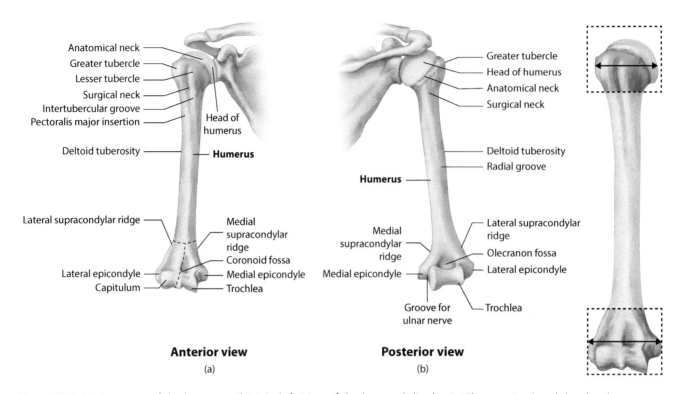

Figure 22.1 **(a)** Anatomy of the humerus. **(b)** AO definition of the humeral diaphysis. The proximal and the distal segments of long bones are defined by a square whose sides have the same length as the widest part of the epiphysis (Adapted from Netter images, Image ID 9183, available at https://www.netterimages.com/osteology-anterior-and-posterior-view-of-the-humerus-labeled-thompson-2e-orthopaedics-frank-h-netter-9183.html).

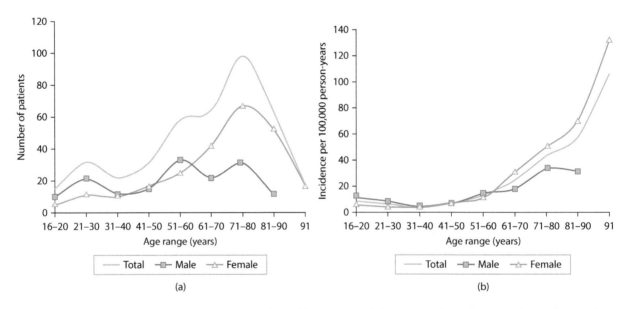

Figure 22.2 **(a)** Age distribution of 401 humeral diaphyseal fractures and **(b)** age- and gender-specific incidence of humeral diaphyseal fractures as reported by Ekholm et al.[1]

The upper extremity is evaluated for swelling, ecchymosis, deformity, open wounds, and neurologic or vascular deficits, with particular attention to the radial nerve. Extensive ecchymosis is common, and typically tracks down the arm as blood pools distally. The classic varus deformity arises due to abduction of the proximal fragment by the deltoid, and adduction and proximal migration of the distal humerus by the biceps and triceps.

Neurovascular injuries should be documented prior to treatment; Sarmiento et al. reported an 11% incidence of radial nerve palsies.[8] The motor component of the radial nerve is best assessed by testing the extensor carpi radialis longus (ECRL) or extensor digitorum communis (EDC). The ECRL can be examined by positioning the patient in approximately 90 degrees of elbow flexion and testing resisted wrist dorsiflexion. Note that interphalangeal joint extension is facilitated by the lumbricals, which are innervated by the ulnar nerve, and therefore does not assess isolated radial nerve function. To examine EDC function, have the patient extend the metacarpophalangeal joints with the proximal interphalangeal joints flexed. All of these tests may be affected by guarding associated with pain from the fracture. The surgeon may need to coach and reassure the patient to get a good examination of motor function.

Although open humeral shaft fractures are uncommon (2–10%),[1,4] any superficial wounds must raise suspicion for open fracture and should accelerate the evaluation and treatment process (Figure 22.3). Due to the relatively loose investing fascia and the large potential spaces within the anterior and posterior compartments of the arm, compartment syndrome is rare, especially after low-energy falls in the elderly.

Imaging

The entire humerus, elbow and shoulder should be visualized on radiographs in at least two planes to evaluate alignment and rotation. In patients who are unable to abduct the arm for a lateral view of the humerus, a transthoracic lateral radiograph may be obtained with the patient standing and the contralateral arm raised above the head to avoid superimposition of both arms (Figure 22.3c). On occasion, computed tomography (CT) can help evaluate rotational deformity, intra-articular extension or potential arterial injury using CT angiography.

Pseudosubluxation refers to the transient inferior subluxation of the humeral head relative to the glenoid, often associated with humerus fractures.[9] This phenomenon occurs due to deltoid and rotator cuff atony, usually as a result of inhibition of the deltoid due to pain, but sometimes related to concomitant axillary nerve palsy. In the setting of a humerus fracture, pseudosubluxation is usually a transient and benign finding that resolves with time and does not require extensive testing, reduction maneuvers or surgical intervention. Active isometric firing of the deltoid, biceps and triceps, combined with

sling support when not exercising, restores the anatomic shoulder joint alignment by approximately 6 weeks in 92% of patients.[9]

Classification

Humeral shaft fractures are commonly classified by location (proximal, middle or distal third) and pattern (transverse, butterfly, comminuted, spiral, oblique). The relatively low incidence of open humeral shaft fractures can be attributed to the low-energy mechanism of injury of most humeral shaft fractures, as well as the extensive muscle coverage throughout the humeral shaft. Wounds can be classified by the Gustilo–Anderson classification.[10]

Goals of treatment

The primary goal of treatment for a humeral shaft fracture is healing with good shoulder and elbow motion. Given the global mobility of the shoulder, deformity has a limited influence on function, and up to 30 degrees of angulation is accepted.

NON-OPERATIVE TREATMENT

Initial splinting

Non-operative treatment of humeral shaft fractures consists of three phases: initial splinting, functional bracing or casting, and rehabilitation.[11]

Initially, the arm is typically immobilized in 90 degrees of elbow flexion with a coaptation splint that extends from the medial aspect of the axilla, around the elbow, over the lateral aspect of the shoulder and to the neck (Figure 22.4a). The purpose of coaptation splinting is to stabilize the fracture and thereby improve patient comfort. Coaptation splinting employs dependency traction and hydrostatic pressure to maintain fracture reduction and is indicated for fractures with minimal shortening, and for short oblique

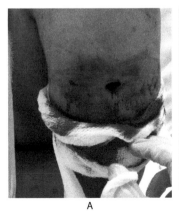
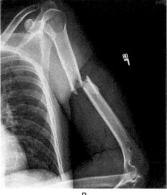
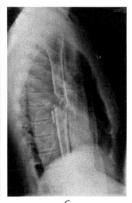

A   B   C

Figure 22.3 Open mid-diaphysis humerus fracture. (a) Open wound on lateral aspect of the arm. (b) Anteroposterior and (c) transthoracic lateral radiographs.

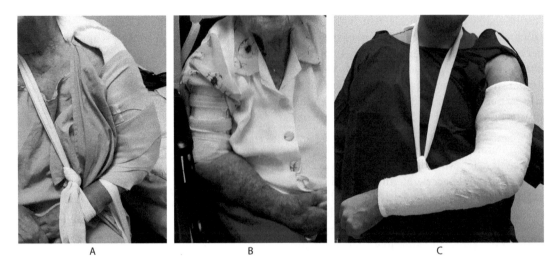

Figure 22.4 Non-operative treatment modalities for humeral diaphysis fractures. **(a)** Coaptation splint. **(b)** Functional (Sarmiento) brace. Note the forearm and hand swelling that may occur with prolonged bracing. **(c)** Hanging arm cast.

or transverse fracture patterns. Coaptation splints are cumbersome for patients and can be associated with pressure ulcers, therefore they should be used only in the initial treatment, as a bridge to either a functional brace or a hanging cast.

Hanging casts were first described by Caldwell in 1933.[12] A cast is applied extending from the proximal humerus to the wrist, with the elbow flexed at 90 degrees and the wrist in neutral position; a sling is passed around the neck and through a loop on the distal aspect of the cast for support (Figure 22.4c). Hanging casts effect and maintain fracture reduction through gravity traction, with the arm hanging freely when the patient is awake. They offer better control of varus angulation in distal third fractures. This approach is a definitive mode of treatment that can be applied immediately, but may be cumbersome for the elderly. Many avoid hanging casts due to concerns about elbow stiffness, although recent data suggest no difference in elbow motion between patients who use casts and those who use functional braces (Jawa A. Personal communication. From Ring D, Boston, MA, 2015).

Functional bracing

Functional bracing was introduced by Sarmiento et al. in 1977[13] and remains the mainstay of non-operative treatment for humeral shaft fractures. The term 'functional bracing' refers to a prefabricated brace that is applied circumferentially around the arm and thereby permits motion of the shoulder and elbow (Figure 22.4b). In theory, a functional brace employs three principles intended to maintain fracture reduction. First, active muscle contraction corrects rotation and angulation. Second, soft tissue compression exerts a 'hydraulic effect', which assists in aligning fracture fragments. Finally, and perhaps most importantly, gravity assists with alignment. The brace consists of two plastic sleeves that encircle the arm and are held in place with two adjustable Velcro straps. The patient

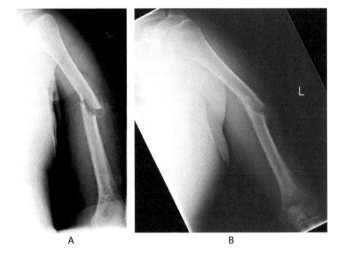

Figure 22.5 **(a)** Simple oblique fracture treated non-operatively in a functional brace. **(b)** Bridging callus with union at 10 weeks.

wears the brace at all times and tightens the straps daily as swelling subsides. The brace may be removed upon clinical and radiographic signs of union, including less pain and bridging callus on radiographs (Figure 22.5). Active, self-assisted shoulder and elbow stretching exercises are initiated as comfort allows.

In Sarmiento's largest case series of 620 humeral shaft fractures treated in a functional brace, over 80% healed in less than 16 degrees of varus and apex anterior angulation, 17% had union with greater deformity and 3% developed a nonunion treated operatively.[8] Shoulder and elbow motion recovered completely in 60% and 76% of patients, respectively. However, this was a young, urban patient population (mean age 36 years), and many patients were lost early in the recovery period (33%).

Other groups have reported 80–89% union of isolated diaphyseal humerus fractures treated non-operatively.[11,14]

Koch et al. report that shoulder and elbow motion at the time of union (mean 10 weeks, range 5–36 weeks) was symmetrical and normal for 59% and 88% of patients, respectively. They noted that patients 40 years and older were more likely to lose shoulder and elbow motion, especially external rotation.

The effect of fracture location on the rate of union is debated. Koch et al. found that six out of nine nonunions were transverse fractures, and that only 73% of transverse fractures achieved union without surgery.[11,15–17] Alternatively, in a retrospective review of 32 humeral shaft nonunions treated with functional bracing, Ring et al. found that only 4 (13%) were transverse, whereas 27 (84%) were spiral or oblique.[18] Of 32 nonunions, 17 involved fractures of the proximal third, whereas only 1 involved a fracture of the distal third of the humerus.

Neuhaus et al. demonstrated that fracture gap is an independent predictor of radiographic and clinical nonunion at 6 weeks; each incremental millimeter of gap on initial in-brace radiographs was associated with a 1.4-fold greater odds of nonunion.[14]

Rehabilitation

In patients treated non-operatively, pendulum exercises for shoulder mobility can be initiated immediately after application of a functional brace if desired, but there is no evidence that this increases final shoulder motion and they are painful and somewhat difficult to do. Active self-assisted wrist and hand range of motion begins immediately, and elbow motion is encouraged as pain subsides. Active and active self-assisted abduction and forward elevation of the shoulder are delayed until union is established.

Some orthopaedic surgeons advocate immediate application of a functional brace in the emergency department, without any period of coaptation splinting (Egol KA. Personal communication. From Wasterlain AS, New York, 2014). The primary advantage of this approach is patient comfort and independence, as coaptation splints are bulky and difficult to manage.

OPERATIVE TREATMENT

Indications

Open reduction and internal fixation (ORIF) is recommended for open fractures (except low velocity gunshot fractures), fractures associated with vascular injury and combined unstable fractures of the arm and forearm (the so-called 'floating elbow'). Surgery is also considered in patients with multiple injuries to allow weight bearing of the affected arm for ambulation with assistive devices.

With respect to the fracture itself, shortening greater than 3 cm, rotation greater than 30 degrees and varus or apex anterior angulation greater than 20 degrees are sometimes cited as surgical indications, although malunion of any degree does not appear to affect function (Figure 22.6).[19] Klenerman noted that despite preservation of limb function, cosmetic deformity becomes visible with apex anterior and varus angulation greater than 20 and 30 degrees, respectively,[20] particularly in thin patients.

Most open fractures and high velocity gunshot wounds should be treated with irrigation and debridement in the operating room, followed by internal fixation. Fractures with intra-articular extension also benefit from surgery, as discussed elsewhere in this book. A fracture with overlying burns should be considered for operative treatment due to the increased risk of compartment syndrome, and because the skin condition may not be ideal for casting or bracing.

The risks and benefits of operative treatment must be discussed and the decision shared with each individual patient. Operative fixation typically permits earlier return to function, however it also carries the risk of nerve injury, infection, implant failure and other surgical complications. Options for operative fixation include plate osteosynthesis, intramedullary nailing and external fixation. Plating options and techniques include open reduction with conventional plates or locking plates and screws and minimally invasive plate osteosynthesis (MIPO).

At the time of writing there are very few high quality prospective studies comparing operative to non-operative treatment for humeral shaft fractures. A 2012 Cochrane review

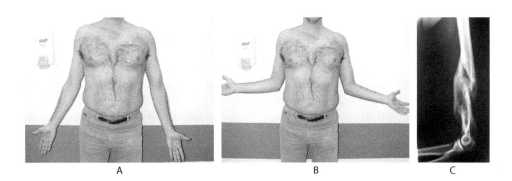

Figure 22.6 Patient with excellent functional outcome despite 'malunion' of greater than 30 degrees. Full and symmetric (a) extension and supination, and (b) external rotation of the affected (right) arm compared to the contralateral side. (c) Hypertrophic callus formation with bony union.

therefore concluded that no recommendations could be made for or against operative treatment for isolated closed diaphyseal fractures of the humerus.[21] A prospective observational study conducted by the HUMMER group is currently underway to compare functional outcomes, measured by the Disabilities of the Arm, Shoulder and Hand (DASH) score, among operatively and non-operatively treated patients with humeral shaft fractures. In a retrospective comparison of functional bracing and compression plating, Denard et al. found no statistical difference in time to union or final range of motion of healed fractures.[22] However, patients treated non-operatively were more prone to non-union (21% vs 9%) and malunion (13% vs 1%).

Surgical approaches

The majority of humeral shaft fractures can be accessed and plated through an anterolateral or posterior approach. Less commonly, a direct medial or direct lateral approach may be used.

ANTEROLATERAL APPROACH

The anterolateral approach[23] is ideal for plating proximal and middle third humeral shaft fractures. Advantages include easy patient positioning and the ability to extend the exposure proximally, with the disadvantage of a prominent scar. Distally, the approach and fixation construct must identify and protect the radial nerve and avoid the coronoid fossa.

The patient is placed in a supine or beach chair position. Prep the entire arm to permit extension of the approach as needed. The skin incision is centred over the fracture and may be extended proximally to the deltopectoral interval, following the lateral edge of the biceps and the anterior edge of the deltoid, and distally along the interval between the freely movable biceps muscle belly, stopping 5 cm proximal to the elbow flexion crease or crossing the elbow flexion crease obliquely when more distal exposure is helpful. The fascia over the biceps and brachialis is divided. Proximally, the plane between the deltoid laterally and the pectoralis major medially is identified by finding the cephalic vein and surrounding fat, which lie relatively superficial between these two muscles. The vein is usually kept medial but can be retracted either medially or laterally.

Proximally a plate will lie just lateral to the biceps tuberosity. The anterior part of the deltoid insertion is elevated to accommodate the plate. At the mid-diaphysis, the biceps is mobilized medially and the brachialis is split longitudinally along its fibers separating its lateral third (radial nerve) and its medial two-thirds (musculocutaneous nerve) (Figure 22.7). Elbow flexion relaxes the brachialis and facilitates dissection. The brachialis split is carried down to periosteum, and the muscle is reflected off the humerus, preserving the periosteum and as much muscle attachment as possible. The radial nerve is vulnerable as it traverses the spiral groove posteriorly in the mid-diaphysis, and as it lies between the brachioradialis and brachialis muscles distally in the anterior compartment.

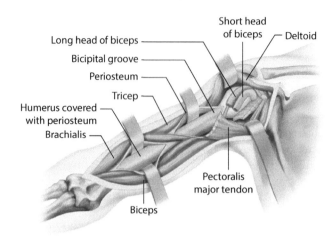

Figure 22.7 Anterolateral approach to the humerus. Proximally the interval is between the deltoid and pectoralis major muscles. The brachialis is split along its fibers at the mid-diaphysis.

Use caution placing anterior-posterior screws mid-shaft and ensure that the nerve is not trapped under the distal lateral corner of the plate. An oscillating drill can help protect the nerve by avoiding the possibility of winding the nerve up in the drill.

POSTERIOR APPROACH

The posterior approach[23] provides excellent exposure for fractures of the distal three-quarters of the humeral shaft and permits plating along the broad posterior surface of the humerus distally. Disadvantages are that the nerve is vulnerable intraoperatively and lies directly over the plate, and that prone or lateral positioning may be difficult in a polytraumatized patient.

The patient is placed prone or in the lateral decubitus position with the arm over a bolster. A tourniquet may be applied during the distal dissection and identification of the radial nerve, and then removed when working more proximally. The incision is centred over the fracture in the posterior midline and may be extended from the olecranon distally to the posterolateral aspect of the acromion proximally. The triceps muscle and fascia are divided sharply, taking care to identify and protect the radial nerve as it lies in the spiral groove of the humerus mid-shaft, and the profunda brachii artery, which travels with the nerve proximally. The approach continues proximally between the long and lateral heads of the triceps until the axillary nerve and posterior humeral circumflex artery are reached at the border of the deltoid (Figure 22.8a). If a plate is applied to the medial column of the distal humerus, identify and protect the ulnar nerve. The elbow joint can be accessed by performing an olecranon osteotomy and reflecting the triceps proximally.

MODIFIED POSTERIOR APPROACH

In the modified posterior approach described by Gerwin et al.,[24] the lower lateral brachial cutaneous nerve, which

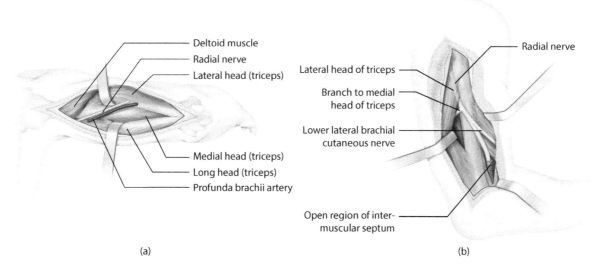

(a)

(b)

Figure 22.8 **(a)** Posterior approach to the humerus. The medial head of the triceps is divided sharply, taking care to protect the radial nerve and profunda brachii artery proximally. **(b)** Modified posterior approach to the humerus.

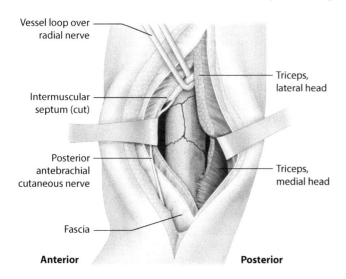

Figure 22.9 Lateral approach to the humerus. Elevation of the triceps from the intermuscular septum and division of the septum permit extensile exposure of the radial nerve.

branches off the radial nerve, is identified. The intermuscular septum is then divided deep to the lower lateral brachial cutaneous nerve, extending distally about 3 cm to reveal and permit mobilization of the radial nerve (Figure 22.8b). The medial and lateral heads of the triceps are elevated off the lateral intramuscular septum and swept medially, permitting exposure of up to 94% of the humeral diaphysis, compared to only 76% with a posterior triceps-splitting approach.

LATERAL APPROACH

The lateral approach[25] allows exposure of the distal two-thirds of the humerus through an intermuscular plane and also permits extensile exposure of the radial nerve (Figure 22.9). A plate can be placed on the anterior, posterior or lateral aspect of the humerus via this approach. The incision is made in line with the centre of the deltoid insertion and the lateral epicondyle. Incise the fascia overlying the lateral head of the triceps, about 1 cm posterior to the intermuscular septum. Sharply elevate the lateral head of the triceps from the intermuscular septum, dissecting down to bone. The radial nerve lies within the investing fat in the proximal aspect of the wound. As in the modified posterior approach, division of the intermuscular septum permits mobilization of the radial nerve distally, where it can be followed into the interval between the brachialis and the mobile extensor wad. The nerve can be traced proximally by dissecting between the deltoid and the lateral head of the triceps.

Plate fixation

Plate osteosynthesis is commonly cited as the preferred surgical treatment due to a simpler technique, lower reoperation rates and fewer shoulder problems compared to intramedullary nailing. Humeral shaft fractures are commonly plated with dynamic compression plates and non-locking cortical screws, applied in compression mode if the fracture is transverse or as a neutralization plate for oblique or spiral fractures that can accept some interfragmentary compression screws.

Locking screws offer biomechanical advantages in osteoporotic bone; a study of humeral shaft fractures in osteoporotic cadavers revealed enhanced torsional cyclic loading with locking plates and screws compared to standard cortical screws.[26] In a retrospective review of 22 humeral shaft nonunions treated with locking plates, no screw loosening or breakage occurred even in cases that continued to demonstrate nonunion.[27] Locking compression plates permit compression while simultaneously enhancing the pull-out strength of the construct.

Tingstad et al. demonstrated that immediate weight bearing after humerus plating is not associated with an increased risk of nonunion or malunion. Therefore, plating remains an effective option for multiply injured patients needing to use crutches or bear weight for any other reason.[28] The decision to allow weight bearing through a humeral shaft fracture should be determined after considering the adequacy of the reduction, stability of the fracture pattern, confidence in the fixation construct, and the needs and compliance of the patient.

SURGICAL TECHNIQUE – PLATE FIXATION

The fracture is exposed via one of the approaches described above.[29] Reduction clamps are used to reduce the fracture. If possible, one or more lag screws should be placed across the major fracture lines. If lag screw fixation is achieved, a large fragment plate and screws should be placed in neutralization mode to protect the lag screws. Transverse fractures are best reduced directly using bone clamps and the compression function of the plate. Prior to surgery, determine

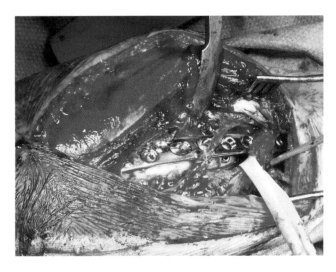

Figure 22.10 Dynamic compression plate. Care must be taken to identify and protect the radial nerve, marked here with a penrose, ensuring that it is not entrapped under the distal lateral aspect of the plate.

the plate length that will allow at least six cortices of fixation proximal and distal to the fracture. When applying a bridge plate across a comminuted fracture, longer plates with fewer screws improve working length and thereby reduce strain across the fracture site. Note that a stress riser occurs at the limit of the plate, which can be minimized by extending the plate longer than might otherwise be necessary. Acceptable plate constructs include a broad or narrow 4.5 mm plate, or one or two 3.5 mm plates in smaller patients. A biomechanical study showed that broad 4.5 mm plates were strongest in posterior-anterior bending and in torsion, but dual 3.5 mm plates offered the best compression and medial-lateral bending strength.[30] Another biomechanical study of plate constructs in humeral shaft nonunions also found that a 4.5 mm narrow compression plate applied perpendicular to a 3.5 mm reconstruction plate was stiffer than single plate constructs.[31] Therefore, dual plating may be useful for patients requiring early weight bearing, for example with crutches. When applying the plate to the bone, keep the position of the radial nerve in mind and check to make sure it does not slip under the corner of a plate (Figure 22.10).

Minimally invasive plate osteosynthesis

MIPO was introduced recently as a method of bridge plating humeral shaft fractures while limiting dissection. The procedure is technically challenging and has a risk of nonunion or malunion with imperfect plate positioning, as well as a potentially higher risk to the radial nerve. The technique can be performed through an anterior or posterior approach. The anterior approach utilizes the deltopectoral interval and is optimal for more proximal fractures. The radial nerve should be identified in both the anterior and posterior approaches (Figure 22.11). Although MIPO has not yet been rigorously compared to traditional plating or intramedullary nailing, the primary advantage appears to be cosmetic, depending on the number and size of the incisions.[32] This potential advantage is debatable since most surgeons still require about 10 cm of total incision length, either as a single large incision through a traditional open approach, or as two or three smaller MIPO incisions. No study to date has demonstrated

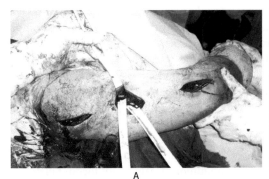
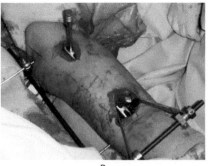

Figure 22.11 Minimally invasive plate osteosynthesis (MIPO). **(a)** Via a posterior approach, the radial nerve is identified in the middle and/or proximal windows. **(b)** A temporary external fixator can be applied to facilitate fracture reduction and plate application, shown here in an anterior approach. (Courtesy of Dr. Bruce Ziran.)

improved function or satisfaction with use of this technique. In elderly patients, the risk of nonunion or nerve entrapment requiring additional surgery may outweigh the benefits of cosmesis, and patients should be involved in the decision regarding surgical approach.

SURGICAL TECHNIQUE – ANTERIOR APPROACH FOR MIPO

The patient is positioned supine on a radiolucent table with image intensification coming from the contralateral side.[32] A narrow 4.5 mm locking compression plate is selected, typically one to two holes longer than for an open technique, and placed over the skin of the anterior arm. The proximal and distal surgical windows are marked; the proximal window is a 3–4 cm incision with a deltopectoral approach, and the distal window is a direct anterior approach to the distal diaphyseal humerus. The biceps muscle is retracted medially and the brachialis muscle is divided longitudinally to expose the anterior cortex of the distal humerus, using caution as the musculocutaneous nerve emerges on the anteromedial aspect of the brachialis. A periosteal elevator is used to create a sub-brachialis extraperiosteal tunnel by blunt dissection. The plate is inserted from the proximal window, through the sub-brachialis tunnel on the anterior aspect of the humerus, taking care to identify and protect the radial nerve in the distal window. A locking tower can be attached proximally to help maneuver the plate. After the proximal fragment is fixed to the plate, the fracture can be reduced indirectly. Screws are then inserted through the plate, which bridges the fracture. Alternatively, some surgeons apply a temporary external fixator at the beginning of the procedure to reduce the fracture and remove it after the plate is secured to bone (Figure 22.11c).

Intramedullary nailing

An intramedullary nail can be inserted into the humerus using an antegrade or retrograde technique, with or without locking screws. A potential advantage of nailing is that it can be performed with less soft tissue injury at the fracture site than plating. It may be preferred in osteoporotic patients as this technique does not rely on screw fixation for fracture stabilization.[2] In patients with pathologic fractures, who often have extensive areas of vulnerable bone, the nail spans and thereby protects the entire diaphysis. A disadvantage is that the nail and locking screw create a stress riser where the intramedullary canal ends above the coronoid and olecranon fossae.[33]

Biomechanical studies of locked humeral nailing suggest optimal mechanics are achieved when the nail is passed from the shorter bone fragment to the longer one.[34] Therefore, antegrade nailing is most appropriate for fractures of the proximal and middle thirds of the diaphysis, whereas distal third fractures should be nailed in a retrograde fashion. A disadvantage of retrograde nailing is the risk of periprosthetic fracture through the nail's entry point above the olecranon fossa.[35]

Modern nails offer distal locking mechanisms with interlocking screws. Biomechanical studies demonstrate that locking screws provide better axial and torsional stability than interference mechanisms.[36,37] Smaller diameter nails (7–9 mm) have minimized the need for reaming and reduced the risk of distraction and iatrogenic comminution at the fracture site. Reaming of the humerus should be minimized because it can harm the endosteal blood supply, causing an extensive zone of necrosis.[38,39] Some surgeons have advocated for an extra-articular entry point 1 cm distal to the crest of the greater tuberosity to avoid damaging the supraspinatus tendon insertion and the humeral head articular surface.[40]

Intraoperative complications occur in as many as 47% of cases and are 1.6 times more frequent when first generation nails are used compared to second generation nails.[35] The most common intraoperative complications are long proximal interlocking screw (8.1%), inadequate nail embedding (7.2%) and iatrogenic fracture propagation (6.3%).[35] Distraction across the fracture site is a common cause of nonunion. Since the distal end of the humeral canal tapers to a blind end, distraction may occur if the nail is too long, causing the distal tip to abut the end of the canal. Alternatively, a long nail may protrude into the subacromial space.

Disadvantages of antegrade intramedullary nailing are the increased incidence of shoulder problems due to violation of the rotator cuff and prominent implants leading to subacromial impingement, the possibility of iatrogenic distal humerus fracture in patients with a narrow canal, the potential for intraoperative breakage of distal locking screws, risk to neurovascular structures with insertion of the distal locking screw, inability to see and protect the radial nerve and greater difficulty with reconstruction if the fracture fails to heal.[35] Approximately 16% of patients treated with antegrade intramedullary nailing experience postoperative shoulder pain, attributed to violation of the rotator cuff and humeral head articular surface, and impingement.[35] Nailing is also associated with restricted shoulder range of motion compared to plating.[41] Antegrade intramedullary nailing violates the rotator cuff, which is already deteriorating in the elderly, and leaves the patient vulnerable to fracture at the end of the rod, particularly at the site of the distal locking screw. An additional insult may increase pain and difficulty with overhead activities such as brushing one's hair or reaching cabinets.[42] However, in patients whose fractures span a large portion of the humerus, nailing may cause less soft tissue trauma than plating (Figure 22.12). In elderly patients, nailing may also lead to more stable fixation than compression plating because it does not rely on screw purchase within osteoporotic bone.

SURGICAL TECHNIQUE – ANTEGRADE LOCKED INTRAMEDULLARY NAILING

The patient is placed in the lateral decubitus, beach chair or supine position with the operative arm against the patient's chest.[43] A 4 cm longitudinal skin incision is made, centred over the greater tuberosity. The deltoid muscle and supraspinatus tendons are carefully split. While protecting the

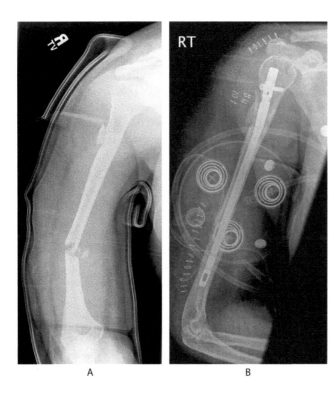

A   B

Figure 22.12 Antegrade intramedullary nail.
(a) Comminuted humeral shaft fracture spanning over
half the length of the humerus in a coaptation splint.
(b) Anatomic alignment achieved after antegrade
intramedullary nailing. (Courtesy of Dr. Jean Yun.)

rotator cuff, a 5 mm drill bit is used to create the entry portal in the humeral canal at the sulcus medial to the greater
tuberosity. Closed reduction of the fracture is achieved
and a 2.5 mm guide wire is passed down the canal across
the fracture site. When necessary, the canal is reamed in 0.5
mm increments, reaming as little as possible, and ensuring
fracture compression to avoid iatrogenic radial nerve injury.
A small incision may be made over the fracture site to identify the radial nerve and ensure it is protected prior to reaming. The nail is inserted over the guide wire until the head
of the nail is countersunk within the humeral head. Manual
compression is applied across the fracture site, and reduction
is confirmed with image intensification. One oblique or two
transverse proximal interlocking screws may be placed from
lateral to medial through the nail insertion handle, avoiding the articular surface and ensuring that screws do not
penetrate too far past the medial cortex. After eliminating
any distraction across the fracture site, distal locking screws
may be inserted using a mini-open technique, staying lateral
to the biceps to avoid radial nerve injury.[44] The rotator cuff
edges are re-approximated and the deltoid muscle is repaired
and the subcutaneous fascia and skin layers are closed.

SURGICAL TECHNIQUE – RETROGRADE LOCKED INTRAMEDULLARY NAILING

The patient is placed in a prone or lateral decubitus position
with the arm over a bolster, and image intensification is

brought in from the ipsilateral side.[23] The incision is made
from the tip of the olecranon, extending 4–5 cm proximally
in the posterior midline. The triceps is split and the olecranon fossa is identified. One of two start points is chosen:
classically 2 cm proximal to the olecranon fossa in the midline or through the superior aspect of the olecranon fossa
itself. Fracture reduction, canal reaming and nail insertion are performed according to the same principles as for
antegrade nailing. The proximal aspect of the nail should be
approximately 1.5 cm from the humeral head articular surface. The nail must be locked proximally to prevent the nail
from backing out distally, with subsequent pain and loss of
elbow motion. After irrigation and removal of bony debris,
the triceps tendon is closed with interrupted sutures. Early
active elbow motion is initiated to prevent stiffness.

Plating versus nailing

Evidence continues to demonstrate fewer complications
associated with plating than with nailing, but the gap
may be narrowing. A 2011 Cochrane review of five trials including 260 patients revealed significantly higher
incidence of shoulder impingement, decreased shoulder
range of motion and higher reoperation rate after locked
intramedullary nailing compared to dynamic compression plating.[41] Reoperations were typically to remove nails
in order to address shoulder impingement. Recent studies suggest that reoperation rates are similar for these two
techniques: 14.3–14.5% for plates compared to 15.4–16.3%
for nails.[2,45] Since functional outcomes and revision rates
for plating are equal to or better than those for nailing,
and since plating systems are approximately half the price
of nailing systems, Chen et al. favor plating as the more
cost-effective technique.

Although data on functional outcomes is limited, no
significant differences in patient-reported function, rates of
infection or iatrogenic radial nerve palsy were detected by
the Cochrane review. A meta-analysis of 14 studies including
727 patients also demonstrated higher shoulder-related complications with nailing, but noted higher infection rate and
higher iatrogenic radial nerve palsy with plating.[46] Similarly,
Ouyang et al. also found impaired shoulder motion after
nailing, but no difference in nonunion rates in their meta-
analysis of 10 randomized controlled trials.[47] Another
meta-analysis by Heineman et al. revealed fewer total complications associated with plates than with nails; when the
analysis was updated to include three new studies, the difference was attenuated but remained statistically significant.[48]

External fixation

External fixation is typically reserved for patients with
severe open fractures, polytrauma, or skin and soft tissue
damage such as burns or high velocity gunshot wounds
(Figure 22.13).[49] When indications were broadened to
include all displaced non-pathologic humeral shaft fractures,
Catagni et al. found good functional shoulder and elbow

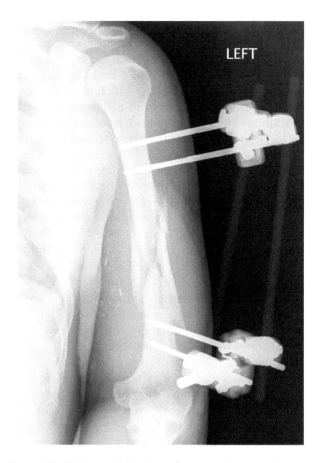

Figure 22.13 External fixation of an open fracture due to a gunshot wound.

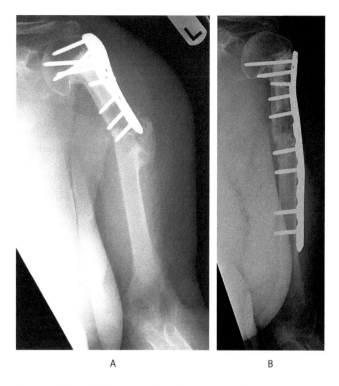

Figure 22.14 (a) Periprosthetic fracture at the distal aspect of a proximal humerus plate with hypertrophic nonunion. (b) The original plate was removed and replaced with a 10-hole metaphyseal plate and with iliac crest bone graft at the nonunion site. Radiographic and clinical union was achieved at 3 months.

motion in 80% and 95% of cases, respectively.[50] External fixation requires inserting pins through soft tissues, which may lead to pin site infections (12%) and restricted motion at the elbow and shoulder; the elderly are especially vulnerable to poor mobility with this treatment modality.

SPECIAL CONSIDERATIONS

Periprosthetic fractures

Periprosthetic humeral shaft fractures include those around a shoulder arthroplasty, total elbow arthroplasty or proximal humerus plate (Figure 22.14). The goals of treatment are to achieve fracture union, maintain prosthesis stability and preserve glenohumeral motion and overall shoulder function.[51] The stability of the implant must be assessed on preoperative radiographs, and with intraoperative stability testing. Minimally displaced fractures with a well-fixed prosthesis can often be managed non-operatively with a functional brace.[51] Revision arthroplasty is generally indicated for fractures around a loose prosthesis, whereas ORIF may be attempted for displaced fractures around a well-fixed implant.[52] Revision arthroplasty requires a long stem to bypass the fracture site, with or without allograft strut reinforcement. Cementless implants are typically preferred because of the

risk of cement extrusion through the fracture site, hindering fracture reduction and potentially placing the radial nerve or other structures at risk. ORIF may require a combination of plates, cerclage cables and allograft struts to achieve adequate fixation.[52]

COMPLICATIONS

Radial nerve palsy

Radial nerve palsy occurs in approximately 2–17% (mean 11.8%) of humeral shaft fractures[8,11,53] and is most commonly associated with fractures in the middle third and at the junction between the middle and distal thirds of the diaphysis. The radial nerve is vulnerable at the mid-diaphysis, where the nerve lies within the spiral groove of the humerus, and at the junction of the middle and distal thirds of the diaphysis, where the nerve is tethered as it pierces the lateral intermuscular septum. Operative exploration of a dysfunctional radial nerve is indicated for sharp penetrating injuries, high velocity gunshot wounds and open fractures.[8] In patients with a normal exam on presentation who subsequently develop radial nerve deficits after closed fracture manipulation, nerve function should be monitored with serial exams; this is not an indication for operative intervention.

Radial nerve injury associated with closed fracture of the humerus is nearly always a neurapraxia or axonotmesis (axonal disruption) and rarely a neurotmesis (disruption of the entire nerve and sheath). Current best evidence suggests exploration may be unnecessary or even harmful. A recent meta-analysis comparing early operative versus nonoperative management of acute radial nerve palsy revealed no difference between the groups in radial nerve function, although surgically treated patients had more complaints.[54] Another meta-analysis also reported equivalent nerve function between surgically and non-surgically treated radial nerve palsies, and found that 71% of patients recover spontaneously without intervention, with an 88% overall recovery rate including those who underwent surgical exploration.[53] Ekholm et al. noted complete recovery in 89% of non-operatively and 73% of operatively treated patients, and partial or complete persistent radial nerve palsy in 13% of operatively treated patients.[55] Complete clinical recovery of a compressive radial neuropathy occurs at a mean of 3.4 months but may take 6 or more months.[56] Nerve conduction studies (NCS) and electromyography (EMG) earlier than 3 weeks after injury (prior to Wallerian degeneration) is not helpful and may be misleading. Thereafter, EMG/NCS cannot distinguish between recoverable and irrecoverable nerve injuries (e.g. neurotmesis). Electrodiagnostic testing can detect electrical signs of muscle function about 4–6 weeks before they are detectable on physical examination.[57] Patients who would be satisfied with tendon transfers generally wait 6 and preferably 12 months for signs of improvement and then proceed with tendon transfers. Patients who prefer more sophisticated hand function might proceed to nerve exploration for potential nerve grafting if there are no clinical or electrophysiological signs of recovery 3–4 months after injury.

Nonunion

Nonunion arises due to both biologic factors, such as impaired blood supply, infection, smoking, osteoporosis and malnutrition, as well as mechanical factors, such as high-energy trauma, inadequate immobilization or distraction across the fracture site.[58,59] Transverse fracture patterns were believed to be associated with nonunion,[60] but others have reported an association with spiral and oblique patterns.[18] Proximal diaphysis fractures may have a higher nonunion rate due to the deforming forces of the deltoid and pectoralis insertions, and the risk of long head of the biceps tendon interposition into the fracture site.[61]

One retrospective study of approximately 10,000 Medicare patients revealed that use of non-steroidal anti-inflammatory drugs (NSAIDs) or opioids 60–90 days after sustaining a humeral shaft fracture was associated with nonunion.[62] However, since there was no relationship between early NSAID use and nonunion, the observed association could reflect increased analgesic use among patients with painful non-healing fractures rather than a direct causal effect.

Diaphyseal humerus fractures that fail to achieve union by 24 weeks meet traditional criteria for nonunion[63]; more recently, nonunion has been defined as failure to progress radiographically for 3 months or continued fracture mobility 6 weeks after injury.[27] Although the review by Sarmiento et al. of 620 patients reported nonunion in only 2% of patients treated with functional bracing, larger more recent studies reveal a 10–23% rate of nonunions.[8,11,15,16,64]

Up to 15% of surgically treated fractures are complicated by nonunion.[65] The majority (70–90%) of humeral diaphyseal nonunions are atrophic, meaning they lack sufficient callus.[60,66] Hypertrophic nonunions are associated with a robust callus, but lack mechanical stability.[67]

Radiographic signs of nonunion include poor fracture consolidation, interfragmentary diastasis or angulation, and hypertrophic callus with persistent pain or instability. Infection must be considered in any open or surgically treated fracture. C-reactive protein (CRP) will typically be elevated in cases of septic nonunion, although erythrocyte sedimentation rate (ESR) may be normal.

Implantable bone stimulators are US Food and Drug Administration (FDA)-approved for use in established nonunions that persist 9 months after injury; however, they may be associated with an increased risk of infection and their efficacy is not yet established.[68]

In the elderly, treatment of nonunion should focus on the patient's functional status and pain. Patients with painless nonunion and acceptable function can sometimes be managed non-operatively (Figure 22.15). Surgical goals in the treatment of nonunion are to provide a stable mechanical construct that allows for early range of motion, and a biological environment conducive to healing. Atrophic nonunion is commonly treated with ORIF with a 4.5 mm compression plate, with or without autologous bone graft. Locked plating is preferred in osteoporotic bone with poor screw purchase. Both autologous iliac crest

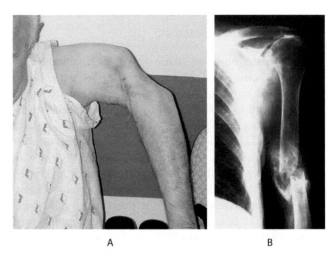

A   B

Figure 22.15 (a) Patient with painless pseudarthrosis and acceptable function, and (b) radiographic evidence of hypertrophic nonunion, managed nonoperatively.

bone graft (ICBG) and demineralized bone matrix (DBM) lead to high union rates, although at the time of writing no human studies have directly and prospectively compared the two.[69,70] A retrospective study on management of atrophic nonunions suggests that DBM leads to equivalent union rates without the donor site morbidity associated with iliac crest autograft.[70] In patients who cannot tolerate donor site morbidity, DBM may be an effective alternative to ICBG.[60,66,67,69]

Hypertrophic nonunion occurs due to a robust biologic healing response in the absence of mechanical stability. Therefore, it can often be treated with plating alone, without bone graft. The nonunion site is debrided down to healthy, bleeding bone and synovial or fibrous tissue is excised. Re- establishing the intramedullary canal provides an excellent source of osteoprogenitor cells. In cases of infected, dysvascular or dead bone, up to 3–4 cm of bone may need to be resected to reach viable bone proximally and distally.[67] Fracture reduction can correct angular deformities, achieve good joint alignment and maximize cortical contact to confer immediate mechanical stability and promote healing. At least six points of fixation (three bicortical screws) should be obtained on either side of the fracture.

Infection

Infection may arise after open or surgically treated fractures and may contribute to nonunion. Treatment involves first eradicating the infection and subsequently achieving bony union. When possible, preoperative aspirates may guide antibiotic treatment. Deep intraoperative cultures should be taken, followed by thorough irrigation and debridement. Immediate internal fixation is appropriate in healthy, non-diabetic, non-smokers with a single nonvirulent organism such as *Staphylococcus epidermidis* and adequate soft tissue coverage.[71] In patients who develop deep infection within 6 weeks after initial operative fixation, over 70% of patients will achieve union with operative debridement, retention of hardware, and culture-specific antibiotic treatment and suppression.[72] Patients who sustained an open fracture or were treated with an intramedullary nail are less likely to achieve union with maintenance of hardware and may require revision ORIF. Fixation may be augmented with antibiotic-impregnated calcium sulfate or methylmethacrylate cement beads.[73] Long-term intravenous antibiotics are initiated based on the cultured organism sensitivities; infectious disease specialists recommend three to five cultures to limit false positives. This single-staged approach is effective in over 70% of clinically aseptic but culture-positive diaphyseal nonunions.[71]

Patients with comorbidities, multiple organisms or virulent organisms such as *Staphylococcus aureus* should undergo staged treatment. Irrigation and debridement with placement of an antibiotic bead pouch is performed first, followed by definitive fixation with compression plating after ESR and CRP have normalized (typically 6–12 weeks later).

REFERENCES

1. Ekholm R, Adami J, Tidermark J, et al. Fractures of the shaft of the humerus. An epidemiological study of 401 fractures. *J Bone Joint Surg Br* 2006;**88**(11):1469–73. doi: 10.1302/0301-620X.88B11.17634.

2. Chen F, Wang Z, Bhattacharyya T. Outcomes of nails versus plates for humeral shaft fractures: A Medicare cohort study. *J Orthop Trauma* 2013;**27**(2):68–72. doi: 10.1097/BOT.0b013e31824a3e66.

3. Court-Brown CM, Caesar B. Epidemiology of adult fractures: A review. *Injury* 2006;**37**(8):691–7. doi: 10.1016/j.injury.2006.04.130.

4. Tytherleigh-Strong G, Walls N, McQueen MM. The epidemiology of humeral shaft fractures. *J Bone Joint Surg Br* 1998;**80**(2):249–53.

5. Chen AL, Koval KJ. Elder abuse: The role of the orthopaedic surgeon in diagnosis and management. *J Am Acad Orthop Surg* 2002;**10**(1):25–31.

6. Sprague S, Bhandari M, Della Rocca GJ, et al. Prevalence of abuse and intimate partner violence surgical evaluation (PRAISE) in orthopaedic fracture clinics: A multinational prevalence study. *Lancet* 2013;**382**(9895):866–76. doi: 10.1016/S0140-6736(13)61205-2.

7. Adili A, Bhandari M, Sprague S, et al. Humeral shaft fractures as predictors of intra-abdominal injury in motor vehicle collision victims. *Arch Orthop Trauma Surg* 2002;**122**(1):5–9.

8. Sarmiento A, Zagorski JB, Zych GA, et al. Functional bracing for the treatment of fractures of the humeral diaphysis. *J Bone Joint Surg Am* 2000;**82**(4):478–86.

9. Pritchett JW. Inferior subluxation of the humeral head after trauma or surgery. *J Shoulder Elbow Surg* 1997;**6**(4):356–9.

10. Gustilo RB, Anderson JT. Prevention of infection in the treatment of one thousand and twenty-five open fractures of long bones: Retrospective and prospective analyses. *J Bone Joint Surg Am* 1976;**58**(4):453–8.

11. Koch PP, Gross DF, Gerber C. The results of functional (Sarmiento) bracing of humeral shaft fractures. *J Shoulder Elbow Surg* 2002;**11**(2):143–50.

12. Caldwell JA. Treatment of fractures in the Cincinnati General Hospital. *Ann Surg* 1933;**97**(2):161–76.

13. Sarmiento A, Kinman PB, Galvin EG, et al. Functional bracing of fractures of the shaft of the humerus. *J Bone Joint Surg Am* 1977;**59**(5):596–601.

14. Neuhaus V, Menendez M, Kurylo JC, et al. Risk factors for fracture mobility six weeks after initiation of brace treatment of mid-diaphyseal humeral fractures. *J Bone Joint Surg Am* 2014;**96**(5):403–7. doi: 10.2106/JBJS.M.00089.

15. Rutgers M, Ring D. Treatment of diaphyseal fractures of the humerus using a functional brace. *J Orthop Trauma* 2006;**20**(9):597–601. doi: 10.1097/01.bot.0000249423.48074.82.

16. Ekholm R, Tidermark J, Tornkvist H, et al. Outcome after closed functional treatment of humeral shaft fractures. *J Orthop Trauma* 2006;**20**(9):591–6. doi: 10.1097/01.bot.0000246466.01287.04.

17. Jawa A, McCarty P, Doornberg J, et al. Extra-articular distal-third diaphyseal fractures of the humerus. A comparison of functional bracing and plate fixation. *J Bone Joint Surg Am* 2006;**88**(11):2343–7. doi: 10.2106/JBJS.F.00334.

18. Ring D, Chin K, Taghinia AH, et al. Nonunion after functional brace treatment of diaphyseal humerus fractures. *J Trauma* 2007;**62**(5):1157–8. doi: 10.1097/01.ta.0000222719.52619.2c.

19. Broadbent MR, Will E, McQueen MM. Prediction of outcome after humeral diaphyseal fracture. *Injury* 2010;**41**(6):572–7. doi: 10.1016/j.injury.2009.09.023.

20. Klenerman L. Fractures of the shaft of the humerus. *J Bone Joint Surg Br* 1966;**48**(1):105–11.

21. Gosler MW, Testroote M, Morrenhof JW, et al. Surgical versus non-surgical interventions for treating humeral shaft fractures in adults. *Cochrane Database Syst Rev* 2012;**1**:CD008832. doi: 10.1002/14651858.CD008832.pub2.

22. Denard A Jr., Richards JE, Obremskey WT, et al. Outcome of nonoperative vs operative treatment of humeral shaft fractures: A retrospective study of 213 patients. *Orthopedics* 2010;**33**(8). doi: 10.3928/01477447-20100625-16.

23. Rockwood CA, Green DP, Bucholz RW. *Rockwood and Green's Fractures in Adults*. 7th ed. Philadelphia, PA: Wolters Kluwer Health, 2010.

24. Gerwin M, Hotchkiss RN, Weiland AJ. Alternative operative exposures of the posterior aspect of the humeral diaphysis with reference to the radial nerve. *J Bone Joint Surg Am* 1996;**78**(11):1690–5.

25. Mills WJ, Hanel DP, Smith DG. Lateral approach to the humeral shaft: An alternative approach for fracture treatment. *J Orthop Trauma* 1996;**10**(2):81–6.

26. Davis C, Stall A, Knutsen E, et al. Locking plates in osteoporosis: A biomechanical cadaveric study of diaphyseal humerus fractures. *J Orthop Trauma* 2012;**26**(4):216–21. doi: 10.1097/BOT.0b013e318220edae.

27. Ring D, Kloen P, Kadzielski J, et al. Locking compression plates for osteoporotic nonunions of the diaphyseal humerus. *Clin Orthop Relat Res* 2004;(425):50–4.

28. Tingstad EM, Wolinsky PR, Shyr Y, et al. Effect of immediate weightbearing on plated fractures of the humeral shaft. *J Trauma* 2000;**49**(2):278–80.

29. Wiesel SW, Miller MD, eds. *Operative Techniques in Orthopaedic Surgery*. Philadelphia, PA: Lippincott Williams & Wilkins, 2011.

30. Kosmopoulos V, Luedke C, Nana AD. Dual small fragment plating improves screw-to-screw load sharing for mid-diaphyseal humeral fracture fixation: A finite element study. *Technol Health Care* 2015;**23**(1):83–92. doi: 10.3233/THC-140875.

31. Rubel IF, Kloen P, Campbell D, et al. Open reduction and internal fixation of humeral nonunions: A biomechanical and clinical study. *J Bone Joint Surg Am* 2002;**84**-A(8):1315–22.

32. Shin SJ, Sohn HS, Do NH. Minimally invasive plate osteosynthesis of humeral shaft fractures: A technique to aid fracture reduction and minimize complications. *J Orthop Trauma* 2012;**26**(10):585–9. doi: 10.1097/BOT.0b013e318254895f.

33. McKee MD, Pedlow FX, Cheney PJ, et al. Fractures below the end of locking humeral nails: A report of three cases. *J Orthop Trauma* 1996;**10**(7):500–4.

34. Lin J, Inoue N, Valdevit A, et al. Biomechanical comparison of antegrade and retrograde nailing of humeral shaft fracture. *Clin Orthop Relat Res* 1998;(351):203–13.

35. Baltov A, Mihail R, Dian E. Complications after interlocking intramedullary nailing of humeral shaft fractures. *Injury* 2014;**45**(Suppl 1):S9–15. doi: 10.1016/j.injury.2013.10.044.

36. Zimmerman MC, Waite AM, Deehan M, et al. A biomechanical analysis of four humeral fracture fixation systems. *J Orthop Trauma* 1994;**8**(3):233–9.

37. Blum J, Machemer H, Baumgart F, et al. Biomechanical comparison of bending and torsional properties in retrograde intramedullary nailing of humeral shaft fractures. *J Orthop Trauma* 1999;**13**(5):344–50.

38. Garnavos C. Diaphyseal humeral fractures and intramedullary nailing: Can we improve outcomes? *Indian J Orthop* 2011;**45**(3):208–15. doi: 10.4103/0019-5413.67117.

39. Ochsner PE, Baumgart F, Kohler G. Heat-induced segmental necrosis after reaming of one humeral and two tibial fractures with a narrow medullary canal. *Injury* 1998;**29**(Suppl 2):B1–10.

40. Dimakopoulos P, Papadopoulos AX, Papas M, et al. Modified extra rotator-cuff entry point in antegrade humeral nailing. *Arch Orthop Trauma Surg* 2005;**125**(1):27–32. doi: 10.1007/s00402-004-0757-3.

41. Kurup H, Hossain M, Andrew JG. Dynamic compression plating versus locked intramedullary nailing for humeral shaft fractures in adults. *Cochrane Database Syst Rev* 2011;(6):CD005959. doi: 10.1002/14651858.CD005959.pub2.

42. Robinson CM, Bell KM, Court-Brown CM, et al. Locked nailing of humeral shaft fractures. Experience in Edinburgh over a two-year period. *J Bone Joint Surg Br* 1992;**74**(4):558–62.

43. Lin J, Hou SM. Antegrade locked nailing for humeral shaft fractures. *Clin Orthop Relat Res* 1999;(365):201–10.

44. Bono CM, Grossman MG, Hochwald N, et al. Radial and axillary nerves. Anatomic considerations for humeral fixation. *Clin Orthop Relat Res* 2000;(373):259–64.

45. Denies E, Nijs S, Sermon A, et al. Operative treatment of humeral shaft fractures. Comparison of plating and intramedullary nailing. *Acta Orthop Belg* 2010;**76**(6):735–42.

46. Dai J, Chai Y, Wang C, et al. Dynamic compression plating versus locked intramedullary nailing for humeral shaft fractures: A meta-analysis of RCTs and nonrandomized studies. *J Orthop Sci* 2014;**19**(2):282–91. doi: 10.1007/s00776-013-0497-8.

47. Ouyang H, Xiong J, Xiang P, et al. Plate versus intramedullary nail fixation in the treatment of humeral shaft fractures: An updated meta-analysis. *J Shoulder Elbow Surg* 2013;**22**(3):387–95. doi: 10.1016/j.jse.2012.06.007.

48. Heineman DJ, Bhandari M, Poolman RW. Plate fixation or intramedullary fixation of humeral shaft fractures—An update. *Acta Orthop* 2012;**83**(3):317–18. doi: 10.3109/17453674.2012.695677.

49. Wisniewski TF, Radziejowski MJ. Gunshot fractures of the humeral shaft treated with external fixation. *J Orthop Trauma* 1996;**10**(4):273–8.

50. Catagni MA, Lovisetti L, Guerreschi F, et al. The external fixation in the treatment of humeral diaphyseal fractures: Outcomes of 84 cases. *Injury* 2010;**41**(11):1107–11. doi: 10.1016/j.injury.2010.09.015.

51. Mineo GV, Accetta R, Franceschini M, et al. Management of shoulder periprosthetic fractures: Our institutional experience and review of the literature. *Injury* 2013;**44**(Suppl 1):S82–5. doi: 10.1016/S0020-1383(13)70018-4.

52. Andersen JR, Williams CD, Cain R, et al. Surgically treated humeral shaft fractures following shoulder arthroplasty. *J Bone Joint Surg Am* 2013;**95**(1):9–18. doi: 10.2106/JBJS.K.00863.

53. Shao YC, Harwood P, Grotz MR, et al. Radial nerve palsy associated with fractures of the shaft of the humerus: A systematic review. *J Bone Joint Surg Br* 2005;**87**(12):1647–52. doi: 10.1302/0301-620X.87B12.16132.

54. Liu GY, Zhang CY, Wu HW. Comparison of initial nonoperative and operative management of radial nerve palsy associated with acute humeral shaft fractures. *Orthopedics* 2012;**35**(8):702–8. doi: 10.3928/01477447-20120725-10.

55. Ekholm R, Ponzer S, Tornkvist H, et al. Primary radial nerve palsy in patients with acute humeral shaft fractures. *J Orthop Trauma* 2008;**22**(6):408–14. doi: 10.1097/BOT.0b013e318177eb06.

56. Arnold WD, Krishna VR, Freimer M, et al. Prognosis of acute compressive radial neuropathy. *Muscle Nerve* 2012;**45**(6):893–5. doi: 10.1002/mus.23305.

57. Kimura J. *Electrodiagnosis in Diseases of Nerve and Muscle: Principles and Practice.* 3rd ed. New York: Oxford University Press, 2001.

58. Cadet ER, Yin B, Schulz B, et al. Proximal humerus and humeral shaft nonunions. *J Am Acad Orthop Surg* 2013;**21**(9):538–47. doi: 10.5435/JAAOS-21-09-538.

59. Ward EF, Savoie FHI, Hughes JLJ. Fractures of the diaphyseal humerus. In: Browner BD, Jupiter JB, Levine AM, et al., eds. *Skeletal Trauma: Fractures, Dislocations, Ligamentous Injuries.* Philadelphia, PA: Saunders, 1998. pp. 1523–47.

60. Healy WL, White GM, Mick CA, et al. Nonunion of the humeral shaft. *Clin Orthop Relat Res* 1987;**219**:206–13.

61. Prasarn ML, Achor T, Paul O, et al. Management of nonunions of the proximal humeral diaphysis. *Injury* 2010;**41**(12):1244–8. doi: 10.1016/j.injury.2010.04.002.

62. Bhattacharyya T, Levin R, Vrahas MS, et al. Nonsteroidal antiinflammatory drugs and nonunion of humeral shaft fractures. *Arthritis Rheum* 2005;**53**(3):364–7. doi: 10.1002/art.21170.

63. Jupiter JB, von Deck M. Ununited humeral diaphyses. *J Shoulder Elbow Surg* 1998;**7**(6):644–53.

64. Papasoulis E, Drosos GI, Ververidis AN, et al. Functional bracing of humeral shaft fractures. A review of clinical studies. *Injury* 2010;**41**(7):e21–7. doi: 10.1016/j.injury.2009.05.004.

65. Rosen H. The treatment of nonunions and pseudarthroses of the humeral shaft. *Orthop Clin North Am* 1990;**21**(4):725–42.

66. Foulk DA, Szabo RM. Diaphyseal humerus fractures: Natural history and occurrence of nonunion. *Orthopedics* 1995;**18**(4):333–5.

67. Pugh DM, McKee MD. Advances in the management of humeral nonunion. *J Am Acad Orthop Surg* 2003;**11**(1):48–59.

68. Nelson FR, Brighton CT, Ryaby J, et al. Use of physical forces in bone healing. *J Am Acad Orthop Surg* 2003;**11**(5):344–54.

69. Marti RK, Verheyen CC, Besselaar PP. Humeral shaft nonunion: Evaluation of uniform surgical repair in fifty-one patients. *J Orthop Trauma* 2002;**16**(2):108–15.

70. Hierholzer C, Sama D, Toro JB, et al. Plate fixation of ununited humeral shaft fractures: Effect of type of bone graft on healing. *J Bone Joint Surg Am* 2006;**88**(7):1442–7. doi: 10.2106/JBJS.E.00332.

71. Amorosa LF, Buirs LD, Bexkens R, et al. A single-stage treatment protocol for presumptive aseptic diaphyseal nonunions: A review of outcomes. *J Orthop Trauma* 2013;**27**(10):582–6. doi: 10.1097/BOT.0b013e31828b76f2.

72. Berkes M, Obremskey WT, Scannell B, et al. Maintenance of hardware after early postoperative infection following fracture internal fixation. *J Bone Joint Surg Am* 2010;**92**(4):823–8. doi: 10.2106/JBJS.I.00470.

73. Fears RL, Gleis GE, Seligson D. Diagnosis and treatment of complications. In: Browner BD, Jupiter JB, Levine AM, et al., eds. *Skeletal Trauma: Fractures, Dislocations, Ligamentous Injuries*. Philadelphia, PA: Saunders, 1998. pp. 567–78.

23

Distal humeral fractures

NATHAN SACEVICH, GEORGE S. ATHWAL AND GRAHAM KING

INTRODUCTION

The objective of treatment for distal humerus fractures in the elderly is to restore a stable, functional and painless elbow, which will enable return to independence for activities of daily living. While the orthopaedic principles of anatomic reduction, stable fixation, preservation of soft tissues and early mobilization remain paramount in the surgical treatment of these injuries, they may often be difficult to achieve. The complex anatomy of the distal humerus, diminished bone quality, fracture comminution and articular involvement present numerous challenges to achieving a successful anatomic reconstruction.

Treatment advances for distal humerus fractures include a better appreciation of the role of non-operative management, the improved availability of computed tomography (CT) with three-dimensional reconstruction, an improved understanding of biomechanically advantageous fixation strategies, the development of periarticular precontoured locking plates and the selective use of elbow arthroplasty.

EPIDEMIOLOGY

Distal humerus fractures account for 1–2% of all fractures in adults.[1] They have a bimodal age distribution with increased incidences occurring between the ages of 12 and 19 years, and in those aged 80 years and older.[2] The first peak in fracture incidence typically occurs in adolescent males and is generally the result of high-energy injuries. The second peak incidence represents the fragility-type distal humerus fracture. These patients are characteristically female and the fractures usually occur as the result of low energy injuries, such as a fall from standing height.[3,4]

The overall incidence of elderly distal humerus fractures is increasing, in parallel to the increasing incidence of other osteoporotic fractures. An increasing activity level among the elderly population is believed to be a contributing factor to this observed trend.[5] An American study performed from 1965 to 1974 identified the incidence of distal humerus fractures in patients greater than 70 years to be 20 per 100,000 persons.[6] Subsequently, a Canadian study by Sheps et al.[7] reported an incidence of 54 per 100,000 persons in the population 80 years or older, with females having an incidence approximately 1.5 times greater than males. A study of osteoporotic distal humerus fractures in Finnish women reported a twofold increase in the age-adjusted incidence of distal humerus fractures from 1970 (12/100,000) to 1995 (28/100,000) and predicted an additional threefold increase by 2030.[8]

When considering treatment options, the importance of patient functional status should be emphasized rather than chronological age. A large combined prospective and retrospective study has noted that greater than 80% of elderly patients presenting with isolated distal humerus fractures were in good general health and were living at home with reasonable independence of activities of daily living.[5] Overall, 41% of men and 69% of women in the retrospective cohort portion of this study demonstrated radiographic signs of osteoporosis. Eighty-nine per cent of patients required surgical treatment and the presence of osteoporosis had a significant negative effect on clinical and radiological outcomes.

Although mortality risk following distal humerus fractures is not well established, it has not been recognized to be as substantial as that reported for other geriatric fractures such as proximal femur fractures.[9,10] Nonetheless, these injuries may result in significant functional deterioration and eventually disability and loss of independence. The economic impact of these injuries may be offset by implementing treatment strategies which yield successful and timely functional outcomes with low complication rates. Furthermore, primary and secondary prevention strategies such as fall prevention and osteoporosis treatment should be implemented.

CLASSIFICATION

The most widely used classification system for distal humerus fractures is that of the AO/Orthopaedic Trauma Association (OTA).[11] In this system, fractures are divided into three principle categories: type A (extra-articular), type B (partial articular) and type C (complete articular). Type A distal humerus fractures are extra-articular and may involve the epicondyles or occur at the distal humerus metaphyseal level. Type B fractures are partial articular with some degree of continuity between the humeral shaft segment and part of the articular segment. Type B fractures include unicondylar fractures and sagittal plane or coronal shear fractures of the articular surface. Type C fractures are complete articular fractures with no continuity between the humeral shaft segment and the articular segments. The AO/OTA system further subclassifies fractures based on fracture line and degree of comminution (types 1–3). Both the AO/OTA type A (extra-articular transcondylar) fractures and the AO/OTA type C fractures have been reported as the most frequent variants identified in geriatric patients.[5,7]

Anatomical considerations

The distal humerus can be considered as a divergent two column structure supporting the distal articular surface. The distal humeral shaft is triangular shaped in cross-section with its apex directed anteriorly. The medial column diverges approximately 45 degrees from the shaft in the coronal plane, whereas the lateral column diverges at approximately 20 degrees from the shaft.[2] The trochlea connects the columns centrally and forms an articulation with the coronoid and olecranon facets of the ulna. The anatomy of the trochlea is analogous to that of a spool. The capitellum is the distal-most portion of the lateral column, which articulates with the radial head. The trochlea is more distal than the capitellum in the coronal plane, which results in a valgus alignment of 4–8 degrees. The distal articular segment of the humerus is internally rotated 3–8 degrees relative to the epicondyles and has 30–40 degrees of anterior angulation relative to the central axis of the humerus.[12] The distal posterior portion of the lateral column is non-articular and permits distal placement of contoured posterolateral plates (Figure 23.1).

The lateral collateral ligament (LCL) consists of the lateral ulnar collateral ligament, the radial collateral ligament and the annular ligament. The lateral ulnar collateral ligament originates on the lateral epicondyle and inserts at the crista supinatoris of the ulna. The radial collateral ligament originates at the lateral epicondyle and merges with the

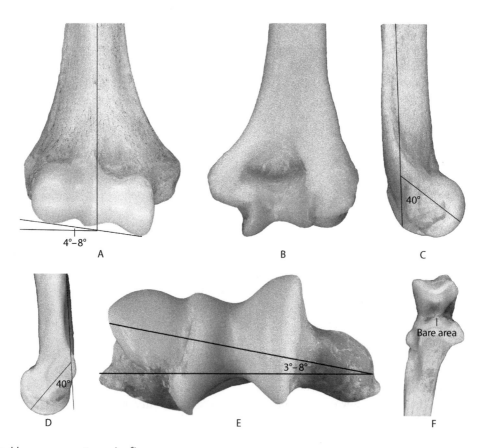

Figure 23.1 Distal humerus anatomy (a–f).

annular ligament distally. The annular ligament attaches to the anterior and posterior margins of the lesser sigmoid notch of the ulna and encircles the radial head. The LCL is considered the primary soft tissue stabilizer of varus angulation and posterolateral rotation and it must be identified and protected during approaches to the radiocapitellar joint and during lateral plate application.

The medial collateral ligament (MCL) originates from the anteroinferior surface of the medial epicondyle and consists of three distinct bundles: anterior, posterior and transverse. The anterior bundle is considered the most important ligamentous stabilizer against valgus stress and posteromedial instability. The anterior bundle of the MCL inserts onto the sublime tubercle on the anteromedial aspect of the coronoid process.[13] The fan-shaped posterior bundle attaches to the medial margin of the trochlear notch and provides secondary valgus stability at higher flexion angles.[14] The medial column and medial epicondyle can accommodate medial plate placement without impinging on the MCL origin.

CLINICAL ASSESSMENT

An accurate history should define the mechanism of injury and identify any possible cardiovascular, neurologic and pharmacologic precipitants of the fall in geriatric distal humeral fractures.[4] A thorough evaluation for associated injuries must be completed. The medical history should identify comorbidities and reversible illnesses that may impact treatment recommendations and perioperative risk. Patient cognitive status and ability to comply with rehabilitation, functional status, pre-existing elbow pathology and social circumstances are important treatment considerations.

The injured extremity should be examined for signs of soft tissue injury and compromise including oedema, bruising, abrasions, fracture blisters, skin tenting and open wounds. The standard open fracture treatment protocol should be initiated in a timely fashion for open distal humerus fractures. A thorough neurologic examination must be performed and accurately documented.

Incomplete ulnar neuropathy has been reported in 26% of patients with type C distal humerus fractures at the time of presentation.[15] Any clinical suggestion of vascular compromise should prompt comprehensive assessment, including brachial-brachial Doppler pressure index and vascular surgeon consultation. Compartment syndrome should always be considered, particularly in the setting of high-energy trauma, and compartment pressures assessed when the clinical examination is inconclusive.

Imaging

Standard anteroposterior and lateral radiographs of the elbow should be performed. Radiographs taken out of immobilization where splint material may impair fracture visualization, as well as traction radiographs, may be beneficial.

Computed tomography imaging is helpful in delineating complex fracture patterns such as coronal plane articular fractures, comminuted or segmental articular fractures, and 'low' transverse extra-articular fractures. Increased interobserver and intraobserver reliability for fracture classification as well as increased intraobserver reliability for treatment decisions has been reported with the use of three-dimensional CT.[16] CT is particularly useful in instances where a less invasive surgical approach for open reduction and internal fixation (ORIF) is being contemplated, such as using a paratricipital approach rather than an olecranon osteotomy. CT may also help to identify highly comminuted articular fractures in the elderly, which may be better treated with primary arthroplasty.

TREATMENT

Non-operative treatment

Complex distal humerus fractures were often historically managed non-operatively with cast immobilization, collar and cuff treatment or early mobilization.[17,18] A number of studies have demonstrated that ORIF yields better outcomes than non-operative treatment.[15,19–22] A pooled analysis of two level III studies, including one that was based exclusively on patients aged 75 years or older, demonstrated that patients treated non-operatively are almost three times more likely to have an unacceptable result.[23] Another retrospective study reported that nonoperatively treated patients were almost six times more likely to have a nonunion and four times more likely to have delayed union than operatively treated patients.[3]

While non-operative management of complex distal humerus fractures in the elderly is generally reserved for patients with limited pre-existing function of their fractured arm or when medical comorbidities preclude operative treatment,[24] it may represent a safe treatment option with satisfactory clinical results.[25]

Cast immobilization is generally the preferred non-operative treatment. A well-padded cast is applied with the elbow at 90 degrees of flexion and the forearm in neutral rotation for 6–8 weeks. Frequent follow-up visits are required to ensure appropriate cast fit and that there has been no development of soft tissue compromise. Once bony union is evident, active range of motion is encouraged. Physiotherapy with static progressive splinting is prescribed in selected patients where the recovery of motion is slow. Collar and cuff immobilization is the recommended non-operative treatment modality for patients with widely displaced fractures and those with cognitive or communicative disability which prevents them from conveying symptoms of an ill-fitting cast and resultant development of pressure ulcers. Despite the prolonged immobilization period often required to achieve union, elbow stiffness is not common in this patient group. A recently published[26] retrospective review of 19 medically unwell and elderly patients treated non-operatively for a fracture of the distal humerus at our institution demonstrated an 81% union rate with an overall 68% good to excellent subjective outcome at final follow-up (Figure 23.2). The mean elbow flexion extension arc was 22–128 degrees, a mean Mayo Elbow Performance Score (MEPS) of 90 and a mean Disabilities of the Arm, Shoulder and Hand (DASH) score of 38. One patient with a distal humeral non-union was sufficiently symptomatic to undergo a total elbow arthroplasty (TEA).

Open reduction and internal fixation

ORIF is recommended for displaced or angulated distal humeral fractures in the elderly. Rigid internal fixation allows for anatomic fracture reduction and permits early range of motion, which is essential in preventing post-traumatic elbow stiffness. Anatomic reduction of the articular surface and overall elbow alignment are prioritized over early motion when stable fixation is unattainable. However, in elderly patients with poor intraoperative fixation stability, consideration should be given to conversion to a primary arthroplasty. A secondary arthroplasty for failed internal fixation has a higher complication rate and a poorer functional outcome than a primary arthroplasty.

POSITIONING AND APPROACHES

The patient can either be positioned in the supine position, with the elbow supported by a sterile bolster or folded sheet placed on the patient's chest. An alternative is the lateral

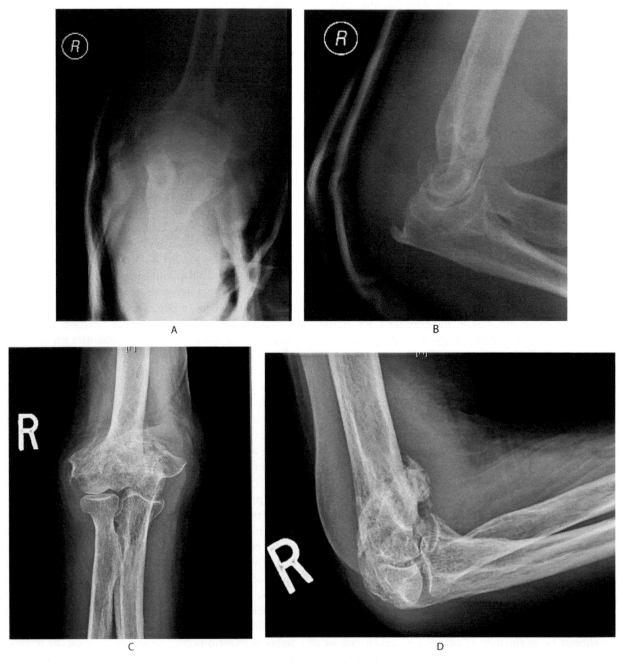

A

B

C

D

Figure 23.2 A 93-year-old man with a type C distal humerus fracture, treated non-operatively with pain free elbow and functional range of motion at last follow-up (a–d).

decubitus position using a bean bag with the elbow supported on an arthroscopy arm holder. A commercially available articulated arm positioner can be used in the supine position when an assistant is unavailable. This device also takes pressure off the patient's chest, which may be important in patients with compromised pulmonary capacity or those undergoing surgery under a regional anaesthetic.

The choice of surgical approach depends on several factors. It must provide adequate exposure to permit anatomic reduction and appropriate fixation while minimizing soft tissue disruption. Fracture pattern, extent of articular involvement, associated soft tissue injury, rehabilitation protocol, surgeon preference and the possibility of intraoperative conversion to arthroplasty must be considered.

In general, a utilitarian posterior skin incision with elevation of full-thickness fasciocutaneous medial and lateral flaps is used to access the distal humerus through one of the posterior approaches or through medial or lateral approaches. Although a direct lateral incision and approach through the Kocher interval, Kaplan interval or a common extensor tendon split can be used for treatment of capitellar fractures and simple partial articular lateral column fractures, the direct midline posterior incision is advantageous as it permits unrestricted access to both the medial and lateral columns and has also been shown to have a decreased risk of cutaneous nerve injury.[27] Furthermore, the same incision can be used for contracture release and for elbow arthroplasty if required secondarily.

The ulnar nerve should be identified and protected throughout the course of the procedure. The necessity for transposition of the ulnar nerve is controversial. If the nerve demonstrates instability or has a tendency to lie over the applied medial plate, anterior transposition should be considered. In the setting of preoperative ulnar nerve dysfunction, transposition has been recommended.[28] In the absence of definitive data, the authors routinely perform an ulnar nerve transposition for all distal humeral fractures requiring medial column fixation.

Posterior approaches include the olecranon osteotomy, the paratricipital 'triceps on' and the 'triceps off' approaches. Triceps off approaches include triceps reflecting, triceps splitting and the triceps tongue approaches. The fracture characteristics, including the degree and complexity of articular involvement, dictate the most appropriate surgical approach.

Visualization of the distal humerus articular segment varies with each approach. The olecranon osteotomy approach has been shown to expose 57% of the distal articular segment, whereas the triceps splitting and triceps reflecting approaches have been shown to expose 35% and 46%, respectively.[29] The latter approaches can generally be used for simple extra-articular fractures. The triceps off approaches require postoperative protective protocols that may be impractical in the geriatric population. These protocols restrict elbow flexion and limit triceps activation, which may compromise the patient's ability to mobilize with ambulatory aids and to perform their activities of daily living.

Potential complications associated with olecranon osteotomy include malunion, nonunion and symptomatic internal fixation. Eight per cent of patients who had undergone olecranon osteotomy required removal of symptomatic osteotomy fixation, regardless of the fixation used.[30] Schmidt-Horlohé et al.[31] reported a 22.5% complication rate, including delayed or nonunion and screw loosening, and 48.4% rate of fixation removal in their series of 31 patients with olecranon osteotomies repaired with one-third semi-tubular hook plates. Ring et al.[32] achieved a 98% union rate at 6 months postoperatively using tension band fixation of the olecranon osteotomy, with 27% of the patients in their series requiring K-wire removal. Hewins et al.[33] reported a 100% union rate with only one of 17 patients requiring fixation removal in their series of olecranon osteotomies repaired with plate fixation. Hewins et al. suggested that plate fixation may provide a more rigid and stable construct by offering more potential points of fixation, increased resistance to tensile forces along the posterior surface of the olecranon and improved resistance of both shear and rotational forces along the osteotomy site.

Olecranon osteotomy

While olecranon osteotomy provides the best visualization of the articular segment,[29] it should be avoided if primary arthroplasty is being considered. The paratricipital approach is preferred for cases where repairability of the fracture is to be determined intraoperatively.

After elevating full-thickness fasciocutaneous flaps, the olecranon bare area is identified through a medial and limited lateral dissection. Predrilling and fixation of a precontoured periarticular locking plate prior to osteotomy simplifies osteotomy reduction and fixation. An apex distal chevron osteotomy provides intrinsic stability though its necessity when using rigid plate fixation is debated. The osteotomy should be cut two-thirds with a saw and the remaining one-third predrilled with a K-wire and completed with osteotomes. This facilitates achieving an anatomic reduction and contact of the fragments[33] (Figure 23.3).

Preserving the innervation of the anconeus by dissecting it from the distal ulna without detaching it from the triceps has been recommended by some authors.[34] The exposure may be extended proximally by continuing into the paratricipital approach.

Paratricipital approach

The triceps sparing paratricipital approach provides limited visualization of the articular segment and is best reserved for extra-articular or simple intra-articular fractures with minimal comminution (Figure 23.4). This approach avoids disruption of the extensor mechanism and skeletonization and devascularization of the proximal ulna. Because the triceps mechanism is preserved, the extensor mechanism does not need to be protected and immediate active triceps function can be initiated in the postoperative rehabilitation program.

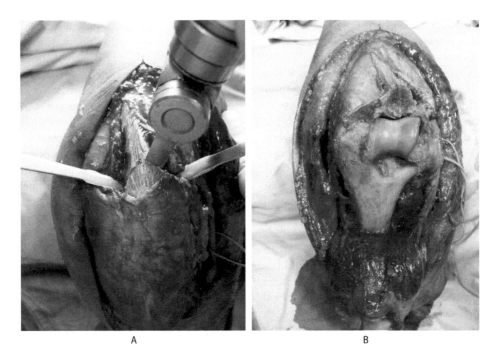

A

B

Figure 23.3 Olecranon osteotomy (a) Apex distal chevron osteotomy. (b) Exposure with olecranon osteotomy reflected.

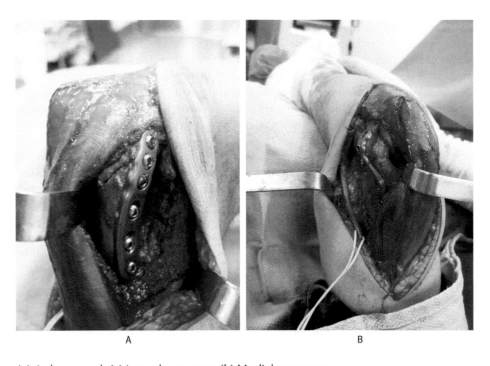

A

B

Figure 23.4 Paratricipital approach (a) Lateral exposure. (b) Medial exposure.

The authors prefer the lateral para-olecranon approach[35] for TEA as it allows improved exposure of the ulna for preparation and placement of the ulnar component relative to the paratricipital approach without detaching the main insertion of the triceps on the olecranon. A description of this approach is outlined below.

After establishing full thickness fasciocutaneous medial and lateral flaps through the posterior skin incision, the ulnar nerve is identified and protected. The medial and lateral borders of the triceps are incised and elevated from the posterior aspect of the distal humerus.

The Kocher interval between the extensor carpi ulnaris and anconeus can be developed and continued distally to increase the distal exposure laterally. On the medial side, the flexor carpi ulnaris can be elevated subperiosteally.[36] Conversion to an olecranon osteotomy may be performed if the exposure is inadequate for fracture fixation. Excellent union rates and good functional outcomes have been reported using a paratricipital approach for the treatment of distal humerus fractures.[37]

Triceps splitting

The triceps splitting approach involves a distal midline triceps tendon split with equal portions of the triceps tendon and its insertion on the olecranon reflected medially and laterally.[38] This approach again provides limited visualization of the articular surface[29] and has not been shown to provide a functional outcome advantage over olecranon osteotomy.[39] Furthermore, there is concern of postoperative triceps weakness. The posterior and posterolateral aspect of the humerus are easily accessible, but true lateral plate positioning is challenging. Meticulous closure of the triceps with transosseous sutures is recommended.[40]

SURGICAL TECHNIQUE

The basic principles of distal humerus ORIF are reconstruction of the articular segment followed by column reconstruction and rigid fixation with a construct that enables immediate initiation of postoperative rehabilitation without external protection. Coronal shear fractures of the capitellum, trochlea or both may occur in association with distal humerus fractures. Internally rotating each condyle may improve visualization of these fragments to facilitate their fixation prior to fixation of the primary sagittal plane articular fracture. Minor comminuted articular fragments can be fixed to major fragments using threaded K-wires, headless compression screws or bioabsorbable pins.

Current plate options include standard 3.5 mm pelvic reconstruction and limited contact dynamic compression (LCDC) plates which are contoured intraoperatively, fracture specific precontoured plates and precontoured locking plates. One-third tubular plates are not recommended. Reconstruction plates are too weak if there is supracondylar comminution or proximal extension of the fractures.

Precontoured locking constructs may offer advantages in the management of osteoporotic fractures[41] where implant fixation in osteoporotic distal fragments is a concern, however the complex geometry of the distal humerus may limit applicability of older plate designs with fixed angle screw constructs. Failure typically occurs at the supracondylar level due to loss of fixation or screw pull-out in the distal fragments.[42] Clinical studies in elderly patients have demonstrated when loss of fixation occurs, it almost always occurs in the lateral column.[43] This may be related in part to biomechanical influences but also the anatomic qualities of bone in various regions of the distal humerus. Diederichs et al.[44] have demonstrated the capitellum to be the region of lowest trabecular bone mineral density and cortical thickness. The trabecular bone mineral density of the medial column in the infra-condylar region was 31% higher than in the lateral column and the cortical thickness 38% higher in the medial distal diaphyseal region when compared to the lateral side.

Double plating has been shown to provide more rigid fixation than a single locked plate for fixation of extra-articular comminuted distal humerus fractures.[45] The most common plating techniques include orthogonal (perpendicular or 90:90) plating and parallel plating. Both techniques have been supported clinically and neither has demonstrated definitive superiority.[46] In the setting of osteoporotic bone, parallel plates are preferred as long screws can be placed from lateral to medial, avoiding plate pull-off due to screw fixation failure from posterior plate fixation. Restoration of a functional articulation requires the anterior aspect of the distal humerus and stability is dependent on the presence of medial trochlea plus either the lateral half of the trochlea or the capitellum.[47]

Orthogonal plating

Provisional reduction and fixation of the articular segment is achieved using K-wires, which are positioned to not interfere with eventual definitive plate and screw insertion. One key element in performing posterolateral plating involves distal application without contacting the posterior articular cartilage of the capitellum.[48] Medial column fixation is achieved using a plate positioned medially along the supracondylar ridge that curves around the medial epicondyle. The sequence of fixation should be tailored for each fracture. Initial stabilization of the larger fragments may permit easier reduction of more comminuted segments. The proximal extent of the plates should be varied to avoid formation of a stress riser in the humeral diaphysis. The drawbacks of orthogonal plating technique, particularly in osteopenic bone, are the limited ability to obtain adequate screw purchase and length in a posteroanterior direction through the posterolateral plate (Figure 23.5a).

Parallel plating

A reliable technique of ORIF for reconstructable distal humerus fractures has been described by Sanchez-Sotelo et al.[49] This technique maximizes fixation of the distal fragments at the supracondylar level and links the medial and lateral columns to form a rigid construct that is similar in concept to that of an arch (Figure 23.5b). The parallel plating technique used by the authors and modified from that of Sanchez-Sotelo et al. is found in Table 23.1. For step 1 of the articular reduction, O'Driscoll has suggested that screws should not be placed into the distal fragment before the plate is applied as independent screws do not contribute to supracondylar stability and do not achieve as much stability as they would if passed through the plate. In our experience, we have often found it useful to place a central spool screw down the axis of the trochlea to fixate the two main fragments to avoid redisplacement during fracture fixation.

MANAGEMENT OF BONE LOSS

Supracondylar compression may not be achievable in the setting of metaphyseal bone loss. In this situation, the humerus can be shortened at the metaphyseal fracture level while preserving overall alignment and geometry of the distal humerus. The olecranon tip is removed and the fossa recreated using a burr to permit impingement-free extension. Slight anterior translation of the distal segment is important to avoid impingement of the coronoid with elbow flexion.

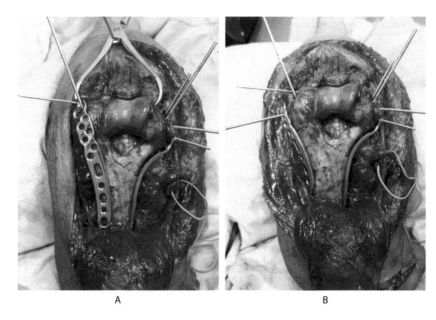

A   B

Figure 23.5 **(a)** Perpendicular plate technique. **(b)** Parallel plate technique.

Table 23.1 Parallel plating technique

Step 1: Articular reduction	Provisional anatomic reduction with temporary K-wire fixation at subchondral level inserted from medial and lateral. A single small diameter screw is inserted down the central axis of the trochlea (medial to lateral) to stabilize the major articular segments. Compression of the intra-articular fracture lines should be performed using large bone clamp prior to screw insertion. Targeted drill guides may simplify placement of these distal articular screws. In the setting of severely comminuted fractures, the proximal ulna and radial head can be used as a reconstruction template.
Step 2: Plate placement and provisional fixation	Medial and lateral precontoured plates selected: • Use caution when placing the lateral plate to protect the radial nerve proximally and avoid detachment of the lateral collateral ligament distally as it inserts on the lateral epicondyle. • Protect the ulnar nerve when placing the medial plate and avoid dissecting anteriorly on the medial epicondyle as this can compromise the integrity of the medial collateral ligament. • A minimum of three medial and lateral screws should be placed proximal and distal to the metaphyseal fracture. • The plates should end at different levels to avoid creation of a stress riser. • Provisionally fix the metaphyseal segment to the diaphysis held using Steinmann pins at level of the medial and lateral epicondyles. Once anatomic reduction of the distal fragments to the shaft at the supracondylar level is confirmed, one cortical screw is loosely placed into a proximal slotted hole to hold each plate in position.
Step 3: Articular fixation	Medial and lateral screws are placed distally to stably fix intra-articular fragments. Screws should: • Pass through the plate where possible. • Be as long as possible. • Pass through as many fragments as possible. • Pass into the opposite column.
Step 4: Supracondylar compression	Plates are fixed proximally under maximal compression at the supracondylar level. • Use a large tenaculum to provide interfragmentary compression. • Insert screws in dynamic compression mode. • Do for both the medial and lateral columns.
Step 5	Remaining proximal screws are placed and full intraoperative motion is confirmed. Bone grafting should be considered if column contact cannot be achieved or if a gap is present in the articular surface.

It has been reported that shortening of less than 1 cm has only a mild effect on triceps strength and that up to 2 cm of humeral shortening can be tolerated without serious disturbance of elbow biomechanics.[50]

POSTOPERATIVE MANAGEMENT

A drain can be used to avoid haematoma formation. Following meticulous layered closure, the elbow is placed in a bulky non-compressive dressing with a plaster slab to maintain the elbow in approximately 30 degrees of extension. The extremity is kept elevated for 3–14 days postoperatively, depending on the severity of soft tissue injury. A physiotherapy program including active range of motion is then initiated once the wound looks safe to do so. Weight bearing through the extremity is restricted until healing is progressing radiographically. A sling may be used for comfort during the day. An anteriorly based night extension splint may be considered to optimize elbow extension. Heterotopic ossification prophylaxis using nonsteroidal anti-inflammatory drugs (NSAIDs e.g. indomethacin) is not recommended in elderly patients due to a higher risk of complications. Radiation has been shown to increase non union rates and is no longer used.[51]

COMPLICATIONS

Wound complications

The incidence of major wound complications after fixation of distal humerus fractures is substantial with rates of 6–16% reported.[15,52] The presence of a grade III open fracture and the use of an olecranon osteotomy stabilized with a plate have been identified as significant risk factors for major wound complications. Fracture healing rates and functional elbow range of motion do not appear to be affected by major wound complications provided they are handled with proper soft tissue coverage techniques.[52] The frequency of wound complications in our practice has decreased with delayed mobilization of the elbow in the elderly; we routinely wait at least 10 days before initiating motion in this population.

Ulnar nerve

The management of ulnar neuropathy, either due to the original trauma or operative intervention, remains controversial. Some authors have advocated for routine anterior transposition, while others have recommended in situ decompression alone. Ruan et al.[28] reported significantly improved outcomes with transposition versus in situ decompression for patients with preoperative ulnar nerve symptoms. Chen et al.[53] found a 33% rate of postoperative ulnar neuritis in patients who had undergone transpositions versus 9% in patients who underwent in situ decompression. In contrast, Vazquez et al.[54] found no significant difference in postoperative ulnar nerve symptoms in patients with no preoperative symptoms who underwent transposition versus no transposition and concluded that anterior transposition was not protective. Based on the available evidence,

neither in situ release nor anterior transposition can be firmly recommended. Subcutaneous anterior transposition is recommended if direct contact with medial hardware is noted intraoperatively following fracture fixation.[55]

Heterotopic ossification

A pooled analysis from a number of studies has demonstrated an 8.6% rate of symptomatic heterotopic ossification when prophylaxis was not used.[23] The indications for routine prophylactic treatment for heterotopic ossification following ORIF of distal humerus fractures remain controversial with insufficient evidence to recommend for or against routine prophylaxis. Risk factors for the development of heterotopic ossification, including central nervous system injury, should be considered and the potential risks of prophylaxis with NSAIDs, including increased non union rates and gastrointestinal bleeding, must be considered. We do not use NSAIDs in elderly patients with distal humeral fractures. Radiation should not be employed due an increased risk of distal humeral non-union.[51]

Contracture

Elbow stiffness is a common complication following trauma and prolonged immobilization. Most patients develop some stiffness following ORIF, however, relatively few require secondary surgery to achieve a functional flexion–extension arc of greater than 100 degrees.

OUTCOMES

Interpretation of reports on the outcome of ORIF for distal humerus fractures is difficult. Much of the published literature consists of small case series with heterogeneity of patient demographics and fracture types, as well as using variable methods of fixation.

Huang et al.[56] have presented the results of intra-articular distal humerus fractures in elderly patients treated by ORIF using inconsistent plating techniques. Of the 23 patients they identified, 14 were available for follow-up at a mean of 51 months postoperatively. They reported a 100% union rate, mean elbow flexion extension arc of 20–120 degrees, mean MEPS of 83, and a mean DASH score of 38. The musculoskeletal functional assessment scores demonstrated disability with a mean total score of 33 (normative 9), hand score of 35 (normative 4) and self-care score of 32 (normative 2). Two patients required subsequent operative intervention, one for stiffness and one for fixation failure.

Another retrospective review of 19 elderly patients with intra-articular distal humerus fractures treated by varying plating techniques at a mean of 97.2 months follow-up reported a 100% union rate, no implant failures, an average flexion arc of 17–128 degrees, with 79% of patients achieving excellent results and 21% good[19] (Figure 23.6).

Although several studies have demonstrated good outcomes with ORIF of distal humerus fractures in the elderly, others have demonstrated poorer outcomes and higher complication rates. Obert et al.[57] have recently reported a 44% complication rate, including neuropathy, mechanical

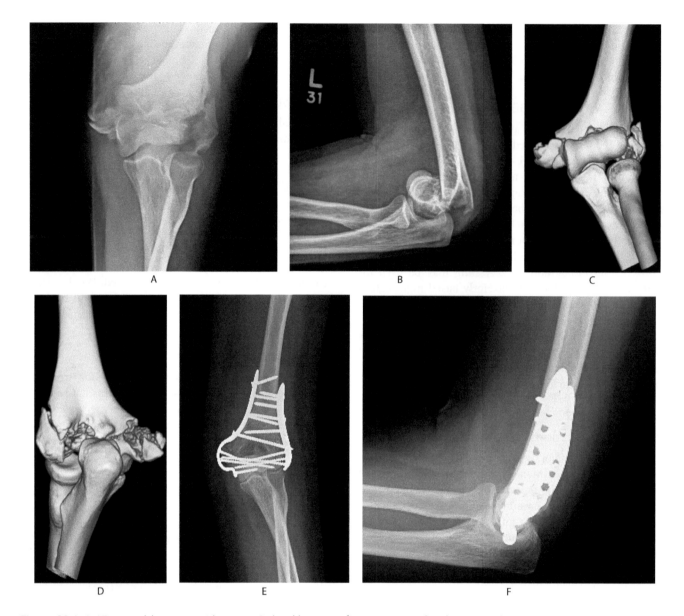

Figure 23.6 A 65-year-old woman with a type C distal humerus fracture treated with open reduction and parallel plating (a–f).

failure and wound dehiscence, in 289 elderly patients who were treated by ORIF. Their data suggested that material failures occur in 7–27% of patients, but this occurred more frequently before 2005. This may be the result of improved fixation techniques with time, including dual plating, the use of anatomically precontoured plates and/or locking screws.

Total elbow arthroplasty

TEA has been recommended by a number of authors as a reasonable primary treatment option for complex distal humerus fractures in the elderly, as well as in the setting of nonunion following failure of internal fixation.[58–60] It provides a number of potential benefits including eliminating non union and post-traumatic arthritis risk and possibly a more expedient return to independent activities of daily living. Proposed indications for primary TEA in the treatment of distal humerus fractures include unreconstructable distal humerus fractures, pre-existing arthritis, severely osteoporotic bone, inflammatory arthritis, pathologic fractures, and reduced life expectancy. Contraindications include infection or infection at a distant site, soft tissue inadequacy, a nonfunctional hand and inability to comply with postoperative lifelong activity restrictions. Arthroplasty should not be considered in young active patients[24] (Figures 23.7 and 23.8).

SURGICAL TECHNIQUE

The patient may be positioned either supine or in the lateral decubitus position with the arm draped free. A posterior skin incision is used and conservative full-thickness fasciocutaneous flaps are developed. The ulnar nerve is identified, protected and transposed. The paratricipital approach is most commonly used. A central triceps split, triceps tongue, elevating from medial to

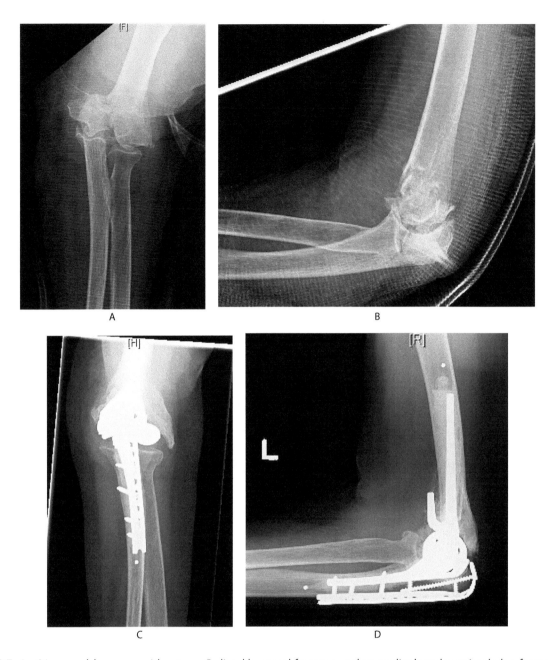

Figure 23.7 An 81-year-old woman with a type C distal humeral fracture and an undisplaced proximal ulna fracture that was treated with a total elbow arthroplasty (TEA) and ORIF of the ulna, complicated by heterotopic ossification (a–d).

lateral (Bryan-Morrey) or from lateral to medial (extended Kocher) should be avoided as triceps strength is compromised and early functional use of the arm delayed.

The authors, however, prefer the lateral para-olecranon approach[35] because it allows improved visualization for accurate placement of the ulnar component. This approach involves developing the interval between the ulna and anconeous (Boyd approach) for the posterolateral arthrotomy. This interval is extended proximally, separating the portion of the triceps tendon that inserts directly on the olecranon tip from the portion that blends with the anconeus fascia to become the lateral cubital retinaculum. The anconeous is subperiosteally elevated from the lateral aspect of the ulna.

The LCL is then released or the lateral epicondylar bone fragments are removed. The lateral cubital retinaculum and the lateral aspect of the triceps tendon with the superficial fascia of the forearm and the anconeus are reflected laterally as a single unit, preserving continuity of the extensor mechanism with the forearm fascia. The triceps tendon inserting on the olecranon tip is maintained. The MCL and the common flexor-pronator origin are released from the medial epicondyle or the medial epicondylar fragment is excised to allow dislocation of the elbow. The distal humerus is delivered through the triceps split. Retraction of the triceps tendon and external rotation of the ulna by hypersupination of the forearm facilitate exposure of the greater sigmoid notch and base of coronoid.

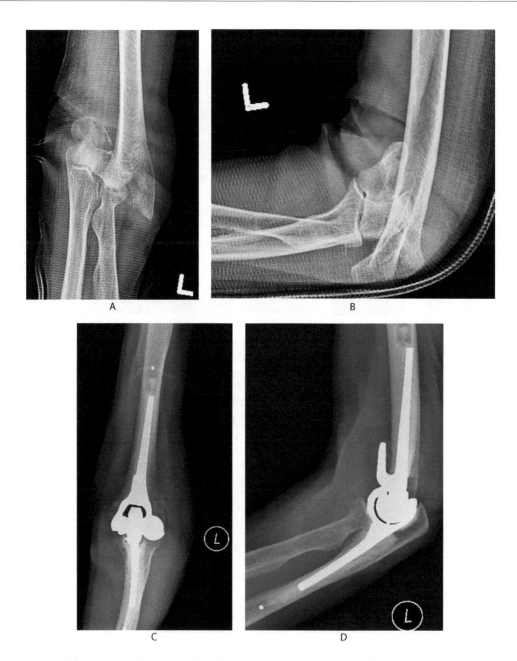

Figure 23.8 An 85-year-old woman with a type A distal humerus fracture treated with total elbow arthroplasty (TEA) **(a–d)**.

With the elbow dislocated, the fractured articular segments are removed. The implant size is best templated from the intact radial head and greater sigmoid notch.

The humeral and ulnar canals are opened, reamed and broached according to the chosen prosthesis instrumentation. The radial head is inspected for arthrosis or associated injury and may be retained, resected or replaced depending on the system employed. Prosthetic trialing is performed to evaluate stability, length, range of motion and alignment. In the setting of extensive comminution, where implant length may be difficult to determine, assessment of soft tissue tension using the trial prosthesis with the elbow positioned in extension may be useful. Placing the yoke of the humeral component and anterior flange at the level of the top of the olecranon fossa is another useful means of assessing length.

The humeral component should be positioned in approximately 14 degrees of internal rotation relative to the posterior flat spot of the distal humerus to re-establish the flexion extension axis.[61] The ulnar component should be oriented parallel to the flat spot of the olecranon. Following placement of intramedullary cement restrictors and canal lavage and drying, antibiotic cement is injected using a third generation technique and the definitive components are inserted and held firmly until the cement is set.

The implants are then linked and the triceps split of the lateral para-olecranon approach is repaired using a side-to-side closure with non-absorbable sutures and buried knots. Transosseous drill tunnels are used if a triceps detaching approach was utilized. The wound is closed in a layered fashion and a drain placed at the surgeon's discretion.

POSTOPERATIVE MANAGEMENT

The elbow is splinted in 30 degrees of extension using a cast and oedema control measures instituted for the first 48 hours. The postoperative splint is removed at 10–14 days and physiotherapy initiated when wound healing is secure. Shoulder, wrist and hand exercises are commenced early. Active elbow flexion and extension may also be started immediately if a triceps preserving approach was used. When a triceps detaching approach is used, an active limited range of flexion is allowed, but active triceps extension is not initiated until the extensor mechanism has healed. This can be problematic in the elderly who often require triceps function to shift in or arise from a chair and it also limits the use of ambulatory aids.

COMPLICATIONS

Soft tissue complications include delayed wound healing, flap necrosis, triceps failure and ulnar neuropathy. Meticulous intraoperative haemostasis and preventing stress on the healing posterior soft tissues are protective measures. Ulnar neuropathy following TEA is typically transient.[62–64] Extensor mechanism failure is a concern particularly when triceps elevating approaches are used. Infection remains a challenging postoperative complication to manage. Irrigation, debridement and antibiotic treatment may be considered for acute postoperative infections. Infections with delayed presentation usually require a staged revision procedure. Implant loosening, peri-prosthetic fracture and polyethylene wear/failure represent additional complications of TEA.

OUTCOMES

Short- and medium-term outcomes of TEA for distal humerus fractures have been reproducibly good with overall good to excellent results.[59,65–68] A few studies have compared the outcomes of distal humerus fractures treated by ORIF versus TEA.

Frankle et al.[58] performed a retrospective review comparing ORIF to elbow arthroplasty in women over the age of 65 years with AO/OTA type C distal humerus fractures and reported improved outcomes in the arthroplasty group at short-term follow-up. The average operative time was 2.5 hours for internal fixation versus 90 minutes for arthroplasty. In the ORIF group there was one deep infection and three elbows with failed internal fixation were salvaged with an arthroplasty. In the arthroplasty group, two elbows required debridement and one elbow failed secondary to uncoupling of the linking mechanism. Eight patients in the arthroplasty group had rheumatoid arthritis (RA), whereas none had RA in the ORIF group.

In 2009, McKee et al.[69] published a prospective, randomized study comparing ORIF to TEA in 42 elderly patients with displaced intra-articular distal humerus fractures. Of the 40 participants followed up for 2 years, five allocated ORIF underwent intraoperative conversion to TEA. MEPS were consistently better in the TEA group at 6 and 12 months, and at 2-year follow-up. There was a non-statistically significant trend of fewer ORIF patients having good or excellent results.

DASH scores were superior for TEA at 6 months but not in the longer term. There were no statistically significant differences between the groups for elbow range of motion, reoperation rate or complication rates.

A recent systematic review and meta-analysis of ORIF versus TEA for the treatment of geriatric distal humerus fractures[70] has suggested that both methods produce similar functional outcome scores and range of motion. The authors of this study advocate for ongoing research including prospective trials and cost analysis assessments to better define the roles of ORIF versus TEA.

Presently, there are no mid-term or long-term studies comparing the outcomes and complications of ORIF to TEA for the treatment of complex distal humerus fractures in the elderly. It has been suggested that there may be an increasing number of failures of distal humerus fractures treated by TEA at mid-term and long-term follow-up with infection seeming to be the main complication in the first 5 years, followed by aseptic loosening and fractures beyond 5 years.[71]

Hemiarthroplasty

Distal humerus hemiarthroplasty for the treatment of complex distal humerus fractures has recently gained favour. This technique replaces the trochlea and capitellum while avoiding the potential for polyethylene wear debris and associated osteolysis, as well as aseptic loosening that is recognized with TEA. Hemiarthroplasty for distal humerus fractures is a technically challenging procedure, which requires the integrity of the medial and lateral columns of the humerus, the collateral ligaments, radial head and coronoid (Figure 23.9).

Specific indications for hemiarthroplasty of distal humerus fractures are evolving but include severely comminuted articular fractures with either a low transcondylar fracture line distal to the collateral origins, and coronal shear fractures or simple condylar fractures that can be plated to effectively stabilize the condyles. It is typically considered for younger and more active patients given the good outcomes established for TEA in elderly low demand patients. It may be considered an intermediary treatment for patients with unreconstructable distal humerus fractures who are deemed too young or active for TEA. Several technical pitfalls are likely to significantly affect patient outcomes including non-anatomic epicondylar reduction with compromised collateral ligament tension, non-rigid fixation of the condyles, inaccurate humeral component sizing and axis malposition.

OUTCOMES

There are a limited number of studies reporting on the outcomes of distal humeral hemiarthroplasty.[72–74] The majority of the studies include a small number of patients with heterogeneous clinical indications and only short-term follow-up. The majority of patients achieve a functional outcome. However, as with ORIF and TEA, complications are not infrequent. Erosion and subsidence of the hemiarthroplasty into the radius and proximal ulna are a concern with longer follow-up.[75]

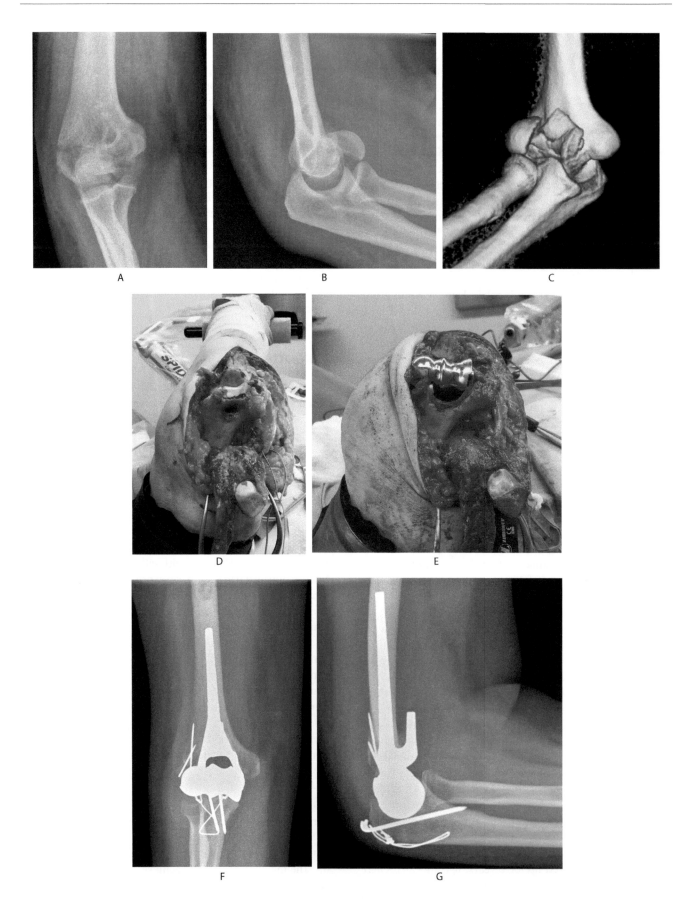

Figure 23.9 Complex intra-articular distal humerus fracture treated with lateral column fixation and hemiarthroplasty using an olecranon osteotomy (a–g).

CONCLUSIONS

Distal humerus fractures in the elderly are increasing in frequency and are some of the most challenging fractures to treat. There is a role for non-operative management of defined fractures in patients with low functional demands and multiple comorbidities. Fracture pattern recognition through advanced imaging techniques, an understanding of biomechanically advantageous fixation strategies and the selective use of elbow arthroplasty have contributed to improved outcomes. Implementation of fracture prevention programs including core strengthening to reduce falls and improved osteoporosis detection and management are critical given our aging population. Improvement of implants, reducing the incidence of postoperative complications and high-level outcome studies are all necessary to advance the management of these complex injuries.

REFERENCES

1. Morrey BF. Fractures of the distal humerus. *Orthop Clin North Am.* 2000;31:145–54.
2. Robinson CM. Fractures of the distal humerus. In: Bucholz RW, Heckman JD, Court-Brown C, Tornetta P, Koval KJ, eds. *Rockwood and Green's Fractures in Adults.* 6th ed. Philadelphia, PA: Lippincott Williams & Wilkins; 2005, pp. 1051–1116.
3. Robinson CM, Hill RM, Jacobs N, et al. Adult distal humeral metaphyseal fractures: Epidemiology and results of treatment. *J Orthop Trauma.* 2003;17:38–47.
4. Palvanen M, Kannus P, Parkkari J, et al. The injury mechanisms of osteoporotic upper extremity fractures among older adults: A controlled study of 287 consecutive patients and their 108 controls. *Osteoporos Int.* 2000;11:822–31.
5. Charissoux J-L, Vergnenegre G, Pelissier M, et al. Epidemiology of distal humerus fractures in the elderly. *Orthop Traumatol Surg Res.* 2013;99:765–9.
6. Rose SH, Melton LJ, Morrey BF, et al. Epidemiologic features of humeral fractures. *Clin Orthop Relat Res.* 1982;168:24–30.
7. Sheps DM, Hildebrand KA. Population-based incidence of distal humeral fractures among adults in a Canadian urban center. *Curr Orthop Pract.* 2011;22:437–42.
8. Palvanen M, Kannus P, Niemi S, et al. Secular trends in distal humeral fractures of elderly women. *Bone.* 2010;46:1355–8.
9. Bliuc D, Nguyen ND, Milch VE, et al. Mortality risk associated with low-trauma osteoporotic fracture and subsequent fracture in men and women. *JAMA.* 2009;301:513–21.
10. Melton LJ, Achenbach SJ, Atkinson EJ, et al. Long-term mortality following fractures at different skeletal sites: A population-based cohort study. *Osteoporos Int.* 2013;24:1689–96.
11. Marsh JL, Slongo TF, Agel J, et al. Fracture and dislocation classification compendium– 2007: Orthopaedic Trauma Association classification, database and outcomes committee. *J Orthop Trauma.* 2007;21(10 Suppl):S1–133.
12. McCarty LP, Ring D, Jupiter JB. Management of distal humerus fractures. *Am J Orthop.* 2005;34:430–8.
13. Morrey BF, ed. Anatomy of the elbow joint. In: *The Elbow and Its Disorders.* Bernard F. Morrey and Joaquin Sanchez-Sotelo. Philadelphia, PA: WB Saunders; 2000, pp. 13–42.
14. Callaway GH, Field LD, Deng XH, et al. Biomechanical evaluation of the medial collateral ligament of the elbow. *J Bone Joint Surg Am.* 1997;79:1223–31.
15. Gofton WT, Macdermid JC, Patterson SD, et al. Functional outcome of AO type C distal humeral fractures. *J Hand Surg Am.* 2003;28(2):294–308.
16. Doornberg J, Lindenhovius A, Kloen P, et al. Two and three dimensional computed tomography for the classification and management of distal humeral fractures. Evaluation of reliability and diagnostic accuracy. *J Bone Joint Surg Am.* 2006;88(8):1795–801.
17. Brown RF, Morgan RG. Intercondylar T-shaped fractures of the humerus: Results in ten cases treated by early mobilisation. *J Bone Joint Surg Br.* 1971;53-B:425–8.
18. Eastwood WJ. The T-shaped fractures of the lower end of the humerus. *J Bone Joint Surg.* 1937;19:364–9.
19. Huang TL, Chiu FY, Chuang TY, et al. The results of open reduction and internal fixation in elderly patients with severe fractures of the distal humerus: A critical analysis of the results. *J Trauma.* 2005;58(1):62–9.
20. Korner J, Lill H, Müller LP, et al. Distal humerus fractures in elderly patients: Results after open reduction and internal fixation. *Osteoporos Int.* 2005;16(Suppl 2):S73–9.
21. Srinivasan K, Agarwal M, Matthews SJ, et al. Fractures of the distal humerus in the elderly: Is internal fixation the treatment of choice? *Clin Orthop Relat Res.* 2005;(434):222–30.
22. John H, Rosso R, Neff U, et al. Operative treatment of distal humeral fractures in the elderly. *J Bone Joint Surg Br.* 1994;76(5):793–6.
23. Nauth A, McKee MD, Ristevski B, et al. Distal humeral fractures in adults. *J Bone Joint Surg Am.* 2011;93:686–700.
24. Lapner M, King GJ. Elbow arthroplasty for distal humeral fractures. *Instr Course Lect.* 2014;63:15–26.
25. Pidhorz L, Alligand-Perrin P, De Keating E, et al. Distal humerus fracture in the elderly: Does conservative treatment still have a role? *Orthop Traumatol Surg Res.* 2013;99:903–7.

26. Desloges W, Faber KJ, King GJ, Athwal GS. Functional outcomes of distal humeral fractures managed nonoperatively in medically unwell and lower-demand elderly patients. *J Shoulder Elbow Surg*. 2015;24(8):1187–96.

27. Dowdy PA, Bain GI, King GJ, et al. The midline posterior elbow incision. An anatomical appraisal. *J Bone Joint Surg Br*. 1995;77(5):696–9.

28. Ruan HJ, Liu JJ, Fan CY, et al. Incidence, management, and prognosis of early ulnar nerve dysfunction in type C fractures of distal humerus. *J Trauma*. 2009;67(6):1397–401.

29. Wilkinson JM, Stanley D. Posterior surgical approaches to the elbow: A comparative anatomic study. *J Shoulder Elbow Surg*. 2001;10(4):380–2.

30. Coles CP, Barei DP, Nork SE, et al. The olecranon osteotomy: A six-year experience in the treatment of intraarticular fractures of the distal humerus. *J Orthop Trauma*. 2006;20(3):164–71.

31. Schmidt-Horlohé K, Wilde P, Bonk A, et al. One-third tubular-hook-plate osteosynthesis for olecranon osteotomies in distal humerus type-C fractures: A preliminary report of results and complications. *Injury*. 2012;43:295–300.

32. Ring D, Gulotta L, Chin K, et al. Olecranon osteotomy for exposure of fractures and nonunions of the distal humerus. *J Orthop Trauma*. 2004;18(7):446–9.

33. Hewins EA, Gofton WT, Dubberly J, et al. Plate fixation of olecranon osteotomies. *J Orthop Trauma*. 2007;21:58–62.

34. Athwal GS, Rispoli DM, Steinmann SP. The anconeus flap transolecranon approach to the distal humerus. *J Orthop Trauma*. 2006;20(4):282–5.

35. Studer A, Athwal GS, MacDermid JC, et al. The lateral para-olecranon approach for total elbow arthroplasty. *J Hand Surg*. 2013;38:2219–26.

36. Patterson SD, Bain GI, Mehta JA. Surgical approaches to the elbow. *Clin Orthop Relat Res*. 2000;370:19–33.

37. Erpelding JM, Mailander A, High R, et al. Outcomes following distal humeral fracture fixation with an extensor mechanism-on approach. *J Bone Joint Surg Am*. 2012;94:548–53.

38. Campbell WC. Incision for exposure of the elbow joint. *Am J Surg*. 1932;15:65–7.

39. McKee MD, Wilson TL, Winston L, et al. Functional outcome following surgical treatment of intra-articular distal humeral fractures through a posterior approach. *J Bone Joint Surg Am*. 2000;82:1701–7.

40. Antuña S, Barco R. *Essentials in Elbow Surgery*. London: Springer; 2014.

41. Schuster I, Korner J, Arzdorf M, et al. Mechanical comparison in cadaver specimens of three different 90-degree double-plate osteosyntheses for simulated C2-type distal humerus fractures with varying bone densities. *J Orthop Trauma*. 2008;22:113–20.

42. O'Driscoll SW. Optimizing stability in distal humeral fracture fixation. *J Shoulder Elbow Surg*. 2005;14:186S–94S.

43. Korner J, Diederichs G, Arzdorf M, et al. A biomechanical evaluation of methods of distal humerus fracture fixation using locking compression plates versus conventional reconstruction plates. *J Orthop Trauma*. 2004;18:286–93.

44. Diederichs G, Issever A-S, Greiner S, et al. Three-dimensional distribution of trabecular bone density and cortical thickness in the distal humerus. *J Shoulder Elbow Surg*. 2009;18:399–407.

45. Tejwani NC, Murthy A, Park J, et al. Fixation of extra-articular distal humerus fractures using one locking plate versus two reconstruction plates: A laboratory study. *J Trauma*. 2009;66:795–9.

46. Shin SJ, Sohn HS, Do NH. A clinical comparison of two different double plating methods for intraarticular distal humerus fractures. *J Shoulder Elbow Surg*. 2010;19(1):2–9.

47. O'Driscoll SW. Parallel plate fixation of bicolumn distal humeral fractures. *Instr Course Lect*. 2009;58:521–8.

48. Goel DP, Pike JM, Athwal GS. Open reduction and internal fixation of distal humerus fractures. *Oper Tech Orthop*. 2010;20:24–33.

49. Sanchez-Sotelo J, Torchia ME, O'Driscoll SW. Complex distal humeral fractures: Internal fixation with a principle-based parallel-plate technique. *J Bone Joint Surg Am*. 2007;89:961–9.

50. Hughes RE, Schneeberger AG, An KN, et al. Reduction of triceps muscle force after shortening of the distal humerus: A computational model. *J Shoulder Elbow Surg*. 1997;6:444–8.

51. Hamid N, Ashraf N, Bosse MJ, et al. Radiation therapy for heterotopic ossification prophylaxis acutely after elbow trauma: A prospective randomized study. *J Bone Joint Surg Am*. 2010;92:2032–8.

52. Lawrence TM, Ahmadi S, Morrey BF, et al. Wound complications after distal humerus fracture fixation: Incidence, risk factors, and outcome. *J Shoulder Elbow Surg*. 2014;23:258–64.

53. Chen RC, Harris DJ, Leduc S, et al. Is ulnar nerve transposition beneficial during open reduction internal fixation of distal humerus fractures? *J Orthop Trauma*. 2010;24:391–4.

54. Vazquez O, Rutgers M, Ring DC, et al. Fate of the ulnar nerve after operative fixation of distal humerus fractures. *J Orthop Trauma*. 2010;24:395–9.

55. Worden A, Ilyas AM. Ulnar neuropathy following distal humerus fracture fixation. *Orthop Clin North Am*. 2012;43:509–14.

56. Huang JI, Paczas M, Hoyen HA, et al. Functional outcome after open reduction internal fixation of intra-articular fractures of the distal humerus in the elderly. *J Orthop Trauma*. 2011;25:259–65.

57. Obert L, Ferrier M, Jacquot A, et al. Distal humerus fractures in patients over 65: Complications. *Orthop Traumatol Surg Res.* 2013;99:909–13.

58. Frankle MA, Herscovici D Jr, DiPasquale TG, et al. A comparison of open reduction and internal fixation and primary total elbow arthroplasty in the treatment of intraarticular distal humerus fractures in women older than age 65. *J Orthop Trauma.* 2003;17(7):473–80.

59. Garcia JA, Mykula R, Stanley D. Complex fractures of the distal humerus in the elderly. The role of total elbow replacement as primary treatment. *J Bone Joint Surg Br.* 2002;84:812–16.

60. Chalidis B, Dimitriou C, Papadopoulos P, et al. Total elbow arthroplasty for the treatment of insufficient distal humeral fractures. A retrospective clinical study and review of the literature. *Injury.* 2009;40:582–90.

61. Sabo MT, Athwal GS, King GJ. Landmarks for rotational alignment of the humeral component during elbow arthroplasty. *J Bone Joint Surg Am.* 2012;94(19):1794–800.

62. Aldridge JM 3rd, Lightdale NR, Mallon WJ, et al., Total elbow arthroplasty with the Coonrad/Coonrad-Morrey prosthesis. A 10- to 31-year survival analysis. *J Bone Joint Surg Br.* 2006;88(4):509–14.

63. Hildebrand KA, Patterson SD, Regan WD, et al. Functional outcome of semiconstrained total elbow arthroplasty. *J Bone Joint Surg Am.* 2000;82-A(10):1379–86.

64. Kasten MD, Skinner HB. Total elbow arthroplasty. An 18-year experience. *Clin Orthop Relat Res.* 1993;(290):177–88.

65. Gambirasio R, Riand N, Stern R, et al. Total elbow replacement for complex fractures of the distal humerus. An option for the elderly patient. *J Bone Joint Surg Br.* 2001;83(7):974–8.

66. Lee KT, Lai CH, Singh S. Results of total elbow arthroplasty in the treatment of distal humerus fractures in elderly Asian patients. *J Trauma.* 2006;61(4): 889–92.

67. Burkhart KJ. Treatment of the complex intraarticular fracture of the distal humerus with the latitude elbow prosthesis. *Oper Orthop Traumatol.* 2010;22(3):279–98.

68. Ali A, Shahane S, Stanley D. Total elbow arthroplasty for distal humeral fractures: Indications, surgical approach, technical tips, and outcome. *J Shoulder Elbow Surg.* 2010;19(2 Suppl):53–8.

69. McKee MD, Veillette CJH, Hall JA, et al. A multicenter, prospective, randomized, controlled trial of open reduction–internal fixation versus total elbow arthroplasty for displaced intra-articular distal humeral fractures in elderly patients. *J Shoulder Elbow Surg.* 2009;18:3–12.

70. Githens M, Yao J, Sox AH, et al. Open reduction and internal fixation versus total elbow arthroplasty for the treatment of geriatric distal humerus fractures: A systematic review and meta-analysis. *J Orthop Trauma.* 2014;28(8):481–8.

71. Desimone LJ, Sanchez-Sotelo J. Total elbow arthroplasty for distal humerus fractures. *Orthop Clin North Am.* 2013;44:381–7.

72. Parsons M, O'Brien, RJ, Hughes JS. Elbow hemiarthroplasty for acute and salvage reconstruction of intra-articular distal humerus fractures. *Tech Shoulder Elbow Surg.* 2005;6(2):87–97.

73. Adolfsson L, Nestorson J. The Kudo humeral component as primary hemiarthroplasty in distal humeral fractures. *J Shoulder Elbow Surg.* 2012;21(4):451–5.

74. Burkhart KJ, Nijs S, Mattyasovszky SG, et al. Distal humerus hemiarthroplasty of the elbow for comminuted distal humeral fractures in the elderly patient. *J Trauma.* 2011;71(3):635–42.

75. Smith GCS, Hughes JS. Unreconstructable acute distal humeral fractures and their sequelae treated with distal humeral hemiarthroplasty: A two-year to eleven-year follow-up. *J Shoulder Elbow Surg.* 2013;22:1710–23.

24

Proximal forearm fractures and elbow dislocations

ANDREW D. DUCKWORTH

INTRODUCTION

Fractures to the proximal forearm account for over 10% of all upper limb fractures, with fractures of the radial head and olecranon the most common fractures occurring around the elbow.[1,2] Recent literature has highlighted an increasing incidence of these fractures occurring in the elderly and an association with osteoporosis has been reported.[3–5] The diagnosis of injuries around the elbow and proximal forearm is routinely made using plain radiographs, with computed tomography (CT) reserved for the more complex fractures and fracture-dislocations.

When assessing and managing fractures and fracture-dislocations around the proximal forearm, a key consideration for all patients is to determine whether it is an isolated osseous injury (stable) or one that is associated with significant soft tissue disruption that could predispose to elbow or forearm instability (unstable). An appreciation of the common injury patterns is useful when determining the appropriate management, in order to restore function and stability to the elbow and forearm.[6]

Non-operative management is the mainstay for isolated non-displaced or minimally displaced fractures of the proximal radius, with a variety of operative interventions available for the more displaced[6–10] and/or unstable fracture patterns.[11–13] However, there is increasing evidence to support the use of conservative methods in isolated displaced proximal radius and olecranon fractures, particularly in the lower-demand elderly patient.[14–17]

EPIDEMIOLOGY

Proximal radial fractures are the most common fractures of the elbow, accounting for over 30% of all elbow fractures and over 50% of all proximal forearm fractures.[1] The literature on the epidemiology of proximal ulna fractures is sparse, despite accounting for 10–20% of all elbow fractures.[6,18] Over 90% of proximal forearm fractures are simple isolated stable injuries that are not associated with an elbow dislocation, forearm instability or another fracture around the elbow.[19–23] With the subcutaneous location of the proximal ulna, open olecranon fractures are more common than for fractures of the proximal radius.[24]

The literature quotes a fairly consistent incidence for radial head fractures of 25–35 per 100,000 adult individuals per year,[23,25] with the incidence of olecranon fractures quoted as 11–12 per 100,000 adult individuals per year.[5,8] An equal gender ratio is reported for both injuries, with the mean age at the time of fracture ranging from 39 to 48 years for proximal radial fractures and almost 60 years for proximal ulna fractures, with figures noted to have increased for both fracture types over the past decade.[3,5,18,23,26]

A recent study from Edinburgh analyzing 285 radial head and neck fractures over a 1-year period found a significantly lower mean age at the time of injury for males, with the incidence of radial head fractures fitting a type D fracture distribution curve (unimodal young male, bimodal female).[3] Radial neck fractures fit a type A distribution (unimodal young male, unimodal older female) with the peak incidence in women more than 80 years of age and the peak incidence in men less than 20 years of age. Kaas et al. performed a retrospective case–control study that compared the peripheral bone mineral density of 35 women ≥50 years of age with a radial head fracture to 57 matched controls and found that the patients who sustained a radial head fracture had an increased risk of osteoporosis (odds ratio 3.4). These two studies have suggested that a proportion of radial head fractures are low energy fragility fractures associated with osteoporosis.[23,27]

Earlier literature analyzing the management of olecranon fractures originally reported a mean age of approximately 45 years.[6,10,28] In a recent prospective epidemiological study of 78 proximal ulna fractures, the reported mean age was 57 years, with the mean age in females (62 vs 51 years) significantly higher and injuries commonly occurring following a low energy fall.[5] This study found a type F fracture distribution (unimodal older male, unimodal older female), with an increasing incidence after the seventh decade (Figure 24.1).

This recent literature has led some to advocate that further investigation with DEXA scanning is potentially indicated in post-menopausal women who present with these injuries, as certain proximal forearm fractures may be an 'index fracture' for poor bone quality.[23,27] Early intervention with appropriate preventative therapy may reduce the risk of future fragility fractures in this patient group. Secondly, given the increasing incidence with age, it has been suggested that further work is needed to investigate the role of non-operative management for simple displaced fractures of the proximal forearm, particular in lower demand elderly patients.

Mechanism of injury

Proximal forearm fractures most commonly occur through either direct or indirect trauma to the elbow following a fall from standing height.[1,8,29] A fall from standing height is found in almost 60% of proximal radial fractures and over two-thirds of proximal ulna fractures.[3,5] Higher energy mechanisms include a fall from height and sports injuries, which are more frequent in men.[23]

Anatomical studies have found that fractures of the olecranon are thought to occur when the elbow is flexed at about 90 degrees, with fractures of the radial head and coronoid occurring at less than 80 degrees of flexion.[30] Fractures of the radial head occur when an axial load, often with a valgus type force, impacts the radial head into the capitellum.[30,31] A study using quantitative 3D CT analysis of Mason type 2 fractures determined that the most common location for injury was the anterolateral quadrant with the forearm in neutral rotation.[32]

A direct blow to the elbow will commonly lead to an injury of the proximal ulna given the subcutaneous location. This leads to impaction of the proximal ulna into the distal humerus resulting in a more comminuted fracture pattern, particularly in the elderly.[7,33,34] Conversely, an indirect traction injury can occur with forceful contraction of the triceps, e.g. following a fall on to the outstretched hand, leading to a short oblique or transverse fracture of the olecranon.[7,33,34] With either mechanism, the complexity and displacement is determined by the force of the injury, the pre-existing bone quality of the patient, disruption of the triceps aponeurosis and the force of the triceps contraction.[30,35]

CLASSIFICATION

AO/OTA classification

The AO/OTA classification combines proximal forearm fractures under one classification system,[36,37] with type A fractures extra-articular of either the radius or ulna, type B fractures intra-articular of the radius or ulna and type C fractures intra-articular of both bones. The implementation of this classification in the clinical setting is questioned due to complexity and reproducibility, with recent studies concluding the interobserver reliability to be poor to fair and the intraobserver reliability to be poor.[38,39] It is felt better suited for the research setting.

There have been studies that have demonstrated an association between the AO/OTA classification and the outcome of proximal radial fractures.[40–42] Ring et al. reported that more than three fragments of comminution (21-B2.3 type injury) had a significantly increased risk of early fixation failure, non-union and loss of forearm rotation following open reduction internal fixation (ORIF).[40]

Radial head fractures

MASON CLASSIFICATION

The original Mason classification classified marginal and non-displaced fractures of the radial head as type 1 and displaced partial fractures as type 2, although the qualitative

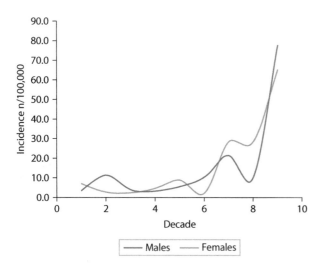

Figure 24.1 The incidence of olecranon fractures, categorized by age and gender.

involvement of the head or displacement were not quantified (Table 24.1 and Figure 24.2).[43] The modified Broberg and Morrey classification suggested that a type 2 fracture involved more than 30% of the articular surface and was more than 2 mm displaced, which was not based on data and has been reported to have moderate reliability.[38,39,44-46] Some have suggested the inclusion of neck fractures and the Mason type 4 fracture (associated elbow dislocation) is not helpful,[35] although there is epidemiological data to suggest neck fractures are predominantly Mason type 1 injuries.[3] The Hotchkiss modification is based on clinical parameters such as mechanical block to forearm rotation and the ability to perform ORIF of the fracture.[47] The main issue with this is the subjective nature of determining a true block to forearm rotation and which fractures are suitable for ORIF.

The clinical value of the Mason classification is questioned by some as it does not reliably predict the management or prognosis of the fracture. Furthermore, systematic review and meta-analysis are felt to be limited due to the wide variety of modifications used and the limited inter- and intraobserver reliability.[48] In a randomized study of 85 orthopaedic surgeons asked to classify 12 radial head

Table 24.1 Description and reliability of the original Mason classification and the three modifications,[38,39,45,46] with reliability data from studies using plain radiograph interpretation

Classification	Type	Description of fracture pattern (management)	Interobserver reliability	Intraobserver reliability
Mason	1	Non-displaced	Satisfactory	Moderate
	2	Displaced partial head		
	3	Displaced entire head		
Johnston	1	Non-displaced	Satisfactory	Moderate
	2	Displaced partial head		
	3	Displaced entire head		
	4	Fracture with elbow dislocation		
Broberg and Morrey	1	<2 mm displacement	Excellent	Moderate
	2	≥2 mm displacement and ≥30% of the articular surface		
	3	Comminuted fracture		
Hotchkiss	1	Non-displaced/displaced marginal fracture No block to forearm motion (non-operative)	–	Moderate
	2	Displaced fracture (ORIF)		
	3	Displaced fracture (excision or replacement)		

Source: Adapted from Table 1 in Duckworth AD et al. Bone Joint J. 2013;95-B(2):151–9.
Note: ORIF, open reduction internal fixation.

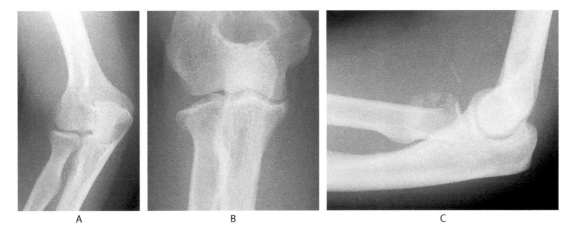

Figure 24.2 Radiographs of the elbow demonstrating Mason type 1 (anteroposterior [AP] view) (a), type 2 (AP view) (b) and type 3 (lateral view) (c) fractures.

fractures using either radiographs and 2D CT, or radiographs and 3D CT, the authors reported that even 3D CT did not significantly improve the interobserver agreement of the Broberg and Morrey modification of the Mason classification.[49]

STABLE VERSUS UNSTABLE INJURIES

For injuries involving a fracture of the radial head, some have suggested that the injury patterns should be considered as stable or unstable[50,51]:

1. Stable isolated radial head fractures are non-displaced or minimally displaced fractures where restoration of elbow and forearm motion is the primary goal of management. Clinically relevant associated injuries are not found, the radiocapitellar contact is preserved and elbow or forearm instability is absent.
2. Unstable fractures are often part of a more complex injury pattern involving associated osseous and/ or ligamentous disruption. In this situation the contact between the radial head and capitellum is often essential to the alignment and stability of the elbow and/or forearm.[51–53] Rineer and colleagues[22] defined unstable fractures as loss of cortical contact of at least one fracture fragment with a gap on radiographs, which they reported in 100% of whole head fractures (Mason type 3).

Proximal ulna fractures

Despite an array of classification systems, the most commonly employed for olecranon fractures is the Mayo classification that incorporates displacement, instability and comminution (Table 24.2 and Figure 24.3).[54] Karlsson et al. found in a study of 315 olecranon fractures that 13% were non-displaced (routinely defined as <2 mm articular displacement) and 22% were comminuted.[8] Recent data would suggest that up to 85% of all olecranon fractures are displaced stable injuries (Mayo type 2).[5,34,55] Alternate

classification systems are summarized in Table 24.2. The Schatzker and Mayo classifications have been found to be prognostic of outcome, with instability and fracture configuration (oblique and comminuted) associated with a poorer result.[6]

The Regan–Morrey classification is used for fractures of the coronoid.[56] Type 1 fractures are defined as an avulsion or tip fracture. Type 2 fractures involve less than or equal to 50% of the coronoid height, with type 3 fractures being greater than 50% of the coronoid height. A recent epidemiological study from Edinburgh reported that only 27% of all coronoid fractures were isolated type 1 fractures, with 73% occurring in association with another significant fracture and/or soft tissue injury.[5]

Table 24.2 The Colton and Schatzker classification systems for olecranon fractures

Classification	Fracture pattern
Mayo	
Type 1A	Undisplaced, stable, no comminution
Type 1B	Undisplaced, stable, comminution
Type 2A	Displaced, stable, no comminution
Type 2B	Displaced, stable, comminution
Type 3A	Displaced, unstable, no comminution
Type 3B	Displaced, unstable, comminution
Colton	
Type 1	Undisplaced and stable
Type 2A	Displaced avulsion
Type 2B	Displaced transverse or oblique
Type 2C	Displaced comminuted
Type 2D	Fracture-dislocation
Schatzker	
Type A	Simple transverse
Type B	Transverse impacted
Type C	Oblique
Type D	Comminuted
Type E	Oblique-distal/extra-articular
Type F	Fracture-dislocation

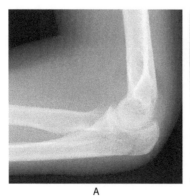 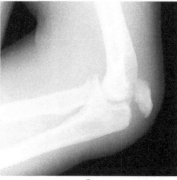 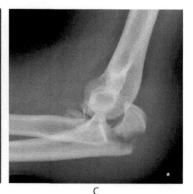

A   B   C

Figure 24.3 Lateral radiographs of the elbow demonstrating Mayo type 1 (a), type 2 (b) and type 3 (c) fractures.

Anatomical considerations

The elbow joint is an intrinsically stable complex hinge joint. There are two osseous stabilizing columns, the radiocapitellar and ulnohumeral articulations, which are reinforced by the soft tissue capsuloligamentous attachments.[35,57,58] Along with the ulnohumeral articulation (sagittal translation), the medial (valgus stress) and lateral (varus stress) collateral ligament complexes act as the primary stabilizers of the elbow.[57-60] Secondary stabilizers include the flexor and extensor muscles that cross the joint, the anterior joint capsule and the radial head.[57-59] These provide stability by limiting posterior translation, as well as rotational and angular stresses, with the radial head a key contributor.[54,61-64]

These is now a strong appreciation for the role of the radial head, in particular radiocapitellar contact, and the coronoid for stable elbow and forearm motion.[54,57,65-67] This concept is essential to consider in all patients, including the elderly, when determining the appropriate management options for all injury patterns involving a fracture of the radial head.[51]

OPERATIVE ANATOMY

For fractures of the radial head, the Kocher exposure utilizes the posterolateral interval between the extensor carpi ulnaris (ECU) and anconeus, and is the most utilized operative approach for fractures of the radial head (Figure 24.4).[35] The vast majority of injuries can be dealt with using this method as it provides good access, particularly given the auto dissection of some of the capsuloligamentous structures that is associated with proximal radius fractures requiring operative management.[40,68,69] For this approach it is best to use the posterior margin of the ECU when dissecting through the joint capsule and the annular ligament, while also protecting the lateral ligamentous complex (if not damaged) and avoiding posterior elevation of the anconeus.[35,58] The posterior interosseous nerve (PIN), as it passes around the radial neck, is protected by pronating the forearm.[70]

A more anterior approach is preferred by some surgeons, which involves either splitting the extensor digitorum communis (EDC) or passing between the EDC and the extensor carpi radialis brevis (ECRB) interval (Figure 24.4).[35,47] It is important in this approach to stay anterior to the anteroposterior midpoint of the capitellum. The perceived advantages to this method are an improved exposure to the coronoid when needed, as well as increased protection for the lateral collateral ligament (LCL). However, the LCL is often only intact when undertaking ORIF of isolated partial radial head fractures, which in all patients, including the elderly, is of debatable benefit over non-operative management.

The approach to the olecranon and proximal ulna often utilizes a posterior longitudinal midline skin incision to allow adequate exposure of the fracture site, with length variable and dependant on the type of fracture and the type of hardware being used.[35] The incision commonly starts proximal to the olecranon and extends over the prominence, continuing distally along the subcutaneous ulna border for usually 3–4 cm past the midpoint of the olecranon.[34,71] A direct midline incision may result in reduced subcutaneous nerve damage,[72] but some surgeons prefer to pass over the medial border of the olecranon to aid with dissecting out the ulnar nerve when required.[35] However, there is no clear indication to dissect out or transpose the ulna nerve in the majority of cases and it can be simply identified with palpation alone.[34,71] Full-thickness subperiosteal dissection is performed as necessary to identify the fracture site and the proximal ulna, with anconeus elevated as required from the lateral aspect of the ulna. The collateral ligaments should be preserved throughout.

The operative approach for unstable complex fractures and fracture-dislocation is often aided by the significant soft tissue disruption associated with these injuries. Avulsion of the origins of the LCL and EDC from the lateral epicondyle is often found, with a small rent in the fascia indicating the interval to be used. These structures are mobilized distally, providing good exposure to the radial head and ulnohumeral joint. Fractures associated with a fracture of the proximal ulna can often be addressed through the posterior rent in the muscle by recreating the deformity. An alternative is the Wrightington approach, which involves elevating the anconeus from the proximal ulna and an osteotomy to remove the insertion of the LCL complex at the crista supinatoris.[73]

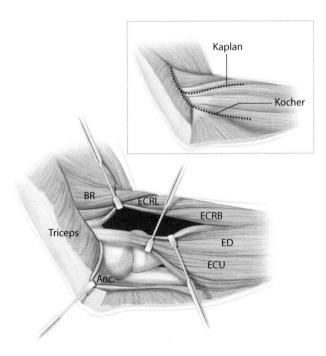

Figure 24.4 The Kocher and Kaplan approaches to the elbow. BR, brachioradialis; ECRB, extensor carpi radialis brevis; ECRL, extensor carpi radialis longus; ECU, extensor carpi ulnaris; ED, extensor digitorum. (Adapted from Bell S. *Current Orthopaedics*. 2008;2(2):90–103)

CLINICAL ASSESSMENT

Patients present after direct or indirect trauma to the elbow, often following a fall from standing height.[1,8,29] Elbow pain (distension of the joint capsule secondary to haemoarthrosis), associated swelling and point tenderness over the proximal forearm are found, often with a reduced range of movement in all directions. The patient will likely be unable to actively extend the elbow and a discontinuity in the extensor mechanism needs to be assessed for. Careful assessment of the skin is necessary to exclude a possible open fracture, particularly in the elderly patient who has sustained direct trauma to the elbow. Distal neurovascular status should always be assessed and documented.

For a fracture of the radial head in particular, an initial and repeated assessment of the arc of motion, forearm rotation, as well as elbow and forearm stability, is often required. Crepitus can sometimes be felt on forearm rotation and/or a frank block to forearm rotation may occur, although the clinical assessment for a bony block to forearm rotation is neither accurate nor reliable as it is very difficult to distinguish a true block to motion secondary to a displaced fragment, from a reluctance to move the forearm secondary to pain. Some authors suggest aspiration of the haemarthrosis to relieve pain and determine if there is a mechanical block to motion that may merit operative treatment.[74-78]

When a proximal forearm fracture is associated with a dislocation of the elbow, deformity and complete loss of elbow motion is seen with associated swelling and ecchymosis. Emergent reduction and assessment of the skin and neurovascular status are paramount.[35,79-81] It is important to be vigilant with a high energy injury mechanism (e.g. a fall from a height) and these patients merit careful evaluation as even minimally displaced fractures and apparently isolated fractures on occasion prove to be unstable and part of a more complex injury pattern.[23,35,82] Widespread tenderness, swelling and ecchymosis may indicate possible forearm or elbow instability, particularly over the medial collateral ligament complex, interosseous ligament of the forearm, and/or the distal radial ulnar joint (DRUJ). Potential clinical tests that can be helpful, but which are difficult to perform in the trauma setting, are:

- Valgus and varus stability with elbow in full extension and at 30 degrees of flexion[53,83]
- Pivot shift test for posterolateral instability[60,83-85]
- Axial compression test for forearm instability[19]

Imaging

A standard anteroposterior (AP) and lateral radiograph of the elbow are the primary investigation, preferably before any potential cast is applied, and should identify fractures of the radial head or neck, the distal humerus, the proximal ulna and any associated elbow dislocation. Initial images may be limited due to pain and repeat imaging once

immobilized may be required. Further imaging modalities are not routinely required for simple isolated fractures of the proximal forearm. CT imaging can aid with both the diagnosis and preoperative planning for the more complex fractures and fracture-dislocations. This may be of use in the elderly patient where complex comminuted fractures are seen, but this should not delay surgery unduly.

Excluding a radioulnar dissociation or distal injury to the forearm can be difficult and if there is any clinical concern then bilateral posterior-anterior (in neutral rotation) and true lateral radiographs of both wrists should be performed.[86-88] A high index of suspicion is advised with increasing fracture complexity and higher energy injuries.[82,89] There is a great deal of debate regarding the amount of radial shortening that is diagnostic of an Essex-Lopresti type lesion.[88,90] MRI can be employed when the diagnosis is in doubt, with cadaveric studies reporting a sensitivity ranging from 88% to 93% and specificity of 100%.[91,92] Intraoperative testing using the push-pull test following radial head excision can be helpful. This uses axial traction and compression of the hand and wrist, with a >3 mm change in the distance between the radial neck and the capitellum felt to be diagnostic of an interosseous ligament injury.[93]

ASSOCIATED INJURIES

Up to 90% of radial head fractures are stable isolated non-displaced or minimally displaced fractures of the neck or the anterolateral portion of the radial head (Mason type 1 and 2), with no clinically relevant associated osseous or ligamentous injury.[3,25,32] A study analyzing the MRIs of 46 radial head fractures (40 Mason type 1 and 2) found evidence of ligamentous injury in over two-thirds of stable fractures, but this did not influence the short-term outcome in terms of elbow motion or the surgeon reported outcome score.[21,94] However, multiple authors have found a clear association between increasing fracture complexity and the rate of associated injuries,[23] with the rate in Mason type 3 fractures 100% in some studies.[21,23,25,26] It has been suggested that these injuries often fit one of the following unstable injury patterns[23,51,95]:

- Radial head fracture with posterior dislocation of the elbow (modified Mason type 4)[44,96]
- Radial head fracture with complete medial collateral ligament (MCL) rupture or capitellum fracture
- Proximal ulna fracture with radial head fracture (Monteggia variants)[97-99]
- Terrible triad injury: radial head fracture, posterior dislocation of the elbow, coronoid fracture[67,96]
- Radioulnar dissociation (Essex-Lopresti variants): radial head fracture plus rupture of the interosseous ligament and rupture of the triangular fibrocartilage complex (TFCC).[100,101]

Associated injuries of the proximal ulna are often variable and need to be assessed and managed on an individual basis. Fractures of the radial head, coronoid, distal humerus and the Monteggia fracture-dislocation (and variants) are seen. Unlike anterior olecranon fracture-dislocations, posterior fracture-dislocations are often associated with radial head and coronoid fractures, as well as an LCL complex injury.[99,102]

Although the average age of patients with more complex injuries is often reported in the literature as being higher than those with simple isolated fractures, no significant association has been found.[3,23] For elderly patients, it is possible to find what would appear to be an unstable displaced and/or comminuted fracture of the radial head, but with no elbow dislocation or proximal ulna fracture. It is essential in these cases to consider these as complex unstable injuries until confirmed otherwise.[35]

TREATMENT

In the elderly patient the aims of treatment for all proximal forearm fractures are to attain a functional and stable elbow and forearm, with minimal associated complications. The management decision should consider the clinical assessment, the fracture complexity and associated injuries, and most importantly the baseline functional status and pre-existing medical comorbidities of the patient. It is also important to consider bone quality, as well as the surgical risks of any proposed surgery. Treatment options include non-operative, ORIF, fracture excision and replacement.

Non-operative

RADIAL HEAD FRACTURES

The vast majority of radial head fractures are isolated stable injuries where non-operative management produces a good or excellent patient reported outcome, with the reported rates of residual pain, stiffness, symptomatic arthritis and re-intervention very low.[14,48,103,104] For elderly patients with an isolated Mason type 1 or type 2 radial head injury, the only clear indication for surgery would be a proven mechanical block to forearm rotation, which is rare.[47,48,105,106]

In a long-term prospective study of 100 (mean age of 46 years; range 17–79 years) stable isolated radial head fractures (57 Mason type 1, 43 Mason type 2) managed with primary non-operative intervention, 92% of patients were satisfied and the median satisfaction score was 10/10 at a mean of 10 years post injury. The mean Disabilities of Arm, Shoulder and Hand (DASH) score was 5.8, 14% of patients reported stiffness and 24% some degree of pain. Only 2% of patients required subsequent surgery for persistent symptoms associated with the original fracture. Although this study reported a worse DASH score in older patients and those with multiple comorbidities, this is not unexpected given the inevitable decline in function with age that is detected in most patient reported outcome scores and has been reported for other injuries.[107]

These findings are supported by data from Sweden. Herbertsson et al. analyzed 32 Mason type 1 fractures at a mean of 21 years after injury and reported full motion and only three patients with occasional pain.[104] In another study from this group, Akesson et al. analyzed 49 patients with an isolated Broberg and Morrey Mason type 2 fracture at a mean of 19 years post injury and reported 82% had no pain, although 12% underwent delayed radial head excision at 4–6 months after injury for unclear reasons.[48]

All studies in this area seem to highlight that the predominant adverse outcome following the non-operative management of these injuries is persistent elbow stiffness and all patients should be counselled regarding this.

PROXIMAL ULNA FRACTURES

The general consensus is that Mayo type 1 stable undisplaced fractures of the olecranon can be managed effectively with non-operative intervention (Table 24.3), with the generally agreed criteria for displacement being <2 mm of articular displacement.[7,29]

With conflicting literature regarding the outcome following surgery for displaced olecranon fractures in elderly patients[108,109] and the rising number of older patients sustaining these injuries, the role of non-operative management has been investigated (Table 24.4). There is now a growing body of evidence supporting the role of non-operative treatment for displaced olecranon fractures in lower demand elderly patients where comorbidities, pre-injury functional status, bone quality and potential complications following surgery need to be considered.[5]

A recent study from Edinburgh reported the outcome of 43 patients with a mean age of 76 years who sustained a displaced fracture of the olecranon that was managed with primary non-operative intervention.[17] At a mean of 4 months following injury the mean Broberg and Morrey score was good, with 72% achieving an excellent or good short-term outcome and no patients requiring further surgery for a symptomatic non-union (Figure 24.5). The long-term outcome was assessed at a mean of 6 years in the 23 patients

Table 24.3 Treatment options for olecranon fractures categorized by the Mayo classification

Mayo classification type	Non-operative	TBW	Plate fixation
1A	Yes	No	No
1B	Yes	No	No
2A	No[a]	Yes	Yes
2B	No[a]	No	Yes
3A	No	No	Yes
3B	No	No	Yes

Source: Adapted from Table 1 in Duckworth AD et al. *Injury.* 2012;43(3):343–6.

Note: TBW, tension-band wire.

[a] In the lower demand elderly patient non-operative treatment may provide a satisfactory outcome.

Table 24.4 Current literature on the non-operative management of isolated displaced olecranon fractures

Author (year)	Patients (n)	Mean age, years (range)	Male/Female	Mean follow-up (months)	Mean elbow flexion arc; mean forearm rotation arc	Outcome	Complications
Parker et al. (1990)[28]	23	48 (13–91)	15/7	26 (5–96)	– –	12 good, 9 fair, 2 poor; 2 loss flexion arc >30°; 3 MRC grading 4+ extension; 16 fibrous union/non-union	None
Veras del Monte et al. (1999)[110]	13	82 (73–90)	3/9	15 (6–33)	129°; 167°	8 good, 3 fair, 1 poor; 92% excellent satisfaction; 67% pain free; 9 fibrous union/non-union	Degenerative arthropathy (n = 1); Skin breakdown (n = 1)
Bruinsma et al. (2012)[111]	10	59 (21–94)	4/6	17 (3–84)	117°; 172°	No angulation or instability; Weakness of extension 4/10; 100% fibrous union/non-union	Painful non-union (n = 2)[a]; Ulnar neuropathy (n = 1)
	6	58 (21–94)	3/3	22 (5–48)	122°; 173°	Mean DASH score 16.8 (n=5); Mean Mayo Elbow Score 88 (n=5); Median VAS score 0	
Duckworth et al. (2014)[b,17]	43	76 (40–98)	15/28	4 (1.5–10)	109°; 159°	Mean Broberg and Morrey score 83; 78% fibrous union/non-union; Mean DASH score 2.9	None
	23	71 (40–87)	8/15	72 (24–180)	– –	91% patient satisfaction; 67% pain free; 83% no subjective extensor weakness	
Gallucci et al. (2014)[16]	28	82 (71–91)	1/27	16 (12–26)	125° (n = 26)	85% fibrous union/non-union; Median DASH score 15; Mean Mayo Elbow Score 95; MRC grading 4 extension 35%; Mean satisfaction score 9/10; Mean VAS score 1	Clicking sensation on movement (n=5)

Note: DASH, Disabilities of Arm, Shoulder and Hand; MRC, Medical Research Council; VAS, visual analogue scale.

a This series was in patients who presented late with an established non-union of a displaced olecranon fracture following no treatment or intentional non-operative management. Of the two patients who required subsequent surgery, this was in younger patients (21 years and 45 years of age). One underwent delayed ORIF for an extension weakness and one underwent excision and advancement of triceps for pain with heavy work.

b Short- and long-term outcome.

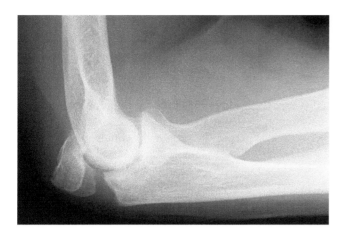

Figure 24.5 An established functional painless non-union at 6 months post injury in a 77-year-old female patient.

who were still alive and it was found that overall patient satisfaction was 91% and the mean DASH score was 2.9. Eighty-three per cent of patients reported no subjective weakness of extensor strength and 78% developed a functional non-union.

Gallucci et al. reported on a retrospective short-term case series of 28 elderly patients (mean age 82 years, all >70 years) treated non-operatively with an above elbow cast for an average of 5 days for a displaced olecranon fracture, which was defined as any articular displacement, or displacement of the posterior cortex of >5 mm.[16] Ten (36%) fractures were comminuted (Mayo type 2B) with articular displacement ranging from 0 to 23 mm (mean 12 mm), but with no fractures open or associated with a dislocation. In 28 patients at a mean of 16 months post injury the mean satisfaction score was 9, the median DASH score was 15 and the mean MEPI score was 95, with 22 outcomes rated excellent and 6 good. Nine (35%) patients had loss of extension strength (Medical Research Council [MRC] grade 4) and 22 (85%) developed a radiographic non-union.

Similar positive short-term results (Table 24.4) have been reported in: (1) an older series of 23 patients with ages ranging from 13 to 91 years,[28] (2) in a case series of 13 elderly patients with a mean age of over 80 years[110] and (3) in a series of 10 patients with a mean age of 59 years who presented with a non-union of a displaced olecranon fracture at a mean of 17 months post injury.[111]

The literature in this area would suggest the predominant adverse outcome following the non-operative management of displaced olecranon fractures is a weakness to elbow extension strength, but which does not appear to markedly affect the patient reported outcome. The only caveat is the rare subtle unstable injury, which may not be apparent on initial radiographs.

COMPLEX ELBOW FRACTURES AND FRACTURE DISLOCATIONS

For some elderly patients non-operative management for complex fractures of the proximal forearm can be used

if it is felt elbow and forearm stability can be maintained without surgery and the patient is willing to accept the possible complications that can occur[44,112–115] which include recurrent instability, pain and loss of function. The type of injury suitable would include radial head fractures associated with a dislocation of the elbow alone, and/or a fracture of the coronoid. Criteria that are commonly used include: (1) a concentric elbow joint on post-reduction AP and lateral elbow radiographs, (2) a partial radial head fracture that does not block forearm rotation, (3) a Regan-Morrey type 1 or 2 fracture of the coronoid and (4) a stable active flexion arc from a minimum of 30 degrees of extension within the first 7–10 days of injury.[114,116,117]

Broberg and Morrey reported the long-term results of cast immobilization with or without acute radial head resection in patients who sustained a Broberg and Morrey type 2 (n = 7) or type 3 (n = 17) fracture of the radial head fracture associated with a dislocation of the elbow.[44] There were associated injuries in 42% (n = 10) of patients, including six coronoid fractures. The authors reported that in patients managed with primary conservative treatment alone, delayed radial head resection was required to improve forearm rotation in those with a Mason type 3 fracture (6/7 patients).

Chan et al. reported a retrospective analysis at a mean of 3 years post injury in 11 patients (mean age 51 years, range 26–76) with a terrible triad injury of the elbow that fit the criteria described above and were managed non-operatively.[116] Three patients had a Mason type 1 fracture and eight were a Mason type 2 (displacement range 2–8 mm), with all coronoid fractures a Regan–Morrey type 2. At final follow-up the mean DASH score was 8 and the mean Mayo Elbow Score was 94. Two patients underwent further surgery – one for surgical stabilization for early recurrent instability and a second for arthroscopic debridement for heterotopic ossification (HO).

Preferred technique

For radial head fractures we would recommend a collar and cuff for comfort, and early active mobilization. We do not routinely undertake aspiration of the joint. The methods of non-operative management have been investigated in patients of all ages. Early mobilization appears to be safe and effective for stable isolated radial head fractures. In a prospective randomized trial of 60 patients comparing immediate active mobilization or 5 days of immobilization followed by active mobilization, the authors reported no differences after the first week of injury and excellent outcomes in both groups.[118] A recent three-arm prospective randomized trial of 180 isolated stable radial head fractures compared immediate mobilization, a sling for 2 days and then active mobilization, and a cast for 1 week prior to mobilization.[119] The authors reported that immediate mobilization was safe and effective, but with a delay of 2 days prior to mobilization potentially advantageous.

For non-displaced olecranon fractures we would recommend splinting the elbow in 45–90 degrees of flexion for approximately 3 weeks, followed by supervised mobilization.[7,35] Check radiographs within the first couple of weeks of injury to ensure there is no displacement of the fracture. From the studies discussed above on the non-operative management of displaced olecranon fractures, the methods of immobilization range from a collar and cuff with early mobilization to an above elbow cast for 4–6 weeks. In our centre, we would generally use an above elbow cast for 2–3 weeks and then allow the patient to mobilize as they are able. If the patient is not in too much pain, a collar and cuff can be used. It is important to perform an AP and lateral radiograph of the elbow within the first 2 weeks to exclude a subtle unstable injury.

For type 4 radial head fractures or terrible triad injuries, a variety of non-operative protocols are suggested in the literature. In the paper by Chan et al.[116] all patients with a terrible triad injury underwent immediate closed reduction and assessment of elbow stability, immobilization and were then reviewed within 1 week of injury for a physical examination and a CT scan of the elbow. Referral to physiotherapy was made within 10 days for protective motion including forearm rotation at 90 degrees of elbow flexion. This protocol is consistent with our approach, although not all patients undergo a CT of the elbow (particularly if there is no associated coronoid fracture) and we do undertake an examination under anaesthesia (EUA) if there is a concern regarding elbow stability or forearm rotation.

ORIF

RADIAL HEAD FRACTURES

Although there are still advocates for ORIF of isolated displaced radial head fractures, in our opinion the role of fixation is diminishing. This is certainly the case in the elderly patient where fixation in osteoporotic bone is challenging. There are some retrospective case series that report good results following ORIF of isolated partially displaced fractures of the radial head, but as has already been discussed, there is a growing body of evidence that a good result would be expected with non-operative management.[106,120–124]

Lindenhovius et al. reported the long-term outcome (mean 22 years) of 16 patients who underwent ORIF for an isolated Mason type 2 fracture and found a complication rate of 31%, a mean DASH score of 12 points and a good or excellent Mayo Elbow Score in 81%.[106] Recently, Yoon et al. reported a retrospective comparative mid-term review of 60 patients with an isolated displaced (2–4.9 mm) fracture of the radial head.[15] Thirty patients were managed with ORIF (mean follow-up 4.5 years) and 30 patients were treated non-operatively (mean follow-up 3 years). Using a combination of surgeon and patient reported outcome measures, superior outcomes were found in favour of non-operative management according to the Mayo Elbow Score (MES), the SF-12 physical component and overall rate of complications. This study found that patients younger than 60 years in both groups had a poorer outcome according to the MES and the Patient Rated Elbow Evaluation questionnaire.

Preferred technique

In our unit, ORIF is now not routinely used for fractures of the radial head, particularly in the elderly patient. If considering fixation, it is important to consider the 90 degree arc ('safe zone') of the radial head that is used to place implants safely so as to avoid impingement at the proximal radioulnar joint. A variety of methods are used for identifying the non-articular part of the proximal radioulnar joint on the radial head:

- Between Lister's tubercle and the radial styloid[125]
- Forearm in neutral rotation, lateral 90 degree arc[126]
- Forearm in full supination, fixation placed posteriorly[127]

PROXIMAL ULNA FRACTURES

The management of a displaced fracture of the olecranon or proximal ulna aims to restore the articular surface with minimal associated complications (Table 24.3).[7,128] The literature would suggest that the risk factors associated with an inferior outcome following surgery are fracture morphology and associated elbow instability and/or fractures.[6,129] A recent Cochrane review of 244 olecranon fractures from six randomized controlled trials concluded that further work is needed in this area to determine the optimal surgical management of simple isolated displaced fractures of the olecranon.[130]

For the stable comminuted displaced fracture (Mayo type 2B) and those fractures associated with other injuries or elbow instability (Mayo type 3), plate fixation is considered to give superior results to tension-band wire (TBW) use.[7,55,128,131–136] For the stable displaced olecranon fracture with minimal or no comminution (Mayo type 2A), although TBW fixation is seen as the gold standard by many and is frequently used, plate fixation is a noted alternative.[6–10,55,71,132,137] For the Mayo type 2 fracture, it is important to consider whether any form of surgical intervention provides a superior outcome to non-operative management in the elderly lower demand patient.

TBW and plate fixation

There is an increasing body of biomechanical evidence to suggest that plate and intramedullary screw fixation confers greater stability at the fracture site than a TBW construct. Wilson et al. performed a biomechanical comparison of TBW and plate fixation in 20 ulna models with identical transverse fractures of the olecranon.[138] They found that the modern pre-contoured location specific plates were significantly better at providing fracture compression, particularly at the articular surface, than the TBW construct. In a more recent study of 12 pairs of simulated olecranon fractures in cadaveric limbs, cyclic loading and assessment of fracture stability following fixation with either a plate or TBW construct demonstrated a median displacement of 0.25 mm for the plate and 1.12 mm for TBW.[139] Whether these findings confer an inferior patient reported outcome is unknown.

There are short- and long-term data reporting good functional outcomes following TBW fixation,[6,71,140–142] although none have specifically analyzed the outcome in the elderly. Flinterman et al. reported the long-term patient reported outcome in 41 patients who sustained a simple transverse displaced fracture of the olecranon. The mean age of the patient group was 35 years (18–73). At a mean of 20 years following surgery, the mean DASH score was 10, the mean MES was 98 and the mean elbow flexion arc was 142 degrees. The only predictor of the DASH score was increasing age at the time of surgery.[143]

The complications documented following TBW fixation are wound breakdown, infection, prominent metalwork, malunion and non-union[6,7,71,133,140,144,145] (Figure 24.6). The most common complication is symptomatic metalwork requiring removal, which is best avoided were possible in the elderly patient. Macko et al. reported the highest re-operation rate at 85% in their 5-year retrospective analysis of 20 patients with a range of displaced olecranon fractures,[140] with symptomatic K-wire prominence most frequent (80%). Proximal wire migration was found in only 15% (n = 3), skin breakdown in 20% (n = 4) and infection in 5% (n = 1).

There is almost no literature exclusively examining the use of plates for the treatment of type 2A fractures specifically in elderly patients (Figure 24.7). There have been recent retrospective comparative studies of TBW versus plate fixation for both simple and comminuted displaced fractures of the olecranon.[146–148] These have consistently reported comparable functional outcomes, a higher rate of metalwork removal following TBW fixation and increased costs with plate fixation. Although it is perceived that plate fixation is associated with symptomatic prominent metalwork given the location of the plate, the literature would suggest the rates of removal are lower than those for TBW, ranging from 5% to 20%.[7,133,134] A recent study by Tarallo et al. compared the outcome of TBW and plate fixation in 78 patients with a Mayo type 2A or 2B fracture.[147]

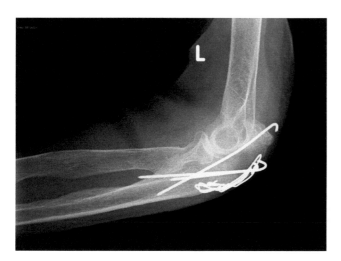

Figure 24.6 A failed TBW fixation at 6 weeks postoperative in a 91-year-old female patient with a stable displaced fracture of the olecranon.

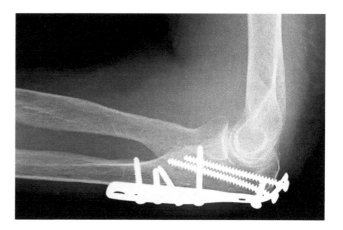

Figure 24.7 Plate fixation of a stable Mayo type 2A olecranon fracture in an 86-year-old woman.

At a mean of 33 months no significant differences were found between groups in terms of functional or clinical outcomes but a higher rate of complications and hardware removal were found following TBW: 38% vs 17% for type 2A fractures and 20% vs 6% for type 2B fractures.

In 1992 Hume et al. performed a prospective randomized trial comparing TBW (n = 19) and plate fixation (n = 22) for displaced olecranon fractures.[133] The authors found that elbow motion at 6 months was comparable but with loss of fracture reduction and prominent symptomatic metalwork significantly more common following TBW. The overall clinical outcome was noted to be far superior in the plate fixation group, with 86% obtaining a good result compared to 47% in the TBW group. Symptomatic metalwork was seen in 42% of patients who underwent TBW fixation, compared to 5% in the plate group.

Intramedullary screw fixation

Despite in vivo biomechanical studies documenting superior fracture stability[149–152] and good results when repairing an olecranon osteotomy for distal humeral fracture fixation,[153–155] there is lack of evidence documenting the efficacy of intramedullary screw primary fixation for displaced fractures of the olecranon, with or without an associated miniplate or TBW construct. There are a small number of studies reporting good results using a locked intramedullary compression nail,[156–158] with Gehr et al. reporting good or excellent short-term results in 93% of 73 (67% comminuted, 33% simple transverse) displaced olecranon fractures.

Suture fixation

To avoid the complications associated with prominent metalwork, some advocate the use of a suture technique to manage displaced fractures of the olecranon in the elderly. Bateman et al. reported that all patients went on to union with no re-operations using a suture anchor fixation technique for both Mayo type 2A and type 2B fractures in eight female patients with a mean age of 74 years.[159] In the six patients available at a mean of 5 years after injury, the mean Oxford Elbow Score (OES) was 47 and the mean DASH was 6.4.

COMPLEX ELBOW FRACTURES AND FRACTURE-DISLOCATIONS

For displaced whole radial head fractures (Mason type 3), there is evidence that ORIF leads to high rates of early failure, non-union and poor functional results.[19,40,160–162] Head fragmentation (>3 fracture fragments including the neck/shaft as a fragment), metaphyseal bone loss, unrepairable fragments and misshapen fragments all make ORIF less appealing.

For proximal ulna fractures associated with other injuries or elbow instability (Mayo type 3), plate fixation is considered to give a superior results to TBW[7,55,128,131–136] but with no specific data in the elderly. Associated coronoid fractures are routinely repaired when they are more than a small avulsion fragment, displaced, or are associated with elbow instability.

Preferred technique

For isolated displaced partial fractures of the radial head, we prefer non-operative management. For isolated displaced fractures of the olecranon in the higher demand elderly patient, we would advocate the use of both plate and TBW fixation. For the lower demand elderly patient, we would recommend non-operative management.

For unstable fractures of the radial head associated with elbow and/or forearm instability we prefer replacement over ORIF (further detail below). For unstable fractures of the proximal ulna, we would advocate the use of plate fixation, with repair of the coronoid when more than an avulsion/type 1 injury. We would routinely repair the coronoid with either sutures placed through drill holes in the proximal ulna or if large enough, screw fixation. For terrible triad injuries requiring operative intervention, we routinely use the protocol described by Pugh et al.[163,164] Monteggia type fracture-dislocations are complex and difficult injuries to manage, particularly in the elderly patient (Figure 24.8). Access is key and we would recommend replacement

of the radial head, fixation of the proximal ulna and then the coronoid, followed by ligament repair.

Excision

RADIAL HEAD FRACTURES AND COMPLEX FRACTURE DISLOCATIONS

Radial head excision has a role in improving forearm rotation and very good long-term outcomes are reported.[165,166] Janssen et al. reported excellent and good results according to the Broberg and Morrey score in 20 of 21 patients who underwent early radial head excision for an isolated Mason type 3 fracture.[167] However, it is essential to ensure there is no ongoing risk of dislocation or subluxation of the elbow or forearm, that is, where restoration of the radiocapitellar contact is essential.[44,112–115] Even partial radial head excision can lead to dislocation or subluxation of the elbow as the key anterolateral part of the head is often involved.[51,59]

In addition to Broberg and Morrey's work,[44] Josefsson et al. analyzed 23 patients with a displaced fracture of the radial head (17 type 2 and 6 type 3) with an associated elbow dislocation and reported that four of eight patients with an associated coronoid fracture suffered a re-dislocation (three acute radial head excision, one non-operative).[96] This would suggest that although non-operative management or radial head excision for the radial head fracture associated with an elbow dislocation is possible, radial head excision alone is not advised when there is a significant coronoid fracture (e.g. terrible triad injury) and is certainly contraindicated when there is a suspected interosseous forearm ligament injury, for example, an Essex-Lopresti injury.[35,165–173] The potential complications of radial head excision in the setting of an unstable complex fracture include proximal radial migration, radioulnar convergence and instability.[87,162,174,175]

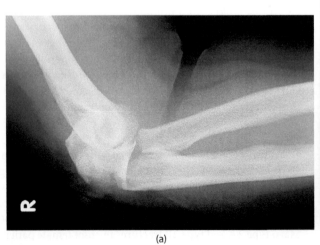
(a)

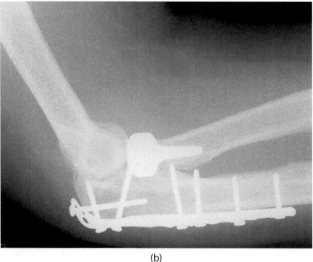
(b)

Figure 24.8 (a) A complex fracture-dislocation of the proximal forearm in an 85-year-old man. (b) Postoperative radiograph following ORIF of the proximal ulna and replacement of the radial head.

Preferred technique

In the acute setting with an elderly patient, if there is any doubt about elbow and/or forearm stability we would recommend replacing the radial head to avoid the possibility of a delay in rehabilitation if further surgery is required. If excision alone is being considered, we would suggest intraoperatively testing:

1. Elbow stability: elbow should not dislocate in full gravity extension after the LCL complex is reattached to the lateral epicondyle.
2. Forearm stability: push–pull test should result in no more than 2–4 mm of translation of the radius.[93]

PROXIMAL ULNA FRACTURES

Although ORIF can be employed in elderly patients with displaced olecranon fractures, complications associated with fixation in osteoporotic bone and wound breakdown are reported.[110] In these elderly patients, although there is an increasing body of evidence to support non-operative management for these injuries, fracture excision with advancement of the triceps is an option.[10,176–178] There are some important requirements for this to work and include: (1) a stable elbow (coronoid and medial collateral ligament intact), (2) a stable forearm (intact interosseous membrane and DRUJ) and (3) the excision involves <50% of the trochlear notch.[7,128,179]

Gartsman et al. reported a large retrospective series of 107 displaced isolated olecranon fractures managed with either excision and advancement (n = 53) or surgical fixation (n = 54).[10] Of the excision group 73% were women and the mean age was 60 years, with 47% women and the mean age 45 years in the fixation group. The rate of complications was higher in the fixation group (24% vs 4%) and included infection, symptomatic metalwork removal, fixation failure, delayed union, skin slough, keloid scarring and intraoperative conversion to excision. At a mean of 3.6 years the functional results were comparable.

Preferred technique

Fracture excision and advancement of the triceps is not a technique we routinely employ. For the stable comminuted fracture in the elderly patient we would suggest non-operative management in the lower demand patients, with fixation in the higher demand patients and in those with evidence of concurrent instability.

Arthroplasty

RADIAL HEAD FRACTURES AND COMPLEX FRACTURE-DISLOCATIONS

Radial head replacement (Figure 24.8) is indicated for proximal forearm fractures associated with elbow or forearm instability that are not suitable for ORIF, which in our experience, is the vast majority of elderly patients. The literature would suggest that replacement is superior to ORIF for an Essex-Lopresti injury, which is associated with chronic forearm pain and instability.[87]

Liu et al. reported a comparison of radial head replacement (n = 37) with ORIF (n = 35) for Mason type 3 radial head fractures in 72 elderly patients with a mean age of 67 years who were followed up for a mean of 1 year.[180] According to the rating of Broberg and Morrey, the mean score in the replacement group was significantly superior to that in the ORIF group (93 vs 81) and the authors concluded that radial head replacement was superior to ORIF in the management of elderly patients with a complex fracture of the radial head (type 3).

Two recent prospective randomized controlled trials have reported superior results following replacement for complex unstable fractures involving the radial head. Chen et al. reported the 2-year follow-up comparing a monopolar fixed neck titanium radial head prosthesis (n = 22) with ORIF (n = 23) and reported superior outcomes (91% good or excellent vs 65%, $P < 0.01$) and a reduced rate of complications (13.6% vs 47.9%, $P < 0.01$) with replacement.[181] These are consistent with the results of another randomized trial by Ruan et al. using a bipolar cemented Tornier© prosthesis.[182]

There is minimal long-term outcome data available. Harrington et al. reported the long-term outcome (mean 12 years) in 20 patients who underwent radial head replacement using a loose and smooth stemmed metal prosthesis for an unstable elbow fracture.[183] In this series, 80% had excellent or good elbow function and the removal rate was 20%, which had no influence on the long-term outcome.

The rate of revision or removal of radial head prosthesis varies (0–32%) in the literature.[183–186] However, increasing age may reduce the risk of requiring further surgery to remove or revise the prosthesis. In a large study from Edinburgh analyzing 105 patients (mean age 50 years, 16–93) who underwent radial head replacement for a complex fracture of the radial head, the overall rate of revision or removal was 27%, with younger age and silastic implants predictive of requiring further surgery to remove or revise the implant.[95]

One of the most significant complications associated with replacement of the radial head is 'over stuffing' the joint.[187–190] There are a variety of techniques to try and avoid this including ensuring that the proximal edge of the replacement does not sit >1 mm proximal to the corner of the coronoid lesser sigmoid notch. Others have suggested using contralateral radiographs of the elbow[191] or intraoperative visualization of the lateral ulnohumeral joint space.[190] The aim is to avoid radiocapitellar erosions, synovitis, ulnohumeral malalignment and arthritis.[188,192–194] Other noted complications include:

- Nerve injury, e.g. PIN, ulnar nerve neuropathy
- Dislocation and/or revision
- Proximal forearm pain: conflicting literature attributing this to radiographic changes secondary to a loose prosthesis,[195,196] particularly when intentionally loose[186,197]

Preferred technique

For complex elbow fracture-dislocations involving the radial head we would routinely undertake replacement. There are advocates for the variety of prostheses available. The replacement is a spacer for maintaining radial head length and restoring the radiocapitellar contact, with the primary aim to restore elbow and forearm stability. Common examples include: (1) a smooth stem replacement that is not rigidly fixed to the neck and (2) a prosthesis with a mobile articulation at the neck (so-called bipolar prostheses).[183–186,198–200] The perceived advantages of the bipolar prostheses are improved capitellar alignment and decreased reaction forces across the joint.[201,202] The potential disadvantages are reduced stability particularly when there is associated soft tissue damage[202–204] and osteolysis related to polyethylene wear.[205,206] We generally favour a monoblock design. These can be rigidly fixed to the neck and there is a reported rate of asymptomatic radial neck bone loss.[184,195] There are comparable short- and medium-term results reported for both implants.[184–186,193,205,207]

ELBOW DISLOCATIONS

Epidemiology

Elbow dislocations account for 3.8% of all dislocations, occur at a mean age of 33–39 years and have an equal gender ratio.[208,209] They account for only 2.7% of dislocations in those ≥65 years of age and 0% of dislocations in those ≥80 years of age.[209] Posterior dislocations are most commonly seen.[209]

The incidence of elbow dislocations ranges in the literature from 2.9 to 7.7 per 100,000 adult individuals per year, with the variation likely due to the inclusion of fracture-dislocations in some series.[208–211] Simple dislocations of the elbow are a rare injury in the elderly, with an overall type C distribution affecting young males and females.[209] Data from Edinburgh have found that elbow fracture-dislocations have a type G distribution curve (bimodal male, unimodal older female), thus fracture-dislocations occur more frequently in the older patient.[209]

MECHANISM OF INJURY

Simple elbow dislocations routinely occur following a fall onto an outstretched hand with the elbow in flexion. This frequently occurs following a fall from standing height, although in males higher energy injuries such as during sporting activities are more common.[208,209]

Clinical assessment

Patients with a dislocation of the elbow will present with elbow pain, deformity and loss of elbow movement, with the elbow often held in flexion. The triangular symmetry of the elbow will be lost. Associated swelling and ecchymosis may also be seen. Emergent reduction and assessment of the skin and neurovascular status are paramount.[35,79–81]

Standard AP and lateral radiographs of the elbow are required before reduction, with check radiographs performed following reduction. These radiographs should identify any associated fractures of the radial head or neck, the distal humerus and the proximal ulna. CT scanning is indicated for complex fractures and fracture-dislocations.

Treatment

Following immediate reduction and immobilization in cast, patients are often seen within 2 weeks of injury to commence mobilization and avoid elbow stiffness. Anakwe et al. reported the long-term outcome of simple elbow dislocations in 110 patients at a mean of 7 years following injury and reported a mean DASH score of 6.7 and a mean satisfaction score of 85.6.[208] Interestingly, 62% reported residual pain, 56% reported subjective elbow stiffness and 8% reported subjective instability. Age was not found to be predictive of outcome according to the DASH or Oxford Elbow Score.

Complications are rare following a simple dislocation but can include instability, stiffness, heterotopic ossification, arthritis and neurovascular injury. Recurrent instability is rare, particularly in the elderly patient. In a case series of 17 patients (mean age 54 years; range 18–86) with an unstable simple elbow dislocation, 15 underwent open reduction and ligament repair (three with concomitant hinged external fixation) and two elderly infirm patients underwent closed reduction and cross pinning of the elbow joint.[212] A stable elbow was achieved in all patients with a mean Broberg and Morrey score of 88.

There are some series that advocate the use of hinged external fixators for complex elbow fracture-dislocations, including in elderly patients.[213–216] This technique is a useful option for the situation of persistent instability despite adequate non-operative or operative methods.

CONCLUSIONS

Recent literature has documented an increasing number of proximal forearm fractures in the elderly population. The important factors to assess when determining the appropriate management are the baseline function of the patient and the stability of the injury. Non-operative management is the mainstay for non-displaced and displaced stable fractures of the radial head. There is increasing evidence to support the non-operative management of isolated displaced olecranon fractures in the older lower demand patient, with TBW and plate fixation alternatives in the higher demand patient.

Although non-operative management may be an option in specific complex fracture or fracture-dislocations in the elderly, it is essential that these are monitored closely to avoid potentially disastrous complications. If there is evidence of elbow and/or forearm instability, replacing the radial head, plate fixation of the proximal ulna and fixation of the coronoid when necessary are recommended.

Further work in this area should aim to determine the longer-term outcome of these injuries and whether an alternative patient reported outcome measure should be used in the elderly patient given the inevitable decline in function with age seen with currently available patient reported outcome scores.

REFERENCES

1. Court-Brown CM, Aitken SA, Forward D, O'Toole RV. The epidemiology of adult fractures. In: Bucholz RW, Court-Brown CM, Heckman JD, Tornetta P, III, editors. *Rockwood and Green's Fractures in Adults*. 7th ed. Philadelphia, PA: Lippincott Williams & Wilkins; 2010. pp. 53–84.

2. Beingessner DM, Pollock JW, King GJ. Elbow fractures and dislocations. In: Court-Brown CM, Heckman JD, McQueen MM, Ricci WMTP, III, editors. *Rockwood and Green's Fractures in Adults*. 8th ed. Philadelphia, PA: Lippincott Williams & Wilkins; 2014. pp. 1179–227.

3. Duckworth AD, Clement ND, Jenkins PJ, Aitken SA, Court-Brown CM, McQueen MM. The epidemiology of radial head and neck fractures. *J Hand Surg Am* 2012;37(1):112–19.

4. Kaas L, Sierevelt IN, Vroemen JP, van Dijk CN, Eygendaal D. Osteoporosis and radial head fractures in female patients: A case-control study. *J Shoulder Elbow Surg* 2012;21(11):1555–8.

5. Duckworth AD, Clement ND, Aitken SA, Court-Brown CM, McQueen MM. The epidemiology of fractures of the proximal ulna. *Injury* 2012;43(3):343–6.

6. Rommens PM, Kuchle R, Schneider RU, Reuter M. Olecranon fractures in adults: Factors influencing outcome. *Injury* 2004;35(11):1149–57.

7. Newman SD, Mauffrey C, Krikler S. Olecranon fractures. *Injury* 2009;40(6):575–81.

8. Karlsson MK, Hasserius R, Karlsson C, Besjakov J, Josefsson PO. Fractures of the olecranon: A 15- to 25-year followup of 73 patients. *Clin Orthop Relat Res* 2002;(403):205–12.

9. Murphy DF, Greene WB, Gilbert JA, Dameron TB, Jr. Displaced olecranon fractures in adults. Biomechanical analysis of fixation methods. *Clin Orthop Relat Res* 1987;(224):210–14.

10. Gartsman GM, Sculco TP, Otis JC. Operative treatment of olecranon fractures. Excision or open reduction with internal fixation. *J Bone Joint Surg Am* 1981;63(5):718–21.

11. Weseley MS, Barenfeld PA, Eisenstein AL. Closed treatment of isolated radial head fractures. *J Trauma* 1983;23(1):36–9.

12. Struijs PA, Smit G, Steller EP. Radial head fractures: Effectiveness of conservative treatment versus surgical intervention. A systematic review. *Arch Orthop Trauma Surg* 2007;127(2):125–30.

13. Pike JM, Athwal GS, Faber KJ, King GJ. Radial head fractures—An update. *J Hand Surg Am* 2009;34(3):557–65.

14. Duckworth AD, Wickramasinghe NR, Clement ND, Court-Brown CM, McQueen MM. Long-term outcomes of isolated stable radial head fractures. *J Bone Joint Surg Am* 2014;96(20):1716–23.

15. Yoon A, King GJ, Grewal R. Is ORIF superior to nonoperative treatment in isolated displaced partial articular fractures of the radial head? *Clin Orthop Relat Res* 2014;472(7):2105–12.

16. Gallucci GL, Piuzzi NS, Slullitel PA, Boretto JG, Alfie VA, Donndorff A, et al. Non-surgical functional treatment for displaced olecranon fractures in the elderly. *Bone Joint J* 2014;96-B(4):530–4.

17. Duckworth AD, Bugler KE, Clement ND, Court-Brown CM, McQueen MM. Nonoperative management of displaced olecranon fractures in low-demand elderly patients. *J Bone Joint Surg Am* 2014;96(1):67–72.

18. Court-Brown CM, McQueen MM, Tornetta P. Proximal forearm fractures and elbow dislocations. In: Court-Brown C, McQueen MM, Tornetta P, editors. *Orthopaedic Surgery Essentials: Trauma*. 1st ed. Philadelphia, PA: Lippincott Williams & Wilkins; 2006. pp. 124–40.

19. Davidson PA, Moseley JB, Jr., Tullos HS. Radial head fracture. A potentially complex injury. *Clin Orthop Relat Res* 1993;297:224–30.

20. Itamura J, Roidis N, Mirzayan R, Vaishnav S, Learch T, Shean C. Radial head fractures: MRI evaluation of associated injuries. *J Shoulder Elbow Surg* 2005;14(4):421–4.

21. Kaas L, Turkenburg JL, van Riet RP, Vroemen JP, Eygendaal D. Magnetic resonance imaging findings in 46 elbows with a radial head fracture. *Acta Orthop* 2010;81(3):373–6.

22. Rineer CA, Guitton TG, Ring D. Radial head fractures: Loss of cortical contact is associated with concomitant fracture or dislocation. *J Shoulder Elbow Surg* 2010;19(1):21–5.

23. Kaas L, van Riet RP, Vroemen JP, Eygendaal D. The epidemiology of radial head fractures. *J Shoulder Elbow Surg* 2010;19(4):520–3.

24. Court-Brown CM, Bugler KE, Clement ND, Duckworth AD, McQueen MM. The epidemiology of open fractures in adults. A 15-year review. *Injury* 2012;43(6):891–7.

25. Kaas L, van Riet RP, Vroemen JP, Eygendaal D. The incidence of associated fractures of the upper limb in fractures of the radial head. *Strategies Trauma Limb Reconstr* 2008;3(2):71–4.

26. van Riet RP, Morrey BF, O'Driscoll SW, van Glabbeek F. Associated injuries complicating radial head fractures: A demographic study. *Clin Orthop Relat Res* 2005;441:351–5.

27. Court-Brown CM, Caesar B. Epidemiology of adult fractures: A review. *Injury* 2006;37(8):691–7.

28. Parker MJ, Richmond PW, Andrew TA, Bewes PC. A review of displaced olecranon fractures treated conservatively. *J R Coll Surg Edinb* 1990;35(6):392–4.

29. Veillette CJ, Steinmann SP. Olecranon fractures. *Orthop Clin North Am* 2008;39(2):229–36, vii.

30. Amis AA, Miller JH. The mechanisms of elbow fractures: An investigation using impact tests in vitro. *Injury* 1995;26(3):163–8.

31. Keon-Cohen BT. Fractures at the elbow. *J Bone Joint Surg Am* 1966;48(8):1623–39.

32. van Leeuwen DH, Guitton TG, Lambers K, Ring D. Quantitative measurement of radial head fracture location. *J Shoulder Elbow Surg* 2012;21(8):1013–17.

33. Sahajpal D, Wright TW. Proximal ulna fractures. *J Hand Surg Am* 2009;34(2):357–62.

34. Baecher N, Edwards S. Olecranon fractures. *J Hand Surg Am* 2013;38(3):593–604.

35. Ring D. Elbow fractures and dislocations. In: Bucholz RW, Court-Brown CM, Heckman JD, Tornetta P, III, editors. *Rockwood and Green's Fractures in Adults.* 7th ed. Philadelphia, PA: Lippincott Williams & Wilkins; 2010, pp. 905–44.

36. Müller ME. *The Comprehensive Classification of Fractures of Long Bones.* Berlin: Springer; 1990.

37. Marsh JL, Slongo TF, Agel J, Broderick JS, Creevey W, DeCoster TA, et al. Fracture and dislocation classification compendium—2007: Orthopaedic Trauma Association classification, database and outcomes committee. *J Orthop Trauma* 2007;21(10 Suppl):S1–133.

38. Sheps DM, Kiefer KR, Boorman RS, Donaghy J, Lalani A, Walker R, et al. The interobserver reliability of classification systems for radial head fractures: The Hotchkiss modification of the Mason classification and the AO classification systems. *Can J Surg* 2009;52(4):277–82.

39. Matsunaga FT, Tamaoki MJ, Cordeiro EF, Uehara A, Ikawa MH, Matsumoto MH, et al. Are classifications of proximal radius fractures reproducible? BMC *Musculoskelet Disord* 2009;10:120.

40. Ring D, Quintero J, Jupiter JB. Open reduction and internal fixation of fractures of the radial head. *J Bone Joint Surg Am* 2002;84-A(10):1811–15.

41. Duckworth AD, Watson BS, Will EM, Petrisor BA, Walmsley PJ, Court-Brown CM, et al. Radial head and neck fractures: Functional results and predictors of outcome. *J Trauma* 2011;71(3):643–8.

42. Duckworth AD, Clement ND, Jenkins PJ, Will EM, Court-Brown CM, McQueen MM. Socioeconomic deprivation predicts outcome following radial head and neck fractures. *Injury* 2012;43(7):1102–6.

43. Mason M. Some observations on fractures of the head of the radius with a review of one hundred cases. *Br J Surg* 1954;42(172):123–32.

44. Broberg MA, Morrey BF. Results of treatment of fracture-dislocations of the elbow. *Clin Orthop Relat Res* 1987;216:109–19.

45. Morgan SJ, Groshen SL, Itamura JM, Shankwiler J, Brien WW, Kuschner SH. Reliability evaluation of classifying radial head fractures by the system of Mason. *Bull Hosp Jt Dis* 1997;56(2):95–8.

46. Doornberg J, Elsner A, Kloen P, Marti RK, van Dijk CN, Ring D. Apparently isolated partial articular fractures of the radial head: Prevalence and reliability of radiographically diagnosed displacement. *J Shoulder Elbow Surg* 2007;16(5):603–8.

47. Hotchkiss RN. Displaced fractures of the radial head: Internal fixation or excision? *J Am Acad Orthop Surg* 1997;5(1):1–10.

48. Akesson T, Herbertsson P, Josefsson PO, Hasserius R, Besjakov J, Karlsson MK. Primary nonoperative treatment of moderately displaced two-part fractures of the radial head. *J Bone Joint Surg Am* 2006;88(9):1909–14.

49. Guitton TG, Ring D. Interobserver reliability of radial head fracture classification: Two-dimensional compared with three-dimensional CT. *J Bone Joint Surg Am* 2011;93(21):2015–21.

50. Duckworth AD, McQueen MM, Ring D. Fractures of the radial head. *Bone Joint J* 2013;95-B(2):151–9.

51. Ring D. Radial head fracture: Open reduction-internal fixation or prosthetic replacement. *J Shoulder Elbow Surg* 2011;20(2 Suppl):S107–12.

52. Ring D. Displaced, unstable fractures of the radial head: Fixation vs. replacement—What is the evidence? *Injury* 2008;39(12):1329–37.

53. Charalambous CP, Stanley JK, Mills SP, Hayton MJ, Hearnden A, Trail I, et al. Comminuted radial head fractures: Aspects of current management. *J Shoulder Elbow Surg* 2011;20(6):996–1007.

54. Morrey BF. Current concepts in the treatment of fractures of the radial head, the olecranon, and the coronoid. *Instr Course Lect* 1995;44:175–85.

55. Buijze G, Kloen P. Clinical evaluation of locking compression plate fixation for comminuted olecranon fractures. *J Bone Joint Surg Am* 2009;91(10):2416–20.

56. Regan W, Morrey B. Fractures of the coronoid process of the ulna. *J Bone Joint Surg Am* 1989;71(9):1348–54.

57. Morrey BF, Tanaka S, An KN. Valgus stability of the elbow. A definition of primary and secondary constraints. *Clin Orthop Relat Res* 1991;(265):187–95.

58. Cohen MS, Hastings H. Rotatory instability of the elbow. The anatomy and role of the lateral stabilizers. *J Bone Joint Surg Am* 1997;79(2):225–33.

59. Morrey BF, An KN. Articular and ligamentous contributions to the stability of the elbow joint. *Am J Sports Med* 1983;11(5):315–19.

60. O'Driscoll SW, Bell DF, Morrey BF. Posterolateral rotatory instability of the elbow. *J Bone Joint Surg Am* 1991;73(3):440–6.

61. Schneeberger AG, Sadowski MM, Jacob HA. Coronoid process and radial head as posterolateral rotatory stabilizers of the elbow. *J Bone Joint Surg Am* 2004;86-A(5):975–82.

62. Beingessner DM, Dunning CE, Gordon KD, Johnson JA, King GJ. The effect of radial head excision and arthroplasty on elbow kinematics and stability. *J Bone Joint Surg Am* 2004;86-A(8):1730–9.

63. Morrey BF, An KN. Stability of the elbow: Osseous constraints. *J Shoulder Elbow Surg* 2005;14(1 Suppl S):174S–8S.

64. Jeon IH, Sanchez-Sotelo J, Zhao K, An KN, Morrey BM. The contribution of the coronoid and radial head to the stability of the elbow. *J Bone Joint Surg Br* 2012;94(1):86–92.

65. Morrey BF. Complex instability of the elbow. *Instr Course Lect* 1998;47:157–64.

66. Ring D, Jupiter JB. Fracture-dislocation of the elbow. *Hand Clin* 2002;18(1):55–63.

67. Ring D, Jupiter JB, Zilberfarb J. Posterior dislocation of the elbow with fractures of the radial head and coronoid. *J Bone Joint Surg Am* 2002;84-A(4):547–51.

68. Ring D, Jupiter JB. Fracture-dislocation of the elbow. *J Bone Joint Surg Am* 1998;80(4):566–80.

69. McKee MD, Schemitsch EH, Sala MJ, O'Driscoll SW. The pathoanatomy of lateral ligamentous disruption in complex elbow instability. *J Shoulder Elbow Surg* 2003;12(4):391–6.

70. Diliberti T, Botte MJ, Abrams RA. Anatomical considerations regarding the posterior interosseous nerve during posterolateral approaches to the proximal part of the radius. *J Bone Joint Surg Am* 2000;82(6):809–13.

71. Chalidis BE, Sachinis NC, Samoladas EP, Dimitriou CG, Pournaras JD. Is tension band wiring technique the "gold standard" for the treatment of olecranon fractures? A long term functional outcome study. *J Orthop Surg Res* 2008;3:9.

72. Dowdy PA, Bain GI, King GJ, Patterson SD. The midline posterior elbow incision. An anatomical appraisal. *J Bone Joint Surg Br* 1995;77(5):696–9.

73. Charalambous CP, Stanley JK, Siddique I, Powell E, Alvi F, Gagey O. The Wrightington approach to the radial head: Biomechanical comparison with the posterolateral approach. *J Hand Surg Am* 2007;32(10):1576–82.

74. Holdsworth BJ, Clement DA, Rothwell PN. Fractures of the radial head—The benefit of aspiration: A prospective controlled trial. *Injury* 1987;18(1):44–7.

75. Dooley JF, Angus PD. The importance of elbow aspiration when treating radial head fractures. *Arch Emerg Med* 1991;8(2):117–21.

76. Carley S. The role of therapeutic needle aspiration in radial head fractures. *J Accid Emerg Med* 1999;16(4):282.

77. Chalidis BE, Papadopoulos PP, Sachinis NC, Dimitriou CG. Aspiration alone versus aspiration and bupivacaine injection in the treatment of undisplaced radial head fractures: A prospective randomized study. *J Shoulder Elbow Surg* 2009;18(5):676–9.

78. Ditsios KT, Stavridis SI, Christodoulou AG. The effect of haematoma aspiration on intra-articular pressure and pain relief following Mason I radial head fractures. *Injury* 2011;42(4):362–5.

79. Sudhahar TA, Patel AD. A rare case of partial posterior interosseous nerve injury associated with radial head fracture. *Injury* 2004;35(5):543–4.

80. Ayel JE, Bonnevialle N, Lafosse JM, Pidhorz L, Al Homsy M, Mansat P, et al. Acute elbow dislocation with arterial rupture. Analysis of nine cases. *Orthop Traumatol Surg Res* 2009;95(5):343–51.

81. Serrano KD, Rebella GS, Sansone JM, Kim MK. A rare case of posterior interosseous nerve palsy associated with radial head fracture. *J Emerg Med* 2012;43(2):e115–17.

82. Helmerhorst GT, Ring D. Subtle Essex-Lopresti lesions: Report of 2 cases. *J Hand Surg Am* 2009;34(3):436–8.

83. Charalambous CP, Stanley JK. Posterolateral rotatory instability of the elbow. *J Bone Joint Surg Br* 2008;90(3):272–9.

84. Nestor BJ, O'Driscoll SW, Morrey BF. Ligamentous reconstruction for posterolateral rotatory instability of the elbow. *J Bone Joint Surg Am* 1992;74(8):1235–41.

85. Lattanza LL, Chu T, Ty JM, Orazov B, Strauss N, O'Reilly OM, et al. Interclinician and intraclinician variability in the mechanics of the pivot shift test for posterolateral rotatory instability (PLRI) of the elbow. *J Shoulder Elbow Surg* 2010;19(8):1150–6.

86. Yeh GL, Beredjiklian PK, Katz MA, Steinberg DR, Bozentka DJ. Effects of forearm rotation on the clinical evaluation of ulnar variance. *J Hand Surg Am* 2001;26(6):1042–6.

87. Jungbluth P, Frangen TM, Arens S, Muhr G, Kalicke T. The undiagnosed Essex-Lopresti injury. *J Bone Joint Surg Br* 2006;88(12):1629–33.

88. Dodds SD, Yeh PC, Slade JF, III. Essex-Lopresti injuries. *Hand Clin* 2008;24(1):125–37.

89. Duckworth AD, Clement ND, Aitken SA, Ring D, McQueen MM. Essex-Lopresti lesion associated with an impacted radial neck fracture: Interest of ulnar shortening in the secondary management of sequelae. *J Shoulder Elbow Surg* 2011;20(6):e19–24.

90. McGinley JC, Kozin SH. Interosseous membrane anatomy and functional mechanics. *Clin Orthop Relat Res* 2001;(383):108–22.

91. Fester EW, Murray PM, Sanders TG, Ingari JV, Leyendecker J, Leis HL. The efficacy of magnetic resonance imaging and ultrasound in detecting disruptions of the forearm interosseous membrane: A cadaver study. *J Hand Surg Am* 2002;27(3):418–24.

92. McGinley JC, Roach N, Hopgood BC, Limmer K, Kozin SH. Forearm interosseous membrane trauma: MRI diagnostic criteria and injury patterns. *Skeletal Radiol* 2006;35(5):275–81.

93. Smith AM, Urbanosky LR, Castle JA, Rushing JT, Ruch DS. Radius pull test: Predictor of longitudinal forearm instability. *J Bone Joint Surg Am* 2002;84-A(11):1970–6.

94. Kaas L, van Riet RP, Turkenburg JL, Vroemen JP, van Niek DC, Eygendaal D. Magnetic resonance imaging in radial head fractures: Most associated injuries are not clinically relevant. *J Shoulder Elbow Surg* 2011;20(8):1282–8.

95. Duckworth AD, Wickramasinghe NR, Clement ND, Court-Brown CM, McQueen MM. Radial head replacement for acute complex fractures: What are the rate and risks factors for revision or removal? *Clin Orthop Relat Res* 2014;472(7):2136–43.

96. Josefsson PO, Gentz CF, Johnell O, Wendeberg B. Dislocations of the elbow and intraarticular fractures. *Clin Orthop Relat Res* 1989;(246):126–30.

97. Penrose JH. The Monteggia fracture with posterior dislocation of the radial head. *J Bone Joint Surg Br* 1951;33-B(1):65–73.

98. Pavel A, Pitman JM, Lance EM, Wade PA. The posterior Monteggia fracture: A clinical study. *J Trauma* 1965;5:185–99.

99. Ring D, Jupiter JB, Simpson NS. Monteggia fractures in adults. *J Bone Joint Surg Am* 1998;80(12):1733–44.

100. Essex-Lopresti P. Fractures of the radial head with distal radio-ulnar dislocation; report of two cases. *J Bone Joint Surg Br* 1951;33B(2):244–7.

101. Edwards GS, Jr., Jupiter JB. Radial head fractures with acute distal radioulnar dislocation. Essex-Lopresti revisited. *Clin Orthop Relat Res* 1988;234(234):61–9.

102. Ring D, Jupiter JB, Sanders RW, Mast J, Simpson NS. Transolecranon fracture-dislocation of the elbow. *J Orthop Trauma* 1997;11(8):545–50.

103. Herbertsson P, Josefsson PO, Hasserius R, Karlsson C, Besjakov J, Karlsson M. Uncomplicated Mason type-II and III fractures of the radial head and neck in adults. A long-term follow-up study. *J Bone Joint Surg Am* 2004;86-A(3):569–74.

104. Herbertsson P, Josefsson PO, Hasserius R, Karlsson C, Besjakov J, Karlsson MK. Displaced Mason type I fractures of the radial head and neck in adults: A fifteen- to thirty-three-year follow-up study. *J Shoulder Elbow Surg* 2005;14(1):73–7.

105. Rosenblatt Y, Athwal GS, Faber KJ. Current recommendations for the treatment of radial head fractures. *Orthop Clin North Am* 2008;39(2):173–85, vi.

106. Lindenhovius AL, Felsch Q, Ring D, Kloen P. The long-term outcome of open reduction and internal fixation of stable displaced isolated partial articular fractures of the radial head. *J Trauma* 2009;67(1):143–6.

107. Court-Brown CM, Cattermole H, McQueen MM. Impacted valgus fractures (B1.1) of the proximal humerus. The results of non-operative treatment. *J Bone Joint Surg Br* 2002;84(4):504–8.

108. Kiviluoto O, Santavirta S. Fractures of the olecranon. Analysis of 37 consecutive cases. *Acta Orthop Scand* 1978;49(1):28–31.

109. Holdsworth BJ, Mossad MM. Elbow function following tension band fixation of displaced fractures of the olecranon. *Injury* 1984;16(3):182–7.

110. Veras Del Monte L, Sirera Vercher M, Busquets Net R, Castellanos Robles J, Carrera Calderer L, Mir Bullo X. Conservative treatment of displaced fractures of the olecranon in the elderly. *Injury* 1999;30(2):105–10.

111. Bruinsma W, Lindenhovius AL, McKee MD, Athwal GS, Ring D. Non-union of non-operatively treated displaced olecranon fractures. *Shoulder Elbow* 2012;4(4):273–6.

112. Josefsson PO, Gentz CF, Johnell O, Wendeberg B. Surgical versus non-surgical treatment of ligamentous injuries following dislocation of the elbow joint. A prospective randomized study. *J Bone Joint Surg Am* 1987;69(4):605–8.

113. Lindenhovius AL, Jupiter JB, Ring D. Comparison of acute versus subacute treatment of terrible triad injuries of the elbow. *J Hand Surg Am* 2008;33(6):920–6.

114. Guitton TG, Ring D. Nonsurgically treated terrible triad injuries of the elbow: Report of four cases. *J Hand Surg Am* 2010;35(3):464–7.

115. Karlsson MK, Herbertsson P, Nordqvist A, Besjakov J, Josefsson PO, Hasserius R. Comminuted fractures of the radial head. *Acta Orthop* 2010;81(2):226–9.

116. Chan K, MacDermid JC, Faber KJ, King GJ, Athwal GS. Can we treat select terrible triad injuries nonoperatively? *Clin Orthop Relat Res* 2014;472(7):2092–9.

117. Mathew PK, Athwal GS, King GJ. Terrible triad injury of the elbow: Current concepts. *J Am Acad Orthop Surg* 2009;17(3):137–51.

118. Liow RY, Cregan A, Nanda R, Montgomery RJ. Early mobilisation for minimally displaced radial head fractures is desirable. A prospective randomised study of two protocols. *Injury* 2002;33(9):801–6.

119. Paschos NK, Mitsionis GI, Vasiliadis HS, Georgoulis AD. Comparison of early mobilization protocols in radial head fractures. A prospective randomized controlled study. The effect of fracture characteristics on outcome. *J Orthop Trauma* 2013;27(3):134–9.

120. Bunker TD, Newman JH. The Herbert differential pitch bone screw in displaced radial head fractures. *Injury* 1985;16(9):621–4.

121. Geel CW, Palmer AK, Ruedi T, Leutenegger AF. Internal fixation of proximal radial head fractures. *J Orthop Trauma* 1990;4(3):270–4.

122. Khalfayan EE, Culp RW, Alexander AH. Mason type II radial head fractures: Operative versus nonoperative treatment. *J Orthop Trauma* 1992;6(3):283–9.

123. Pearce MS, Gallannaugh SC. Mason type II radial head fractures fixed with Herbert bone screws. *J R Soc Med* 1996;89(6):340P–4P.

124. Zarattini G, Galli S, Marchese M, Mascio LD, Pazzaglia UE. The surgical treatment of isolated Mason type 2 fractures of the radial head in adults: Comparison between radial head resection and open reduction and internal fixation. *J Orthop Trauma* 2012;26(4):229–35.

125. Caputo AE, Mazzocca AD, Santoro VM. The nonarticulating portion of the radial head: Anatomic and clinical correlations for internal fixation. *J Hand Surg Am* 1998;23(6):1082–90.

126. Smith GR, Hotchkiss RN. Radial head and neck fractures: Anatomic guidelines for proper placement of internal fixation. *J Shoulder Elbow Surg* 1996;5(2 Pt 1):113–17.

127. Soyer AD, Nowotarski PJ, Kelso TB, Mighell MA. Optimal position for plate fixation of complex fractures of the proximal radius: A cadaver study. *J Orthop Trauma* 1998;12(4):291–3.

128. Hak DJ, Golladay GJ. Olecranon fractures: Treatment options. *J Am Acad Orthop Surg* 2000;8(4):266–75.

129. Villanueva P, Osorio F, Commessatti M, Sanchez-Sotelo J. Tension-band wiring for olecranon fractures: Analysis of risk factors for failure. *J Shoulder Elbow Surg* 2006;15(3):351–6.

130. Matar HE, Ali AA, Buckley S, Garlick NI, Atkinson HD. Surgical interventions for treating fractures of the olecranon in adults. *Cochrane Database Syst Rev* 2014;11:CD010144.

131. Horne JG, Tanzer TL. Olecranon fractures: A review of 100 cases. *J Trauma* 1981;21(6):469–72.

132. Fyfe IS, Mossad MM, Holdsworth BJ. Methods of fixation of olecranon fractures. An experimental mechanical study. *J Bone Joint Surg Br* 1985;67(3):367–72.

133. Hume MC, Wiss DA. Olecranon fractures. A clinical and radiographic comparison of tension band wiring and plate fixation. *Clin Orthop Relat Res* 1992;(285):229–35.

134. Bailey CS, MacDermid J, Patterson SD, King GJ. Outcome of plate fixation of olecranon fractures. *J Orthop Trauma* 2001;15(8):542–8.

135. Buijze GA, Blankevoort L, Tuijthof GJ, Sierevelt IN, Kloen P. Biomechanical evaluation of fixation of comminuted olecranon fractures: One-third tubular versus locking compression plating. *Arch Orthop Trauma Surg* 2010;130(4):459–64.

136. Erturer RE, Sever C, Sonmez MM, Ozcelik IB, Akman S, Ozturk I. Results of open reduction and plate osteosynthesis in comminuted fracture of the olecranon. *J Shoulder Elbow Surg* 2011;20(3):449–54.

137. Murphy DF, Greene WB, Dameron TB, Jr. Displaced olecranon fractures in adults. Clinical evaluation. *Clin Orthop Relat Res* 1987;(224):215–23.

138. Wilson J, Bajwa A, Kamath V, Rangan A. Biomechanical comparison of interfragmentary compression in transverse fractures of the olecranon. *J Bone Joint Surg Br* 2011;93(2):245–50.

139. Gruszka D, Arand C, Nowak T, Dietz SO, Wagner D, Rommens P. Olecranon tension plating or olecranon tension band wiring? A comparative biomechanical study. *Int Orthop* 2015;39(5):955–60.

140. Macko D, Szabo RM. Complications of tension-band wiring of olecranon fractures. *J Bone Joint Surg Am* 1985;67(9):1396–401.

141. Karlsson MK, Hasserius R, Besjakov J, Karlsson C, Josefsson PO. Comparison of tension-band and figure-of-eight wiring techniques for treatment of olecranon fractures. *J Shoulder Elbow Surg* 2002;11(4):377–82.

142. Rommens PM, Schneider RU, Reuter M. Functional results after operative treatment of olecranon fractures. *Acta Chir Belg* 2004;104(2):191–7.

143. Flinterman HJ, Doornberg JN, Guitton TG, Ring D, Goslings JC, Kloen P. Long-term outcome of displaced, transverse, noncomminuted olecranon fractures. *Clin Orthop Relat Res* 2014;472(6):1955–61.

144. Ishigaki N, Uchiyama S, Nakagawa H, Kamimura M, Miyasaka T. Ulnar nerve palsy at the elbow after surgical treatment for fractures of the olecranon. *J Shoulder Elbow Surg* 2004;13(1):60–5.

145. De Carli P, Gallucci GL, Donndorff AG, Boretto JG, Alfie VA. Proximal radio-ulnar synostosis and nonunion after olecranon fracture tension-band wiring: A case report. *J Shoulder Elbow Surg* 2009;18(3):e40–4.

146. Amini MH, Azar FM, Wilson BR, Smith RA, Mauck BM, Throckmorton TW. Comparison of outcomes and costs of tension-band and locking-plate osteosynthesis in transverse olecranon fractures: A matched-cohort study. *Am J Orthop (Belle Mead NJ)* 2015;44(7):E211–15.

147. Tarallo L, Mugnai R, Adani R, Capra F, Zambianchi F, Catani F. Simple and comminuted displaced olecranon fractures: A clinical comparison between tension band wiring and plate fixation techniques. *Arch Orthop Trauma Surg* 2014;134(8):1107–14.

148. Schliemann B, Raschke MJ, Groene P, Weimann A, Wahnert D, Lenschow S, et al. Comparison of tension band wiring and precontoured locking compression plate fixation in Mayo type IIA olecranon fractures. *Acta Orthop Belg* 2014;80(1):106–11.

149. Hutchinson DT, Horwitz DS, Ha G, Thomas CW, Bachus KN. Cyclic loading of olecranon fracture fixation constructs. *J Bone Joint Surg Am* 2003;85-A(5):831–7.

150. Molloy S, Jasper LE, Elliott DS, Brumback RJ, Belkoff SM. Biomechanical evaluation of intramedullary nail versus tension band fixation for transverse olecranon fractures. *J Orthop Trauma* 2004;18(3):170–4.

151. Nowak TE, Mueller LP, Burkhart KJ, Sternstein W, Reuter M, Rommens PM. Dynamic biomechanical analysis of different olecranon fracture fixation devices—Tension band wiring versus two intramedullary nail systems: An in-vitro cadaveric study. *Clin Biomech (Bristol, Avon)* 2007;22(6):658–64.

152. Nowak TE, Burkhart KJ, Mueller LP, Mattyasovszky SG, Andres T, Sternstein W, et al. New intramedullary locking nail for olecranon fracture fixation—An in vitro biomechanical comparison with tension band wiring. *J Trauma* 2010;69(5):E56–61.

153. Wadsworth TG. Screw fixation of the olecranon after fracture or osteotomy. *Clin Orthop Relat Res* 1976;(119):197–201.

154. Cannada L, Loeffler B, Zadnik MB, Eglseder AW. Treatment of high-energy supracondylar/intercondylar fractures of the distal humerus. *J Surg Orthop Adv* 2011;20(4):230–5.

155. Coles CP, Barei DP, Nork SE, Taitsman LA, Hanel DP, Bradford HM. The olecranon osteotomy: A six-year experience in the treatment of intraarticular fractures of the distal humerus. *J Orthop Trauma* 2006;20(3):164–71.

156. Gehr J, Friedl W. Intramedullary locking compression nail for the treatment of an olecranon fracture. *Oper Orthop Traumatol* 2006;18(3):199–213.

157. Edwards SG, Argintar E, Lamb J. Management of comminuted proximal ulna fracture-dislocations using a multiplanar locking intramedullary nail. *Tech Hand Up Extrem Surg* 2011;15(2):106–14.

158. Nijs S, Graeler H, Bellemans J. Fixing simple olecranon fractures with the Olecranon Osteotomy Nail (OleON). *Oper Orthop Traumatol* 2011;23(5):438–45.

159. Bateman DK, Barlow JD, VanBeek C, Abboud JA. Suture anchor fixation of displaced olecranon fractures in the elderly: A case series and surgical technique. *J Shoulder Elbow Surg* 2015;24(7):1090–7.

160. King GJ, Evans DC, Kellam JF. Open reduction and internal fixation of radial head fractures. *J Orthop Trauma* 1991;5(1):21–8.

161. Heim U. [Surgical treatment of radial head fracture]. *Z Unfallchir Versicherungsmed* 1992;85(1):3–11.

162. Lindenhovius AL, Felsch Q, Doornberg JN, Ring D, Kloen P. Open reduction and internal fixation compared with excision for unstable displaced fractures of the radial head. *J Hand Surg Am* 2007;32(5):630–6.

163. McKee MD, Pugh DM, Wild LM, Schemitsch EH, King GJ. Standard surgical protocol to treat elbow dislocations with radial head and coronoid fractures. Surgical technique. *J Bone Joint Surg Am* 2005;87(Suppl 1; Pt 1):22–32.

164. Pugh DM, Wild LM, Schemitsch EH, King GJ, McKee MD. Standard surgical protocol to treat elbow dislocations with radial head and coronoid fractures. *J Bone Joint Surg Am* 2004;86-A(6):1122–30.

165. Broberg MA, Morrey BF. Results of delayed excision of the radial head after fracture. *J Bone Joint Surg Am* 1986;68(5):669–74.

166. Herbertsson P, Josefsson PO, Hasserius R, Besjakov J, Nyqvist F, Karlsson MK. Fractures of the radial head and neck treated with radial head excision. *J Bone Joint Surg Am* 2004;86-A(9):1925–30.

167. Janssen RP, Vegter J. Resection of the radial head after Mason type-III fractures of the elbow: Follow-up at 16 to 30 years. *J Bone Joint Surg Br* 1998;80(2):231–3.

168. Coleman DA, Blair WF, Shurr D. Resection of the radial head for fracture of the radial head. Long-term follow-up of seventeen cases. *J Bone Joint Surg Am* 1987;69(3):385–92.

169. Ikeda M, Sugiyama K, Kang C, Takagaki T, Oka Y. Comminuted fractures of the radial head. Comparison of resection and internal fixation. *J Bone Joint Surg Am* 2005;87(1):76–84.

170. Herbertsson P, Hasserius R, Josefsson PO, Besjakov J, Nyquist F, Nordqvist A, et al. Mason type IV fractures of the elbow: A 14- to 46-year follow-up study. *J Bone Joint Surg Br* 2009;91(11):1499–504.

171. Antuna SA, Sanchez-Marquez JM, Barco R. Long-term results of radial head resection following isolated radial head fractures in patients younger than forty years old. *J Bone Joint Surg Am* 2010;92(3):558–66.

172. Iftimie PP, Calmet Garcia J, de Loyola Garcia Forcada I, Gonzalez Pedrouzo JE, Gine Goma J. Resection arthroplasty for radial head fractures: Long-term follow-up. *J Shoulder Elbow Surg* 2011;20(1):45–50.

173. Faldini C, Nanni M, Leonetti D, Capra P, Bonomo M, Persiani V, et al. Early radial head excision for displaced and comminuted radial head fractures: Considerations and concerns at long-term follow-up. *J Orthop Trauma* 2012;26(4):236–40.

174. Jungbluth P, Frangen TM, Muhr G, Kalicke T. A primarily overlooked and incorrectly treated Essex-Lopresti injury: What can this lead to? *Arch Orthop Trauma Surg* 2008;128(1):89–95.

175. Schiffern A, Bettwieser SP, Porucznik CA, Crim JR, Tashjian RZ. Proximal radial drift following radial head resection. *J Shoulder Elbow Surg* 2011;20(3):426–33.

176. McKeever FM, Buck RM. Fracture of the olecranon process of the ulna; treatment by excision of fragment and repair of triceps tendon. *J Am Med Assoc* 1947;135(1):1–5.

177. Inhofe PD, Howard TC. The treatment of olecranon fractures by excision or fragments and repair of the extensor mechanism: Historical review and report of 12 fractures. *Orthopedics* 1993;16(12):1313–17.

178. Iannuzzi N, Dahners L. Excision and advancement in the treatment of comminuted olecranon fractures. *J Orthop Trauma* 2009;23(3):226–8.

179. An KN, Morrey BF, Chao EY. The effect of partial removal of proximal ulna on elbow constraint. *Clin Orthop Relat Res* 1986;(209):270–9.

180. Liu R, Liu P, Shu H, Gong J, Sun Q, Wu J, et al. Comparison of primary radial head replacement and ORIF (open reduction and internal fixation) in Mason type III fractures: A retrospective evaluation in 72 elderly patients. *Med Sci Monit* 2015;21:90–3.

181. Chen X, Wang SC, Cao LH, Yang GQ, Li M, Su JC. Comparison between radial head replacement and open reduction and internal fixation in clinical treatment of unstable, multi-fragmented radial head fractures. *Int Orthop* 2011;35(7):1071–6.

182. Ruan HJ, Fan CY, Liu JJ, Zeng BF. A comparative study of internal fixation and prosthesis replacement for radial head fractures of Mason type III. *Int Orthop* 2009;33(1):249–53.

183. Harrington IJ, Sekyi-Otu A, Barrington TW, Evans DC, Tuli V. The functional outcome with metallic radial head implants in the treatment of unstable elbow fractures: A long-term review. *J Trauma* 2001;50(1):46–52.

184. Moro JK, Werier J, MacDermid JC, Patterson SD, King GJ. Arthroplasty with a metal radial head for unreconstructible fractures of the radial head. *J Bone Joint Surg Am* 2001;83-A(8):1201–11.

185. Grewal R, MacDermid JC, Faber KJ, Drosdowech DS, King GJ. Comminuted radial head fractures treated with a modular metallic radial head arthroplasty. Study of outcomes. *J Bone Joint Surg Am* 2006;88(10):2192–200.

186. Doornberg JN, Parisien R, van Duijn PJ, Ring D. Radial head arthroplasty with a modular metal spacer to treat acute traumatic elbow instability. *J Bone Joint Surg Am* 2007;89(5):1075–80.

187. van Glabbeck F, van Riet RP, Baumfeld JA, Neale PG, O'Driscoll SW, Morrey BF, et al. Detrimental effects of overstuffing or understuffing with a radial head replacement in the medial collateral-ligament deficient elbow. *J Bone Joint Surg Am* 2004;86-A(12):2629–35.

188. van Riet RP, van Glabbeek F, Verborgt O, Gielen J. Capitellar erosion caused by a metal radial head prosthesis. A case report. *J Bone Joint Surg Am* 2004;86-A(5):1061–4.

189. Rowland AS, Athwal GS, MacDermid JC, King GJ. Lateral ulnohumeral joint space widening is not diagnostic of radial head arthroplasty overstuffing. *J Hand Surg Am* 2007;32(5):637–41.

190. Frank SG, Grewal R, Johnson J, Faber KJ, King GJ, Athwal GS. Determination of correct implant size in radial head arthroplasty to avoid overlengthening. *J Bone Joint Surg Am* 2009;91(7):1738–46.

191. Athwal GS, Rouleau DM, MacDermid JC, King GJ. Contralateral elbow radiographs can reliably diagnose radial head implant overlengthening. *J Bone Joint Surg Am* 2011;93(14):1339–46.

192. Doornberg JN, Linzel DS, Zurakowski D, Ring D. Reference points for radial head prosthesis size. *J Hand Surg Am* 2006;31(1):53–7.

193. Burkhart KJ, Mattyasovszky SG, Runkel M, Schwarz C, Kuchle R, Hessmann MH, et al. Mid- to long-term results after bipolar radial head arthroplasty. *J Shoulder Elbow Surg* 2010;19(7):965–72.

194. van Riet RP, Morrey BF. Delayed valgus instability and proximal migration of the radius after radial head prosthesis failure. *J Shoulder Elbow Surg* 2010;19(7):e7–10.

195. van Riet RP, Sanchez-Sotelo J, Morrey BF. Failure of metal radial head replacement. *J Bone Joint Surg Br* 2010;92(5):661–7.

196. O'Driscoll SW, Herald JA. Forearm pain associated with loose radial head prostheses. *J Shoulder Elbow Surg* 2012;21(1):92–7.

197. Ring D, King G. Radial head arthroplasty with a modular metal spacer to treat acute traumatic elbow instability. Surgical technique. *J Bone Joint Surg Am* 2008;90(Suppl 2; Pt 1):63–73.

198. Harrington IJ, Tountas AA. Replacement of the radial head in the treatment of unstable elbow fractures. *Injury* 1981;12(5):405–12.

199. Knight DJ, Rymaszewski LA, Amis AA, Miller JH. Primary replacement of the fractured radial head with a metal prosthesis. *J Bone Joint Surg Br* 1993;75(4):572–6.

200. Markolf KL, Tejwani SG, O'Neil G, Benhaim P. Load-sharing at the wrist following radial head replacement with a metal implant. A cadaveric study. *J Bone Joint Surg Am* 2004;86-A(5):1023–30.

201. Stuffmann E, Baratz ME. Radial head implant arthroplasty. *J Hand Surg Am* 2009;34(4):745–54.

202. Moungondo F, El Kazzi W, van Riet R, Feipel V, Rooze M, Schuind F. Radiocapitellar joint contacts after bipolar radial head arthroplasty. *J Shoulder Elbow Surg* 2010;19(2):230–5.

203. Moon JG, Berglund LJ, Zachary D, An KN, O'Driscoll SW. Radiocapitellar joint stability with bipolar versus monopolar radial head prostheses. *J Shoulder Elbow Surg* 2009;18(5):779–84.

204. Chanlalit C, Shukla DR, Fitzsimmons JS, Thoreson AR, An KN, O'Driscoll SW. Radiocapitellar stability: The effect of soft tissue integrity on bipolar versus monopolar radial head prostheses. *J Shoulder Elbow Surg* 2011;20(2):219–25.

205. Dotzis A, Cochu G, Mabit C, Charissoux JL, Arnaud JP. Comminuted fractures of the radial head treated by the Judet floating radial head prosthesis. *J Bone Joint Surg Br* 2006;88(6):760–4.

206. Zunkiewicz MR, Clemente JS, Miller MC, Baratz ME, Wysocki RW, Cohen MS. Radial head replacement with a bipolar system: A minimum 2-year follow-up. *J Shoulder Elbow Surg* 2012;21(1):98–104.

207. Smets S, Govaers K, Jansen N, van Riet R, Schaap M, van Glabbeek F. The floating radial head prosthesis for comminuted radial head fractures: A multicentric study. *Acta Orthop Belg* 2000;66(4):353–8.

208. Anakwe RE, Middleton SD, Jenkins PJ, McQueen MM, Court-Brown CM. Patient-reported outcomes after simple dislocation of the elbow. *J Bone Joint Surg Am* 2011;93(13):1220–6.

209. Hindle P, Davidson EK, Biant LC, Court-Brown CM. Appendicular joint dislocations. *Injury* 2013;44(8):1022–7.

210. Stoneback JW, Owens BD, Sykes J, Athwal GS, Pointer L, Wolf JM. Incidence of elbow dislocations in the United States population. *J Bone Joint Surg Am* 2012;94(3):240–5.

211. Yang NP, Chen HC, Phan DV, Yu IL, Lee YH, Chan CL, et al. Epidemiological survey of orthopedic joint dislocations based on nationwide insurance data in Taiwan, 2000–2005. *BMC Musculoskelet Disord* 2011;12:253.

212. Duckworth AD, Ring D, Kulijdian A, McKee MD. Unstable elbow dislocations. *J Shoulder Elbow Surg* 2008;17(2):281–6.

213. Cheung EV, O'Driscoll SW, Morrey BF. Complications of hinged external fixators of the elbow. *J Shoulder Elbow Surg* 2008;17(3):447–53.

214. Schep NW, De Haan J, Iordens GI, Tuinebreijer WE, Bronkhorst MW, De Vries MR, et al. A hinged external fixator for complex elbow dislocations: A multicenter prospective cohort study. *BMC Musculoskelet Disord* 2011;12:130.

215. Maniscalco P, Pizzoli AL, Renzi BL, Caforio M. Hinged external fixation for complex fracture-dislocation of the elbow in elderly people. *Injury* 2014;45(Suppl 6):S53–7.

216. Iordens GI, Den Hartog D, Van Lieshout EM, Tuinebreijer WE, De Haan J, Patka P, et al. Good functional recovery of complex elbow dislocations treated with hinged external fixation: A multicenter prospective study. *Clin Orthop Relat Res* 2015;473(4):1451–61.

25

Radius and ulnar diaphyseal fractures

TAYLOR A. HORST, DAVID C. RING AND JESSE B. JUPITER

INTRODUCTION

Diaphyseal forearm fractures are uncommon in the elderly. Most fractures are treated operatively, especially if both the ulna and the radius are fractured. Stabilization with plates and screws enhances union, provides better alignment, allows immediate functional use of the arm and is safe for most open fractures. In the elderly, a locked plate might be useful when the plate extends into the metaphysis. It is not clear that intramedullary nailing can accurately restore the radial bow and control rotation in comminuted fractures. Bone grafting is not necessary when comminution is bridged and periosteal and muscle attachments are preserved. Complications such as infection, nerve damage, malunion and nonunion from operative treatment are uncommon.

EPIDEMIOLOGY

Diaphyseal fractures of the forearm usually result from an axial load applied to the forearm through the hand.[1] The incidence and prevalence of diaphyseal forearm fractures decrease with age. The average age of an adult with a forearm fracture is 35 years.[2] Court-Brown and Caesar studied a population of over 5900 fractures and noted a prevalence of 24% in individuals over 50 years of age, 13% in those over 65 years of age and 12% in those over 75 years of age.[2] Among various categories of patients grouped by age and sex in patients aged 60 or greater, Singer et al. reported an incidence of forearm diaphyseal fractures ranging from no fractures to 4.3 fractures per 10,000 population per year (Table 25.1).[3]

EVALUATION AND DIAGNOSIS

Diaphyseal fractures of both forearm bones are usually obvious due to the inherent instability created by the injury. Individual fractures of the radius or ulnar may be less obvious. As with any skeletal injury, physical examination should include the entire extremity, paying particular attention to the joints and soft tissues as well as the bone. Look for skin lacerations indicating an open fracture. When only one forearm bone is fractured, evaluate the proximal and distal radioulnar joints. It is also important to check the neurovascular status of the limb by documenting pulses and neurologic function distal to the injury. Examination of the surrounding soft tissues is important not only to rule out concurrent acute issues such as compartment syndrome but also to judge appropriate timing for surgical intervention.

Radiographs are usually sufficient for the evaluation of diaphyseal forearm fractures. Computed tomography (CT) scans may be used on occasion to evaluate radioulnar joint alignment.

ANATOMY AND BIOMECHANICS OF THE FOREARM

The proximal radioulnar joint is stabilized by the annular ligament, while the distal radioulnar joint is stabilized by the triangular fibrocartilage complex (the dorsal and volar radioulnar ligaments in particular), the wrist capsule and the interosseous ligament (perhaps a distal band in particular). These structures have the potential to be damaged with forearm trauma and are at particular risk when only one forearm bone is broken.

Table 25.1 Incidence of diaphyseal forearm fractures per 10,000 population per annum by age and gender

Age (years)	Men	Women
60–64	0.29	1.77
65–69	0.32	0.52
70–74	0.46	3.15
75–79	0.58	0.68
80–84	1.03	1.86
85–89	0.00	4.31
90–94	0.00	1.95

Source: Data from Singer BR, et al. 1998. *J Bone Joint Surg Br* 80(2): 243–248.

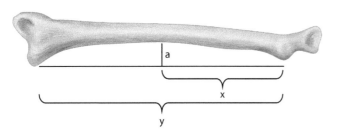

Figure 25.1 Illustration showing measurement of radial bow. Maximal radial bow is located at position 'a'. Location of maximal radial bow is equal to x/y times 100.

The ulna is a relatively straight bone around which the bowed radius rotates. Full pronation and supination depend on the bow of the radius away from the ulna. This bow allows for clearance of the ulna and the forearm muscles (Figure 25.1).[4] The oblique grouping of fibres which connect the two bones is referred to as the interosseous ligament. This broad ligament functions as a longitudinal support of the radius and also prevents separation of the two bones.

Disruption of the bones at particular levels may result in specific deformities due to soft tissue attachments. With proximal third fractures, the biceps and supinator muscles flex and supinate the proximal fragment, while the distal fragment is pronated by the pronator teres and the pronator quadratus. Fractures involving the middle third of the forearm have the supinator, biceps and the pronator muscles maintaining the proximal fragment in a neutral position, while the pronator quadratus pronates the distal fragment. The brachioradialis dorsiflexes and radially deviates the distal segment in distal third fractures while the pronator quadratus, wrist flexors and extensors and thumb abductors can add additional deformities depending on the location of the fracture.[5] Understanding these deforming forces enables the physician to treat fractures amendable to closed treatment with the forearm supinated for proximal third fractures, neutral for middle third fractures and pronated for distal third fractures. This knowledge can also help facilitate open reduction.

PRINCIPLES BEHIND SURGICAL FIXATION

Strain is defined as the change in the length of a fracture gap under a load divided by resting length of the fracture gap, also known as the percentage of a deformation of a material or zone. Primary bone healing occurs when the strain is kept to less than 2%.[6] A strain of 2–10% has been found to be ideal to induce secondary healing through callus formation.[7] Both bone forearm fractures that do not involve comminution can be treated with rigid fixation using compression. This method creates a minimal strain environment allowing direct primary bone healing. For transverse fractures the plate is slightly pre-bent and placed on the tension side of the fracture so that the far cortex compresses first (Figure 25.2).[8] For oblique or spiral fractures, interfragmentary compression screws can be placed outside the plate and then supported with a neutralization plate.

Fragmented forearm fractures are managed with bridge plating, which relies on secondary bone healing (healing by callus) (Figure 25.3). If there is more than a simple butterfly fragment, it is better to not perform precise reduction of each fragment. Rather it is important to preserve the periosteal sleeve and muscle attachments and restore length and alignment. The plate maintains alignment by providing relative stability, and higher strain, leading to healing by callus (Figure 25.4).

Plates with screws that lock to the plate are not usually necessary or helpful for diaphyseal fractures because diaphyseal bone maintains good quality even in the later years. Cadaveric studies looking at plate and screw constructs have found that the length of the plate used is more important than the number of screws used. Sanders et al. found that with four-point mechanical testing, longer plates with two screws in the outermost holes and two screws in the inner most holes were stronger than a six-hole plate with six screws used when tested in medial-lateral and tension band modes.[9] When a fracture is relatively proximal or distal and when important screws for fixation will be in the metaphysis, locked screws can help gain better fixation of osteoporotic bone in the elderly.[6] In these circumstances the locked plates can enhance fracture fixation where fracture configuration or bone quality do not provide sufficient screw purchase to achieve the plate-bone compression necessary to minimize the gap strain with unlocked plate screw constructs (Figure 25.5).[6]

Studies looking at angular malalignment have found that forearm rotation is limited with angulation of the ulnar or radius greater than 20 degrees.[10] Restoration of the normal bow of the radius helps maintain forearm rotation and grip strength. The radial bow is assessed on an anteroposterior (AP) radiograph with the forearm in neutral rotation, the shoulder abducted 90 degrees and the elbow flexed 90 degrees. The bow is quantified by drawing a line from the radial tuberosity to the most ulnar edge of the distal radius. A perpendicular line is then drawn at the point of maximal radial bow with the length of this line then being measured (Figure 25.1).[4] It can be helpful in comminuted

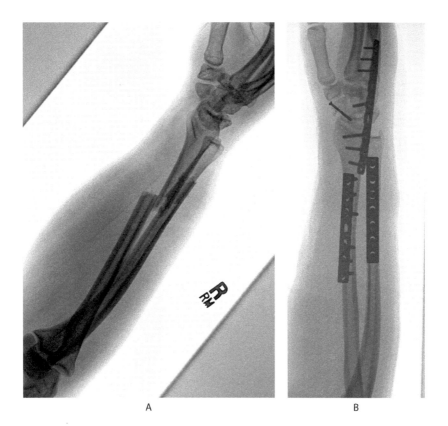

Figure 25.2 (a) Preoperative radiograph depicting transverse fractures of radius and ulna. (b) Postoperative radiographs showing the ideal method for treating transverse fractures with the plate slightly pre-bent and placed on the tension side of the fracture so that the far cortex compresses.

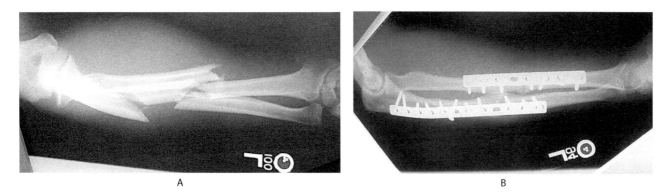

Figure 25.3 (a) Preoperative segmental both bone forearm fracture. (b) Bridge plate technique used to treat segmental both bone forearm fractures. Bridge plating relies on secondary bone healing.

fractures involving both bones to obtain radiographs of the uninjured forearm to help guide surgical treatment of the injured side. Determining the appropriate radial bow is essential to properly stabilizing the fracture for functional use of the extremity.

MANAGEMENT

Initial and nonoperative management

Most diaphyseal forearm fractures in adults are unstable and benefit from splint immobilization for comfort prior to surgery. Because diaphyseal bone fractures and isolated radial shaft fractures are usually unstable there is little role for nonoperative treatment. Regaining length can be difficult, particularly if the patient has a muscular forearm, so surgery should be scheduled within a few days.

Isolated fractures of the ulna with fewer than 10 degrees of angulation and at least 50% apposition can be treated nonoperatively. Nonoperative treatment in a short arm cast or removable brace may be sufficient and it is used essentially to treat the symptoms associated with the injury (Figure 25.6). Sarmiento et al. have demonstrated that even with up to 50% displacement of the

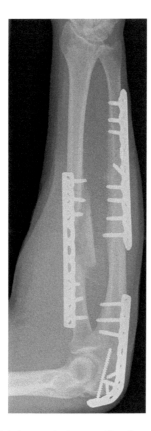

Figure 25.4 Bridging technique utilized to restore length rather than precise segmental fixation.

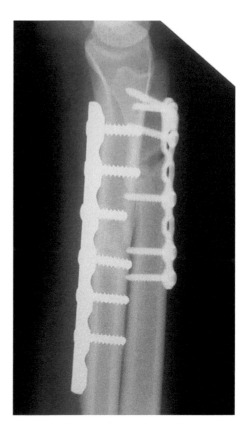

Figure 25.5 Locked plating enhancing fracture fixation due to location of fracture and poor bone quality.

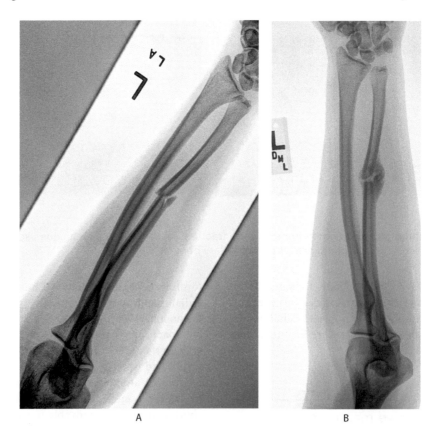

A

B

Figure 25.6 (a) Pretreatment imaging of isolated ulnar shaft fracture. (b) Isolated ulnar shaft fracture after treatment with a removable brace.

shaft, stabilization with a functional fracture brace with a good interosseous mold can maintain alignment and allow healing.[11]

Operative fixation

Regional anesthesia may be a good option for patients with declining health. It can provide anesthesia while avoiding hemodynamic instability and airway instrumentation. It also provides superb and intraoperative and postoperative analgesia.[12] A recent review of the literature covering over 74,000 non-cardiac surgery patients showed regional anesthesia to be associated with reduced early mortality and morbidity.[13] The decision regarding the type of anesthesia should always take into account the overall health of the patient and the goals of surgery. Patients who may be at increased risk for compartment syndrome or neurologic compromise during or following surgery may be better candidates for general anesthesia to more easily monitor acute postoperative neurovascular status.

APPROACHES

The surgical approach to the ulnar shaft is between the extensor carpi ulnaris (ECU) and flexor carpi ulnaris (FCU). The fascial separation of these two muscles is most evident distally. Care should be taken to avoid the dorsal cutaneous branch of the ulnar nerve as it crosses at the level of or just proximal to the ulnar styloid. The periosteum is preserved and the muscle is elevated only from the side of the bone where the plate will lie. Based on the rationale of trying to avoid the interosseous ligament, plate placement on the flexor surface of the ulnar may be ideal.

Henry's approach to the radius in the mid-forearm[14] between the flexor carpi radialis and the brachioradialis is the favored approach to the diaphyseal radius for internal fixation. The superficial radial nerve is kept with the brachioradialis and the radial artery with the flexor carpi radialis. More proximal exposure puts the posterior interosseous nerve at risk. Care should be taken to fully supinate the forearm in order to move the posterior interosseous nerve dorsal and lateral. Follow the biceps tendon down to bone and sweep the supinator off the radius from the biceps laterally. If the anatomy is distorted and uncertain, pronate the forearm, dissect the supinator and find the nerve to be sure it is safe.

Thompson's[15] approach to the radius between the extensor carpi radialis brevis (ECRB) tendon and extensor digitorum communis (EDC) can be used for more proximal fractures in the radius. Proximally, the approach lies between the internervous plane of the ECRB and the EDC. Distally the plane is more obvious between the abductor pollicis longus (APL) and the extensor pollicis brevis (EPB). This approach is used infrequently because of the risk to the posterior interosseous nerve proximally and the crossing of the first dorsal compartment muscles over the plate distally.

Reduction techniques

When both diaphyseal forearm bones are fractured the surgeon is working against all of the finger and wrist motors to realign the fracture. Indirect reduction with an external fixator or using the plate via a push screw are useful techniques to facilitate reduction and limit handling of the bone and damage to the soft tissues (Figure 25.7).

Fixation methods

When the fracture pattern is amenable, standard compression plating technique can be used with a 3.5 mm dynamic compression (DC) plate or limited contact dynamic compression (LCDC) type plate. Screw purchase should engage six cortices above and below the fracture in order to minimize strain.[8] Elderly diaphyseal forearm fractures are more likely to involve osteoporotic bone and locking plates may be useful if the plate extends to the metaphysis.

Other modifications to standard plate and screw fixation such as using fewer screws, near and far screws only, or unicortical screws seem unwise given that plate and screw fixation essentially solved the problem of diaphyseal forearm fractures. These modifications seem risky and meddlesome. A greater number of screws provide more rotational stability and more points of fixation in case a screw loosens or was inadvertently placed in the fracture site.[16]

Intramedullary nailing is periodically attempted for diaphyseal forearm fractures (including isolated fractures of the ulna),[17-20] but to date has not met the standards set by plate and screw fixation. Potential advantages include less soft tissue dissection[21] and decreased blood loss. Disadvantages may include inadequate restoration of the radial bow and inadequate control of rotation, especially for comminuted or segmental fractures. The use of locked nails should be considered experimental[20] and more data and experience are needed before one can say that they are an alternative to the reliable method of plate and screw fixation.[22]

Bone grafting

Anderson et al. used 4.5 mm plates and subperiosteal stripping and recommended application of bone graft in fractures with disruption of more than one third of the cortical circumference.[23] With 3.5 mm plates, preservation of the periosteal and muscle attachments, and greater use of bridge plating for comminution, bone graft is no longer considered helpful. Wright et al. described 101 comminuted forearm fractures that did not receive bone grafting and which went on to achieve a 98% union rate.[24] Likewise, several studies have demonstrated that the union rates of closed diaphyseal comminuted fractures are similar whether or not they are treated with bone grafting.[25-27] While certain fractures may necessitate the use of bone grafting, its use is not required in routine diaphyseal forearm fractures in the elderly.

Bone augmentation may be more applicable in the elderly population with a periprosthetic ulnar fracture around a total

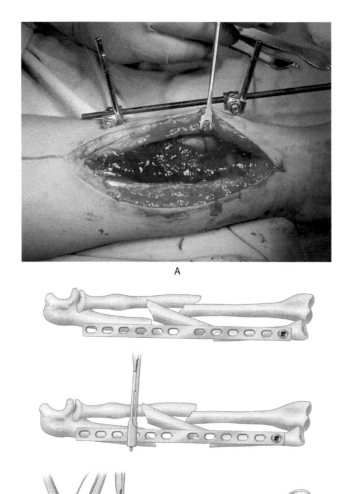

A

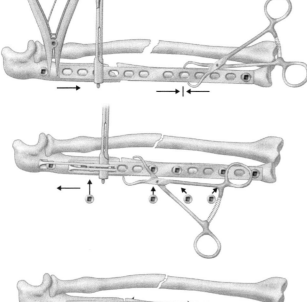

B

Figure 25.7 Two methods that can assist with fracture reduction while minimizing the damage to the bone and surrounding soft tissues. (a) Fracture reduction with an external fixation device. (b) Illustration of the push screw technique.

elbow. In this population the fracture around the component is often due to bone loss from a loose component. Revision of the ulnar component may benefit from additional strut allografts, allograft-prosthetic composites or impaction grafting to augment the deficient bone.[28] A variety of fixation techniques can be utilized, in addition to using a longer ulnar implant to bypass the fracture.

POSTOPERATIVE MANAGEMENT

Initial postoperative splinting may be used for comfort. Elderly patients may be less physically resilient and getting the arm free the day after surgery to assist with self-care is important. For healthy patients without any surrounding soft tissue or skin healing concerns, active, self-assisted elbow, forearm, wrist and hand motion is encouraged immediately.

The long-term symptoms and disability associated with both bone forearm fractures are minimal.[29] Disability has been found to correlate better with subjective and psychosocial aspects of illness, such as pain and pain catastrophizing, than with the objective measurements of impairment recorded by Bot et al.[29] Likewise, Droll et al. reported that after an average of 5 years, arm-specific and general disability correlated with pain rather than with the limited residual impairments and motion and grip strength.[30]

COMPLICATIONS

Many adverse events that are associated with high energy open forearm fractures are uncommon in the elderly. For instance, cross union, or synostosis, between the fractured bones of the forearm is an uncommon complication that is unlikely in low energy injuries in the elderly.[31] Open fractures with high energy trauma, infection, delayed fixation and associated head injury are more commonly associated with synostosis.

Neurovascular injury is uncommon in forearm fractures in the elderly. Most nerve injuries associated with the injury in diaphyseal forearm fractures are associated with a transient neuropraxia from nerve traction or contusion and often recover spontaneously.[32] Iatrogenic surgical complications can occur with injury to the posterior interosseous nerve and superficial radial sensory nerve depending on the approach used for fixation. Identification and protection of these nerves is important.

Deep infections are uncommon,[23,25,29] even with immediate internal fixation of open fractures.[33] Nonunion of diaphyseal forearm fractures is uncommon and when it does occur, is often associated with technical deficiencies in fixation, bone loss and infection (Figure 25.8).[23,25,29]

One of the more likely complications following fixation of diaphyseal forearm fractures may be failure of the hardware bone interface due to poor biology of the bone from osteoporosis or metabolic bone disease like osteomalacia. Revision procedures should take care to utilize fixed angle constructs like locked plating if they were not used initially. If unicortical locked screws were present, bicortical locked

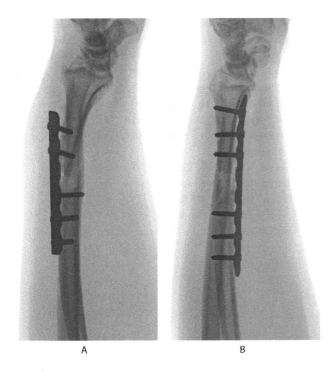

Figure 25.8 **(a)** Nonunion of radial shaft fracture likely due to inadequate fixation. **(b)** Adequate fixation and cancellous bone graft for defects usually achieve union.

screws should be used to decrease the torsional stresses on the bone.[34,35] Augmentation with polymethyl methacrylate or calcium phosphate cement can help create a stronger composite for fixation when bone quality is so poor that modifications to routine techniques still fail to provide stability.[36]

Routine plate removal is unnecessary. A subcutaneous ulnar plate or long screws that irritate tendons might be considered for removal. If a plate is bothersome enough to consider surgery, one should wait 18 months to allow adequate fracture healing and limit the risk of refracture.[37,38]

SUMMARY

Diaphyseal forearm fractures are treated with plate and screw fixation to restore alignment and provide sufficient stability to allow immediate functional use of the arm. In elderly patients, locking plates can be helpful for relatively distal or proximal fractures where the plate will extend into the metaphysis. With good technique and sound fixation, adverse events are uncommon and the elderly patient can regain near normal function of the upper extremity.

REFERENCES

1. Means, K. & Graham, T. 2010. Disorders of the forearm axis. In: *Green's Operative Hand Surgery*, 6th ed., edited by Wolfe, S.W., Pederson, W. C., Hotchkiss, R. N. & Kozin, S. H. Philadelphia, PA: Elsevier, pp. 837–868.

2. Court-Brown, C. M. & Caesar, B. 2006. Epidemiology of adult fractures: A review. *Injury* 37: 691–697.

3. Singer, B., Mclauchlan, G., Robinson, C. & Christie, J. 1998. Epidemiology of fractures in 15 000 adults. The influence of age and gender. *J Bone Jt Surg Br* 80: 243–248.

4. Schemitsch, E. H. & Richards, R. R. 1992. The effect of malunion on functional outcome after plate fixation of fractures of both bones of the forearm in adults. *J Bone Joint Surg Am* 74(7): 1068–1078.

5. Cruess, R. 1973. Importance of soft tissue evaluation in both hand and wrist trauma: Statistical evaluation. *Orthop Clin North Am* 4: 969.

6. Egol, K. A., Kubiak, E. N., Fulkerson, E., Kummer, F. J. & Koval, K. J. 2004. Biomechanics of locked plates and screws. *J Orthop Trauma* 18: 488–493.

7. Perren, S. M. 2002. Evolution of the internal fixation of long bone fractures: The scientific basis of biological internal fixation: Choosing a new balance between stability and biology. *J Bone Jt Surg Br* 84-B: 1093–1110.

8. Ruedi, T. P. & Murphy, W. M. (eds.) 2000. *AO Principles of Fracture Management*. Stuttgart: Thieme.

9. Sanders, R., Haidukewych, G. J., Milne, T., Dennis, J. & Latta, L. L. 2002. Minimal versus maximal plate fixation techniques of the ulna: The biomechanical effect of number of screws and plate length. *J Orthop Trauma* 16: 166–171.

10. Matthews, L. S., Kaufer, H., Garver, D. F. & Sonstegard, D. A. 1982. The effect on supination-pronation of angular malalignment of fractures of both bones of the forearm. *J Bone Joint Surg Am* 64(1): 14–17.

11. Sarmiento, A., Cooper, J. S. & Sinclair, W. F. 1975. Forearm fractures. Early functional bracing—A preliminary report. *J Bone Joint Surg Am* 57: 297–304.

12. Mirza, F. & Brown, A. R. 2011. Ultrasound-guided regional anesthesia for procedures of the upper extremity. *Anesthesiol Res Pract* 2011: 579824.

13. Luger, T. J., Kammerlander, C., Luger, M. F., Kammerlander-Knauer, U. & Gosch, M. 2014. Mode of anesthesia, mortality and outcome in geriatric patients. *Z Gerontol Geriatr* 47: 110–124.

14. Henry, A. 1970. *Extensile Exposures*. Baltimore, MD: Williams & Wilkins.

15. Thompson, J. 1918. Anatomical methods of approach in operations on the long bones of the extremities. *Ann Surg* 68: 309–329.

16. Lindvall, E. M. & Sagi, H. C. 2006. Selective screw placement in forearm compression plating: Results of 75 consecutive fractures stabilized with 4 cortices of screw fixation on either side of the fracture. *J Orthop Trauma* 20: 157–162.

17. Gao, H., Luo, C. F., Zhang, C. Q., Shi, H. P., Fan, C. Y. & Zen, B. F. 2005. Internal fixation of diaphyseal fractures of the forearm by interlocking intramedullary nail: Short-term results in eighteen patients. *J Orthop Trauma* 19: 384–391.

18. Hong, G., Cong-Feng, L., Hui-Peng, S., Cun-Yi, F. & Bing-Fang, Z. 2006. Treatment of diaphyseal forearm nonunions with interlocking intramedullary nails. *Clin Orthop Relat Res* 450: 186–192.

19. Kose, A., Aydin, A., Ezirmik, N., Can, C. E., Topal, M. & Tipi, T. 2014. Alternative treatment of forearm double fractures: New design intramedullary nail. *Arch Orthop Trauma Surg* 134: 1387–1396.

20. Saka, G., Saglam, N., Kurtulmus, T., Avci, C. C., Akpinar, F., Kovaci, H. & Celik, A. 2014. New interlocking intramedullary radius and ulna nails for treating forearm diaphyseal fractures in adults: A retrospective study. *Injury* 45(Suppl 1): S16–S23.

21. Street, D. M. 1986. Intramedullary forearm nailing. *Clin Orthop Relat Res* 212: 219–230.

22. Ozkaya, U., Kilic, A., Ozdogan, U., Beng, K. & Kabukcuoglu, Y. 2009. Comparison between locked intramedullary nailing and plate osteosynthesis in the management of adult forearm fractures. *Acta Orthop Traumatol Turc* 43: 14–20.

23. Anderson, L. D. 1975. Compression-plate fixation in acute diaphyseal fractures. *J Bone Joint Surg Am* 57: 287.

24. Wright, R. R., Schmeling, G. J. & Schwab, J. P. 1997. The necessity of acute bone grafting in diaphyseal forearm fractures: A retrospective review. *J Orthop Trauma* 11: 288–294.

25. Chapman, M., Gordon, J. & Zissimos, A. 1989. Compression-plate fixation of acute fractures of the diaphyses of the radius and ulna. *J Bone Joint Surg Am* 71: 159–169.

26. Wei, S. Y., Born, C. T., Abene, A., Ong, A., Hayda, R. & Delong, W. G., Jr. 1999. Diaphyseal forearm fractures treated with and without bone graft. *J Trauma* 46: 1045–1048.

27. Ring, D., Rhim, R., Carpenter, C. & Jupiter, J. B. 2005. Comminuted diaphyseal fractures of the radius and ulna: Does bone grafting affect nonunion rate? *J Trauma Acute Care Surg* 59: 436–440.

28. Foruria, A. M., Sanchez-Sotelo, J., Oh, L. S., Adams, R. A. & Morrey, B. F. 2011. The surgical treatment of periprosthetic elbow fractures around the ulnar stem following semiconstrained total elbow arthroplasty. *J Bone Joint Surg Am* 93: 1399–1407.

29. Bot, A. G. J., Doornberg, J. N., Lindenhovius, A. L. C., Ring, D., Goslings, J. C. & Van Dijk, C. N. 2011. Long-term outcomes of fractures of both bones of the forearm. *J Bone Joint Surg Am* 93A: 527–532.

30. Droll, K. P., Perna, P., Potter, J., Harniman, E., Schemitsch, E. H. & Mckee, M. D. 2007. Outcomes following plate fixation of fractures of both bones of the forearm in adults. *J Bone Joint Surg Am* 89: 2619–2624.

31. Vince, K. G. & Miller, J. 1987. Cross-union complicating fracture of the forearm. *J Bone Joint Surg Am* 69: 640–653.

32. Seigel, D. & Gelberman, R. 1991. Peripheral nerve injuries associated with fractures and dislocations. In: *Operative Nerve Repair and Reconstruction*, edited by Gelberman, R. Philadelphia, PA: J.B. Lippincott, p. 619.

33. Jones, J. A. 1991. Immediate internal fixation of high-energy open forearm fractures. *J Orthop Trauma* 5: 272–279.

34. Fulkerson, E., Egol, K. A., Kubiak, E. N., Liporace, F., Kummer, F. J. & Koval, K. J. 2006. Fixation of diaphyseal fractures with a segmental defect: A biomechanical comparison of locked and conventional plating techniques. *J Trauma* 60: 830–835.

35. Roberts, J. W., Grindel, S. I., Rebholz, B. & Wang, M. 2007. Biomechanical evaluation of locking plate radial shaft fixation: Unicortical locking fixation versus mixed bicortical and unicortical fixation in a sawbone model. *J Hand Surg* 32: 971–975.

36. Collinge, C., Merk, B. & Lautenschlager, E. P. 2007. Mechanical evaluation of fracture fixation augmented with tricalcium phosphate bone cement in a porous osteoporotic cancellous bone model. *J Orthop Trauma* 21: 124–128.

37. Hidaka, S. & Gustilo, R. B. 1984. Refracture of bones of the forearm after plate removal. *J Bone Jt Surg* 66: 1241–1243.

38. Deluca, P., Lindsey, R. & Ruwe, P. 1988. Refracture of bones of the forearm after the removal of compression plates. *J Bone Jt Surg* 70: 1372–1376.

26

Distal radius and ulnar fractures

MARGARET M. McQUEEN

INTRODUCTION

Fracture of the distal radius is the most common fracture encountered by orthopaedic trauma surgeons. There are around 120,000 fractures per year in the United Kingdom and 607,000 annually in the United States[1,2] with a peak in incidence in the older patient, particularly in females. Recently there has been more interest in the outcome of treatment in the older patient as awareness of the possible impact on the patient's independence has increased. Although Abraham Colles is famously associated with stating that if a distal radius fracture malunited it would 'at some remote period again enjoy perfect freedom in all its motions, and be completely exempt from pain', in the same publication he also stated that if a fracture was allowed to malunite 'the patient is doomed to endure for many months considerable lameness and stiffness of the limb, accompanied by severe pain on attempting to bend the hand and fingers'. He clearly appreciated the possible impact of a poorly treated fracture on function. Correction of the displacement in a distal radius fracture is aimed at improving the ability of the patient to complete tasks requiring some strength in the hand and wrist which may have little impact on the functional ability of the frail elderly patient. Careful judgement must be employed in making treatment decisions in these cases. This chapter aims to inform the orthopaedic trauma surgeon making treatment decisions in the older patient.

CLASSIFICATION

Before deciding the appropriate management for an elderly patient with a distal radius fracture it is important to understand the range of fracture types which can occur.

Many classification systems have been proposed for fractures of the distal radius and ulna over the years, the majority of which are morphological and consider in varying degrees the presence or absence of displacement, comminution and articular involvement. The simplest and probably clinically most used is differentiation between intra- and extra-articular fractures and the presence or absence of comminution. For research purposes the most commonly used is the AO/OTA classification system.

The AO/OTA system (Figure 26.1) is an alphanumeric classification and has 27 different subgroups. Three different types (A, extra-articular; B, partial articular; C, complete articular) are divided into nine main groups and 27 different subtypes depending on comminution and direction of displacement. The system is not used frequently in clinical practice because of its complexity but is commonly used for research purposes.

Although classification systems are widely used for distal radius fractures, their reliability has not been established. At best inter- or intraobserver reliability has been demonstrated for the AO/OTA system[3] when only type A, B or C is considered. Undue reliance should not be placed on classification systems especially when considering treatment and prognosis. For research purposes it is preferable to classify distal radius fractures by consensus amongst authors.

EPIDEMIOLOGY

Fracture of the distal radius is the most common fracture encountered by the orthopaedic trauma surgeon. It accounts for around 17.5% of all fractures and recent reports of its annual incidence range from 20.6 to 27 per 100,000/year.[4-7] In all studies, the incidence in females is

A = Extra-articular fracture   B = Partial-articular fracture   C = Complete-articular fracture

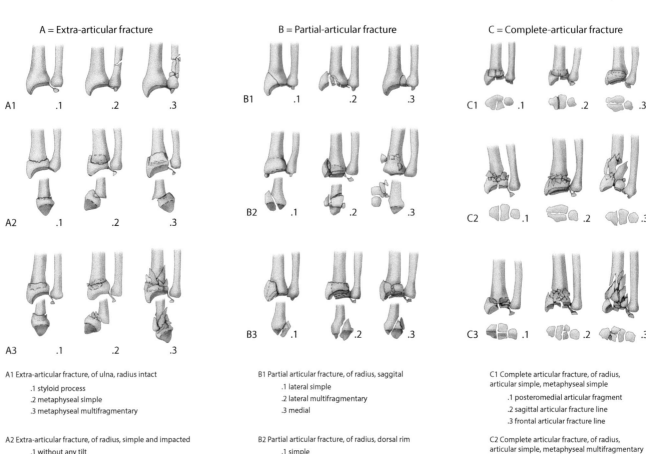

A1   .1   .2   .3   B1   .1   .2   .3   C1   .1   .2   .3

A2   .1   .2   .3   B2   .1   .2   .3   C2   .1   .2   .3

A3   .1   .2   .3   B3   .1   .2   .3   C3   .1   .2   .3

A1 Extra-articular fracture, of ulna, radius intact

   .1 styloid process

   .2 metaphyseal simple

   .3 metaphyseal multifragmentary

A2 Extra-articular fracture, of radius, simple and impacted

   .1 without any tilt

   .2 with dorsal tilt (Pouteau-Colles)

   .3 with volar tilt (Goyrand-Smith)

A3 Extra-articular fracture, of radius, multifragmentary

   .1 impacted with axial shortening

   .2 with a wedge

   .3 complex

B1 Partial articular fracture, of radius, saggital

   .1 lateral simple

   .2 lateral multifragmentary

   .3 medial

B2 Partial articular fracture, of radius, dorsal rim

   .1 simple

   .2 with lateral sagittal fracture

   .3 with dorsal dislocation of the carpus

B3 Partial articular fracture, of radius, volar rim

   .1 simple, with a small fragment

   .2 simple, with a large fragment

   .3 multifragmentary

C1 Complete articular fracture, of radius, articular simple, metaphyseal simple

   .1 posteromedial articular fragment

   .2 sagittal articular fracture line

   .3 frontal articular fracture line

C2 Complete articular fracture, of radius, articular simple, metaphyseal multifragmentary

   .1 sagittal articular fracture line

   .2 frontal articular fracture line

   .3 extending into diaphysis

C3 Complete articular fracture, of radius, multifragmentary

   .1 metaphyseal simple

   .2 metaphyseal multifragmentary

   .3 extending into diaphysis

Figure 26.1 The AO/OTA classification of fractures of the distal radius.

higher than in males by a factor of two to three with a type A age/gender distribution.[8]

There are no publications specifically detailing the epidemiology of distal radius fractures in the elderly. In Edinburgh a study of all distal radius fractures presenting in a 1-year period between July 2007 and June 2008 was undertaken. A total of 1124 fractures were identified, 508 (45%) of which were in patients aged 65 years or over. Of these 508 patients, 441 (86.8%) were female and 67 (13.2%) were male. The median age was 77 years, ranging from 65 years to 98 years. The median age was 78 years for females and 75 years for men. The annual age- and gender-related incidence is shown in Figure 26.2 and demonstrates an increasing incidence for women with age peaking at 125/10,000 of the population in the 85–89-year-old age group. The incidence is much lower for men and shows a modest peak at the same age of 33.7/10,000 of the population.

These figures are consistent with other data.[7,9] One of these studies also showed a rising incidence of distal radius fractures in older patients over a 19-year period. Data from Edinburgh show an increase in the incidence of distal radius fractures over a 17-year period, mainly attributable to an increase in incidence in both younger and older men and in women over 75 years of age. It is of interest, however, that the percentage of patients who were independent for the activities of daily living increased significantly over the period, confirming that although getting older, individuals were also getting fitter.[5]

Of the 508 fractures, 448 (88%) were caused by a fall from standing height, while 28 were caused by higher energy injury, with small numbers of other causes. Extra-articular fractures (OTA/AO type A) accounted for 62%, complete intra-articular fractures (type C) for 23.8% and partial articular fractures (type B) for 14.2% of the total. Overall, 70% of fractures had metaphyseal comminution and 68% were displaced at presentation. Although the vast majority of fractures in older patients occur in lower energy injury, they have a high prevalence of comminuted, displaced fractures. Along with the evidence of increasing incidence in

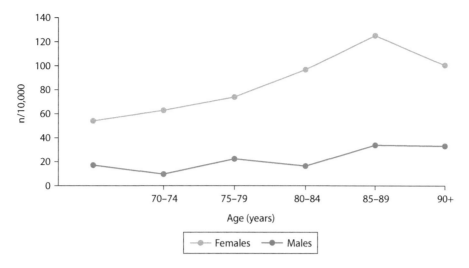

Figure 26.2 The annual age and gender related incidence of distal radius fractures in patients aged 65 years or over.

older patients, this suggests that there will be an increasing burden on orthopaedic trauma services in the years to come.

RISK FACTORS

Reported lifetime risks of distal radius fractures from the age of 50 onwards range from 12% to 52.7% for women[10,11] and from 2.4% to 6.2% for men.[10,12] The wide range, particularly in women, may be real but could also be a result of differences in the methods of ascertainment of the fractures.

Low bone mineral density (BMD) is an important predictor of future fracture risk but there is also evidence that increasing falls, especially with aging, are a significant risk factor.[13,14] The risk of distal radius fracture increases with the higher the level of activity[15] implying that individuals who sustain distal radius fractures are in the fitter cohort of older people.

ASSESSMENT

Assessment of a patient with a distal radius fractures is particularly important in the elderly patient as treatment decisions are often complex and have to consider many factors. These include assessment of the clinical and radiological aspects of the fracture and of the patient's general state of fitness. The latter may require multidisciplinary input from care of the elderly physicians and anaesthetic staff (see Chapters 3 and 4)

Clinical assessment of the fracture

The history of injury is usually straightforward with the patient or carers reporting a fall onto the outstretched hand or occasionally a higher energy injury. Pain and swelling around the wrist are invariable features and where there is displacement a deformity can be seen. Specific questioning should exclude any median or ulnar nerve injury and the

presence of pain elsewhere in the arm which may indicate an ipsilateral injury.

Radiological assessment

Posteroanterior (PA), lateral and oblique X-ray views are required and there is usually little doubt about the diagnosis.
PA views allow assessment of:

- Radial length/ulnar variance (Figure 26.3b)
- Extent of metaphyseal comminution
- Ulnar styloid fracture location (tip/waist/base)
- Presence, orientation and displacement of articular fractures.

Lateral views allow assessment of:

- Dorsal/palmar tilt (Figure 26.3a)
- Extent of metaphyseal comminution
- Carpal alignment (Figure 26.3c)
- Displacement of the volar cortex
- Position of the distal radioulnar joint (DRUJ)
- Presence, orientation and displacement of articular fractures.

It is important to appreciate that significant discrepancy regarding intra- and interobserver reliability has been demonstrated in the measurement of standard radiographic criteria. For extra-articular fractures the mean standard deviation between surgeons was 3.2 degrees for radial angle, 3.6 degrees for conventional lateral palmar tilt and 2.1 degrees for 15 degrees of lateral palmar tilt.[16]

Assessment of outcome

Outcome measures for distal radius fracture may use either a combination of objective and subjective factors including pain, range of motion, grip strength, ability to undertake the activities of daily living and radiological measurements

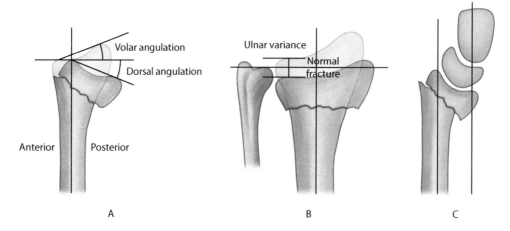

Figure 26.3 (a) A lateral diagram of the distal radius showing measurement of dorsal and volar angulation. **(b)** A diagrammatic representation of a posteroanterior (PA) view showing measurement of ulnar variance. **(c)** Assessment of carpal alignment. The perpendicular line down the radius does not intersect within the area of the carpus with a perpendicular line drawn along the long axis of the capitate indicating carpal malalignment.

or patient related outcome measurements (PROMS). The most frequently used physician based scores for distal radius fractures are the Mayo wrist score,[17] the Gartland and Werley score[18] and the Green and O'Brien[19] score. None have been examined to determine their reliability, responsiveness or validity and although these measurements are theoretically objective the effort applied can be influenced by the patient's psychological state.[20]

There have been a number of PROMS developed ranging from generic measures assessing the impact of injury on the patient's health and well-being (e.g. Short Form 36 [SF36], Sickness Impact Profile [SIP]) to more specific measures of outcome focused on the wrist itself. The latter include the Disability of Arm, Shoulder and Hand (DASH) score which is a 30 item disability/symptom score from zero (no disability) to 100 (severe disability). The normal DASH score is less than 15. The Patient Related Wrist Evaluation (PRWE) is also in frequent use and is specific to the wrist rather than the whole upper extremity.

TREATMENT

The main treatment options for fracture of the distal radius in the elderly are non-operative management, external fixation or internal fixation using either closed reduction (CRIF) or open reduction (ORIF). The decision as to which to use in the elderly is based on the demands which the individual places on their hand and wrist, the mental and physical state of the patient and the type of fracture. To allow an informed decision it is useful to be able to predict the likely outcome of treatment.

Prediction of instability

As many distal radius fractures are treated non-operatively in the elderly it is important to be able to predict the radiological outcome of such treatment. If operative treatment is

being considered then a knowledge of the likely radiological outcome will also inform that decision.

Several factors have been associated with redisplacement following closed manipulation of a distal radius fracture.

AGE

Increasing age results in increasing metaphyseal instability of a distal radius fracture. Patients over 80 years of age with a displaced fracture of the distal radius are three times more likely to have instability than those under 30 years of age. This is even more striking in patients with minimally or undisplaced fractures when the risk of instability increases tenfold in older patients.[21] It is important to be vigilant for later redisplacement in fractures in elderly patients with osteopenic bones.

INITIAL FRACTURE DISPLACEMENT

The greater the degree of initial displacement (particularly radial shortening), the more energy has been imparted to the fracture resulting in a higher likelihood that closed treatment will be unsuccessful.[21]

METAPHYSEAL COMMINUTION

The presence of a metaphyseal defect or comminution as evidenced by either plain radiographs or computerized tomography increases the chance of instability.[21,22]

DISPLACEMENT FOLLOWING CLOSED TREATMENT

Displacement following closed treatment is a predictor of instability as repeat manipulation is unlikely to result in a successful radiographic outcome.[23,24]

In a study of the natural history of over 3500 distal radius fractures, Mackenney and his co-authors[21] reported the independently significant predictors of early instability (redisplacement before 2 weeks), late instability (redisplacement between 2 weeks and fracture union) and malunion for both undisplaced and displaced fractures. Mathematical formulae were constructed to give a percentage chance of redisplacement or malunion for individual patients. The authors gave an example of an independent 85-year-old woman with a dorsally displaced fracture of the distal radius with metaphyseal comminution and a positive ulnar variance of 2 mm. The calculated probability of malunion is 82%. Clinical application of these formulae is likely to allow informed decision-making when considering the appropriate treatment for an elderly patient, encourage early treatment in appropriate cases and reduce the prevalence of malunion.

Prediction of function

The aim of treatment of a distal radius fracture is to restore normal function of the wrist and hand and it is critical that treatment has a realistic chance of achieving that goal. There are many influences on function, including age, psychological state and anatomical position, and it is important to achieve a balance between them to achieve the maximum possible function. With increasing age as demands upon the wrist become less, the symptoms from a malunion are likely to reduce and the importance of normal anatomy declines.

There is as yet no consensus on how patients should be treated as the definition of an elderly patient is not clear. Physiological and actual age may vary greatly but the surgeon usually makes a judgement on a subjective impression. The use of more objective measures available in the geriatric and epidemiological literature such as the Physical Activity Scale of the Elderly (PASE) score may be of value.

Lessening demands may account for reports of malunion of the distal radius in older people being compatible with good function. In 74 older patients with distal radius fractures treated non-operatively, 71% had at least one unacceptable radiographic deformity but at review 6 months after fracture the authors reported that self-reported disability was low and patient satisfaction high despite a mean DASH score of 24 and a patient dissatisfaction rate of 28%. Mean DASH scores were higher if the radiological deformity was outside the acceptable range but this was not statistically significant.[25] In another study, 25 low demand patients over 60 years of age were treated non-operatively. Overall, 32% of patients had fair or poor radiographic results but only 12% had fair or poor functional outcomes. The authors concluded that non-operative treatment yields satisfactory results in low demand patients.[26] No relationship between anatomy and function was found in a group of 74 older patients with conservatively managed distal radius fractures 6 months after injury although only 59% of patients were satisfied with the outcome.[27] Grewal and MacDermid found that the relative risk of a poor outcome with malalignment of the distal radius showed a decreasing trend with increasing age.[28] Functional outcome in malunited fractures in the super-elderly (defined as those aged 80 years or over) was compared with a similar group without malunion. No differences in functional outcome were found, even in those living independently.[29]

In contrast to these studies, Brogren and her co-authors[30] examined 143 patients 1 year after distal radius fracture and classified them into three groups: no malunion, single malunion (either dorsal tilt of 10 degrees or positive ulnar variance) and combined malunion (both dorsal tilt of 10 degrees and positive ulnar variance). The average age was 65 years, younger than that in some of the previously quoted studies. With regression analysis the relative risk of higher disability was 2.5 with single malunion and 3.7 with a combined malunion. There was no difference in these results when adjusted for age or gender. The authors concluded that malunion with a dorsal angle greater than 10 degrees or a positive ulnar variance leads to higher arm related disability after distal radius fracture, regardless of age or gender.

The individual measures of anatomical reduction have also been examined in an attempt to clarify which are important in restoring function. Correction of ulnar variance appears to be important in restoration of grip strength and DRUJ function.[23,30,31] Loss of the normal palmar tilt may also have a deleterious effect on function causing worsening incongruence of the DRUJ, increased tightness of the interosseous membrane and limited rotation. In addition, loss of the normal palmar tilt positions the carpus in a dorsal collapse alignment. A number of studies have implicated residual dorsal tilt in poorer grip strength and DRUJ function.[30,32] Resultant carpal malalignment (Figure 26.4) has been implicated as the strongest negative influence on function and prognosis.[23,33,34]

Articular damage may be influenced by the initial insult to the articular cartilage and the effects of residual

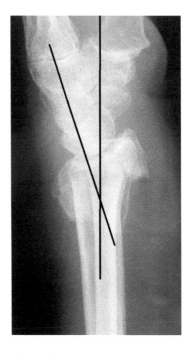

Figure 26.4 A lateral view of a distal radius fracture. Perpendicular lines down the long axes of the radius and the capitate do not intersect within the area of the carpus. The carpus is therefore malaligned.

incongruity and its end result is degenerative change. The relationship between the three and their influence on function remains uncertain, especially in the older patient. This is illustrated by the difficulty in demonstrating consistent relationships between articular incongruity, osteoarthrosis and significant functional compromise. In 1986 Knirk and Jupiter correlated patient outcome with residual intra-articular incongruity. They found a 91% prevalence of radiographically apparent arthrosis with any measurable intra-articular step-off and a 100% prevalence with over 2 mm of articular step-off. However, only one patient with bilateral fractures had to stop working as a direct result of the injuries and 61% reported an excellent or good outcome.[35] Long-term reviews of younger patients have failed to show a significant relationship between radiological degenerative change and functional outcome[36] so it is unlikely that residual articular malalignment will have a significant impact on function for the older patient.

In treatment of the elderly patient where biological and chronological age may vary significantly, it is difficult to know whether age, level of comorbidity and pre-injury function or a combination of those is the most important factor in deciding whether there will be benefit in correcting the anatomical position. At present we cannot predict the outcome of a distal radius fracture with any degree of confidence but can only recommend levels of displacement which can be accepted in the fit, active and fully functioning patient regardless of age (Table 26.1). These should not be applied to the frail elderly patient when it may be preferable to accept a malunion. These levels are more stringent than those recommended by the American Academy of Orthopedic Surgeons (AAOS) as the AAOS publication does not consider the effect of carpal malalignment. If the carpus is malaligned and the dorsal tilt is beyond neutral then correction should be undertaken. Some dorsal tilt can be accepted if the carpus is aligned.[37] Palmar tilt can be accepted provided the carpus is aligned.

Non-operative treatment

Non-operative treatment remains the most common treatment method for fractures of the distal radius and consists of plaster or splint management with or without closed reduction. Rates of non-operative treatment are probably around 70%[38] in the UK and vary from 60% to 96% with geographic location in the United States.[1,39] Rates of

non-operative treatment have been shown to increase with increasing age and comorbidities.[39,40] Non-operative treatment is also less likely to be employed by hand surgeons compared to orthopaedic trauma surgeons.[1,40]

Trends in the use of non-operative treatment of distal radius fractures have changed over the years. In the 1950s just over 95% of distal radius fractures were treated non-operatively in the United States[41] in comparison to as few as 60% in some areas of the United States in this millennium.[39] Recent evidence shows an increase from 3% to 16% in the use of ORIF and an accompanying decrease from 82% to 70% in non-operative management in the elderly since 2000,[1] a change attributed to the introduction of locking plates despite a lack of evidence showing clear benefit.

INDICATIONS FOR NON-OPERATIVE TREATMENT

Non-operative treatment is indicated for undisplaced stable fractures or displaced fractures which are stable after reduction. Stability after reduction may be assessed by observation over time or by predictive algorithms.[21]

Manipulative reduction is indicated where the radiological position falls outside acceptable limits (Table 26.1) and non-operative treatment is predicted to be successful, that is, if the fracture is likely to be stable. It is also used when there is an impending complication which may be averted by early reduction even if further treatment may be necessary. In some situations manipulative treatment is not necessary. These include fracture with a high risk of instability where more definitive primary treatment should be used. Manipulative reduction should not be used where the fracture is displaced and unstable but the patient is not considered suitable for surgical treatment, for example in a low demand or very elderly patient. In a series of 59 low demand patient who had undergone manipulative reduction and who had a mean age of 82 years, 53 patients ultimately had a malunion. The authors concluded that primary reduction was ineffective in elderly frail patients and recommend that it should only be performed where there is a specific indication such as median nerve symptoms.[42]

TECHNIQUE OF MANIPULATIVE REDUCTION

Reduction of a displaced distal radius fracture requires adequate analgesia or pain relief, which can be achieved by haematoma block, regional or general anaesthesia or intravenous sedation although the latter two should be avoided if possible in the elderly. In a number of comparative studies

Table 26.1 The radiological limits beyond which reduction is advised

Radiological measurement	Recommended limits
Positive ulnar variance (mm)	2–3
Carpal malalignment	None
Dorsal tilt	Neutral if carpus malaligned <10° if carpus aligned
Palmar tilt	No limit if carpus aligned
Gap or step in joint (mm)	2

there is a consensus that Bier's block is a safe, effective and practical procedure and superior to haematoma block.[43,44]

Reduction of distal radius fractures is usually straightforward, with longitudinal traction disengaging the fracture and direct pressure or wrist flexion restoring volar tilt. Care must be taken in the elderly as excessive traction may produce shearing of the skin. Excessive wrist flexion, the Cotton-Loder position, should be avoided as it increases carpal tunnel pressures and therefore the risk of acute carpal tunnel syndrome (CTS).

CAST IMMOBILIZATION

Once the reduction manoeuvres have been performed, a plaster cast is applied. There are a number of controversies around the use of plaster casts including the type of cast, the use of bracing, the position of immobilization and the length of time required in cast.

Type of cast

The initial cast is usually a back slab or sugar tong splint which is completed when swelling has reduced. It is important to allow free finger movement within a cast by ensuring that the cast ends proximal to the metacarpophalangeal joints.

Although it has been suggested that holding the forearm in supination prevents redisplacement from the deforming force of brachioradialis, randomized studies have shown no benefit of above elbow immobilization compared to forearm casts in maintaining the fracture reduction[45,46] with some showing a disadvantage because of long-term rotational contracture with above elbow casts.[47] No advantage has been demonstrated by the use of braces rather than casts.

Position of immobilization

Extreme positions of the wrist should be avoided. Slight flexion and ulnar deviation is commonly used but neutral or even dorsiflexed positions do not seem to affect the final radiological position. It is likely that fracture and patient factors rather than the wrist position determine the stability of a distal radius fracture.[21]

Length of time in cast

Undisplaced fractures need a very limited or no immobilization time with some evidence that functional recovery is faster than when conventional cast immobilization is used.[48] If immobilization is used, removable wrist splints may be more acceptable to the older patient than a cast. In displaced fractures, which have required manipulative reduction, the accepted length of time in a cast is 5–6 weeks. However in a randomized controlled trial (RCT), no significant anatomical differences but less pain was reported in patients over 60 years of age whose casts were retained for 3 rather than 5 weeks.[49]

Radiological and clinical review following fracture reduction should be undertaken at regular intervals. All fractures should be reviewed at 1 week as even minimally displaced fractures which have not required initial reduction may displace (Figure 26.5). Instability more than 2 weeks after reduction has been reported in almost half of cases[21] indicating that fracture review should also be undertaken at 2 and 3 weeks after injury.

OUTCOME OF NON-OPERATIVE MANAGEMENT

The majority of reports of outcomes after non-operative treatment are in cohorts of older patients. In a review of the outcome of non-operative management in 66 patients, Foldhazy and his co-authors reported a high rate of radiological deformity with a mean dorsal angle of 13 degrees in patients less than 60 years of age and 18 degrees in the older patients at 9–13 years after injury. Overall, 52 cases were rated as excellent or good according to the modified Green and O'Brien score. The authors noted a slower recovery in older patients and concluded that some patients with non-operatively treated distal radius fractures still experience some impairment a decade after injury.[50] In other reports concentrating on older patients significant numbers of malunited fractures are found.[25–27,51] Function does not return to normal with mean DASH scores of 15.7 to 24[25,51,52] and patient satisfaction ranging from 59% to 92%.[25,27,51]

Operative treatment

The decision to treat the elderly patient with surgery is a complex one and should be based primarily on the functional ability of the patient pre-injury and the requirements after surgery. The main effect of correcting the anatomical position of the distal radius is to restore the ability to perform the activities of daily living which require strength and endurance. It therefore follows that if the individual no longer requires to perform these activities then surgery will not improve their quality of life. The discussion on operative treatment in this chapter assumes that the patient is active and performing these activities.

There are a number of methods of operative treatment available for distal radius fractures including closed reduction and percutaneous pinning, ORIF, different types of external fixation or combinations of each type of treatment. Once the decision is made that a patient is a suitable candidate for surgery the choice of the treatment type should be guided by the fracture type and the relative outcomes of the treatment methods.

Around 60% of distal radius fractures are extra-articular and almost one-half are likely to have metaphyseal instability. One-third are articular fractures but fewer than 5% are complex articular fractures. A small proportion are volar displaced fractures including volar shearing fractures. For the purposes of making decisions about surgical treatment, four groups should be considered: metaphyseal unstable, extra or minimal articular fractures, displaced articular fractures and volar displaced fractures.

METAPHYSEAL UNSTABLE, EXTRA OR MINIMAL ARTICULAR FRACTURES

These are the most common fractures requiring surgical treatment in the older patient. Metaphyseal instability

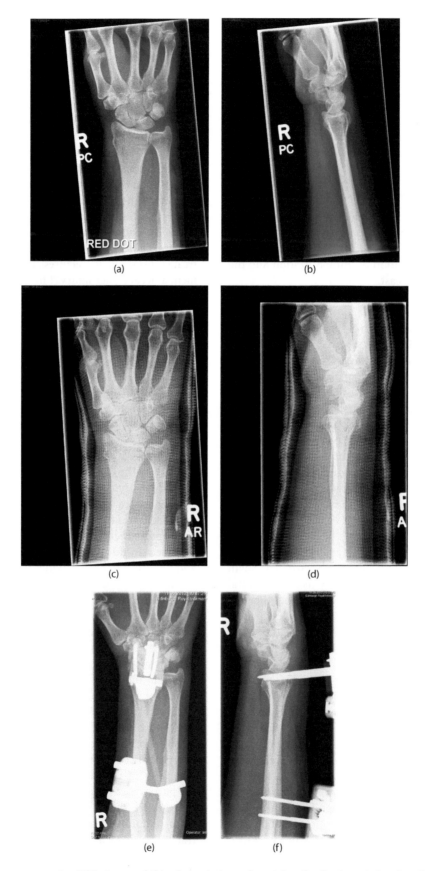

Figure 26.5 (a) An anteroposterior (AP) view and (b) a lateral view of a minimally displaced distal radius fracture in a fit 72-year-old woman. There is loss of the normal volar tilt but no dorsal angulation and the carpus is aligned. (c,d) The fracture was treated in a cast without manipulation. At 1 week after injury the fracture has collapsed into dorsal angulation with a malaligned carpus. (e,f) The fracture has been rereduced and held with a non-bridging external fixator.

may be predicted or actual. A minimal articular fracture is one which has an articular component and which does not require articular reduction (Figure 26.6). In active older patients with these fractures, reduction and stabilization is indicated to maximize the chance of good recovery. Metaphyseal unstable fractures can be stabilized by closed reduction and percutaneous pinning, ORIF or external fixation. Closed re-manipulation and plaster management was

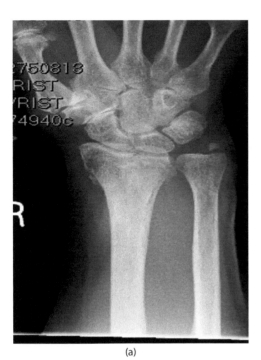

(a)

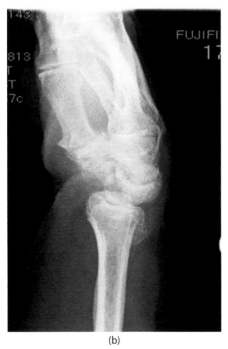

(b)

Figure 26.6 A metaphyseal displaced fracture with an undisplaced vertical fracture extending into the radiocarpal joint. During treatment this fracture will behave as an extra-articular fracture.

popular a number of years ago but has been shown to be ineffective by a number of authors.[23,24,53] This practice should be abandoned in favour of more stable fixation techniques.

Percutaneous pinning

Percutaneous pinning of fractures of the distal radius is an appealing technique as it is minimally invasive. It has been widely used for the treatment of unstable extra-articular or minimal articular distal radius fractures as well as for intra-articular fractures.

There are three basic constructs for percutaneous pinning:

1. Distal radius pinning where pins are placed across the fracture in the distal radius. These may be only radial styloid pins or may also include a pin from the dorsal ulnar aspect to the volar aspect of the radius.
2. Ulnar radial pinning where the pins are placed from the radius across the ulna.
3. Intra-focal pinning or the Kapandji technique where the pins are inserted into the fracture, used as reduction tools and then driven into the proximal radius (Figure 26.7).

Whichever technique is used it is important to avoid damage to the dorsal sensory branch of the radial nerve or tendons which are close to the insertion points of both radial styloid and dorsal ulnar wires by using open pin placement techniques. Pins may be left protruding from the skin for ease of removal but a small RCT demonstrated lower pin track infection rates in wires buried below the skin.[54] This has the disadvantage of requiring a further minor procedure to remove the wires. Most authors recommend a short arm cast for up to 6 weeks after percutaneous pinning. An RCT of 60 patients compared 1 and 6 weeks in a cast after percutaneous pinning and found no differences between the groups. However only 24 patients had metaphyseal comminution so the likelihood is that the majority were stable fractures.[55]

Despite a number of comparative studies, no differences between the different types of percutaneous pinning have been demonstrated although the results are difficult to interpret as many of the fractures had no comminution and are therefore unlikely to have been unstable.[56,57]

Complications of percutaneous pinning

The most common complication of percutaneous pinning is damage to the superficial branch of the radial nerve which occurs in up to 15% of cases[55,56] and may occur after pin removal.[55,56] Placement of the pins should be done under direct visualization using small skin incisions and blunt dissection down to bone. Care should be taken when removing buried pins that the incisions are large enough to ensure protection of the nerve.

Pin track infection is a frequently ignored complication of percutaneous pinning and is often poorly defined. It is important to differentiate between minor and major pin track infections. Major pin track infection occurs when further surgery is required to eradicate the problem or the pins

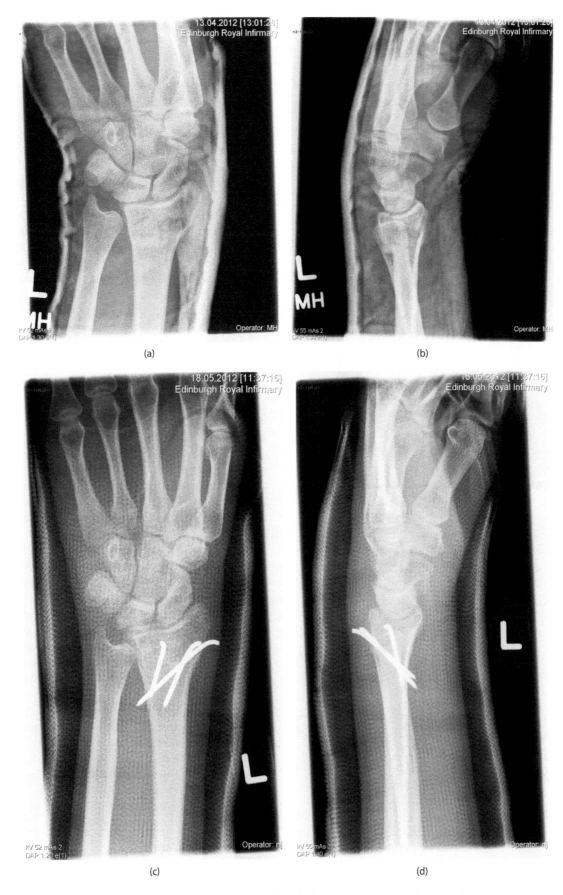

(a)

(b)

(c)

(d)

Figure 26.7 An unstable fracture of the distal radius treated with three pins inserted through the fracture site using the Kapandji technique.

have to be removed early. The majority of pin track infections are minor after percutaneous pinning with rates recorded from 1.7% to 70%.[54–56,58,59] Major pin track infection occurs rarely with most authors reporting none. Burial of pins subcutaneously may contribute to avoidance of pin track infection, especially if the pins are in place for prolonged periods.[54]

External fixation

There are two different methods of external fixation: bridging or spanning fixation and non-bridging or non-spanning fixation. For bridging external fixation pins are placed in the second metacarpal and the radial shaft thus bridging the radiocarpal, intercarpal and carpometacarpal joints (Figure 26.8). This technique depends on ligamentotaxis and may be static, dynamic (allowing some wrist movement) or augmented (with internal fixation, bone graft or bone substitute or a fifth pin in the distal fragment). For non-bridging external fixation pins are placed in the distal fragment of the fracture and in the radial shaft allowing direct fixation of the fracture without immobilizing any joints (Figure 26.9).

Bridging external fixation

The most common indication for bridging external fixation is actual or predicted instability in the dorsally displaced extra-articular or minimal articular fracture of the distal radius, especially where the distal fragment is too small to accommodate pins for non-bridging fractures and open injuries.

Two pins are inserted in the second metacarpal by hand after predrilling at about 45 degrees to the frontal plane. Pins should be placed through open incisions and engage both cortices. The proximal pins are placed in the mid lateral position in the radial diaphysis in the plane between the brachioradialis muscle and superficial radial nerve and the extensor carpi radialis tendons. The pins are then connected by a bar and clamps. The fracture is reduced with the fixator in position and the clamps are then tightened. Care must be taken not to over-distract the wrist as this may increase the load required to generate metacarpophalangeal joint flexion and result in hand stiffness. Release of pin tracks may be required at the end of the procedure to eliminate tension on the skin which may lead to pin track infection. Physiotherapy may be required if hand stiffness develops. The fixator can usually be removed at 5–6 weeks after application. Anaesthesia is not required for removal.

Non-bridging external fixation

Indications for non-bridging external fixation are similar to those for bridging external fixation but there must be sufficient space (1 cm of intact volar cortex) in the distal fragment to site the pins. The technique can also be used for displaced articular fractures if there is sufficient space for pins once the joint surface has been reduced and fixed. Non-bridging external fixation can also be used for distal radial osteotomy for dorsal malunion.

Two distal pins are placed from dorsal to volar, although some fixators use radial sided pins. Fluoroscopy is essential. The pins are placed midway between the fracture and the

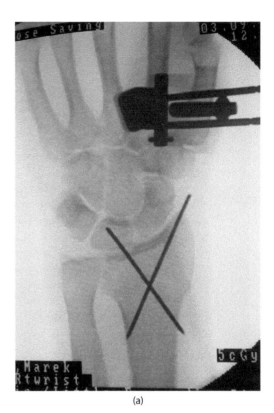

(a)

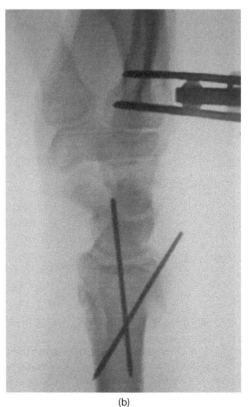

(b)

Figure 26.8 An unstable distal radius fracture treated with bridging external fixation. The fixation has been augmented with percutaneous pins. PA (a) and lateral (b) views of and unstable distal radius fracture treated with bridging external fixation. The fixation has been augmented with percutaneous pins.

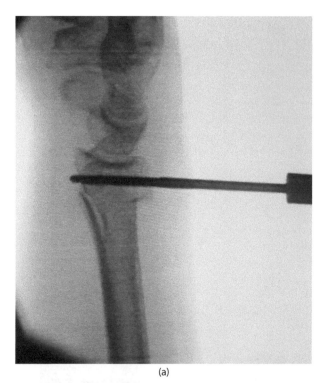

(a)

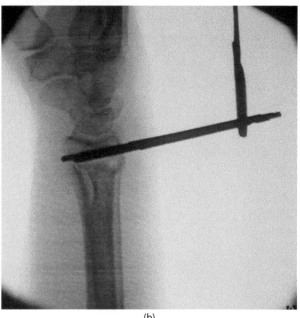

(b)

Figure 26.9 (a) Distal pin placement for a non-bridging external fixator. The pins have been placed parallel to the radiocarpal joint between the fracture and the joint with the fracture still displaced. Note that the pins penetrate the volar cortex. (b) The pins have been used as a joystick to reduce the fracture. There is a metaphyseal defect, the likely cause of instability.

radiocarpal joint, parallel to the joint surface on the lateral view (Figure 26.9) and on either side of Lister's tubercle and the extensor pollicis longus (EPL) tendon and should penetrate the volar cortex. Open pin placement and careful retraction will protect the extensor tendons. The forearm

is then rotated to confirm free rotation and images are obtained to exclude penetration of the distal radioulnar or radiocarpal joint. Two proximal pins are then placed in the radius proximal to the fracture in a similar fashion to that used for bridging external fixation except that their position is usually more dorsal to volar than mid-lateral. The fracture is reduced by using the distal pins as a 'joystick' to control the position of the distal fragment (Figure 26.9b). Care should be taken to avoid over-reduction where there is volar comminution. As the distal pins move with the reduction, they should move into the centre of correctly placed skin incisions but each pin track should be released if there is any residual tension.

Pin track care is carried out as for bridging external fixation. No other form of immobilization is necessary and the patient is encouraged to move the hand and wrist fully. Physiotherapy is not usually required unless finger stiffness develops. The fixator is usually removed after 5–6 weeks. Anaesthesia is not required for removal.

Complications of external fixation

Pin Track Complications

The most common complication of external fixation is pin track infection. It is important to differentiate between those which compromise the final outcome by early removal of the fixator or an added surgical procedure (major pin track infections) and those which do not, merely requiring treatment with antibiotics and increased frequency of dressing changes (minor pin track infection).[60]

Rates of pin track infection reported in the literature vary from 0% to 39% for minor pin track infections.[34,61–68] Major pin track infections are rare in external fixation of the distal radius even in the elderly with none in most reports[62–67,69] and sporadic single cases in others.[23,34,68] In the biggest series of external fixation of distal radius fractures reported in the literature, minor pin track infection occurred in 126 of 588 cases (21%). Major pin track infection requiring early removal of the fixator or further surgery occurred in only 12 cases (2%).[60]

Other pin track complications including pin track fracture, pin pull-out or loosening and skin adherence are rare. The largest prevalence of pin track fracture was reported by Ahlborg et al. with 11 pin track fractures in 314 cases of bridging external fixation. The authors found no relationship with pin track infection and no increased prevalence in the elderly.[70] In 588 cases, Hayes et al. reported only three pin track fractures (0.5%), all in the second metacarpal.[60] Pin track fractures which occur during treatment can be managed by re-siting the pin; those occurring outside this time should be treated by standard methods for the specific fracture.

Pin pull-out was originally cited as a potential problem for pins placed in the distal fragment with non-bridging external fixation but these fears have proven to be unfounded with only occasional cases occurring in both bridging and non-bridging external fixators.[60]

Pin loosening has been attributed to osteoporotic bone with one study reporting an increased rate in women older than 75 years. However this did not lead to an increase in the number of fixators requiring early removal.[70]

Tethering of the skin can occur after healing of the pin tracks but is poorly documented. Ahlborg et al. reported a 1% rate of surgery to correct skin tethering.[70] This procedure is simple and can be done using local anaesthetic.

Radial Nerve Damage

The superficial branch of the radial nerve runs deep to the brachioradialis muscle in the forearm and around 5 cm proximal to the radial styloid it emerges dorsally from beneath the brachioradialis tendon. At this point it is vulnerable to damage with insertion of the proximal pins of an external fixator. This is a preventable complication if care is taken to place pins using open incisions and protection of the nerve.

The rate of damage to the radial nerve is reported to occur in 0–13% of cases.[60–62, 66–68,70–73] No study reports any difference in the rate of radial nerve injury between different types of external fixation.

Joint Distraction

There is a risk that bridging external fixation will cause over-distraction of the radiocarpal and mid-carpal joints with excessive force being applied in attempts to reduce a fracture. Initial concerns were raised that distraction of the wrist might lead to complex regional pain syndrome or hand stiffness and that outcome was compromised more with a longer duration of distraction. In a study of 42 patients with augmented external fixation for unstable distal radial fractures, moderately increased distraction resulted in improved clinical outcome and did not cause subsequent joint stiffness but caution against extreme distraction, which could induce carpal malalignment, worsen intercarpal ligament injury and induce finger stiffness, was advised.[74]

Volar locked plating

The main indication for volar locked plating in extra-articular or minimal articular displaced fractures is similar to that for non-bridging external fixation, namely for fractures with actual or predicted instability and sufficient space for pins in the distal fragment. This technique is therefore contraindicated in cases with a very small distal fragment. Volar locked plating can be used for corrective osteotomy for malunion of the distal radius. It is advisable to use locking plates for volar displaced fractures in the older patient who is likely to be osteoporotic.

The approach used for the majority of distal radius fractures is the modified Henry's approach between the radial artery and flexor carpi radialis (FCR) tendon. If access is required to the ulnar side of the radius, for example when there is a volar ulnar corner fracture or for carpal tunnel decompression, an approach between the flexor tendons and ulnar neurovascular bundle can be used. The technique of volar plating for extra-articular or minimal articular

fractures depends on whether the surgeon wishes to reduce the fracture manually or with the plate. Reduction with the plate using the 'lift' technique allows easier restoration of the volar tilt (Figure 26.10) but in volar displaced fractures the fracture must be reduced prior to plate application. It is important to avoid screw penetration of the radiocarpal or DRUJs or the dorsal cortex. The plate should not be placed distal to the watershed line as this risks flexor pollicis longus (FPL) rupture. In elderly patients with osteoporotic bone and a large metaphyseal defect there is a risk of

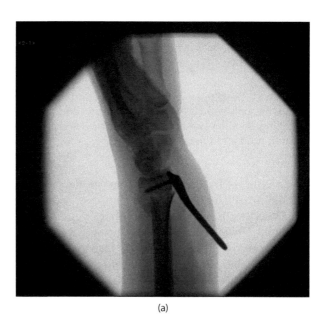

(a)

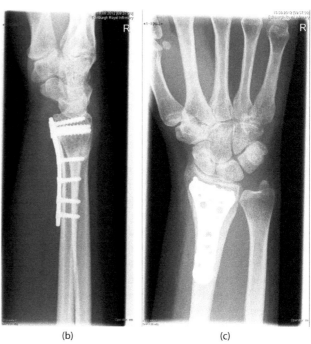

(b)   (c)

Figure 26.10 **(a)** A locked volar plate has been applied to a displaced fracture with the screws parallel to the joint. **(b)** The plate shaft has been applied to bone thereby reducing the fracture. Care should be taken with this technique to prevent cut-out of screws.

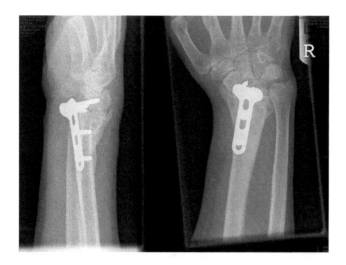

Figure 26.11 Despite an initial good reduction this fracture has collapsed into dorsal angulation and radial shortening. As the plate is a fixed angle device the screws have migrated into the radiocarpal joint.

subsidence of the fracture and migration of the screws into the radiocarpal joint (Figure 26.11). This may be prevented by augmentation by either bone substitute or grafting.[75]

Theoretically after volar plating whether locked or not, there is no need for immobilization of the wrist as the fixation is very stable. However, in practice a plaster or splint is frequently used in the first few weeks. Early finger motion is encouraged and wrist motion when comfort allows but certainly by 3–4 weeks after fracture.

Complications of volar locked plating

Reported rates of complications after volar locked plating are high, ranging from 5.9% to 48%[68,75–78] with the majority of complications being hardware related. The main hardware related complications are tendon rupture or irritation and screw penetration into the radiocarpal joint or DRUJ which frequently result in high re-operation rates.[68,75–79]

Screw penetration

Screw penetration into the radiocarpal joint or DRUJ is reported in a number of studies and ranges from 3% to 57%.[75,76,79–81] Although screws may inadvertently be placed into a joint at the time of surgery this should largely be avoidable with the use of suitable imaging such as oblique and tilted lateral views. However, especially in elderly patients with poor bone who may have significant metaphyseal comminution, collapse around the plate is a concern with rates of collapse of up to 57% being reported.[75,81,82] As the plate is a fixed angle device the screws penetrate the radiocarpal joint as the fracture collapses (Figure 26.11) which is more likely in a fracture with a small distal fragment as screws are of necessity close to the subchondral bone.[75] In intra-articular fractures there is also a danger of screws being placed in sagittal fracture lines allowing their migration into the joint.[79] Such penetration of the radiocarpal joint usually requires

removal of the metalwork. Augmentation of the defect with bone substitutes may prevent collapse.[75,79]

Tendon complications

Hardware related tendon problems are either tendon irritation or tendon rupture and may involve flexor or extensor tendons with EPL and FPL being most commonly affected. A wide range of prevalences are reported from 0.8% to 19.6%.[75,76,80,83]

Extensor tendon pathology is likely to be related to screw prominence dorsally which can be difficult to visualize using radiographs because of the irregularity of the dorsal surface of the radius and the prominence of Lister's tubercle. To reduce the chance of dorsal penetration the measured length of the distal screws should be reduced by 2 mm and symptoms of tenosynovitis should prompt hardware removal. Flexor tendon irritation or rupture usually affects the FPL tendon although it has been reported in other flexor tendons.[83] It has been attributed to plate prominence, especially with placement distal to the watershed and was rarely reported as a complication of distal radius fractures before the advent of locked plating.

OUTCOME OF OPERATIVE TREATMENT

Cohort studies

Percutaneous pinning

There have been a number of cohort studies examining the outcome of percutaneous pinning for distal radius fractures. Although some earlier papers were optimistic about the outcome of the technique more recent papers have reported significant loss of position at final review,[58,84] particularly in older patients, patients with poor bone stock and comminuted fractures.[55,58,85]

Bridging external fixation

Most authors agree that with bridging external fixation alone unstable fractures of the distal radius will redisplace by varying degrees. In 14 of 60 cases with an average age of 63 years significant loss of reduction was reported[23]; furthermore, 10 of the 60 cases did not fully reduce with closed reduction. In total, 24 of 60 patients were considered to have malunion. At 1 year grip strength was around two-thirds of the opposite normal side, although recovery of movement was an average of 89% of the opposite wrist. In a series of 641 distal radius fractures, 230 cases with an average age of 58 years were treated with bridging fixators, and 24% had a malunion at final review despite successful initial reduction.[60] Wilcke et al. treated 30 patients with distal radius fractures with bridging external fixation but excluded those with severe comminution, which are the most likely to be unstable. Even so nine patients had residual dorsal angulation after healing. The mean DASH score at 1 year after injury was 11 but the patients were all under 70 years of age.[86]

Augmentation of bridging external fixation may reduce loss of reduction. In a series of 70 cases treated with bridging external fixation augmented with percutaneous pins, half of the fractures lost more than 5 degrees of initially reduced volar tilt. However, no cases deteriorated sufficiently to be considered radiologically unacceptable.[87] In a retrospective comparison of 20 cases treated with bridging external fixation without augmentation and 36 cases with augmentation of the bridging external fixator using percutaneous pins, bridging external fixation alone did not regain volar tilt but augmentation was better at retaining the initial reduction and provided a better range of movement and grip strength.[88]

Bone grafting or insertion of bone substitutes into the metaphyseal defect after reduction and bridging external fixation can assist in maintenance of the reduction and may allow earlier removal of the fixator at 3 weeks without loss of reduction. Bone substitutes seem to be equally effective as autograft and are probably preferable to avoid graft donor site complications.

Non-bridging external fixation

There is a consensus that non-bridging external fixation restores and maintains volar tilt[34, 60,64,69,89] and carpal alignment[34,60, 64,89] in patients of varying ages. Radial length is restored with a small increase in ulnar variance after removal of the fixator.[34,60, 64,69,89] In a retrospective radiological comparison of 588 bridging or non-bridging external fixators Hayes et al. reported a 6.2 times increased chance of dorsal malunion in bridging external fixation compared to non-bridging external fixation and a 2.5 times increased chance of radial shortening in the bridging group.[60]

Functional results in cohort studies are equally good. Andersen et al. reported 88% excellent or good results with the Gartland and Werley score and concluded that non-bridging external fixation is a reliable method of maintaining radiological reduction with a good functional outcome after 1 year.[69] Flinkkila and his co-authors reported 90% restoration of grip strength and up to 97% restoration of movement at a mean of 16 months after fracture and concluded that non-bridging external fixation is an easy, minimally invasive and reliable method that restores the anatomy and function after unstable fracture of the distal forearm. The authors consider it their treatment of choice for these fractures.[64]

The ease of the technique was demonstrated by Hayes et al. who reported on the success of the technique in the hands of surgeons in training thus confirming its generalizability.[60]

Volar locked plating

Despite initial enthusiasm, the radiological and functional outcomes of volar locked plating for extra-articular and minimal articular distal radius fractures are similar to other techniques. Reported radiological results indicate that volar locked plating is successful in restoring volar tilt and radial length[75,81,82] even in older patients.[90,91]

Functional outcome with volar locked plating is generally good with DASH scores ranging from 13 to 28.[75,81,82,91]

Some of the differences are probably explained by the age of the patient with the oldest cohorts having the highest DASH scores.[91] Variations in the length of follow-up may also explain some of the differences. When other outcome measures are used, the percentages of good and excellent scores are usually high.

Comparative studies of the outcome of non-operative and operative treatment

Analysis of any RCT for the treatment of distal radius fractures is frequently hampered by varying definitions of instability, with widely varying inclusion and exclusion criteria, which makes comparisons difficult. Instability for these purposes should be defined as a fracture which has redisplaced in plaster or which can be predicted to have a chance of instability of more than 70%.[21]

Percutaneous pinning versus cast

Stoffelen et al. examined 98 patients with distal radius fractures randomized to Kapandji pinning and cast for 1 week or plaster cast for 6 weeks after closed reduction. The authors found no significant differences in the two groups for either functional or radiological outcome.[92] Azzopardi and his co-authors found marginal radiographic advantage and no functional advantage in the use of percutaneous pinning.[93] Wong et al. studied older patients and found small radiological advantages in dorsal angulation but not in ulnar variance with the use of percutaneous pinning. They found no functional differences.[94] The only study to report anatomical and functional advantages of percutaneous pinning compared to cast management was in patients under 65 years of age[59] suggesting that in the older patient pinning is compromised by poor bone quality.

Bridging external fixation versus cast

There seems to be a consensus amongst authors of randomized or pseudo-RCTs, which compare bridging external fixation with cast management. All authors agree that bridging external fixation results in a better anatomical position than non-operative management[23,95–98] but most reported that improvement is not reflected in the functional results.[97,98,23] For patient orientated measures the only series which reported DASH scores showed no differences[95] while Christensen et al. reported improvement in the Gartland and Werley scores for external fixation at 3 and 9 months after injury.[96] Some authors reported either a trend towards better function[98] or improvement in a small number of objective surgeon orientated outcomes.[95] However, these advantages in anatomy and function were usually accompanied by an increase in early complications,[97] usually because of minor pin track infection or radial nerve irritation.

Non-bridging external fixation versus cast

The only randomized study comparing non-bridging external fixation with cast compared 30 cases treated with non-bridging external fixation with 26 cases treated in plaster but in patients under 60 years of age. The authors concluded that a non-bridging external fixator was highly effective in maintaining the reduced position of distal radial fractures.[99] The following year the same group published a similar RCT containing 106 patients and confirmed the superiority of the external fixator in maintaining the reduced position. They reported better grip strength and a higher proportion of excellent results both subjectively and objectively in the external fixation groups although each group achieved similar proportions of satisfactory results.[100]

Volar locked plating versus cast

There is only one RCT comparing volar locked plating and non-operative management, comparing 90 patients over 65 years of age with unstable distal radius fractures treated with a volar locked plate or manipulation under anaesthetic and plaster management. Radiological results were superior in the plated group. The DASH and PRWE scores showed early advantages in the plated group but this was not sustained at later follow-up. The operative group had a higher complication rate (36% vs 11%) with a 22% tendon complication rate and a 31% secondary surgery rate.[76]

External fixation versus percutaneous pinning

Three studies have compared the outcome of external fixation to percutaneous pinning. Ludvigsen et al.[101] examined 60 patients with distal radius fractures with metaphyseal comminution randomized to bridging external fixation (average age 61 years) or percutaneous pinning (average age 58 years) reviewed at 6 months after injury. There were no significant differences in radiological outcome, complication rates or function as measured by the modified Gartland and Werley score. In a series of 50 younger patients aged less than 65 years and randomized to augmented bridging external fixation or percutaneous pinning, there were no differences in the radiological outcome or DASH scores except for better articular surface reduction in the external fixation group.[102] In a randomized study of 40 patients non-bridging external fixation (median age 59.5 years) allowed more rapid early rehabilitation than percutaneous pinning (median age 61.4 years) but there were no longer term advantages.[103]

Percutaneous pinning versus locked plating

In the last few years there have been two retrospective comparisons and a number of prospective randomized comparisons of percutaneous pinning and ORIF with volar locking plates. The two retrospective studies studied older patients and found a greater loss of reduction with percutaneous pinning,[104,105] particularly for ulnar variance and in patients with lower bone density measurements.[105] Locked plating demonstrated a faster recovery time and a better final grip strength in one study[105] but no significant differences in function in the other.[104] In two randomized studies there were no demonstrable differences in the radiological outcomes[106,107] but the study which recruited older patients

warned against over-reduction with pinning in the presence of volar comminution.[106] Both showed a consistent advantage in DASH scores for plating up to 6 months after injury. A further study showed no differences in outcome between the two groups but the inclusion criteria and fractures were heterogeneous rendering the results of limited use in clinical practice.[108]

Bridging external fixation versus plating

Of the seven RCTs published in the last 5 years none concentrate on the elderly patient, with all recruiting a wide range of patient ages. Four studies showed no differences between bridging external fixation and volar locked plating in the patient orientated scores (DASH and PRWE) at any time period[61, 71,77,109] and three showed subjective improvement for the first few months after surgery, which was not sustained by 6 months.[68,72,73] Early improvement in recovery of range of movement with plates was reported by some authors[61,68,73,77] but in all of these studies, the patients treated with plates were allowed to mobilize their wrist early in the postoperative period while the external fixation device immobilized the wrist until its removal. Landgren et al.[109] extended the outcome studies on a previously reported study[61] to 5 years and found no differences in function between external fixation and plating.

Radiological results were equivalent between plating and augmented external fixation in most studies,[61,71-73,77] with poorer radiological results occurring when the bridging external fixator was not augmented in all cases.[68] Only two studies reported malunion rates of around 30% for both groups.[61,73]

Complication rates were similar for the two methods of treatment in most studies.[61,68,71,73,77] Egol et al. reported a higher re-operation rate for plates with most re-operations being due to hardware problems.[77] Grewal and her co-authors found more tendon complications in their ORIF group, a number of which would be deemed major complications. All but one complication (acute compartment syndrome) in the external fixation group were minor, mainly minor pin track infections.[71]

Esposito et al. undertook a meta-analysis of nine studies and concluded that overall there was very little clinical difference between the two methods of treatment. They cite lower DASH scores for plates but the difference did not reach the acknowledged clinically important difference of 10. They found that overall complication rates were similar but that external fixation had a higher rate of infection, although this was minor.[110] However the mean age of the participants was over 55 years in only two of the included studies.

Bridging versus non-bridging external fixation

McQueen reported on an RCT of non-bridging versus bridging external fixation in 60 patients with redisplaced fractures of the distal radius and an average age of 61 years. Because they had all redisplaced and all had metaphyseal comminution, there was little heterogeneity in the fractures.

Anatomical results were statistically significantly better in the non-bridging group throughout the period of review. Functional results were superior throughout the period of review although pain scores did not differ at 1 year after treatment. The author concluded that non-bridging external fixation was significantly better than bridging external fixation and should be the treatment of choice for unstable distal radius fractures where external fixation is contemplated and where there is space for pins in the distal fragment.[34]

Since then, three further RCTs comparing bridging and non-bridging external fixation in patients with extra-articular or minimal articular fractures of the distal radius have been reported.[62,66,111] All demonstrated better reduction in the non-bridging groups. The DASH score was used in two studies with no differences in one[62] and better DASH scores in the non-bridging group in the other.[66] The former study reported better early SF12 physical health scores for the non-bridging group but no differences in pain scores.

Non-bridging external fixation versus plating

There has been one report of an RCT comparing non-bridging external fixation to volar locked plating[78] which recruited 102 patients with an average age of 63 years. Surgery time was less and restoration of volar tilt was superior in the non-bridging external fixation group. At 1 year after surgery there were no differences in range of movement, grip strength, pain or PROMS. However differences are evident in the analysis of complications. Although the overall complication rate was similar in each group (20% external fixation versus 21% volar locked plate) the more serious nature of the complications in the volar locked plate group is reflected in the re-operation rate of 36.5% in that group compared to 6% in the external fixation group.[78]

DISPLACED INTRA-ARTICULAR FRACTURES

Although severe articular fractures account for less than 5% of distal radius fractures, they are the most challenging to treat especially in the older patient with poor bone stock. There remains debate about the effect of articular incongruity on the development of post-traumatic osteoarthritis but this may be less relevant in the older patient. There is a consensus that 2 mm of articular displacement should be reduced in the fit active patient but the application of this to the elderly has not been established. Reduction of the articular surface is not required in the frail elderly who should be treated in a cast for comfort.

Surgical treatment must address both the intra-articular displacement and any accompanying metaphyseal displacement and instability so a combination of techniques may be required. Each fracture must be assessed to ascertain the fracture pattern and displacement of the fragments and a treatment strategy defined on this basis. Two techniques are used for the surgical treatment of displaced articular fractures: closed or percutaneous reduction of the articular surface with bridging external fixation or ORIF. The first requires initial application of a bridging external fixator and

then manipulation and fixation of articular fragments percutaneously with the use of imaging. ORIF is performed using an approach tailored to the fracture type and may require all the fixation techniques in the surgeon's armamentarium. In practice, closed reduction and percutaneous fixation is possible in the less severe fractures, particularly when there is no volar ulnar fragment displacement or rotation.

Outcome

Restoration of articular congruity may be less relevant in the older patient because a shorter life expectancy may prevent the development of post-traumatic arthritis. There are a limited number of reports of the outcome of both methods of treatment and these are in cohorts with a range of ages but mostly in younger patients. These demonstrate that results are satisfactory provided reduction of the joint is achieved and that radiological arthritis and other complications occur in substantial numbers of cases.[112–114] Functional outcome scores rarely revert to baseline and complication rates are high, reflecting the complexity of the fractures treated.

An RCT of the two techniques[115] demonstrated that if indirect reduction and percutaneous fixation was possible then better functional outcome was achieved compared to ORIF, provided the joint was reduced. If the closed method did not reduce the joint, the authors proceeded to ORIF. The authors recommended that open reduction be preceded by an attempt at a minimally invasive percutaneous reduction and if a good reduction is achieved then ORIF is unnecessary.

In a small number of cases it may not be possible to restore articular congruity or metaphyseal alignment because of severe articular or metaphyseal comminution, poor bone quality or any combination of the three. In these circumstances a salvage procedure may be required. Distraction plating may be useful particularly in cases with poor bone stock.[116] Arthrodesis is rarely required in the elderly patient.

PARTIAL ARTICULAR FRACTURES

Partial articular fractures of the distal radius are either volar shearing or volar lip (volar Barton's), dorsal shearing or dorsal lip (Barton's) or radial styloid (Chauffeur's) fractures and usually result from impaction of the scaphoid and lunate complex onto the distal radius.

Volar shearing fractures

Volar shearing fractures are the AO type B3 fracture (Figure 26.1) and are categorized by the size and comminution of the volar fragment and whether the sigmoid notch is involved. They have long been recognized as being inherently unstable and non-operative treatment is therefore reserved for the elderly, frail patient or the rare undisplaced fracture.

Operative treatment is with a palmar buttress plate with an emphasis on reduction of the articular surface, including the sigmoid notch. The plate should be slightly under contoured to apply compression across the fracture against the intact dorsal cortex. Care should be taken to place the plate sufficiently ulnar to support an ulnar-sided volar lip

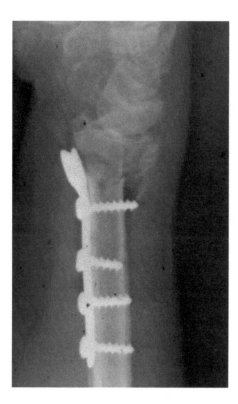

Figure 26.12 This fracture was initially displaced in a volar direction. The plate has been undercontoured and dorsal displacement has occurred. Note the dorsal comminution which has allowed dorsal displacement.

fracture which may be occult. The surgeon should examine the pre-operative imaging carefully to exclude subtle fracture lines extending into the dorsal cortex which may otherwise be unrecognized, risking dorsal malunion if an under contoured plate is used[117] (Figure 26.12).

Most reports of the outcome of volar shearing fractures of the distal radius include a majority of cases with high energy injury which may not reflect the true epidemiology of these injuries. Reported radiological results are good provided the risk of dorsal malunion is avoided.[117–119] Functional results are reported with a high proportion of excellent and good results[118] and restoration of near normal DASH scores up to 25 years after injury.[119,120]

Radial styloid fractures

Radial styloid fractures are the most common type of partial articular fracture. These are usually undisplaced and generally benign injuries but careful examination of the carpus is mandatory to exclude scaphoid fracture or carpal ligamentous injury. In most cases in the elderly they may be treated in a cast or splint for pain relief and the wrist mobilized when symptoms allow. Only rarely is surgical intervention necessary where there is severe displacement and comminution when radial buttress plating may be necessary.

FRACTURES OF THE DISTAL ULNA

Fractures of the distal ulna are a common association with distal radius fractures. They may involve the ulnar shaft, neck, head or ulnar styloid or a combination of several of these.

Extra-articular fractures of the distal ulna associated with distal radius fractures are either diaphyseal or in the neck or distal part of the ulna. Many of these fractures will be realigned once the distal radius is reduced in which case cast immobilization is sufficient. However, if the ulna remains malaligned or unstable after distal radius stabilization then ORIF is required in the fit elderly patient. Malalignment has been defined as more than 10 degrees of angulation and instability as more than 50% translation with forearm rotation.[121]

There is only one study comparing operative and non-operative treatment for extra-articular ulnar fractures which was a prospective non-randomized study of 61 unstable or malaligned fractures of the distal ulna with associated distal radius fractures. The patients were all over 64 years of age. At an average review period of 34 months there were no significant differences in the radiological or functional outcome.[121] For the older patient it seems that non-operative management of extra-articular ulnar fractures is satisfactory but if ORIF is deemed necessary it will achieve union with few complications and good functional result.

Intra-articular distal ulnar fractures may occur in isolation or in association with distal radius fractures when they may occur with ulnar neck or styloid fractures. Treatment should follow the general principals of the treatment of intra-articular fractures as residual displacement is likely to cause a block to forearm rotation. Where there is significant displacement ORIF with headless screws or K-wires may be necessary, supplemented with plating where appropriate.

In a study of 14 older patients with intra-articular ulnar fractures in association with distal radius fractures the distal radius was fixed with a volar plate and the ulna managed non-operatively. At a mean of 18-month review, all the ulnar fractures had healed and all had good or excellent results using the modified Gartland and Werley score. The authors concluded that satisfactory results can be achieved by non-operative management of an ulnar fracture, especially in older patients who may have osteoporotic bone.[122]

Ulnar styloid fractures

Ulnar styloid fractures are the most common ulnar-sided injury associated with distal radius fractures, being reported to occur in 40–60% of distal radius fractures. There is conflicting evidence about the effect of an ulnar styloid fracture on outcome. Older publications examine ulnar styloid fractures in association with a non-operatively managed distal radius fracture and mostly conclude that an ulnar styloid fracture compromises the outcome. More recent studies evaluate series of distal radius fractures treated with volar plating and ulnar styloid fractures without intraoperative DRUJ instability. None show any correlation between functional outcomes and the presence, level or displacement of an ulnar styloid fracture.[31,123,124] Where the ulnar styloid fracture is basal and associated with DRUJ instability most authorities agree that ORIF should be used to stabilize the DRUJ.

COMPLICATIONS

Complications of distal radius fractures are relatively common and are reported to occur in a wide range of 5–31% of mixed series of fractures.[125,126] Some of these complications are associated with treatment of the fracture and are reported elsewhere in this chapter.

Fracture specific complications

NERVE INJURY

Median nerve

The most common nerve injury associated with distal radius fracture is median nerve injury presenting as CTS. It has been reported as occurring in 3–17% of fractures.[126–128] Suggested contributory causes of early CTS after distal radius fracture are swelling and haematoma extending into the carpal canal or deep to the fascia at the level of the fracture, direct nerve contusion, haematoma block and the Cotton-Loder position. Later CTS has been attributed to callus formation and malunion.

Although CTS can present at any time after fracture the most common is the subacute group which is defined as occurring 1–12 weeks after fracture.[128] This occurs in older patients with lower energy injury, with malunion being a possible contributory factor and has a negative influence on functional outcome after distal radius fracture. Decompression is successful in the majority of patients but it should be noted that compression may occur proximal to the wrist crease at the level of the fracture and release should be extended to this area. Acute onset CTS (within a week of fracture) can occur in the older patient although it is commoner in younger patients with high energy injuries. It should first be treated with reduction of a displaced fracture as the symptoms may resolve. Progressively worsening symptoms are an indication for urgent decompression.

Ulnar nerve

Ulnar nerve injury is less common than median injury with prevalence reported as being 0.5–4.2%.[127,129] It is thought that the mobility of the ulnar nerve at the wrist and in the forearm protects it from injury. Reported risk fractures are instability of the DRUJ, open fractures, high energy injury and severe fracture displacement. Most of these injuries are neuropraxias which recover spontaneously. Exploration is recommended where there is complete ulnar palsy with an open wound or concurrent acute CTS.

TENDON INJURY

Tendon injury occurs with distal radius fractures treated both operatively and non-operatively. The most common tendon injury involves the EPL and is usually reported as occurring in less than 1% of fractures[126] but has been reported in up to 5% of fractures.[130] A number of mechanisms for EPL injury after distal radius fracture have been proposed and may be either fracture or hardware related. Hardware related rupture most commonly occurs with plating and is discussed in the relevant section of this chapter.

Attrition and ischaemia have both been cited as the cause of tendon rupture after distal radius fracture. EPL ruptures have been reported as occurring more commonly in undisplaced or minimally displaced distal radius fractures[130] and at various times after injury. It is likely that fracture related ruptures occur earlier after injury at an average of around 6 weeks while later ruptures may be more likely to be related to attritional problems on hardware.[83]

If the patient has symptoms causing a functional problem after EPL rupture then tendon transfer, usually with the extensor indicis proprius, should be considered. This is reported as achieving satisfactory outcomes with low DASH scores,[83] minimal loss of thumb extension and restoration of around 70% of grip and tip pinch strength by 8 weeks after surgery.

Fracture related flexor tendon injuries are much rarer possibly because the muscle belly of the pronator quadratus acts as a cushioning layer between the flexor tendons and bone. Before the early 1990s only 12 cases of flexor tendon rupture had been reported in the world literature. However a literature search for flexor tendon rupture in distal radius fracture in the last 25 years identifies 19 studies specifically relating to flexor tendon rupture, mainly FPL, after volar plating indicating that this is a hardware related problem.

MALUNION

Malunion of fractures of the distal radius (Figure 26.13) remains common although it is frequently not reported as a complication of distal radius fracture. When reported the prevalence is difficult to assess as there is considerable controversy around the definition of malunion. Treatment of malunion should not be considered because of radiological deformity alone but only in the symptomatic patient.

Typical symptoms of malunion are:

1. DRUJ, carpal or radiocarpal pain
2. Weakness of grip
3. Reduced range of movement, especially rotation
4. Deformity

Treatment of malunion

In the fit independent patient the treatment of symptomatic malunion is surgical. It is usual practice that correction of malunion be delayed as this allows a clear definition of residual problems and may prevent unnecessary surgery. However delay leads to an increased period of disability and more difficulty in defining the plane of deformity at surgery. Delay may also lead to soft tissue contracture and more

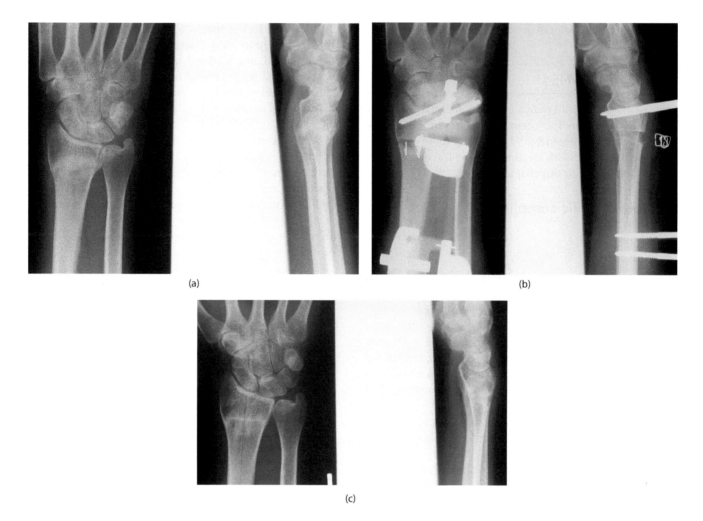

Figure 26.13 (a) A dorsal malunion of a distal radius fracture. If symptomatic in the older patient distal radial osteotomy should be considered. (b) An opening wedge osteotomy with bone grafting. (c) The osteotomy has healed with excellent correction.

challenging correction of the deformity with the potential for more added ulnar procedures. Contraindications to distal radial osteotomy include significant osteoarthritis of the radiocarpal joint when fusion may be necessary, intra-articular osteotomy in the presence of less than 2 mm of displacement and the presence of complex regional pain syndrome.

Dorsal malunion usually requires a dorsal approach although some surgeons may utilize a volar approach if a volar locking plate is to be used. A closing or opening wedge may be used although an opening wedge osteotomy is more frequently used as it generates additional radial length. It can be tailored to correct both frontal and sagittal deformity (Figure 26.13) but usually requires bone grafting to fill the resultant defect.

Many types of fixation have been described to stabilize distal radial osteotomy. Dorsal plating has been the most popular although more recently volar locked plates have been used for dorsal deformity. Cited advantages over dorsal plating are fewer tendon problems than with dorsal

plates and the use of morselized bone grafting as the volar locked plate does not need structural support and in some cases no bone graft but these advantages have not yet been proven. The use of non-bridging external fixation to stabilize the osteotomy (Figure 26.13) has a number of potential advantages. These include a minimally invasive technique, easy control and correction of the distal fragment, the use of non-structural cancellous bone graft and the ease of removal of the implant which does not require hospital admission.[131]

The consensus view on the outcome of osteotomy for a dorsal extra-articular malunion is that the procedure improves both radiological and functional outcomes but rarely to normal.[132–134] The technique is reliable in improving the radiological outcome although volar tilt is not consistently restored with plating techniques.[132–134] Volar tilt is reliably restored and maintained using non-bridging external fixation, perhaps because of the control obtained by the distal pins.[131] Functional outcomes show consistent improvement in both objective and patient related outcome measures.[131,135,] Complication rates are generally high with substantial re-operation rates in some series.[132–135]

Volar malunion of the distal radius is less common than dorsal malunion, probably because the prevalence of volar displacement is less and because there is a general recognition that volar displaced fractures are unstable and undergo primary fixation. The approach is volar and plating is the treatment of choice. Volar malunion is frequently a translational deformity with little angular deformity or bone loss. Where this is the case an oblique sliding osteotomy can be performed and bone grafting is not required.[136] If an angular deformity is present an opening wedge osteotomy and bone graft is required.[137] Good radiographic and functional results have been reported with both techniques although residual DRUJ symptoms limit its success.[136,137]

There are a number of ulnar-sided procedures for distal radius malunion. Ulnar-sided procedures are indicated for persistent pain, rotational contracture or instability of the DRUJ and may be performed in conjunction with distal radial osteotomy, at a later stage or in isolation if there is no malunion of the distal radius. After distal radial osteotomy the range of forearm rotation should always be assessed. If rotation remains significantly compromised then an ulnar-sided procedure, ranging from excisional hemiarthroplasty of the DRUJ to an excision of the distal ulna with or without replacement,[138] should be considered.

COMPLEX REGIONAL PAIN SYNDROME

Complex regional pain syndrome (CRPS) is a serious and often debilitating complication of a number of injuries but is most commonly seen after distal radius fracture. Its aetiology is unknown and it is characterized by a number of symptoms and signs including pain, swelling, colour and temperature change and joint contracture. The subject is considered in detail in Chapter 25.

REFERENCES

1. Chung KC, Shauver MJ, Yin H, et al. Variations in the use of internal fixation for distal radial fracture in the United States Medicare population. *J Bone Joint Surg Am*, 2011;93:2154–62.
2. Court-Brown CM, Caesar B. Epidemiology of adult fractures: A review. *Injury*, 2006;37:691–7.
3. Kreder HJ, Hanel DP, McKee M, et al. Consistency of AO fracture classification for the distal radius. *J Bone Joint Surg Br*, 1996;78:726–31.
4. Flinkkila T, Sirnio K, Hippi M, et al. Epidemiology and seasonal variation of distal radius fractures in Oulu, Finland. *Osteoporos Int*, 2011;22:2307–12.
5. McQueen MM. Fractures of the distal radius and ulna. In: Court-Brown CM, Heckman JD, McQueen MM, et al., editors. *Rockwood and Green's Fractures in Adults*. 8th ed. Philadelphia, PA: Wolters Kluwer; 2015. pp. 1057–120.
6. Orces CH, Martinez FJ. Epidemiology of fall related forearm and wrist fractures among adults treated in US hospital emergency departments. *Inj Prev*, 2011;17:33–6.
7. Sigurdardottir K, Halldorsson S, Robertsson J. Epidemiology and treatment of distal radius fractures in Reykjavik, Iceland, in 2004. Comparison with an Icelandic study from 1985. *Acta Orthop*, 2011;82:494–8.
8. Court-Brown CM. The epidemiology of fractures and dislocations. In: Court-Brown CM, Heckman JD, McQueen MM, et al., editors. *Rockwood and Green's Fractures in Adults*. 8th ed. Philadelphia, PA: Wolters Kluwer; 2015. pp. 59–108.
9. Brogren E, Petranek M, Atroshi I. Incidence and characteristics of distal radius fractures in a southern Swedish region. *BMC Musculoskelet Disord*, 2007;8:48.
10. Ahmed LA, Schirmer H, Bjornerem A, et al. The gender- and age-specific 10-year and lifetime absolute fracture risk in Tromso, Norway. *Eur J Epidemiol*, 2009;24:441–8.
11. Cooley H, Jones G. A population-based study of fracture incidence in southern Tasmania: Lifetime fracture risk and evidence for geographic variations within the same country. *Osteoporos Int*, 2001;12:124–30.
12. Cummings SR, Black DM, Rubin SM. Lifetime risks of hip, Colles', or vertebral fracture and coronary heart disease among white postmenopausal women. *Arch Intern Med*, 1989;149:2445–8.
13. Nguyen TV, Center JR, Sambrook PN, et al. Risk factors for proximal humerus, forearm, and wrist fractures in elderly men and women: The Dubbo Osteoporosis Epidemiology Study. *Am J Epidemiol*, 2001;153:587–95.
14. Nordvall H, Glanberg-Persson G, Lysholm J. Are distal radius fractures due to fragility or to falls? A consecutive case-control study of bone mineral density, tendency to fall, risk factors for osteoporosis, and health-related quality of life. *Acta Orthop*, 2007;78:271–7.
15. Ivers RQ, Cumming RG, Mitchell P, et al. Risk factors for fractures of the wrist, shoulder and ankle: The Blue Mountains Eye Study. *Osteoporos Int*, 2002;13:513–18.
16. Johnson PG, Szabo RM. Angle measurements of the distal radius: A cadaver study. *Skeletal Radiol*, 1993;22:243–6.
17. Cooney WP, Bussey R, Dobyns JH, et al. Difficult wrist fractures. Perilunate fracture-dislocations of the wrist. *Clin Orthop Relat Res*, 1987;(214):136–47.
18. Gartland JJ Jr., Werley CW. Evaluation of healed Colles' fractures. *J Bone Joint Surg Am*, 1951;33-A:895–907.
19. Green DP, O'Brien ET. Open reduction of carpal dislocations: Indications and operative techniques. *J Hand Surg Am*, 1978;3:250–65.

20. Souer JS, Lozano-Calderon SA, Ring D. Predictors of wrist function and health status after operative treatment of fractures of the distal radius. *J Hand Surg Am*, 2008;33:157–63.

21. Mackenney PJ, McQueen MM, Elton R. Prediction of instability in distal radial fractures. *J Bone Joint Surg Am*, 2006;88:1944–51.

22. Wadsten MA, Sayed-Noor AS, Englund E, et al. Cortical comminution in distal radial fractures can predict the radiological outcome: A cohort multicentre study. *Bone Joint J*, 2014;96-B:978–83.

23. McQueen MM, Hajducka C, Court-Brown CM. Redisplaced unstable fractures of the distal radius: A prospective randomised comparison of four methods of treatment. *J Bone Joint Surg Br*, 1996;78:404–9.

24. McQueen MM, MacLaren A, Chalmers J. The value of remanipulating Colles' fractures. *J Bone Joint Surg Br*, 1986;68:232–3.

25. Jaremko JL, Lambert RG, Rowe BH, et al. Do radiographic indices of distal radius fracture reduction predict outcomes in older adults receiving conservative treatment? *Clin Radiol*, 2007;62:65–72.

26. Young BT, Rayan GM. Outcome following nonoperative treatment of displaced distal radius fractures in low-demand patients older than 60 years. *J Hand Surg Am*, 2000;25:19–28.

27. Anzarut A, Johnson JA, Rowe BH, et al. Radiologic and patient-reported functional outcomes in an elderly cohort with conservatively treated distal radius fractures. *J Hand Surg Am*, 2004;29:1121–7.

28. Grewal R, MacDermid JC. The risk of adverse outcomes in extra-articular distal radius fractures is increased with malalignment in patients of all ages but mitigated in older patients. *J Hand Surg Am*, 2007;32:962–70.

29. Clement ND, Duckworth AD, Court-Brown CM, et al. Distal radial fractures in the superelderly: Does malunion affect functional outcome? *ISRN Orthop*, 2014;2014:189803.

30. Brogren E, Hofer M, Petranek M, et al. Relationship between distal radius fracture malunion and arm-related disability: A prospective population-based cohort study with 1-year follow-up. *BMC Musculoskelet Disord*, 2011;12:9.

31. Zenke Y, Sakai A, Oshige T, et al. The effect of an associated ulnar styloid fracture on the outcome after fixation of a fracture of the distal radius. *J Bone Joint Surg Br*, 2009;91:102–7.

32. McQueen M, Caspers J. Colles fracture: Does the anatomical result affect the final function? *J Bone Joint Surg Br*, 1988;70:649–51.

33. Gupta A, Batra S, Jain P, et al. Carpal alignment in distal radial fractures. *BMC Musculoskelet Disord*, 2002;3:14.

34. McQueen MM. Redisplaced unstable fractures of the distal radius. A randomised, prospective study of bridging versus non-bridging external fixation. *J Bone Joint Surg Br*, 1998;80:665–9.

35. Knirk J, Jupiter J. Intraarticular fractures of the distal end of the radius in young adults. *J Bone Joint Surg*, 1986;68A:647–59.

36. Forward DP, Davis TR, Sithole JS. Do young patients with malunited fractures of the distal radius inevitably develop symptomatic post-traumatic osteoarthritis? *J Bone Joint Surg Br*, 2008;90:629–37.

37. Ng CY, McQueen MM. What are the radiological predictors of functional outcome following fractures of the distal radius? *J Bone Joint Surg Br*, 2011;93:145–50.

38. Court-Brown CM, Aitken S, Hamilton TW, et al. Nonoperative fracture treatment in the modern era. *J Trauma*, 2010;69:699–707.

39. Fanuele J, Koval KJ, Lurie J, et al. Distal radial fracture treatment: What you get may depend on your age and address. *J Bone Joint Surg Am*, 2009;91:1313–19.

40. Chung KC, Shauver MJ, Birkmeyer JD. Trends in the United States in the treatment of distal radial fractures in the elderly. *J Bone Joint Surg Am*, 2009;91:1868–73.

41. Emmett JE, Breck LW. A review and analysis of 11,000 fractures seen in a private practice of orthopaedic surgery, 1937–1956. *J Bone Joint Surg Am*, 1958;40-A:1169–75.

42. Beumer A, McQueen MM. Fractures of the distal radius in low-demand elderly patients: Closed reduction of no value in 53 of 60 wrists. *Acta Orthop Scand*, 2003;74:98–100.

43. Abbaszadegan H, Jonsson U. Regional anesthesia preferable for Colles' fracture. Controlled comparison with local anesthesia. *Acta Orthop Scand*, 1990;61:348–9.

44. Cobb AG, Houghton GR. Local anaesthetic infiltration versus Bier's block for Colles' fractures. *Br Med J (Clin Res Ed)*, 1985;291:1683–4.

45. Bong MR, Egol KA, Leibman M, et al. A comparison of immediate postreduction splinting constructs for controlling initial displacement of fractures of the distal radius: A prospective randomized study of long-arm versus short-arm splinting. *J Hand Surg Am*, 2006;31:766–70.

46. Grafstein E, Stenstrom R, Christenson J, et al. A prospective randomized controlled trial comparing circumferential casting and splinting in displaced Colles fractures. *CJEM*, 2010;12:192–200.

47. Pool C. Colles's fracture. A prospective study of treatment. *J Bone Joint Surg Br*, 1973;55:540–4.

48. Stoffelen D, Broos P. Minimally displaced distal radius fractures: Do they need plaster treatment? *J Trauma*, 1998;44:503–5.

49. McAuliffe TB, Hilliar KM, Coates CJ, et al. Early mobilisation of Colles' fractures. A prospective trial. *J Bone Joint Surg Br*, 1987;69:727–9.

50. Foldhazy Z, Tornkvist H, Elmstedt E, et al. Long-term outcome of nonsurgically treated distal radius fractures. *J Hand Surg Am*, 2007;32:1374–84.

51. Synn AJ, Makhni EC, Makhni MC, et al. Distal radius fractures in older patients: Is anatomic reduction necessary? *Clin Orthop Relat Res*, 2009;467:1612–20.

52. Amorosa LF, Vitale MA, Brown S, et al. A functional outcomes survey of elderly patients who sustained distal radius fractures. *Hand (N Y)*, 2011;6:260–7.

53. Schmalholz A. Closed rereduction of axial compression in Colles' fracture is hardly possible. *Acta Orthop Scand*, 1989;60:57–9.

54. Hargreaves DG, Drew SJ, Eckersley R. Kirschner wire pin tract infection rates: A randomized controlled trial between percutaneous and buried wires. *J Hand Surg Br*, 2004;29:374–6.

55. Allain J, le Guilloux P, Le Mouël S, et al. Trans-styloid fixation of fractures of the distal radius. A prospective randomized comparison between 6- and 1-week postoperative immobilization in 60 fractures. *Acta Orthop Scand*, 1999;70:119–23.

56. Lenoble E, Dumontier C, Goutallier D, et al. Fracture of the distal radius. A prospective comparison between trans-styloid and Kapandji fixations. *J Bone Joint Surg Br*, 1995;77:562–7.

57. Strohm PC, Muller CA, Boll T, et al. Two procedures for Kirschner wire osteosynthesis of distal radial fractures. A randomized trial. *J Bone Joint Surg Am*, 2004;86-A:2621–8.

58. Brady O, Rice J, Nicholson P, et al. The unstable distal radial fracture one year post Kapandji intrafocal pinning. *Injury*, 1999;30:251–5.

59. Rodriguez-Merchan EC. Plaster cast versus percutaneous pin fixation for comminuted fractures of the distal radius in patients between 46 and 65 years of age. *J Orthop Trauma*, 1997;11:212–17.

60. Hayes AJ, Duffy PJ, McQueen MM. Bridging and non-bridging external fixation in the treatment of unstable fractures of the distal radius: A retrospective study of 588 patients. *Acta Orthop*, 2008;79:540–7.

61. Abramo A, Kopylov P, Geijer M, et al. Open reduction and internal fixation compared to closed reduction and external fixation in distal radial fractures: A randomized study of 50 patients. *Acta Orthop*, 2009;80:478–85.

62. Atroshi I, Brogren E, Larsson GU, et al. Wrist-bridging versus non-bridging external fixation for displaced distal radius fractures: A randomized assessor-blind clinical trial of 38 patients followed for 1 year. *Acta Orthop*, 2006;77:445–53.

63. Egol KA, Paksima N, Puopolo S, et al. Treatment of external fixation pins about the wrist: A prospective, randomized trial. *J Bone Joint Surg Am*, 2006;88:349–54.

64. Flinkkila T, Ristiniemi J, Hyvonen P, et al. Nonbridging external fixation in the treatment of unstable fractures of the distal forearm. *Arch Orthop Trauma Surg*, 2003;123:349–52.

65. Hove LM, Krukhaug Y, Revheim K, et al. Dynamic compared with static external fixation of unstable fractures of the distal part of the radius: A prospective, randomized multicenter study. *J Bone Joint Surg Am*, 2010;92:1687–96.

66. Krukhaug Y, Ugland S, Lie SA, et al. External fixation of fractures of the distal radius: A randomized comparison of the Hoffman compact II non-bridging fixator and the Dynawrist fixator in 75 patients followed for 1 year. *Acta Orthop*, 2009;80:104–8.

67. Westphal T, Piatek S, Schubert S, et al. Outcome after surgery of distal radius fractures: No differences between external fixation and ORIF. *Arch Orthop Trauma Surg*, 2005;125:507–14.

68. Wilcke MK, Abbaszadegan H, Adolphson PY. Wrist function recovers more rapidly after volar locked plating than after external fixation but the outcomes are similar after 1 year. *Acta Orthop*, 2011;82:76–81.

69. Andersen JK, Hogh A, Gantov J, et al. Colles' fracture treated with non-bridging external fixation: A 1-year follow-up. *J Hand Surg Eur Vol*, 2009;34:475–8.

70. Ahlborg HG, Josefsson PO. Pin-tract complications in external fixation of fractures of the distal radius. *Acta Orthop Scand*, 1999;70:116–18.

71. Grewal R, MacDermid JC, King GJ, et al. Open reduction internal fixation versus percutaneous pinning with external fixation of distal radius fractures: A prospective, randomized clinical trial. *J Hand Surg Am*, 2011;36:1899–906.

72. Jeudy J, Steiger V, Boyer P, et al. Treatment of complex fractures of the distal radius: A prospective randomised comparison of external fixation 'versus' locked volar plating. *Injury*, 2012;43:174–9.

73. Wei DH, Raizman NM, Bottino CJ, et al. Unstable distal radial fractures treated with external fixation, a radial column plate, or a volar plate. A prospective randomized trial. *J Bone Joint Surg Am*, 2009;91:1568–77.

74. Capo JT, Rossy W, Henry P, et al. External fixation of distal radius fractures: Effect of distraction and duration. *J Hand Surg Am*, 2009;34:1605–11.

75. Knight D, Hajducka C, Will E, et al. Locked volar plating for unstable distal radial fractures: Clinical and radiological outcomes. *Injury*, 2010;41:184–9.

76. Arora R, Lutz M, Deml C, et al. A prospective randomized trial comparing nonoperative treatment with volar locking plate fixation for displaced and unstable distal radial fractures in patients sixty-five years of age and older. *J Bone Joint Surg Am*, 2011;93:2146–53.

77. Egol K, Walsh M, Tejwani N, et al. Bridging external fixation and supplementary Kirschner-wire fixation versus volar locked plating for unstable fractures of the distal radius: A randomised, prospective trial. *J Bone Joint Surg Br*, 2008;90:1214–21.

78. Gradl G, Gradl G, Wendt M, et al. Non-bridging external fixation employing multiplanar K-wires versus volar locked plating for dorsally displaced fractures of the distal radius. *Arch Orthop Trauma Surg*, 2013;133:595–602.

79. Sahu A, Charalambous CP, Mills SP, et al. Reoperation for metalwork complications following the use of volar locking plates for distal radius fractures: A United Kingdom experience. *Hand Surg*, 2011;16:113–18.

80. Drobetz H, Kutscha-Lissberg E. Osteosynthesis of distal radial fractures with a volar locking screw plate system. *Int Orthop*, 2003;27:1–6.

81. Rozental TD, Blazar PE. Functional outcome and complications after volar plating for dorsally displaced, unstable fractures of the distal radius. *J Hand Surg Am*, 2006;31:359–65.

82. Arora R, Lutz M, Zimmermann R, et al. [Limits of palmar locking-plate osteosynthesis of unstable distal radius fractures]. *Handchir Mikrochir Plast Chir*, 2007;39:34–41.

83. White BD, Nydick JA, Karsky D, et al. Incidence and clinical outcomes of tendon rupture following distal radius fracture. *J Hand Surg Am*, 2012;37:2035–40.

84. Kennedy C, Kennedy MT, Niall D, et al. Radiological outcomes of distal radius extra-articular fragility fractures treated with extra-focal kirschner wires. *Injury*, 2010;41:639–42.

85. Oskam J, Kingma J, Bart J, et al. K-wire fixation for redislocated Colles' fractures. Malunion in 8/21 cases. *Acta Orthop Scand*, 1997;68:259–61.

86. Wilcke MK, Abbaszadegan H, Adolphson PY. Patient-perceived outcome after displaced distal radius fractures. A comparison between radiological parameters, objective physical variables, and the DASH score. *J Hand Ther*, 2007;20:290–8.

87. Dicpinigaitis P, Wolinsky P, Hiebert R, et al. Can external fixation maintain reduction after distal radius fractures? *J Trauma*, 2004;57:845–50.

88. Lin C, Sun JS, Hou SM. External fixation with or without supplementary intramedullary Kirschner wires in the treatment of distal radial fractures. *Can J Surg*, 2004;47:431–7.

89. McQueen MM, Simpson D, Court-Brown CM. Use of the Hoffman 2 compact external fixator in the treatment of redisplaced unstable distal radial fractures. *J Orthop Trauma*, 1999;13:501–5.

90. Chung KC, Squitieri L, Kim HM. Comparative outcomes study using the volar locking plating system for distal radius fractures in both young adults and adults older than 60 years. *J Hand Surg Am*, 2008;33:809–19.

91. Figl M, Weninger P, Liska M, et al. Volar fixed-angle plate osteosynthesis of unstable distal radius fractures: 12 months results. *Arch Orthop Trauma Surg*, 2009;129:661–9.

92. Stoffelen DV, Broos PL. Kapandji pinning or closed reduction for extra-articular distal radius fractures. *J Trauma*, 1998;45:753–7.

93. Azzopardi T, Ehrendorfer S, Coulton T, et al. Unstable extra-articular fractures of the distal radius: A prospective, randomised study of immobilisation in a cast versus supplementary percutaneous pinning. *J Bone Joint Surg Br*, 2005;87:837–40.

94. Wong TC, Chiu Y, Tsang WL, et al. Casting versus percutaneous pinning for extra-articular fractures of the distal radius in an elderly Chinese population: A prospective randomised controlled trial. *J Hand Surg Eur Vol*, 2010;35:202–8.

95. Aktekin CN, Altay M, Gursoy Z, et al. Comparison between external fixation and cast treatment in the management of distal radius fractures in patients aged 65 years and older. *J Hand Surg Am*, 2010;35:736–42.

96. Christensen OM, Christiansen TC, Krasheninnikoff M, et al. Plaster cast compared with bridging external fixation for distal radius fractures of the Colles' type. *Int Orthop*, 2001;24:358–60.

97. Horne JG, Devane P, Purdie G. A prospective randomized trial of external fixation and plaster cast immobilization in the treatment of distal radial fractures. *J Orthop Trauma*, 1990;4:30–4.

98. Kreder HJ, Agel J, McKee MD, et al. A randomized, controlled trial of distal radius fractures with metaphyseal displacement but without joint incongruity: Closed reduction and casting versus closed reduction, spanning external fixation, and optional percutaneous K-wires. *J Orthop Trauma*, 2006;20:115–21.

99. Jenkins NH, Jones DG, Johnson SR, et al. External fixation of Colles' fractures. An anatomical study. *J Bone Joint Surg Br*, 1987;69:207–11.

100. Jenkins NH, Jones DG, Mintowt-Czyz WJ. External fixation and recovery of function following fractures of the distal radius in young adults. *Injury*, 1988;19:235–8.

101. Ludvigsen TC, Johansen S, Svenningsen S. [Unstable fractures of the distal radius. External fixation or percutaneous pinning?]. *Tidsskr Nor Laegeforen*, 1996;116:3093–7.

102. Harley BJ, Scharfenberger A, Beaupre LA, et al. Augmented external fixation versus percutaneous pinning and casting for unstable fractures of the distal radius—A prospective randomized trial. *J Hand Surg Am*, 2004;29:815–24.

103. Franck WM, Dahlen C, Amlang M, et al. [Distal radius fracture—Is non-bridging articular external fixator a therapeutic alternative? A prospective randomized study]. *Unfallchirurg*, 2000;103:826–33.

104. Lee YS, Wei TY, Cheng YC, et al. A comparative study of Colles' fractures in patients between fifty and seventy years of age: Percutaneous K-wiring versus volar locking plating. *Int Orthop*, 2012;36:789–94.

105. Oshige T, Sakai A, Zenke Y, et al. A comparative study of clinical and radiological outcomes of dorsally angulated, unstable distal radius fractures in elderly patients: Intrafocal pinning versus volar locking plating. *J Hand Surg Am*, 2007;32:1385–92.

106. Marcheix PS, Dotzis A, Benko PE, et al. Extension fractures of the distal radius in patients older than 50: A prospective randomized study comparing fixation using mixed pins or a palmar fixed-angle plate. *J Hand Surg Eur Vol*, 2010;35:646–51.

107. Rozental TD, Blazar PE, Franko OI, et al. Functional outcomes for unstable distal radial fractures treated with open reduction and internal fixation or closed reduction and percutaneous fixation. A prospective randomized trial. *J Bone Joint Surg Am*, 2009;91:1837–46.

108. Costa ML, Achten J, Parsons NR, et al. Percutaneous fixation with Kirschner wires versus volar locking plate fixation in adults with dorsally displaced fracture of distal radius: Randomised controlled trial. *BMJ*, 2014;349:g4807.

109. Landgren M, Jerrhag D, Tagil M, et al. External or internal fixation in the treatment of non-reducible distal radial fractures? *Acta Orthop*, 2011;82:610–13.

110. Esposito J, Schemitsch EH, Saccone M, et al. External fixation versus open reduction with plate fixation for distal radius fractures: A meta-analysis of randomised controlled trials. *Injury*, 2013;44:409–16.

111. Uchikura C, Hirano J, Kudo F, et al. Comparative study of nonbridging and bridging external fixators for unstable distal radius fractures. *J Orthop Sci*, 2004;9:560–5.

112. Bini A, Surace MF, Pilato G. Complex articular fractures of the distal radius: The role of closed reduction and external fixation. *J Hand Surg Eur Vol*, 2008;33:305–10.

113. Gavaskar AS, Muthukumar S, Chowdary N. Fragment-specific fixation for complex intra-articular fractures of the distal radius: Results of a prospective single-centre trial. *J Hand Surg Eur Vol*, 2012;37:765–71.

114. Konstantinidis L, Helwig P, Strohm PC, et al. Clinical and radiological outcomes after stabilisation of complex intra-articular fractures of the distal radius with the volar 2.4 mm LCP. *Arch Orthop Trauma Surg*, 2010;130:751–7.

115. Kreder HJ, Hanel DP, Agel J, et al. Indirect reduction and percutaneous fixation versus open reduction and internal fixation for displaced intra-articular fractures of the distal radius: A randomised, controlled trial. *J Bone Joint Surg Br*, 2005;87:829–36.

116. Richard MJ, Katolik LI, Hanel DP, et al. Distraction plating for the treatment of highly comminuted distal radius fractures in elderly patients. *J Hand Surg Am*, 2012;37:948–56.

117. Keating JF, Court-Brown CM, McQueen MM. Internal fixation of volar-displaced distal radial fractures. *J Bone Joint Surg Br*, 1994;76:401–5.

118. Jupiter JB, Fernandez DL, Toh CL, et al. Operative treatment of volar intra-articular fractures of the distal end of the radius. *J Bone Joint Surg Am*, 1996;78:1817–28.

119. Souer JS, Ring D, Jupiter JB, et al. Comparison of AO Type-B and Type-C volar shearing fractures of the distal part of the radius. *J Bone Joint Surg Am*, 2009;91:2605–11.

120. Bolmers A, Luiten WE, Doornberg JN, et al. A comparison of the long-term outcome of partial articular (AO Type B) and complete articular (AO Type C) distal radius fractures. *J Hand Surg Am*, 2013;38:753–9.

121. Cha SM, Shin HD, Kim KC, et al. Treatment of unstable distal ulna fractures associated with distal radius fractures in patients 65 years and older. *J Hand Surg Am*, 2012;37:2481–7.

122. Namba J, Fujiwara T, Murase T, et al. Intra-articular distal ulnar fractures associated with distal radial fractures in older adults: Early experience in fixation of the radius and leaving the ulna unfixed. *J Hand Surg Eur Vol*, 2009;34:592–7.

123. Buijze GA, Ring D. Clinical impact of united versus nonunited fractures of the proximal half of the ulnar styloid following volar plate fixation of the distal radius. *J Hand Surg Am*, 2010;35:223–7.

124. Kim JK, Koh YD, Do NH. Should an ulnar styloid fracture be fixed following volar plate fixation of a distal radial fracture? *J Bone Joint Surg Am*, 2010;92:1–6.

125. Diaz-Garcia RJ, Oda T, Shauver MJ, et al. A systematic review of outcomes and complications of treating unstable distal radius fractures in the elderly. *J Hand Surg Am*, 2011;36:824–35.

126. McKay SD, MacDermid JC, Roth JH, et al. Assessment of complications of distal radius fractures and development of a complication checklist. *J Hand Surg Am*, 2001;26:916–22.

127. Aro H, Koivunen T, Katevuo K, et al. Late compression neuropathies after Colles' fractures. *Clin Orthop Relat Res*, 1988;(233):217–25.

128. Stewart HD, Innes AR, Burke FD. The hand complications of Colles' fractures. *J Hand Surg Br*, 1985;10:103–6.

129. Bacorn RW, Kurtzke JF. Colles' fracture; a study of two thousand cases from the New York State Workmen's Compensation Board. *J Bone Joint Surg Am*, 1953;35-A:643–58.

130. Roth KM, Blazar PE, Earp BE, et al. Incidence of extensor pollicis longus tendon rupture after non-displaced distal radius fractures. *J Hand Surg Am*, 2012;37:942–7.

131. McQueen MM, Wakefield A. Distal radial osteotomy for malunion using non-bridging external fixation: Good results in 23 patients. *Acta Orthop,* 2008;79:390–5.

132. Buijze GA, Prommersberger KJ, Gonzalez del Pino J, et al. Corrective osteotomy for combined intra- and extra-articular distal radius malunion. *J Hand Surg Am,* 2012;37:2041–9.

133. Flinkkila T, Raatikainen T, Kaarela O, et al. Corrective osteotomy for malunion of the distal radius. *Arch Orthop Trauma Surg,* 2000;120:23–6.

134. Lozano-Calderon SA, Brouwer KM, Doornberg JN, et al. Long-term outcomes of corrective osteotomy for the treatment of distal radius malunion. *J Hand Surg Eur Vol,* 2010;35:370–80.

135. Jupiter JB, Ring D. A comparison of early and late reconstruction of malunited fractures of the distal end of the radius. *J Bone Joint Surg Am,* 1996;78:739–48.

136. Thivaios GC, McKee MD. Sliding osteotomy for deformity correction following malunion of volarly displaced distal radial fractures. *J Orthop Trauma,* 2003;17:326–33.

137. Shea K, Fernandez DL, Jupiter JB, et al. Corrective osteotomy for malunited, volarly displaced fractures of the distal end of the radius. *J Bone Joint Surg Am,* 1997;79:1816–26.

138. Gaebler C, McQueen MM. Ulnar procedures for post-traumatic disorders of the distal radioulnar joint. *Injury,* 2003;34:47–59.

27

Carpal fractures and dislocations

ANDREW D. DUCKWORTH

INTRODUCTION

There is a dearth of literature relating to carpal fractures and dislocations in the elderly patient. This is to be expected, given that the vast majority of carpal injuries occur in a young and active population. The diagnosis of carpal injuries can be challenging in all patients, irrespective of age, with the diagnosis of suspected scaphoid fractures a continuing dilemma despite the various advanced imaging modalities now available. The diagnosis and management of carpal injuries in the elderly patient can be particularly challenging. Degenerative changes may potentially mask acute pathology and the demands of the patient are different to those of the younger population who normally present with these injuries.

The most common injury of the carpus is a fracture of the scaphoid. Although there are advocates for percutaneous fixation over casting for non- and minimally displaced scaphoid waist fractures in the younger patient, there is no evidence to suggest that this would be of benefit in the elderly population. Given the potential issues with carpal instability and non-union, displaced fractures and proximal pole fractures routinely require operative intervention. One of the most devastating carpal injuries is a perilunate dislocation or fracture-dislocation. Again, these are rare in the elderly and operative intervention is routinely necessary to try and regain wrist function and prevent disability.

The elderly patient will potentially attend with the chronic sequelae of a previous carpal injury, for example, the scaphoid non-union advanced collapse (SNAC) wrist. The management options in this situation can be difficult, as the customary treatment in the younger patient may not be appropriate or necessary in the elderly.

EPIDEMIOLOGY

There is limited literature documenting the epidemiology of all carpal injuries, with most of the data related to the epidemiology of scaphoid fractures. The literature consistently suggests that carpal fractures account for 2–3% of all fractures with an incidence of 37.5 per 100,000 adult individuals per year.[1,2] The overall mean age ranges from 35 to 40 years with a male predominance.[3-5] Data from Edinburgh suggest carpal fractures have a type A fracture curve with a bimodal distribution of younger males and older females.[2] Only 7.7% of carpal fractures occur at ≥65 years of age and 1.5% in those ≥80 years of age.[2] Alsawadi and Stanton reviewed the available epidemiological literature to determine the characteristics of scaphoid fractures in patients over 70 years of age and found the incidence in the literature ranged from 0.2 to 14 per 100,000 adult individuals per year.[6] Previously published data from Edinburgh found there were 9 (total 151) fractures in patients over 70 years of age with an incidence of 12.9 per 100,000 adult individuals per year (Figure 27.1).[7]

Scaphoid and triquetral fractures make up more than 90% of all fractures of the carpus.[3-5] Triquetral fractures are the second most common carpal fracture[3-5] and commonly occur in an older population, with a mean age of 51 years and a type A fracture distribution curve. Fractures of the scaphoid, trapezium, hamate and pisiform occur at a mean age ranging from 29 to 43 years, the male predominance is 66–100% and a type B fracture distribution curve is seen (unimodal younger male).[2] Studies have found that risk factors for a scaphoid fracture are youth and male gender.[5,7,8]

Hey et al. reported that 7% of patients sustain multiple carpal fractures, with almost 50% a perilunate fracture-dislocation.[5] Fracture-dislocations are twice as common as a perilunate dislocation and displace dorsally in 97% of cases.[9] Data from Edinburgh reported that perilunate dislocations have an incidence of 0.5 per 100,000 adult individuals per year, with a male predominance and occur in the younger patient with a mean age of 26 years.[10] None were found in those ≥65 years of age. Open carpal fractures are known to be very rare.[5,11]

Mechanism of injury

Carpal fractures and dislocations are routinely secondary to an axial compression force to the wrist that results in hyperextension, causing shear forces across the dorsal structures and exerting tension to the palmar wrist structures.[12–14] A fall from standing height onto the outstretched hand

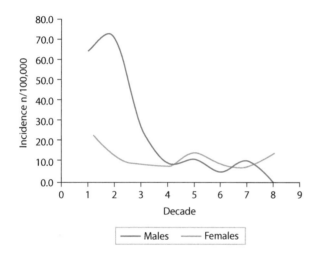

Figure 27.1 The incidence of scaphoid fractures in Edinburgh, 2007–2008. (Adapted from Duckworth AD, et al. *J Trauma Acute Care Surg* 2012;72(2):E41–5.)

accounts for almost two-thirds of all injuries, with high energy mechanisms less common and more frequently seen in males, e.g. sports, assault and motor vehicle collision.[3–5] As would be expected, high energy injuries are a risk factor for sustaining an associated injury with a carpal fracture, for example, a perilunate dislocation or fracture-dislocation.[5,7] Hook of hamate fractures occur with racket sports and golf related injuries, while body or coronal fractures often occur in young men following a punch injury.[15,16] It is proposed that carpal instability results from a high energy force to the wrist associated with hyperextension, ulnar deviation and intercarpal supination.[12,17]

CLASSIFICATION

Scaphoid fractures

Although there are numerous classifications for a fracture of the scaphoid, a constant criticism is that there is a lack of consideration given to the significant associated soft tissue injuries potentially seen. Furthermore, it is unknown whether these classifications are applicable to the assessment and management of the elderly patient.

One of the most commonly employed classifications within the literature is the Herbert and Fisher classification (Table 27.1),[18] which aims to identify the fracture types that require fixation. Other classifications include the:

- AO/OTA classification,[19,20] which divides fractures into location (distal pole, waist, proximal pole) and comminution
- Russe classification,[21] which uses the inclination of the fracture line to guide the risk of fracture instability
- Mayo classification,[22,23] which sets out criteria aimed at predicting instability and guiding management and includes fracture malalignment, >1 mm of fracture

Table 27.1 The Herbert and Fisher scaphoid fracture classification

Type	Prevalence (%)[7]	General comments
Type A: stable acute fractures	31.1	High union rate
A1 (tuberosity)	14.6	Non-operative management
A2 (unicortical waist)	16.5	
Type B: unstable acute fractures	68.9	Most common type
B1 (distal oblique/pole)	21.2	Bicortical fractures that are unstable
B2 (complete waist)	36.4	Common in younger patients and following a high energy injury
B3 (proximal pole)	6	
B4 (trans-scaphoid PLFD)	2	Operative management likely required
B5 (comminuted)	3.3	
Type C: Delayed union	Unclear	
Type D: Non-union	Unclear	
D1 (fibrous)		
D2 (sclerotic)		

Source: Adapted from Duckworth AD, Ring D. Carpus fractures and dislocations (Table 31.10). In: Tornetta P, Court-Brown CM, Heckman JD, McKee M, McQueen MM, Ricci WM, *Rockwood and Green's Fractures in Adults.* 8th ed. Philadelphia, PA: Lippincott Williams & Wilkins; 2014. pp. 991–1056.
Note: PLFD, perilunate fracture-dislocation.

displacement,[24,25] proximal pole fracture, perilunate fracture-dislocation, bone loss and/or comminution, a lateral intrascaphoid angle of >35 degrees and/or a dorsal intercalated segment instability (DISI) deformity.[26]

SCAPHOID NON-UNION

The Herbert and Fisher classification (Table 27.1)[18] defines two types of scaphoid non-union:

1. Type D1: fibrous non-union, often with minimal deformity, symptoms and signs variable, risk of wrist arthritis small
2. Type D2: established sclerotic non-union, unstable, progressive (often humpback) deformity leading to SNAC.[27]

Lunate fractures and Kienböck's disease

Acute fractures of the lunate were classified into five groups by Teisen and Hjarback[28] according to the involvement of the palmar or dorsal pole, the body of the lunate and the character of the fracture, for example, horn avulsion, transverse, frontal or transarticular. Avulsion fractures frequently occur in the radial corner and body fractures are frequently transverse in the coronal plane.

Kienböck's disease is the idiopathic avascular necrosis (AVN) of the lunate,[29,30] which can sometimes be mistaken for a fracture on radiographs. Some have suggested that neglected lunate fractures[29,30] or ischaemia following a perilunate dislocation or fracture-dislocation[26] result in Kienböck's, while others postulate that venous congestion is responsible.[31] The Lichtman classification divides Kienböck's disease into four stages with an aim to help guide treatment[32]:

1. No changes on plain radiographs
2. Increased density of the lunate
3. Lunate collapse ± fragmentation (subdivided according to position of scaphoid)
4. Radiocarpal arthritis

Carpal ligament injuries

The three systems commonly used for describing carpal instability are inherently related and can be useful in understanding the mechanism of injury and the treatment necessary. They can involve purely ligamentous, or ligamentous and bony pathologies. The three systems are:

1. Intercalated segment instability[33,34] was originally described by Linscheid et al.[33] and this system is based on the position of the lunate and related intercalated segment on standard lateral radiographs of the wrist:
   a. DISI with lunate extension and capitate displacement dorsally:
      i. Scapholunate angle >60 degrees, capitolunate and radiolunate angle >15 degrees

ii. Causes – Scapholunate dissociation (SLD) and displaced scaphoid fractures
   b. Volar intercalated segment instability (VISI) with lunate flexion and capitate displacement volarly (less common):
      i. Scapholunate angle <30 degrees, capitolunate angle >30 degrees and radiolunate angle >15 degrees in volar direction
      ii. Causes – Lunotriquetral dissociation and complex multi-ligamentous disruption
2. Static versus dynamic[35]:
   a. Static: Carpal instability is apparent on standard non-stressed radiographs of the wrist and is associated with multiple ligament disruption.
   b. Dynamic: Carpal instability is apparent on stress testing and stress radiographs, with normal routine radiographs.
3. Dissociative versus non-dissociative (can be combined):
   a. Dissociative instability results from an isolated injury to a major intrinsic ligament of the carpus, for example, scapholunate disruption or scaphoid fracture.[36–38]
   b. Non-dissociative instability occurs when there is an injury between the carpal rows, that is, extrinsic ligament injury, for example, radiocarpal instability, Barton fracture-dislocation.[38]

SCAPHOLUNATE DISSOCIATION

SLD is the most common carpal ligament injury and involves a range of injuries to the scapholunate interosseous ligament, from simple sprains to scaphoid dislocation. Injury to the ligament results in dyskinesia between the scaphoid and lunate articulation, leading to progressive widening of the joint over time.[39] Any classification system for SLD needs to consider the chronicity of the injury and whether it is a static or dynamic instability. Static scapholunate instability is often defined as the characteristic increase in the scapholunate gap and a scapholunate angle of greater than 60 degrees in a non-loaded wrist.[40] Geissler et al. classified four grades of ligament injury based upon arthroscopic assessment[41]:

1. Ligament in continuity with normal carpal alignment but attenuated (midcarpal space) – non-operative management
2. Carpal malalignment (midcarpal space) – arthroscopic reduction and fixation
3. Carpal malalignment (both carpal spaces) with a 1 mm (probe) gap between bones – arthroscopy ± open reduction and fixation
4. Carpal malalignment (both carpal spaces), unstable with 2.7 mm scope passable between bones – open reduction internal fixation (ORIF)

An alternative classification by Kuo and Wolfe[42,43] classifies the disruption into occult, dynamic, complete SLD, DISI deformity and a SLAC (scapholunate advanced collapse) wrist with an aim to guide management.

LUNATOTRIQUETRAL DISSOCIATION

Lunatotriquetral dissociation (LTD) is often stable and is less common than SLD.[44] It includes:

- Ligament sprains
- Partial or complete ligament injury
- Part of perilunate injury
- Ulnocarpal impingement
- Triangular fibrocartilage complex (TFCC) injury

Although LTD is not normally associated with degenerative changes over time, carpal kinematics are affected and a VISI deformity can occur, with chronic ulnar-sided wrist pain a cause of notable disability.[45] It has been suggested that concomitant injury to the dorsal radiotriquetral ligament or palmar ulnocarpal ligaments needs to occur before a severe fixed deformity results.[46]

PERILUNATE DISLOCATIONS AND FRACTURE-DISLOCATIONS

These rare but devastating injuries are commonly classified according to the Mayfield classification and in terms of the greater (fracture-dislocation) or lesser (dislocation) arc injury patterns,[12,17,47] with a dorsal trans-scaphoid perilunate fracture-dislocation most common.[9,48,49] Lesser-arc perilunate dislocations are a pure ligamentous disruption around the lunate, while a greater-arc injury involves ligamentous injuries with an associated fracture of one or more of the bones around the lunate. Injury to the ligaments around the lunate normally starts radially and propagates to the ulnar side, with the distal row displaced in a dorsal or dorso-radial direction.[26] Alternate classifications are the Witvoet and Allieu[50] and Herzberg et al.[9] classification systems. The Mayfield classification breaks the injury down into four stages according to the carpal keystone (the lunate)[12,51]:

1. Scaphoid fracture and/or SLD
2. Lunocapitate disruption
3. Lunotriquetral disruption
4. Perilunate dislocation

ANATOMICAL CONSIDERATIONS

Two rows of eight bones make up the carpus, with the proximal row including the scaphoid, lunate and triquetrum. The distal row is made up of the trapezium, trapezoid, capitate, hamate and pisiform. The proximal carpal row is known as the key intercalated segment, bridging between the bones of the forearm and the distal row of the carpus and the metacarpals[33,52-54] which delivers movement, congruency and force transmission at the wrist joint.[26,55,56] The intrinsic and extrinsic ligaments of the wrist are essential to allowing a degree of movement while maintaining stability.[35,55,56] The intrinsic ligaments connect individual carpal bones to one another, while

the extrinsic ligaments connect the carpal bones to the forearm bones and the metacarpals.[26] Defining these ligaments can be difficult clinically as they often merge with the articular surface and capsule of the wrist, and a recent review of 58 anatomical studies found that all but one of the carpal ligaments are not described consistently.[57]

The oval ring theory[53,58] considers the proximal intercalated segment, the variable geometry of the carpus with the lunate at the keystone that is anchored by interosseous ligaments to the scaphoid (radially) and triquetrum (ulnarly),[33,52-54,59] along with the synchronous and reciprocating motion of the proximal and distal rows.[26] The older and alternative columnar theory first put forward by Navarro breaks the carpus into radial (scaphoid, trapezium and trapezoid), central (lunate, capitate and hamate) and ulnar (triquetrum and pisiform) columns.[60] Although this concept aids with the understanding of load transmission in the wrist, it is limited when considering the concept of synchronous motion.[26]

Neurovascular supply

The carpus is innervated by the anterior and posterior interosseous nerves, with the blood supply coming from intraosseous and extraosseous vessels from the dorsal and palmar vascular systems.[61,62] An understanding of the vasculature of the carpus is essential when considering the risks of non-union and AVN, particularly when attempting to preserve the blood supply during surgical approaches to the wrist. As the blood supply to the carpus is thought to enter distally, this leaves the proximal carpal row vulnerable to an interruption of blood supply and potentially AVN.[61,62] The risk of AVN is increased due to the single vessel supply of the scaphoid, capitate and 20% of the lunate, while the trapezoid and about half of all hamates do not have an intraosseous anastomosis.[61-63,26] The risk of scaphoid AVN and non-union is associated with the predominantly retrograde blood supply from soft tissue attachments that supply two vascular pedicles originating from the scaphoid branches of the radial artery.[26,61,64] Although the vasculature to the lunate is potentially compromised when performing a dorsal approach to the wrist, this is limited by the concurrent supply from the palmar radiocarpal arch.[26]

Operative anatomy: scaphoid

The scaphoid is located within the wrist joint at a 45-degree angle to the longitudinal and horizontal axes of the wrist.[26] The ligamentous attachments are primarily found on the non-articular dorso-radial surface.[26,57,65] For the volar approach to the scaphoid, an incision is made in line with the flexor carpi radialis (FCR) tendon from proximal to the scaphoid and extending approximately 5 cm across the transverse wrist crease to just distal to the distal pole of the scaphoid and is about 5 cm in length.[26] The FCR is mobilized in an ulnar direction and the superficial radial artery is retracted. The wrist capsule should now be visible and is cut along the line of the scaphoid, with care taken to preserve as much of the radioscaphocapitate ligament as possible.

An open dorsal approach to the scaphoid is normally used for fractures of the proximal pole[66] and utilizes a straight 3–4 cm incision over the dorsum of the wrist at the level of the scapholunate.[26] The extensor pollicis longus (EPL) is normally left alone and the dorsal wrist capsule is then incised, with care taken throughout to preserve the dorsal ridge vasculature.

CLINICAL ASSESSMENT

A clear history is important when assessing carpal injuries as untreated fractures can present late with an established non-union, particularly with regard to the scaphoid. Wrist pain is the primary presenting feature of carpal fractures and dislocations. It is noted that the most reliable sign of carpal injury is well-localized tenderness, for example, injury to the scaphoid often presents with radial sided wrist pain and tenderness in the anatomical snuffbox (ASB).[26,67] Associated swelling and ecchymosis of the carpus, with a reduced range of movement, is sometimes found in the acute phase following injury. A general guide suggests ligament injuries can be acute (within a month of injury), subacute (1–6 months after injury) or chronic (>6 months after injury) and is important when considering treatment options.

Injuries associated with carpal instability and/or dislocation may present with an obvious deformity to the wrist. Other potential signs of ligament instability include an audible click or clunk on moving/stressing the wrist and diminished strength with repetitive grip strength testing.[26] Assessment of the contralateral wrist can be helpful, particularly in elderly patients who present with long-standing problems associated with instability. Although associated with poor diagnostic performance characteristics due to their infrequency, Table 27.2 presents some of the special tests that can be used in the diagnosis of carpal ligament injuries.

Although open injuries are exceedingly rare, assessment of the skin should always be carried out in the elderly patient. Distal neurovascular status should be assessed and documented, which is of particular importance following a dislocation or fracture-dislocation to the carpus. Anything from 15–50% of perilunate injuries will have symptoms and signs of median neuropathy,[69] although ulnar neuropathy, arterial injury and/or tendon injury do occur.[9,48] In the elderly patient, chronic presentations may be seen and these will likely present with increasing problems with nerve compression or tendon rupture.[70] Tendon ruptures can also occur with a chronic presentation of a hamate fracture, for example, little finger flexor,[71,72] while a lesion of the deep branch of the ulnar nerve can occur following a hook of hamate fracture or pisiform fracture.[15,73,74]

Scaphoid fractures

There continue to be numerous studies analysing the diagnostic performance characteristics of the various clinical signs employed in the diagnosis of scaphoid fractures, as no single sign has been reported to be sufficiently sensitive and specific.[26,75,76] The literature initially reported the diagnostic performance characteristics of individual clinical signs,[77] as well as subsequently documenting the change in these characteristics when clinical signs are combined.[75] Mallee et al. reported the results of a systematic review and meta-analysis of 13 studies analysing 25 different clinical tests for a suspected fracture of the scaphoid and found that ASB tenderness was the most sensitive of the clinical signs but with poor specificity that results in the over-treatment of a number of patients.[78] Other high-sensitivity tests were axial compression of the thumb, scaphoid tubercle tenderness and ASB pain on ulnar deviation of the wrist (Table 27.3). There are an insufficient number of scaphoid fractures in the elderly to determine if comparable results would be found in the older population.

Recent studies have attempted to develop clinical prediction rules combing demographic and clinical

Table 27.2 Clinical signs used in the detection of carpal fractures and carpal instability

Condition and signs	Description
Scapholunate	
Scaphoid shift test	Pressure to scaphoid tubercle with wrist moving in ulnar-radial deviation, a clunk will be found with subluxation of the scaphoid from the fossa. Positive in up to 30% of uninjured wrists (low specificity).[68]
Lunotriquetral	
Ballottement test	Fix lunate with one hand and displace triquetram in the volar-dorsal plane with the other hand, with pain experienced indicative of instability or osteoarthritis.
Shear test	Dorsal pressure is applied over the pisiform and palmar pressure over the lunate, with pain and possibly clicking/crepitus found if there is instability. Most sensitive test for lunotriquetral disruption.
Midcarpal	
Midcarpal shift test	Dorsal pressure to the capitate with wrist moving in ulnar-radial deviation, a clunk will be found with reduction of the lunate.

Table 27.3 The sensitivity and specificity for various clinical signs as determined by Mallee et al. for suspected fractures of the scaphoid

Clinical sign	Studies (n)	Patients (n)	Sensitivity (%)	Specificity (%)
Anatomical snuffbox tenderness	8	1164	87–100	3–98
Axial compression of the thumb	8	961	48–100	22–97
Scaphoid tubercle tenderness	4	879	82–100	17–57
Pain on ulnar deviation	4	394	67–100	17–60
Pain on radial deviation	3	316	67–90	31–42
Reduced range of movement of the thumb	2	412	65–66	38–59
Thumb–index finger pinch	2	264	75–79	44–76

Source: Adapted from Mallee WH, et al., J Hand Surg Am 2014;39(9):1683–91, Table 2.

characteristics predictive of a true fracture.[79,80] A recent large prospective study of 223 confirmed and suspected scaphoid fractures reported that that the strongest predictor of a true scaphoid fracture within 72 hours of injury was the absence of ASB pain on ulnar deviation of the wrist and pain on thumb–index finger pinch, with scaphoid tubercle tenderness most predictive at approximately 2 weeks post injury.[80]

IMAGING

Standard four view radiographs of the scaphoid will identify the vast majority of carpal injuries and static instability of the wrist.[81,82] These are:

- Neutral posteroanterior (PA)
- Lateral
- 45-Degree radial oblique (supinated anteroposterior [AP])
- 45-Degree ulnar oblique (pronated AP)

Important radiographic signs that can aid in the detection of carpal fractures and carpal instability are found in Table 27.4. PA and lateral views are useful in the assessment of fractures and fracture-dislocations of the carpus, as well as for determining carpal alignment and/or collapse (Figures 27.2 and 27.3). The neutral PA view is limited in the diagnosis of[26]:

- Scaphoid fractures due to the overhang of the tubercle[82,83]
- Triquetral avulsion fractures secondary to the normal superimposition of the lunate dorsal lip
- Lunate fractures due to the palmar cortical line of the radial styloid

For suspected fractures of the scaphoid, the Ziter view, and carpal box or tunnel views can be helpful given that up to 30–40% of scaphoid fractures are not diagnosed on primary assessment and investigation with four view radiographs.[14,26,81,84] An oblique pronated lateral view will move the triquetrum dorsal to the lunate and aid with diagnosis of triquetral fractures.[85] Carpal tunnel views can aid

in the diagnosis of tuberosity fractures of the trapezium,[86] hamate hook fractures[87,88] and pisiform fractures.[87] The standard lateral view is useful for assessment of displacement and head rotation for fractures of the capitate. Trapezoid fractures, particularly coronal fractures, are rarely detected on standard plain radiographs[89] and further imaging is used in more than 80% of cases.[89] Always be sure to exclude a perilunate dislocation or fracture-dislocation as the evidence would indicate that 16–25% of perilunate injuries are initially missed,[9,90,91] particularly the lesser-arc injury, commonly due to the lack of a bony injury and often the inexperience of the initial assessor (Figure 27.4). Delay in the management of these injuries is associated pain, stiffness, carpal tunnel syndrome and secondary osteoarthritis.[9,90,91]

Additional views that can help detect carpal ligament instability are flexion-extension and radio-ulnar stress views, and clenched fist views.[38] Some would also advocate comparative radiographs of the contralateral uninjured wrist.[92] It is important to assess the intercarpal, carpometacarpal and radiocarpal joint spaces, particularly on the neutral PA view and stress views as indicated. Although the normal distance is debated, a normal space is said to be ≤2 mm, with ligament disruption diagnostic at >5 mm (Figure 27.3).

Standard four view radiographs can be used in the assessment of carpal fracture displacement regarding step-off, translation, rotation and angulation.[23] The lateral view is of particular importance (Table 27.4). Despite only moderate interobserver reliability reported using this technique,[93–95] the prevalence of displacement and instability is low and it would seem sensible that in the elderly patient with no gapping or translation at the fracture site and no lunate dorsal angulation, further imaging is rarely required.

Advanced imaging

Advanced imaging is predominantly used for the diagnosis of suspected scaphoid fractures, assessing fracture displacement, and in the diagnosis of ligamentous injuries to the wrist. The need for such imaging in the elderly patient will likely be limited to displaced carpal fractures, symptomatic carpal instability and the assessment of symptomatic

Table 27.4 Plain radiographic signs used in the detection of carpal fractures and carpal instability

Sign	Description
Inter- and intracarpal angles	*Neutral lateral view*
Scapholunate angle	Normal 45°, range 30–60°
	DISI >60° and VISI <30°
	>60–80° = scapholunate instability/SLD
Radiolunate angle	Normal <15°
	>15–0° = carpal instability
Capitolunate angle	Normal <15°
	>15–20° = carpal instability
Gilula's lines	*Neutral PA view*
	Three carpal arcs create smooth curves:
	1. *Proximal articular surface of the proximal carpal row*
	2. *Distal articular surface of the proximal carpal row*
	3. *Proximal cortical margins of hamate and capitate*
	Broken arc indicates a carpal fracture and/or instability
	Can be useful in subtle perilunate injuries and lunotriquetral disruption
Carpal height ratio	*Neutral PA view*
	Carpal height/third metacarpal length (Figure 27.2)
	Normal ratio is 45–60%
	Carpal collapse defined as <45%
	Can be seen with perilunate injuries
Terry Thomas sign	*Neutral PA view* (Figure 27.3)
	Increased gap between scaphoid and lunate
	>3 mm diagnostic of SLD or >5 mm if positive cortical ring sign
	SLD with a normal scapholunate angle is most likely atraumatic
Cortical ring sign	*Neutral PA view*
	Scaphoid tubercle viewed end-on due to scaphoid flexion
	Suggestive of SLD
Spilled teapot sign	*Lateral view*
	Palmar rotation of lunate
	Suggestive of a perilunate dislocation or fracture-dislocation
Ulnocarpal translation	*Neutral PA and radial deviation views*
	Increased translation and defined as >50% of lunate being uncovered
	Suggestive of a perilunate fracture or fracture-dislocation
Soft tissue signs of fracture	*PA view in ulnar deviation:* Scaphoid fat pad sign
	Lateral view: Pronator fat pad/stripe sign

Note: Some authors advocate contralateral wrist views to aid in determining the normal alignment and spacing of the patient's carpus. DISI, dorsal intercalated segment instability; PA, posteroanterior; SLD, scapholunate dissociation; VISI, volar intercalated segment instability.

non-unions. The most commonly employed modalities include ultrasound, bone scintigraphy, CT, MRI and wrist arthroscopy. Fluoroscopy using stress manoeuvres is advocated by some for suspected ligamentous disruption,[96,97] with arthrography very limited due to the high false positive and false negative rate.[98,99]

The efficacy and necessity of the use of these imaging modalities in the elderly patient, particularly for the suspected scaphoid fracture, is unknown. Furthermore, there are two key issues regarding the interpretation of diagnostic performance characteristics for the various imaging modalities available for suspected scaphoid fractures. The first is the low prevalence of true scaphoid fractures among suspected fractures (5–20%), which dramatically lowers the probability that a positive test will correspond with a true fracture as false positives are nearly as common as true positives.[8,14,26,100]

A proposed solution to this is the use of clinical prediction rules, which have been documented to effectively guide patient management throughout medicine.[101,102] The development and use of such rules for the suspected scaphoid fracture, including a combination of demographic and

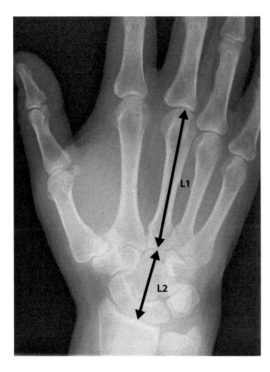

Figure 27.2 Carpal height ratio (L2/L1).

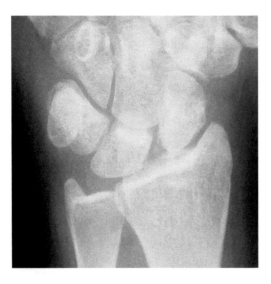

Figure 27.3 Terry Thomas sign with widening of the scapholunate distance, indicative of scapholunate dissociation.

clinical risk factors, could potentially increase the prevalence of true fractures among suspected fractures.[103,104] This would result in the use of advanced secondary imaging in higher risk patients, which may improve the diagnostic performance characteristics currently reported. The substantial influence of clinical prediction rules on the probability of a suspected scaphoid fracture has been already demonstrated in studies from Holland[79] and Edinburgh.[80] The second issue is the lack of a consensus reference standard for confirming a fracture,[105,106] which means that an alternative

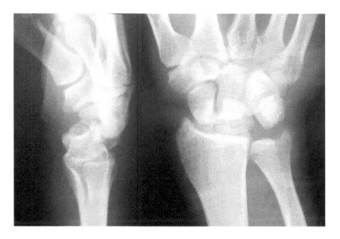

Figure 27.4 A trans-scaphoid perilunate fracture–dislocation of the carpus, with obvious disruption of Gilula's lines on the posteroanterior view (see Table 27.4).

method for calculating diagnostic performance characteristics (latent class analysis) is required.[78,107]

Ultrasound

Ultrasound can be used in the diagnosis of suspected scaphoid fractures and ligament injuries.[26] It is non-invasive and inexpensive but is operator dependent. It has lower diagnostic performance characteristics than the other available methods when diagnosing a suspected scaphoid fracture, with sensitivity ranging from 37% to 93% and specificity ranging from 61% to 91%.[8,108–110]

Bone scintigraphy

Bone scintigraphy is used in the diagnosis of suspected carpal fractures and avulsion injuries.[26] There are authors who advocate the use of bone scintigraphy for the suspected scaphoid fracture.[111,112] However, it is felt by many that use is limited given the lower specificity when compared to both CT and MRI.[113–116] This was recently confirmed in a Cochrane meta-analysis of six studies (11 studies in total) that reported a sensitivity of 99% but a specificity of 86% (Table 27.5).[117]

Computed tomography

CT is used in the diagnosis of suspected carpal fractures, for determining fracture displacement, and in the diagnosis of carpal malunion and non-union, and dynamic CT is used by some for determining the presence of ligamentous injuries.[26,118,119] Scaphoid fracture displacement can be assessed on CT imaging using the lateral intrascaphoid angle, the AP intrascaphoid angle, the dorsal cortical angle and the scaphoid height to length ratio.[120,121] The recent Cochrane review mentioned above analysed four studies to determine the diagnostic performance characteristics of CT for suspected scaphoid fractures and reported the lowest sensitivity at 72%, but with a specificity of 99% (Table 27.5).[117] Studies have reported that CT is superior to standard radiographs for the diagnosis of scaphoid fracture displacement,[122,123]

Table 27.5 The sensitivity and specificity for various imaging modalities as determined by Mallee et al. for suspected fractures of the scaphoid

Imaging modality (number of studies assessed)	Sensitivity (%)	Specificity (%)
Bone scintigraphy (n = 6)	99	86
CT (n = 4)	72	99
MRI (n = 5)	88	100

Source: Adapted from Mallee et al. *Cochrane Database Syst Rev* 2015;6:CD010023.

with a step of ≥1 mm at the dorsal or radial cortices and a gap of ≥1 mm on sagittal or coronal views quoted.[24,25]

Magnetic resonance imaging

MRI is used for suspected carpal fractures, the diagnosis of AVN of the carpus and diagnosing ligamentous injuries.[26] It is suggested by some that MRI is the gold standard investigation for suspected scaphoid fractures, with practical limitations including limited access and cost efficiency.[8,116,124,125] Furthermore, given all these imaging modalities are being used in low prevalence situations such as the suspected scaphoid fracture, the positive predictive value of these tests is lower than expected and false positive MRI scans in healthy individuals have been reported in one study.[103,126] Mallee et al. in their Cochrane review analysed five studies to determine the diagnostic performance characteristics of MRI for suspected scaphoid fractures and reported a sensitivity of 88% and the highest specificity at 100% (Table 27.5).[117]

WRIST ARTHROSCOPY

Wrist arthroscopy can be used in the diagnosis of suspected scaphoid fractures and fracture displacement, the assessment and management of non-union, as well as for determining the presence and grade of carpal ligamentous injuries and associated degenerative changes in the wrist.[127–130] It is generally agreed that arthroscopy is the reference standard for diagnosing carpal ligament injuries. Buijze et al. reported on 58 consecutive scaphoid fractures that were managed with arthroscopy assisted operative fracture fixation and found a significant correlation between radiographic comminution and displacement, and instability found at the time of surgery.[131] Use in the elderly patient is limited.

Associated injuries

Much of the literature regarding associated injuries is in relation to fractures of the scaphoid and it is not known if associated injuries are more common in elderly patients. Approximately 1 in 10 of all scaphoid fractures has a related injury and are associated with a high energy mechanism of injury.[7,132] Almost 80% of associated upper limb fractures are of the proximal or distal radius. Radial

head fractures are most commonly found,[7,132] with distal radius fractures, perilunate dislocations and trans-scaphoid perilunate fracture-dislocations also seen.[5,7]

The literature has reported an increasing incidence of concomitant ligamentous injuries using wrist arthroscopy,[133] although the clinical relevance of these injuries is unknown. An associated distal radius fracture can be indicative of a ligamentous injury and potential carpal instability.[134] Hamate fractures or fracture-dislocations have been reported to be associated with a fracture of the metacarpals.[135] Almost 25% of perilunate dislocations or fracture-dislocations will be seen in a multiply injured patient, with approximately 10% having a concomitant upper limb injury.[9]

TREATMENT

In the elderly patient, the aims of management for all carpal fractures and dislocations are to achieve a functional and stable wrist with minimal associated complications. Given that the vast majority of the carpal fractures and dislocations occur in younger patients, there is a scarcity of literature in relation to the elderly patient. As with all elderly trauma, the treatment choice should consider the clinical assessment of the patient and the complexity of the injury, but primarily should consider the baseline functional status and the pre-existing medical comorbidities of the patient, as well as the risks attached to any suggested surgery. Management options include non-operative, ORIF, fracture excision and fusion.

Non-operative

SCAPHOID FRACTURES

For *suspected fractures of the scaphoid* there are advocates for repeated clinical examination and radiographs at 10–14 days post injury, while others recommended early advanced imaging for example, CT or MRI, despite the potential issues with this. As has already been discussed, a few authors have promoted the use of clinical prediction rules that combine demographic and clinical risk factors that could target advanced secondary imaging in higher risk patients.[79,80] Whatever pathway is employed, and pending the diagnosis being confirmed or refuted, a below elbow forearm cast (with or without thumb immobilization) or wrist splint with thumb immobilization is routinely applied.

Good results can be expected with the non-operative treatment of *tubercle fractures of the scaphoid* as they are normally benign avulsion fractures (Figure 27.5).[136–138] There are advocates for a wrist splint for 1 month followed by mobilization, while others favour casting. Fractures managed without immobilization have been found to be associated with displacement and a fibrous union but are not associated with disability.[139]

For *non-displaced or minimally displaced waist fractures* (Figure 27.6) that are stable, non-operative management will attain a union rate of 95–99%,[140] has a 3–20% rate of

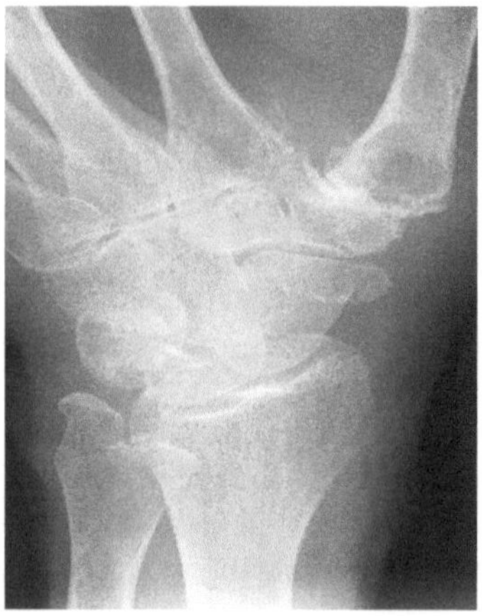

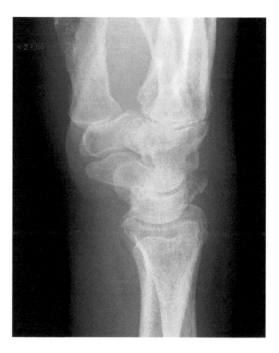

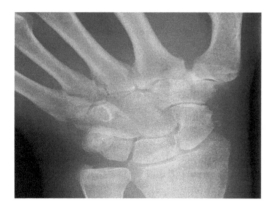

Figure 27.5 An oblique radiograph of the wrist demonstrating a displaced scaphoid tubercle fracture in a 72-year-old woman.

Figure 27.6 A posteroanterior (PA) radiograph demonstrating a non-displaced scaphoid waist fracture in a 65-year-old woman.

Figure 27.7 A lateral radiograph demonstrating a triquetral fracture in a 68-year-old woman.

displacement while in cast,[141,142] and is certainly seen by some as the management of choice for these injuries,[136–138] particularly in the elderly patient. There are several systematic reviews and meta-analysis that have not found early surgery for these fractures to be superior to non-operative management.[138,143–145]

For *displaced fractures of the scaphoid* there is some evidence to suggest that non-operative management in a cast may be appropriate,[146–148] particularly in the elderly patient with multiple comorbidities and low functional demands where the risk of surgery outweighs the benefit.[149] The primary risk of cast treatment is non-union, with the union rate ranging from 70% to 90%[25,150,151] and the risk of secondary wrist osteoarthritis being 16–31%.[137,151] The consequences of malunion are discussed later. Ultimately, the outcome in such cases is not completely clear and it may be that in the elderly patient conservative treatment provides a comparable outcome to surgery.

Preferred technique

For suspected fractures we would routinely use either a below elbow forearm cast or wrist splint with thumb extension for 2 weeks, at which point the patient is reviewed with repeat clinical assessment and radiographs to ascertain the diagnosis. If a fracture is confirmed we would use a below elbow forearm cast until the fracture has united, which can take from 6 to 12 weeks or longer. The use of further imaging in the elderly patient is limited in our practice. Several systematic reviews have been found to advocate one form of immobilization over another.[144,145,152] There are two randomized trials reporting no significant benefit to above elbow casts,[150,153] and two large prospective randomized trials reporting no advantage to a scaphoid cast over a Colles-type below elbow cast.[142]

OTHER CARPAL FRACTURES

Avulsion triquetral fractures account for over 90% of all triquetral injuries (Figure 27.7). Cast immobilization for approximately 1 month is used for isolated lunate fractures as non-union is rare.[154,155] Good or excellent results are reported following the non-operative management of non-displaced or minimally displaced trapezium[89,156,157] and hamate fractures.[135,158,159]

Preferred technique

The vast majority of other carpal fractures are isolated non-displaced or minimally displaced fractures where we would recommend non-operative management. The method is primarily dependant on the patient and we would routinely use a wrist splint or standard below elbow or scaphoid cast for approximately 1 month followed by routine mobilization. For simple triquetral avulsion fractures we would recommend a wrist splint for comfort with immediate mobilization as able.

LIGAMENTOUS INJURIES

The issue with ligamentous injuries in the elderly is that it is often difficult to distinguish between a partial disruption and age-related changes,[26] although non-operative management would often be the mainstay in an elderly patient with a subtle or partial injury. For *acute SLD* grade 1 injury and no evidence of carpal instability, non-operative management with cast immobilization can be used.[26] For an *acute lunotriquetral dissociation* with minimal deformity and no evidence of instability, conservative management in a below elbow cast is possible,[160] with surgery reserved for refractory cases. For *perilunate dislocations and fracture-dislocations* conservative and/or delayed intervention has been found to give poor results and is not recommended.[9,161-163] Although there are suggestions of stable perilunate dislocations post closed reduction that can be managed successfully in a scaphoid cast with the wrist in a neutral position, these patients need to be monitored very closely due to the unpredictable nature of these injuries and the tendency to lose reduction[69,162] even several months following the injury.[48] Given the high risk of late reduction loss and subsequent deformity, many advocate early operative intervention as described below.[26,69,162]

Operative

SCAPHOID FRACTURES

For *non-displaced or minimally displaced waist fractures* there is an increasing amount of data supporting early percutaneous screw fixation of these injuries due a decreased time to union and a more rapid return to sports and work; however all these trials have been in a predominantly young and active population (mean age range in studies of 24–33 years) and it is unlikely these benefits would balance out the risks of surgery in elderly patients.[151,164-169]

Displaced and/or comminuted fractures, proximal pole fractures, as well as those associated with increasing displacement and carpal instability, are routinely managed with ORIF due to the risks of re-displacement[142] and non-union[170,171] when treated non-operatively. However, the outcome in the elderly population is unknown, primarily because these injuries are less common in older patients. These should be managed on a case-by-case basis, with the aim to minimise the risk of developing carpal instability and a painful disabled wrist.

Preferred technique

ORIF of the scaphoid requires anatomic reduction of the fracture under direct vision, which can be aided with manoeuvres or K-wire joy sticking of each fracture fragment. There are advocates for both volar and dorsal approaches, with the volar approach limiting the risk to the vascular supply, while the dorsal approach gives you better access to proximal fractures.[23,172,173]

OTHER CARPAL FRACTURES

Although very rarely required, particularly in the elderly, the indications for ORIF of other carpal fractures include displacement and/or associated carpal instability. Fractures of the body of the triquetrum rarely occur as part of a perilunate dislocation or secondary to an impaction-type injury, for example, ulnar impaction,[26] while displaced lunate fractures frequently occur as part of a perilunate injury.[3-5] All these fractures may require ORIF in elderly patients, with excision with or without grafting reserved for select cases and for non-union.[72,174] In the rare case where there is an ulnar nerve lesion secondary to a fracture of the hamate or pisiform, decompression of Guyon's canal may be required.

Preferred technique

For the other displaced carpal fractures that are often associated with other bony or soft tissue injuries of the carpus, we would recommend closed or open reduction as the injury pattern allows and internal fixation when feasible. In elderly patients, we would suggest that surgery should be considered on a case-by-case basis.

LIGAMENTOUS INJURIES

As many of the carpal ligament injuries occur in and much of the literature concentrates on the younger patient, it is largely unknown how to effectively manage such injuries in the elderly patient. It is likely that when elderly patients do present with such injuries they will be chronic in nature with associated degenerative changes, and fusion with or without denervation rather than repair will be required.

Scapholunate dissociation

For *SLD* an early diagnosis and appropriate management with reduction is important in restoring the normal kinematics of the wrist and preventing progression to a SLAC wrist that is painful and progressively arthritic.[39] For acute partial tears of ≤3 mm but associated with instability, closed reduction and K-wire fixation is used (scaphoid-lunate, scaphoid-capitate),[26] with good results reported in the majority of patients.[175,176] Open repair and fixation is recommended in acute cases when reduction and stability cannot be achieved closed, with repair reportedly giving superior results to ligament reconstruction.[177-179] This is most likely related to the increasing use of intraosseous suture retaining anchors.[180-182] In patients who present with a subacute SLD, ligament repair augmented with local soft tissue, e.g. Blatt's technique (proximal dorsal capsular flap), is recommended.[183,184] A dorsal, palmar or combined approach can be used and it is essential that a robust repair of the capsule is performed.

Partial or complete wrist fusion is often required for chronic scapholunate instability, particularly in elderly patients, where there will likely be an irreparable ligament, a fixed carpal deformity and/or associated degenerative changes to the wrist.[26] A scaphotrapeziotrapezoidal (STT) fusion can be used for chronic instability as it provides effective pain relief and good functional results,[149,185,186] although it is associated with adjacent joint arthritis in the longer term.[187] Scaphoid excision and four corner fusion is often reserved for younger patients.[26] Despite the use of fusion, there are a variety of ligament reconstruction techniques including a dorsal capsular flap, a palmar ligament reefing technique or combined palmar and dorsal surgeries that incorporate flexor and/or extensor tendons.[183,188–190] The latter soft tissue procedures leave the patient with a superior range of movement but the suitability of such procedures in the elderly patient is doubtful.[189]

Lunotriquetral dissociation

For an acute displaced and unstable *lunotriquetral dissociation*, closed reduction and percutaneous fixation are commonly employed, with open procedures reserved for acute cases where closed reduction has failed and there is a residual deformity, e.g. VISI. For subacute and chronic cases where repair and reconstruction is indicated, part of the extensor carpi ulnaris tendon can be used.[45] Partial fusion, e.g. lunotriquetral joint, proximal row carpectomy or total wrist fusion, is reserved for failed cases and/or progressive radiological signs of wrist arthritis, with wrist denervation potentially useful for controlling pain.

Perilunate injuries

Perilunate dislocations and fracture-dislocations are exceedingly rare in the elderly due to the force required. However, prompt early closed reduction and subsequent open operative stabilization is routinely required to limit swelling and damage to the median nerve, as well as to optimize outcome.[26,191] In patients with clinical median nerve compression at presentation, urgent closed reduction will resolve symptoms in a large number of patients.[69,192] Urgent open reduction in theatre is necessary when a closed reduction is not possible,[191] with carpal tunnel decompression required when there is no resolution of symptoms following reduction or symptoms subsequently develop.[193]

For pure dislocations (lesser-arc injuries), K-wire fixation is recommended as it reduces the rate of loss of reduction, with stable reductions requiring percutaneous wires from the scaphoid to the lunate and the scaphoid to the capitate. For unstable or irreducible dislocations, open fixation is required[162,194] as superior results when compared to closed methods are consistently reported.[162,195] For fracture-dislocations (greater-arc injuries), ORIF of the fracture(s) and repair and stabilization of ligamentous injuries is required,[48] with scaphoid screw fixation often used.[196–198] The literature consistently reports the severity of these injuries, with long-term radiographic arthritis common and return to baseline function rare.[9,195,196,198,199]

For chronic injuries less than 3 months old, ORIF may still be possible although it is associated with poorer outcomes.[9,200] However, once bone ischaemia and soft tissue contracture are evident, salvage procedures such as a proximal row carpectomy (lunate and fossa and head of capitate need to be maintained)[191,201,202] or a total wrist fusion are required.[192]

Preferred technique

Elderly patients with carpal ligament injuries and instability need to be managed symptomatically and the indications for surgery are often different to those in their younger counterparts. If ligament repair and/or reconstruction is very likely to be successful and not associated with excessive risks, this can be considered in a select group of patients. Otherwise, patients should be managed symptomatically and wrist denervation and fusion procedures will be the mainstay of treatment. We would recommend that all patients with perilunate injuries be managed with early closed reduction and surgical stabilization, using a combination of the techniques described above. A dorsal or a volar approach can be used, but a combined approach is often needed for the more severe injuries where a closed reduction is not possible[192,203,204] and in those patients with median nerve compression.[196,205]

COMPLICATIONS

Non-union: scaphoid

Non-union of the scaphoid can result in SNAC and debilitating arthrosis of the wrist.[206] Proposed risk factors for non-union are displaced fractures, proximal pole fractures and a delay in the diagnosis and/or management of the patient.[147,171,207–209]

As with younger patients, the non-union may have been asymptomatic for some time and the patient will present either due to a new injury that uncovers the diagnosis, or due to progressive symptoms associated with SNAC.[210] Common symptoms include radial sided wrist pain, a reduced range of motion at the wrist with pain particularly at the extremes of movement, and reduced grip strength.[148,210,211] Symptoms will often be related to the degree of deformity, collapse and degenerative arthrosis.[206]

DIAGNOSIS

Radiographs are the first line investigation for non-union and potential findings include an established and persistent gap between fracture fragments, bone cysts and sclerosis along the fracture lines[148,212,213] (Figure 27.8). SNAC is the end stage of this process when left untreated (Figure 27.9). Although some would suggest that clinical assessment and radiographs alone can confirm union of the scaphoid,[93] further imaging can be invaluable in corroborating the diagnosis, as well as assessing the degree and extent of collapse and arthrosis of the wrist. Further imaging commonly employs CT rather than MRI, with sagittal images optimal for assessing the non-union and the extent of any associated collapse.[26,214,215] This may not always be necessary in the older patient but can be helpful in preoperative planning.

MANAGEMENT

The often quoted aims of scaphoid non-union management are to improve the clinical symptoms of the patient by achieving union and correcting any associated deformity, which will potentially impede the onset of wrist arthrosis.[26,148] In the elderly patient an established non-union will be the common presentation, with any chance

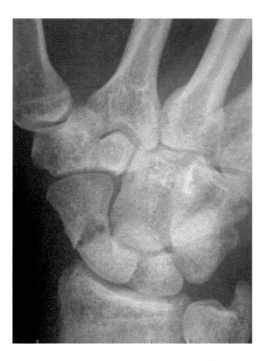

Figure 27.8 An established scaphoid waist fracture non-union.

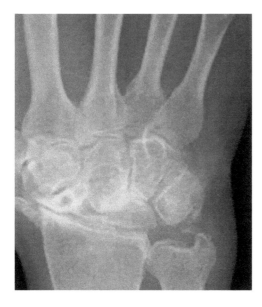

Figure 27.9 Severe scaphoid non-union advanced collapse.

of delaying or prevent wrist arthritis by achieving union probably doubtful. More commonly, a wrist salvage procedure will be employed in the elderly symptomatic patient, although there are limited data on which procedure to use and in which clinical scenarios they are most effective in.[148] Wrist salvage procedures include[26]:

- Wrist denervation: Provides effective pain relief but can be short term.[216]
- Partial or total scaphoid excision: Can be effective but often requires excision of sizable fragments, with

>8 mm associated with wrist weakness and a poor outcome.[217]
- Proximal row carpectomy: A systematic review reported comparable results to a four corner fusion, although a proximal row carpectomy is associated with a better range of movement and lower complication rates but with an increased rate of secondary arthritis.[218]
- Wrist fusion (partial or complete): Good results reported for radiocarpal and midcarpal arthritis that causes severe pain, weakness and a reduced range of movement. Pain relief is the primary benefit, but also improved strength is also reported.[219]

On the infrequent occasions when trying to achieve union is felt to be beneficial, the union rates have recently been quoted to be 80% for bone grafting alone and 84% for bone grafting and internal fixation,[220] although much of the work is in a younger patient population. The surgical management of stable non-unions in the elderly patient is less clear as the primary aims are to manage symptoms, prevent instability and delay the onset of wrist arthritis. Although there are reports of good results using percutaneous or open techniques for stable non-unions,[221,222] the role in the elderly patient is not clearly defined. The union rates for unstable non-unions alone are 60–95% using bone grafting and internal fixation,[223,224] with smoking a noted risk factor for union not being achieved.[224,225] Key to a good outcome and prevention of arthritis is correcting the deformity,[226] which was difficult with the once commonly used Matti-Russe inlay graft.[227] Screw fixation[148,228] and anterior wedge grafting with vascularized or non-vascularized grafts are now used.[229,230] Despite there being advocates for the many different methods of grafting, none has been reported to be better in gaining union.[148,223,231] A volar approach is commonly used to preserve the blood supply, although a dorsal approach may be necessary for proximal non-unions. A randomized controlled trial of vascularized (distal radius) versus non-vascularized (iliac crest) bone grafting for scaphoid non-union reported no significant difference in time to union or postoperative function, with 100% union in the non-vascularized arm compared with 85% in the vascularized arm.[232]

Non-union: lunate

The management of an isolated non-union of the lunate is rare following a body fracture, as the majority will present as Kienböck's disease, particularly in the elderly patient. The management options at this stage depend on the severity of the disease but include radial shortening, radial wedge osteotomy and ulnar lengthening, with a wrist fusion reserved for established disease and arthrosis.[26,233–235]

Malunion

It is debated whether a malunion of the scaphoid, often with the classical humpback deformity, leads to disability and loss of wrist function.[120,236] Improved function has been reported in case series of scaphoid osteotomy to correct malunion,[237] while non-union studies where the fracture has united in a malaligned position have reported no association with the short- and long-term outcome.[238,239]

There are also short- and long-term retrospective studies that have found no association between radiological malunion and outcome.[238,239] The short-term outcome at 1 year post injury in 42 consecutive patients managed non-operatively with a malunited scaphoid waist fracture reported no significant association between any functional and patient reported outcome measures and any of the radiological characteristics of malunion.[239]

Although there is no clear evidence, the risks of any surgery to correct a malunion in the elderly patient will outweigh the likely minimal benefit in a lower demand patient, particularly as the literature in this area suggests the main aim of surgery is to delay the onset of wrist osteoarthritis in younger active patients.[26]

Avascular necrosis

The most common presentation of carpal AVN is in the scaphoid as it is the most commonly injured, with proximal pole fractures particularly at risk. Other causes include scapholunate ligament injury and Preiser's disease (idiopathic). AVN of the lunate is surprisingly rarely reported following perilunate dislocation and fracture-dislocations, which is proposed to be due to the preservation of the palmar radiocarpal arch as the dislocation occurs through the space of Poirier.

Radiographs are the first line investigation, with some questioning the usefulness of MRI as an effective secondary imaging modality. Treatment options are debated but include vascularized bone graft[146,240,241] and arthroscopic debridement,[242] although in the elderly patient these will be seldom indicated.

CONCLUSIONS

Carpal fractures and instability are less common in the elderly population, with the diagnosis of most injuries made on routine four view scaphoid radiographs. The difficulty surrounding the diagnosis of carpal injuries in the elderly is predominantly related to differentiating degenerative changes in the wrist from acute injuries. However, there are consistent issues regarding the definition of fracture displacement and the importance of diagnosing and managing complex injuries early, for example, perilunate fracture-dislocations. Although young patients with displaced and/or unstable injuries of the carpus undergo operative intervention, it is unknown whether surgery in the elderly patient is always indicated and if this provides a superior outcome to conservative management.

The vast majority of isolated stable carpal fractures can be managed non-operatively in the elderly patient. Although percutaneous fixation is advocated by some for non- or minimally displaced fractures of the scaphoid in the younger patient, as with other carpal fractures, non-operative management would seem appropriate in the elderly population where the potential benefits of surgery will likely not outweigh the risks of any surgery. For displaced carpal fractures and proximal pole scaphoid fractures, operative management should be considered on a case-by-case basis, as conservative treatment is certainly an option in some elderly patients.

Little is known about the management of carpal instability in the elderly patient. Advances have been made in the diagnosis of these injuries with the use of advanced imaging modalities and wrist arthroscopy. Although exceedingly rare in the elderly population, immediate reduction and operative intervention is still recommended for all patients who sustain a perilunate dislocation or fracture-dislocation. A more frequent presentation in the elderly patient, however, is likely with the chronic sequelae of carpal instability. The appropriate management of the posttraumatic and/or degenerative wrist in the elderly patient is an area of future research. It is necessary to contemplate if with the growing number of elderly people in society this will influence the assessment and management of carpal injuries, as these patients present a new set of challenges given the limited literature currently available.

REFERENCES

1. Emmett JE, Breck LW. A review and analysis of 11,000 fractures seen in a private practice of orthopaedic surgery, 1937–1956. *J Bone Joint Surg Am* 1958;40-A(5):1169–75.
2. Court-Brown CM. The epidemiology of fractures and dislocations. In: Court-Brown CM, Heckman JD, McQueen MM, Ricci WMTP, III, editors. *Rockwood and Green's Fractures in Adults*. 8th ed. Philadelphia, PA: Lippincott Williams & Wilkins; 2014. pp. 59–108.
3. Hove LM. Fractures of the hand. Distribution and relative incidence. *Scand J Plast Reconstr Surg Hand Surg* 1993;27(4):317–19.
4. van Onselen EB, Karim RB, Hage JJ, Ritt MJ. Prevalence and distribution of hand fractures. *J Hand Surg Br* 2003;28(5):491–5.
5. Hey HW, Chong AK, Murphy D. Prevalence of carpal fracture in Singapore. *J Hand Surg Am* 2011;36(2):278–83.
6. Alsawadi A, Stanton J. Scaphoid fracture in the elderly: A review. *Hand Surg* 2012;17(2):295–8.
7. Duckworth AD, Jenkins PJ, Aitken SA, Clement ND, Court-Brown CM, McQueen MM. Scaphoid fracture epidemiology. *J Trauma Acute Care Surg* 2012;72(2):E41–5.
8. Jenkins PJ, Slade K, Huntley JS, Robinson CM. A comparative analysis of the accuracy, diagnostic uncertainty and cost of imaging modalities in suspected scaphoid fractures. *Injury* 2008;39(7):768–74.

9. Herzberg G, Comtet JJ, Linscheid RL, Amadio PC, Cooney WP, Stalder J. Perilunate dislocations and fracture-dislocations: A multicenter study. *J Hand Surg Am* 1993;18(5):768–79.

10. Hindle P, Davidson EK, Biant LC, Court-Brown CM. Appendicular joint dislocations. *Injury* 2013;44(8): 1022–7.

11. Court-Brown CM, Bugler KE, Clement ND, Duckworth AD, McQueen MM. The epidemiology of open fractures in adults. A 15-year review. *Injury* 2012;43(6):891–7.

12. Mayfield JK. Mechanism of carpal injuries. *Clin Orthop Relat Res* 1980;(149):45–54.

13. Linscheid RL, Dobyns JH. The unified concept of carpal injuries. *Ann Chir Main* 1984;3(1):35–42.

14. Kozin SH. Incidence, mechanism, and natural history of scaphoid fractures. *Hand Clin* 2001;17(4):515–24.

15. Futami T, Aoki H, Tsukamoto Y. Fractures of the hook of the hamate in athletes. 8 cases followed for 6 years. *Acta Orthop Scand* 1993;64(4):469–71.

16. Evans MW, Jr. Hamate hook fracture in a 17-year-old golfer: Importance of matching symptoms to clinical evidence. *J Manipulative Physiol Ther* 2004;27(8):516–18.

17. Mayfield JK. Wrist ligamentous anatomy and pathogenesis of carpal instability. *Orthop Clin North Am* 1984;15(2):209–16.

18. Herbert TJ, Fisher WE. Management of the fractured scaphoid using a new bone screw. *J Bone Joint Surg Br* 1984;66(1):114–23.

19. Marsh JL, Slongo TF, Agel J, Broderick JS, Creevey W, DeCoster TA, et al. Fracture and dislocation classification compendium—2007: Orthopaedic Trauma Association classification, database and outcomes committee. *J Orthop Trauma* 2007;21(10 Suppl):S1–133.

20. Müller ME. *The Comprehensive Classification of Fractures of Long Bones*. Berlin: Springer; 1990.

21. Russe O. Fracture of the carpal navicular. Diagnosis, non-operative treatment, and operative treatment. *J Bone Joint Surg Am* 1960;42-A:759–68.

22. Cooney WP, III. Scaphoid fractures: Current treatments and techniques. *Instr Course Lect* 2003;52:197–208.

23. Dias JJ, Singh HP. Displaced fracture of the waist of the scaphoid. *J Bone Joint Surg Br* 2011;93(11):1433–9.

24. Eddeland A, Eiken O, Hellgren E, Ohlsson NM. Fractures of the scaphoid. *Scand J Plast Reconstr Surg* 1975;9(3):234–9.

25. Cooney WP, Dobyns JH, Linscheid RL. Fractures of the scaphoid: A rational approach to management. *Clin Orthop Relat Res* 1980;(149):90–7.

26. Duckworth AD, Ring D. Carpus fractures and dislocations. In: Court-Brown CM, Heckman JD, McQueen MM, Ricci WMTP, III, editors. *Rockwood and Green's Fractures in Adults*. 8th ed. Philadelphia, PA: Lippincott Williams & Wilkins; 2014. pp. 991–1056.

27. Fisk GR. Carpal instability and the fractured scaphoid. *Ann R Coll Surg Engl* 1970;46(2):63–76.

28. Teisen H, Hjarbaek J. Classification of fresh fractures of the lunate. *J Hand Surg Br* 1988;13(4):458–62.

29. Beckenbaugh RD, Shives TC, Dobyns JH, Linscheid RL. Kienbock's disease: The natural history of Kienbock's disease and consideration of lunate fractures. *Clin Orthop Relat Res* 1980;(149):98–106.

30. Gelberman RH, Bauman TD, Menon J, Akeson WH. The vascularity of the lunate bone and Kienbock's disease. *J Hand Surg Am* 1980;5(3):272–8.

31. Schiltenwolf M, Wrazidlo W, Brocai DR, Schneider S, Lederer W. [A prospective study of early diagnosis of lunate necrosis by means of MRI]. *Rofo* 1995;162(4):325–9.

32. Lichtman DM, Degnan GG. Staging and its use in the determination of treatment modalities for Kienbock's disease. *Hand Clin* 1993;9(3):409–16.

33. Linscheid RL, Dobyns JH, Beabout JW, Bryan RS. Traumatic instability of the wrist. Diagnosis, classification, and pathomechanics. *J Bone Joint Surg Am* 1972;54(8):1612–32.

34. Linscheid RL, Dobyns JH, Beckenbaugh RD, Cooney WP, III, Wood MB. Instability patterns of the wrist. *J Hand Surg Am* 1983;8(5 Pt 2):682–6.

35. Taleisnik J. The ligaments of the wrist. *J Hand Surg Am* 1976;1(2):110–18.

36. Cooney WP, Dobyns JH, Linscheid RL. Arthroscopy of the wrist: Anatomy and classification of carpal instability. *Arthroscopy* 1990;6(2):133–40.

37. Wright TW, Dobyns JH, Linscheid RL, Macksoud W, Siegert J. Carpal instability non-dissociative. *J Hand Surg Br* 1994;19(6):763–73.

38. Gelberman RH, Cooney WP, III, Szabo RM. Carpal instability. *Instr Course Lect* 2001;50:123–34.

39. Tang JB, Ryu J, Omokawa S, Wearden S. Wrist kinetics after scapholunate dissociation: The effect of scapholunate interosseous ligament injury and persistent scapholunate gaps. *J Orthop Res* 2002;20(2):215–21.

40. Mitsuyasu H, Patterson RM, Shah MA, Buford WL, Iwamoto Y, Viegas SF. The role of the dorsal intercarpal ligament in dynamic and static scapholunate instability. *J Hand Surg Am* 2004;29(2):279–88.

41. Geissler WB, Freeland AE, Savoie FH, McIntyre LW, Whipple TL. Intracarpal soft-tissue lesions associated with an intra-articular fracture of the distal end of the radius. *J Bone Joint Surg Am* 1996;78(3):357–65.

42. Kuo CE, Wolfe SW. Scapholunate instability: Current concepts in diagnosis and management. *J Hand Surg Am* 2008;33(6):998–1013.

43. Kitay A, Wolfe SW. Scapholunate instability: Current concepts in diagnosis and management. *J Hand Surg Am* 2012;37(10):2175–96.

44. Jorgsholm P, Thomsen NO, Bjorkman A, Besjakov J, Abrahamsson SO. The incidence of intrinsic and extrinsic ligament injuries in scaphoid waist fractures. *J Hand Surg Am* 2010;35(3):368–74.

45. Sammer DM, Shin AY. Wrist surgery: Management of chronic scapholunate and lunotriquetral ligament injuries. *Plast Reconstr Surg* 2012;130(1):138e–56e.

46. Li G, Rowen B, Tokunaga D, Ryu J, Kato H, Kihira M. Carpal kinematics of lunotriquetral dissociations. *Biomed Sci Instrum* 1991;27:273–81.

47. Johnson RP. The acutely injured wrist and its residuals. *Clin Orthop Relat Res* 1980;(149):33–44.

48. Cooney WP, Bussey R, Dobyns JH, Linscheid RL. Difficult wrist fractures. Perilunate fracture-dislocations of the wrist. *Clin Orthop Relat Res* 1987;(214):136–47.

49. Chou YC, Hsu YH, Cheng CY, Wu CC. Percutaneous screw and axial Kirschner wire fixation for acute transscaphoid perilunate fracture dislocation. *J Hand Surg Am* 2012;37(4):715–20.

50. Witvoet J, Allieu Y. [Recent traumatic lesions of the semilunar bone]. *Rev Chir Orthop Reparatrice Appar Mot* 1973;59(Suppl 1):98–125.

51. Mayfield JK. Patterns of injury to carpal ligaments. A spectrum. *Clin Orthop Relat Res* 1984;(187):36–42.

52. Weber ER. Concepts governing the rotational shift of the intercalated segment of the carpus. *Orthop Clin North Am* 1984;15(2):193–207.

53. Linscheid RL. Kinematic considerations of the wrist. *Clin Orthop Relat Res* 1986;(202):27–39.

54. Trumble TE, Bour CJ, Smith RJ, Glisson RR. Kinematics of the ulnar carpus related to the volar intercalated segment instability pattern. *J Hand Surg Am* 1990;15(3):384–92.

55. Mayfield JK, Johnson RP, Kilcoyne RF. The ligaments of the human wrist and their functional significance. *Anat Rec* 1976;186(3):417–28.

56. Berger RA. The anatomy of the ligaments of the wrist and distal radioulnar joints. *Clin Orthop Relat Res* 2001;(383):32–40.

57. Buijze GA, Lozano-Calderon SA, Strackee SD, Blankevoort L, Jupiter JB. Osseous and ligamentous scaphoid anatomy: Part I. A systematic literature review highlighting controversies. *J Hand Surg Am* 2011;36(12):1926–35.

58. Lichtman DM, Schneider JR, Swafford AR, Mack GR. Ulnar midcarpal instability – Clinical and laboratory analysis. *J Hand Surg Am* 1981;6(5):515–23.

59. Kauer JM. The mechanism of the carpal joint. *Clin Orthop Relat Res* 1986;(202):16–26.

60. Navarro A. Luxaciones del carpo. *An Fac Med (Lima)* 1921;6:113–41.

61. Gelberman RH, Menon J. The vascularity of the scaphoid bone. *J Hand Surg Am* 1980;5(5):508–13.

62. Gelberman RH, Panagis JS, Taleisnik J, Baumgaertner M. The arterial anatomy of the human carpus. Part I: The extraosseous vascularity. *J Hand Surg Am* 1983;8(4):367–75.

63. Botte MJ, Pacelli LL, Gelberman RH. Vascularity and osteonecrosis of the wrist. *Orthop Clin North Am* 2004;35(3):405–21, xi.

64. Berger RA. The anatomy of the scaphoid. *Hand Clin* 2001;17(4):525–32.

65. Buijze GA, Dvinskikh NA, Strackee SD, Streekstra GJ, Blankevoort L. Osseous and ligamentous scaphoid anatomy: Part II. Evaluation of ligament morphology using three-dimensional anatomical imaging. *J Hand Surg Am* 2011;36(12):1936–43.

66. Slade JF, III, Jaskwhich D. Percutaneous fixation of scaphoid fractures. *Hand Clin* 2001;17(4):553–74.

67. Botte MJ, Gelberman RH. Fractures of the carpus, excluding the scaphoid. *Hand Clin* 1987;3(1):149–61.

68. Easterling KJ, Wolfe SW. Scaphoid shift in the uninjured wrist. *J Hand Surg Am* 1994;19(4):604–6.

69. Adkison JW, Chapman MW. Treatment of acute lunate and perilunate dislocations. *Clin Orthop Relat Res* 1982;(164):199–207.

70. Takami H, Takahashi S, Ando M, Masuda A. Open reduction of chronic lunate and perilunate dislocations. *Arch Orthop Trauma Surg* 1996;115(2):104–7.

71. Milek MA, Boulas HJ. Flexor tendon ruptures secondary to hamate hook fractures. *J Hand Surg Am* 1990;15(5):740–4.

72. Yamazaki H, Kato H, Nakatsuchi Y, Murakami N, Hata Y. Closed rupture of the flexor tendons of the little finger secondary to non-union of fractures of the hook of the hamate. *J Hand Surg Br* 2006;31(3):337–41.

73. Foucher G, Schuind F, Merle M, Brunelli F. Fractures of the hook of the hamate. *J Hand Surg Br* 1985;10(2):205–10.

74. Smith P, III, Wright TW, Wallace PF, Dell PC. Excision of the hook of the hamate: A retrospective survey and review of the literature. *J Hand Surg Am* 1988;13(4):612–15.

75. Parvizi J, Wayman J, Kelly P, Moran CG. Combining the clinical signs improves diagnosis of scaphoid fractures. A prospective study with follow-up. *J Hand Surg Br* 1998;23(3):324–7.

76. Powell JM, Lloyd GJ, Rintoul RF. New clinical test for fracture of the scaphoid. *Can J Surg* 1988;31(4):237–8.

77. Freeland P. Scaphoid tubercle tenderness: A better indicator of scaphoid fractures? *Arch Emerg Med* 1989;6(1):46–50.

78. Mallee WH, Henny EP, van Dijk CN, Kamminga SP, van Enst WA, Kloen P. Clinical diagnostic evaluation for scaphoid fractures: A systematic review and meta-analysis. *J Hand Surg Am* 2014;39(9):1683–91.

79. Rhemrev SJ, Beeres FJ, van Leerdam RH, Hogervorst M, Ring D. Clinical prediction rule for suspected scaphoid fractures: A prospective cohort study. *Injury* 2010;41(10):1026–30.

80. Duckworth AD, Buijze GA, Moran M, Gray A, Court-Brown CM, Ring D, et al. Predictors of fracture following suspected injury to the scaphoid. *J Bone Joint Surg Br* 2012;94(7):961–8.

81. Gabler C, Kukla C, Breitenseher MJ, Trattnig S, Vecsei V. Diagnosis of occult scaphoid fractures and other wrist injuries. Are repeated clinical examinations and plain radiographs still state of the art? *Langenbecks Arch Surg* 2001;386(2):150–4.

82. Cheung GC, Lever CJ, Morris AD. X-ray diagnosis of acute scaphoid fractures. *J Hand Surg Br* 2006;31(1):104–9.

83. Compson JP. The anatomy of acute scaphoid fractures: A three-dimensional analysis of patterns. *J Bone Joint Surg Br* 1998;80(2):218–24.

84. Barton NJ. Twenty questions about scaphoid fractures. *J Hand Surg Br* 1992;17(3):289–310.

85. de Beer JD, Hudson DA. Fractures of the triquetrum. *J Hand Surg Br* 1987;12(1):52–3.

86. Hsu KY, Wu CC, Wang KC, Shih CH. Simultaneous dislocation of the five carpometacarpal joints with concomitant fractures of the tuberosity of the trapezium and the hook of the hamate: Case report. *J Trauma* 1993;35(3):479–83.

87. Lacey JD, Hodge JC. Pisiform and hamulus fractures: Easily missed wrist fractures diagnosed on a reverse oblique radiograph. *J Emerg Med* 1998;16(3):445–52.

88. Kato H, Nakamura R, Horii E, Nakao E, Yajima H. Diagnostic imaging for fracture of the hook of the hamate. *Hand Surg* 2000;5(1):19–24.

89. Kain N, Heras-Palou C. Trapezoid fractures: Report of 11 cases. *J Hand Surg Am* 2012;37(6):1159–62.

90. Altissimi M, Mancini GB, Azzara A. Perilunate dislocations of the carpus. A long-term review. *Ital J Orthop Traumatol* 1987;13(4):491–500.

91. Kozin SH. Perilunate injuries: Diagnosis and treatment. *J Am Acad Orthop Surg* 1998;6(2):114–20.

92. Abdel-Salam A, Eyres KS, Cleary J. Detecting fractures of the scaphoid: The value of comparative X-rays of the uninjured wrist. *J Hand Surg Br* 1992;17(1):28–32.

93. Dias JJ, Brenkel IJ, Finlay DB. Patterns of union in fractures of the waist of the scaphoid. *J Bone Joint Surg Br* 1989;71(2):307–10.

94. Bhat M, McCarthy M, Davis TR, Oni JA, Dawson S. MRI and plain radiography in the assessment of displaced fractures of the waist of the carpal scaphoid. *J Bone Joint Surg Br* 2004;86(5):705–13.

95. Bernard SA, Murray PM, Heckman MG. Validity of conventional radiography in determining scaphoid waist fracture displacement. *J Orthop Trauma* 2010;24(7):448–51.

96. Nielsen PT, Hedeboe J. Posttraumatic scapholunate dissociation detected by wrist cineradiography. *J Hand Surg Am* 1984;9A(1):135–8.

97. Pliefke J, Stengel D, Rademacher G, Mutze S, Ekkernkamp A, Eisenschenk A. Diagnostic accuracy of plain radiographs and cineradiography in diagnosing traumatic scapholunate dissociation. *Skeletal Radiol* 2008;37(2):139–45.

98. Tirman RM, Weber ER, Snyder LL, Koonce TW. Midcarpal wrist arthrography for detection of tears of the scapholunate and lunotriquetral ligaments. *AJR Am J Roentgenol* 1985;144(1):107–8.

99. Walsh JJ, Berger RA, Cooney WP. Current status of scapholunate interosseous ligament injuries. *J Am Acad Orthop Surg* 2002;10(1):32–42.

100. Adey L, Souer JS, Lozano-Calderon S, Palmer W, Lee SG, Ring D. Computed tomography of suspected scaphoid fractures. *J Hand Surg Am* 2007;32(1):61–6.

101. Reilly BM, Evans AT. Translating clinical research into clinical practice: Impact of using prediction rules to make decisions. *Ann Intern Med* 2006;144(3):201–9.

102. Llewelyn H. Assessing properly the usefulness of clinical prediction rules and tests. *BMJ* 2012;344:e1238.

103. Ring D, Lozano-Calderon S. Imaging for suspected scaphoid fracture. *J Hand Surg Am* 2008;33(6):954–7.

104. Duckworth AD, Ring D, McQueen MM. Assessment of the suspected fracture of the scaphoid. *J Bone Joint Surg Br* 2011;93(6):713–19.

105. Altman DG, Bland JM. Diagnostic tests. 1: Sensitivity and specificity. *BMJ* 1994;308(6943):1552.

106. Altman DG, Bland JM. Diagnostic tests. 2: Predictive values. *BMJ* 1994;309(6947):102.

107. Buijze GA, Mallee WH, Beeres FJ, Hanson TE, Johnson WO, Ring D. Diagnostic performance tests for suspected scaphoid fractures differ with conventional and latent class analysis. *Clin Orthop Relat Res* 2011;469(12):3400–7.

108. DaCruz DJ, Taylor RH, Savage B, Bodiwala GG. Ultrasound assessment of the suspected scaphoid fracture. *Arch Emerg Med* 1988;5(2):97–100.

109. Munk B, Bolvig L, Kroner K, Christiansen T, Borris L, Boe S. Ultrasound for diagnosis of scaphoid fractures. *J Hand Surg Br* 2000;25(4):369–71.

110. Senall JA, Failla JM, Bouffard JA, van Holsbeeck M. Ultrasound for the early diagnosis of clinically suspected scaphoid fracture. *J Hand Surg Am* 2004;29(3):400–5.

111. Tiel-van Buul MM, Broekhuizen TH, van Beek EJ, Bossuyt PM. Choosing a strategy for the diagnostic management of suspected scaphoid fracture: A cost-effectiveness analysis. *J Nucl Med* 1995;36(1):45–8.

112. Beeres FJ, Rhemrev SJ, den Hollander P, Kingma LM, Meylaerts SA, le Cessie S, et al. Early magnetic resonance imaging compared with bone scintigraphy in suspected scaphoid fractures. *J Bone Joint Surg Br* 2008;90(9):1205–9.

113. Fowler C, Sullivan B, Williams LA, McCarthy G, Savage R, Palmer A. A comparison of bone scintigraphy and MRI in the early diagnosis of the occult scaphoid waist fracture. *Skeletal Radiol* 1998;27(12):683–7.

114. Breederveld RS, Tuinebreijer WE. Investigation of computed tomographic scan concurrent criterion validity in doubtful scaphoid fracture of the wrist. *J Trauma* 2004;57(4):851–4.

115. Rhemrev SJ, de Zwart AD, Kingma LM, Meylaerts SA, Arndt JW, Schipper IB, et al. Early computed tomography compared with bone scintigraphy in suspected scaphoid fractures. *Clin Nucl Med* 2010;35(12):931–4.

116. Yin ZG, Zhang JB, Kan SL, Wang XG. Diagnosing suspected scaphoid fractures: A systematic review and meta-analysis. *Clin Orthop Relat Res* 2010;468(3):723–34.

117. Mallee WH, Wang J, Poolman RW, Kloen P, Maas M, de Vet HC, et al. Computed tomography versus magnetic resonance imaging versus bone scintigraphy for clinically suspected scaphoid fractures in patients with negative plain radiographs. *Cochrane Database Syst Rev* 2015;6:CD010023.

118. Cruickshank J, Meakin A, Breadmore R, Mitchell D, Pincus S, Hughes T, et al. Early computerized tomography accurately determines the presence or absence of scaphoid and other fractures. *Emerg Med Australas* 2007;19(3):223–8.

119. Mallee W, Doornberg JN, Ring D, van Dijk CN, Maas M, Goslings JC. Comparison of CT and MRI for diagnosis of suspected scaphoid fractures. *J Bone Joint Surg Am* 2011;93(1):20–8.

120. Amadio PC, Berquist TH, Smith DK, Ilstrup DM, Cooney WP, III, Linscheid RL. Scaphoid malunion. *J Hand Surg Am* 1989;14(4):679–87.

121. Bain GI, Bennett JD, MacDermid JC, Slethaug GP, Richards RS, Roth JH. Measurement of the scaphoid humpback deformity using longitudinal computed tomography: Intra- and interobserver variability using various measurement techniques. *J Hand Surg Am* 1998;23(1):76–81.

122. Nakamura R, Imaeda T, Horii E, Miura T, Hayakawa N. Analysis of scaphoid fracture displacement by three-dimensional computed tomography. *J Hand Surg Am* 1991;16(3):485–92.

123. Lozano-Calderon S, Blazar P, Zurakowski D, Lee SG, Ring D. Diagnosis of scaphoid fracture displacement with radiography and computed tomography. *J Bone Joint Surg Am* 2006;88(12):2695–703.

124. Hansen TB, Petersen RB, Barckman J, Uhre P, Larsen K. Cost-effectiveness of MRI in managing suspected scaphoid fractures. *J Hand Surg Eur Vol* 2009;34(5):627–30.

125. Patel NK, Davies N, Mirza Z, Watson M. Cost and clinical effectiveness of MRI in occult scaphoid fractures: A randomised controlled trial. *Emerg Med J* 2013;30(3):202–7.

126. de Zwart AD, Beeres FJ, Ring D, Kingma LM, Coerkamp EG, Meylaerts SA, et al. MRI as a reference standard for suspected scaphoid fractures. *Br J Radiol* 2012;85(1016):1098–101.

127. Ruch DS, Smith BP. Arthroscopic and open management of dynamic scaphoid instability. *Orthop Clin North Am* 2001;32(2):233–40, vii.

128. Ruch DS, Chang DS, Yang CC. Arthroscopic evaluation and treatment of scaphoid nonunion. *Hand Clin* 2001;17(4):655–62, x.

129. Schadel-Hopfner M, Iwinska-Zelder J, Braus T, Bohringer G, Klose KJ, Gotzen L. MRI versus arthroscopy in the diagnosis of scapholunate ligament injury. *J Hand Surg Br* 2001;26(1):17–21.

130. Buijze GA, Jorgsholm P, Thomsen NO, Bjorkman A, Besjakov J, Ring D. Diagnostic performance of radiographs and computed tomography for displacement and instability of acute scaphoid waist fractures. *J Bone Joint Surg Am* 2012;94(21):1967–74.

131. Buijze GA, Jorgsholm P, Thomsen NO, Bjorkman A, Besjakov J, Ring D. Factors associated with arthroscopically determined scaphoid fracture displacement and instability. *J Hand Surg Am* 2012;37(7):1405–10.

132. Wildin CJ, Bhowal B, Dias JJ. The incidence of simultaneous fractures of the scaphoid and radial head. *J Hand Surg Br* 2001;26(1):25–7.

133. Caloia MF, Gallino RN, Caloia H, Rivarola H. Incidence of ligamentous and other injuries associated with scaphoid fractures during arthroscopically assisted reduction and percutaneous fixation. *Arthroscopy* 2008;24(7):754–9.

134. Hove LM. Simultaneous scaphoid and distal radial fractures. *J Hand Surg Br* 1994;19(3):384–8.

135. Wharton DM, Casaletto JA, Choa R, Brown DJ. Outcome following coronal fractures of the hamate. *J Hand Surg Eur Vol* 2010;35(2):146–9.

136. Dias JJ, Wildin CJ, Bhowal B, Thompson JR. Should acute scaphoid fractures be fixed? A randomized controlled trial. *J Bone Joint Surg Am* 2005;87(10):2160–8.

137. Dias JJ, Dhukaram V, Abhinav A, Bhowal B, Wildin CJ. Clinical and radiological outcome of cast immobilisation versus surgical treatment of acute scaphoid fractures at a mean follow-up of 93 months. *J Bone Joint Surg Br* 2008;90(7):899–905.

138. Ibrahim T, Qureshi A, Sutton AJ, Dias JJ. Surgical versus nonsurgical treatment of acute minimally displaced and undisplaced scaphoid waist fractures: Pairwise and network meta-analyses of randomized controlled trials. *J Hand Surg Am* 2011;36(11):1759–68.

139. Mody BS, Belliappa PP, Dias JJ, Barton NJ. Nonunion of fractures of the scaphoid tuberosity. *J Bone Joint Surg Br* 1993;75(3):423–5.

140. Bohler L, Trojan E, Jahna H. The results of treatment of 734 fresh, simple fractures of the scaphoid. *J Hand Surg Br* 2003;28(4):319–31.

141. Leslie IJ, Dickson RA. The fractured carpal scaphoid. Natural history and factors influencing outcome. *J Bone Joint Surg Br* 1981;63-B(2):225–30.

142. Clay NR, Dias JJ, Costigan PS, Gregg PJ, Barton NJ. Need the thumb be immobilised in scaphoid fractures? A randomised prospective trial. *J Bone Joint Surg Br* 1991;73(5):828–32.

143. Buijze GA, Doornberg JN, Ham JS, Ring D, Bhandari M, Poolman RW. Surgical compared with conservative treatment for acute nondisplaced or minimally displaced scaphoid fractures: A systematic review and meta-analysis of randomized controlled trials. *J Bone Joint Surg Am* 2010;92(6):1534–44.

144. Symes TH, Stothard J. A systematic review of the treatment of acute fractures of the scaphoid. *J Hand Surg Eur Vol* 2011;36(9):802–10.

145. Alshryda S, Shah A, Odak S, Al-Shryda J, Ilango B, Murali SR. Acute fractures of the scaphoid bone: Systematic review and meta-analysis. *Surgeon* 2012;10(4):218–29.

146. Pao VS, Chang J. Scaphoid nonunion: Diagnosis and treatment. *Plast Reconstr Surg* 2003;112(6):1666–76.

147. Wong K, von Schroeder HP. Delays and poor management of scaphoid fractures: Factors contributing to nonunion. *J Hand Surg Am* 2011;36(9):1471–4.

148. Buijze GA, Ochtman L, Ring D. Management of scaphoid nonunion. *J Hand Surg Am* 2012;37(5):1095–100.

149. Gaebler C, McQueen MM. Carpus fractures and dislocations. In: Bucholz RW, Court-Brown CM, Heckman JD, Tornetta P, editors. *Rockwood and Green's fractures in adults.* 7th ed. Philadelphia, PA: Lippincott Williams & Wilkins; 2010. pp. 781–828.

150. Alho A, Kankaanpaa. Management of fractured scaphoid bone. A prospective study of 100 fractures. *Acta Orthop Scand* 1975;46(5):737–43.

151. Saeden B, Tornkvist H, Ponzer S, Hoglund M. Fracture of the carpal scaphoid. A prospective, randomised 12-year follow-up comparing operative and conservative treatment. *J Bone Joint Surg Br* 2001;83(2):230–4.

152. Doornberg JN, Buijze GA, Ham SJ, Ring D, Bhandari M, Poolman RW. Nonoperative treatment for acute scaphoid fractures: A systematic review and meta-analysis of randomized controlled trials. *J Trauma* 2011;71(4):1073–81.

153. Gellman H, Caputo RJ, Carter V, Aboulafia A, McKay M. Comparison of short and long thumb-spica casts for non-displaced fractures of the carpal scaphoid. *J Bone Joint Surg Am* 1989;71(3):354–7.

154. Cetti R, Christensen SE, Reuther K. Fracture of the lunate bone. *Hand* 1982;14(1):80–4.

155. Hsu AR, Hsu PA. Unusual case of isolated lunate fracture without ligamentous injury. *Orthopedics* 2011;34(11):e785–9.

156. Nagumo A, Toh S, Tsubo K, Ishibashi Y, Sasaki T. An occult fracture of the trapezoid bone. A case report. *J Bone Joint Surg Am* 2002;84-A(6):1025–7.

157. Gruson KI, Kaplan KM, Paksima N. Isolated trapezoid fractures: A case report with compilation of the literature. *Bull NYU Hosp Jt Dis* 2008;66(1):57–60.

158. Whalen JL, Bishop AT, Linscheid RL. Nonoperative treatment of acute hamate hook fractures. *J Hand Surg Am* 1992;17(3):507–11.

159. Walsh JJ, Bishop AT. Diagnosis and management of hamate hook fractures. *Hand Clin* 2000;16(3):397–403, viii.

160. Reagan DS, Linscheid RL, Dobyns JH. Lunotriquetral sprains. *J Hand Surg Am* 1984;9(4):502–14.

161. Weil WM, Slade JF, III, Trumble TE. Open and arthroscopic treatment of perilunate injuries. *Clin Orthop Relat Res* 2006;445:120–32.

162. Apergis E, Maris J, Theodoratos G, Pavlakis D, Antoniou N. Perilunate dislocations and fracture-dislocations. Closed and early open reduction compared in 28 cases. *Acta Orthop Scand Suppl* 1997;275:55–9.

163. Gellman H, Schwartz SD, Botte MJ, Feiwell L. Late treatment of a dorsal transscaphoid, trans-triquetral perilunate wrist dislocation with avascular changes of the lunate. *Clin Orthop Relat Res* 1988;(237):196–203.

164. Haddad FS, Goddard NJ. Acute percutaneous scaphoid fixation. A pilot study. *J Bone Joint Surg Br* 1998;80(1):95–9.

165. Bond CD, Shin AY, McBride MT, Dao KD. Percutaneous screw fixation or cast immobilization for nondisplaced scaphoid fractures. *J Bone Joint Surg Am* 2001;83-A(4):483–8.

166. Yip HS, Wu WC, Chang RY, So TY. Percutaneous cannulated screw fixation of acute scaphoid waist fracture. *J Hand Surg Br* 2002;27(1):42–6.

167. Papaloizos MY, Fusetti C, Christen T, Nagy L, Wasserfallen JB. Minimally invasive fixation versus conservative treatment of undisplaced scaphoid fractures: A cost-effectiveness study. *J Hand Surg Br* 2004;29(2):116–19.

168. McQueen MM, Gelbke MK, Wakefield A, Will EM, Gaebler C. Percutaneous screw fixation versus conservative treatment for fractures of the waist of the scaphoid: A prospective randomised study. *J Bone Joint Surg Br* 2008;90(1):66–71.

169. Iacobellis C, Baldan S, Aldegheri R. Percutaneous screw fixation for scaphoid fractures. *Musculoskelet Surg* 2011;95(3):199–203.

170. Singh HP, Taub N, Dias JJ. Management of displaced fractures of the waist of the scaphoid: Meta-analyses of comparative studies. *Injury* 2012;43(6):933–9.

171. Eastley N, Singh H, Dias JJ, Taub N. Union rates after proximal scaphoid fractures; meta-analyses and review of available evidence. *J Hand Surg Eur Vol* 2013;38(8):888–97.

172. Herbert TJ. Open volar repair of acute scaphoid fractures. *Hand Clin* 2001;17(4):589–99, viii.

173. Martus JE, Bedi A, Jebson PJ. Cannulated variable pitch compression screw fixation of scaphoid fractures using a limited dorsal approach. *Tech Hand Up Extrem Surg* 2005;9(4):202–6.

174. Scheufler O, Radmer S, Erdmann D, Germann G, Pierer G, Andresen R. Therapeutic alternatives in nonunion of hamate hook fractures: Personal experience in 8 patients and review of literature. *Ann Plast Surg* 2005;55(2):149–54.

175. Whipple TL. The role of arthroscopy in the treatment of wrist injuries in the athlete. *Clin Sports Med* 1992;11(1):227–38.

176. Whipple TL. The role of arthroscopy in the treatment of scapholunate instability. *Hand Clin* 1995;11(1):37–40.

177. Cohen MS, Taleisnik J. Direct ligamentous repair of scapholunate dissociation with capsulodesis augmentation. *Tech Hand Up Extrem Surg* 1998;2(1):18–24.

178. Beredjiklian PK, Dugas J, Gerwin M. Primary repair of the scapholunate ligament. *Tech Hand Up Extrem Surg* 1998;2(4):269–73.

179. Minami A, Kato H, Iwasaki N. Treatment of scapholunate dissociation: Ligamentous repair associated with modified dorsal capsulodesis. *Hand Surg* 2003;8(1):1–6.

180. Bickert B, Sauerbier M, Germann G. Scapholunate ligament repair using the Mitek bone anchor. *J Hand Surg Br* 2000;25(2):188–92.

181. Baczkowski B, Lorczynski A, Kabula J, Camilleri R. Scapholunate ligament repair using suture anchors. *Ortop Traumatol Rehabil* 2006;8(2):129–33.

182. Rosati M, Parchi P, Cacianti M, Poggetti A, Lisanti M. Treatment of acute scapholunate ligament injuries with bone anchor. *Musculoskelet Surg* 2010;94(1):25–32.

183. Blatt G. Capsulodesis in reconstructive hand surgery. Dorsal capsulodesis for the unstable scaphoid and volar capsulodesis following excision of the distal ulna. *Hand Clin* 1987;3(1):81–102.

184. Muermans S, De Smet L, Van Ransbeeck H. Blatt dorsal capsulodesis for scapholunate instability. *Acta Orthop Belg* 1999;65(4):434–9.

185. Eckenrode JF, Louis DS, Greene TL. Scaphoid-trapezium-trapezoid fusion in the treatment of chronic scapholunate instability. *J Hand Surg Am* 1986;11(4):497–502.

186. Watson HK, Belniak R, Garcia-Elias M. Treatment of scapholunate dissociation: Preferred treatment—STT fusion vs other methods. *Orthopedics* 1991;14(3):365–8.

187. Fortin PT, Louis DS. Long-term follow-up of scaphoid-trapezium-trapezoid arthrodesis. *J Hand Surg Am* 1993;18(4):675–81.

188. Schweizer A, Steiger R. Long-term results after repair and augmentation ligamentoplasty of rotatory subluxation of the scaphoid. *J Hand Surg Am* 2002;27(4):674–84.

189. Szabo RM, Slater RR, Jr., Palumbo CF, Gerlach T. Dorsal intercarpal ligament capsulodesis for chronic, static scapholunate dissociation: Clinical results. *J Hand Surg Am* 2002;27(6):978–84.

190. Almquist EE, Bach AW, Sack JT, Fuhs SE, Newman DM. Four-bone ligament reconstruction for treatment of chronic complete scapholunate separation. *J Hand Surg Am* 1991;16(2):322–7.

191. Jones DB, Jr., Kakar S. Perilunate dislocations and fracture dislocations. *J Hand Surg Am* 2012;37(10):2168–73.

192. Hildebrand KA, Ross DC, Patterson SD, Roth JH, MacDermid JC, King GJ. Dorsal perilunate dislocations and fracture-dislocations: Questionnaire, clinical, and radiographic evaluation. *J Hand Surg Am* 2000;25(6):1069–79.

193. DiGiovanni B, Shaffer J. Treatment of perilunate and transscaphoid perilunate dislocations of the wrist. *Am J Orthop (Belle Mead NJ)* 1995;24(11):818–26.

194. Green DP, O'Brien ET. Classification and management of carpal dislocations. *Clin Orthop Relat Res* 1980;(149):55–72.

195. Herzberg G, Forissier D. Acute dorsal trans-scaphoid perilunate fracture-dislocations: Medium-term results. *J Hand Surg Br* 2002;27(6):498–502.

196. Kremer T, Wendt M, Riedel K, Sauerbier M, Germann G, Bickert B. Open reduction for perilunate injuries—Clinical outcome and patient satisfaction. *J Hand Surg Am* 2010;35(10):1599–606.

197. Souer JS, Rutgers M, Andermahr J, Jupiter JB, Ring D. Perilunate fracture-dislocations of the wrist: Comparison of temporary screw versus K-wire fixation. *J Hand Surg Am* 2007;32(3):318–25.

198. Knoll VD, Allan C, Trumble TE. Trans-scaphoid perilunate fracture dislocations: Results of screw fixation of the scaphoid and lunotriquetral repair with a dorsal approach. *J Hand Surg Am* 2005;30(6):1145–52.

199. Forli A, Courvoisier A, Wimsey S, Corcella D, Moutet F. Perilunate dislocations and transscaphoid perilunate fracture-dislocations: A retrospective study with minimum ten-year follow-up. *J Hand Surg Am* 2010;35(1):62–8.

200. Komurcu M, Kurklu M, Ozturan KE, Mahirogullari M, Basbozkurt M. Early and delayed treatment of dorsal transscaphoid perilunate fracture-dislocations. *J Orthop Trauma* 2008;22(8):535–40.

201. Rettig ME, Raskin KB. Long-term assessment of proximal row carpectomy for chronic perilunate dislocations. *J Hand Surg Am* 1999;24(6):1231–6.

202. Inoue G, Miura T. Proximal row carpectomy in perilunate dislocations and lunatomalacia. *Acta Orthop Scand* 1990;61(5):449–52.

203. Trumble T, Verheyden J. Treatment of isolated perilunate and lunate dislocations with combined dorsal and volar approach and intraosseous cerclage wire. *J Hand Surg Am* 2004;29(3):412–17.

204. Lutz M, Arora R, Kammerlander C, Gabl M, Pechlaner S. [Stabilization of perilunate and transscaphoid perilunate fracture-dislocations via a combined palmar and dorsal approach]. *Oper Orthop Traumatol* 2009;21(4–5):442–58.

205. Sotereanos DG, Mitsionis GJ, Giannakopoulos PN, Tomaino MM, Herndon JH. Perilunate dislocation and fracture dislocation: A critical analysis of the volar-dorsal approach. *J Hand Surg Am* 1997;22(1):49–56.

206. Mack GR, Bosse MJ, Gelberman RH, Yu E. The natural history of scaphoid non-union. *J Bone Joint Surg Am* 1984;66(4):504–9.

207. Cooney WP. Failure of treatment of ununited fractures of the carpal scaphoid. *J Bone Joint Surg Am* 1984;66(7):1145–6.

208. Ruby LK, Stinson J, Belsky MR. The natural history of scaphoid non-union. A review of fifty-five cases. *J Bone Joint Surg Am* 1985;67(3):428–32.

209. Langhoff O, Andersen JL. Consequences of late immobilization of scaphoid fractures. *J Hand Surg Br* 1988;13(1):77–9.

210. Kawamura K, Chung KC. Treatment of scaphoid fractures and nonunions. *J Hand Surg Am* 2008;33(6):988–97.

211. Burgess RC. The effect of a simulated scaphoid malunion on wrist motion. *J Hand Surg Am* 1987;12(5 Pt 1):774–6.

212. Dias JJ, Taylor M, Thompson J, Brenkel IJ, Gregg PJ. Radiographic signs of union of scaphoid fractures. An analysis of inter-observer agreement and reproducibility. *J Bone Joint Surg Br* 1988;70(2):299–301.

213. Dias JJ. Definition of union after acute fracture and surgery for fracture nonunion of the scaphoid. *J Hand Surg Br* 2001;26(4):321–5.

214. Schmitt R, Christopoulos G, Wagner M, Krimmer H, Fodor S, van Schoonhoven J, et al. Avascular necrosis (AVN) of the proximal fragment in scaphoid nonunion: Is intravenous contrast agent necessary in MRI? *Eur J Radiol* 2011;77(2):222–7.

215. Megerle K, Worg H, Christopoulos G, Schmitt R, Krimmer H. Gadolinium-enhanced preoperative MRI scans as a prognostic parameter in scaphoid nonunion. *J Hand Surg Eur Vol* 2011;36(1):23–8.

216. Strauch RJ. Scapholunate advanced collapse and scaphoid nonunion advanced collapse arthritis—Update on evaluation and treatment. *J Hand Surg Am* 2011;36(4):729–35.

217. Garcia-Elias M, Lluch A. Partial excision of scaphoid: Is it ever indicated? *Hand Clin* 2001;17(4):687–95, x.

218. Mulford JS, Ceulemans LJ, Nam D, Axelrod TS. Proximal row carpectomy vs four corner fusion for scapholunate (Slac) or scaphoid nonunion advanced collapse (Snac) wrists: A systematic review of outcomes. *J Hand Surg Eur Vol* 2009;34(2):256–63.

219. Houshian S, Schroder HA. Wrist arthrodesis with the AO titanium wrist fusion plate: A consecutive series of 42 cases. *J Hand Surg Br* 2001;26(4):355–9.

220. Munk B, Larsen CF. Bone grafting the scaphoid nonunion: A systematic review of 147 publications including 5,246 cases of scaphoid nonunion. *Acta Orthop Scand* 2004;75(5):618–29.

221. Mahmoud M, Koptan W. Percutaneous screw fixation without bone grafting for established scaphoid nonunion with substantial bone loss. *J Bone Joint Surg Br* 2011;93(7):932–6.

222. Reigstad O, Grimsgaard C, Thorkildsen R, Reigstad A, Rokkum M. Long-term results of scaphoid nonunion surgery: 50 patients reviewed after 8 to 18 years. *J Orthop Trauma* 2012;26(4):241–5.

223. Trezies AJ, Davis TR, Barton NJ. Factors influencing the outcome of bone grafting surgery for scaphoid fracture non-union. *Injury* 2000;31(8):605–7.

224. Dinah AF, Vickers RH. Smoking increases failure rate of operation for established non-union of the scaphoid bone. *Int Orthop* 2007;31(4):503–5.

225. Little CP, Burston BJ, Hopkinson-Woolley J, Burge P. Failure of surgery for scaphoid non-union is associated with smoking. *J Hand Surg Br* 2006;31(3):252–5.

226. Trumble T, Nyland W. Scaphoid nonunions. Pitfalls and pearls. *Hand Clin* 2001;17(4):611–24.

227. Schneider LH, Aulicino P. Nonunion of the carpal scaphoid: The Russe procedure. *J Trauma* 1982;22(4):315–19.

228. Merrell GA, Wolfe SW, Slade JF, III. Treatment of scaphoid nonunions: Quantitative meta-analysis of the literature. *J Hand Surg Am* 2002;27(4):685–91.

229. Tomaino MM, King J, Pizillo M. Correction of lunate malalignment when bone grafting scaphoid nonunion with humpback deformity: Rationale and results of a technique revisited. *J Hand Surg Am* 2000;25(2):322–9.

230. Eggli S, Fernandez DL, Beck T. Unstable scaphoid fracture nonunion: A medium-term study of anterior wedge grafting procedures. *J Hand Surg Br* 2002;27(1):36–41.

231. Tambe AD, Cutler L, Murali SR, Trail IA, Stanley JK. In scaphoid non-union, does the source of graft affect outcome? Iliac crest versus distal end of radius bone graft. *J Hand Surg Br* 2006;31(1):47–51.

232. Braga-Silva J, Peruchi FM, Moschen GM, Gehlen D, Padoin AV. A comparison of the use of distal radius vascularised bone graft and non-vascularised iliac crest bone graft in the treatment of non-union of scaphoid fractures. *J Hand Surg Eur Vol* 2008;33(5):636–40.

233. Allan CH, Joshi A, Lichtman DM. Kienbock's disease: Diagnosis and treatment. *J Am Acad Orthop Surg* 2001;9(2):128–36.

234. Daecke W, Lorenz S, Wieloch P, Jung M, Martini AK. Lunate resection and vascularized Os pisiform transfer in Kienbock's Disease: An average of 10 years of follow-up study after Saffar's procedure. *J Hand Surg Am* 2005;30(4):677–84.

235. Mehrpour SR, Kamrani RS, Aghamirsalim MR, Sorbi R, Kaya A. Treatment of Kienbock disease by lunate core decompression. *J Hand Surg Am* 2011;36(10):1675–7.

236. Nakamura P, Imaeda T, Miura T. Scaphoid malunion. *J Bone Joint Surg Br* 1991;73(1):134–7.

237. Lynch NM, Linscheid RL. Corrective osteotomy for scaphoid malunion: Technique and long-term follow-up evaluation. *J Hand Surg Am* 1997;22(1):35–43.

238. Raudasoja L, Rawlins M, Kallio P, Vasenius J. Conservative treatment of scaphoid fractures: A follow up study. *Ann Chir Gynaecol* 1999;88(4):289–93.

239. Forward DP, Singh HP, Dawson S, Davis TR. The clinical outcome of scaphoid fracture malunion at 1 year. *J Hand Surg Eur Vol* 2009;34(1):40–6.

240. Waters PM, Stewart SL. Surgical treatment of non-union and avascular necrosis of the proximal part of the scaphoid in adolescents. *J Bone Joint Surg Am* 2002;84-A(6):915–20.

241. Arora R, Lutz M, Zimmermann R, Krappinger D, Niederwanger C, Gabl M. Free vascularised iliac bone graft for recalcitrant avascular non-union of the scaphoid. *J Bone Joint Surg Br* 2010;92(2):224–9.

242. Menth-Chiari WA, Poehling GG. Preiser's disease: Arthroscopic treatment of avascular necrosis of the scaphoid. *Arthroscopy* 2000;16(2):208–13.

28

Metacarpal fractures

MARK HENRY

INTRODUCTION

Elderly patients with metacarpal fractures have thinner cortices and a higher likelihood of fixation failure. On the other hand, the fractures are typically due to low energy injuries and may less frequently benefit from fixation. Older patients often have lower functional demands and are more accepting of deformity. Preserving independence in an older person with a metacarpal fracture means avoiding cumbersome methods of hand immobilization.

EPIDEMIOLOGY

The annual incidence of hand fractures ranges from 61 per 10,000 people younger than 20 years of age to 29 per 10,000 people older than 20 years of age and from 37 per 10,000 males to 13 per 10,000 females.[1,2] After age 65, women are at greater risk than men likely due to osteoporosis.[3] More than a third of metacarpal fractures involve the small finger.[3]

CLASSIFICATION

There is no well-accepted or widely used classification system for metacarpal fractures. The AO/OTA universal fracture classification system can be applied to the metacarpals but has an interobserver kappa coefficient of 0.44 and an intraobserver kappa coefficient of 0.62.[4] To permit comparison between study cohorts and facilitate communication between providers, metacarpal fractures are largely categorized by the location within the bone combined with the pattern of the fracture. Further distinction is given to degrees of comminution, intra-articular extension and open fractures. Metacarpal fractures are commonly divided into head, neck, shaft and base. Head and base fractures are intra-articular injuries; neck and shaft are extra-articular. Shaft fractures can be grouped as transverse/short oblique and spiral/long oblique. Transverse/short oblique fractures tend to angulate in the sagittal plane, apex dorsal (Figure 28.1). Conversely, displacement of long oblique/spiral fractures is characterized more by axial shortening and rotational deformity than sagittal plane angulation (Figure 28.2). At first glance, it can be difficult to distinguish a spiral from a long oblique fracture, but a spiral fracture always has one component of the fracture interface that runs in a pure longitudinal direction. The importance of distinguishing the two patterns relates simply to predicting the likelihood of malrotation, which is theoretically greater for the spiral fracture induced by a rotational mechanism of injury as opposed to the axial shearing mechanism of the long oblique fracture.

TREATMENT

Clinical evaluation

Comorbidities and activity level are important considerations in the elderly. Details about social support and living situation relate directly to the elderly patient's capacity for self-care with an injured hand, the degree to which different types of splints may interfere with function and the availability of transportation to receive associated care such as hand therapy.[1] Specific attention should be given to the mechanism of injury, including the direction of the applied force and the level of energy imparted, as this information will be used to estimate the probability of further displacement when selecting treatment.

Although shortening, translation and angular deformity can all be easily discerned on radiographs, axial rotation of the metacarpal is more difficult to evaluate. Ask

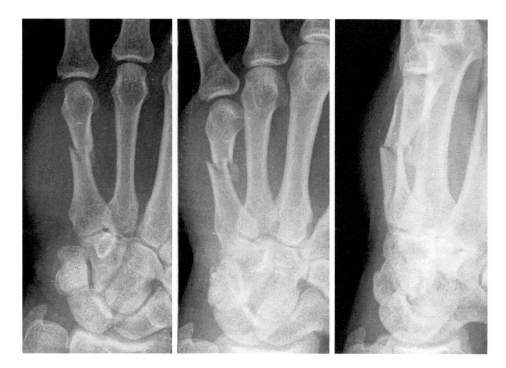

Figure 28.1 Transverse/short oblique fractures of the metacarpal shaft tend to angulate apex dorsal rather than shorten or axially rotate in comparison to long oblique/spiral fractures. The features of translation and the volar third fragment indicate a higher degree of inherent instability and periosteal disruption in this 68-year-old male.

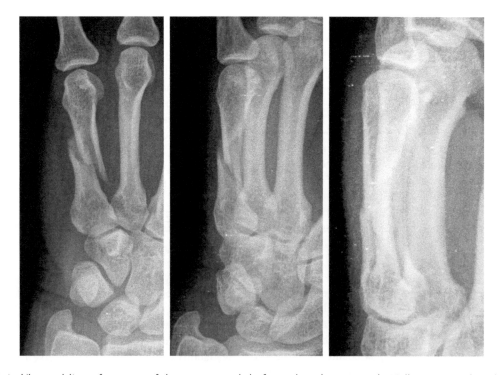

Figure 28.2 Spiral/long oblique fractures of the metacarpal shaft tend to shorten and axially rotate rather than angulate in the sagittal plane in comparison to transverse/short oblique fractures.

the patient to actively flex the metacarpophalangeal (MP) joints as far as possible and examine the alignment of the digits relative to each other, viewing down the axis of the metacarpals (Figure 28.3). Axial malrotation of the meta-carpal will cause the involved proximal phalanx to project radially or ulnarly, out of alignment with neighbouring digits. The often cited examination of nail plate alignment is unreliable for evaluation of axial rotation. The inher-ent stability of the fracture can be assessed by asking the patient to actively flex and extend within her comfort zone.

Excessive axial shortening or apex dorsal angulation at the fracture site theoretically poses the long-term threat of functionally limiting extensor lag. In cadaver studies, each 2 mm of axial shortening produced a corresponding 7 degrees of extensor lag.[5] Reduced flexor efficiency has also been cited for angulations over 30 degrees at the small metacarpal neck.[6,7] These cadaveric observations have not been borne out in clinical practice. A study of 42 patients with

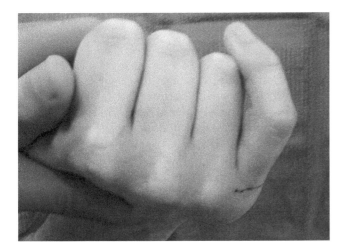

Figure 28.3 Malrotation at the metacarpal level is best assessed by flexing the metacarpophalangeal (MP) joints and viewing down the axis of the metacarpal. The projection of the proximal phalanges (parallel or divergent) represents the rotation status of the metacarpal.

initial extensor lag from shortening all corrected the deficit by 1 year and achieved 94% of contralateral grip strength.[8]

Radiographic evaluation requires at least three different views of the hand (Figure 28.4). The standard anteroposterior (AP) view is useful for evaluating relative shortening and revealing sagittal fracture planes. Oblique coronal fractures without translation or angulation are easily obscured on the AP view by fragment overlap and are better visualized on the oblique. A true lateral view offers little useful information at the head or shaft level as the metacarpal shadows overlap each other. If the lateral view is slightly supinated, it can at least show the index and long finger carpometacarpal (CMC) joint profile and rule out fracture dislocations. The most broadly useful third view is an oblique, pronated around 35 degrees. This gives sufficient pronation to overcome the problem of overlap seen on the lateral, but still facilitates reasonably accurate measurement of sagittal plane angulation and demonstrates the CMC profiles of the ring and small fingers.[9] Multiple specialty views have been described but are rarely necessary.

Treatment planning

There are three categories of metacarpal fracture treatment: non-operative, closed reduction and pinning, and open reduction with internal fixation (ORIF). The non-operative category ranges from no immobilization of any kind to hard splints or casts spanning forearm to hand. In between are multiple designs for strapping or splinting

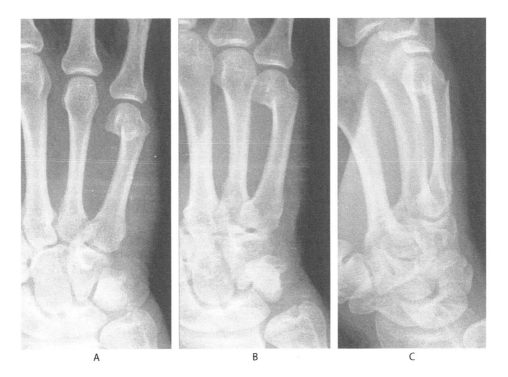

A   B   C

Figure 28.4 Characteristic features of small finger metacarpal neck fracture demonstrating: (a) shortening and radial translation of the distal fragment on posteroanterior (PA) view, (b) apex dorsal angulation, volar impaction of the neck and supination deformity seen best on the oblique view and (c) apex dorsal deformity, volar translation and neck impaction and the extension proximally into the shaft best seen on the lateral view.

that attempt to provide comfort and influence the position of the fracture while allowing motion. The pinning category includes transverse pinning to adjacent metacarpals, intramedullary pinning with one or more wires and interfragmentary/intrafocal pinning at the fracture interface. ORIF potentially includes any type of fixation device but, with modern systems, is largely confined to screws alone or plate and screws (Figure 28.5). The most successful outcomes result from matching the individual fracture and patient characteristics to the treatment strategy.[10] Several differences between elderly and younger adult patients are worth considering:

- Cortical thickness is reduced, limiting the purchase of both Kirschner wires (K-wires) and screws, but with a greater relative impact on screws.
- Cortical bone is weaker and more likely to fail adjacent to an implant, propagating new fracture lines from the point of implant penetration to nearby fracture edges or other implants.
- Fixed angle screws near a joint can cut out of osteoporotic cancellous bone.
- The adjacent small joints, MP and proximal interphalangeal (PIP) may have deformity and reduced motion from pre-existing osteoarthritis.
- Infirm older patients may benefit from independent exercises when it is difficult to get to a hand therapist's office.
- Less active elderly patients may accept more deformity and stiffness than healthier, more active patients. Older generations may also be more adaptive.

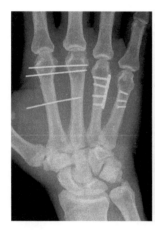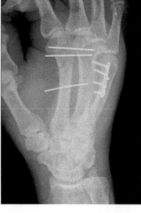

Figure 28.5 A very active working man with metacarpophalangeal (MP) osteoarthritis sustained heavy crush trauma with multiple metacarpal fractures (open at the ring finger, and small and closed at the index finger). Mixed fixation methods, tailored to match the fracture characteristics and associated soft tissue injuries, allowed immediate therapy that yielded a final result of range of motion (ROM) equivalent to contralateral. No one method of fixation is universally superior to another; the selection should simply correlate the advantages and disadvantages with the clinical features of the injury pattern.

- Elderly patients with metacarpal fractures may be less prone to stiffness, perhaps due to relatively low energy injuries and diminished scarring.
- Comorbidities such as coronary artery disease, congestive heart failure and chronic obstructive pulmonary disease increase the risks of anaesthesia.
- Comorbidities such as diabetes and peripheral vascular disease may increase the complications of surgery.
- Older patients may have lower physiological reserve when adverse events occur.

Non-surgical treatment

Non-surgical treatment is appropriate for fractures with acceptable alignment and fractures that can be reduced to an acceptable position, provided that position can be effectively maintained. The most difficult displacement to reduce and control is translation and angulation in the coronal plane. High degrees of axial malrotation can be improved by neighbour strapping (particularly for the long and ring fingers) but cannot be reliably controlled without direct bony fixation. Sagittal plane translation and angulation is easily reduced but often tends to gradually drift back towards the position demonstrated in the original injury films.

Patients love to hear that the fracture will definitely heal. To decide if the alignment is acceptable to the patient, the surgeon can point out where prominences are expected, what the knuckle will look like and rotational deformity (especially when great enough to result in full digital overlap). Most patients, the elderly in particular, are unlikely to rate angular deformity or shortening displeasing enough to request more invasive treatment from a cosmetic standpoint alone. Once patients understand that the fracture will heal, the hand will function well and arthritis is not an issue, deformity is often quite acceptable.

The most relevant functional issue is an active extensor lag at the MP or PIP joint.[5] If the patient does not demonstrate an extensor lag when acutely injured, then good final function can be anticipated without correction of the angular deformity or shortening. If a slight extensor lag is present acutely, correction through rebalancing after healing is anticipated.[8] Rotational deformity is less well-tolerated but should be interpreted in the context of existing deformity patterns for the elderly hand. Subtle degrees that do not result in digital overlap are easy to adapt to. A moderate degree of initial rotational abnormality can be reduced and maintained by the influence of adjacent digits, particularly the long or ring finger.

If non-surgical treatment has been selected, the next decision concerns the method of immobilization or positional control. If the presenting posture is considered acceptable and no formal reduction was performed, then there is little need for splinting. Patients fare well with early motion, using side strapping for rotational control and prevention of catching the injured digit on clothing and furniture.[11]

If an unstable metacarpal fracture was reduced, then the patient may benefit from 3–4 weeks of initial intrinsic plus splinting.[12] The MP joints are flexed around 70 degrees with the distal extent of the hard splint terminating at the level of the PIP joints, allowing full PIP motion. Hand based intrinsic plus splints are smaller and lighter to wear, but without the wrist support, some patients tend to flex the wrist, which drives MP extension and PIP flexion, counteracting the intended benefits of intrinsic plus splinting (Figure 28.6). Flexion of the MP joints reduces flexor and intrinsic tone and theoretically the tendency to pull the distal metacarpal fragment into flexion. An MP extension block with active flexion of the PIP joints might also help guide the injured ray into better rotational alignment. It is not clear that earlier

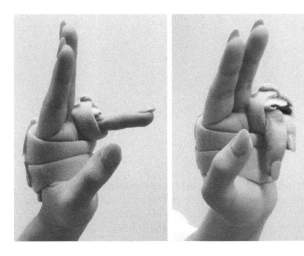

Figure 28.6 When a hard splint (intrinsic plus) is judged to be necessary, treatment related morbidity can be minimized by including only the fractured digit and its neighbour, allowing freedom of proximal interphalangeal (PIP) and wrist motion (provided the patient lacks the guarding response that encourages a wrist flexion posture).

performance of motion exercises necessarily achieves better final motion or alignment.[13]

For stable fractures or when the deformity is accepted, less cumbersome immobilization such as a removable wrist splint has higher patient satisfaction.[14] Immobilization of the fingers is particularly cumbersome in elderly patients (Figure 28.7). A fractured finger can be strapped to an adjacent finger (buddy taping) to provide support and comfort while allowing motion.

Closed reduction and pinning

Manipulative reduction and pinning can often restore angulation, translation, rotation and length adequate for good aesthetics and function. No one method of pinning is superior to others.[15] Options include transverse pinning to an adjacent intact metacarpal, intramedullary pinning (antegrade or retrograde), intramedullary headless screw fixation, and interfragmentary/intrafocal pinning at the fracture site. Intra-articular fractures at the base of the thumb metacarpal can be stabilized using a combination of interfragmentary pinning (to maintain articular reduction) and intermetacarpal pinning to the index (to prevent axial subsidence).[16]

Transverse pinning is best suited for transverse or short oblique fractures at any level in the metacarpal, from head to base, that can be realigned with closed manipulation (Figure 28.8). The strategy is modelled after the principles of external fixation with the adjacent intact metacarpal replacing the external fixator bar (Figure 28.9). Three 0.045-inch K-wires are placed: one as distal as possible without interfering with the sagittal bands, one just distal to the fracture site and one just proximal to the fracture site; the strong intermetacarpal/CMC ligaments serve as

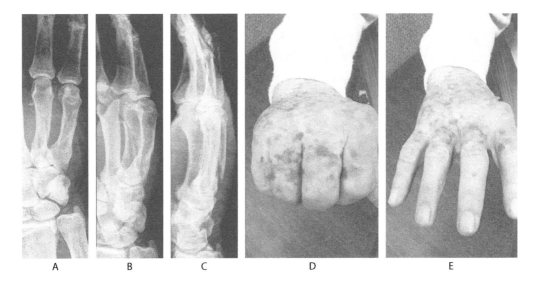

A   B   C   D   E

Figure 28.7 A 94-year-old man in assisted living. (a–c) Long oblique ring and small metacarpal fractures experienced shortening of less than 5 mm, angulation of less than 20 degrees in the sagittal plane and no rotational deformity. (d–e) An unsupervised home program of immediate active mobilization without splinting led to no further displacement and minimized treatment induced stiffness. Total utilization of medical resources was three office visits.

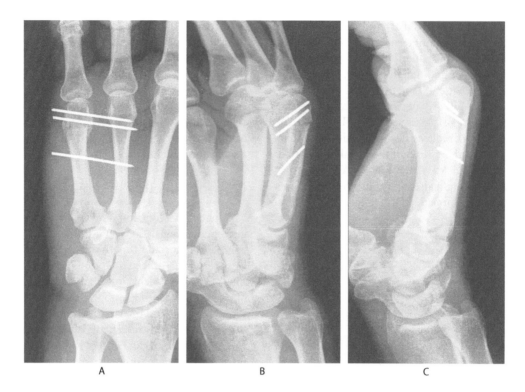

A   B   C

Figure 28.8 A male manual labourer whose preoperative films are shown in Figure 28.4. **(a)** Posteroanterior (PA) view shows the correction of radial translation – often requires percutaneous instrumentation to push the distal fragment into position. The goal is to keep the transverse pins proximal to the sagittal bands and the collateral ligaments (ring finger axis) but with a distal fragment (small finger axis) obligatory transgression of the collateral ligament fibres for 3 weeks is unavoidable with this technique. **(b)** Oblique and **(c)** lateral views show placement of the proximal pin immediately proximal to the shaft extension of the fracture, and full correction of the original deformities regarding angulation, length and translation.

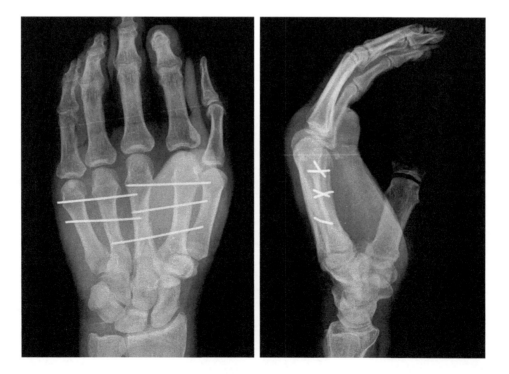

Figure 28.9 Although the pattern of comminuted fractures in adjacent metacarpals represents an overall more unstable injury, the four metacarpals can be divided into a radial column (index and long) and an ulnar column (ring and small). As long as one bone in each column is intact, reliable stabilization is still achieved with the minimally invasive strategy of transverse pinning in this working man.

the fourth, most proximal point of stabilization.[17] One advantage of transverse pinning is that the construct directly controls all possible directions and modes of displacement.[18] Other advantages are that the pins do not transgress or interfere with the extensor tendons or joints (MP or CMC) and the buried pin tips reside in well-vascularized and well-padded intrinsic muscles. The primary disadvantage is transgression of an otherwise unaffected anatomic structure, the adjacent metacarpal, with an extremely low risk of sustaining a subsequent fracture or infection through the residual pin tract. Pins are left protruding for ease of subsequent removal or buried in the intrinsic muscles to reduce the risk of pin tract infection (12% if left out through the skin).[19] Pins are removed 3 or 4 weeks after surgery. With the added stability of pinning, gentle active full range motion can begin as soon as tolerated, but some surgeons will reserve motion therapy until after pin removal to limit pin irritation or infection. Supplementary splints of any type can be used prior to pin removal (most commonly intrinsic plus splinting) followed by neighbour strapping or nothing after pin removal. Twenty-eight patients with transverse pinning for small metacarpal neck fractures experienced no complications and achieved a final Disabilities of the Arm, Shoulder and Hand (DASH) score of 5 with full flexion.[20]

Intramedullary pinning can be accomplished with single or multiple wires, entering antegrade at the margin of the CMC joint or retrograde through the MP joint (Figure 28.10). The advantage compared to transverse pinning is containment of the fixation to just the injured bone. The disadvantage is that the entry points directly transgress the extensor tendons and MP joint (retrograde) or are immediately adjacent to the CMC joint, the extensor tendons and cutaneous nerve branches (antegrade). Rotational malalignment is not directly controlled. The quality of angular control is dependent on the fill of the wire(s) in the canal, less precise than the purchase of four cortices with each wire in transverse pinning. Wires can migrate into joints, tendons and nerves, with the cut edge of metal abrading these structures during early motion therapy. If the surgeon places the wires entirely within bone and no subsequent migration occurs, then no removal is required. Compared to plate and screw fixation, intramedullary nailing patients had a higher rate of loss of reduction (5/38), wire penetration into the MP joint (3/38), and tendon to hardware friction necessitating wire removal (15/38).[21]

Open reduction with internal fixation

The indication for ORIF of a metacarpal fracture in a patient of any age is an inherently unstable fracture incapable of being reduced and maintained in an acceptable position by closed means, with or without pinning. Such circumstances represent the minority of cases in the general population and an extremely small percentage of all metacarpal fractures in the elderly. The lower energy mechanisms of injury seen in the elderly rarely create the highly unstable, dramatically displaced fracture patterns seen after punching walls or using power tools (Figure 28.11). Wider latitude exists

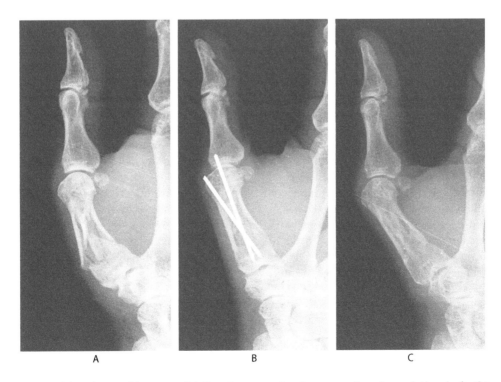

A   B   C

Figure 28.10 A 66-year-old active working man. (a) Despite comminution extending through the shaft, (b) reduction can be maintained with temporary intramedullary K-wire fixation. (c) Even at 4 months, long after complete clinical healing and full use by the patient, radiographic lucency can still be seen at the original fracture site – a common finding.

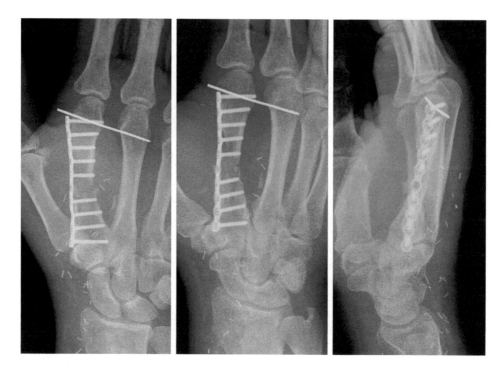

Figure 28.11 Even the elderly can sustain injury patterns more often seen in the younger patient such as this self-induced point blank gunshot wound through the index metacarpal. Immediate debridement and autogenous bone grafting accompany lateral plating so that the sagittal plane forces of rehabilitation are borne by the width of the plate not the thickness. The plate is kept just shy of the collateral ligaments at the metacarpophalangeal (MP) joint, and the simple addition of a temporary distal transverse intermetacarpal wire shields the transmission of force to the weak link of the plate segment that spans the bone defect until graft incorporation improves the inherent strength of the construct.

for a functionally acceptable reduction in the elderly than in actively working younger patients with higher demands. Even when the fracture pattern and degree of displacement lend themselves to an ORIF strategy, the chances of implant loosening are increased in the elderly, offsetting the benefits. One pattern, even in the elderly, that represents an ideal indication for ORIF is a displaced intra-articular fracture of the metacarpal head (Figure 28.12). Seven patients with an average age of 28 years achieved a mean arc of MP joint motion of 79 degrees with lag screw fixation.[22] The one older patient in the series, a 59-year-old man, reached only a 60 degree arc.

A spiral/long oblique fracture of the midshaft in good quality bone is another well-matched pattern for lag screw fixation only without a plate (Figure 28.13). Excellent fixation is achieved because of strong interfragmentary compression exerted by tightening down the head of the lag screw into the countersunk cortex. In the elderly patient with poor bone quality the same degree of interfragmentary compression will not be realized and substantial risk exists for the screw head to propagate a secondary fracture line to the fracture edge or between screw tracts. Even when the fixation appears sound at the time of surgery, screw threads may strip out from thin cortices during early rehabilitation. Lag screw fixation is an acceptable strategy in an elderly patient, but only after careful assessment of the fracture with a realistic appraisal of bone quality. An alternative is to reduce the fracture and compress it

with forceps or a bone reduction clamp and then use position screws (no gliding hole).

Other internal fixation options include fine caliber (24–28 gauge) steel wire in a cerclage, interosseous or composite (combined with K-wire) construct. Bioabsorbable fixation has demonstrated higher complication rates but no evidence of superiority over titanium plates and screws; a poor choice for the elderly patient.[23] Plate and screw systems for the hand have become more refined and versatile. However, elderly patients require modified application of the technology, with the caveat that age has proven to be an independent predictor of reduced motion following plate and screw fixation.[24]

In younger patients undergoing ORIF, the majority of fractures can be secured with screws only, with the minority requiring plates. In the elderly, the opposite is true. Although seemingly the application of a 'more invasive' strategy to an already compromised patient, it is exactly this state of compromise that calls for the distribution of force across a wider section of bone (Figure 28.14). As long as the plates are not applied dorsally (which should almost never be the case), there is really no detriment to a laterally applied plate compared to lag screws. Use of a plate distributes the load over a greater length of bone.

Small plates with screws that lock to the plate are available in the hand now, but their role is debated. A nonlocking screw compresses the plate against the bone. If used through the plate and across the fracture site, the screw

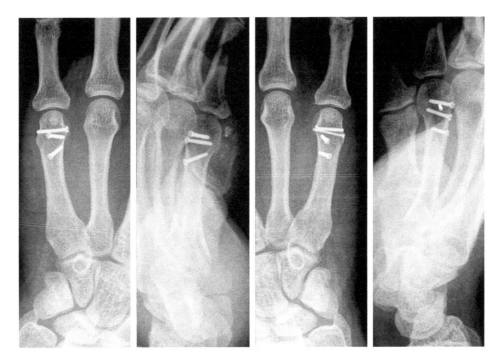

Figure 28.12 Bilateral simultaneous intra-articular fractures of the metacarpal head making countersunk lag screws the fixation of choice. Screws should be placed in different planes to resist all patterns of potential displacement.

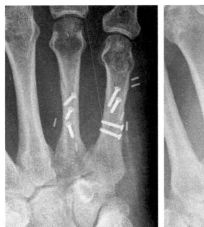
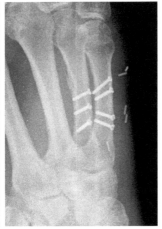
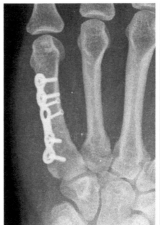
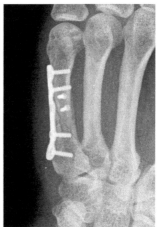

Figure 28.13 Good bone quality in this actively working man made lag screw only fixation the most appropriate treatment, permitting immediate unrestricted motion therapy through which he achieved full active range coincident to clinical healing of the fractures.

Figure 28.14 Bone quality and comminution in the shaft of this female patient who desired immediate functional use of her hand was inappropriate for lag screw only fixation (preoperative films shown in Figure 28.2). Supplemental plating permitted side strap only protection postoperatively without hard splinting. Her immediate use promoted achievement of full active motion including composite hyperextension by 3 weeks postoperatively and a Disabilities of the Arm, Shoulder and Hand (DASH) score of 0 by 8 weeks postoperatively.

compresses both the plate and the near fragment against the opposing fragment. For a non-locking screw to be most effective, the leading threads need to achieve purchase in the bone fragment near the tip of the screw. This should be possible in cortical bone, even the cortical bone of an elderly patient in the midshaft region. As one moves from the mid-shaft towards either metaphysis and the cortices thin, the capacity for screw tip purchase may disappear. Particularly in elderly patients, locking screws may provide more secure fixation in the metaphysis. In a younger patient where plate to bone compression is desired, it would be preferable to use

non-locking screws all the way into the metaphyseal regions, except when the plate is being used for juxta-articular support in the absence of metaphyseal integrity.

After ORIF, the patient should begin active, self-assisted stretching exercises within a week of surgery. Once MP joint effusions capable of inducing an intrinsic minus posture are no longer a concern, commensurate with the degree of stability achieved at the time of surgery, patients can eliminate any hard intrinsic plus splints in favour of side strapping only. A retrospective review of 19 patients with 43 fractures (closed adjacent multiple metacarpals) and a mean age of 24 studied the outcomes following plate fixation with mostly 2.0 mm plates (included were cases with 1.5 mm and 2.4 mm plates) and the initiation of active and assisted range of motion (ROM) by 3–5 days postoperatively. One patient was lost to follow-up; the remaining 18 patients achieved full motion (total active motion >230 degrees) and returned to their full employment within 2 months of surgery. Only two requested implant removal.[25]

Surgical technique: ORIF

To limit the potential for wound to tendon adhesions, a longitudinal incision can be placed as far away from the paths of the zone 6 extensor tendons as possible. For instance, index and small finger metacarpals are approached from the mid-axial border of the hand. For central metacarpals, the incision can be equidistant from the bordering tendon pathways, not directly overlying the metacarpal axis. Identify and protect branches of the superficial radial or dorsal ulnar cutaneous nerves. Limit handling of the extensor tendons. The metacarpal is exposed by elevating the interosseous fascia, muscle and periosteum together. Minimize periosteal stripping and remove any clot or loose tissue from the fracture surfaces. Hold the provisional reduction either manually (Brown-Adson forceps work well), with specialized bone holding clamps, or using the plate fixed to one of the fracture fragments as a reduction aid.

Plan the location of all lag screws before drilling the first one; each screw must have adequate placement away from the fracture edge and from adjacent screws. A bone fragment that appears to be a single, solid fragment may actually contain subtle non-displaced fissures. Although fixation of a plate to bone at the metacarpal level should use 2.0 mm diameter screws, interfragmentary screw fixation is best performed with 1.5–1.7 mm screws. A screw that connects a plate to the bone is transferring load from the bone to the plate, bearing greater load and thus requiring a larger caliber. Lag screws direct and maintain the reduction of the fracture fragments that transfer load from one fragment to another, placing less stress on the screws that can be of smaller caliber without risk of breakage.

Small intercalary comminuted fragments are not reduced. Maintain periosteum, muscle and fascia attachments. Medium sized fragments can be fixed to the neighbouring larger fragment with small (e.g. 1.2 mm) lag or position screws to create a unified fragment group. Eventually, one must develop a proximal fragment group and a distal fragment group. The final reduction between groups is manually positioned and held so that the plate can be properly contoured in all planes. The plane of the cortex changes along the length of the bone, necessitating axial twist contouring of plates. Failure to do so will induce a rotational deformity when the final screws are tightened. Placing the plate laterally may limit irritation and adhesion to the overlying extensor tendons. As the plate position becomes more proximal for the long or ring finger, lateral placement is more technically difficult but not impossible for all but some intra-articular fractures of the CMC joint (Figure 28.15). If lag screws are to be placed

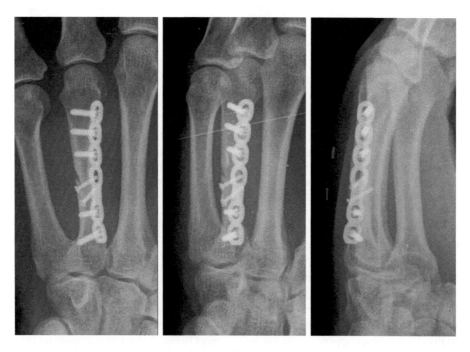

Figure 28.15 The short fracture interface does not permit sufficient fixation with lag screws alone despite good bone quality. Avoid dorsal plate placement whenever possible, as drilling and screw placement can be performed in the coronal plane all the way down to the intermetacarpal joint proximally; stay proximal to the collateral ligaments distally.

prior to plate application, the exact location of the plate must be planned before drilling for the lag screws. Failure to mark all the screw positions in advance can result in a lag screw obstructing the path of a plate fixation screw, leaving an insufficient number of screws on one side of the plate – there should be a minimum of two. Adequacy of the reduction and implant placement must be checked by three means that are cross-referenced: direct observation of the fracture interface, clinical assessment of digital alignment and rotation, and fluoroscopic imaging in multiple planes.

Recovery

Patients are encouraged to actively move the fingers and assist in stretching the hand with their other hand. Most patients find this straightforward and prefer to do it on their own, but some enjoy the coaching and camaraderie of a certified hand therapist. There is little role for pure passive motion. At 4 weeks after injury, splints are discarded in favour of either neighbour strapping or nothing. Strengthening will come with return to normal use and a formal strengthening program is optional.

After pinning, local scar adhesions may tether the tendons. One method to break the tendon free from local adhesions is a specific pattern of exercise after pin removal: the tendon is actively contracted with the MP joint in flexion, but held in check by the thumb over the proximal phalanx. The thumb suddenly releases the tendon that is already 'pre-loaded' by the active contraction, resulting in a rapid excursion of the tendon, separating the scar adhesion before the scar tissue has the opportunity to creep and move with the tendon.[26] Patients should be reminded to think of following through the motion into full hyperextension of the MP joint past neutral just as a baseball batter follows through his swing. Scar massage can separate the skin layer of the wound from the tendon, improving tendon excursion.

COMPLICATIONS

The most common adverse outcome of a metacarpal fracture is stiffness. Excessive immobilization and invasive surgical treatment can contribute to stiffness. Limited sagittal plane malalignment is commonly accepted, and is rarely problematic. Delayed or nonunion at the metacarpal level is uncommon. Risk factors include devitalized fragments, fixation that maintains a gap between fragments and infection. Nonunion occurs four times as often at the narrower interface of transverse fractures compared to a broader oblique interface.[27]

Other complications specific to metacarpal fixation (up to 15%) include broken or migrating K-wires that may necessitate early removal, potentially lose fixation or cause pin tract infection.[28,29] Only an exposed K-wire can become infected. Cutting off K-wires below the skin surface at the time of surgery minimizes, but does not eliminate, the risk

of pin tract infection. A previously buried wire can become exposed through the reduction of swelling or with migration. The appearance is similar for skin irritation around an exposed pin and a true pin tract infection. The former can be managed with local pin site care and prophylactic oral antibiotics at the surgeon's discretion. An infected wire at the skin surface only is treated by pin removal with or without oral antibiotics. If the fracture is not yet healed, the pin can be retained and oral antibiotics prescribed. If a deep abscess has developed or the pin is loose and the infection seems to be in the bone, formal operative debridement is warranted. Soft tissue infections should need no more than 7–10 days of oral antibiotics. If acute osteomyelitis has already developed, the duration of treatment is 4–6 weeks on either oral or parenteral antibiotics depending on culture and sensitivity results.

Tendon attrition and rupture can occur over cut ends of wires or against permanent hardware placed on the dorsal surface of the metacarpal (plates belong lateral not dorsal). Rarely a concern in the younger patient, pressure necrosis from a splint can occur in the thin delicate skin of the elderly.

SUMMARY

Metacarpal fractures heal and shortening and sagittal plane angulation are largely aesthetic concerns. Substantial axial rotation deformity is less well-tolerated by patients. Elderly patients are bothered less by deformity than younger patients and are more concerned about retaining mobility particularly in the early recovery period. Most patients are happy with supportive splints allowing finger motion. When operative treatment is chosen, temporary pinning is usually adequate. When planning internal fixation, fractures that might otherwise be treated well with screws alone may benefit from plate fixation in the elderly due to unexpected fragmentation, the risk of fragmenting through a screw track and thin cortices.

REFERENCES

1. Anakwe RE, Aitken SA, Cowie JG, Middleton SD, Court-Brown CM. The epidemiology of fractures of the hand and the influence of social deprivation. *Journal of Hand Surgery* 36(1) (2011): 62–65.
2. Feehan LM, Sheps SB. Incidence and demographics of hand fractures in British Columbia, Canada: A population-based study. *Journal of Hand Surgery* 31(7) (2006): 1068–1074.
3. Stanton JS, Dias JJ, Burke FD. Fractures of the tubular bones of the hand. *Journal of Hand Surgery* 32(6) (2007): 626–636.
4. Szwebel JD, Ehlinger V, Pinsolle V, Bruneteau P, Pelissier P, Salmi LR. Reliability of a classification of fractures of the hand based on the AO comprehensive classification system. *Journal of Hand Surgery* 35(5) (2010): 392–395.

5. Strauch RJ, Rosenwasser MP, Lunt JG. Metacarpal shaft fractures: The effect of shortening on the extensor tendon mechanism. *Journal of Hand Surgery* 23 (1998): 519–523.

6. Ali A, Hamman J, Mass DP. The biomechanical effects of angulated boxer's fractures. *Journal of Hand Surgery* 24 (1999): 835–844.

7. Birndorf MS, Daley R, Greenwald DP. Metacarpal fracture angulation decreases flexor mechanical efficiency in human hands. *Plastic and Reconstructive Surgery* 99 (1997): 1079–1083.

8. Al-Qattan MM. Outcome of conservative management of spiral/long oblique fractures of the metacarpal shaft of the fingers using a palmar wrist splint and immediate mobilisation of the fingers. *Journal of Hand Surgery* 33(6) (2008): 723–727.

9. Leung YL, Beredjiklian PK, Monaghan BA, Bozentka DJ. Radiographic assessment of small finger metacarpal neck fractures. *Journal of Hand Surgery* 27 (2002): 443–448.

10. Henry MH. Fractures of the proximal phalanx and metacarpals in the hand: Preferred methods of stabilization. *Journal of the American Academy of Orthopedic Surgeons* 16 (2008): 320–329.

11. Braakman M. Functional taping of fractures of the fifth metacarpal results in a quicker recovery. *Injury* 29 (1998): 5–9.

12. Debnath UK, Nassab RS, Oni JA, Davis TR. A prospective study of the treatment of fractures of the little finger metacarpal shaft with a short hand cast. *Journal of Hand Surgery* 29(3) (2004): 214–217.

13. Harding IJ, Parry D, Barrington RL. The use of a moulded metacarpal brace versus neighbour strapping for fractures of the finger metacarpal neck. *Journal of Hand Surgery* 26(3) (2001): 261–263.

14. Strub B, Schindele S, Sonderegger J, Sproedt J, von Campe A, Gruenert JG. Intramedullary splinting or conservative treatment for displaced fractures of the little finger metacarpal neck? A prospective study. *Journal of Hand Surgery* 35(9) (2010): 725–729.

15. Wong T-C, Ip FK, Yeung SH. Comparison between percutaneous transverse fixation and intramedullary K-wires in treating closed fractures of the metacarpal neck of the little finger. *Journal of Hand Surgery* 31(1) (2006): 61–65.

16. Lutz M, Sailer R, Zimmerman R, Gabl M, Ulmer H, Pechlaner S. Closed reduction transarticular Kirshner wire fixation versus open reduction internal fixation in the treatment of Bennett fracture dislocation. *Journal of Hand Surgery* 28(2) (2003): 142–147.

17. El-Shennawy M, Nakamura K, Patterson RM, Viegas SF. Three-dimensional kinematic analysis of the second through fifth carpometacarpal joints. *Journal of Hand Surgery* 26 (2001): 1030–1035.

18. Galanakis I, Aliquizakis A, Katonis P, Papadokostakis G, Stergiopoulos K, Hadjipavlou A. Treatment of closed unstable metacarpal fractures using percutaneous transverse fixation with Kirschner wires. *Journal of Trauma* 55 (2003): 509–513.

19. Sletten IN, Nordsletten L, Husby T, Odegaard RA, Hellund JC, Kvernmo HD. Isolated, extra-articular neck and shaft fractures of the 4th and 5th metacarpals: A comparison of transverse and bouquet (intramedullary) pinning in 67 patients. *Journal of Hand Surgery* 37 (2012): 387–395.

20. Potenza V, Caterini R, De Maio F, Bisicchia S, Farsetti P. Fractures of the neck of the fifth metacarpal bone. Medium-term results in 28 cases treated by percutaneous transverse pinning. *Injury* 43 (2012): 242–245.

21. Ozer K, Gillani S, Williams A, Peterson SL, Morgan S. Comparison of intramedullary nailing versus plate-screw fixation of extra-articular metacarpal fractures. *Journal of Hand Surgery* 33 (2008): 1724–1731.

22. Tan JS, Foo AT, Chew WC, Teoh LC. Articularly placed interfragmentary screw fixation of difficult condylar fractures of the hand. *Journal of Hand Surgery* 36 (2011): 604–609.

23. Sakai A, Oshige T, Zenke Y, Menuki K, Murai T, Nakamura T. Mechanical comparison of novel bioabsorbable plates with titanium plates and small-series clinical comparisons for metacarpal fractures. *Journal of Bone and Joint Surgery* 94 (2012): 1597–1604.

24. Shimzu T, Omokawa S, Akahane M, Murata K, Nakano K, Kawamura K, Tanaka Y. Predictors of the postoperative range of finger motion for comminuted periarticular metacarpal and phalangeal fractures treated with a titanium plate. *Injury* 43 (2012): 940–945.

25. Souer JS, Mudgal CS. Plate fixation in closed ipsilateral multiple metacarpal fractures. *Journal of Hand Surgery* 33(6) (2008): 740–744.

26. Henry MH, Stutz C, Brown H. Technique for extensor tendon acceleration. *Journal of Hand Therapy* 19 (2006): 421–424.

27. Fusetti C, Della Santa DR. Influence of fracture pattern on consolidation after metacarpal plate fixation. *Chirurgie de la Main* 23 (2004): 32–36.

28. Hsu LP, Schwartz EG, Kalainov DM, Chen F, Makowiec RL. Complications of K-wire fixation in procedures involving the hand and wrist. *Journal of Hand Surgery* 36 (2011): 610–616.

29. Stahl S, Schwartz O. Complications of K-wire fixation of fractures and dislocations in the hand and wrist. *Archives Orthopedic and Trauma Surgery* 121 (2001): 527–530.

29

Phalangeal fractures and dislocations

GUANG YANG, EVAN P. McGLINN AND KEVIN C. CHUNG

INTRODUCTION

Phalanx fractures and dislocations are some of the most common musculoskeletal injuries. The goal of treatment is to optimize hand function and minimize adverse outcomes. Elderly patients are, in general, more accepting of deformity, have lower functional demands and adapt less well to cumbersome treatments. This chapter addresses the management of phalanx fractures in the elderly.

EPIDEMIOLOGY

In 1998, approximately 0.84% of all patients visiting an emergency room in the United States had a hand fracture, most often a phalanx fracture.[1,2] Finger fractures are most common in childhood. The incidence of finger fracture is 16/100,000 patients in a year among people aged 55–64 years and 35/100,000 in people aged 65–74 years, which is much less than the 185/100,000 in children aged 5–14 years.[1] Phalanx fractures are more common after falls in elderly women and during sports among boys and young men.[3,4]

ANATOMY

Final hand function after phalanx fracture is influenced by the condition of the skin, tendons and nerves. There are three phalanges in each finger that are connected by the proximal interphalangeal (PIP) joint and the distal interphalangeal (DIP) joint (Figure 29.1). The thumb has two phalanges and only one interphalangeal (IP) joint.

The distal phalanx is the smallest of the phalanges. The tip of the distal phalanx is horseshoe shaped and referred to as the tuft. The central, thinner part of the distal phalanx is called the shaft and has a smooth surface.

The proximal portion of the distal phalanx is called the base and along with the distal portion of the middle phalanx constitutes the DIP joint. The middle phalanges and proximal phalanges have similar shape, although the proximal phalanges are larger in size. Each of them has a base, shaft, neck and head from proximal to distal. The heads of these phalanges enlarge as two condyles separated by a shallow groove.

The DIP joint can hyperextend. The capsule is reinforced by the collateral ligaments and volar plate. Movement and stability are enhanced by the terminal extensor tendon and flexor digitorum profundus (FDP) tendon.

The head of the proximal phalanx and base of the middle phalanx constitute the bony structures of the PIP joint. The PIP joint is a hinge joint that has flexion and extension motions. The collateral ligaments originate from the proximal phalangeal head and insert on the base of the middle phalanx. The length of the collateral ligaments changes little as the proximal phalanx is flexed and extended.[5] Accessory collateral ligaments (ACLs) originate slightly proximal and volar to the collateral ligaments and insert on the volar plate and flexor sheath. These ligaments provide lateral stability as the joint moves. The volar plate is a fibrocartilaginous structure that is attached proximally to the neck of the proximal phalanx and distally to the base of the middle phalanx. The volar plate limits hyperextension of the joint.

The metacarpophalangeal (MCP) joint is a condylar joint that can move along two axes including flexion/extension and radial/ulnar deviation.[6] The soft tissue boundaries of the joint are also made up of the articular capsule, the collateral ligaments and volar plate. The volar plate is more flexible and mobile than the PIP volar plate. Unlike the PIP joint, there is a pear-shaped metacarpal head in the MCP joint. The collateral ligaments

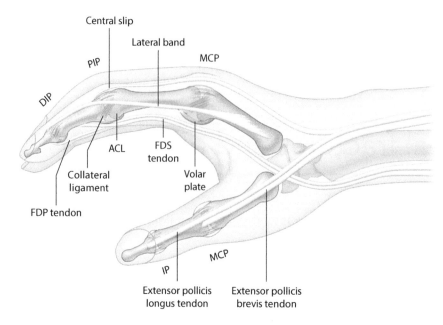

Figure 29.1 A simplified diagram illustrating the phalanges and joints of the digits.

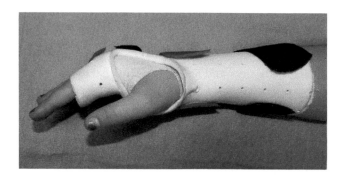

Figure 29.2 Safe position of the hand. The wrist is in 30 degrees of extension, the metacarpophalangeal joint is in 70–90 degrees of flexion and the proximal interphalangeal joint is in full extension.

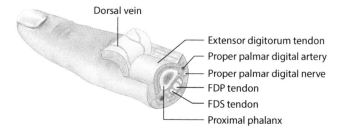

Figure 29.3 Cross-sectional anatomy of the proximal phalanx of the finger.

are longest in flexion and shortest in extension because of the 'cam effect' produced by the larger radius of curvature on the volar part of the head as well as the pear shape in the coronal plane. To limit the chances that the collateral ligaments will contract at the shorter position in extension, the MCP joint is typically immobilized in 70–90 degrees of flexion (Figure 29.2).

The dorsal extensor apparatus, FDP tendon, flexor digitorum superficialis (FDS) tendon and the flexor sheath are close-knit to the phalanges and joints. One-half of the dorsal distal phalanx is covered by nail bed and nail (Figure 29.3).

TREATMENT CONSIDERATIONS FOR ELDERLY PATIENTS

Some chronic hand diseases such as rheumatoid disease, osteoarthritis and Dupuytren disease are common in

elderly patients. Three radiographic views are usually sufficient to define the location, orientation, displacement and fragmentation of the fracture as well as pre-existing arthritis (Figure 29.4). The goals of treatment are adequate alignment and motion and a durable articulation.

Most closed non-displaced fractures as well as some displaced fractures after closed reduction are stable. They can be managed with a splint or buddy taping to adjacent fingers (Figure 29.5). Irreducible fractures and fractures that lose alignment after reduction are considered for operative treatment.

Rotation and angulation of a phalanx fracture can cause the finger to overlap or diverge. Angulation of the fracture apex volar or dorsal will result in a bone–tendon length discrepancy leading to an extension lag. It is difficult to judge rotational alignment on radiographs.[7] Measurements of the angle of the nail plate relative to the horizontal plane are not accurate for malrotation because there is substantial variation from person to person and finger to finger.[8] Soft tissue swelling and pain can affect accuracy, but observation of the fingers during passive or active flexion is the most reliable test of malrotation. The overlapping or

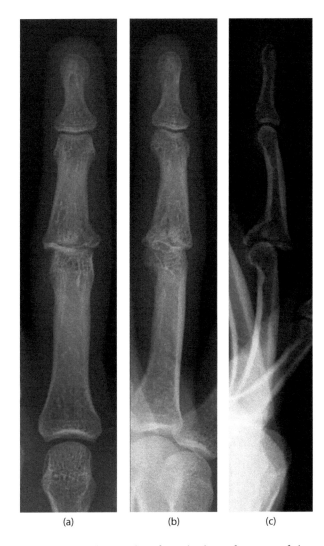

(a)   (b)   (c)

Figure 29.4 Radiographs of a volar base fracture of the ring finger middle phalanx. **(a,b)** Anteroposterior and oblique views show a narrow joint space and incongruent surface of the proximal interphalangeal (PIP) joint, but the intra-articular fracture with dislocation of the PIP joint is not apparent. **(c)** The lateral view demonstrates the intra-articular fracture and dorsal dislocation of the joint.

divergence of the finger indicates rotation or angulation deformities of the fractures (Figure 29.6). It is also used to address whether the deformities are corrected after fracture reduction.

Immobilization of fingers for more than 4 weeks has been shown to increase joint stiffness as a result of extensor tendon and joint capsular scarring.[9] Rigid internal fixation allows early mobilization to prevent finger stiffness. However, open reduction and internal fixation (ORIF) causes additional soft tissue injury, which may result in more adhesions that may limit motion and cause complications. The surgeon should strive to balance bony stability and tissue injury, using an individualized approach based on fracture type and injury configuration.

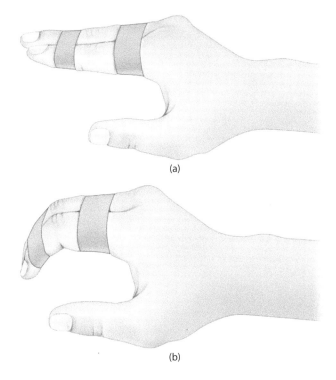

(a)

(b)

Figure 29.5 **(a,b)** Buddy taping allows the injured finger to move with the adjacent finger that provides support.

PHALANGEAL FRACTURES

Distal phalangeal fractures

The distal phalanx is most the commonly fractured phalanx.[10] The long finger distal phalanx is the most common because its length makes it more vulnerable.[11] Distal phalanx fractures can be divided into tuft fractures, shaft fractures and base fractures.

Typically, tuft fractures are caused by crush injuries to the fingertips. These fractures can be longitudinal or transverse, but most of them are comminuted fractures with associated nail bed injuries. Closed tuft fractures are usually stable owing to the volar soft tissues and dorsal nail plate. Symptomatic treatment, sometimes including protective splinting of the DIP, is sufficient for closed tuft fractures.[12] Even with displacement, open reduction is not helpful if the fracture fragments are too small for fixation. Non-union of the comminuted tuft fractures is often asymptomatic owing to fibrous union. The roles of subungual haematoma decompression for pain relief and nail bed repair for improved aesthetics are both debated and are unnecessary in older patients. For open fractures with nail bed injury, small devitalized fracture fragments can be removed during debridement followed by nail bed and soft tissue repair. Substantial displacement on radiographs often indicates severe soft tissue injury. Adequate reduction of the fracture often restores vascularity to an initially dysvascular tip that is widely displaced.

Non-displaced shaft and base fractures of the distal phalanx can be immobilized by splinting the DIP for 3 weeks

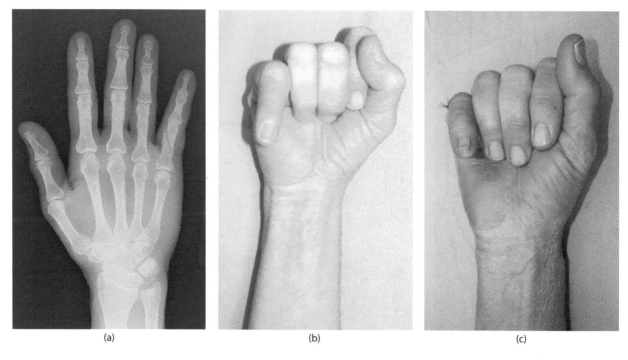

Figure 29.6 **(a)** Radiograph demonstrating a spiral fracture of the small finger of a 63-year-old woman. **(b)** Rotation of the fracture results in divergence of the small finger while making a fist. **(c)** Correction of the divergence of the small finger after open reduction of the fracture.

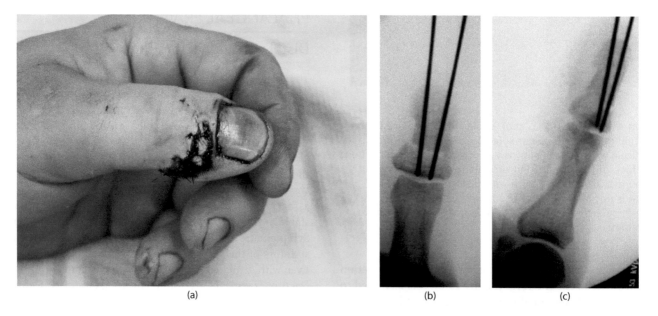

Figure 29.7 **(a)** A 68-year-old man sustained a crush injury to his left thumb. **(b,c)** Intraoperative fluoroscopies show the distal phalanx fracture of the thumb is fixed by two K-wires after closed reduction.

for comfort or allowed protected active mobilization. Most displaced fractures of the shaft of the distal phalanx are open fractures with a transverse laceration of the nail matrix. If the fracture does not stay aligned after reduction, suture of the skin and nail bed, and replacement of the nail plate with a piece of suture pack foil, the fracture can be fixed with one or two Kirschner wires (K-wires) (Figure 29.7). Fractures that realign well can be splinted with the DIP joint extension

for 4–6 weeks with regularly scheduled radiographs to confirm fracture reduction.

Intra-articular fractures at the dorsal base of the distal phalanx are called mallet fractures. The finger presents with a flexion deformity with inability to extend the DIP joint (Figure 29.8). Although mallet fractures are displaced intra-articular fractures, the role of ORIF is debated. Some authors suggest that less than one-third of the articular

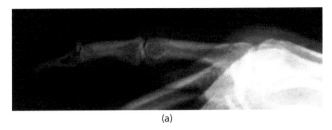

(a)

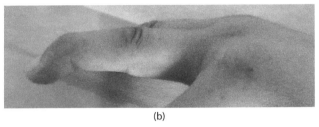

(b)

Figure 29.8 Mallet fracture. (a) Lateral radiograph demonstrates a dorsal articular avulsion fracture of the extensor tendon insertion of the middle finger. (b) The patient presented with a flexion deformity of the distal interphalangeal joint.

surface of the DIP joint can be treated with a splint.[13] Other authors state that non-operative treatment yields good results even when the displaced fragment of the fracture is greater than one-third of the articular surface of the distal phalanx unless there is volar subluxation of the remaining intact joint.[14] The DIP joint of the affected digit is immobilized in extension or slight hyperextension for 4–6 weeks. A variety of splints are available that can be applied along the dorsal or volar aspect of the DIP joint or both. In the study of Wehbe and Schneider, 21 patients aged 5–56 years old were followed for a mean of 3 years.[15] Six were treated surgically and the others were splinted. All but one regained a near normal range of painless motion of the DIP joint. Wehbe concluded that ORIF offered no advantage over non-operative treatment and surgical treatment had more problems. Kalainov et al. retrospectively reviewed 22 closed mallet fractures in 21 patients (20–69 years old) who were treated by a DIP joint extension splint.[16] The sizes of all fractures were greater than one-third of the articular surface, and 13 of them presented with volar subluxation of the DIP joint. At 2-year follow-up evaluation, all patients reported minimal difficulties with activities of daily living and work, and the patients expressed relatively high satisfaction with finger function. Considering that surgical treatment of mallet fractures is difficult and unreliable, we recommend non-operative treatment for elderly patients.

Intra-articular fractures at the volar base of the distal phalanx are often caused by avulsion of the terminal FDP tendon. They occur most commonly in sports activities and are uncommon in the elderly. If operative treatment is favored, fixation depends on the size of the fragment: pull-out suture technique, K-wire, screw or suture anchors are options.

Lateral fractures of bases are due to lateral ligament avulsion, and the fragments are usually small. Splinting the DIP joint in extension for 3–4 weeks is sufficient treatment.

Middle and proximal phalangeal fractures

NON-ARTICULAR FRACTURES

Stable and minimally displaced extra-articular fractures of the middle and proximal phalanges can be immobilized in a splint for 3–4 weeks, or mobilized immediately by strapping the injured finger to an adjacent finger (buddy strapping).

Displaced transverse fractures of one finger with little or no soft tissue injury are treated with closed reduction under local anesthesia. Most displaced transverse fractures displace with an apex angulation configuration, because the fragments are pulled by the interosseous muscles, lumbricals and extensor tendons. For reduction of the fractures, longitudinal traction is applied in the distal direction, and then the distal fragment is flexed to correct the angulation deformity. Both radiographic and clinical alignment should be checked after reduction, rotation in particular. For stable fractures, a short arm cast is used to immobilize the hand in safe position. If a fracture is stable only when the IP joints are in flexion, then the fracture is considered to be unstable. The unstable transverse fractures after reduction will be pinned to keep alignment. The cast or pin is maintained for approximately 3 weeks; buddy taping is continued for an additional 2 weeks after that.

Displaced oblique, spiral and comminuted fractures are often considered unstable fractures. In these cases, percutaneous or internal fixation will be performed. A wide variety of fixation methods is available, and selection of the technique is largely based on surgeon experience and preference.

K-wires

K-wires are commonly used for fixation usually after closed reduction but sometimes after open reduction. For short oblique and transverse fractures, the finger is distracted and reduced under fluoroscopy guidance. One 0.045-inch (1.1 mm) K-wire is inserted through the flexed MCP joint and down the medullary canal of the proximal phalanx to stabilize the fracture. Another crossed 0.045 K-wire can then be placed near the mid-lateral line of the finger to limit rotation (Figure 29.9). For open reduction, the K-wires can be inserted antegrade and then passed retrograde through the fracture site after reduction.

For long oblique fractures, K-wires are inserted perpendicular to the fracture line. A pointed reduction forceps is helpful to maintain reduction of the spiral oblique fracture while K-wires are inserted.[17] The PIP joint is not usually immobilized, but crossing the DIP joint can limit the potential for extensor lag in the treatment of middle phalanx fractures. The patient is placed in a splint and gentle limited active PIP motion exercises are initiated 1 week postoperatively. The wires are removed in the office 3–4 weeks after insertion.

The major advantage of pin fixation is minimal soft tissue damage. Favourable outcomes are reported in some studies.[17,18] Green and Anderson achieved full range of motion in 18 of 22 patients with long oblique fractures of the proximal phalanx treated by closed reduction and two or three

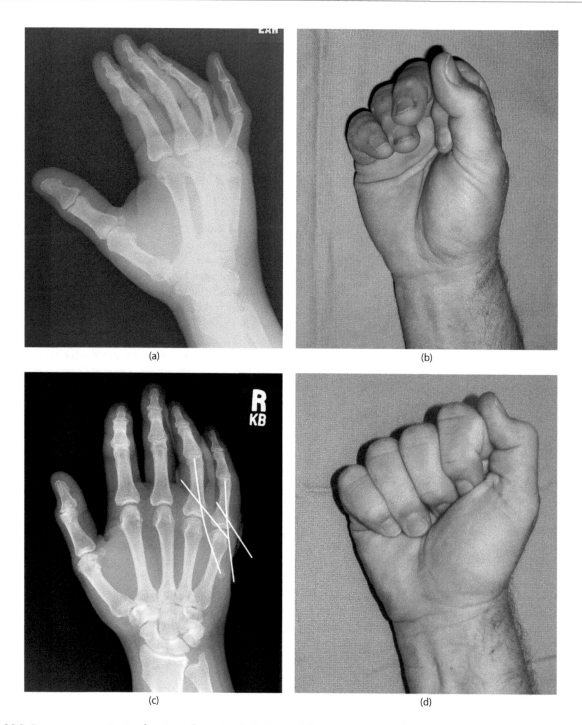

Figure 29.9 Percutaneous K-wire fixation of proximal phalangeal fractures. **(a)** The fractures at the base of the proximal phalanges of the ring and little fingers of a 65-year-old man are shown on the radiograph. **(b)** The flexion function of the hand preoperatively. **(c)** Radiograph shows two cross K-wires were used to fix the fractures after closed reduction, and the proximal interphalangeal (PIP) joints are not pinned. **(d)** The final flexion function of the hand after the K-wires were removed.

percutaneous pins.[18] Belsky and colleagues used transverse K-wire fixation for 100 patients with long oblique phalangeal fractures.[17] Good and excellent results were reported in 90% of fractures, and a total active movement of 215 degrees or more was achieved in 61% of fractures. Other studies have less optimal results. Faruqui et al. reviewed 338 patients with the base of the proximal phalanx fractures treated by closed reduction and percutaneous pinning.[19] Nearly half of the patients had flexion loss averaging 20 degrees and a third of patients had fixed flexion contracture greater than 15 degrees at the PIP joint.

Pin loosening is the most common complication of pin fixation.[20] Other complications include pin track infection, nerve injury and tendon rupture.

Plate and screw fixation

ORIF can provide much more stable fixation that allows early initiation of mobilization to limit tendon adhesion and joint stiffness. Because ORIF results in additional soft tissue injury with the potential for increased scarring and stiffness, it is generally reserved for articular fractures and fractures associated with wounds and tendon, nerve or blood vessel injury.

Lag screws placed perpendicular to the fracture line are suggested in long oblique or spiral phalangeal fractures if the fracture size can accommodate screws. For fracture of the shaft, the size of fracture fragment is three times as wide as the diameter of the screw and at least two screws are required. Significantly good outcomes can be expected, because lag screws can provide sufficient stability to allow early mobilization; moreover the effect on tendon sliding is minimum (Figure 29.10).[21] Furthermore, screw fixation of phalangeal fractures is not as technically challenging as fixation of metacarpal fractures.

Plating is used for comminuted phalangeal fractures (Figure 29.11).[22] Kurzen et al. reported 54 patients aged 26–83 years with phalangeal fractures treated by open reduction and plate fixation.[23] One or more major complications were detected in 33 patients. Overall, 22 patients experienced functionally limiting stiffness with an average range of motion at the PIP joint of 154 degrees.

ARTICULAR FRACTURES

Because the articular surface is damaged along with soft tissue structures such as the volar plate and collateral ligaments, the outcomes of articular fractures are often not as satisfying as those of non-articular fractures. Long-term problems including pain and stiffness greatly reduce range of motion, and arthritis and recurrent subluxation are not uncommon.

Condylar fractures

Condylar fractures may occur as the result of avulsion through the collateral ligament when a shearing force is applied to the joint. Most condylar fractures are displaced and unstable fractures that benefit from ORIF. There are two popular approaches to expose the fractures: the dorsal longitudinal incision or the mid-axial approach on the

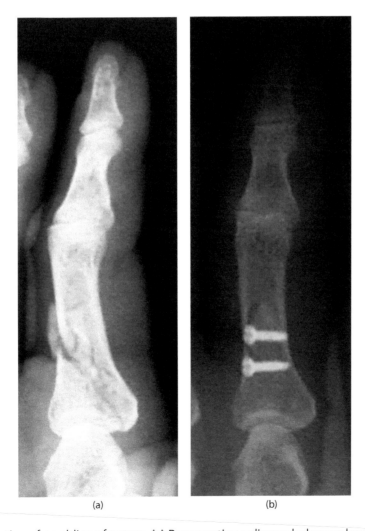

(a)   (b)

Figure 29.10 Lag screw fixation of an oblique fracture. **(a)** Preoperative radiograph shows a long oblique fracture of the proximal phalanx of the index finger. **(b)** Postoperative radiograph of fixation with two lag screws.   *(Continued)*

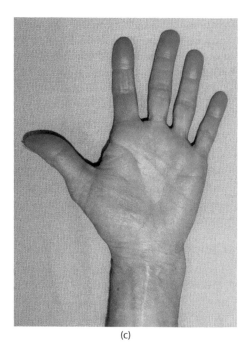
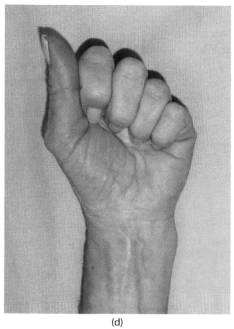

(c)

(d)

Figure 29.10 (Continued) Lag screw fixation of an oblique fracture. **(c,d)** At 20-year follow-up, the patient had excellent extension and flexion function of the hand.

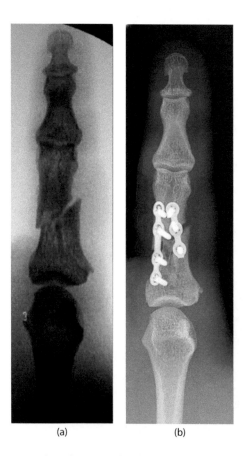

(a)

(b)

Figure 29.11 Plate fixation of open comminuted fractures of the proximal phalanx. **(a)** Intraoperative fluoroscopy shows the comminuted fractures of the proximal phalanx. **(b)** Open reduction and internal fixation (ORIF) was performed using two dorsally placed plates.

radial or ulnar side. For the dorsal approach, the joint is exposed between the central tendon and lateral band. It is important to be careful not to injure the insertion of the central tendon and collateral ligament when exposing the fracture fragments. When a mid-lateral approach is used, the vertical retinacular fibers are incised to expose the collateral ligament. It is important to preserve the collateral ligament attachments that may be the only blood supply of the fracture.[24] Once reduced, one or two K-wires or screws are used for fixation depending on the size of the fracture fragment (Figure 29.12). The reduction and stability should be confirmed by radiographs after moving the joint.

Base fractures

Dorsal intra-articular base fractures of the middle phalanx may be avulsions of the insertion of the central tendon. ORIF through the dorsal approach can be considered if the fragment is large enough to be secured. Smaller displaced fragments can be excised followed by reattachment of the insertion of the central slip. It is helpful to pin the PIP joint in extension for 3–4 weeks to protect the repair. Exercises can help maintain the mobility of the DIP joint.

Fractures of the lateral base of the middle phalanx are often caused by the collateral ligament avulsion injuries. Fractures with lateral instability of the joint may benefit from operative treatment, but most of these are minimally displaced and treated non-operatively. A dorsolateral approach is often used to expose the fracture, and the lateral and central bands of the extensor mechanism are elevated.[25] The capsule is then incised to expose the fracture site. Wire sutures, lag screws and K-wires are all options for fixation of these fractures.

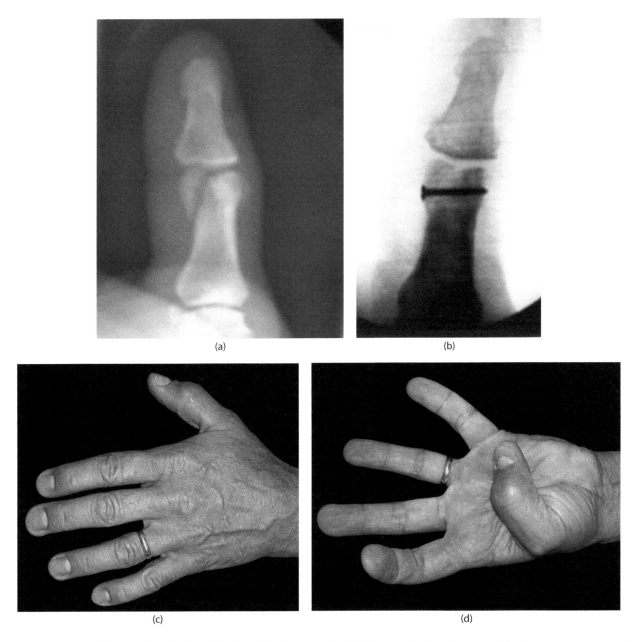

Figure 29.12 Screw fixation of a displaced unicondylar fracture. (a) An intra-articular, ulnar condylar fracture at the proximal phalanx of the left thumb is shown on a preoperative radiograph. (b) The fracture was treated with open reduction and internal fixation (ORIF) using one screw. (c,d) The 2-month clinical results show good extension and flexion of the interphalangeal (IP) joint of the thumb.

Fractures of the middle phalanx involving less than 40% of the volar joint surface with or without PIP joint subluxation are often stable after closed reduction.[26] They can be treated by closed reduction with 3 weeks of 30-degree dorsal extension block splinting (Figure 29.13). In less reliable patients or for injuries with borderline joint stability, extension block pinning is an option. In this technique, a K-wire is inserted into the head of the proximal phalanx just over the dorsal lip of the middle phalanx, blocking extension past a given point. The pin is removed 3 weeks later. In the study by Maalla et al., extension block pinning was applied for 22 PIP joints with

fracture-dislocations.[27] The mean final arc of motion of the PIP joints was 85 degrees, and no pain in 12 cases with a mean follow-up period of 2 years and 7 months.

Volar base fractures of the middle phalanx with large (>40%) fragments and dorsal dislocation or subluxation of the PIP joint are often comminuted. A 'V' sign (space between the joint surfaces at the dorsal joint) indicates subluxation of the joint on lateral radiographs (Figure 29.14). Options are ORIF, hemi-hamate autograft or external fixation.

To expose the volar fracture of the base of the middle phalanx, a volar Brunner incision is made. The A3 pulley is removed, the flexor tendons moved aside and the collateral

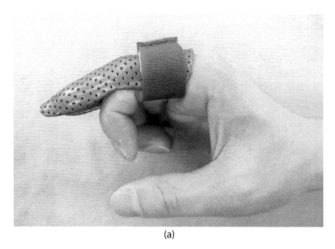

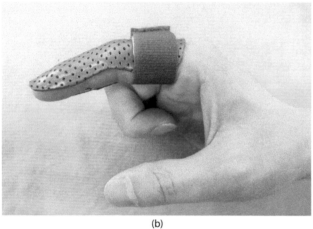

Figure 29.13 Dorsal extension blocking splint. (a,b) Splint applied to the dorsal surface of the injured finger. The proximal interphalangeal (PIP) joint is able to flex, but extension is limited by the splint position.

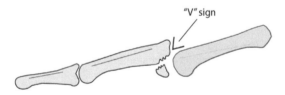

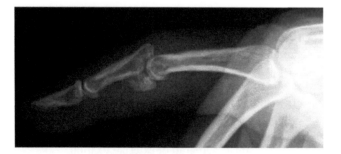

Figure 29.14 Diagram demonstrating the dorsal 'V' sign of the volar base fracture of the middle phalanx with proximal interphalangeal (PIP) joint dorsal dislocation.

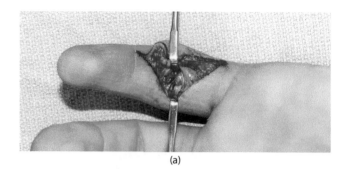

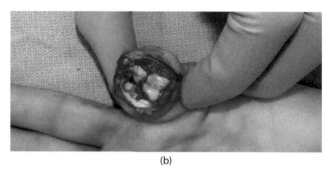

Figure 29.15 Shotgun approach to the proximal interphalangeal (PIP) joint. (a) The flexor tendons and volar plate are retracted to expose the joint. (b) The joint is hyperextended and shotgunned open to visualize the articular fracture.

ligaments incised to open up the PIP joint with a 'shotgun' approach either retracting the flexor tendons laterally or splitting the FDS proximally to allow one slip to fall to each side (Figure 29.15). The volar plate is detached from the base of the middle phalanx and either left detached or sutured back to the FDS insertion upon closure. Impacted fragments are pushed back into position (consider bone graft for support because a defect is created) and the volar lip of the middle phalanx is replaced. K-wires, screws or a small plate are used for fixation. The patient is placed in a dorsal blocking splint for 4 weeks postoperatively.

If the fracture is too complex to repair or partially or fully healed in malreduction, hemi-hamate reconstruction can be considered as a primary procedure. The dorsal distal hamate articular surface is removed and shaped to replace the excised fracture of the volar base of the middle phalanx. Afendras et al. examined eight patients with a mean age of 49 years who had hemi-hamate reconstruction a minimum of 4 years after injury.[28] The arc of motion was 67 degrees (45–95 degrees) at the PIP joint and grip strength was 91% of the uninjured side. Four patients had arthritis, but only one of them had troublesome pain.

Dynamic external fixation devices have been used to treat complex articular fractures of the base of the middle phalanx.[29-32] The external fixator is typically comprised of pins or wires placed through the middle and proximal phalanges with elastic bands or the wires themselves supplying the force of distraction. They provide distraction across the PIP joint to provide fracture and joint reduction

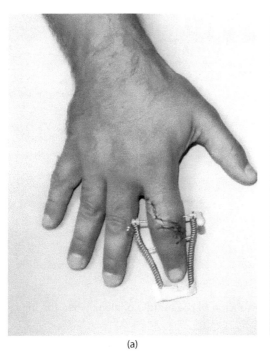
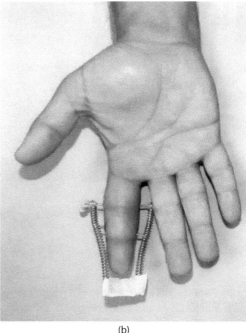

(a)   (b)

Figure 29.16 Dorsal **(a)** and volar **(b)** views of external fixation. The external fixation provides distraction across the injured proximal interphalangeal (PIP) joint.

and stabilize the alignment during healing (Figure 29.16). Motion of the PIP joint helps limit adhesions or contractures and encourages the fractures to heal in a configuration allowing motion (so-called 'secondary congruence').[30] Morgan et al. described 14 patients with more than 50% articular involvement treated with dynamic digital traction for an average of 34 days.[32] An average of 24 months after surgery, all the patients including one 63-year-old man were pain-free during rest and usual activity.

Intra-articular base fractures of the proximal phalanx with substantial displacement or malalignment can be treated with ORIF. The extensor tendon is split in the midline and repaired upon closure. These fractures usually feature impaction of the articular surface that may benefit from bone grafting (e.g. cancellous bone from the distal radius) after realignment of the fragments. Fixation is usually with a plate and screws.

DISLOCATIONS IN THE DIGITS

Dislocations of the finger DIP joint

Simple dislocations of the finger DIP joint and thumb IP joint are usually dorsal dislocations and are uncommonly irreducible. After fractures are excluded by radiographs, closed reduction can be performed under digital block anesthesia. These are readily reduced by traction in the distal longitudinal direction, flexing or extending the distal phalanx, and pushing the dislocated bone back in place. Radiographs confirm successful reduction. Although injury to tendon insertions is uncommon, the joint should be tested to ensure active motion is restored and that the

joint is stable with active motion. The joint is immobilized for 2–3 weeks before starting active, self-assisted stretching exercises.

Dislocations of the PIP joint

Dorsal dislocations of the PIP joint are common and at risk primarily for stiffness. Splint immobilization for comfort is reasonable for a few days, but no longer. A small volar plate avulsion fracture should not influence treatment. Patients are encouraged to move and stretch PIP dislocations immediately. Buddy tapes or straps can be used for comfort.

The less common volar (central slip) and lateral (radial collateral ligament incarceration) dislocations have the potential for associated problems. Central slip injures are evaluated by the Elson test after reduction (Figure 29.17).[33] The patient's injured PIP joint is passively flexed to 90 degrees over the edge of a table. The examiner resists extension when the patient actively extends the PIP joint. No extension power felt at the PIP joint or a tendency to extension at the DIP joint indicates the complete rupture of the central slip. This test is best performed under a digital block to eliminate the effects of pain.[34] The Elson test may not be positive acutely, so it should be checked again after a few weeks. If the central slip is ruptured, the joint is usually splinted in full extension for 6 weeks.

The irreducible PIP dislocation is usually due to incarceration of a collateral ligament in the joint. A slight widening on the side of the joint is often seen on radiographs. Open reduction is the only way to remove the collateral ligament from the joint. The reduced joint is managed with buddy taping for about 3 weeks.

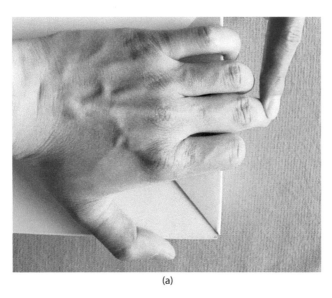
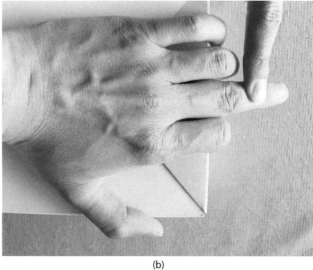

(a)   (b)

Figure 29.17 **(a,b)** Elson test. The examiner resists the active extension of the middle phalanx while the injured proximal interphalangeal (PIP) joint is flexed to 90 degrees.

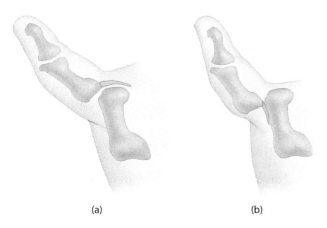

(a)   (b)

Figure 29.18 Two types of dorsal dislocations of the thumb metacarpophalangeal (MCP) joint. **(a)** The proximal phalanx is in a hyperextended position and the volar plate is not interposed in the joint space in the simple dislocation. **(b)** In the complex dislocation, the proximal phalanx and the metacarpal are parallel with the volar plate interposed in the joint space.

Dislocation and ligament injury of the MCP joint

Most dislocations of the MCP joint of the finger as well as thumb are dorsal dislocations presented with the joints held in extension. They are commonly divided into two types: simple (reducible) dislocations and complex (irreducible) dislocations (Figure 29.18). Simple dislocation is characterized by subluxation of the joint (the articular surfaces are still partially apposed) and the base of the phalanx is locked in hyperextension. The volar plate is not interposed in the joint space. The method of reduction for the simple dislocation is to flex the wrist in order to relax the flexor tendons first. Then the dislocated proximal phalanx is flexed

as pressure is applied in a distal direction. If longitudinal traction is applied in the distal direction prior to flexion, the volar plate will be interposed in the joint space, which transfers the simple dislocation into a complex dislocation. After reduction, a dorsal blocking splint will be applied for 1 week, followed by buddy taping.

In a complex MCP dislocation, the joint is in slight hyperextension, the dorsally displaced proximal phalanx lies above the metacarpal on radiographs and the volar plate is interposed in the joint space. Complex dislocations are treated with open reduction via a dorsal or volar approach. The dorsal approach is simple and safe. Just expose the joint through a midline split or by partially incising one of the sagittal bands. The volar plate will distort the anatomy as it is over the top of the metacarpal head. Divide the volar plate longitudinally and the volar plate can then go around the metacarpal head allowing reduction.

Care should be taken to protect the digital nerve during a volar approach because the prominent metacarpal head makes it vulnerable during skin incision. For a volar approach, after exposure, an incision between the volar plate and collateral ligament is made to reduce the interposed volar plate. Then the proximal phalangeal base is gently reduced onto the metacarpal head. The MCP joint is splinted in slight flexion and terminal extension is prevented for up to 2 weeks depending on joint stability.[35]

Collateral ligament injuries of the MCP joint are diagnosed based on local tenderness and instability. Stability is tested by flexing the MCP joints (placing them where the collateral ligament should be most taut). Compare to the adjacent ligaments. Greater opening and pain make the diagnosis. Radiographs are normal or show small avulsion fractures. The treatment is with buddy strapping for at least 1 month. Patients have discomfort from this injury for 6–12 months—make sure they know this or they will think something is wrong.

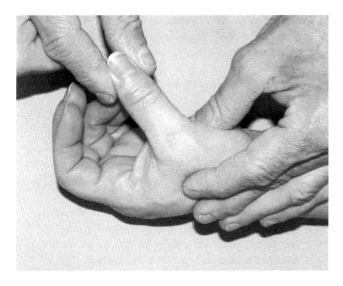

Figure 29.19 Stress test of the thumb shows more than 30-degree angulation of the metacarpophalangeal (MCP) joint which increases the probability of complete ulnar collateral ligament rupture.

The diagnosis of ligament injuries of the thumb MCP joint depends on the mechanism of injury and clinical findings. The role of MRI and ultrasound are debated. Joint deviation of more than 30 degrees total or 15 degrees more than the contralateral uninjured thumb increases the likelihood of complete rupture (Figure 29.19).[36] This test should be done under local anaesthesia if the patient cannot cooperate because of pain. Partial tears (sprains) can be treated non-operatively with immobilization for 4 weeks followed by range of motion exercises.[37] Complete ruptures of the ulnar collateral ligament of the thumb MP ('gamekeeper' or 'skiier' thumb) are at risk for a Stener lesion (displacement of the collateral ligament superficial to the adductor aponeurosis preventing healing) and are considered for operative treatment. An alternative is to splint the thumb for 3–4 weeks and re-examine. Thumbs that are stable after a few weeks do not have Stener lesions. Various techniques for repair of the ligament avulsion from the proximal phalanx base are described including reattachment of ligament with a pull-out suture or bone anchor, and screw fixation of larger avulsion fracture fragments. Studies show that acute surgical management yields a stable, mobile joint.[38] The role of operative treatment for the less common complete radial collateral ligament injury is less clear.

Arthrodesis of the MCP joint is recommended for elderly patients with pain and degenerative arthritis rather than reconstruction using tendon graft in chronic injury.

CONCLUSIONS

The treatment of phalangeal fractures and dislocations aims for adequate alignment and motion, and a durable articulation. Appropriate treatment requires understanding of the anatomy of the hand, types of injury and injury mechanisms. Most fractures and dislocations can be treated non-operatively in elderly patients, particularly those who are infirm or low demand. Non-operative treatments should consist of light-weight splints and buddy taping when possible, leaving as much of the hand free for use as possible. Operative treatment is used selectively, and with a shared decision based on knowledge of the potential risks.

REFERENCES

1. Chung, K. C., and S. V. Spilson. The frequency and epidemiology of hand and forearm fractures in the United States. *J Hand Surg Am* 26 (2001): 908–915.
2. Feehan, L. M., and S. B. Sheps. Incidence and demographics of hand fractures in British Columbia, Canada: A population-based study. *J Hand Surg Am* 31 (2006): 1068–1074.
3. De Jonge, J. J., J. Kingma, B. van der Lei, and H. J. Klasen. Phalangeal fractures of the hand. An analysis of gender and age-related incidence and aetiology. *J Hand Surg Br* 19 (1994): 168–170.
4. van Onselen, E. B., R. B. Karim, J. J. Hage, and M. J. Ritt. Prevalence and distribution of hand fractures. *J Hand Surg Br* 28 (2003): 491–495.
5. Loubert, P. V., T. J. Masterson, M. S. Schroeder, and A. M. Mazza. Proximity of collateral ligament origin to the axis of rotation of the proximal interphalangeal joint of the finger. *J Orthop Sports Phys Ther* 37 (2007): 179–185.
6. Schultz, R. J., A. Storace, and S. Krishnamurthy. Metacarpophalangeal joint motion and the role of the collateral ligaments. *Int Orthop* 11 (1987): 149–155.
7. Bansal, R., and M. A. Craigen. Rotational alignment of the finger nails in a normal population. *J Hand Surg Eur Vol* 32 (2007): 80–84.
8. Tan, V., T. Kinchelow, and P. K. Beredjiklian. Variation in digital rotation and alignment in normal subjects. *J Hand Surg Am* 33 (2008): 873–878.
9. Oetgen, M. E., and S. D. Dodds. Non-operative treatment of common finger injuries. *Curr Rev Musculoskelet Med* 1 (2008): 97–102.
10. Jupiter, J. B., and M. R. Belsky. Fractures and dislocations of the hand. In *Skeletal Trauma: Fractures, Dislocations, Ligamentous Injuries*, edited by B. D. Browner, J. B. Jupiter, A. M. Levine, and P. G. Trafton. Philadelphia, PA: Saunders, 1992, pp. 925–1024.
11. Cannon, N. M. Rehabilitation approaches for distal and middle phalanx fractures of the hand. *J Hand Ther* 16 (2003): 105–116.
12. Schneider, L. H. Fractures of the distal phalanx. *Hand Clin* 4 (1988): 537–547.
13. Wang, Q. C., and B. A. Johnson. Fingertip injuries. *Am Fam Physician* 63 (2001): 1961–1966.
14. Weber, P., and H. Segmuller. [Non-surgical treatment of mallet finger fractures involving more than one third of the joint surface: 10 cases]. *Handchir Mikrochir Plast Chir* 40 (2008): 145–148.

15. Wehbe, M. A., and L. H. Schneider. Mallet fractures. *J Bone Joint Surg Am* 66 (1984): 658–669.

16. Kalainov, D. M., P. E. Hoepfner, B. J. Hartigan, C. Carroll 4th, and J. Genuario. Nonsurgical treatment of closed mallet finger fractures. *J Hand Surg Am* 30 (2005): 580–586.

17. Belsky, M. R., R. G. Eaton, and L. B. Lane. Closed reduction and internal fixation of proximal phalangeal fractures. *J Hand Surg Am* 9 (1984): 725–729.

18. Green, D. P., and J. R. Anderson. Closed reduction and percutaneous pin fixation of fractured phalanges. *J Bone Joint Surg Am* 55 (1973): 1651–1654.

19. Faruqui, S., P. J. Stern, and T. R. Kiefhaber. Percutaneous pinning of fractures in the proximal third of the proximal phalanx: Complications and outcomes. *J Hand Surg Am* 37 (2012): 1342–1348.

20. Stahl, S., and O. Schwartz. Complications of K-wire fixation of fractures and dislocations in the hand and wrist. *Arch Orthop Trauma Surg* 121 (2001): 527–530.

21. Ford, D. J., S. el-Hadidi, P. G. Lunn, and F. D. Burke. Fractures of the phalanges: Results of internal fixation using 1.5mm and 2mm A. O. screws. *J Hand Surg Br* 12 (1987): 28–33.

22. Kawamura, K., and K. C. Chung. Fixation choices for closed simple unstable oblique phalangeal and metacarpal fractures. *Hand Clin* 22 (2006): 287–295.

23. Kurzen, P., C. Fusetti, M. Bonaccio, and L. Nagy. Complications after plate fixation of phalangeal fractures. *J Trauma* 60 (2006): 841–843.

24. Khouri, J. S., J. M. Bloom, and W. C. Hammert. Current trends in the management of proximal interphalangeal joint injuries of the hand. *Plast Reconstr Surg* 132 (2013): 1192–1204.

25. Bekler, H., A. Gokce, and T. Beyzadeoglu. Avulsion fractures from the base of phalanges of the fingers. *Tech Hand Up Extrem Surg* 10 (2006): 157–161.

26. Merrell, G., and Slade J. F. Dislocations and ligament injuries in the digits. In *Green's Operative Hand Surgery*, edited by S. W. Wolfe, R. N. Hotchkiss, W. C. Pederson, and S. H. Kozin. Philadelphia, PA: Elsevier/Churchill Livingstone, 2011, pp. 291–332.

27. Maalla, R., M. Youssef, G. Ben Jdidia, C. Khimiri, and H. Essadam. Extension-block pinning for fracture-dislocation of the proximal interphalangeal joint. *Orthop Traumatol Surg Res* 98 (2012): 559–563.

28. Afendras, G., A. Abramo, A. Mrkonjic, M. Geijer, P. Kopylov, and M. Tagil. Hemi-hamate osteochondral transplantation in proximal interphalangeal dorsal fracture dislocations: A minimum 4 year follow-up in eight patients. *J Hand Surg Eur Vol* 35 (2010): 627–631.

29. Badia, A., F. Riano, J. Ravikoff, R. Khouri, E. Gonzalez-Hernandez, and J. L. Orbay. Dynamic intradigital external fixation for proximal interphalangeal joint fracture dislocations. *J Hand Surg Am* 30 (2005): 154–160.

30. Ellis, S. J., R. Cheng, P. Prokopis, A. Chetboun, S. W. Wolfe, E. A. Athanasian, and A. J. Weiland. Treatment of proximal interphalangeal dorsal fracture-dislocation injuries with dynamic external fixation: A pins and rubber band system. *J Hand Surg Am* 32 (2007): 1242–1250.

31. Kiefhaber, T. R., and P. J. Stern. Fracture dislocations of the proximal interphalangeal joint. *J Hand Surg Am* 23 (1998): 368–380.

32. Morgan, J. P., D. A. Gordon, M. S. Klug, P. E. Perry, and P. S. Barre. Dynamic digital traction for unstable comminuted intra-articular fracture-dislocations of the proximal interphalangeal joint. *J Hand Surg Am* 20 (1995): 565–573.

33. Elson, R. A. Rupture of the central slip of the extensor hood of the finger. A test for early diagnosis. *J Bone Joint Surg Br* 68 (1986): 229–231.

34. Strauch, R. J. Extensor tendon injury. In *Green's Operative Hand Surgery*, edited by R. N. Hotchkiss, S. W. Wolfe, W. C. Pederson, and S. H. Kozin. Philadelphia, PA: Elsevier/Churchill Livingstone, 2011.

35. Calfee, R. P., and T. G. Sommerkamp. Fracture-dislocation about the finger joints. *J Hand Surg Am* 34 (2009): 1140–1147.

36. Greenleaf R. M., and T. B. Hughes. Thumb ulnar collateral ligament repair techniques. In *Hand and Upper Extremity Reconstruction*, edited by K. C. Chung. Philadelphia, PA: Elsevier/Churchill Livingstone, 2009, pp. 79–87.

37. Lee, A. T., and M. G. Carlson. Thumb metacarpophalangeal joint collateral ligament injury management. *Hand Clin* 28 (2012): 361––370, ix–x.

38. Melone, C. P., Jr., S. Beldner, and R. S. Basuk. Thumb collateral ligament injuries. An anatomic basis for treatment. *Hand Clin* 16 (2000): 345–357.

30

Cervical spine fractures

PAUL A. ANDERSON

INTRODUCTION

The geriatric population is expanding, experiencing a longer lifespan and becoming more vigorous later into life with activities such as driving and recreation. With this increase in an active elderly population, cervical spine injuries are becoming a more important part of trauma care. Morbidity and mortality can be decreased with improved awareness of cervical spine injuries and the initiation of appropriate treatment more rapidly. Also, recognition of the unique characteristics of the geriatric spine will help clinicians discern acute injury and provide appropriate care and treatment.

This chapter will review the epidemic of cervical spine injuries in the elderly. The methods of evaluation and radiologic examination will be discussed emphasizing the best available medical evidence. Common classification systems and how they can be applied to geriatric fractures are presented with discussion of how common fracture types behave differently in the geriatric population. These include fractures in patients with ankylosed spine, type 2 odontoid fractures and central cord syndrome. Finally, complications are discussed.

EPIDEMIOLOGY

The geriatric population is increasing by 6% per annum in the United States, while the incidence of cervical fractures in patients above 65 years of age is growing by 21%

per annum or 3.5 times faster. The rate of increase was linearly proportional to age so that older groups (>85 years) had even higher fracture rates.[1] Further, in a retrospective review of high energy trauma, cervical spine injuries were associated with the highest mortality rates of all orthopaedic injuries with a mortality rate of 47% for cervical spine fractures with neurological deficit and 44% for C2 fractures.[2] In a review of another level 1 trauma centre, the mortality rate was 24% for geriatric cervical spine fractures and less than a third were able to return home after injury.[3] For fractures that had a neurological deficit the mortality rate was 50%.[3]

The most common mechanism for trauma in the elderly population is falls, occurring in up to 75% of cases.[4] Other common mechanisms include motor vehicle collisions in which the patient is a driver, passenger or pedestrian. Patients commonly have pre-existing comorbidities including hypertension, congestive heart failure, diabetes, dementia, stroke, arrhythmias and chronic obstructive pulmonary disease (COPD), although this association does not imply causality.[4] Geriatric patients having ground level falls are more likely to have intracranial haemorrhage, and alcohol intoxication is not as likely as compared to younger patients.[5]

COMPLEXITY OF GERIATRIC FRACTURES

Geriatric patients tolerate trauma poorly and have much lower survival rates and greater complications than younger patients with similar levels of trauma. Many complexities account for this problem including medical comorbidities, declining cognitive abilities, osteoporosis, pre-existing disability and poor social networking (Table 30.1).

Geriatric patients sustaining cervical spine injuries have significantly more medical comorbidities such as hypertension, heart disease, diabetes, lung disease and cognitive medical problems than younger patients.[6] Treatment requires balancing treatment of medical comorbidities with spinal care. It is recommended that a multidisciplinary team be created to co-manage these patients similar to programs established for hip fractures.[6,7] The medical comorbidities are significant risk factors for the morbidity and mortality associated with spinal fractures in the elderly.

Osteoporosis

Poor bone mineral density (BMD) (whether diagnosed or undiagnosed) predisposes to injury and may complicate surgical reconstruction. It is important to assess the quality

Table 30.1 Special considerations in geriatric cervical spine fractures

Epidemiology	Increasing incidence relative to population growth
	Mechanisms: fall from standing height
	Predominance of C2 fractures
Assessment	Less sensitivity to pain
	Pre-existing spinal disease
	Cognitive changes (acute and chronic)
	Medical comorbidities
	Osteoporosis
	Ankylosis and instability
	Less sensitive clearance protocols
Surgery	Osteoporosis
	Long lever arms from ankylosis (more fixation)
	Difficulty with imaging
	Greater risk of hardware failure
Non-operative care	Poorly tolerant of bracing
	Dysphagia in orthoses
	Halo vest associated with increased mortality
	Poor compliance
Complications	Increased mortality
	Increased surgical site infection
	Dysphagia
	Pulmonary complications
	Venous thromboembolism
	Mental status changes

of bone in planning treatment as well as for long-term management to prevent further fractures. Surgical strategies to reduce risk of hardware failure include use of more fixation levels and correct balancing to achieve proper alignment, thus reducing unwanted bending moments. Combined anteroposterior surgery, although not desirable, may be needed. Similarly, external mobilization may be required despite its risk of complications.

Cognitive changes are commonly seen in geriatric cervical spine patients which may be a major factor producing the fall. If possible, these should be addressed before discharge to avoid future falls. Careful attention to medications, in particular avoiding benzodiazepine and opioids, should be considered. Physical and occupational therapy should focus on balance and fall prevention programs.

ASSESSMENT OF THE GERIATRIC CERVICAL SPINE

Geriatric patients require similar diagnostic protocols to evaluate the cervical spine as all other patients. However, important differences may make the process more difficult and less precise in this population. In general, geriatric patients have less pain, making clinical assessment by history and palpation less sensitive. Further, they are more likely to have long-standing cognitive changes or acute mental status changes reducing clinical discrimination by clinical examination. Medical comorbidities and pre-existing spinal disease require experienced physicians to differentiate these from injury processes.

Screening

Current guidelines by the Eastern Association for the Surgery of Trauma (EAST) recommend that patients meeting National Emergency X-Radiography Utilization Study (NEXUS) criteria do not require radiologic screening.[8] The NEXUS criteria are based on a normal cognitive state, no neck pain or tenderness, no neurologic signs or symptoms and no distracting injuries. Distracting injuries include craniofacial trauma, burns, long bone and pelvic fractures, large joint dislocations, thoracic trauma and shock. Distracting injuries significantly reduce the sensitivity of the NEXUS criteria.[9] Patients meeting all the criteria are considered low risk and do not require radiographic evaluation. Touger et al. evaluated 2943 elderly patients and compared these to 31,000 non-elderly patients using NEXUS criteria.[8] Cervical spine injury was twice as common in the elderly patients. The percentage of patients cleared clinically (meeting NEXUS criteria) was similar between the two groups. The predominant geriatric fracture type was a C2 fracture. Two geriatric patients who were low risk based on NEXUS criteria had occult C2 lateral mass fractures and were treated successfully non-operatively. More recently, Goode et al. questioned the effectiveness of NEXUS criteria in geriatric patients with blunt (high energy) trauma as compared to falls from standing height (low energy).[10] They found a significantly higher incidence of cervical spine injury in high energy trauma: 12.8% compared to 4.5%. The sensitivity and positive predictive value of NEXUS criteria in elderly patients were low (65.9% and 19.3%, respectively) and significantly lower than in non-geriatric patients. The authors concluded that NEXUS criteria should not be used in blunt trauma geriatric patients and these patients should undergo CT evaluation regardless of whether they meet NEXUS criteria.

Clinical assessment

The clinical evaluation of the geriatric trauma patient includes special attention given to identifying spinal injuries. The mechanism of injury gives clues to the potential risk of cervical spine injury. However, with concurrent stiffening of the spine from aging and low BMD in elderly patients, even low energy mechanisms may result in significant spinal injuries. The presence or absence of pain and transient or persistent neurologic changes should be noted. The patient's ability to ambulate after the trauma may give some insight into spinal stability. Physical exam should include observation for signs of cranial or facial trauma which is common in patients with ground level falls. These include contusion about the head and face and facial fractures. The cervical spine is assessed by palpation for tenderness in the midline and then along each lateral mass.

Patients with low-energy falls who meet NEXUS criteria may be cleared without further radiologic imaging.[8] After it has been determined that the patient meets NEXUS criteria, they can be checked for pain with neck range of motion. This is best tested using the Canadian C-Spine Rule where right and left rotation is performed actively by the patient under physician supervision.[11] Keep in mind that geriatric patients have a high predominance of fractures at C2 and, therefore, may have pain or be unable to perform rotational maneuvers.

Neurologic assessment of all patients should be performed according to criteria described in the Guide to the Neurologic Evaluation of the Spinal Injury Patient by the American Spinal Injury Association (ASIA) (Figure 30.1).[12] The neurologic exam includes cranial nerve assessment, motor and sensory tests in the lower and upper extremities, and examination of the perineum. Reflexes are less helpful in geriatric patients unless there are signs of hyperreflexia which may indicate an upper motor neuron lesion from spinal cord compression or injury. In patients with neurologic deficits, the degree of spinal cord impairment is recorded using the ASIA Impairment Scale (Table 30.2). The neurologic exam should be recorded as in Figure 30.1.

Spinal cord injuries are devastating, especially to the elderly where the chance of mortality is greater than 80%. Various spinal cord injury patterns are seen. A complete cord injury is where there is no motor sensory function below the level of injury. Incomplete patterns include anterior cord, Brown-Sequard, central cord and posterior cord syndromes. Anterior cord syndrome causes loss of function of distal motor and pain and temperature functions due to injury of the anterior two-thirds of the spinal cord. Only posterior cord function remains. The prognosis is extremely poor. Brown-Sequard syndrome is a hemi-cord injury where there is ipsilateral loss of motor function and contralateral loss of sensory function. Central cord syndrome is a common injury pattern seen in elderly patients due to pre-existing cervical stenosis. In this syndrome there is greater loss of upper extremity function than lower extremity function. This pattern of neurologic injury is due to the lamination of axonal tracks where the upper extremities are more medial and thus affected to a greater degree in central cord syndrome than the more laterally placed lower extremity tracts. This prognosis is variable and many patients can make a significant recovery. Posterior cord syndrome is rare; there is only loss of dorsal column function and thus light touch, proprioception and vibration.

The severity of neurologic injury is classified by the ASIA motor score and the ASIA impairment scale.[12] The ASIA motor score is based on muscle examination of five key muscle groups in both the upper and lower extremities (Figure 30.1). Each muscle group is scored from 0 to 5. The bilateral sum of all scores ranges from 0 to 100. The ASIA impairment scale is important for prognosis (Table 30.2). An ASIA A is a complete motor sensory quadriplegia, while an ASIA E is normal. ASIA B–ASIA D are incomplete injuries with ASIA B being complete motor loss below the zone of injury but spared distal sensory function. ASIA C and D have retained motor and sensory function with the former having <grade 3 function and the latter ≥grade 3 function.

Radiologic imaging

Radiologic imaging is indicated in patients who fail NEXUS criteria, that is, patients who are symptomatic with pain or neurologic dysfunction, have cognitive impairment or have distracting injuries. Multidetector CT is the diagnostic procedure of choice when evaluating the cervical spine in geriatric patients. Reformations can be created in the axial, sagittal and coronal planes. The overall sensitivity is 99% in identifying cervical spine injury and far better than plain radiography.[9] MRI is not useful as a screening tool but is indicated to evaluate soft tissues such as the posterior ligamentous complex, the presence of spinal cord compression or extent of spinal cord injury, progressive neurologic deterioration, and for preoperative planning.[13] Many radiographic findings are age related and in these cases MRI can be useful to differentiate these from acute injuries. In addition, in patients with a facet dislocation, a herniated disc may be present and MRI should be used prior to reduction in the neurologically intact patient.

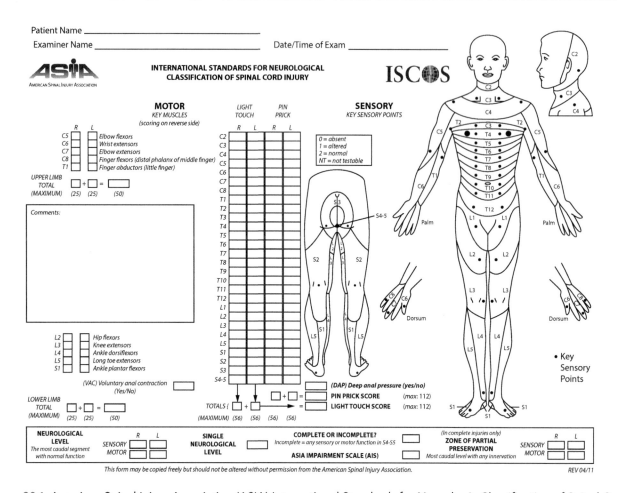

Figure 30.1 American Spinal Injury Association (ASIA) International Standards for Neurologic Classification of Spinal Cord Injury. (Reprinted with permission from American Spinal Injury Association.)

Table 30.2 American Spinal Injury Association Impairment Scale (AIS)

A	No sensory or motor function is preserved in the sacral segments S4–5.
B	Motor loss complete, retained sensory function below level of injury including sacral region.
C	Motor function is preserved below the neurological level and more than half of key muscle functions have a muscle grade less than 3.
D	Motor function is preserved below the neurological level and more than half of key muscle functions have a muscle grade ≥3.
E	Normal motor and sensory function.

The interpretation of spine imaging is problematic in geriatric patients. Age related changes may be difficult to differentiate from subtle acute trauma. It is not uncommon for patients to have severe facet degenerative change, especially at C3–4 and C4–5 and have small amounts of anterior subluxation which could be thought secondary to trauma. Further, pre-existing kyphotic changes need to be differentiated from posterior ligamentous injuries. Bony erosive change especially about the dens may predispose to fracture or may even be associated with chronic fracture creating concern for the presence of a new fracture.[14] Ankylosed segments from diffuse idiopathic spinal hyperostosis (DISH), surgery or ankylosing spondylitis are predisposed to fracture. Even minor incomplete fractures may be associated with significant instability. Hyperextension injuries may occur through the disc space which may show a normal appearing disc height but which is abnormal for that patient. Differentiating such pre-existing changes from acute trauma is difficult and requires careful examination, experience, interpretation of imaging and patience. Often the patient is immobilized in a collar allowing time to pass until further evaluation as the clinical course may ultimately dictate the status of the cervical spine. MRI may be indicated for specific areas of concern, such as disc or posterior ligamentous injury.

Assessment of bone quality

All geriatric patients with fractures should have assessment of bone quality. This is consistent with the American Orthopedic Association's 'Own the Bone' initiative where orthopaedic surgeons are trained in diagnosing and beginning basic treatment of metabolic bone disease in fragility fracture patients. In most geriatric cervical spine patients, CT has been performed including the thoracolumbar spine. These imaging studies can provide an opportunity to estimate whether patients have osteopenia or osteoporosis. The World Health Organization's criterion for osteoporosis is a DEXA T score of less than –2.5, while osteopenia is between –1 and –2.5. Normal bone density is T scores greater than –1. However, patients having fragility fractures, including those of the cervical spine, are diagnosed as osteoporotic, despite T scores being greater than –2.5.

If available, thoracolumbar CT can be used to estimate BMD. All CT determines the X-ray attenuation coefficient for each voxel of tissue scanned. This is termed the Hounsfield unit (HU) and is the amount of X-ray energy absorbed per voxel of tissue. For bone, HU is directly related to the BMD. HUs are scaled with air equal to –1000 and water equal to 0. Cortical bone is generally 300–500, while normal cancellous bone is greater than 125.

HUs can be measured using the tool platform of most picture archiving and communication systems (PACS). An elliptical region of interest (ROI) is drawn as large as possible on an axial section of the mid-body of a nonfractured lumbar spine vertebral body (Figure 30.2). The ROI should include only trabecular bone without degenerative changes or bony defects. The PACS tool will report an average HU. Schreiber et al. reported HUs in patients with normal BMD based on DEXA T score.[15] Normal T scores (greater than –1.0) had HU >118 while osteopenic patients (T score less than –1 to more than –2.5) had thresholds between 93 and 108, and osteoporotic had HU <95. Patients with an abnormal HU should be considered

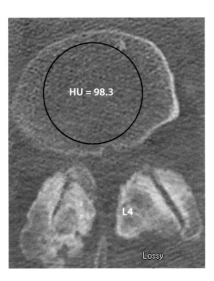

Figure 30.2 A region of interest (ellipse) is drawn in the L4 mid-vertebral body of an 84-year-old man with a C2 fracture. The picture archiving and communication systems (PACS) software reports mean Hounsfield units of 98.3 which is low indicating, at a minimum, osteopenia.

for further evaluation of their metabolic bone disease, including DEXA.

Another important consideration is calcium and vitamin D serum levels. After trauma, these values change due to production of acute phase reactive proteins and may not be reliable indicators of normal steady state conditions. Although recent recommendations are to check these levels during initial hospitalization, it may be more appropriate to evaluate them 4–6 weeks later. In the majority of patients, it is safe to simply prescribe calcium supplementation (1200 mg/day) based on dietary conditions and 2000 units of vitamin D3.

Sarcopenia is the loss of muscle mass from aging and is strongly correlated with BMD and risk of falls. Sarcopenia is increasingly being identified as a potential cause of fracture and an opportunity for treatment. Evaluation of nutrition and counseling may be considered to aid management of osteoporosis and also for fracture healing.

DEXA is the gold standard to diagnose osteoporosis and osteopenia. While useful to definitively diagnose and monitor treatment, it has no role during the acute hospitalization of patients with geriatric fractures and should be delayed until follow-up. Vertebral fracture assessment and trabecular bone scores are new quantitative techniques that may aid in evaluating quality of bone.

Vertebral artery injury

The vertebral arteries arise from the subclavian artery and ascend into the neck. The cervical components of vertebral arteries are divided into four segments. Segment one (V1) is the extra spinal part extending from the subclavian artery to where the vertebral artery enters the spine at the C6 foramen transversarium. Part V2 is where the vertebral artery ascends within the subaxial spine in the foramen transversarium up to C2. In the V3 segment, the vertebral artery ascends vertically from the C2 transversarium to the C1 foramen transversarium and then turns posteriorly and medially lying on the cranial surface of the lateral arch of the atlas. Segment V4 of the vertebral artery turns rostrally, penetrates the dura and passes anteriorly to the medulla combining with the contralateral vertebral artery to form the basilar artery. Normally, the left side is more dominant than the right side.

In geriatric patients, atherosclerosis and poor vessel compliance can create anomalies of the vertebral artery and make the vessels more prone to injury during blunt trauma. Additionally, pre-existing cerebrovascular disease may compromise cranial blood flow in patients with blunt cervical trauma associated with cervical spine fractures. Blunt head and neck trauma has recently been identified as a potential factor for stroke from vertebral artery injury and screening protocols have been developed.[16,17] Cervical spine fractures are a significant risk factor for vertebral artery injury. Specific fracture types include any fracture of C1, C2 or C3, occipito-cervical dissociation, subaxial fracture dislocation, subluxations and fractures that involve the foramen transversarium. It is recommended that patients having these fractures undergo cerebrovascular imaging, preferably with CT angiography (CTA). MRA may be performed alternatively, but is not as sensitive as CTA.

The diagnosis and treatment of vertebral artery injuries is controversial among spine surgeons. Although up to 25% of patients with cervical spine fractures may have a vertebral artery injury, it is not clear if these are clinically significant or result in neurologic injury (stroke).[17] Therefore a question remains if these should be diagnosed and treated. Neurologic injuries from the vertebral artery in cervical spine patients include death from brain stem stroke, 'locked-in' syndrome and asymptomatic cerebellar strokes. However, the majority of patients with vertebral artery injuries associated with cervical spine fractures are asymptomatic without evidence of stroke or have incidental cerebellar or small brain stem lesions on imaging.[18] It is felt that in the majority of symptomatic patients, vertebral artery injuries were caused directly from the initial blunt trauma.[18] No information is available that provides evidence that treatment of a vertebral artery injury associated with cervical spine fracture is beneficial. Recent guidelines recommend patients at high risk for vertebral artery injury should undergo CTA. If the patient is asymptomatic then it is recommended that anti-platelet therapy be administered if not contraindicated.[18]

CLASSIFICATION OF INJURY

Cervical spine injuries are classified similarly to those in non-geriatric patients. Common names are assigned based on morphologic features. After a morphologic description, the severity of injury is estimated. Because of the unique anatomic features, the cervical spine will be divided into cranio-cervical, atlanto-axial and subaxial.

Cranio-cervical injury

Cranio-cervical injuries include occipital condyle fractures and occipital cervical disassociation. Occipital condyle fractures are secondary to head impaction and are usually associated with traumatic brain injury and/or cranial nerve (CN) injury especially CN VI, VII, IX, XI and XII.[19]

Occipital condyle fractures are classified based on morphology.[19] However, the stability is determined by the status of the alar ligaments. The alar ligaments extend from the lateral tip of the dens to the anterior medial aspect of the occipital condyle and are essential for cranio-cervical stability. Just lateral to this is the hypoglossal neuroforamen containing the CN XII which explains the higher incidence of this CN palsy in association with cranio-cervical injuries.

The type I occipital condyle fractures are comminuted fractures of the occipital condyle and are generally stable. Type II is the extension of a basilar skull fracture to involve the occipital condyle. Rarely, the entire occipital condyle is displaced resulting in an unstable fracture. Type III are avulsion fractures at the attachment of the alar ligaments. These

are stable if the occipital C1 articulations are congruous and non-displaced. If displaced, then patients have craniocervical disassociation, which is present in about one-third of type III cases. Bilateral type III fractures have significant potential for instability.

Cranio-cervical disassociation is injury to the alar ligament, tectorial membrane and bony attachments so that the cranium is separated from the upper cervical spine. Other terms used are cranio-cervical instability and atlanto-axial instability. In geriatric patients cranio-cervical disassociation is rare and when associated with neurologic injury is usually fatal. The classification of cranial cervical disassociation is now functionally based on severity of injury.[20] Type I are injuries where alignment on CT between the occipital condyle C1 lateral masses is normal but on MRI abnormal edema is present in the alar ligaments and tectorial membrane. Type II injuries have normal CT alignment, but displace under a diagnostic trial of traction. Type III are displaced between the occiput condyles in C1 greater than 2 mm.

Atlanto-axial injury

The atlanto-axial spine is highly mobile accounting for 50% of axial rotation and 10–15 degrees of flexion-extension. It is the most common location of injury in geriatric patients. The most common mechanisms are falls from standing height where the patient strikes the face or cranium. This produces hyperextension forces in the upper cervical spine. The hyperextension force may cause impingement between the occiput and C1–C2 spinal process and result in C1 posterior arch fracture. If the impact is more cranial, then axial directed forces are created which can cause a comminuted atlas fracture or so-called 'Jefferson's fracture'. Further, in hyperextension the anterior arch of C1 impinges on the dens which can cause an odontoid fracture. These may be predisposed by erosive changes secondary to degenerative changes which are common in approximately 50% of geriatric odontoid fractures. Many odontoid fractures in geriatric patients are actually acute injuries superimposed on chronic insufficiency fractures.[14,21] These are associated with neurologic injuries in about 30% of patients.[22] From similar mechanisms, forces may be directed more posteriorly, causing fracture in the posterior body or in the posterior elements of C2. These are referred to as hangman's fractures or traumatic spondylolisthesis of the axis. Comminuted fractures, especially in the C1/C2 lateral masses and C2 body, are much more common than in younger patients.

ATLAS INJURIES

Atlas injuries are classified by location, including anterior and posterior arch fractures, bursting fractures (Jefferson) and lateral mass fractures. In the latter two patterns, stability is determined by the status of the transverse ligament which connects the two lateral masses behind the dens. When disrupted, the lateral masses can be unstable relative to each other and displace laterally over time. This is present when greater than 7 mm of combined displacement of the C1 lateral mass relative to C2 is seen on coronal CT or open mouth radiographs.

AXIS FRACTURES

The axis is the most common cervical vertebra injured in geriatric patients.[3] The most common mechanism of injury is forced hyperextension usually from ground level falls. The patterns of axis injuries include odontoid fractures, traumatic spondylolisthesis of the axis and axis body fractures.

Odontoid fractures are classically classified by Anderson and D'Alonzo.[23] Type I are avulsion fractures from the alar ligaments attachment at the tip of the dens. Unless associated with cranio-cervical injuries, these are stable. Type II are fractures to the waist of the dens and in general have a poorer prognosis (Figure 30.3). Type III are fractures of the dens extending into the C2 vertebral body (Figure 30.4). Grauer et al. further refined the classification of the type II fracture into a non-displaced, oblique pattern which is

favourable for screw fixation, that is, the obliquity goes from anterior superior to inferior to posterior inferior, and type III which is unfavourable for screw fixation with the opposite oblique pattern or comminution of the C2 body.[24]

Traumatic spondylolisthesis of the axis represents a continuum of injury. Initially, bending forces create a fracture in the pars interarticularis or pedicle or even posterior body of C2. Further loading causes a C2–3 disco-ligamentous injury. The fractures can be non-displaced or displaced with subluxation or translation through the C2–3 disc space. A rare, but more severe, injury is the traumatic spondylolisthesis associated with C2–3 facet dislocation. Atypical fractures are more common in the elderly where the fracture extends more anteriorly into the vertebral body rather than the pars. Also, fractures may occur at different locations on each side, but in all cases there is separation of the posterior elements from the C2 body (Figure 30.5).

A more common injury in geriatric patients is C2 body fractures which are often comminuted. Benzel proposed three types but each have many variations. Type I

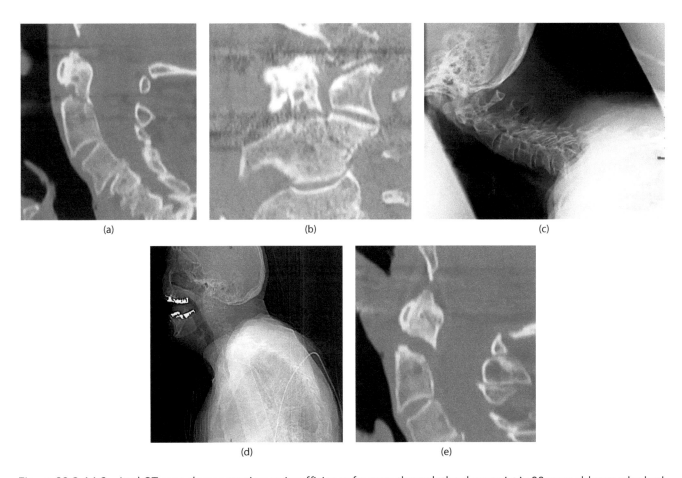

(a) (b) (c)

(d) (e)

Figure 30.3 **(a)** Sagittal CT scan demonstrating an insufficiency fracture through the dens waist in 88-year-old man who had a ground level fall. Note erosions at the odontoid base which predispose to fracture. **(b)** Coronal reconstruction demonstrating erosive disease around the dens. A fracture through the dens waist and a left-sided C2 lateral mass fracture. **(c)** Upright radiograph taken in brace. Notice the patient's difficulty holding his head up and he has progressively increased sagittal plane imbalance with his cervical spine alignment almost perpendicular to the weight-bearing axis. This increases shear forces making displacement more likely. **(d)** A scout film from CT scan shows this patient having severe spinal imbalance. Note the anterior translation of his head and neck due to thoracic and lumbar kyphosis. **(e)** At 12 months, the patient has a clear non-union as seen in the sagittal CT scan. He had minimal symptoms and was treated non-operatively.

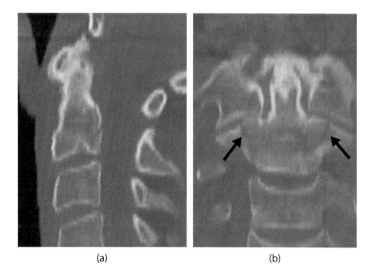

(a) (b)

Figure 30.4 A 72-year-old man who fell striking his forehead. He was neurologically intact. (a) Sagittal CT scan shows a non-displaced type III dens fracture. (b) On the coronal CT the fracture lines extend from the body out into both lateral masses and into the C1–2 articulations. He was treated successfully in a hard collar for 6 weeks.

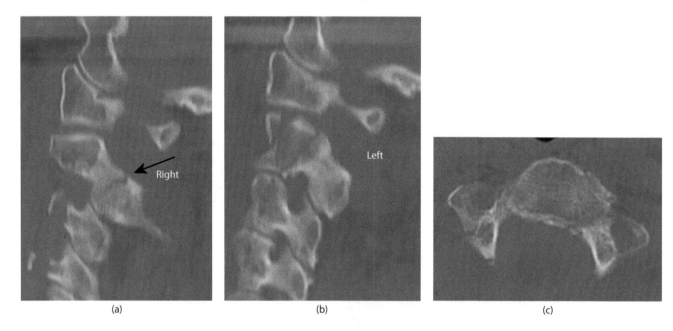

(a) (b) (c)

Figure 30.5 A 78-year-old woman who sustained a fall down the stairs presented with severe neck pain. She was found to have a comminuted C2 fracture. (a) The sagittal CT through the left lateral masses shows a non-displaced fracture in the area of the pars. (b) A more anteriorly placed fracture in the left base of the pinnacle. (c) Axial CT showing an oblique fracture that starts on the left side at the base of the pedicle and extends into the posterior elements on the right side. The patient was treated non-operatively with a hard collar for 6 weeks.

are coronal-oriented vertical fractures. A type II is a sagittal-oriented vertical fracture. A type III fracture is a horizontally-oriented low transverse body fracture. In many cases, the fracture patterns will extend into the lateral masses and across the body of the vertebra (Figure 30.6).

Subaxial cervical spine

Subaxial injuries are classified by common names based on fracture morphology and location. Fracture types involving anterior structures are compression fractures, burst fractures, flexion axial loading fractures and extension avulsion fractures. The extension avulsion type includes disco-ligamentous injuries, as well as extension tear-drop fractures. With the exception of spinous process fractures, isolated posterior element fractures are rare. Posterior element fractures are usually associated with other more serious injuries. Injuries to the lateral masses are common and include a spectrum from superior or inferior facet fractures, lateral mass fractures, to facet subluxations and dislocations. The facets and lateral masses are essential to prevent anterior shear and thus any of these injuries may be unstable and lead to anterior

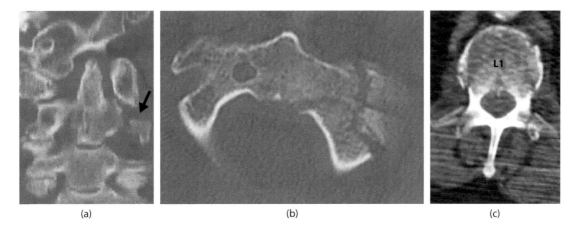

Figure 30.6 (a) A coronal CT scan of an 88-year-old man who was involved in a motor vehicle accident and was found to have a lateral mass fracture of C2. On the left side there is a split compression fracture much like a tibial plateau fracture. The vertebral artery was injured and the patient was placed on aspirin, but had no neurological consequences. (b) Axial CT scan showing a comminuted lateral mass fracture. (c) In addition the patient was found to have an L1 burst fracture which was treated non-operatively. The CT axial section shows minimal retropulsion and extreme bone demineralization. Non-contiguous spine fractures are common in geriatric patients, especially in those with higher energy mechanism or severe osteoporosis.

subluxation. The prediction models used to determine stability do not appear to be accurate in these injuries.

SUBAXIAL FRACTURE TYPES

Geriatric patients have similar patterns to younger patients. However, they have a tendency for more comminution and being multilevel. In addition, since extension forces are common mechanisms due to ground level falls, fractures in the lateral masses and posterior elements and disc disruptions in elderly patients are more frequent. Spinal cord injuries are more likely in those patients who have central canal stenosis. Fracture stability may be increased in patients who have significant amounts of pre-existing ankylosis.

Anterior column injuries

Anterior column injuries from axial loading and flexion are compression fractures, bursting fractures, and flexion axial loading injuries or so-called tear-drop fractures. Compression fractures should be viewed suspiciously as they may be associated with posterior ligamentous injury, making them very unstable. An MRI may be useful to assess this, especially in the elderly. Bursting fractures are characterized by comminution of the vertebral body with a retropulsed fragment from the posterior superior corner of the vertebral body into the spinal canal. The flexion axial loading injury, often seen in diving-type accidents, is a shear injury to the vertebral body with avulsion of the inferior anterior corner creating the tear drop. The vertebral body then displaces posteriorly into the spinal canal. There may be a significant flexion component as indicated by wide separation or fracturing in the posterior element. These fractures are typically unstable and may be associated with anterior cord injuries. Hyperextension may result in disc disruption or small avulsion fractures of the annulus and there is occasionally posterior translation of the cranial vertebra resulting in canal stenosis (Figure 30.7).

Posterior column injuries

Posterior element fractures are often seen in combination with other more serious fractures in the lateral masses or anterior columns. However, isolated fractures of the spinous process and lamina can be seen due to both hyperextension and hyperflexion forces. Hyperextension injuries are usually quite stable, although hyperflexion injuries may result in significant injury of the posterior ligamentous complex and are best evaluated with MRI.

Lateral mass column injuries

Injuries to the lateral masses are quite common. These include isolated fractures to the superior and/or inferior facets, entire lateral mass fractures including lateral mass fracture separation and subluxations and dislocations of the facets. These can be unilateral or, more commonly, bilateral (Figure 30.8).

ASSESSMENT OF SEVERITY IN SUBAXIAL INJURIES

More recently attention has been directed to predicting stability and the need for surgery based on scoring systems.[25,26] The Subaxial Cervical Spine Injury Classification (SLIC) was developed to quantitatively assess stability combined with neurologic injury.[25] Three domains are evaluated: injury morphology, integrity of the disco-ligamentous complex and neurologic state. Each domain is scored using an ordinal scale and is shown in Table 30.3. The total SLIC score is quantitatively based on the sum of each individual domain. SLIC scores less than or equal to 3 are generally treated non-operatively while scores greater than or equal to 5 are treated surgically.[27] SLIC scores equal to 4 are common and may be treated either operatively or non-operatively. An alternative is to attempt non-operative treatment and if failure occurs then perform surgery. Several limitations of the SLIC system should be noted. The system has not been evaluated in geriatric patients and it may behave differently than in

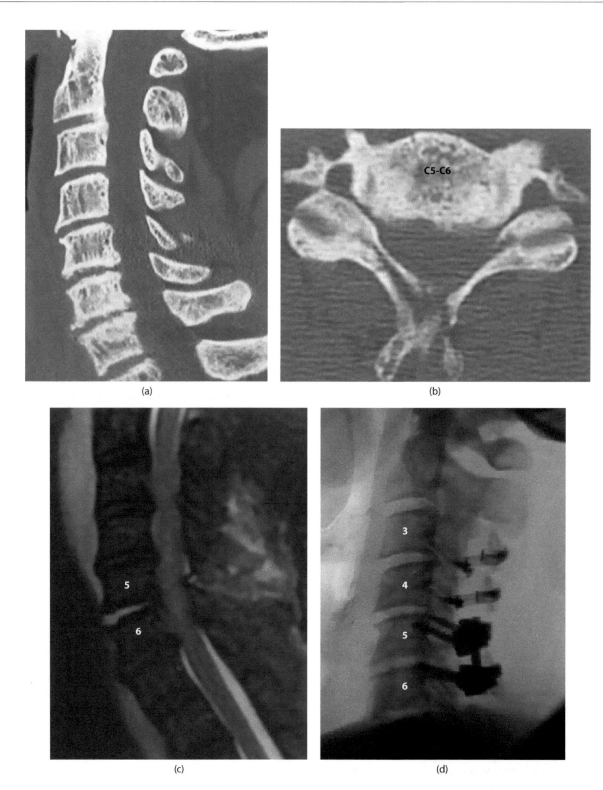

(a)

(b)

C5-C6

(c)

(d)

Figure 30.7 **(a)** This is a 76-year-old man who was in a motor vehicle accident sustaining multiple facial injuries and presented with a central cord syndrome. Sagittal CT scan shows mild spinal stenosis but no other osseous lesions. **(b)** Axial CT scan shows fractures in the posterior elements and severe foraminal narrowing. **(c)** Sagittal T2 MRI sequence showing increased signal throughout the disc as well as increased signal in the anterior retropharyngeal space. This indicates a C5–6 disco-ligamentous injury which is not appreciated on the CT scan. There is also significant posterior soft tissue injury, particularly at C5–6, indicating probable ligamentous disruption. There is severe spinal stenosis with cord signal changes from C3 through C7. **(d)** The patient was treated with laminoplasty C3 through C6 and posterior fusion at C5–6. Patient overall made a good recovery, but has persistent loss of hand function due to impairment of sensation.

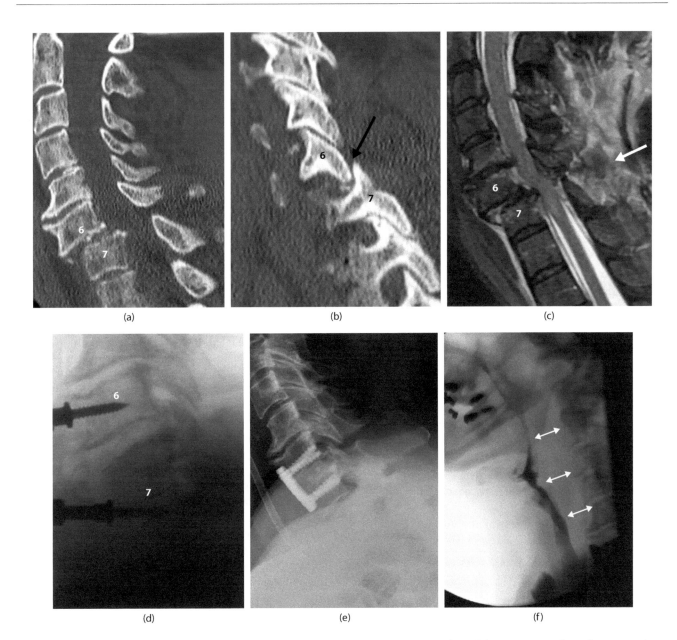

Figure 30.8 (a) A 77-year-old alcoholic fell down a flight of stairs. She sustained a mild ASIA D spinal cord injury with weakness in both upper extremities. Sagittal CT scan shows a fracture dislocation at C6–7. (b) Right sagittal reconstruction through the lateral masses showing dislocation. A similar finding was present on the left side. (c) T2 MRI sequence shows minimal spinal stenosis despite subluxation with cord signal changes. There is high intensity signal in posterior ligaments at C6–7 indicating significant ligamentous injury (arrow). (d) Reduction was obtained by closed means intraoperatively. Discectomy was performed and distraction pins were inserted in the cervical spine to help allow manual manipulation and reduction. Although reduction was achieved, the distraction pins stripped out of the bone. (e) Postoperative lateral radiograph showing excellent reduction after discectomy and interbody fusion. The patient made a full neurological recovery and healed her fusion. (f) The postoperative swallowing study 5 days after surgery showed persistent retropharyngeal swelling (arrows).

younger patients. The behavior of facet fractures does not appear to be predictive of the SLIC or other scoring systems due to the tendency for increased displacement over time.

The Allen-Ferguson classification defines injury force vectors and provides severity grades for each vector.[28] Six injury vectors were described and each vector is rated between 0–5 points. No surgical decision tree was provided.

Another quantitative system is the Cervical Spine Injury Severity Score (CSISS).[26] In this system, the spine is divided into four columns: the anterior column, two lateral columns and the posterior column. Each column is assessed on an analog scale of 0 to 5, where 0 is no injury and 5 is the worst injury of that segment. This takes into account both bony and ligamentous factors.

Table 30.3 Subaxial Cervical Spine Injury Classification (SLIC)

Domain		Score
Morphology (0–4)	Compression	1
	Burst	2
	Distraction	3
	Translation/rotation	4
Disco-ligamentous complex (0–3)	Intact	0
	Indeterminate	1
	Ruptured	2
Neurological	Intact	0
	Root injury	1
	Complete cord injury	2
	Incomplete cord injury	3
	Continuous cord compression in setting of neurological deficits	+1

Table 30.4 Principles of non-operative care in the geriatric patient

Assure proper fit by orthotist
Foam padding that can wick away moisture
Avoid rigid braces such as halo vest, CTO and C-TLSO
Skin check twice daily
Swallow study before oral intake
Upright radiographs to assure maintenance of alignment
Occupational therapy for assessment of ADL
Radiographic rechecks biweekly

Note: ADL, activities of daily living; C-TLSO, cervico-thoracolumbosacral orthosis; CTO, cervical thoracic orthosis.

The CSISS score is the sum of all individual scores for the sections. In a validity study, the CSISS score was highly predictive of surgical treatment when the CSISS was greater than 7 and of non-operative care when it was less than 5.[26] The scores between 5 and 7 were similar to the SLIC scores of 4 and are, in reality, surgeon and patient preference. The reliability of these systems has been evaluated for inter- and intraobserver reliability. The SLIC and CSISS inter- and intraobserver reliabilities were excellent while the Allen-Ferguson was poor.[29] With respect to surgical management, the interobserver agreement of the SLIC and CSISS was moderate.

GENERAL PRINCIPLES OF NON-OPERATIVE TREATMENT

Geriatric patients often have medical comorbidities and therefore non-operative care is often recommended to avoid surgical morbidity and mortality. Use of non-operative care, however, is not without significant risk in terms of skin breakdown from the orthosis, lack of compliance (especially in cognitively impaired patients), dysphagia associated with bracing, aspiration pneumonitis and overall failure of treatment. To avoid these adverse events a methodical approach to non-operative care should be used (Table 30.4). The authors recommend that the most rigid brace to be applied in geriatric patients is a hard cervical collar. The collar should be fitted by an orthotist and should have foam padding to wick away fluid. It is recommended that the patient has skin checks at least twice daily in an attempt to avoid decubitus ulceration. The use of the halo vest is associated with increased mortality and should be avoided if possible. Another important principle is to ensure that the brace is effective. In this case, upright radiographs are taken immediately after brace application and assessed for alignment, and the clinical response is noted. Severe pain while upright in bracing is indicative of fracture subluxation or neurological compression and should be critically evaluated. If the brace is successful, then initially biweekly lateral radiographs are obtained until fracture healing.

Bracing can significantly reduce the patient's ability to swallow and protect their airway. Many patients require head and neck motion to initiate swallowing and impairing this may lead to aspiration pneumonitis. In geriatric patients, prior to oral intake, a speech pathology consult and a bedside swallowing examination is performed. If the patient fails this they then undergo a full radiographic swallowing examination by the speech pathologist. On occasion this may require the use of a feeding tube or altered diets per recommendations from speech pathologists. Elderly patients in cervical braces have reduced ability to care for themselves and therefore occupational therapy should be consulted.

PRINCIPLES OF SURGICAL TREATMENT

The goals of surgery are to adequately decompress the neural elements and provide stability and long-term healing of the injured segments. Both anterior and posterior approaches may be utilized depending on fracture type and the location of neural compression. The anterior approach to the subaxial spine is well known and provides direct access to ventral compressive pathology such as vertebral body fractures or disc herniations. Reconstruction is performed using allograft and plating. Several problems are present in using the anterior approach in geriatric patients. Postoperatively, an increase in swelling may lead to further difficulties in swallowing and a possibility of aspiration pneumonitis. This would be especially true when more rostral levels are treated and for multilevel fusions. Fixation is dependent on relatively short screws in potentially osteoporotic bone which are therefore more likely to fail. Further, anterior fixation has a significant biomechanical disadvantage compared to posterior instrumentation for flexion and axial loading which are the most common postoperative deforming forces.

The posterior approach involves turning a patient prone, which could be problematic in patients with unstable spines or with significant pre-existing deformity. The posterior approach does allow access to multiple levels. Reduction of facet dislocations is more easily performed from a posterior approach than an anterior approach as well. However, the posterior approach may cause more risk of pulmonary complications due directly to surgery, haemodynamic instability during surgery and a far greater risk of postoperative wound infection. Current practice is to use 1 gram of vancomycin powder in the wound posteriorly for trauma patients.

Cranio-cervical fixation is performed using occipital plates and screws and then combinations of C1 lateral mass screws, C2 screws and lateral mass screws in the subaxial spine as required. Atlanto-axial fixation is performed by several approaches. Jeanneret and Magerl described posterior C1–2 transarticular screws combined with posterior spinous process wiring.[30] Another method is to utilize C1 lateral mass crews and C2 pedicle screws. In cases where the vertebral artery is at risk C2 laminar screws may be used. In the subaxial spine, fixation is obtained using pedicle screws at C2, lateral mass screws from C3 to C6 and pedicle screws in C7 and the thoracic spine. An important goal is to achieve satisfactory fixation and that may involve multiple levels of fixation. Avoiding excessive fusion length is less of an issue in the geriatric patient than a younger patient and it is always better to have better fixation than reducing the number of levels permanently fused. It is important to obtain fusion and therefore proper bone grafting techniques should be applied. It is our preference to use allograft bone material in geriatric patients.

Combined anterior/posterior fusions may be considered in highly unstable and comminuted fractures. Our preference is to avoid these if at all possible in the geriatric patient to reduce risk of surgical morbidity.

TREATMENT OF CRANIO-CERVICAL INJURIES

Occipital condyle fractures

Type I and type II occipital condyle fractures can be treated with a hard collar for 6 weeks (Table 30.5). The type III occipital condyle (an avulsion fracture from the alar ligaments) is treated in a collar if it is non-displaced. Displaced type III occipital condyle fractures are highly unstable and should be treated with posterior occipito-cervical fusion.

Cranio-cervical disassociation

Type I cranio-cervical disassociation (non-displaced) and type II (displaced under traction test) are treated initially non-operatively in a collar (Table 30.5). Type II injuries are diagnosed by a traction test and if reduced spontaneously may be treated non-operatively initially, but need careful follow-up to ensure that adequate alignment is maintained. Type III (displaced on initial examination) are treated operatively with an occipital cervical fusion.

TREATMENT OF ATLANTO-AXIAL INJURIES

Atlas fractures

Anterior/posterior arch injuries without subluxation are treated in a collar (Table 30.6). The treatment of Jefferson's type fracture remains controversial. The authors currently recommend non-operative treatment in geriatric patients with a collar. If the displacement is increasing over time, then one may consider a posterior occipital cervical fusion. The new technique of osteosynthesis using lateral mass screws and a transverse rod of the C1 arch is not recommended for geriatric patients. Lateral mass fractures of the atlas should be viewed suspiciously as they often will

Table 30.5 Summary of treatment of cranio-cervical injuries

	Type		Treatment
Occipital condyle fracture	I		*Collar*
	II	Non-displaced	*Collar*
		Displaced	Collar
			Occipito-cervical fusion
	II	Non-displaced	*Collar*
		Displaced	*Occipito-cervical fusion*
Cranio-cervical disassociation	I		*Collar*
	II		*Collar*
			Occipito-cervical fusion
	III		*Occipito-cervical fusion*

Note: Italics indicate preferred treatment.

Table 30.6 Summary of treatment of atlanto-axial injuries

	Type	Treatment
Atlas fracture	Arch fractures	*Collar*
	Jefferson's	*Collar*
		Possible occipito-cervical fusion
	Lateral mass	*Collar*
		Possible occipito-cervical fusion
Odontoid fracture	I	*Collar*
	II	*Collar*
		Posterior C1–2 fusion
		Odontoid screw
	III	*Collar*
Traumatic spondylisthesis of axis	Non-displaced	*Collar*
	Displaced	*Collar*
		Posterior C1–3 fusion
		Anterior C2–3 fusion
	Associated C2–3 facet dislocation	*Posterior C2–3 fusion*
C2 body fracture	1	*Collar*
	2	*Collar*
	3	*Collar*

Note: Italics indicate preferred treatment.

displace laterally, resulting in torticollis. Careful scrutiny of open mouth radiographs is needed. This is usually tolerated in geriatric patients. But if the patient has chronic pain or a significant deformity, then reduction via traction and occipital cervical fusion may be warranted.

Axis fractures

ODONTOID FRACTURES

Type I and type III odontoid fractures have a good prognosis and should be treated in a hard collar (Figure 30.3). Patients may be immobilized immediately and upright X-ray radiographs obtained to assure alignment. Displacement may occur but is usually well tolerated due to the large canal size at C2.

The treatment of type II odontoid fractures remains difficult without consensus. The goals of treatment are similar to those when treating hip fractures. Patients should be mobilized as quickly as possible and complications avoided.

The AOSpine North America performed a multi-center prospective observational study of 159 geriatric patients with type II odontoid fractures.[31] Surgery was performed in 101 and non-operative care in 58 patients. Death occurred in 18% of patients by 1 year. Mortality was statistically associated with non-operative care (odds ratio (OR) 2.9), greater age (OR 1.07), male sex (OR 4.3) and poor baseline and cognitive function.[32] Concerns

regarding non-operative treatment are its high risk of nonunion, chronic pain and late neurologic injury. In this study, 30% of non-operatively treated patients developed nonunion, of whom 11 of 15 had subsequent surgery.[33] However, at 12 months there was no difference in health related quality of life in patients having union or nonunion. No patient with nonunion developed late neurologic symptoms.

Functional outcomes for both operative and non-operative groups were estimated at baseline and compared with those at 12 months. Surgical patients had a 5-point deterioration in neck disability which was significantly less than the 14-point deterioration in the non-operative group.[31] Mortality was 26% in the non-operative and 14% in the operative group, which was not statistically significant. Although baseline demographics showed equipoise between the two treatment groups, significant selection bias may have contributed to the differences in mortality and outcomes observed; therefore, comparison between these two groups should be carried out with caution. Dysphagia, pneumonia and airway complications are much more common in operatively treated patients, especially those treated with anterior odontoid screws while nonunion was seen in non-operative cases.[23]

Robinson et al. performed a meta-analysis of management of odontoid type II dens fractures in the elderly.[34] They identified 38 articles with a total of 1284 cases. They concluded that mortality was lower in patients aged 65–80 treated surgically, posterior fixation has a higher union rate than anterior fixation or non-operative treatment, nonunion is not associated with poor outcome and complications are similar between operative and non-operative treatment methods. The authors recommended surgical treatment of odontoid fractures in the elderly.

AUTHOR'S RECOMMENDATION

Type II fractures are treated either non-operatively in a hard collar with rapid mobilization or by surgery. Physiologically, younger geriatric patients are best treated surgically (Figure 30.9). Physiologically older, frail or patients with significant dementia are treated non-operatively (Figure 30.3). The halo vest should at all times be avoided due to the potential complications of skin breakdown, aspiration, pneumonia and death.[35] Treatment decisions are best made in consultation with the patient and their family to understand their preferences. The balance between operative risks and nonoperative care should be explained. Patients with significant pre-existing cognitive disorders are usually best treated non-operatively.

The best surgical approach for geriatric patients with type II odontoid fractures is posterior fusion with rigid instrumentation. This can be performed with C1–2 transarticular screws (Magerl) or C1 lateral mass screws and C2 screw fixation (Harms).[30,36] Fixation into C2 needs to be determined by local anatomy with particular attention to the course of the vertebral artery. The author does not recommend anterior odontoid screw fixation as that is associated with severe dysphagia, higher mortality and higher failure rates than posterior fixation.[37]

Traumatic spondylolisthesis of the axis

Traumatic spondylolisthesis of the axis, whether the fractures are located in the pedicle, pars interarticularis or posterior vertebral body, is initially treated non-operatively regardless of initial displacement (Figure 30.4). If alignment can be reasonably maintained then these fractures have a high propensity for healing even in geriatric patients. Patients with neurologic injuries associated with these should have reduction and fixation. It is recommended that a C1 to C3 or C4 posterior fusion be performed. Alternatively, an anterior C2–3 discectomy and fusion can be performed but this is poorly tolerated in geriatric patients.

C2 BODY FRACTURES

C2 body fractures tend to be comminuted and involve the body and extend into the lateral masses including the C1–2 articulations (Figure 30.6a–c). These are treated non-operatively with a collar. Careful attention to the open mouth or anterior/posterior view radiographs should be paid as fractures may lead to progressive torticollis, which may require posterior C1 to C3 or C4 fusion.

TREATMENT OF SUBAXIAL SPINE INJURIES

In general treatment for geriatric subaxial cervical spine injuries is similar to that in younger patients (Table 30.7). First, the fracture is analyzed descriptively based on morphology as described above. Then the SLIC score is

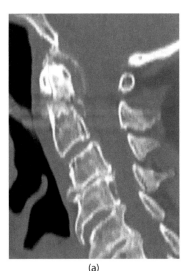
(a)

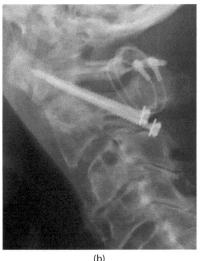
(b)

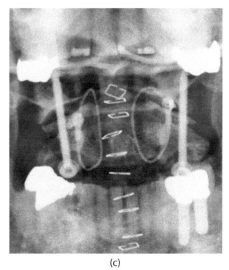
(c)

Figure 30.9 **(a)** An 88-year-old active man who fell while on ice sustaining a type II odontoid fracture. Notice the significant amount of calcification erosions in and around the dens which predispose to fracture. Non-operative treatment was attempted but failed due to severe pain and inability to mobilize. He was treated successfully with C1–2 posterior fusion using C1–2 transarticular screw technique. **(b)** Lateral radiograph after C1–2 transarticular screws with excellent reduction. Posterior fusion is added with allograft iliac crest wired to C1–2 spinous processes. **(c)** Postoperative AP showing the C1–2 transarticular screws crossing the C1–2 articulation.

Table 30.7 Summary of treatment of subaxial cervical spine injuries

Type			Treatment
Anterior column	Compression fracture	Intact PLC	*Collar*
		Disrupted PLC	Collar
			Posterior fusion
	Burst fracture	Intact PLC	
		Disrupted PLC	*Collar*
			Anterior corpectomy and fusion
			Posterior fusion
	Flexion axial loading injury		*Anterior corpectomy and fusion*
			Posterior fusion
	Disc distraction	Non-displaced	*Collar*
		Displaced or deficit	*Anterior corpectomy and fusion*
Posterior column	Isolated lamina and spinous process		*Collar*
Lateral mass column	Superior and inferior facet fracture	SLIC≤3	*Collar*
		SLIC=4	*Collar*
			Anterior or posterior fusion
		SLIC≥5	*Anterior or posterior fusion*
	Lateral mass fractures	SLIC≤3	*Collar*
		SLIC=4	*Collar*
			Anterior or posterior fusion
		SLIC≥5	*Anterior or posterior fusion*
			Collar
	Unilateral facet dislocation	Non-displaced	Collar
		Displaced	*Anterior discectomy and fusion*
			Posterior fusion
	Bilateral facet dislocation		*Anterior discectomy and fusion*
			Posterior fusion
Central cord syndrome		No compression	*Collar*
		Residual compression and deficit	Anterior decompression and fusion
			Laminoplasty
			Laminectomy and fusion
Fractures in patients with ankylosed spines			*Posterior instrumentation and fusion*

Note: Italics indicate preferred treatment. PLC, posterior ligamentous complex; SLIC, Subaxial Cervical Spine Injury Classification.

determined. For cases where a SLIC score is less than or equal to 3, a non-operative treatment is chosen. For cases with SLIC scores of more than 5, operative treatment should be considered. In the geriatric patient this may be more complicated based on medical comorbidities as well as other injuries. Patients with an indeterminate SLIC score (4) should have individualized care based on surgeon and patient preference.

Anterior column injuries

The compression fracture can be successfully treated non-operatively. However, the posterior ligamentous complex should be carefully scrutinized. The author's opinion is that these patients should all undergo MRI imaging prior to deciding on a treatment approach. If there is significant posterior ligamentous injury then a posterior cervical fusion should be recommended. Burst fractures of the subaxial spine in geriatric patients in the absence of neurologic changes are treated non-operatively in a collar. If there is significant posterior ligamentous complex injury then a surgical procedure should be performed. This can be either an anterior corpectomy and reconstruction with a plate or posterior lateral mass fixation. This particular injury pattern as well as the flexion axial loading injury may require an anterior and posterior fusion if there is relatively poor bone quality. Most flexion axial loading injuries will have a concomitant posterior element to the injury and therefore are treated surgically, similar to bursting fractures as described above.

Discoligamentous injuries from hyperextension injuries are generally stable and may be treated non-operatively. When associated with small amounts of retrolisthesis or with neurologic deficits they are treated with an anterior discectomy and fusion. Alternatively, a posterior fixation with or without decompression could be performed (Figure 30.7).

POSTERIOR ELEMENT FRACTURES

Isolated fractures to the spinous processes and lamina are treated non-operatively. More serious injuries associated with facet column or anterior injuries are usually unstable, will have high SLIC scores and are treated operatively.

LATERAL MASS COLUMN INJURIES

Treatment of lateral mass injuries remains problematic. Even experienced surgeons will have difficulty determining which fractures will displace or result in pain or even later neurologic findings despite quantitative scoring systems and the best medical imaging. Therefore all of these fractures, when treated non-operatively, need careful follow-up. There is an increasing tendency to treat these more aggressively with surgery. Fractures of the superior and inferior facets result in potential for progressive anterior subluxation. The larger the amount of facet that is fractured, the more likely the fracture will undergo displacement. This may be an important parameter when deciding treatment. When more than 50% of the facet is fractured there is a loss of shear restraint and the patient may develop progressive anterior subluxation. In younger patients these fractures are commonly treated surgically. Whether the same is true for geriatric patients is not known, but it is the preference of the author to treat these surgically. Fractures involving the entire lateral mass involve both cranial and caudal motion segments and therefore late subluxation may occur at either facet articulation. This so-called fracture separation of lateral masses occurs when the base of the pedicle and the lamina are fractured isolating the lateral mass. This allows the lateral mass to rotate anteriorly, allowing subluxation of both the cranial and caudal level. The majority of these fractures will undergo displacement over time. The surgical decision making depends on discussion with the patient on the relative risks of surgery versus non-operative care and it may be best in the geriatric patient to attempt non-operative treatment and operate only after failure.

Unilateral facet dislocations result in up to 25% vertebral body subluxation and are associated with fractures in the majority of geriatric patients. These injuries tend to displace with non-operative treatment and the author recommends an anterior discectomy and fusion with instrumentation. Bilateral facet dislocations are highly unstable and should undergo surgical treatment (Figure 30.8). First, reduction should be obtained and then fusion performed. Either an anterior or posterior approach can be utilized. Because of the risk of a disc herniation concomitant with the bilateral facet dislocations in patients who are neurologically intact, a pre-reduction MRI should be obtained (Figure 30.8c). If there is a large disc herniation behind the vertebral body of the cranial segment then an open reduction via an anterior approach is recommended.

SPINAL CORD INJURY

Spinal cord injuries in geriatric patients are devastating and have a high mortality rate. Fasset et al. reviewed a single spinal cord injury center's experience, including 7481 patients.[38] Of these, 412 were greater than 70 years of age and were found to have a 10-fold higher (27.2% compared to 3.2%) mortality within 12 months of injury than younger patients. Unfortunately, the mortality rate in geriatric patients has not changed over a 20-year period. Given the poor expected quality of life and prognosis, geriatric patients with complete spinal cord injuries may be candidates for palliative care rather than surgical treatment and rehabilitation.

The acute management of spinal cord injury in geriatric patients is no different than in younger patients. After evaluation, the goals are to protect against further injury, reduce fracture dislocations and provide long-term stability. Prevention of further spinal cord injury is achieved by accurate diagnosis, care and handling. Specifically, the neck and head should be immobilized with a collar, and proper lifting and rolling techniques should be utilized. Shock should be aggressively treated. In a spinal cord injury patient hypotension may be from neurogenic shock due to the loss of vascular tone and this form of shock responds best to vasopressors rather than fluids or blood products. It should be rapidly corrected and mean arterial blood pressure maintained at 85 mm Hg and continued for 5 days. Supplemental oxygen to maintain an oxygen saturation of at least 90% is essential. Neuroprotective agents, such as methylprednisolone, should be used with caution in geriatric patients. The use of methylprednisolone in younger patients is controversial at best and recent guidelines recommend against its routine use due to the lack of proven efficacy and the variety of complications that are seen including pneumonia, sepsis, gastrointestinal hemorrhage and death.[39] These complications are more common in elderly patients.[39]

Tong traction may be an effective means to achieve spinal cord decompression by realignment and reduction of retropulsed bone fragments. This may be effectively used in geriatric patients, but several cautions should be considered. Many injuries occur at C2 which are less well managed using tong traction. Ligamentous injuries may be occult and therefore over-distraction is a possibility. Alignment should be carefully checked on serial radiographs while weights are being adjusted. Traction should only be used for a short time and early definitive treatment performed to avoid complications associated with recumbency.

Geriatric patients have a high incidence of hyperextension injuries and pre-existing spinal canal stenosis which results in a central cord syndrome where the upper extremities have poorer function than the lower extremities. Although the prognosis is generally for improvement, the long-term results still show significant reduction in quality of life.[40,41] No consensus as to whether surgery is warranted or the timing of such surgery is available. A study evaluating the effect of the timing of surgical treatment on neurologic recovery in all types of cervical cord injuries showed greater neurologic improvement when surgery was performed within 24 hours.[42] This has been extrapolated to central cord syndrome but proven benefits remain elusive. It is the author's preference to perform an early (<24 hours) decompression in patients with central cord syndrome who have ongoing compression unless they are making a rapid recovery. The choice of surgical procedure depends upon location, number of levels of cord compression, presence of segmental instability, bone quality and pre-existing kyphotic angulation. In the typical patient with multilevel stenosis and no instability a laminoplasty is preferred (Figure 30.10).

FRACTURES IN PATIENTS WITH ANKYLOSED SPINES

Geriatric patients are at increased risk of spinal fracture due to progressive stiffening of the spine with resultant loss of viscoelastic properties of the intervertebral disc. A stiffer spine cannot distribute loads making fractures more likely. In addition, disease processes, such as DISH, ankylosing spondylitis and even surgical arthrodesis, create multilevel spinal fusions. In these cases, the spine is at up to a fivefold increase risk for fractures.[43] When fractures occur they are almost always unstable. The risk of neurologic deficits, in particular delayed neurologic deficits after hospitalization, is common.

DISH, also known as Forestier's disease, is characterized by flowing syndesmophytes with a relatively normal disc height (Figure 30.11).[20] These osteophytes flow laterally and then cranial-wards rather than straight cranially as in ankylosing spondylitis. They are much more common on the right than on the left side. Additionally, geriatric patients will have spontaneous arthrodesis of multiple segments from degenerative changes with concomitant loss of disc height.

The biomechanical effect of fusion or stiffening regardless of cause is well known. There is loss of viscoelastic properties so that energy cannot be dissipated after loading or trauma. As the number of fused levels increases, the lever arms increase in length predisposing to higher fracture risk. Further, the longer the lever arm, the greater the increased risk of neurologic injury and the greater the instability of the spine. In addition, in ankylosing spondylitis and in many geriatric patients, osteoporosis further weakens the spine making fracture risk greater. Epidural hematomas are much more common in ankylosing spondylitis patients than normal and may expand to many segments. Finally, the biomechanical effects of aging where patients have generally increased kyphosis and forward bending, particularly of their head and neck, predispose them to hyperextension injuries during a ground level fall where the face is the first part to strike the ground.

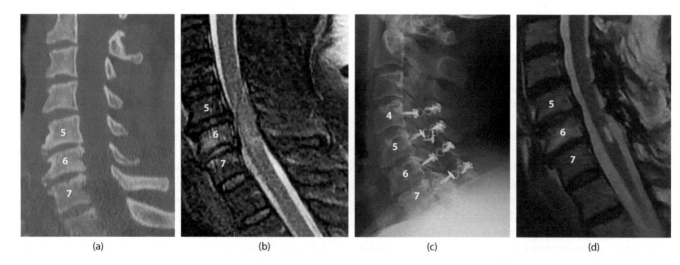

(a) (b) (c) (d)

Figure 30.10 This is a 70-year-old man who fell off of a ladder striking his face and forehead. He presented with an ASIA C quadriplegia. He had a toe flicker bilaterally. Sensation was decreased but was present in both lower and upper extremities. He had no motor function in the upper extremities. (a) Sagittal CT reconstruction showed diffuse spondylosis with narrowing of the spinal canal. He was treated by laminoplasty C4–7. At 2 years he had regained all strength but had poor hand and lower extremity coordination due to muscle spasticity. (b) The sagittal MRI scan shows oedema in the vertebral bodies of C6–7 and severe spinal stenosis C5–6 to C6–7 with significant cord signal change. (c) Lateral radiograph following laminoplasty and reconstruction with plates from C4 to C7. (d) MRI following injury showing open spinal canal without cord compression. There is a focal high intensity cord signal indicative of significant cord trauma.

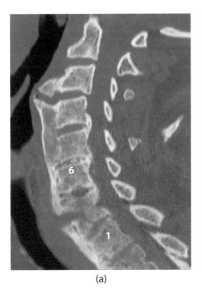
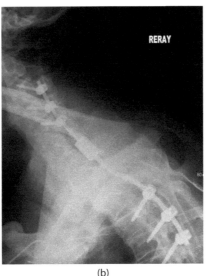
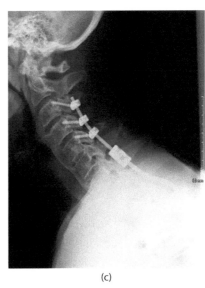

(a)   (b)   (c)

Figure 30.11 An 83-year-old man with severe diffuse idiopathic spinal hyperostosis (DISH) who sustained a hyperextension injury. He was neurologically intact. **(a)** On sagittal CT scan large anterior osteophytes are seen bridging from C4 to the thoracic spine. There is a hyperextension injury at C7. **(b)** Postoperative lateral cervical spine radiograph showing excellent alignment. **(c)** Lateral thoracic radiograph showing pedicle screws and overall good alignment.

The prognosis for patients with fractures and ankylosing spondylitis is poor unless quickly identified and treated (Figure 30.12). A delay in diagnosis is common. Caron et al. reported that out of 122 patients with ankylosing spondylitis, 19% had a delay in diagnosis of whom 81% had progressive neurologic deterioration.[44] Non-contiguous fractures occur in at least 15% of patients and therefore it is essential that the entire spinal column be carefully scrutinized. The most common fracture is a transdiscal injury at C6–7. Morbidities are common and are significantly increased in patients with ankylosed spines. Mortality rate as reported by Robinson et al. is 15% at 1 year after injury.[45]

The treatment of patients having cervical fractures with ankylosed spines is almost always surgical stabilization. Non-operative treatment is poorly tolerated and is usually ineffective (Figure 30.12). Early treatment is recommended to avoid the potential for displacement. Higher mortality and morbidity, especially pneumonia, has been reported in cases treated non-operatively with orthosis.[44] Traction or the halo vest should not be used as displacement is likely and the benefit of ligamentotaxis to realign and stabilize the segmental spine is not possible due to loss of any elasticity of these ligaments.

Surgical intervention is best performed posteriorly. The goals are to achieve reduction, to provide decompression if needed and to stabilize the spine. The reduction is achieved by careful positioning (which can be complex in patients with large deformities) and by use of instrumentation which aligns the spine along the lateral masses. Laminectomy can be performed as needed. Stabilization is performed using lateral mass screws from C3 to C6 and pedicle screws at C2, C7 and in the upper thoracic spine. If possible, at least three levels above and below the site of injury should be instrumented (Figure 30.13).[44] Using this method, Caron et al.

reported they had no mechanical failures of fixation in ankylosing spondylitis patients.[44] Odontoid fractures will occasionally occur in patients with subaxial ankylosis and are most likely to have a worse prognosis. These are best treated with atlanto-axial fusion.

Complications in both nonoperatively and operatively treated ankylosed patients occur in over 50% of patients.[45] The patients, in general, have a restrictive pulmonary deficit from their stiffness making aspiration, pneumonia and respiratory failure more likely. In addition, the inflammatory process of ankylosing spondylitis increases the risk of coronary artery disease as well as aneurysm of the proximal aorta. Wound infections appear much more common so precautions such as installation of vancomycin powder may be warranted.

COMPLICATIONS

Fractures of the cervical spine in the elderly result in higher mortality than even hip fractures. Although the causes are similar as in those patients, aspiration pneumonitis, sepsis and recurrent falls in particular are common problems. It is recommended that co-management of geriatric spine fractures in a comprehensive program be instituted similar to the fracture care program recommended by O'Malley and Kates.[7]

Dysphagia

All geriatric patients having cervical spine injuries should be assessed for dysphagia. Swallowing is significantly impaired by any retropharyngeal swelling due to the fracture as well from immobilization in orthoses. Before allowing oral intake in geriatric cervical spine injured patients,

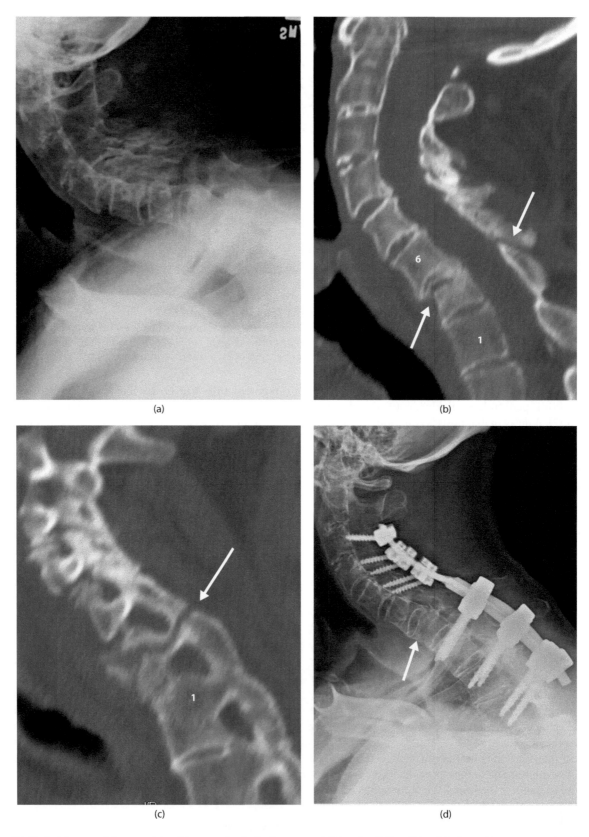

(a)

(b)

(c)

(d)

Figure 30.12 A 69-year-old man with a history of ankylosing spondylitis who fell striking his face. He presented with neck pain and plain radiographs were misinterpreted as no injury. (a) The lateral radiograph shows a wedge fracture with a posterior opening through the posterior elements. (b) One month later he presented with a chin-on-chest deformity and increasing pain. A sagittal CT scan shows ankylosing spondylitis with a wedge compression fracture at T1 and a fracture through the posterior elements. (c) Sagittal CT in lateral mass plane showing the transverse fracture through the C7–T1 facet. (d) Postoperative lateral radiograph at 3 months showing good healing of the fracture.

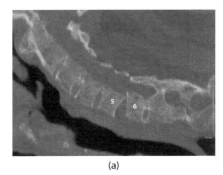

(a)

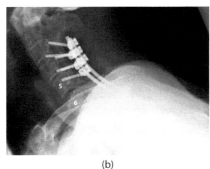

(b)

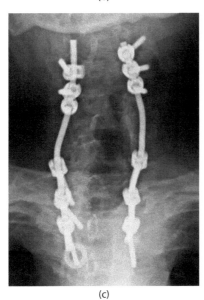

(c)

Figure 30.13 A 77-year-old woman with ankylosing spondylitis sustained a hyperextension injury. (a) Sagittal CT shows the fracture through the disc space of the posterior elements at C5–6 with 4 mm anterior translation. The patient was an ASIA B quadriplegic with an anterior cord syndrome. She was treated with open reduction and posterior instrumentation from C3 to T3. (b) Lateral view shows overall good alignment. (c) Postoperative anteroposterior radiograph.

a swallowing examination should be performed and any dietary restrictions adhered to per speech pathology. Patients may need to have repeat examinations as conditions change with time. Other considerations to reduce the risk of aspiration are to have the patient sitting upright while eating, avoid distractions and eating under nursing supervision.

Venous thromboembolism

Patients with spine fractures, unless kept immobilized or have neurologic deficits, are at a relatively low risk for venous thromboembolic disease. In general, prophylactic anticoagulation is not recommended for geriatric patients with isolated cervical spine injuries unless other risk factors are present. These include history of venous thromboembolic disease, family history of thromboembolism or abnormal coagulation, history of cancer, expected immobility and multiple injuries. Because of the risk of epidural haematoma, if anticoagulation is to be used it is also recommended that it not start until 48 hours. We initially use a fractionated heparin which is continued for 2–6 weeks depending on the mobility of the patient, as well as other risk factors. Patients with spinal cord injuries should have anticoagulation started within 48 hours if possible.

Wound infection

Older age and a posterior approach are significant risk factors for wound infection in all spine and trauma patients. Therefore geriatric patients are specifically at high risk. Prevention of surgical site infection is done by proper selection of perioperative antibiotics and discontinuing them within 24 hours of surgery to avoid risk of *Clostridium difficile* infection. Further, in posterior procedures, the author recommends the use of 1 gram of vancomycin powder which a recent meta-analysis has shown to reduce surgical site infection compared to historical controls.[46]

Hardware failure

Hardware failure is much more common in geriatric patients, and therefore special considerations are required during surgery. Specifically, the use of screws as long as possible with a larger diameter is necessary. The screw pull-out strength is proportional to the length of the screw and to the square of the diameter of the screw. Further, extending fixation over more segments may be needed, which is more easily accomplished using a posterior rather than anterior approach. At the cervical thoracic junction, pedicle screws have significantly greater holding power than lateral mass screws. Postoperative bracing may be required in geriatric patients but should be limited to a soft or hard collar.

Pulmonary events

Geriatric patients with cervical fractures are significantly at risk for pulmonary complications such as pneumonia. This may be related to aspiration pneumonitis or atelectasis. In geriatric patients, a rapid decision should be made regarding a course of treatment and performed at an early date. These patients should be prioritized if surgery is warranted and treatment should be performed as soon as possible to avoid the risks of recumbency. Postoperatively it is important to use incentive spirometer treatment and rapid mobilization to reduce the risk of pulmonary complications.

Decubitus ulceration

Geriatric patients have fragile skin and if there is presence of cognitive deficits that are pre-existing or amplified from hospitalization the risk of decubitus ulceration significantly increases. Rigid braces such as cervico-thoracic or halo vests are poorly tolerated and in the cognitively impaired patient are associated with too high a risk of skin breakdown to warrant their use. When applying a brace, we recommend the use of a certified orthotist and skin integrity checks three times a day. In addition, the patients need to be log-rolled at least twice hourly to avoid decubitus ulceration in the back and sacrum. Significant pre-existing deformity, such as kyphosis, may make bracing ineffective and increase the risk of skin decubitus ulceration. Imaginative methods in consultation with the orthotist need to be used to obtain reasonable bracing. It may be best in these patients to perform surgical stabilization to avoid complications related to skin ulceration.

Cognitive function

Impaired cognitive function is a significant risk factor for mortality after cervical spine injury in the elderly. The baseline cognitive fracture function may not be alterable. However, in hospital cognitive function can be worsened with the use of medication. Benzodiazepines should be avoided and attention to haemodynamic status to avoid orthostatic hypotension is necessary. Further, although the use of opioids may be required for pain control, these should be limited as much as possible. A balance between cognitive impairment and pain relief needs to be obtained. It is our preference to use limited opioids and to make sure the family understands the problems of opioids, cognitive impairment, and risk of falls compared to pain relief. Multimodal pain relief with the use of acetaminophen, non-steroidal anti-inflammatory agents and lidoderm patches may be helpful. Also, achieving spinal stability may actually reduce opioid consumption.

CONCLUSIONS

Geriatric cervical spine injuries are increasing in incidence and result in significant morbidity and mortality. Further, like hip fractures, long-term changes in health related quality of life and independence occur. Although the treatment is based on principles similar to those for younger patients, important differences are present. Rapid decision making is important to allow early mobilization regardless of treatment method. Medical comorbidities and bone quality need to be assessed and optimized, if possible. Careful consideration of these factors needs to occur when planning and executing surgical procedures. Complications may be decreased with the use of comprehensive management strategies similar to those being introduced for hip fracture patients.

REFERENCES

1. Zusman NL, Ching AC, Hart RA, Yoo JU. Incidence of second cervical vertebral fractures far surpassed the rate predicted by the changing age distribution and growth among elderly persons in the United States (2005–2008). *Spine.* 2013;38(9):752–756.
2. Keller JM, Sciadini MF, Sinclair E, O'Toole RV. Geriatric trauma: Demographics, injuries, and mortality. *J Orthop Trauma.* 2012;26(9):e161–e165.
3. Damadi AA, Saxe AW, Fath JJ, Apelgren KN. Cervical spine fractures in patients 65 years or older: A 3-year experience at a level I trauma center. *J Trauma.* 2008;64(3):745–748.
4. Labib N, Nouh T, Winocour S, et al. Severely injured geriatric population: Morbidity, mortality, and risk factors. *J Trauma.* 2011;71(6):1908–1914.
5. Wang H, Coppola M, Robinson RD, et al. Geriatric trauma patients with cervical spine fractures due to ground level fall: Five years experience in a level one trauma center. *J Clin Med Res.* 2013;5(2):75–83.
6. Kammerlander C, Zegg M, Schmid R, Gosch M, Luger TJ, Blauth M. Fragility fractures requiring special consideration: Vertebral fractures. *Clin Geriatr Med.* 2014;30(2):361–372.
7. O'Malley NT, Kates SL. Co-managed care: The gold standard for geriatric fracture care. *Curr Osteoporos Rep.* 2012;10(4):312–316.
8. Touger M, Gennis P, Nathanson N, et al. Validity of a decision rule to reduce cervical spine radiography in elderly patients with blunt trauma. *Ann Emerg Med.* 2002;40(3):287–293.
9. Anderson PA, Muchow RD, Munoz A, Tontz WL, Resnick DK. Clearance of the asymptomatic cervical spine: A meta-analysis. *J Orthop Trauma.* 2010;24(2):100–106.
10. Goode T, Young A, Wilson SP, Katzen J, Wolfe LG, Duane TM. Evaluation of cervical spine fracture in the elderly: Can we trust our physical examination? *Am Surg.* 2014;80(2):182–184.
11. Stiell IG, Wells GA, Vandemheen KL, et al. The Canadian C-spine rule for radiography in alert and stable trauma patients. *JAMA.* 2001;286(15):1841–1848.
12. Kirshblum SC, Waring W, Biering-Sorensen F, et al. Reference for the 2011 revision of the International Standards for Neurological Classification of Spinal Cord Injury. *J Spinal Cord Med.* 2011;34(6):547–554.
13. Muchow RD, Resnick DK, Abdel MP, Munoz A, Anderson PA. Magnetic resonance imaging (MRI) in the clearance of the cervical spine in blunt trauma: A meta-analysis. *J Trauma.* 2008;64(1):179–189.

14. Shinseki MS, Zusman NL, Hiratzka J, Marshall LM, Yoo JU. Association between advanced degenerative changes of the atlanto-dens joint and presence of dens fracture. *J Bone Joint Surg Am.* 2014;96(9):712–717.

15. Schreiber JJ, Anderson PA, Rosas HG, Buchholz AL, Au AG. Hounsfield units for assessing bone mineral density and strength: A tool for osteoporosis management. *J Bone Joint Surg Am.* 2011;93(11):1057–1063.

16. Bromberg WJ, Collier BC, Diebel LN, et al. Blunt cerebrovascular injury practice management guidelines: The Eastern Association for the Surgery of Trauma. *J Trauma.* 2010;68(2):471–477.

17. Hagedorn JC 2nd, Emery SE, France JC, Daffner SD. Does CT angiography matter for patients with cervical spine injuries? *J Bone Joint Surg Am.* 2014;96(11):951–955.

18. Harrigan MR, Hadley MN, Dhall SS, et al. Management of vertebral artery injuries following non-penetrating cervical trauma. *Neurosurgery.* 2013;72(Suppl 2):234–243.

19. Anderson PA, Montesano PX. Morphology and treatment of occipital condyle fractures. *Spine.* 1988;13(7):731–736.

20. Bransford RJ, Koller H, Caron T, et al. Cervical spine trauma in diffuse idiopathic skeletal hyperostosis: Injury characteristics and outcome with surgical treatment. *Spine.* 2012;37(23):1923–1932.

21. Julien TP, Schoenfeld AJ, Barlow B, Harris MB. Subchondral cysts of the atlantoaxial joint: A risk factor for odontoid fractures in the elderly. *Spine J.* 2009;9(10):e1–e4.

22. Kepler CK, Vaccaro AR, Dibra F, et al. Neurologic injury because of trauma after type II odontoid nonunion. *Spine J.* 2014;14(6):903–908.

23. Anderson LD, D'Alonzo RT. Fractures of the odontoid process of the axis. *J Bone Joint Surg Am.* 1974;56(8):1663–74.

24. Grauer JN, Shafi B, Hilibrand AS, et al. Proposal of a modified, treatment-oriented classification of odontoid fractures. *Spine J.* 2005;5(2):123–129.

25. Vaccaro AR, Hulbert RJ, Patel AA, et al. The subaxial cervical spine injury classification system: A novel approach to recognize the importance of morphology, neurology, and integrity of the disco-ligamentous complex. *Spine.* 2007;32(21):2365–2374.

26. Anderson PA, Moore TA, Davis KW, et al. Cervical spine injury severity score. Assessment of reliability. *J Bone Joint Surg Am.* 2007;89(5):1057–1065.

27. Dvorak MF, Fisher CG, Fehlings MG, et al. The surgical approach to subaxial cervical spine injuries: An evidence-based algorithm based on the SLIC classification system. *Spine.* 2007;32(23):2620–2629.

28. Allen BL Jr., Ferguson RL, Lehmann TR, O'Brien RP. A mechanistic classification of closed, indirect fractures and dislocations of the lower cervical spine. *Spine.* 1982;7(1):1–27.

29. Stone AT, Bransford RJ, Lee MJ, et al. Reliability of classification systems for subaxial cervical injuries. *Evid Based Spine Care J.* 2010;1(3):19–26.

30. Jeanneret B, Magerl F. Primary posterior fusion C1/2 in odontoid fractures: Indications, technique, and results of transarticular screw fixation. *J Spinal Disord.* 1992;5(4):464–475.

31. Vaccaro AR, Kepler CK, Kopjar B, et al. Functional and quality-of-life outcomes in geriatric patients with type-II dens fracture. *J Bone Joint Surg Am.* 2013;95(8):729–735.

32. Fehlings MG, Arun R, Vaccaro AR, Arnold PM, Chapman JR, Kopjar B. Predictors of treatment outcomes in geriatric patients with odontoid fractures: AOSpine North America multi-centre prospective GOF study. *Spine.* 2013;38(11):881–886.

33. Smith JS, Kepler CK, Kopjar B, et al. Effect of type II odontoid fracture nonunion on outcome among elderly patients treated without surgery: Based on the AOSpine North America geriatric odontoid fracture study. *Spine.* 2013;38(26):2240–2246.

34. Robinson Y, Robinson AL, Olerud C. Systematic review on surgical and nonsurgical treatment of type II odontoid fractures in the elderly. *Biomed Res Int.* 2014;2014:231948.

35. Kuntz C 4th, Mirza SK, Jarell AD, Chapman JR, Shaffrey CI, Newell DW. Type II odontoid fractures in the elderly: Early failure of nonsurgical treatment. *Neurosurg Focus.* 2000;8(6):e7.

36. Harms J, Melcher RP. Posterior C1–C2 fusion with polyaxial screw and rod fixation. *Spine.* 2001;26(22):2467–2471.

37. Smith HE, Kerr SM, Maltenfort M, et al. Early complications of surgical versus conservative treatment of isolated type II odontoid fractures in octogenarians: A retrospective cohort study. *J Spinal Disord Tech.* 2008;21(8):535–539.

38. Fassett DR, Harrop JS, Maltenfort M, et al. Mortality rates in geriatric patients with spinal cord injuries. *J Neurosurg Spine.* 2007;7(3):277–281.

39. Hurlbert RJ, Hadley MN, Walters BC, et al. Pharmacological therapy for acute spinal cord injury. *Neurosurgery.* 2013;72(Suppl 2):93–105.

40. Aarabi B, Alexander M, Mirvis SE, et al. Predictors of outcome in acute traumatic central cord syndrome due to spinal stenosis. *J Neurosurg Spine.* 2011;14(1):122–130.

41. Aarabi B, Hadley MN, Dhall SS, et al. Management of acute traumatic central cord syndrome (ATCCS). *Neurosurgery.* 2013;72(Suppl 2):195–204.

42. Fehlings MG, Vaccaro A, Wilson JR, et al. Early versus delayed decompression for traumatic cervical spinal cord injury: Results of the Surgical Timing in Acute Spinal Cord Injury Study (STASCIS). *PLoS One.* 2012;7(2):e32037.

43. Prieto-Alhambra D, Munoz-Ortego J, De Vries F, et al. Ankylosing spondylitis confers substantially increased risk of clinical spine fractures: A nationwide case-control study. *Osteoporos Int* 2015;26(1):85–91.

44. Caron T, Bransford R, Nguyen Q, Agel J, Chapman J, Bellabarba C. Spine fractures in patients with ankylosing spinal disorders. *Spine.* 2010;35(11):E458–E464.

45. Robinson Y, Robinson AL, Olerud C. Complications and survival after long posterior instrumentation of cervical and cervicothoracic fractures related to ankylosing spondylitis or diffuse idiopathic skeletal hyperostosis. *Spine.* 2015;40(4):E227–E233.

46. Chiang HY, Herwaldt LA, Blevins AE, Cho E, Schweizer ML. Effectiveness of local vancomycin powder to decrease surgical site infections: A meta-analysis. *Spine J.* 2014;14(3):397–407.

31

Thoracolumbar and sacral fractures

S. RAJASEKARAN, RISHI MUGESH KANNA, AJOY PRASAD SHETTY AND
ANUPAMA MAHESH

THORACOLUMBAR FRACTURES

Introduction

People's life expectancy across the world has increased and the number of elderly in the population is expected to increase considerably in the years to come. In the United States, the fastest growing age group is those above 85 years and this segment of the population is expected to double by 2025.[1] Osteoporosis is very common in the elderly population and the spine is the most common site for osteoporotic fractures.[2] Injuries of the vertebral column in the elderly population are increasingly being recognized as an important healthcare issue. These fractures can be multiple and spontaneous and can result in significant morbidity and mortality. Adverse outcomes after spinal injury in elderly patients, including poorer chest function and increased in-hospital and post-discharge mortality, have been described. Patients who sustain an osteoporotic vertebral fracture are at a high risk of future fractures of the spine and the proximal femora. To prevent complications of inactivity it is essential that these patients are returned to functional activities as early as possible.

Management of vertebral fractures in the elderly requires a thorough understanding of geriatric physiology, the natural history of osteoporotic fractures and their treatment principles. Management can be complex because of their altered physiology, poor functional reserve, presence of comorbidities, cognitive dysfunction, polypharmacy and other factors. Although the majority of injuries can be managed conservatively, operative treatment is indicated in unstable fractures, polytraumatized patients, chronic painful post-traumatic deformities and pseudarthroses. Conservative care using bracing is cumbersome particularly because of poor bone quality, pre-existing spinal deformity, fragile skin, restrictive lung disorders, cognition abnormalities and restrictions in the usage of analgesics. On the other hand, surgical management is difficult for all the above reasons and the co-existing occurrence of osteoporosis and degenerative spinal diseases including diffuse idiopathic skeletal hyperostosis, ankylosing spondylitis and degenerative spondylosis which make instrumentation difficult. This chapter will focus on the injuries affecting the thoracolumbar and sacral regions in the elderly, with special emphasis on osteoporotic vertebral fractures.

OSTEOPOROTIC VERTEBRAL FRACTURES

Epidemiology

With improvements in preventive and therapeutic medical care life expectancy has increased throughout the world. The number of elderly people (aged 65 and above) has increased by approximately 1.7 million in the last 25 years.[3] It is expected that 23% of the population will be aged 65 years and above by 2034.[4] With increasing age, gradual bone loss due to osteoporosis, cognitive dysfunction, decreased muscle tone and medications that affect balance increase the risk of the elderly sustaining fractures, especially of the spine, hip and the wrist. The estimated lifetime risk of developing a spine, hip or wrist fracture after the age of 50 years is 40% in women and 13% in men.

Most of our knowledge regarding the demographics of osteoporotic fractures has been derived from studies of the Caucasian population. In the United States, it is estimated that approximately 10 million people suffer from osteoporosis and an additional 18 million have osteopenia.[5] Approximately 1.5 million osteoporosis-related fractures occur in the United States each year. The most commonly affected regions are the vertebrae with approximately 750,000 fractures each year, wrist (250,000 fractures) and hip (250,000 fractures).[6] Few studies have assessed the prevalence and incidence of vertebral fractures in non-white ethnic groups. It is notable that the estimated prevalence of vertebral fractures in Hispanic American or Japanese American women is approximately one-half of that of white women, and it is even lower in African Americans.[7] Apart from the morbidity caused by these fractures, management of these fractures places significant socioeconomic stress on the family and society. In a study of the management of osteoporotic fractures, it was observed that approximately US$14 billion was spent on the care of patients in whom osteoporosis-related complications developed.[6]

Clinical features

Osteoporotic vertebral fractures typically occur at the thoracolumbar junction (T12–L1) and in the mid-thoracic region. Only about 30% of vertebral fractures are recognized at the time of injury because the diagnosis depends on the patient reporting back pain of sufficient severity to warrant a radiograph. Most of the remaining 'clinically silent' fractures heal without untoward sequelae but may also result in progressive vertebral deformities which may have a significant impact on health and quality of life. Gehlbach et al. observed that one or more asymptomatic vertebral fractures were noted in 132 (14%) of 934 chest X-ray films obtained in women age 60 years and older.[8] The prevalence of radiographically identified vertebral deformities increases from 5% between the ages of 50 and 54 to 50% between the ages of 80 and 84.[9]

Most osteoporotic vertebral fractures occur following trivial day-to-day activities. In cases of severe osteoporosis, the cause of trauma can be as simple as coughing, stepping out of a bathtub, vigorous sneezing, lifting a trivial object or even sudden muscle contraction. In some patients with less severe osteoporosis, more force may be required such as falling off a chair or slipping on the floor. In the acute stage, there is pain in the affected region which is aggravated by activity. The pain may radiate along the thoracic or abdominal wall and is felt as a constricting band by the patient. The acute pain usually improves in 2–3 weeks and most patients are able to perform their daily activities once the acute pain subsides.

As the collapsed anterior part of the vertebral body heals, the spine gradually bends forward causing a kyphotic deformity. Multiple fractures may result in significant loss of height (Figure 31.1). Progressive kyphosis and sagittal imbalance results in shortening of the paraspinal musculature and imposes significant stress on the muscles resulting in muscle fatigue and pain. This chronic pain is typically worse with ambulation and relieved or improved with bed rest. The pain may continue long after the acute fracture has healed.

The kyphotic deformity also affects the general functioning of the patient. The increasing thoracic kyphosis is compensated for by exaggerated lumbar lordosis, retroversion of the pelvis and knee flexion (Figure 31.2). This abnormal

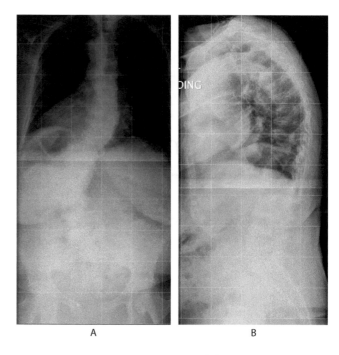

Figure 31.1 (a) Anteroposterior and (b) lateral radiographs in a 74-year-old patient who presented with chronic low back pain. The radiographs show a degenerative scoliosis and multi-level osteoporotic compression fractures that had resulted in global kyphosis.

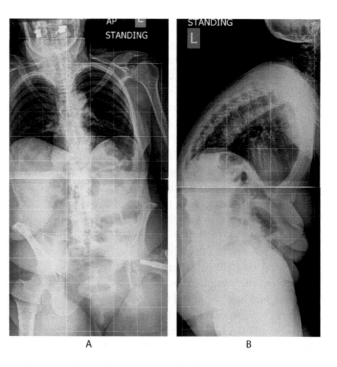

Figure 31.2 (a) Anteroposterior (AP) and (b) lateral standing radiographs of an 80-year-old patient with multiple osteoporotic fractures of the thoracolumbar spine. Note the exaggerated kyphosis at the thoracolumbar region, straight lumbar spine, retroverted pelvis and a high positive sagittal balance. The soft tissue shadow of the abdomen shows the compressed abdominal contents and reduced thoracic volume.

posture places significant stress on the hip musculature resulting in early fatigue. With increasing kyphosis, the rib cage presses down on the pelvis, reducing the thoracic and abdominal space. In severe cases, this can lead to impaired pulmonary function, a protuberant abdomen and early satiety leading to weight loss. In a prospective study of osteoporotic fractures it was observed that the overall function declined in patients with vertebral fractures similarly to those with hip fractures. Apart from chronic pain, sleep disturbance, anxiety due to fear of falling, depression due to decreased mobility and lack of self-esteem, and poor quality of life are the other sequelae that follow vertebral fractures. Recent studies have observed a relationship between osteoporotic kyphotic deformity and gastroesophageal reflux disease (GERD) in the elderly.[10] Although the exact mechanism is unclear decreased lumbar lordosis, poor sagittal balance, a high intake of oral medications and decreased back muscle strength were observed to be important risk factors for GERD.[10]

Vertebral deformities are associated with a 2.8-fold increase in the risk of hip fracture and a fivefold increase in the risk of another vertebral fracture within 3 years.[11,12] Early detection of vertebral fractures has tremendous importance because it has been shown that early treatment with antiosteoporotic medications reduces the risk of future fractures of the spine and hip. Vertebral fractures are also associated with increased mortality. The reasons for increased mortality are not clear but are presumed to be due to pulmonary disease, decreased mobility and cardiovascular disease. In one study, vertebral fractures were associated with a 16% reduction in expected 5-year survival.[13] A prospective study found that women with clinical vertebral fractures had an 8.6-fold increased 4-year mortality, compared with a 6.7-fold increase among those with hip fractures.[14]

Usually neurological symptoms are very rare, both in the acute stage and the chronic deformity phase. Because the majority of the damage is limited to the anterior column, the fracture is usually stable and rarely associated with spinal canal compromise. However a chronic kyphosis, with an unfused retropulsed bone fragment following an osteoporotic fracture can indent the spinal cord resulting in myelopathy in some patients. This post-traumatic vertebral collapse is described as Kummell's disease and can result in delayed neurological deficit (Figure 31.3). The classic clinical presentation of Kummell's disease includes a 'trivial' trauma to the spine where patients are essentially asymptomatic for weeks to months, but then develop instability type back pain, angular kyphosis and sometimes a neurological deficit. Radiographs show an area of bone destruction and radiolucency within the collapsed vertebral body. Kummell's disease is considered to represent delayed, post-traumatic vertebral body collapse secondary to osteonecrosis.[15]

Investigations

In all patients with vertebral fractures, the clinician should consider secondary causes of osteoporosis such

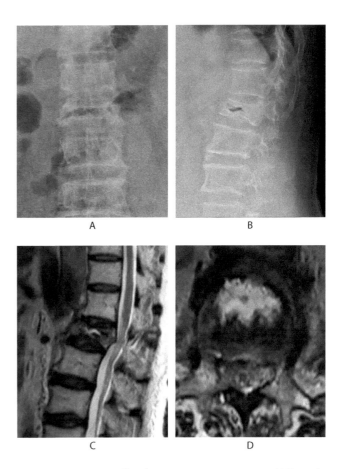

A   B

C   D

Figure 31.3 Kummell's disease. Anteroposterior (AP) and lateral radiographs (a,b) show a linear gas shadow within the fractured L1 vertebral body. Sagittal and axial T2 MRI images (c,d) show a corresponding fluid signal within the body indicative of osteonecrosis.

as osteomalacia, multiple myeloma, hyperthyroidism, hyperparathyroidism and renal failure. Initial tests should include a complete blood count, serum calcium, phosphorus, alkaline phosphatize and renal parameters. If clinically indicated, further testing should include serum 25-hydroxyvitamin D and parathyroid hormone levels, protein electrophoresis, thyroid function tests and levels of sex steroids.

Plain anteroposterior (AP) and lateral radiographs are the initial images obtained for a suspected compression fracture. The AP view will show a decrease in the height of the vertebral body, mild widening of interpedicular distance and osteoporosis. The lateral view is diagnostic and shows compression of the anterior aspect of the vertebra resulting in the classic wedge-shaped vertebral body. Typical features include generalized osteoporosis or osteopenia and a fracture involving the anterior vertebral body with intact pedicles and posterior elements. Healed vertebral collapse may be seen in other vertebrae. Compression fractures usually occur at the thoracolumbar junction, usually at T8–L1 and rarely at T6–T8 and L2–L4. It is important to image the entire spine because 20–30% of vertebral compression fractures are multiple. In some patients, the acute fracture is not well visualized and serial plain films taken 2–3 weeks later can show the vertebral injury because the deformity can take days to weeks to develop.

Three broad types of vertebral collapse are described: anterior wedge, biconcave and crush deformities. Sugita et al. proposed a classification system for osteoporotic vertebral fractures based on their study of 135 fractures in 73 patients.[16] The fractures were classified into five types based on the initial lateral radiographs. These are: (a) the swelled-front type, in which 50% of the anterior wall of the vertebral body is swollen; (b) the bow type, in which the anterior wall is pinched in and the endplate is falling in, resembling the bow of a ship; (c) the projecting type, in which 50% of the anterior wall of the vertebral body is projecting and which appears as a small bulge without a fracture line; (d) the concave type, in which the endplate is falling in and the anterior wall is intact; and (e) the dented type, in which the centre of the anterior wall of the vertebral body is dented and a fracture line is seen in the vertebral body. They observed that of the five types, the swelled-front type, bow-shaped type and projecting type fractures had a poor prognosis with late collapse and they often showed a vacuum cleft. On the other hand, concave type and dented type fractures had a better prognosis and almost always achieved fusion.

Computed tomography (CT) and magnetic resonance imaging (MRI) are not regularly performed. CT scans have been helpful in identifying fractures that are not well visualized on plain films, distinguishing a compression fracture from a burst fracture, demonstrating posterior vertebral wall integrity and in evaluation of the integrity of the posterior elements. CT also can reveal spinal canal narrowing and the presence of retropulsion of bone fragments (Figure 31.4). MRI is recommended when patients are suspected to have spinal cord compression or other neurologic symptoms. Malignancy should be considered as the first diagnosis in patients younger than 55 years

with a compression fracture without trauma, or only minimal trauma. A complete past medical history including any treatment for malignancy or swelling in the neck or breast, should be taken and MRI should be part of the initial investigation in these patients (Figures 31.5 and 31.6). In osteoporotic fractures, the affected vertebra will appear bright in T1 and T2 images because of fatty replacement of the marrow. In acute fractures, a dark marrow oedema line can be seen in T1 images. Malignant vertebral collapse will appear dark in T1 and bright in T2 images. Contrast enhancement of the affected vertebra will be present. Another important differentiating feature is the status of the posterior cortex. In malignant collapse, the posterior cortex will be bulging into the spinal canal whereas in benign fractures, the posterior wall will appear intact or can have a sharp angulated fracture. Follow-up MRI in patients with persistent pain will show typical fluid signal within the vertebral body diagnostic of pseudarthrosis. Table 31.1 details the MRI features of both benign and malignant fractures.

Bone density studies are useful for evaluating the severity of osteoporosis and in advising patients of the likelihood of subsequent fractures. A T score of –2.5 indicates severe osteoporosis and warrants appropriate treatment as explained below. It is important to recognize that bone mineral density measured at the lumbar spine in those over 70 years of age may be falsely elevated due to end plate sclerosis, aortic calcification or spondyloarthropathy. In general, a low bone mineral density (T score <–1) is an independent predictor of fractures and hence it is recommended that all women aged 65 years or older, regardless of additional risk factors, have a bone mineral density measurement. A nuclear medicine bone scan is useful when surveying the entire skeleton for osteoporotic fractures, especially when symptoms are atypical. It is particularly helpful in diagnosing sacral insufficiency fractures, which are common in osteoporosis but difficult to visualize

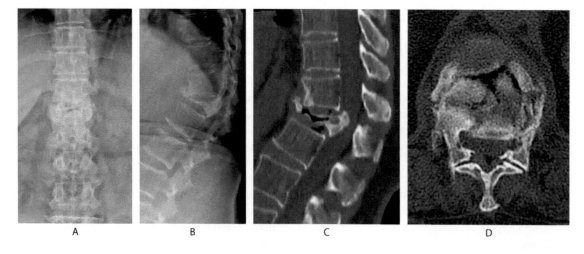

A   B   C   D

Figure 31.4 (a) Anteroposterior (AP) and (b) lateral radiographs depict an osteoporotic compression fracture of T12. (c) Sagittal and (d) axial CT shows posterosuperior corner retropulsion of the fractured vertebra and an intravertebral vacuum phenomenon.

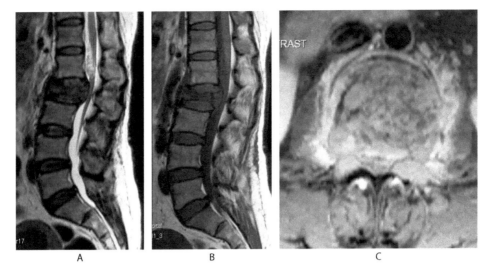

Figure 31.5 **(a)** Sagittal T2 images show iso- to hypointense signals, **(b)** T1 images show hypointense signals with a bulging posterior vertebral cortex. **(c)** Axial contrast enhanced images show enhancement and involvement of the pedicles by the tumour infiltration.

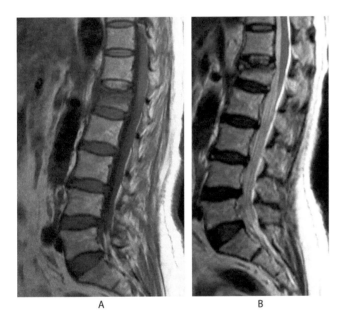

Figure 31.6 Sagittal **(a)** T1 MR image shows hypointense signals, whereas the **(b)** T2 image shows an isointense body with an intact posterior vertebral wall suggestive of a benign fracture.

on radiographs. Bone scans also can differentiate between an acute or healed compression fracture because new fractures will appear as 'hot' spots.

Management

The care of patients with vertebral fractures includes pain management, rehabilitation and prevention of further fractures. Acute pain due to vertebral fractures may last 2–3 weeks but rarely beyond 10 weeks. Most compression fractures are stable and can be treated by conservative methods.

Patients are treated with a short period, of no more than a few days, of bed rest. Prolonged inactivity should be avoided, especially in elderly patients.

Oral analgesics are administered for pain control. Standard analgesics include acetaminophen 50–60 mg/kg body weight per day in divided doses, tramadol 50 mg/dose, codeine 30 mg/dose and non-steroidal anti-inflammatory drugs (NSAIDs). Acetaminophen is avoided in patients with hepatic derangement. Opiate analgesics can cause constipation, gastric distension, nausea, vomiting and drowsiness, which are discomforting and potentially harmful in the elderly patient. NSAIDs (diclofenac, aceclofenac, ibuprofen, ketorolac) provide good analgesia but can be potentially nephrotoxic and induce gastritis. These are used judicially in consultation with a geriatrician and based on the patient's analgesic needs. Generally, analgesic needs can be met with therapeutic doses of acetaminophen and breakthrough pain can be managed with codeine 30–60 mg every 6 hours.

Calcitonin, by subcutaneous or intranasal administration, can be beneficial in reducing pain from acute vertebral fractures. It is recommended that a calcitonin dose of 50–100 IU be given subcutaneously, or 200 IU intranasally, for pain due to vertebral fractures. Several short-term randomized trials have demonstrated that calcitonin has a rapid analgesic effect.[17,18] Physical modalities for pain relief such as heat, cold and ultrasound and massage therapy are used for osteoporotic fracture pain but have not been studied for efficacy.

With progressive kyphosis, the patient's centre of gravity shifts forward which can affect the normal gait pattern. Walking aids such as four-post walkers, elbow crutches or walking sticks can provide stability and help in preventing falls. Controversy exists regarding the role of bracing. A hyperextension orthosis or a thoracolumbar sacral orthosis (TLSO) is usually prescribed for these fractures, as it is believed to offer pain relief, correct posture and help

Table 31.1 MRI differentiation of benign and malignant fractures in the osteoporotic spine

MRI features	Osteoporotic benign fracture	Malignant collapse
T1 intensity	Hypointense	Shows complete replacement of normal bone marrow with low signal intensity in the whole vertebral body.
T2 intensity	Hyperintense initially because of haemorrhage and oedema and then is essentially isointense with adjacent non-collapsed vertebrae once the oedema subsides.	On T2 weighted images, iso- to high-signal intensity is seen in the collapsed vertebra.
Contrast enhancement	Absent	Abnormal enhancement is seen in the vertebrae on post-contrast medium enhanced images particularly those obtained after fat suppression. Enhancement is usually non-homogeneous in a diffuse or patchy distribution.
Posterior vertebral wall	Retropulsion of a posterior fragment (often posterosuperior) is one of the morphological features and is very characteristic of benign fractures. Acute or sharp posterior angulation of cortex, instead of a convex posterior wall, is typical of benign fractures. A vacuum cleft in a collapsed vertebra is indicative of avascular necrosis and is suggestive of benign aetiology.	Posterior bulging or break present. The presence of an epidural mass is said to have an 80% sensitivity and 100% specificity for malignant fractures.
Posterior spinal elements	Intact, normointense	Involvement of the pedicles is pathognomonic. May show similar T1, T2 intensity changes in the posterior elements due to tumour infiltration.
Other vertebra	Normal, or may show chronic collapse (normointense bones).	Multiple vertebral involvement.

immobilization of the spine. However various authors have shown that external support has no mechanical stabilizing effect on the spine.[19,20] In a systematic review, Giele et al. concluded that there is no evidence for the effectiveness of bracing in patients with traumatic thoracolumbar fractures.[20] If used chronically, bracing may lead to weakness of the paravertebral muscles and cause disuse osteoporosis and worsening of back pain.

Once the acute pain improves, patients are advised to undertake core strengthening exercises. Exercise programs for elderly patients after a vertebral fracture have demonstrated decreased use of analgesics, improved quality of life, and increased bone mineral density. A randomized controlled trial in elderly women with vertebral fractures found that an exercise program consisting of balance and muscle strengthening exercises, resulted in reduced use of analgesics and pain level.[21] Most patients perceive significant improvements in their pain and functional capacity after 6–12 weeks and can return to a normal exercise program once the fracture has fully healed. Regular activity and muscle strengthening exercises have been shown to decrease future vertebral fractures and chronic back pain.[22]

In 20–30% of patients, the fracture may not heal completely, resulting in painful pseudarthrosis. Such patients who continue to have severe pain and who do not respond to conservative treatment may be candidates for percutaneous vertebral augmentation procedures such as vertebroplasty and kyphoplasty. Percutaneous vertebroplasty involves injecting acrylic cement into the collapsed vertebra to stabilize and strengthen the fractured vertebral body. This procedure does not restore the shape or height of the compressed vertebra. Kyphoplasty involves an initial insertion of an inflatable balloon through the pedicle into the vertebral body to re-expand the collapsed vertebra. With these procedures, pain relief has been reported in 60–100% of cases.[23,24] The procedures can be performed under local or regional anaesthesia as a day case procedure.

To assess the safety and efficacy of vertebroplasty for osteoporotic fractures, Buchbinder et al. performed a multicentre, randomized, double-blind, placebo-controlled trial in which participants with one or two painful osteoporotic vertebral fractures that were of less than 1-year duration were randomly assigned to undergo vertebroplasty or a sham procedure. Out of 78 participants, they observed that vertebroplasty did not result in a significant advantage in any measured outcome at 1 week or at 1, 3 or 6 months. There were significant reductions in overall pain and also improvement in rest pain, physical functioning and quality of life in both study groups.[25] In another study by Kallmes et al., 131 patients, who had one to three painful osteoporotic vertebral compression fractures, were assigned to undergo either vertebroplasty or a simulated procedure without cement (control group). The authors observed that at 1 month, there was no significant difference between the vertebroplasty group and the control group in either the disability score or the pain rating. Both groups had immediate improvement in disability and pain scores after the intervention. The authors also noted that there was a trend towards a higher rate of improvement in pain in the vertebroplasty group (64% vs 48%, $P = 0.06$) and at 3 months, there was a higher crossover rate in the control group than in the vertebroplasty group (51% vs 13%, $P<0.001$).[26] While these two randomized trials questioned the efficacy of vertebroplasty for osteoporotic fractures, the methodology of the trials was criticized by Boszczyk.[27] He observed that the results of these trials contradict previously published clinical series on vertebroplasty which have shown good clinical efficacy. He analysed the procedural details of the two randomized controlled trials (RCTs) specifically with regard to injected polymethylmethacrylate (PMMA) volumes which was an average fill volume of 2.8±1.2 mL per level. He noted that the existing data indicate that a minimum fill volume of 13–16% of the vertebral body volume is necessary for a relevant biomechanical effect on restoration of vertebral strength. This would be a minimum of 4 mL PMMA for any thoracic or lumbar vertebra (average 30 mL volume). Hence he concluded that the treatment arm of the two studies included patients who were not treated in a reasonably effective manner and hence the information provided is insufficient to conclusively disprove the clinical efficacy of vertebroplasty.[27]

Vertebroplasty

Although percutaneous vertebroplasty was performed first by Galibert and Deramond in 1987, the technique only gained popularity in the treatment of osteoporotic vertebral fractures in the last decade. The procedure can be performed under local or general anaesthesia. The patient is positioned prone on a series of soft pillows placed to support the head, chest, pelvis and the knee joints or on two longitudinal bolsters under the chest and pelvis. A radiolucent table is mandatory and after positioning the patient, AP and lateral images are taken to check the adequacy of the imaging.

The procedure starts with an AP image of the target vertebra. The arm of the fluoroscope is tilted cranially or caudally until the vertebral endplates of the involved vertebra are seen parallel to each other. The arm is then rotated in the mediolateral plane until the spinous process of the affected vertebra is seen exactly midway between the two pedicles. A small skin incision is made horizontally starting from the lateral wall of the pedicle and extending laterally along the transverse process. A Jamshidi needle is then passed through the fascia and the paraspinal muscles, with medial angulation towards the spine. The needle tip is aimed towards the lateral pedicle wall in the upper lateral quadrant of the pedicle eye and confirmed with an AP image. Under fluoroscopy guidance, the needle is gently tapped into the pedicle with slight medial angulation until the medial pedicle wall is reached. A lateral fluoroscopy image is now taken to locate the position of the needle tip. When the tip is at the lateral margin of the pedicle in the AP view, the tip of the needle should be at the posterior point of the pedicle in the lateral view. As the needle progresses to the centre of the pedicle in the lateral view, the tip of the needle must be seen in the centre of the pedicle in the AP view. When the tip has crossed the pedicle and enters the vertebral body in the lateral view, the tip of the needle can cross the medial margin of the pedicle in the AP view (Figure 31.7). Once the needle is confirmed to be in the ideal position (anterior one-third of the vertebra in the lateral view and the middle of the vertebra in the AP view), cementing can be started to perform a unipedicular vertebroplasty. If the needle is lateralized on the AP view, then a bipedicular vertebroplasty (Jamshidi needle into both pedicles) is performed to ensure an adequate fill. A biopsy should be performed in case of suspected pathological fractures.

When the cement has the consistency of toothpaste, it is injected through the needle under continuous lateral fluoroscopic control in order to observe and prevent any cement leakage (Figure 31.8). By adjusting the position of the needle, one can avoid cement leakage into the disc space. If there is any leakage into the canal cementing should be stopped. The cement is allowed to set for some more time and the needle is re-directed to start cementing. If there is any further leakage, then cementing should be abandoned.

The actual volume of cement to be injected is not clear. While small amounts of cement (<2 mL) will have no appreciable effect, excessive cement can harden the vertebral body beyond its original state and may have an adverse effect on adjacent osteoporotic vertebrae. Biomechanical studies have shown that the minimum volume required for achieving restoration of compressive strength or stress distribution ranges between 13 and 16% of the original vertebral body volume.[27,28] The average vertebral body volume is estimated to range from 12 mL, at T6, to 45 mL at L5 depending on the size of the vertebral body.[27,28] This would indicate that for the 16% cement fill required to restore vertebral strength, a minimum of 2–3 mL is required in lower thoracic vertebrae and 3.5–7 mL is required in the thoracolumbar and lumbar vertebrae.

If there is a need for vertebroplasty at more than one level, caution should be exercised to avoid injecting more than 20–30 mL cement in a single stage. Augmentation of more than one vertebral body can be associated with fat embolism from the vertebral marrow. The reasons for embolism are probably related to the increase in intraosseous pressure during cement injection forcing the bone marrow contents into the circulation. In a retrospective study

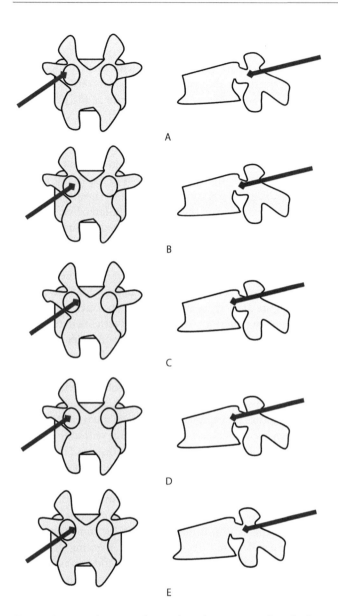

Figure 31.7 Technique of vertebroplasty. **(a–c)** The ideal needle entry point is in the upper and lateral corner of the pedicle. Medial angulation is maintained as it traverses the pedicle. When it reaches the medial pedicle wall, it should have crossed the posterior vertebral border. **(d)** Possible error 1: The needle has been inserted with less medial angulation. In the anteroposterior (AP) view, it is still well away from the medial pedicle wall but in the lateral view, the tip is already beyond the posterior vertebral wall. **(e)** Possible error 2: The needle has been inserted with too much medial angulation. In the AP view, the tip is touching the medial pedicle cortex but in the lateral view, the tip has not traversed the pedicle fully. This is a dangerous error as it is associated with a risk of canal breach and neurological complications.

of 78 patients, Kaufmann et al. reported a significant drop in oxygen saturation for 10 minutes after vertebroplasty.[29] Based on this, it has been recommended that the maximum volume of injected cement should not exceed 30 mL or three levels per session.

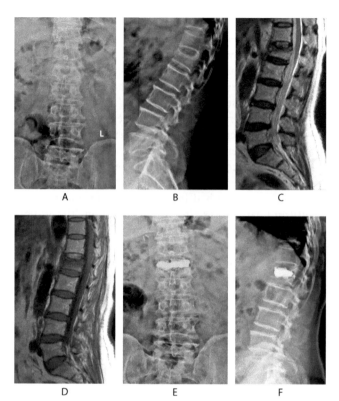

Figure 31.8 Management of a painful osteoporotic vertebral fracture with bipedicular vertebroplasty. The anteroposterior (AP) and lateral radiographs depict a compression fracture of the L1 vertebra **(a,b)**. Sagittal T2 and T1 images **(c,d)** show oedema and collapse of the L1 vertebra. The patient was treated by vertebroplasty. Note the good fill of the cement within the body in the AP and lateral views **(e,f)**.

Vertebroplasty in the acutely fractured vertebral body is not advised for two reasons: first because of the favourable outcomes with conservative care in most patients and second the high risk of cement leakage in the presence of acute fractures. Use of continuous fluoroscopy while injecting the cement and using the cement only when the consistency has become like toothpaste can reduce the chances of cement leakage. In patients with a suspected defect in the posterior vertebral wall, a small amount of contrast dye can be injected into the vertebral body to look for extravasation into the spinal canal. The cement diffuses into osseous space and after it solidifies it stabilizes the vertebral body. Pain relief is enabled by two probable mechanisms. First, the cement combines the individual bone fragments in a single block avoiding the painful micro-movements between individual fragments. The second mechanism may be related to the exothermic process that accompanies the polymerization of PMMA which results in 'thermal neurolysis' of the painful nerve endings within the vertebral body. In addition, the PMMA results in significant strengthening of osteoporotic bone, reducing the risk of subsequent fractures.

After vertebroplasty, it has been reported that a marked improvement in pain symptoms can occur in 90% of cases.

But the procedure can be associated with complications including bleeding at the site of needle insertion, transient fever, cement leakage into the disk or into the paravertebral soft tissues, epidural space or paravertebral veins, leading to pulmonary embolism, new fractures in adjacent vertebrae, infection and rarely cerebral embolism and even death (Figure 31.9). The incidence of complications ranges from 1% to 3%.[30] Cement leakage into the spinal canal is the most feared complication. Although leakage of cement into the spinal canal is asymptomatic in most cases, it can potentially lead to serious neurological complications (Figure 31.10). Although intraforaminal leakage is less common, it can be more bothersome for the patient. In a study by Cotten et al., it was found that while leakage from the spinal canal was well tolerated, two of the eight patients with foraminal leakage had significant radiculopathy. In most cases, the symptoms are transient and respond well to nerve-root blocks or oral medication.[31]

A number of reports have indicated an increased risk of secondary vertebral fractures adjacent to the augmented vertebra.[32–36] Several factors have been considered to be risk elements for developing adjacent vertebral level fractures. These include the degree of augmentation of the treated vertebra (i.e. more cement fill), location of the adjacent vertebra at the thoracolumbar junction, leakage of cement into the disc space and a decreased vertebral stiffness secondary to severe osteoporosis. Lin et al. studied 38 patients who underwent vertebroplasty over a 12-month period and observed that vertebral bodies adjacent to a disc with leakage of cement had a 58% chance of developing a new fracture compared with 12% of vertebral bodies adjacent to a disc without leakage.[37] Leakage into the disc can restrict the flexibility of the adjacent vertebral body and thus may increase the risk of a secondary fracture. This factor appears more important in vertebrae where the initial strength of the vertebral body is very low. Heini et al. and Tomita et al. observed that the lower the initial bone mineral density, the more pronounced the augmentation effect.[38–40] In strong non-osteoporotic bone, cement augmentation does not produce any significant changes.

Other authors have suggested that adjacent fracture risk is part of the disease process as patients with vertebral fractures develop fractures at adjacent levels even while on conservative treatment. The rates of new fracture after cement augmentation procedures vary between vertebroplasty (0–52%), kyphoplasty (5.8–36.8%) and conservatively

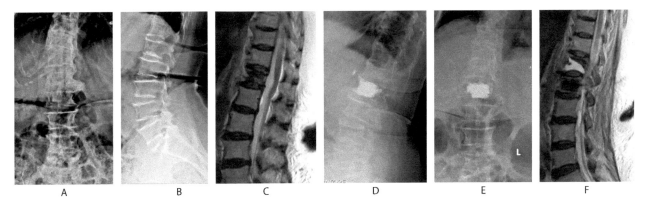

Figure 31.9 Complication of vertebroplasty. The patient presented with a T12 osteoporotic collapse as seen in the anteroposterior (AP), lateral and sagittal MR images (a–c). Despite vertebroplasty (d,e), the patient had severe pain postoperatively and a repeat MRI (f) revealed a frank pseudarthrosis at T12 and incorrect cementing at the L1 level.

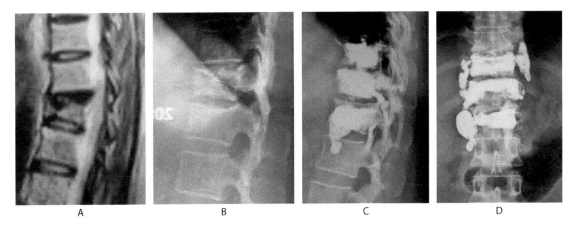

Figure 31.10 An osteoporotic fracture at the T12 level is seen in the sagittal MR and lateral radiographs (a,b). The patient has been incorrectly managed by vertebroplasty at three levels. Note that the cement has extravasated into the spinal canal and paravertebral regions (c,d). Fortunately the patient maintained her normal neurology.

treated patients (19.2–58%) but these are not comparable due to the varied scientific designs of the studies.[41] Several authors have suggested that kyphoplasty could reduce the risk of adjacent fractures. With the development of a kyphotic deformity, the body's centre of gravity shifts forward resulting in an increased forward bending moment and may predispose the adjacent vertebrae to have secondary fractures. Hence partial reduction of kyphotic deformity with kyphoplasty can decrease the risk of new fractures.[42] In a comparative study, Kasperk et al. found that at a mean follow-up of 6 months, seven (35%) out of 20 conservatively treated patients developed secondary fractures, while 12.5% of 40 patients who had undergone kyphoplasty developed adjacent level fractures.[42]

Kyphoplasty

Kyphoplasty is similar to vertebroplasty and can be performed in the thoracic and lumbar vertebrae (Figure 31.11). In addition to the pain relief in patients with vertebral osteoporotic fractures, kyphoplasty enables a partial recovery of the height of the vertebral body. To restore sagittal vertebral anatomy after a fracture, the vertebral endplates must be reduced to their correct anatomic position, which can be potentially achieved by kyphoplasty. The technique involves the inflation of a percutaneously inserted balloon into the vertebral body through either or both the pedicles. Upon inflation, the balloon restores the vertebral body height in addition to creating a cavity. The balloon is removed and PMMA is injected into the cavity created by the balloon. The risk of cement extravasation is probably reduced as compared to vertebroplasty due to the space produced by the newly created vertebral cavity, thus resulting in lower injection pressures while injecting the cement. In the systematic review by Akbar et al., cement leakage was significantly higher with vertebroplasty (40%) than with kyphoplasty (8%), and 3% of vertebroplasty leaks were symptomatic whereas no kyphoplasty leaks were reported to be symptomatic.[43]

Biomechanically kyphoplasty achieves better restoration of vertebral height (97%) as compared to vertebroplasty (30%).[44] But this gain appears transient, as with repetitive cyclical loading, there is a four times greater loss in vertebral height in kyphoplasty patients as compared to vertebroplasty patients.[45] It is hypothesized that the repetitive loading crushes the cancellous bone around the cement bolus, whereas in vertebroplasty the cement is injected under more pressure, thus allowing it to interdigitate in the cancellous bone resisting further compression. As far as clinical outcomes are concerned, direct comparisons between vertebroplasty and kyphoplasty are not possible because of a lack of comparative and controlled studies between the two approaches. Meta-analyses have shown that vertebroplasty and kyphoplasty reduce pain comparably and show similar improvement in patient function in most series.[46–49] On the economic side, kyphoplasty is 10–20 times more expensive than a vertebroplasty procedure due to additional costs

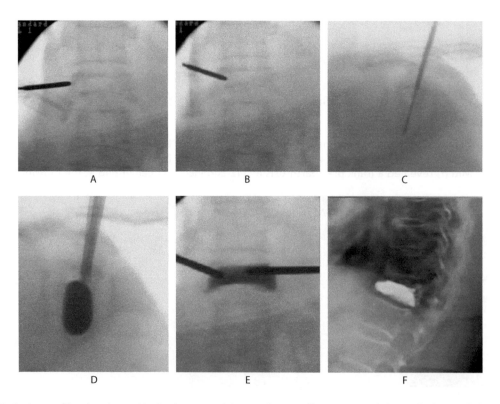

Figure 31.11 Technique of kyphoplasty. Under image guidance, the needle is inserted through the pedicles into the vertebral body (a,b). A special drill is then passed to create a track into the body. The balloon in a collapsed state is inserted into the drilled track (c) and gently inflated to elevate the collapsed vertebral body (d). The balloon is deflated and withdrawn following which cementing is performed (e,f).

incurred by the device, duration of the procedure and in-patient hospitalization.[50,51]

Internal fixation in osteoporotic fractures

Internal fixation with rods, sublaminar wires and pedicle screws are rarely required in the management of osteoporotic fractures. However patients who have a chronic vertebral pseudarthrosis can develop a neurological deficit and spinal instrumentation is necessary in such situations. Various operative techniques have been reported to be successful in the management of neurological deficits due to osteoporotic vertebral collapse including posterior stabilization alone, posterior stabilization and decompression (Figure 31.12) and combined anterior and posterior stabilization.[52,53] Anterior decompression and reconstruction alone is not advised due to the risks of implant related complications and pseudarthrosis as reported by some authors who recommend additional posterior reinforcement to increase the rate of arthrodesis.[54] An anterior approach is also considered to have significant morbidity in elderly patients.

Shikata et al. showed good results with posterolateral decompression, reconstruction and stabilization in osteoporotic fractures with neurological deficit.[53] Ataka et al. postulated that the instability at the fracture site rather than neural compression is the major factor causing neurological disorders in patients with osteoporotic thoracolumbar vertebral collapse. They studied 14 consecutive patients who had incomplete neurological deficits following vertebral collapse in the osteoporotic thoracolumbar spine and performed posterior instrumented fusion without neural decompression. In an average follow-up period of 25 months, there was no implant failure, and in all patients, back pain was relieved, and neurological improvement of at least one modified Frankel grade was obtained.[55] A posterior closing wedge osteotomy, where the posterior elements are shortened along with neural decompression, and correction of kyphotic deformity has been postulated to decrease the stress on the spinal instrumentation.[56,57]

The presence of degenerative changes such as facet arthropathy, hypertrophied joints, osteophytes and diffuse idiopathic spinal hyperostosis (DISH)-like changes

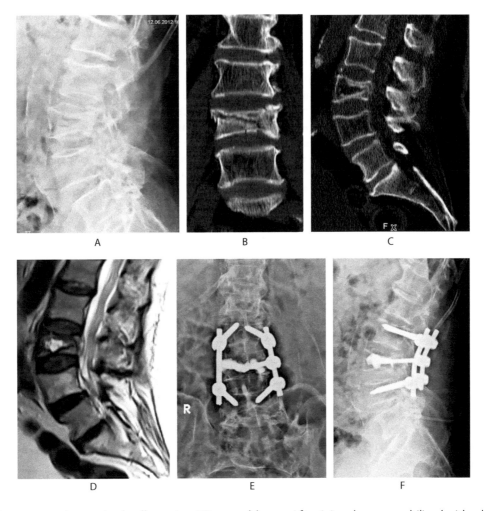

Figure 31.12 L3 osteoporotic vertebral collapse in a 73-year-old man. After injury he was mobilized with a brace. However, 4 weeks later he developed persistent instability type back pain and sudden buckling of the knees while walking. A lateral radiograph and coronal, sagittal CT and MRI images (a–d) revealed osteonecrosis in the L3 body, evident by gas shadow and fluid in the vertebra. The patient was treated by posterior stabilization and vertebroplasty at L3 (e,f).

pose difficulties during surgical exposure, identification of standard anatomical landmarks and pedicle screw insertion. Degenerative spondylosis also involves changes like disc space collapse, osteophytosis and ligamentum flavum buckling which results in stenosis of the canal and spinal cord compression. This needs consideration while planning the surgical treatment. Spondylosis also leads to increased rigidity which results in the creation of a rigid lever arm so that long segment fixation is needed to decrease the stress on the implants. A major concern in internal fixation of osteoporotic spines performed for various conditions like osteoporotic fractures with neurological deficit, traumatic spinal injuries and other degenerative conditions, is the strength of the implant fixation. Several authors have suggested that long segment fixation of the spine at least two to three segments from the affected level is preferred.[58,59] Additionally, correction of kyphotic deformity, restoration of sagittal anatomic alignment and reconstruction of the anterior vertebral defect may reduce instrumentation failure. Pedicle screws should be long enough to have adequate purchase within the pedicle and anterior part of the vertebral body. The screw width should be a minimum of 6.5 mm and 7–8 mm in the lumbar vertebra. The screws should be directed towards the subchondral zone to achieve good purchase in the cortical part of the vertebra. For additional supplementation, sublaminar wires can be used which provide enhanced stability to the construct. The lamina, being the thickest part of the osteoporotic bone, has significant pull-out strength. Despite being the most rigid form of posterior instrumentation, pedicle screws can have poor fixation in patients with osteoporosis. To improve the hold of the pedicle screws in osteoporotic spines, pedicle augmentation using materials such as PMMA, calcium phosphate or calcium hydroxyapatite have been suggested.[60] Although various biomechanical studies on osteoporotic spines have demonstrated improved pull-out strength of pedicle screws augmented with bone cement, application of PMMA carries risks of cement leakage, embolic insults and irremovable hardware.[61]

Prevention of future vertebral fractures

Calcium and vitamin D deficiency is commonly present in the elderly due to reduced intake of these nutrients and impaired gastrointestinal absorption. The prevalence of vitamin D deficiency in the elderly patients is quoted to range from 5 to 18%.[62] Apart from deficiencies which increase the chances that the elderly will sustain vertebral osteoporotic fractures, a combination of calcium and vitamin D supplementation also has beneficial effects in vertebral fracture healing. In a 3-year randomized trial in community living people with a mean age of 71 years, those treated with calcium and vitamin D had a 54% reduction in non-vertebral fractures compared with a placebo.[63] In another study, treatment with calcium and vitamin D led to 32% fewer non-vertebral fractures and 43% fewer hip fractures in an elderly population.[64]

Several other drugs are effective in reducing vertebral fractures in patients who have experienced a vertebral fracture. Randomized trials have shown that bisphosphonates reduce the risk of vertebral and non-vertebral fractures, including hip fractures, whereas selective estrogen receptor modulators such as raloxifene and perhaps calcitonin have only shown beneficial effects on vertebral fractures.[65] Bisphosphonates are administered weekly (alendronate, risedronate), monthly (ibandronate) or yearly (zoledronate). They can cause significant reflux oesophagitis and hence it should be explained to the patient that they should avoid recumbency for 30 minutes after taking the medication. Bisphosphonates, which include etidronate, alendronate and risedronate, must be taken well before food intake to ensure adequate absorption.

Calcitonin, administered by nasal spray, is shown to provide immediate pain relief for osteoporotic fractures.[66] Raloxifene is an estrogen receptor modulator with modest effects on bone mineral density. It has been shown to reduce vertebral fracture in post-menopausal female patients.[67] Hormonal replacement therapy with estrogen has beneficial effects on bone mineral density, but its effects on future prevention of vertebral fractures are uncertain. Recombinant parathyroid hormone is currently used in patients with severe osteoporosis and is considered to be effective in decreasing the risk of vertebral and non-vertebral fractures in post-menopausal women.[68] The drug is administered daily by subcutaneous injection. Studies have shown that the bone mineral density increases within 6 months and the incidence of subsequent fractures decreases.[69] In a study by Bouxsein et al., of 1226 post-menopausal women with one or more vertebral fractures recombinant parathyroid hormone reduced the risk of any new, new adjacent and new non-adjacent vertebral fractures by 72%, 75% and 70%, respectively, compared with the rates in the placebo group.[70]

Conclusion

The prevalence of vertebral compression fractures steadily increases with advancing age. They affect approximately 25% of all post-menopausal women. Although less common in older men, compression fractures are a major health concern in this group. Most fractures heal well with conservative care such as rest, analgesics, anti-osteoporotic medications and bracing. More severe fractures can cause significant pain, leading to inability to perform activities of daily living. Patients with persistent pain and progressive deformity may require interventions like vertebroplasty and kyphoplasty. Prevention of index compression fractures and future vertebral and non-vertebral fractures is key and involves diagnosing and treating predisposing factors, identifying high-risk patients and educating patients about osteoporosis and preventing falls.

TRAUMATIC THORACOLUMBAR INJURIES

Apart from osteoporotic fractures which occur following trivial injuries in individuals with low bone mass, severe thoracolumbar injury in the geriatric population may occur after high energy trauma. The evaluation of spinal injury in this population requires a heightened level of suspicion, especially in an ankylosed or spondylotic spine, because the incidence of missed injuries and non-contiguous fractures is higher than reported in the general population. Since elderly patients have reduced physiological reserve, it is essential that serious injuries to the chest, abdomen and pelvis, long bones and head are looked for and managed with priority. For patients with predominant injury to the thoracolumbar spine, the stability of the fracture and the neurological status of the patient must be carefully assessed.

Epidemiology

Although severe spinal trauma causing spinal cord injury (SCI) is uncommon in the elderly, it is of considerable concern because of the high peri-injury morbidity and mortality in the elderly. Contrary to popular belief, the incidence of severe spinal trauma and SCI is increasing in the elderly population. In a research survey on SCI patients conducted by the Spinal Injury Association, it was observed that 32% of respondents were greater than 60 years of age. Another study conducted in 2007 showed that annual admissions for older persons with SCI have increased approximately five-fold in the last 25 years.[71] The percentage of older persons with SCI has increased from 4.2% in the early 1980s to 15.4% in recent years. The US database on SCI further confirms that the mean age of patients with SCI is increasing and the percentage of persons older than 60 years has increased from 4.7% before 1980 to 10.9% since 2000.

The increased incidence possibly results from the rise in the number of the elderly population and because of the success of accident prevention efforts targeted at younger people. A Finnish study on fall-induced, fracture-associated spinal cord injuries in adults older than 50 years observed that the incidence increased at a rate that could not be explained merely by demographic changes, such as increased life expectancy, over that time period.[72] Although many initiatives such as sterner traffic laws including the use of helmets and seat belts may have decreased the rate of SCI and head injury among younger individuals, the mean age of SCI has increased, indicating that a higher number of injuries are now seen among older adults.

A recent study also showed that the mechanisms of injury in older persons with SCI differ significantly from those in younger persons. Unlike younger individuals, older people were much more likely to sustain an SCI secondary to a fall (74%) followed by road traffic accidents (13%).[73] SCI in elderly patients is associated with high morbidity and mortality. In a study that analysed early clinical outcomes, the overall mortality in patients above 50 years of age with SCI was 23% in the first 4 months.[74] While patients with American Spinal Injury Association (ASIA) grade A (complete) injury had a 60% mortality, in patients over 65 years of age with complete cord injuries, the mortality was 100%. Jackson et al. studied 74 cases in which older persons were treated surgically for spinal injuries and reported that the mortality rate during initial hospitalization was fivefold higher in patients older than 65 years of age.[75]

The pattern of injury also differs in the elderly. Patients older than 60 years were significantly more likely to have cervical SCI.[76] In older adults, cervical injuries accounted for 94% of SCIs, compared with only 70% of SCIs in patients younger than 60 years.[77] Prasad et al. observed that after the sixth decade, patients were significantly more likely to have upper cervical trauma, compared with lower cervical trauma in younger patients.[78] In another epidemiological study in Canada, it was observed that patients older than 60 years were likely to have significantly more injuries above C5.[77]

Clinical presentation

Acute fractures present as axial, non-radiating back pain of stabbing or aching quality. Pain may not be midline in distribution and it can be referred to the ribs, hip, groin or buttocks. Midline tenderness corresponding to the radiographic level of injury is present in most of the cases. The presence of a palpable gap in between spinous processes indicates rupture of the posterior ligamentous complex (PLC) suggestive of an unstable injury. Compression and burst fractures are stable injuries and these fractures may heal in kyphosis without symptoms depending on the extent of kyphosis, status of adjacent vertebrae and bone quality. The diagnosis and management of compression fractures of the thoracolumbar spine have been explained in the previous section. Burst injuries to the thoracolumbar spine can be either inherently stable or unstable. Unstable injuries include Chance fractures, flexion distraction injuries and fracture-dislocations. There are no specific classification systems for the thoracolumbar injuries in the elderly. Different classification systems of thoracolumbar fractures exist and the most popular ones are McAfee's classification, the Thoracolumbar Injury Classification and Severity Score (TLICS) and the AO classification.

McAfee's simplified system of classifying injuries to the thoracolumbar spine is as follows:

1. *Wedge compression fractures* result from isolated failure of the anterior column due to forward flexion. They rarely are associated with neurological deficit except when multiple adjacent vertebral levels are affected.
2. In *stable burst fractures,* the anterior and middle columns fail because of a compressive load, with no loss of integrity of the posterior elements.
3. In *unstable burst fractures,* the anterior and middle columns fail in compression, and the posterior column is disrupted. The posterior column can fail in compression, lateral flexion or rotation.
4. *Chance fractures* are horizontal avulsion injuries of the vertebral bodies caused by flexion around an axis anterior to the anterior longitudinal ligament. The entire vertebra is pulled apart by a strong tensile force.

5. In *flexion distraction injuries,* the flexion axis is posterior to the anterior longitudinal ligament. The anterior column fails in compression, whereas the middle and posterior columns fail in tension.
6. *Translational injuries* are characterized by malalignment of the neural canal, which has been totally disrupted. Usually all three columns have failed as the result of a shear force.

The TLICS is based on three major injury characteristics: mechanism of injury, integrity of the PLC and neurological status. Based on the severity scores within these three categories, a total score is calculated that can be used to guide treatment. Recently the AOSpine Knowledge Forum proposed a comprehensive modified AO classification including morphology of the fracture, neurological status and description of relevant patient-specific modifiers.[79] The fracture morphology is assessed based on three main injury patterns: type A (compression injury to the vertebral body without PLC involvement), type B (tension band disruption – the failure of posterior (PLC) or anterior (anterior longitudinal ligament) constraints) and type C (displacement/translation) injuries. Neurological status is classified as follows: no neurological injury (N1), radicular symptoms or deficits (N2), incomplete SCI or any kind of cauda equina injury (N3), complete SCI (N4) and unknown neurological status (NX). The classification appears much simpler and equally comprehensive when compared with the previous AO classification and includes important information about neurology and posterior ligamentous structures. The inter- and intraobserver reliability of this classification is yet to be studied, other than by the originators.

Alhough there are no specific classifications for fractures in elderly patients, the above can be used to help guide our treatment strategy. The presence of a neurological injury and/or severe ligamentous injury suggests an unstable fracture pattern. The presence of ankylosing spondylitis, diffuse idiopathic skeletal hyperostosis or other ankylosing conditions increases the risk of spinal instability as well as posing a potential risk for neurological injury. These fractures are associated with significant instability.

Radiographic evaluation

Standard radiographic evaluation includes AP and lateral radiographs. Radiographic evaluation should include assessment of the kyphosis angle, loss of anterior vertebral height and interspinous distance on lateral radiographs. In the AP view, vertebral collapse, translation and interpedicular widening can be seen. Disruption of the PLC implies a three column injury; these are unstable injuries requiring surgical management. CT scan of the injured area may be obtained to characterize the fracture further and evaluate the degree of canal compromise. CT scans provide finer details about the bony involvement, the extent of canal compromise and occult posterior element fractures. MRI is required for patients with a neurological deficit to identify possible spinal cord, cauda equina or root injury, cord oedema and haemorrhage or epidural haematoma. The advantages of MRI are its ability to evaluate injury to the discs and PLC, screening of the whole spine and evaluation of epidural haematoma and cord injury. An important issue in the elderly population is adequate knowledge about contraindications to MRI scanning such as the presence of foreign bodies like pacemakers and metallic stents.

Management

Managing elderly patients after spinal injury is multifaceted. The initial step in management is assessment of the patient's general physical status and this includes accounting for their physical health, mental health and cognitive function. Decision-making in the elderly patient population should include the patients, the patient's family members and a geriatrician. Stable compression and burst fractures can be managed conservatively similar to the management for osteoporotic fractures. Unstable injuries and those with neurological deficit require surgical stabilization. When planning surgical care, poor bone quality, underlying spinal deformity, pre-existing spinal stenosis and ankylosing spinal disorders should be considered. These factors might necessitate the need for long segment fixation, thus preparing the surgeon for prolonged surgical time, blood loss and costs (Figure 31.13). The use of rigid internal fixation allows for early patient mobilization, thereby minimizing potential perioperative complications, including pneumonia, thromboembolic disease and pressure ulceration.

There are relatively few absolute indications for emergency surgery. They are usually progressively deteriorating neurology and open spine injures. In the absence of the above indications, the patient can be nursed on a firm mattress with frequent log rolls to avoid pressure sores and meticulous attention to bowel, bladder and skin care. There is no evidence that early surgery can improve neurological outcomes. On the other hand, undue delayed surgical management may increase the risk of complications, including pneumonia, bed sores, nerve injury, paralysis, epidural hematoma formation and death. The rate of postoperative complications in patients undergoing extensive thoracolumbar surgery remains high as demonstrated by Cloyd et al.[80,81] The authors demonstrated that increasing age and increasing levels of fusion were associated with an elevated risk for major postoperative complications. The number of comorbidities was associated with a greater risk for perioperative complications in elderly patients. Given the published poorer outcomes and increased complications of elderly patients after spinal surgery, it is imperative that we involve geriatric care physicians in the management of elderly patients in the early stages to reduce perioperative medical complications.

In patients with neurological deficit and spinal instability, the goals of surgery are to achieve decompression of the spinal cord and stabilization of the unstable segments. Stabilization and fusion through the posterior approach

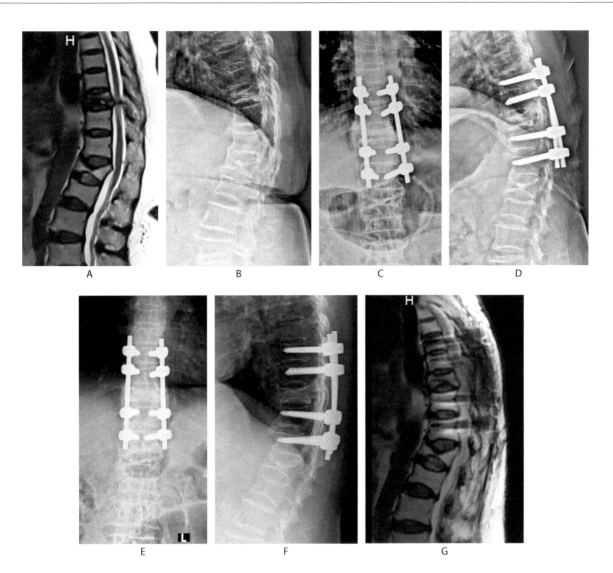

Figure 31.13 This 72-year-old patient presented with an osteoporotic fracture at the T8 level and a neurological deficit. A sagittal MR image (a) shows an acute fracture at T8 associated with ligamentum flavum hypertrophy causing cord compression. Another healed fracture at T11 is noted in the lateral radiograph (b). The patient has been treated by long segment fixation from T6 to T10 and posterior decompression (c). Follow-up radiographs at 2 years show a stable fixation with fracture healing (e,f). MRI shows complete fracture healing and a clear canal (g).

is the most popular and widely employed surgical method for management of unstable fractures. The familiarity of approach, the ease of decompression and stabilization, and the decreased rate of complications in the elderly make this approach a favoured one for most surgeons. Long segment pedicle screw fixation is the preferred technique in view of osteoporosis and spinal rigidity. Short segment fixations can be associated with implant failure (Figure 31.14). In patients with significant collapse of the vertebral body, in an effort to decrease the stress on the posterior instrumentation, the posterior column can be shortened, or the vertebral body can be reinforced with vertebroplasty, kyphoplasty, calcium phosphate or transpedicular bone grafts.

In patients with severe comminution of the vertebra and retropulsion into the spinal canal causing cord compression, decompression and reconstruction with a titanium cage

may be necessary to prevent an anterior collapse. Although combined anterior/posterior approaches maintain better kyphosis correction, it is not clear if this difference is clinically relevant. The advantages of combined surgical approaches are improved sagittal alignment, thorough spinal canal and neural decompression for optimum recovery of neural function, and stabilization of the disrupted PLC.

Conclusion

The incidence of elderly patients with SCI is increasing. Patients' medical comorbidities, associated injuries, primary injury pattern, the presence of neurological injury, bone quality, pre-existing spinal degenerative conditions and the patient's general physical and cognitive function are important issues to be considered when planning the management. It should be remembered that the mortality is high

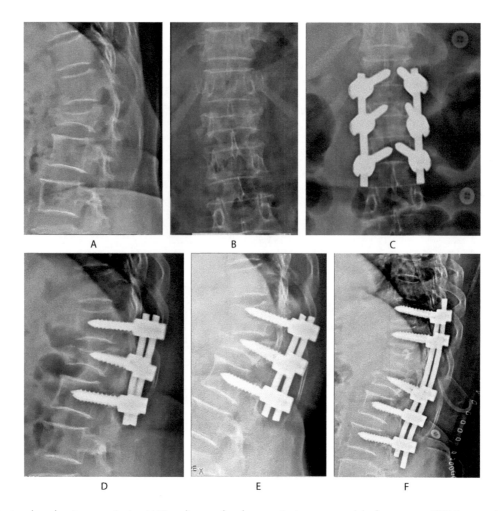

Figure 31.14 Lateral and anteroposterior (AP) radiographs demonstrate an unstable fracture at T12 in a patient with osteoporosis **(a,b)**. The fracture has been treated by short segment fixation from T11 to L1 **(c,d)**. However, 2 months after surgery, the lateral radiograph shows pull-out of proximal screws and worsening kyphosis **(e)**. This was treated by extension of instrumentation and fixation from T9 to L2 **(f)**.

in patients with complete SCI and that surgical treatment is associated with complications.

SACRAL FRACTURES

Introduction

Osteoporotic fracture of the sacrum was a previously underrecognized entity but it is being increasingly identified now. In a Finnish study, the incidence of osteoporotic fractures of the pelvis in women above 60 years of age was observed to have increased fivefold from 1970 to 1997.[82] It is expected that this number will triple by the year 2030. This increase in incidence is probably due to the increased awareness among patients and doctors, increased life expectancy and the availability of better diagnostic facilities.

Osteoporotic fractures of the sacrum are denoted as sacral insufficiency fractures (SIF) and were first described by Lourie in 1982.[83] The true prevalence and the financial costs related to SIF are not known. In a 2-year prospective study by Weber et al., the frequency of SIFs in women aged

over 55 years who presented to hospital with low back pain was 1.8%.[84] Dasgupta et al. observed that 7 out of 10 patients with SIF were admitted for a mean 20 days as in-patients at a cost comparable to that of hip fractures.[85] This shows that significant cost is involved in the management of SIFs.

Denis et al. have classified traumatic sacral fractures according to their location into three different zones.[86] According to the Denis classification, zone 1 fractures involve the sacral ala, which lies lateral to the sacral foramina and the central sacral canal. Zone 2 fractures involve one or several sacral foramina but do not enter the central sacral canal. These fractures are associated with unilateral radiculopathy along the sacral nerve root. Zone 3 fractures occur through the body of the sacrum and involve the central sacral canal. Fractures in this region are associated with displacement and compromise of the central sacral nerve roots resulting in bilateral neurological deficit, saddle anaesthesia and lax sphincters. Although there is no specific classification for SIF, the Denis classification system is used to describe the fractures. The vast majority of SIFs occur in zone 1 running vertically along the ala parallel to the sacroiliac (SI) joints. Some patients can have an additional transverse fracture connecting the two vertical fracture lines. The transverse fracture line can be either in the middle ('H'-shaped fracture) or in the lower end of the vertical fractures ('U'-shaped fracture).

Similar to osteoporotic vertebral fractures, SIFs often arise insidiously without any significant trauma, resulting from axial stresses transmitted from the lumbar spine to the sacral ala. In a meta-analysis by Finiels et al., no history of trauma was identified in two-thirds of 493 patients.[87] Apart from senile and post-menopausal osteoporosis, other causes that can predispose to SIF include corticosteroid induced osteopenia, radiation therapy, hyperparathyroidism, osteomalacia, renal osteodystrophy, transient osteoporosis associated with pregnancy and lactation, rheumatoid arthritis, lumbosacral fusion, Paget's disease and organ transplantation and limb reconstruction surgeries.

Clinical features

Typical features include sudden onset, intractable, low back and buttock pain. The symptoms are exacerbated by weight-bearing and generally improve with rest. Changes in posture from supine to lateral position or getting up from lying down can produce acute exacerbations of pain. Depending on the location of the fracture, the patient can have radicular symptoms in the lower limbs, neurological symptoms such as saddle anaesthesia and sphincter disturbances. SIFs are often associated with pubic rami fractures and can present with groin pain. A thorough history to elicit all the secondary causes of osteoporosis and SIF should be taken. Physical examination will reveal direct tenderness and pain over the SI joint on lateral compression. SI joint stress tests may be misleadingly positive in patients with SIF. This is due to stress transmission from the SI joint to the sacral fracture. Neurological examination is often normal but SIFs involving zone 3 have lax sphincters and associated lower limb and saddle paraesthesia. The clinician should be aware of SIFs and vertebral osteoporotic fractures as a cause of persistent low back pain.

Evaluation

In patients with evident osteoporosis, blood investigations are not required. In doubtful situations, initial tests should include a complete blood count, serum calcium, phosphorus, alkaline phosphatize and renal parameters. These are performed to rule out secondary causes of osteoporosis. If clinically indicated, further testing should include serum vitamin D, parathyroid hormone levels, electrophoresis for myeloma, serum T3, T4 levels and sex steroids.

Plain AP and lateral radiographs of the pelvis are the initial investigations performed in all patients. Unless displaced, most SIF are not visualized in standard radiographs but there can be associated fractures of the pubic ramus. The curved anatomy of the sacrum, osteoporosis and overlying bowel gas shadows make identification of fracture lines difficult. Although CT is useful in delineating the fracture line, MRI is the most sensitive screening investigation as it can show the typical bone marrow oedema in the sacral ala and body. T1 weighted images demonstrate low signal intensity while T2 weighted images demonstrate high signal intensity. T2 weighted fat suppression images are particularly sensitive to demonstrate a fracture line. Coronal T1 and T2 images demonstrate H- and U-shaped fractures very well by depicting the horizontal fracture line. MRI is also useful to show epidural haematomata, displaced fractures into the sacral canal and neural compression. A technetium-99m bone scan is also a very sensitive investigation to demonstrate SIFs when radiographs appear normal. Two parallel hot spots near the SI joint or the classic 'H' pattern may be visualized. The presence of SI arthritis also shows high signal uptake in a bone scan and can confuse the observer. Bone mineral density assessment through DEXA scanning of the lumbar spine, hip and radius is performed in all patients to quantify the severity of osteopenia. Based on the T score, appropriate medical management of osteoporosis is provided.

Management

Akin to osteoporotic vertebral fractures, the majority of SIFs are treated conservatively with bed rest and analgesics (acetaminophen, codeine or NSAIDs) followed by gradual mobilization as tolerated by the patient. Patients are also started on anti-resorptive medications, calcium and vitamin D supplementation (refer to medical management of osteoporotic vertebral fractures). Once the patient is able to move out of the bed, early rehabilitation and moderate weight-bearing exercises can be initiated. This induces muscle and bone healing and helps prevent disuse osteoporosis and other problems of immobilization including deep vein thrombosis, loss of muscle strength, impaired cardiac and respiratory functions, urinary tract complications, gastrointestinal tract complications and pressure sores.

Sacroplasty

Sacroplasty involves injection of cement into the fracture site under fluoroscopy guidance. The principle is similar to vertebroplasty where the cement is expected to provide stability to the fracture and ablate painful nerve endings. Several case series have demonstrated immediate pain relief and improved quality of life following sacroplasty.[88] The procedure aims to limit the need for analgesics and lessen the period of bed rest.

Sacroplasty is performed under either local anaesthetic or general anaesthesia. The patient is placed prone on a radiolucent table. Under fluoroscopic guidance, a bone biopsy needle is percutaneously inserted through the posterior sacral cortex into the sacral ala near the fracture site in a plane parallel to the SI joint. It is crucial to avoid inadvertent penetration into the spinal canal or anterior to the sacrum. Once the safe needle position is confirmed, the cement is injected under fluoroscopy guidance. In a prospective study of 52 patients treated with sacroplasty for SIF, a 50% reduction in the visual analogue scale (VAS) score for back pain at 2 days, a 80% reduction at 2 weeks and a 90% reduction at 1 year was observed.[89] The authors also observed a reduction in the use of narcotic analgesics after sacroplasty. Complications of sacroplasty involve the leakage of PMMA cement outside of the fractured sacrum, and so far two cases of cement leakage into the neural foramen have been described, which resolved with steroid root block.

Apart from sacroplasty, balloon augmentation or sacral kyphoplasty has been described. So far, two case reports have demonstrated the feasibility of this method for osteoporotic fractures.[90] The technique is similar to sacroplasty but there is a theoretical advantage of a lower risk of cement extravasation. Similarly transiliosacral screws have also been reported as an alternative method of sacral stabilization in patients with SIF.

Conclusion

Although not as common as vertebral osteoporotic fractures, SIF are an important and curable cause of low back pain. They usually present as instability, like low back pain in elderly patients, often without a history of trauma. Radiographs may demonstrate the fracture but if strongly suspected, MRI is the most sensitive investigation to clearly show the fracture. Most fractures heal well with rest, analgesia and treatment for osteoporosis. Recently, percutaneous cement injection (sacroplasty) has been shown to have good results in reducing the pain.

REFERENCES

1. Chapman J, Smith JS, Kopjar B, Vaccaro AR, Arnold P, Shaffrey CI, Fehlings MG. (2013). The AOSpine North America Geriatric Odontoid Fracture Mortality Study: A retrospective review of mortality outcomes for operative versus nonoperative treatment of 322 patients with long-term follow-up. *Spine (Phila Pa 1976)* 38:1098–1104. doi: 10.1097/BRS.0b013e318286f0cf.

2. O'Neill TW, Cockerill W, Matthis C, Raspe HH, Lunt M, Cooper C, Banzer D, et al. (2004). Back pain, disability, and radiographic vertebral fracture in European women: A prospective study. *Osteoporos Int* 15:760–765. doi: 10.1007/s00198-004-1615-4.

3. Miller KE, Zylstra RG, Standridge JB. (2000). The geriatric patient: A systematic approach to maintaining health. *Am Fam Physician* 61:1089–1104.

4. Dodds C, Foo I, Jones K, Singh SK, Waldmann C. (2013). Peri-operative care of elderly patients – An urgent need for change: A consensus statement to provide guidance for specialist and non-specialist anaesthetists. *Perioper Med (Lond)* 2:6. doi: 10.1186/2047-0525-2-6.

5. Riggs BL, Melton LJ 3rd. (1995). The worldwide problem of osteoporosis: Insights afforded by epidemiology. *Bone* 17:505S–511S.

6. Ray NF, Chan JK, Thamer M, Melton LJ 3rd. (1997). Medical expenditures for the treatment of osteoporotic fractures in the United States in 1995: Report from the National Osteoporosis Foundation. *J Bone Miner Res* 12:24–35. doi: 10.1359/jbmr.1997.12.1.24.

7. Genant HK. (1995). Current assessment of osteoporosis: Proceedings of an international symposium convened during ECR '95 in Vienna, Austria. *Eur J Radiol* 20:163–164.

8. Gehlbach SH, Bigelow C, Heimisdottir M, May S, Walker M, Kirkwood JR. (2000). Recognition of vertebral fracture in a clinical setting. *Osteoporos Int* 11:577–582. doi: 10.1007/s001980070078.

9. Melton LJ 3rd, Kan SH, Frye MA, Wahner HW, O'Fallon WM, Riggs BL. (1989). Epidemiology of vertebral fractures in women. *Am J Epidemiol* 129:1000–1011.

10. Imagama S, Hasegawa Y, Wakao N, Hirano K, Hamajima N, Ishiguro N. (2012). Influence of lumbar kyphosis and back muscle strength on the symptoms of gastroesophageal reflux disease in middle-aged and elderly people. *Eur Spine J* 21:2149–2157. doi: 10.1007/s00586-012-2207-1.

11. Ross PD, Davis JW, Epstein RS, Wasnich RD. (1991). Pre-existing fractures and bone mass predict vertebral fracture incidence in women. *Ann Intern Med* 114:919–923.

12. Ross PD, Genant HK, Davis JW, Miller PD, Wasnich RD. (1993). Predicting vertebral fracture incidence from prevalent fractures and bone density among non-black, osteoporotic women. *Osteoporos Int* 3:120–126.

13. Center JR, Nguyen TV, Schneider D, Sambrook PN, Eisman JA. (1999). Mortality after all major types of osteoporotic fracture in men and women: An observational study. *Lancet* 353:878–882. doi: 10.1016/S0140-6736(98)09075-8.

14. Bliuc D, Nguyen ND, Milch VE, Nguyen TV, Eisman JA, Center JR. (2009). Mortality risk associated with low-trauma osteoporotic fracture and subsequent fracture in men and women. *JAMA* 301:513–521. doi: 10.1001/jama.2009.50.

15. Gorsch RV. (1921). Compression fracture of the first lumbar vertebra with delayed symptoms (Kuemmel's disease). *Ann Surg* 73:360–361.

16. Sugita M, Watanabe N, Mikami Y, Hase H, Kubo T. (2005). Classification of vertebral compression fractures in the osteoporotic spine. *J Spinal Disord Tech* 18:376–381.

17. Lyritis GP, Ioannidis GV, Karachalios T, Roidis N, Kataxaki E, Papaioannou N, Kaloudis J, Galanos A. (1999). Analgesic effect of salmon calcitonin suppositories in patients with acute pain due to

recent osteoporotic vertebral crush fractures: A prospective double-blind, randomized, placebo-controlled clinical study. *Clin J Pain* 15:284–289.

18. Lyritis GP, Paspati I, Karachalios T, Ioakimidis D, Skarantavos G, Lyritis PG. (1997). Pain relief from nasal salmon calcitonin in osteoporotic vertebral crush fractures. A double blind, placebo-controlled clinical study. *Acta Orthop Scand Suppl* 275:112–114.

19. Jellema P, van Tulder MW, van Poppel MN, Nachemson AL, Bouter LM. (2001). Lumbar supports for prevention and treatment of low back pain: A systematic review within the framework of the Cochrane Back Review Group. *Spine (Phila Pa 1976)* 26:377–386.

20. Giele BM, Wiertsema SH, Beelen A, van der Schaaf M, Lucas C, Been HD, Bramer JA. (2009). No evidence for the effectiveness of bracing in patients with thoracolumbar fractures. *Acta Orthop* 80:226–232. doi: 10.3109/17453670902875245.

21. Malmros B, Mortensen L, Jensen MB, Charles P. (1998). Positive effects of physiotherapy on chronic pain and performance in osteoporosis. *Osteoporos Int* 8:215–221. doi: 10.1007/s001980050057.

22. Wolff I, van Croonenborg JJ, Kemper HC, Kostense PJ, Twisk JW. (1999). The effect of exercise training programs on bone mass: A meta-analysis of published controlled trials in pre- and postmenopausal women. *Osteoporos Int* 9:1–12. doi: 10.1007/s001980050109.

23. Watts NB. (2003). Is percutaneous vertebral augmentation (vertebroplasty) effective treatment for painful vertebral fractures? *Am J Med* 114:326–328.

24. Watts NB, Harris ST, Genant HK. (2001). Treatment of painful osteoporotic vertebral fractures with percutaneous vertebroplasty or kyphoplasty. *Osteoporos Int* 12:429–437. doi: 10.1007/s001980170086.

25. Buchbinder R, Osborne RH, Ebeling PR, Wark JD, Mitchell P, Wriedt C, Graves S, Staples MP, Murphy B. (2009). A randomized trial of vertebroplasty for painful osteoporotic vertebral fractures. *N Engl J Med* 361:557–568. doi: 10.1056/NEJMoa0900429.

26. Kallmes DF, Comstock BA, Heagerty PJ, Turner JA, Wilson DJ, Diamond TH, Edwards R, et al. (2009). A randomized trial of vertebroplasty for osteoporotic spinal fractures. *N Engl J Med* 361:569–579. doi: 10.1056/NEJMoa0900563.

27. Boszczyk B. (2010). Volume matters: A review of procedural details of two randomised controlled vertebroplasty trials of 2009. *Eur Spine J* 19:1837–1840. doi: 10.1007/s00586-010-1525-4.

28. Molloy S, Mathis JM, Belkoff SM. (2003). The effect of vertebral body percentage fill on mechanical behavior during percutaneous vertebroplasty. *Spine (Phila Pa 1976)* 28:1549–1554.

29. Kaufmann TJ, Jensen ME, Ford G, Gill LL, Marx WF, Kallmes DF. (2002). Cardiovascular effects of polymethylmethacrylate use in percutaneous vertebroplasty. *AJNR Am J Neuroradiol* 23:601–604.

30. Wardlaw D, Cummings SR, Van Meirhaeghe J, Bastian L, Tillman JB, Ranstam J, Eastell R, Shabe P, Talmadge K, Boonen S. (2009). Efficacy and safety of balloon kyphoplasty compared with non-surgical care for vertebral compression fracture (FREE): A randomised controlled trial. *Lancet* 373:1016–1024. doi: 10.1016/S0140-6736(09)60010-6.

31. Cotten A, Boutry N, Cortet B, Assaker R, Demondion X, Leblond D, Chastanet P, Duquesnoy B, Deramond H. (1998). Percutaneous vertebroplasty: State of the art. *Radiographics* 18:311–320; discussion 320–313. doi: 10.1148/radiographics.18.2.9536480.

32. Legroux-Gerot I, Lormeau C, Boutry N, Cotten A, Duquesnoy B, Cortet B. (2004). Long-term follow-up of vertebral osteoporotic fractures treated by percutaneous vertebroplasty. *Clin Rheumatol* 23:310–317. doi: 10.1007/s10067-004-0914-7.

33. Baroud G, Heini P, Nemes J, Bohner M, Ferguson S, Steffen T. (2003). Biomechanical explanation of adjacent fractures following vertebroplasty. *Radiology* 229:606–607; author reply 607–608. doi: 10.1148/radiol.2292030378.

34. Baroud G, Vant C, Wilcox R. (2006). Long-term effects of vertebroplasty: Adjacent vertebral fractures. *J Long Term Eff Med Implants* 16:265–280.

35. Berlemann U, Ferguson SJ, Nolte LP, Heini PF. (2002). Adjacent vertebral failure after vertebroplasty. A biomechanical investigation. *J Bone Joint Surg Br* 84:748–752.

36. Boger A, Heini P, Windolf M, Schneider E. (2007). Adjacent vertebral failure after vertebroplasty: A biomechanical study of low-modulus PMMA cement. *Eur Spine J* 16:2118–2125. doi: 10.1007/s00586-007-0473-0.

37. Lin EP, Ekholm S, Hiwatashi A, Westesson PL. (2004). Vertebroplasty: Cement leakage into the disc increases the risk of new fracture of adjacent vertebral body. *AJNR Am J Neuroradiol* 25:175–180.

38. Heini PF, Berlemann U, Kaufmann M, Lippuner K, Fankhauser C, van Landuyt P. (2001). Augmentation of mechanical properties in osteoporotic vertebral bones – A biomechanical investigation of vertebroplasty efficacy with different bone cements. *Eur Spine J* 10:164–171.

39. Tomita S, Kin A, Yazu M, Abe M. (2003). Biomechanical evaluation of kyphoplasty and vertebroplasty with calcium phosphate cement in a simulated osteoporotic compression fracture. *J Orthop Sci* 8:192–197. doi: 10.1007/s007760300032.

40. Tomita S, Molloy S, Abe M, Belkoff SM. (2004). Ex vivo measurement of intravertebral pressure during vertebroplasty. *Spine (Phila Pa 1976)* 29:723–725.

41. Hadjipavlou AG, Tzermiadianos MN, Katonis PG, Szpalski M. (2005). Percutaneous vertebroplasty and balloon kyphoplasty for the treatment of osteoporotic vertebral compression fractures and osteolytic tumours. *J Bone Joint Surg Br* 87:1595–1604. doi: 10.1302/0301-620X.87B12.16074.

42. Kasperk C, Grafe IA, Schmitt S, Noldge G, Weiss C, Da Fonseca K, Hillmeier J, et al. (2010). Three-year outcomes after kyphoplasty in patients with osteoporosis with painful vertebral fractures. *J Vasc Interv Radiol* 21:701–709. doi: 10.1016/j.jvir.2010.01.003.

43. Akbar M, Eichler M, Hagmann S, Lehner B, Hemmer S, Kasperk C, Wiedenhofer B. (2012). [Role and limitations of vertebroplasty and kyphoplasty in the management of spinal metastases]. *Orthopade* 41:640–646. doi: 10.1007/s00132-012-1909-8.

44. Belkoff SM, Mathis JM, Deramond H, Jasper LE. (2001). An ex vivo biomechanical evaluation of a hydroxyapatite cement for use with kyphoplasty. *AJNR Am J Neuroradiol* 22:1212–1216.

45. Kim MJ, Lindsey DP, Hannibal M, Alamin TF. (2006). Vertebroplasty versus kyphoplasty: Biomechanical behavior under repetitive loading conditions. *Spine (Phila Pa 1976)* 31:2079–2084. doi: 10.1097/01.brs.0000231714.15876.76.

46. Kim KH, Kuh SU, Chin DK, Jin BH, Kim KS, Yoon YS, Cho YE. (2012). Kyphoplasty versus vertebroplasty: Restoration of vertebral body height and correction of kyphotic deformity with special attention to the shape of the fractured vertebrae. *J Spinal Disord Tech* 25:338–344. doi: 10.1097/BSD.0b013e318224a6e6.

47. Kim SB, Jeon TS, Lee WS, Roh JY, Kim JY, Park WK. (2010). Comparison of kyphoplasty and lordoplasty in the treatment of osteoporotic vertebral compression fracture. *Asian Spine J* 4:102–108. doi: 10.4184/asj.2010.4.2.102.

48. Mudano AS, Bian J, Cope JU, Curtis JR, Gross TP, Allison JJ, Kim Y, et al. (2009). Vertebroplasty and kyphoplasty are associated with an increased risk of secondary vertebral compression fractures: A population-based cohort study. *Osteoporos Int* 20:819–826. doi: 10.1007/s00198-008-0745-5.

49. Shen MS, Kim YH. (2006). Vertebroplasty and kyphoplasty: Treatment techniques for managing osteoporotic vertebral compression fractures. *Bull NYU Hosp Jt Dis* 64:106–113.

50. Mathis JM. (2006). Percutaneous vertebroplasty or kyphoplasty: Which one do I choose? *Skeletal Radiol* 35:629–631. doi: 10.1007/s00256-006-0145-x.

51. Mathis JM, Ortiz AO, Zoarski GH. (2004). Vertebroplasty versus kyphoplasty: A comparison and contrast. *AJNR Am J Neuroradiol* 25:840–845.

52. Hu SS. (1997). Internal fixation in the osteoporotic spine. *Spine (Phila Pa 1976)* 22:43S–48S.

53. Shikata J, Yamamuro T, Iida H, Shimizu K, Yoshikawa J. (1990). Surgical treatment for paraplegia resulting from vertebral fractures in senile osteoporosis. *Spine (Phila Pa 1976)* 15:485–489.

54. Suk SI, Kim JH, Lee SM, Chung ER, Lee JH. (2003). Anterior-posterior surgery versus posterior closing wedge osteotomy in posttraumatic kyphosis with neurologic compromised osteoporotic fracture. *Spine (Phila Pa 1976)* 28:2170–2175. doi: 10.1097/01.BRS.0000090889.45158.5A.

55. Ataka H, Tanno T, Yamazaki M. (2009). Posterior instrumented fusion without neural decompression for incomplete neurological deficits following vertebral collapse in the osteoporotic thoracolumbar spine. *Eur Spine J* 18:69–76. doi: 10.1007/s00586-008-0821-8.

56. Uchida K, Kobayashi S, Matsuzaki M, Nakajima H, Shimada S, Yayama T, Sato R, Baba H. (2006). Anterior versus posterior surgery for osteoporotic vertebral collapse with neurological deficit in the thoracolumbar spine. *Eur Spine J* 15:1759–1767. doi: 10.1007/s00586-006-0106-z.

57. Uchida K, Nakajima H, Yayama T, Miyazaki T, Hirai T, Kobayashi S, Chen K, Guerrero AR, Baba H. (2010). Vertebroplasty-augmented short-segment posterior fixation of osteoporotic vertebral collapse with neurological deficit in the thoracolumbar spine: Comparisons with posterior surgery without vertebroplasty and anterior surgery. *J Neurosurg Spine* 13:612–621. doi: 10.3171/2010.5.SPINE09813.

58. Saita K, Hoshino Y, Higashi T, Yamamuro K. (2008). Posterior spinal shortening for paraparesis following vertebral collapse due to osteoporosis. *Spinal Cord* 46:16–20. doi: 10.1038/sj.sc.3102052.

59. Saita K, Hoshino Y, Kikkawa I, Nakamura H. (2000). Posterior spinal shortening for paraplegia after vertebral collapse caused by osteoporosis. *Spine (Phila Pa 1976)* 25:2832–2835.

60. Verlaan JJ, Dhert WJ, Verbout AJ, Oner FC. (2005). Balloon vertebroplasty in combination with pedicle screw instrumentation: A novel technique to treat thoracic and lumbar burst fractures. *Spine (Phila Pa 1976)* 30:E73–E79.

61. Peh WC, Gilula LA. (2003). Percutaneous vertebroplasty: Indications, contraindications, and technique. *Br J Radiol* 76:69–75.

62. Liu BA, Gordon M, Labranche JM, Murray TM, Vieth R, Shear NH. (1997). Seasonal prevalence of vitamin D deficiency in institutionalized older adults. *J Am Geriatr Soc* 45:598–603.

63. Dawson-Hughes B, Harris SS, Krall EA, Dallal GE. (2000). Effect of withdrawal of calcium and vitamin D supplements on bone mass in elderly men and women. *Am J Clin Nutr* 72:745–750.

64. Chapuy MC, Arlot ME, Duboeuf F, Brun J, Crouzet B, Arnaud S, Delmas PD, Meunier PJ. (1992). Vitamin D3 and calcium to prevent hip fractures in the elderly women. *N Engl J Med* 327:1637–1642. doi: 10.1056/NEJM199212033272305.

65. Harris ST. (2001). Bisphosphonates for the treatment of postmenopausal osteoporosis: Clinical studies of etidronate and alendronate. *Osteoporos Int* 12(Suppl 3):S11–S16.

66. Chestnut CH 3rd. (1993). Calcitonin in the prevention and treatment of osteoporosis. *Osteoporos Int* 3(Suppl 1):206–207.

67. Barrett-Connor E, Mosca L, Collins P, Geiger MJ, Grady D, Kornitzer M, McNabb MA, Wenger NK. (2006). Effects of raloxifene on cardiovascular events and breast cancer in postmenopausal women. *N Engl J Med* 355:125–137. doi: 10.1056/NEJMoa062462.

68. Neer RM, Arnaud CD, Zanchetta JR, Prince R, Gaich GA, Reginster JY, Hodsman AB, et al. (2001). Effect of parathyroid hormone (1–34) on fractures and bone mineral density in postmenopausal women with osteoporosis. *N Engl J Med* 344:1434–1441. doi: 10.1056/NEJM200105103441904.

69. Finkelstein JS, Hayes A, Hunzelman JL, Wyland JJ, Lee H, Neer RM. (2003). The effects of parathyroid hormone, alendronate, or both in men with osteoporosis. *N Engl J Med* 349:1216–1226. doi: 10.1056/NEJMoa035725.

70. Bouxsein ML, Chen P, Glass EV, Kallmes DF, Delmas PD, Mitlak BH. (2009). Teriparatide and raloxifene reduce the risk of new adjacent vertebral fractures in postmenopausal women with osteoporosis. Results from two randomized controlled trials. *J Bone Joint Surg Am* 91:1329–1338. doi: 10.2106/JBJS.H.01030.

71. Fassett DR, Harrop JS, Maltenfort M, Jeyamohan SB, Ratliff JD, Anderson DG, Hilibrand AS, Albert TJ, Vaccaro AR, Sharan AD. (2007). Mortality rates in geriatric patients with spinal cord injuries. *J Neurosurg Spine* 7:277–281. doi: 10.3171/SPI-07/09/277.

72. Kannus P, Niemi S, Palvanen M, Parkkari J. (2000). Continuously increasing number and incidence of fall-induced, fracture-associated, spinal cord injuries in elderly persons. *Arch Intern Med* 160:2145–2149.

73. Hagen EM, Aarli JA, Gronning M. (2005). The clinical significance of spinal cord injuries in patients older than 60 years of age. *Acta Neurol Scand* 112:42–47. doi: 10.1111/j.1600-0404.2005.00430.x.

74. Alander DH, Parker J, Stauffer ES. (1997). Intermediate-term outcome of cervical spinal cord-injured patients older than 50 years of age. *Spine (Phila Pa 1976)* 22:1189–1192.

75. Jackson AP, Haak MH, Khan N, Meyer PR. (2005). Cervical spine injuries in the elderly: Acute postoperative mortality. *Spine (Phila Pa 1976)* 30:1524–1527.

76. Koyanagi I, Iwasaki Y, Hida K, Akino M, Imamura H, Abe H. (2000). Acute cervical cord injury without fracture or dislocation of the spinal column. *J Neurosurg* 93:15–20.

77. Pickett GE, Campos-Benitez M, Keller JL, Duggal N. (2006). Epidemiology of traumatic spinal cord injury in Canada. *Spine (Phila Pa 1976)* 31:799–805. doi: 10.1097/01.brs.0000207258.80129.03.

78. Prasad VS, Schwartz A, Bhutani R, Sharkey PW, Schwartz ML. (1999). Characteristics of injuries to the cervical spine and spinal cord in polytrauma patient population: Experience from a regional trauma unit. *Spinal Cord* 37:560–568.

79. Vaccaro AR, Oner C, Kepler CK, Dvorak M, Schnake K, Bellabarba C, Reinhold M, et al. (2013). AOSpine thoracolumbar spine injury classification system: Fracture description, neurological status, and key modifiers. *Spine (Phila Pa 1976)* 38:2028–2037. doi: 10.1097/BRS.0b013e3182a8a381.

80. Cloyd JM, Acosta FL Jr., Ames CP. (2008). Effect of age on the perioperative and radiographic complications of multilevel cervicothoracic spinal fusions. *Spine (Phila Pa 1976)* 33:E977–E982. doi: 10.1097/BRS.0b013e31818e2ad7.

81. Cloyd JM, Acosta FL Jr., Ames CP. (2008). Complications and outcomes of lumbar spine surgery in elderly people: A review of the literature. *J Am Geriatr Soc* 56:1318–1327. doi: 10.1111/j.1532-5415.2008.01771.x.

82. Kannus P, Palvanen M, Niemi S, Parkkari J, Jarvinen M. (2000). Epidemiology of osteoporotic pelvic fractures in elderly people in Finland: Sharp increase in 1970–1997 and alarming projections for the new millennium. *Osteoporos Int* 11:443–448. doi: 10.1007/s001980070112.

83. Lourie H. (1982). Spontaneous osteoporotic fracture of the sacrum. An unrecognized syndrome of the elderly. *JAMA* 248:715–717.

84. Weber M, Hasler P, Gerber H. (1993). Insufficiency fractures of the sacrum. Twenty cases and review of the literature. *Spine (Phila Pa 1976)* 18:2507–2512.

85. Dasgupta B, Shah N, Brown H, Gordon TE, Tanqueray AB, Mellor JA. (1998). Sacral insufficiency fractures: An unsuspected cause of low back pain. *Br J Rheumatol* 37:789–793.

86. Denis F, Davis S, Comfort T. (1988). Sacral fractures: An important problem. Retrospective analysis of 236 cases. *Clin Orthop Relat Res* 227:67–81.

87. Finiels H, Finiels PJ, Jacquot JM, Strubel D. (1997). [Fractures of the sacrum caused by bone insufficiency. Meta-analysis of 508 cases]. *Presse Med* 26:1568–1573.

88. Pommersheim W, Huang-Hellinger F, Baker M, Morris P. (2003). Sacroplasty: A treatment for sacral insufficiency fractures. *AJNR Am J Neuroradiol* 24:1003–1007.

89. Frey ME, Depalma MJ, Cifu DX, Bhagia SM, Carne W, Daitch JS. (2008). Percutaneous sacroplasty for osteoporotic sacral insufficiency fractures: A prospective, multicenter, observational pilot study. *Spine J* 8:367–373. doi: 10.1016/j.spinee.2007.05.011.

90. Uemura A, Matsusako M, Numaguchi Y, Oka M, Kobayashi N, Niinami C, Kawasaki T, Suzuki K. (2005). Percutaneous sacroplasty for hemorrhagic metastases from hepatocellular carcinoma. *AJNR Am J Neuroradiol* 26:493–495.

32

Pelvic fractures

JOHN KEATING

INTRODUCTION

Pelvic fractures in the elderly are most commonly low energy osteoporotic fractures or pelvic insufficiency fractures. Although these fractures are actually the most common traumatic pelvic injuries the literature on them is sparse in comparison to that devoted to the management of higher energy pelvic disruptions, which are relatively uncommon by comparison. It is worth noting that 73% of all pelvic fractures occur in older patients.[1] Osteoporosis is a reduction in the volume of normally mineralized bone and renders bone susceptible to fracture from low energy trauma. Insufficiency fractures of the pelvis are fractures which occur spontaneously without obvious trauma in response to normal physiological loads. Although higher energy major pelvic disruptions do occur, they are less common but obviously life-threatening injuries in the older patient. The majority of pelvic fractures encountered in the elderly are stable and amenable to non-operative treatment but they do incur a substantial demand on healthcare resources since they are often associated with a prolonged hospital stay and requirement for rehabilitation.[2]

EPIDEMIOLOGY

Low energy osteoporotic fractures are the most frequent pattern of pelvic injury encountered in elderly patients. It has been estimated that two-thirds of pelvic fractures in older patients are due to low energy trauma, most commonly a result of simple falls.[3,4] Pelvic fracture incidence does increase with age. The overall incidence of pelvic fractures has been estimated to be between 20 and 37/100,000 per year.[5,6] However this incidence increases to 92/100,000 per year in patients over 60 years of age[7] and

rises to 446/100,000 per year in patients over 85 years of age.[8] More than 90% of pelvic fractures in patients over the age of 60 years can be considered osteoporotic.[7] In addition to this, the actual incidence of pelvic fractures in the elderly is increasing. Clement and Court-Brown[9] reported an increase from 7.9/100,000 to 13.1/100,000 over a 10-year period. Kannus et al.[7] reported a threefold increase in osteoporotic pelvic fractures over the period 1970–1997 in Finland. The increase in actual numbers of fractures can be explained to some extent by the increasing number of elderly patients in the population, but there is also evidence that the age specific incidence of pelvic fractures is increasing in European epidemiological studies[9,10] although the explanation for this is not certain.

Pelvic fractures in the elderly are associated with an increase in the standardized mortality ratio at 1 year, even when they are isolated injuries. Higher energy pelvic fractures in the elderly can be a result of a motor vehicle accident but falls from a height or down stairs are a more frequent cause of unstable pelvic fracture patterns in patients over the age of 65 years.[11] Acetabular fractures are much less common and account for less than 20% of osteoporotic pelvic fractures.[3,4]

ASSESSMENT

There is generally a history of a fall in the majority of patients but in those with cognitive impairment the history may be unreliable. High energy trauma does occur but is much less common than in younger patients.[4,12] Unstable fracture patterns in the elderly are more likely to occur as a consequence of higher energy falls than road traffic accidents.[1] The patients most commonly complain of anterior groin pain, often associated with posterior pelvic pain. Patients complaining of posterior pain may have a posterior fracture and these patients should be considered for further imaging by computed tomography (CT) or magnetic resonance imaging (MRI). In low energy trauma resulting in the most common pelvic injury, an isolated pubic ramus fracture, physical signs are limited. In the majority of cases there is no external rotation or shortening of the leg, as would commonly be found in hip fractures.

For the small number of patients involved in higher energy trauma who present with multiple trauma, an assessment according to Advanced Trauma Life Support (ATLS) guidelines is appropriate. High energy pelvic fractures are uncommon in older patients but are associated with higher mortality rates than in younger patients. It is recognized that even mechanically stable patterns (e.g. lateral compression injury) are associated with a risk of significant bleeding.[13–15] Assessment of older patients can be difficult – the presence of a normal blood pressure may actually represent hypotension in a patient with pre-existing hypertension.[16] Development of a physiological tachycardia in response to blood loss may be impaired in patients on β-blockers or other anti-arrhythmic agents.[13] Patients on warfarin for atrial fibrillation or other indications are more susceptible to serious haemorrhage.

IMAGING

Plain radiography will identify most anterior fractures but posterior injuries are often missed on these radiographs. Lau and Leung[17] reported a prevalence of 59% of posterior ring fractures in patients presenting with an apparently isolated pubic ramus fracture. Other authors have reported an even higher incidence. Scheyerer et al.[18] described a case series of patients with a pubic ramus fracture and found that 96.8% of patients had a posterior ring injury on CT scan, although their series had a proportion of higher energy injuries with a younger mean age than would be typically associated with isolated ramus fractures. On MRI, the posterior pelvic ring is involved in over 90% of patients with pelvic injuries.[19] However, in elderly patients after falls, even a completely normal plain radiograph does not rule out a fracture. Ohishi et al.[10] reported on 113 elderly patients with negative pelvic radiographs after falls and recorded that over 90% had some bone or soft tissue abnormality and one-third had occult pelvic ring fractures on MRI scan. Occult fractures of the pelvic ring are therefore quite common and the absence of radiographic abnormality on the plain radiographs does not rule out a fracture.

Patients who present with hip fractures should be evaluated carefully for the presence of an associated pelvic fracture. The incidence of occult pelvic fractures among in-patients with suspected hip fractures has been reported with incidence varying from 11% to 51%.[20–28] Apart from the anterior ring, the most common site of fracture is the sacrum.[10]

Although pelvic inlet and outlet views can be obtained, they are not commonly used in modern orthopaedic practice, particularly in elderly patients following low

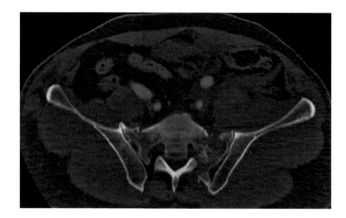

Figure 32.1 CT scan of the sacrum showing bilateral osteoporotic sacral alar fractures.

energy falls. The most common situation is either to find a pubic ramus fracture with a suspected posterior injury or a negative plain radiograph in a patient with pelvic pain after a fall. A CT scan will identify the majority of bony injuries either occult or in association with anterior ramus fractures (Figure 32.1). If this investigation is negative, then an MRI scan will usually pick up associated soft tissue injuries which may the source of pain. Clearly, not all elderly patients with stable low energy pubic ramus fractures require additional imaging. However a CT scan should be considered if the mechanism of injury was not a low energy fall. Other relative indications are suspicion of a significant posterior lesion or patients who have significant persistent pain.

CLASSIFICATION

Patients with high energy pelvic ring disruptions are commonly described using two radiological classification systems: the AO/OTA classification mainly devised by Tile[29,30] and the Young-Burgess classification developed in Baltimore.[31] The Tile/OTA[32] system is a morphological system based on pelvic ring stability and in particular the integrity of the posterior ligament complex. Injuries are divided into stable (type A), rotationally unstable (type B) and vertically unstable patterns. The rotationally unstable types are classified as open book patterns (B1), lateral compression (B2) or combinations of these two patterns (B3). Vertical shear patterns are either unilateral (C1), combined with contralateral rotational injury (C2) or bilateral vertical shear (C3). This is the most comprehensive classification system with the ability to describe most patterns of injury in detail with the use of subgroups under each main category.

The most common pattern of injury in the elderly is the isolated pubic ramus fracture. In this system this injury is considered a stable fracture of the ring and is termed an A2.2 injury. Considering the high incidence of occult posterior lesions which can be detected by CT or MRI scanning, there is an argument for classifying these fractures as lateral compression injuries (B2). However the posterior injury is

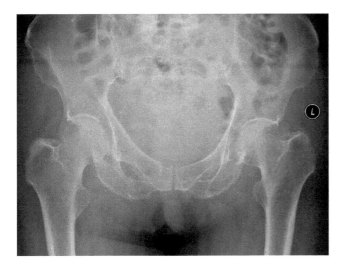

Figure 32.2 Anteroposterior (AP) view of the pelvis showing right-sided pubic ramus fractures, the most common pattern of pelvic fracture in elderly patients.

Table 32.1 Classification of fragility fractures of the pelvis

Category	Type	Radiographic features
Isolated anterior injury	1a	Isolated unilateral disruption
	1b	Isolated bilateral disruption
Non-displaced posterior injury	2a	Isolated sacral fracture; no anterior lesion
	2b	Non-displaced sacral crush fracture with anterior ring fracture
	2c	Non-displaced sacral, iliosacral or ilium fracture with anterior disruption
Displaced unilateral posterior injury	3a	Displaced unilateral iliac fracture
	3b	Displaced unilateral iliosacral disruption
	3c	Displaced unilateral displaced sacral fracture
Displaced bilateral posterior injury	4a	Bilateral iliac fracture or bilateral iliosacral disruption
	4b	Bilateral sacral fracture, spinopelvic dissociation
	4c	Combination of different dorsal instabilities

Source: From Rommens PM, Hofmann A. Injury 2013;44(12): 1733–1744.

generally a minor anterior sacral ala compression and this will not influence management. In a study of elderly patients with pelvic fractures using this classification,[9] 85% were isolated pubic ramus fractures which are termed A2.2 injuries using this classification system (Figure 32.2). Of the remainder 8% were other type A patterns and therefore stable pelvic ring injuries and only 7% were type B or C mechanically unstable pelvic ring disruptions.

The Young–Burgess[31] system was devised for use with high energy pelvic ring disruptions. It relates the mechanism of injury to the pattern of ring disruption, and the expected injuries. It is a simpler classification, dividing fracture patterns into anteroposterior compression (APC), lateral compression, vertical shear and combined mechanical injury (CMI). This system does not really pertain to low energy osteoporotic fractures. Its application is therefore really limited to the small percentage of older patients who sustain higher energy pelvic trauma, which will be less than 10% of cases. Although it does guide the treating surgeon to the expected injuries (e.g. the association of APC injuries with transfusion requirement and urethral/bladder injury), the associations are not particularly sensitive or specific. Both classification systems are widely used and reported in published studies but the levels of interobserver agreement for both systems are moderate to poor.[33–35]

A key difference in the pattern of pelvic fracture in the older patients is the relative infrequency of ligamentous injury and the higher prevalence of lower energy trauma, which results in a very different spectrum of injury than that covered by the foregoing systems of classification. On this basis Rommens and Hofmann[36] recently proposed a new classification for fragility fractures of the pelvis (FFP; Table 32.1). This was based on an analysis of pelvic ring fractures in a population of 245 patients with a mean age of 80 years. Their classification divides these fractures into four groups with increasing instability. A summary of the classification is given in Table 32.1. Additional imaging by means of CT or MRI scanning is required for accurate use of this classification.

Types I and II where there was an isolated anterior injury or an associated undisplaced posterior injury were the most common and amenable to non-operative management. However they do suggest percutaneous fixation needs to be considered in some type 2 injuries. In type 3 and type 4 there are unilateral or bilateral displaced posterior injuries, respectively. They suggest these are much more unstable fractures and best treated by standard methods of internal fixation. One of the interesting observations in their study was that unlike younger adults, where transforaminal sacral fractures are very common, they are very rare in elderly patients where the fractures are almost always localized to the sacral ala (Figure 32.1). Use of this classification and the associated treatment recommendations will need to be supported by prospective clinical studies.

For the majority of patients plain radiographs of the pelvis will be sufficient to make the diagnosis and plan treatment, which is generally non-operative. Additional imaging by CT or MRI scanning is indicated in patients presenting with:

- Haemodynamic instability
- Mechanically unstable pelvic fracture patterns
- Suspicion of posterior ring involvement
- Persistent pelvic pain after 2 weeks

TREATMENT

Low energy pelvic fractures

PUBIC RAMUS FRACTURES

Although pubic ramus fractures can occur at any age, they are comparatively uncommon in younger patients. Hill et al.[37] reported an overall incidence of 6.9/100,000/year but this rose to 25.9/100,000/year in patients over the age of 60 years. The majority of these are due to falls on the side, resulting in lateral compression injuries. They are often associated with posterior ring injuries but in the majority these consist of a type I alar compression fracture, which is stable and does not require operative intervention. Isolated fractures of the pubic ramus, classified as a type A2.2 injury, account for 85% of pelvic fractures in the elderly (Figure 32.2). The most common pattern of injury is unilateral with fractures involving both the superior and inferior pubic ramus. Management is almost invariably non-operative with a short period of initial bed rest and analgesia with mobilization as soon as pain allows. Although as indicated there is a high incidence of occult posterior fractures, these are almost invariably stable and their presence does not alter management or the prognosis.[17] For this reason routine imaging by means of CT or MRI scanning in all of these patients is not indicated.

Both non-union and displacement (Figure 32.3) can occur but are very rare complications of these fractures.[38,39] In order to facilitate rehabilitation it is important to achieve adequate analgesia. Failure to do so will hamper regaining mobility, increase the risk of complications and prolong the hospital stay. Patients with cognitive impairment may find it difficult to communicate analgesic needs and this should be taken into account in their management. Some care in choosing analgesic management is

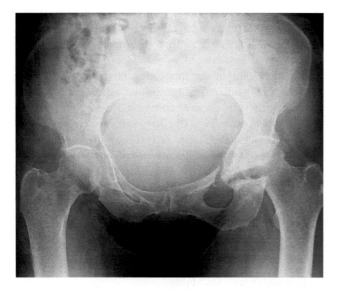

Figure 32.3 Anteroposterior (AP) view of the pelvis 2 years after injury showing pubic ramus non-union, an uncommon complication of low energy ramus fractures.

required – opioid medication can increase confusion and non-steroidal analgesics are best avoided due to renal and cardiovascular side-effects.

Some authors have recommended interventions in selected patients. Tosounidis et al.[40] reported the use of external fixation in patients with pubic ramus fractures with associated sacral fractures if pain persisted for longer than 2 weeks. Percutaneous fixation with retrograde medullary ramus screws and iliosacral screws is also an option. Winkelhagen et al.[41] reported on a series of six patients with persistent pain following isolated pubic ramus fractures treated by medullary ramus screws. They noted significant improvement in pain which facilitated mobilization and discharge. The technique had the advantage of being minimally invasive, and biomechanically is equivalent to plating.[42] Injection of methyl methacrylate cement into ramus fractures to relieve pain has also been reported.[38] These techniques have only been reported in small numbers of patients and are probably only applicable to a subset of patients with these fractures where there is a posterior lesion and pain control is a significant problem.

Lau and Leung[17] reported on a series of patients with pubic ramus fractures and recommended internal fixation in type II lateral compression fractures where there was an associated posterior iliac wing crescent fracture. Other fracture patterns were treated non-operatively and healed. Other authors have reported relatively high rates of operative intervention. Scheyerer et al.[18] reported on a series of patients with isolated ramus fractures on plain radiographs with a 96.8% incidence of posterior fractures on CT scans and a 30% operative rate. However the mean age of their patients was 56 years, the series included many lateral compression fractures and it can be assumed therefore that their findings would not apply to the elderly population who present with low energy ramus fractures after a simple fall.

Pharmacological measures may have a role to play in accelerating healing. Peichl et al.[43] reported on the use of parathyroid hormone (PTH 1-84) in patients with low energy pubic ramus pelvic fractures. In 21 patients who received PTH 1-84 injections, fractures healed at a mean time of 7.8 weeks compared to 12.6 weeks in a control group of 44 patients, which was significantly faster. The relief of pain as measured by visual analogue scores and function as measured by the timed up and go test were also significantly better in the treatment group. Although the data are encouraging, corroboration of the findings in other studies would be useful.

The main issue with most pubic ramus fractures is the burden imposed on the healthcare system. The duration of hospital stay has been reported to vary from 9 to 17 days.[2,9,37] Shorter lengths of stay are associated with younger age and independent mobility prior to fracture.

Once the patient has been discharged, routine follow-up of these fractures is not required – the majority are united 6–8 weeks after injury. Although most patients do recover and regain their previous level of mobility, the fracture is a hallmark of frailty. However in their study Hill et al.[37] reported a mean hospital stay of 9 days and 78% of patients were discharged to their original residence. The overall survival rates at 1 and 5 years were reported as 86.7% and 45.6%, respectively.[37] In another study[44] of pubic ramus fractures and sacral insufficiency fractures the mortality was 23% at 1 year and 47% at 3 years. Male gender appears to be associated with a much poorer survival. Clement and Court-Brown[9] reported a 40% 1-year mortality in male patients, which was significantly higher than in female patients.

Iliac wing fractures

Isolated osteoporotic fractures of the iliac wing are relatively uncommon (Figure 32.4). The literature on their management is very limited and mainly relates to higher energy fractures in younger patients.[45,46] They tend to occur as a result of a direct traumatic blow to the iliac wing itself, which is an uncommon mechanism of injury in the older patient. When they do occur they are often relatively comminuted without extensive displacement and can usually be treated non-operatively in the expectation that the majority will unite uneventfully. Surgical fixation of these comminuted fractures would be technically challenging in any event. Occasionally a two part fracture may rotate or displace significantly and in these cases non-union is a risk. Plate fixation is the method of choice for these fractures.

Pelvic and sacral insufficiency fractures

Pelvic insufficiency fractures are a well-recognized but under-diagnosed clinical entity in older patients presenting with pelvic pain. Patients present with lower lumbar back and pelvic pain. There is a history of injury in two-thirds of patients.[47] Pain is exacerbated by physical activity. They often occur in the presence of other comorbidities particularly osteoporosis, rheumatoid arthritis and metabolic bone disorders including Paget's disease, hyperparathyroidism and osteomalacia. Physical findings are limited – stress tests of the sacroiliac joints however do tend to provoke increased pain. This would include compression of the sacroiliac joints and the flexion abduction external rotation test (FABER test). Neurological impairment is rare but has been reported. Sacral insufficiency fractures often occur in association with pubic ramus fractures, and in one report 78% of cases had concomitant ramus fractures.[48]

These injuries are frequently not apparent on plain radiographs and the pain is often misdiagnosed as mechanical back pain. A delay in diagnosis of between 1 and 2 months is therefore common.[47,49] In both of these studies the sensitivity of plain radiographs in establishing the diagnosis was less than 40%.

Supplementary imaging is usually required to establish the diagnosis. Bone scintigraphy will demonstrate increased uptake, but it may be 48–72 hours after injury before the scan is positive. Bone scans typically show a characteristic H-shaped pattern of radionuclide uptake across the sacrum and sacroiliac joints.[50] CT scanning will reveal the diagnosis in most cases with either fresh fracture lines in early cases or sclerotic healing fractures in later presentations. Even on CT scans, the findings may be quite subtle. However the main differential diagnosis is either osteomyelitis or bone malignancy and the CT scan will usually rule these out. MRI scan is the most useful and sensitive investigation for establishing the diagnosis, particularly T2 weighted short tau inversion recovery (STIR) images and T2 weighted images with fat suppression.

Sacral fractures were classified by Denis et al.[51] based on location. Type I fractures are lateral to the sacral foramena, type II are transforamenal and type III are medial to the sacral foramena. Sacral insufficiency fractures are most commonly located in the ala of the sacrum and are therefore type I injuries.

Treatment consists of bed rest followed by mobilization. In general the prognosis for healing is good with the majority of patients progressing to bone union with complete pain resolution, although this may take 2–4 months.[48,52,53] Although the published studies support non-operative treatment as the method of choice in the first instance, it is recognized that in some patients there may be prolonged healing times with concomitant disability. These patients merit further investigation to determine if there is a reversible underlying metabolic cause contributing to the delayed or non-union.

A number of operative interventions have been proposed for patients with insufficiency fractures and these include percutaneous iliosacral screw fixation, transiliac bar fixation[12] and sacroplasty[54–56] with injection of polymethylmethacrylate cement. The published literature concerning the outcome of these techniques is limited and all of these interventions have a recognized rate of complications, some of which are major. At the present time the recommended option for these

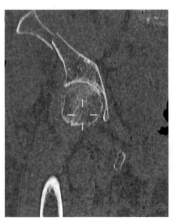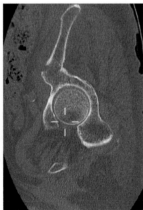

Figure 32.4 Two-dimensional CT reconstruction image of an isolated iliac blade fracture. These can be managed without surgery as long as there is good bony apposition, as in this case.

fractures is for non-operative intervention with fixation being considered for that small group of patients in whom the fracture fails to unite and pain persists.

Unstable pelvic fractures

Management of unstable pelvic fractures in the elderly is a particular challenge. These injuries are difficult to treat in younger patients with good quality bone and who are physiologically better equipped to withstand the effects of the injury. The problems are of greater magnitude in the older patient. High energy pelvic disruptions are associated with a very poor prognosis in the older patient for a variety of reasons. Hypotension in association with the pelvic fracture or associated injuries is poorly tolerated, particular if it lasts for a long period of time. The associated soft tissue injury around the pelvis is often more severe with very extensive bruising and degloving. Considerable fracture comminution is usual and may render restoration of skeletal stability very difficult (Figure 32.5a–c).

ACUTE PHASE

There have been some significant changes in the acute phase of management of patients in recent years. In particular there has been considerable evolution of approaches to initial resuscitation of patients with haemodynamic instability in association with an unstable pelvic fracture pattern. Formerly there was a vogue in the unstable patient to undertake aggressive fluid resuscitation with crystalloids, reduce pelvic volume by application of external fixation and consider pelvic angiography and embolization in patients who were non-responders to these measures. These interventions all have a rational basis but some very specific drawbacks. Overenthusiastic fluid resuscitation with crystalloids may be detrimental in a number of ways – it can exacerbate hypothermia, dilute clotting factors and promote continued haemorrhage if the source of bleeding has not been controlled.

Application of anterior external fixators to reduce pelvic volume is most effective in patients with open book fractures (APC or AO type B1 patterns of injury). However the procedure is far from straightforward, particularly if the patient is obese or the abdomen is distended. Technical errors in application are very common unless the operator is experienced in pelvic external fixation and the procedure can be time consuming. Furthermore, anterior frames although effective in closing up the anterior elements may actually increase posterior displacement and since the posterior area of the pelvis is often a source of blood loss, this may be very detrimental. In the older patient iliac wing comminution is a common feature of pelvic fracture and may preclude application in this location (Figure 32.6a–d).

Finally although angiography and embolization has been reported to be an effective intervention, in most of these patients the major source of blood loss is venous in origin and will not be affected by an arterial embolization. The procedure

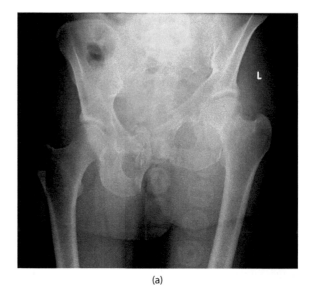

(a)

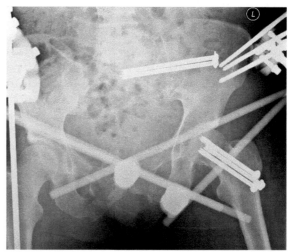

(b)

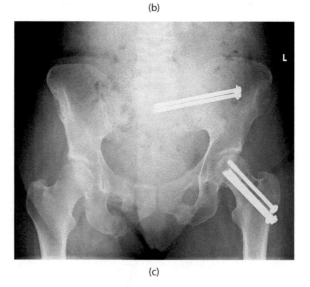

(c)

Figure 32.5 **(a)** Vertical shear injury in an elderly female with comminuted ramus fractures and a left sided sacral alar fracture. There is an associated left sided femoral neck fracture. **(b)** Combined internal and external fixation with an anterior frame and percutaneous iliosacral screws. **(c)** Healed fracture after frame removal. There is a degree of pelvic malunion.

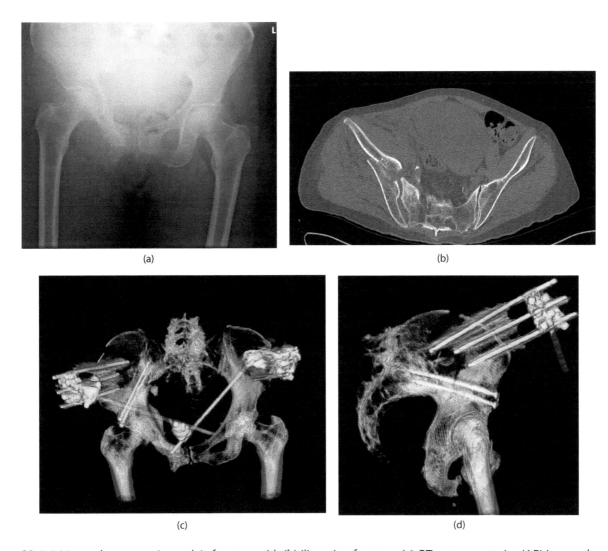

Figure 32.6 **(a)** Lateral compression pelvic fracture with **(b)** iliac wing fracture. **(c)** CT anteroposterior (AP) image showing external fixation and percutaneous screw fixation of the iliac wing fracture. **(d)** CT lateral view.

is also invariably time consuming and therefore may simply not be practical in a patient with life-threatening hypotension. Hou et al.[57] in a recent study reported a high mortality rate with the use of angiography to control haemorrhage in pelvic fractures and recommended against use of this intervention as part of the acute phase of resuscitation.

The modern approach to resuscitation has been modified to address these drawbacks in the following way:

- Early application of a pelvic binder
- Development of permissive hypotension and massive transfusion protocols
- Pelvic packing for selected cases with severe unresponsive hypotension

PELVIC BINDER

The use of pelvic binders has largely supplanted use of external fixation in the acute phase of management of haemodynamically unstable patients with pelvic fractures. These have a number of advantages and particularly in elderly patients. These include:

- Very quick to apply
- Can be applied at a very early stage of the resuscitation process
- Limited technical expertise necessary
- Apply circumferential pressure around pelvis and will therefore close anterior and posterior elements of the pelvic ring
- Applied at the level of the trochanters so leave abdomen exposed

The pelvic binder can be left in situ while other investigations and interventions are undertaken. It is clearly not a method for provision of definitive pelvic stabilization, and soft tissue compromise may be exacerbated if it is left in situ for prolonged periods.

FLUID RESUSCITATION

Until 2006 the conventional approach to fluid resuscitation was to use crystalloids, colloids and red blood cells in the early phase and plasma and platelets in later phases.[58] As already indicated, vigorous resuscitation with large volumes of crystalloid is no longer considered the most effective strategy in these patients. In the early stages the concept of 'permissive hypotension' is now popular. The underlying concept is to restore blood pressure to a safe level but one below normal to limit the volume of crystalloid used and minimizing the risk of exacerbating further blood loss. A systolic blood pressure of between 80 mmHg and 100 mmHg is considered to be appropriate, a level at which the radial pulse is still palpable. However there is no general agreement as regards the exact level and exact evidence of which patient subgroups would benefit most from this approach is lacking as yet.[59,60] Although the approach has some logic, good evidence from clinical trials that it is associated with improved survival is lacking.[61]

For the older patients there may be some definite hazards in this technique of resuscitation. Many older patients have hypertension and the level of 'permissive hypotension' which is safe may be impossible to estimate with any certainty. Some degree of renal impairment is also common in these patients and even modest degrees of hypotension may exacerbate this. The technique is also contraindicated in the presence of a head injury where it may compromise cerebral perfusion.[62]

Early fluid resuscitation has changed in favour of what is termed 'haemostatic resuscitation'. This involves much earlier introduction of blood products in the acute resuscitation phase. This change has occurred as result of a number of studies which have indicated more favourable survival rates in patients with life-threatening haemorrhage in military practice.[63–65] Major transfusion protocols are now used where red blood cells, fresh frozen plasma and platelets are given from the outset, with minimal use of crystalloids and colloids. It has been suggested that a ratio of 1:1:1 or 2:1:1 should be used but the optimal ratio of these blood products remains to be determined and is still a source of some controversy, with some authors suggesting there may be a survival bias in the results of the published studies.[66,67]

Monitoring of coagulation in bleeding patients has also changed. It was recognized that traditional laboratory tests including prothrombin time and partial thromboplastin time only test selected components of the coagulation process.[68] They also have the salient disadvantage that they are time consuming and therefore not available at the point of care when the patient is still haemodynamically unstable. The old cascade model of coagulation has now been replaced with a newer cell based model which emphasizes the role of cellular elements, particularly platelets, in haemostasis. This cell based model is in three phases: initiation, amplification and propagation, and the quality of haemostasis is dependent on the quantity of thrombin production. Tests have been developed to reflect this newer concept of haemostasis and include viscoelastic haemostatic assays of thromboelastography and rotational thromboelastometry.[69] These tests have a number of advantages over older investigations: they can be performed much more quickly so results are available during the resuscitation phase. They can also reveal low fibrinogen, poor platelet function and hyperfibrinolysis and so are a much better guide to blood product requirement and type of product needed.

SURGICAL CONTROL OF HAEMORRHAGE

Patients with unstable pelvic fractures tend to fall into two main groups: those who are haemodynamically stable at presentation or rapidly respond to initial resuscitation or a second group with potentially life-threatening hypotension unresponsive to initial fluid resuscitation. It is the latter group that is at most risk of mortality in the early stages after presentation. Death may result from uncontrolled haemorrhage shortly after presentation. Patients with serious life-threatening haemorrhage are a relatively small subset of the pelvic fracture population – about 10% of the total. Blood loss in pelvic fractures is mainly from the pelvic venous plexus. Arterial sources of blood loss are found in 15–20% of cases. Bone bleeding also occurs but is less important. Reduction of the pelvic volume will help control blood loss and achieve haemodynamic stability. The most effective method for doing this in modern practice is by application of a pelvic binder. This is much more rapid and much safer to apply than use of external fixation which is much less frequently used now than in the past. A pelvic binder will apply circumferential pressure around the pelvis which is preferable in patients with a posterior element to the injury.

Vigorous early resuscitation with blood products as outlined above is the next step but in a proportion of these patients these measures may not be adequate and hypotension persists. In these patients additional sources of bleeding should be ruled out by either a rapid CT scan or alternatively an abdominal ultrasound. Of these the CT scan is preferable because it is a more accurate investigation and it is possible to scan the patient from the skull vertex to the pubic symphysis in order to identify injuries to other body areas. If there are no other sources of blood loss identified then the alternatives are either pelvic packing or angiography and embolization. Pelvic packing can be done rapidly and is the more appropriate intervention in a patient with severe hypotension. This is probably best accomplished by an extraperitoneal approach to the pelvis in patients without a source of intra-peritoneal blood loss.[70] This can be done via a low infra-umbilical incision or a Pfannenstiel incision.

The alternative of pelvic angiography is more time consuming[71] but may be a rational alternative in patients who demonstrate a transient response to resuscitation with recurrent but non-life-threatening hypotension, where the time available is a less critical consideration. With the advent of pelvic binders, early haemostatic resuscitation and pelvic packing angiography is probably used less now than formerly. It still has a limited role in control of pelvic haemorrhage but it is associated with a risk of significant soft tissue complications such as gluteal necrosis, particularly if major vessels are embolized.[44]

DEFINITIVE ORTHOPAEDIC TREATMENT

Major unstable fracture patterns are uncommon in older patients but when they do occur they can pose particular difficulties in comparison to younger patients with similar injuries. The main differences are:

- Greater fracture comminution
- Osteoporotic bone with greater difficulty in achieving stable reduction and fixation
- A lower incidence of pelvic ligament disruption
- Poor soft tissues, increasing the risk of wound breakdown and other complications

Accepted indications for fixation of pelvic fractures include:

- Open book fractures with >2.5 cm pubic symphysis diastasis
- Vertical shear patterns with >1 cm displacement of the hem-pelvis
- Lateral compression patterns with a locked symphysis or tilt fracture
- Lateral compression patterns with displaced crescent fractures
- Combinations of the above

At the outset, the decision to perform fixation depends on the nature of the injury and the associated pattern of disruption. Many pelvic fractures in this age group occur as a consequence of lower energy trauma and there is a high incidence of lateral compression patterns. These fractures can be considered stable in almost all cases because the pelvic ligaments are intact. Consequently the majority are amenable to non-operative treatment.

The indications for operative treatment in the older patient are the same as for younger patients. However there are some modifications in the management of unstable fracture patterns taking into account the difficulties of managing these fractures in osteoporotic bone. The timing of fixation has also been modified in recent years. It is apparent that subjecting patients to prolonged major surgery to fix fractures is probably best carried out when correction of physiological derangements common in major trauma has been achieved. Patients who present with the so-called lethal triad of hypothermia, coagulopathy and acidosis benefit from correction of these abnormalities prior to surgery. Stable patients who do not have these features can safely have surgery but there is accumulating evidence that patients with these physiological abnormalities do better with surgery being staged to allow reversal of abnormal physiology.

External fixation

External fixation has the advantage of being minimally invasive but has many drawbacks particularly in older patients. These patients often have comminution of the iliac wing in the most common region of external fixator pin placement which may make this pin site location impossible to use. Other disadvantages include pin track infection, limitation of patient mobility and a very high rate of malunion particularly in more unstable patterns of injury. For vertical shear injuries malunion rates of 95% have been reported when external fixation is used as the definitive treatment (Figure 32.5c).

A good alternative may well be the anterior subcutaneous fixator device.[72,73] This is applied in a minimally invasive approach to the supra-acetabular region. The pins are placed in this region and the bar connecting the pins is positioned subcutaneously. This has the advantage of placing pins in much better bone and the device is not percutaneous, so there is no problem with pin track infection. This may be advantageous in the older patient where comminution or poor bone quality makes the traditional iliac wing location more prone to complications including pin loosening and pin track infection. It is also more comfortable and allows the patient to sit and ambulate more readily than with a conventional external fixator applied.

Percutaneous fixation

The use of percutaneous iliosacral screws and retrograde medullary ramus screws may be very useful in limiting the extent of surgery in an older patient. These techniques require high quality imaging in theatre, the ability to achieve a closed reduction, and they can be technically demanding to insert safely. However for patients with ramus fractures and type I or II sacral fractures they are very useful alternatives to more extensive surgical procedures in the older patient.

COMPLICATIONS

Mortality

Older patients with major pelvic fractures might be expected to have a higher mortality but there is conflicting data in the literature regarding this. Holstein et al.[74] analysed risk factors for mortality in over 5000 pelvic fracture patients from the German Pelvic Trauma Registry. They did not find any relationship between age and mortality. Patients over the age of 70 years comprised about 40% of survivors and non-survivors. However in contrast to these findings, Gabbe et al.[75] reviewed the mortality in an Australian population and identified age over 65 years to be associated with an increase in the mortality rate. Patients over the age of 65 years had an eightfold increase in mortality compared to patients aged between 15 and 34 years. Bible et al.[76] reviewed 70 patients over the age of 60 years with isolated unstable type B and type C pelvic fractures and reported a 1-year mortality rate of 12.9% which they concluded was lower than the expected rate of mortality in hip fractures or in patients with concurrent injuries. Dong et al.[77] reported on 40 older patients with unstable pelvic fractures and noted that an Injury Severity Score over 25 was associated with a significant increase in mortality. Additional injuries were present in 70%, and 52% of patients had a reduced level of independence 15 months after injury.

General medical complications

As might be expected, medical complications in elderly patients are not infrequent following low energy pelvic fractures. Mears and Berry[78] reported on medical complications in these patients. The incidence varied from 15% to 50% with a higher incidence being associated with bilateral displaced fractures and a lower incidence with unilateral undisplaced ramus or sacral insufficiency fractures. Complications included urinary tract infection, pneumonia, delirium, urinary retention, decubitus ulcer and atrial fibrillation.

Major pelvic fractures are a well-recognized risk factor for development of deep venous thrombosis and pulmonary embolism.[79–81] These are not uncommon after pelvic fractures in general but studies have suggested the incidence of these fractures is age related with increasing age being associated with a higher risk.[8,82] Kim et al.[24] reported that patients over the age of 50 years were a higher risk group for this complication. In general, more severe degrees of pelvic fracture instability and the requirement for surgical fixation are associated with an increased risk.

For the more common low energy pelvic fractures that are considerably more frequent in the elderly, there is little guidance in the literature regarding the incidence of thromboembolic complications. However these fractures are invariably associated with a period of immobility and it seems reasonable to conclude that there will be an increased risk of deep vein thrombosis in the early stages following injury. The current accepted clinical practice is to prescribe some form of recognized thromboembolic prophylaxis.

Functional outcome

Unstable pelvic fractures are associated with significant rates of morbidity and disability. In general more severe injuries with greater degrees of instability are associated with worse outcomes. Lateral compression patterns of injury are the most frequent unstable pelvic fracture pattern particularly in the elderly. Although these can generally be treated non-operatively, they are associated with functional impairment. Hoffman et al.[83] reported on functional outcome after fixation of lateral compression fractures as measured by the Short Musculoskeletal Function Assessment (SMFA) questionnaire. Even at 2 years there were significant differences from population norms with persistent disability evident in the pelvic fracture patients.

In another study looking at functional outcome using the EuroQol disability questionnaire[84] more severe patterns of disruption and increasing age were associated with poorer functional outcomes.

Lower energy pelvic fractures in the elderly might be expected to have a more benign outcome but there is evidence that even these injuries are associated with adverse functional outcomes. Mears and Berry[78] reported on functional outcomes after low energy pelvic fractures in patients over 65 years of age. Their series included patients with pubic ramus fractures and sacral insufficiency fractures. They reported a significant deterioration in mobility and independent living following the fracture. Other authors have reported these fractures are also associated with diminished levels of mobility and independence. Hill et al.[37] reported that 60% of patients regained their previous level of mobility and 81% returned to their pre-injury accommodation after pubic ramus fracture.

REFERENCES

1. Court-Brown CM, Caesar B. Epidemiology of adult fractures: A review. *Injury* 2006;37:691–697.
2. Koval KJ, Aharonoff GB, Schwartz MC, et al. Pubic rami fracture: A benign pelvic injury? *J Orthop Trauma* 1997;11:7–9.
3. Boufous S, Finch C, Lord S, et al. The increasing burden of pelvic fractures in older people, New South Wales, Australia. *Injury* 2005;36:1323–1329.
4. Callaway DW, Wolfe R. Geriatric trauma. *Emerg Med Clin North Am* 2007;25:837–860.
5. Melton LJ, Sampson JM, Morrey BF, et al. Epidemiologic features of pelvic fractures. *Clin Orthop Relat Res* 1981;155:43–47.
6. Ragnarsson B, Jacobsson B. Epidemiology of pelvic fractures in a Swedish county. *Acta Orthop Scand* 1992;63:297–300.
7. Kannus P, Palvanen M, Niemi S, et al. Epidemiology of osteoporotic pelvic fractures in elderly people in Finland: Sharp increase in 1970–1997 and alarming projections for the new millennium. *Osteoporos Int* 2000;11:443–448.
8. Montgomery KD, Potter HG, Helfet DL. The detection and management of proximal deep venous thrombosis in patients with acute acetabular fractures: A follow-up report. *J Orthop Trauma* 1997;11:330–336.
9. Clement ND, Court-Brown CM. Elderly pelvic fractures: The incidence is increasing and patient demographics can be used to predict the outcome. *Eur J Orthop Surg Traumatol* 2014;24(8):1431–1437.
10. Ohishi T, Ito T, Suzuki D, et al. Occult hip and pelvic fractures and accompanying muscle injuries around the hip. *Arch Orthop Trauma Surg* 2012;132:105–112.
11. Clement ND, Aitken S, Duckworth AD, et al. Multiple fractures in the elderly. *J Bone Joint Surg Br* 2012;94-B:231–236.
12. Vanderschot P. Treatment options of pelvic and acetabular fractures in patients with osteoporotic bone. *Injury* 2007;38:497–508.

13. Henry SM, Pollak AN, Jones AL, et al. Pelvic fracture in geriatric patients: A distinct clinical entity. *J Trauma* 2002;53:15–20.

14. Kimbrell BJ, Velmahos GC, Chan LS, et al. Angiographic embolization for pelvic fractures in older patients. *Arch Surg* 2004;139:728–732.

15. Velmahos GC, Toutouzas KG, Vassiliu P, et al. A prospective study on the safety and efficacy of angiographic embolization for pelvic and visceral injuries. *J Trauma* 2002;53:303–308.

16. Demetriades D, Sava J, Alo K, et al. Old age as a criterion for trauma team activation. *J Trauma* 2001;51:754–756.

17. Lau T, Leung F. Occult posterior pelvic ring fractures in elderly patients with osteoporotic pubic rami fractures. *J Orthop Surg* 2010;18(2):153–157.

18. Scheyerer MJ, Osterhoff G, Wehrle S, et al. Detection of posterior pelvic injuries in fractures of the pubic rami. *Injury* 2012;43:1326–1329.

19. Cosker TD, Ghandour A, Gupta SK, et al. Pelvic ramus fractures in the elderly: 50 patients studied with MRI. *Acta Orthop* 2005;76:513–516.

20. Bogost GA, Lizerbram EK, Crues JV 3rd. MR imaging in evaluation of suspected hip fracture: Frequency of unsuspected bone and soft-tissue injury. *Radiology* 1995;197:263–267.

21. Chana R, Noorani A, Ashwood N, et al. The role of MRI in the diagnosis of proximal femoral fractures in the elderly. *Injury* 2006;37:185–189.

22. Frihagen F, Nordsletten L, Tariq R, et al. MRI diagnosis of occult hip fractures. *Acta Orthop* 2005;76:524–530.

23. Galloway HR, Meikle GR, Despois M. Patterns of injury in patients with radiographic occult fracture of neck of femur as determined by magnetic resonance imaging. *Australas Radiol* 2004;48:21–24.

24. Kim KC, Ha YC, Kim TY, Choi JA, Koo KH. Initially missed occult fractures of the proximal femur in elderly patients: Implications for need of operation and their morbidity. *Arch Orthop Trauma Surg* 2010;130:915–920.

25. Lee KH, Kim HM, Kim YS, et al. Isolated fractures of the greater trochanter with occult intertrochanteric extension. *Arch Orthop Trauma Surg* 2010;130:1275–1280.

26. Lim KB, Eng AK, Chng SM, et al. Limited magnetic resonance imaging (MRI) and the occult hip fracture. *Ann Acad Med Singapore* 2002;31:607–610.

27. Oka M, Monu JU. Prevalence and patterns of occult hip fractures and mimics revealed by MRI. *AJR Am J Roentgenol* 2004;182:283–288.

28. Sankey RA, Turner J, Lee J, et al. The use of MRI to detect occult fractures of the proximal femur. *J Bone Joint Surg* 2009;91-B:1064–1068.

29. Tile M. Pelvic ring fractures: Should they be fixed? *J Bone Joint Surg Br* 1988;70:1–12.

30. Tile M. Acute pelvic fractures: I: Causation and classification. *J Am Acad Orthop Surg* 1996;4:143–151.

31. Dalal SA, Burgess AR, Siegel JH, et al. Pelvic fracture in multiple trauma: Classification by mechanism is key to pattern of organ injury, resuscitative requirements, and outcome. *J Trauma* 1989;29:981–1000.

32. Fracture and dislocation compendium. Orthopaedic Trauma Association Committee for Coding and Classification. *J Orthop Trauma* 1996;10(Suppl 1): v–ix, 1–154.

33. Furey AJ, O'Toole RV, Nascone JW, et al. Classification of pelvic fractures: Analysis of inter- and intraobserver variability using the Young-Burgess and Tile classification systems. *Orthopedics* 2009;32:401–406.

34. Gabbe BJ, Esser M, Bucknill A, et al. The imaging and classification of severe pelvic ring fractures: Experiences from two level 1 trauma centres. *Bone Joint J* 2013;95-B:1396–1401.

35. Koo H, Leveridge M, Thompson C, et al. Interobserver reliability of the Young-Burgess and Tile classification systems for fractures of the pelvic ring. *J Orthop Trauma* 2008;22:379–384.

36. Rommens PM, Hofmann A. Comprehensive classification of fragility fractures of the pelvic ring: Recommendations for surgical treatment. *Injury* 2013;44(12):1733–1744.

37. Hill RM, Robinson CM, Keating JF. Fractures of the pubic rami. Epidemiology and five-year survival. *J Bone Joint Surg Br* 2001;83:1141–1144.

38. Beall DP, D'Souza SL, Costello RF, et al. Percutaneous augmentation of the superior pubic ramus with polymethyl methacrylate: Treatment of acute traumatic and chronic insufficiency fractures. *Skelet Radiol* 2007;36:979–983.

39. Steinitz D, Guy P, Passariello A, et al. All superior pubic ramus fractures are not created equal. *Can J Surg* 2004;47:422–425.

40. Tosounidis G, Wirbel R, Culemann U, et al. Misinterpretation of anterior pelvic ring fractures in the elderly. *Unfallchirurg* 2006;109:678–680.

41. Winkelhagen J, van den Bekerom MPJ, Bolhuis HW, et al. Preliminary results of cannulated screw fixation for isolated pubic ramus fractures. *Strategies Trauma Limb Reconstr* 2012;7:87–91.

42. Simonian PT, Routt ML Jr, Harrington RM, et al. Internal fixation of the unstable anterior pelvic ring: A biomechanical comparison of standard plating techniques and the retrograde medullary superior pubic ramus screw. *J Orthop Trauma* 1994;8:476–482.

43. Peichl P, Holzer LA, Maier R, Holzer G. Parathyroid hormone 1-84 accelerates fracture-healing in pubic bones of elderly osteoporotic women. *J Bone Joint Surg Am* 2011;93:1583–7.

44. Matityahu A, Marmor M, Elson JK, et al. Acute complications of patients with pelvic fractures after pelvic angiographic embolization. *Clin Orthop Relat Res* 2013;471:2906–2911.

45. Abrassart S, Stern R, Peter R. Morbidity associated with isolated iliac wing fractures. *J Trauma* 2009;66(1):200–203. doi: 10.1097/TA.0b013e31814695ba.

46. Switzer JA, Nork SE, Routt ML Jr. Comminuted fractures of the iliac wing. *J Orthop Trauma* 2000;14(4):270–276.

47. Finiels H, Finiels PJ, Jacquot JM, et al. Fractures of the sacrum caused by bone insufficiency. Meta-analysis of 508 cases. *Presse Med* 1997;26:1568–1573.

48. Aretxabala I, Fraiz E, Perez-Ruiz F, et al. Sacral insufficiency fractures. High association with pubic rami fractures. *Clin Rheumatol* 2000;19:399–401.

49. Soubrier M, Dubost JJ, Boisgard S, et al. Insufficiency fracture. A survey of 60 cases and review of the literature. *Joint Bone Spine* 2003;70:209–218.

50. Ries T. Detection of osteoporotic sacral fractures with radionuclides. *Radiology* 1983;146:783–5.

51. Denis F, Davis S, Comfort T. Sacral fractures: An important problem. Retrospective analysis of 236 cases. *Clin Orthop Relat Res* 1988; 227:67–81.

52. Gotis-Graham I, McGuigan L, Diamond T, et al. Sacral insufficiency fractures in the elderly. *J Bone Joint Surg Br* 1994;76:882–886.

53. Weber M, Hasler P, Gerber H. Insufficiency fractures of the sacrum. Twenty cases and review of the literature. *Spine* 1993;18:2507–2512.

54. Garant M. Sacroplasty: A new treatment for sacral insufficiency fracture. *J Vasc Interv Radiol* 2002;13:1265–1267.

55. Lever M, Lever E, Lever EG. Rethinking osteoporotic sacral fractures. *Injury* 2009;40: 466–467.

56. Pommersheim W, Huang-Hellinger F, Baker M, et al. Sacroplasty: A treatment for sacral insufficiency fractures. *Am J Neuroradiol* 2003;24:1003–1007.

57. Hou Z, Smith WR, Strohecker KA, et al. Hemodynamically unstable pelvic fracture management by Advanced Trauma Life Support guidelines results in high mortality. *Orthopedics* 2012;35(3):319–324.

58. American Society of Anesthesiologists Task Force on Perioperative Blood Transfusion and Adjuvant Therapies. Practice guidelines for perioperative blood transfusion and adjuvant therapies: An updated report by the American Society of Anesthesiologists Task Force on Perioperative Blood Transfusion and Adjuvant Therapies. *Anesthesiology* 2006;105(1):198–208.

59. Pieracci FM, Biffl WL, Moore EE. Current concepts in resuscitation. *J Intensive Care Med* 2012;27(2):79–96.

60. Stahel PF, Moore EE, Schreier SL, et al. Transfusion strategies in postinjury coagulopathy. *Curr Opin Anaesthesiol* 2009;22(2):289–298.

61. Jansen JO, Thomas R, Loudon MA, et al. Damage control resuscitation for patients with major trauma. *BMJ* 2009;338:b1778.

62. Stahel PF, Smith WR, Moore EE. Hypoxia and hypotension, the "lethal duo" in traumatic brain injury: Implications for prehospital care. *Intensive Care Med* 2008;34(3):402–404.

63. Borgman MA, Spinella PC, Perkins JG, et al. The ratio of blood products transfused affects mortality in patients receiving massive transfusions at a combat support hospital. *J Trauma* 2007;63(4):805–813.

64. Holcomb JB, Jenkins D, Rhee P, et al. Damage control resuscitation: Directly addressing the early coagulopathy of trauma. *J Trauma* 2007;62(2):307–310.

65. Johansson PI, Hansen MB, Sørensen H. Transfusion practice in massively bleeding patients: Time for a change? *Vox Sang* 2005;89(2):92–96.

66. Rajasekhar A, Gowing R, Zarychanski R, et al. Survival of trauma patients after massive red blood cell transfusion using a high or low red blood cell to plasma transfusion ratio. *Crit Care Med* 2011;39(6):1507–1513.

67. Snyder CW, Weinberg JA, McGwin G Jr, et al. The relationship of blood product ratio to mortality: Survival benefit or survival bias? *J Trauma* 2009;66(2):358–362.

68. Segal JB, Dzik WH, Transfusion Medicine/Hemostasis Clinical Trials Network. Paucity of studies to support that abnormal coagulation test results predict bleeding in the setting of invasive procedures: An evidence-based review. *Transfusion* 2005;45(9):1413–1425.

69. Johansson PI. Coagulation monitoring of the bleeding traumatized patient. *Curr Opin Anaesthesiol* 2012;25(2):235–241.

70. Smith WR, Moore EE, Osborn P, et al. Retroperitoneal packing as a resuscitation technique for hemodynamically unstable patients with pelvic fractures: Report of two representative cases and a description of technique. *J Trauma* 2005;59:1510–1514.

71. Osborn PM, Smith WR, Moore EE, et al. Direct retroperitoneal pelvic packing versus pelvic angiography: A comparison of two management protocols for haemodynamically unstable pelvic fractures. *Injury* 2009;40(1):54–60.

72. Vaidya R, Colen R, Vigdorchik J, Tonnos F, Sethi A. Minimally invasive treatment of unstable pelvic ring injuries with an internal anterior fixator and posterior iliosacral screw. *J Orthop Trauma* 2012;26(1):1–8.

73. Vaidya R, Kubiak EN, Bergin PF, et al. Complications of anterior subcutaneous internal fixation for unstable pelvis fractures: A multicenter study. *Clin Orthop Relat Res* 2012;470:2124–2131.

74. Holstein JH, Culemann U, Pohlemann T. What are predictors of mortality in patients with pelvic fractures? *Clin Orthop Relat Res* 2012;470:2090–2097.

75. Gabbe BJ, de Steiger R, Esser M, Bucknill A, Russ MK, Cameron PA. Predictors of mortality following severe pelvic ring fracture: Results of a population-based study. *Injury* 2011;42(10):985–991.

76. Bible JE, Kadakia RJ, Wegner A, et al. One-year mortality after isolated pelvic fractures with posterior ring involvement in elderly patients. *Orthopedics* 2013;36(6):760–764. doi: 10.3928/01477447-20130523-21.

77. Dong J, Hao W, Wang B, et al. Management and outcome of pelvic fractures in elderly patients: A retrospective study of 40 cases. *Chin Med J* 2014;127(15):2802–2807.

78. Mears SC, Berry DJ. Outcomes of displaced and nondisplaced pelvic and sacral fractures in elderly adults. J Am Geriatr Soc 2011;59:1309–1312.

79. Greets WH, Code KI, Jay RM, et al. A prospective study of venous thromboembolism after major trauma. *N Engl J Med* 1994;331:1601–1606.

80. Hill J, Treasure T, Guideline Development Group. Reducing the risk of venous thromboembolism (deep vein thrombosis and pulmonary embolism) in patients admitted to hospital: Summary of the NICE guideline. *Heart* 2010;96:879–882.

81. O'Malley KF, Ross SE. Pulmonary embolism in major trauma patients. *J Trauma* 1990;30:748–750.

82. Kim JW, Oh CW, Oh JK, et al. The incidence and the risk factors of venous thromboembolism in Korean patients with pelvic or acetabular fractures. *J Orthop Sci* 2014;19:471–477.

83. Hoffmann MF, Jones CB, Sietsema DL. Persistent impairment after surgically treated lateral compression pelvic injury. *Clin Orthop Relat Res* 2012;470:2161–2172.

84. Holstein JH, Pizanis A, Köhler D, et al. What are predictors for patients' quality of life after pelvic ring fractures? *Clin Orthop Relat Res* 2013;471:2841–2845.

33

Acetabular fractures

SAMEER JAIN AND PETER V. GIANNOUDIS

INTRODUCTION

Background

Fractures of the acetabulum in elderly patients are becoming increasingly common due to a progressively ageing population. Elderly patients represent the fastest growing subset of the UK population as a consequence of improved healthcare, better living standards and greater general health awareness.[1] As well as an increasing life expectancy, these patients remain more active and have greater physical demands. Acetabular fractures in this group of patients are challenging to manage as they frequently consist of complex fracture patterns in the presence of reduced bone mineral density, pre-existing hip disease and medical comorbidities. Due to greater expectations from treatment, there is a higher demand on healthcare resources with clear socioeconomic implications. Whereas older age once represented a contraindication to surgical treatment, an increasingly active and socially demanding elderly population has caused a paradigm shift in practice towards operative management of these complex injuries. Conservative management traditionally involves prolonged bed rest, which is strongly associated with higher rates of mortality and morbidity due to the risk of nosocomial infection, pressure sores and venous thromboembolism.[2] In addition, recent advances in surgical techniques and implant technology make operative treatment a more feasible option with more predictable outcomes.

Anatomy

The word 'acetabulum' is etymologically derived from Latin and literally means 'vinegar cup'. It forms the proximal part of the hip girdle and articulates with the head of the femur within a synovial ball-and-socket joint. It is formed by a confluence of the ilium, ischium and pubis which make up the innominate bone. It is further divided into the anterior and posterior columns which have an inverted 'Y' configuration (Figure 33.1). The anterior column is comprised of the anterior half of the ilium superiorly and extends to the pubic symphysis inferiorly. The posterior column is comprised of the posterior half of the ilium superiorly and extends to the ischium inferiorly. The cotyloid fossa is a recessed non-articular part of the floor of the acetabulum which provides the attachment of the ligamentum teres. The medial wall of the acetabulum is known as the quadrilateral plate, which is thinner than the superior weight-bearing surface and is therefore more susceptible to fracture in the elderly population. A thick labrum normally circumscribes the edge of the acetabulum and contributes to stability of the hip joint. Running inferiorly is the transverse acetabular ligament which acts as a tension band during loading of the hip joint.[3] The acetabulum has a natural inclination of 40–48 degrees and is anteverted by 18–21 degrees. The vascular supply is provided by the corona mortis which is an anastomosis of the external iliac and internal iliac arteries via the epigastric and obturator arteries, respectively.

Mechanism of injury

Acetabular fractures have a bimodal distribution. High energy blunt trauma accounts for the majority of fractures in young patients, while low energy trauma is primarily responsible for these injuries in elderly patients. These most often occur following a fall onto the side of the hip with forces transmitted via the greater trochanter through the femoral neck. These forces are then conveyed to the acetabulum usually leading to atypical fracture patterns. While simple falls from standing height are the most common presentation in older patients, fractures of the acetabulum may

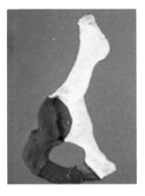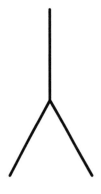

Figure 33.1 Inverted Y representing column theory. Red: posterior column; white: anterior column.

also be the result of high energy trauma, for example, road traffic accidents. These may involve concomitant injures to the ipsilateral intertrochanteric region, femoral neck or pelvis. In the absence of trauma, insufficiency fractures of the acetabulum may occur in the presence of reduced bone mineral density and may be difficult to diagnose. A high index of suspicion can lead to an early diagnosis and improve outcomes in these patients who can usually be successfully managed conservatively.[4] Pathological fractures of the acetabulum most often occur in the presence of metastatic deposits in this age group and can be extremely disabling.[5] A full narrative on the management of pathological fractures is outside the scope of this chapter but it is important to treat these patients with a multidisciplinary team approach involving orthopaedic bone tumour surgeons, oncologists, occupational therapists and physiotherapists in order to provide a full assessment of treatment goals and reconstructive options.

Aims and objectives

Following clinical and radiological assessment, certain factors must be considered before selecting an appropriate management strategy. These include analysis of fracture displacement and available bone stock for reconstructive surgery as well as a thorough assessment of the patient's cognitive status and functional demands. Due to the great variability in patient characteristics and expectations from treatment, the management plan must be individualized according to the patient's personal requirements. This can be challenging as many elderly patients have complex medical comorbidities and social needs. In addition, certain fracture characteristics specific to the elderly population can make surgical management extremely demanding. The aim of this chapter is to provide an overview of the epidemiology, classification, radiological assessment and treatment of acetabular fractures in the geriatric population.

EPIDEMIOLOGY

The epidemiology of acetabular fractures has rarely been investigated and is therefore difficult to accurately describe.

Accounting for all age groups, the annual incidence of acetabular fractures in the UK population has been estimated by Laird and Keating to be three patients per 100,000 per year.[6] The dataset in this epidemiological study involved a total of 351 patients over a 16-year period of whom 231 (65.8%) were males and 120 (34.2%) were females. Over time, there was an increase in the mean age of the patients from 46.8 years to 53.7 years but this did not reach statistical significance. An increase in simple falls as the mechanism of injury was also observed and this may have been a due to the increasing mean age at which these injuries were seen. There was also an increase in the proportion of females with these injuries and importantly, there was a significant reduction in mortality.

A prospective epidemiological database study of 1,309 displaced acetabular fractures gathered over 27 years in the United States revealed that 235 (17.9%) patients were aged over 60 years.[7] During the first half of the study period, 62 (10%) patients were over 60 years while during the second half, 174 (24%) patients were in this age group. This reflects a 2.4-fold increase in the prevalence of acetabular fractures in elderly patients. In this group, simple low energy falls were the mechanism of injury in 117 (49.8%) patients while high energy injuries, such as road traffic accidents, were responsible for injury in 88 (37.4%) patients. It is noteworthy that while acetabular fractures were associated with other injuries, such as chest and abdominal injuries, in 527 (49.1%) patients less than 60 years of age, only 70 (29.8%) of the older patient group sustained a concurrent injury. This may be explained by the fact that elderly patients with acetabular fractures usually have low energy injuries and are therefore less likely to suffer from polytrauma. Of those who did present with a concurrent injury, older patients were more likely to suffer coexisting limb injuries rather than the visceral injuries seen in their younger counterparts.

CLASSIFICATION

Letournel classification

Numerous classification systems have been used to describe fractures of the acetabulum but the most well known is that of Letournel.[8,9] This anatomical classification is based on the radiographic evaluation of the anterior and posterior columns of the acetabulum. It is useful in describing and communicating fracture patterns and also aids in planning the surgical approach. Multiplanar computed tomography (CT) scanning offers substantially improved interobserver agreement when compared to plain radiography.[10] According to this system, fractures can be divided into two main groups with each group further divided into five subtypes (Table 33.1). In general, the position of the femoral head at the time of impact dictates the type of fracture. If the hip is in a position of external rotation then the anterior column is likely to be injured, while in internal rotation an injury to the posterior column is more likely to occur. In the abducted position a low transverse fracture is more

Table 33.1 Letournel classification

Main group	Subtypes
Elementary	Posterior wall
	Posterior column
	Anterior wall
	Anterior column
	Transverse
Associated	T-shaped fracture
	Posterior column and posterior wall fracture
	Transverse and posterior wall fractures
	Anterior column or anterior wall fracture associated with a posterior hemitransverse fracture
	Associated both-column fracture

Table 33.2 AO comprehensive classification

Type	Description	Subtypes
A	Partial articular fractures, one column	A1 Posterior wall fracture
		A2 Posterior column fracture
		A3 Anterior wall or column fracture
B	Partial articular fractures, both columns	B1 Transverse fracture
		B2 T-shaped fracture
		B3 Anterior column plus posterior hemitransverse fractures
C	Complete articular fractures, both columns with separation of the articular surface from pelvis	C1 High
		C2 Low
		C3 Involving the sacroiliac joint

common, while in the adducted position a high transverse fracture is more likely to occur. With respect to the so-called associated fracture patterns, it is important to understand the key principles behind their nomenclature. If both columns are fractured, this is known as a transverse fracture (separating the innominate bone into two segments, that is, superior iliac and inferior ischiopubic) but if both columns are fractured and separated from one another, this is called a T-shaped fracture. This is in contrast to the complex both-column fracture in which both columns are fractured and separated from each other but there is also dissociation of the articular surface from the innominate bone and central dislocation of the femoral head. A radiological analysis of 647 acetabular fractures revealed that posterior wall fractures (24.2%) were the most common of the elementary patterns while transverse and posterior wall fractures (20.7%) and both-column fractures (20.2%) were the most common of the associated patterns.[9]

AO comprehensive classification

In order to standardize the nomenclature regarding acetabular fractures and introduce factors which could influence surgical decision-making, Tile modified this system to include a number of prognostic indicators such as subluxation, dislocation, intra-articular comminution and articular surface involvement. In this description, three main groups of fracture are categorized alphabetically according to the AO comprehensive classification (Table 33.2).[11] Type A injuries are partial articular fractures which involve a single column and are further subdivided into posterior wall fractures, posterior column fractures and anterior wall or anterior column fractures. Type B injuries are also partial articular fractures but these involve both columns and are further subdivided into transverse fractures, T-shaped fractures and anterior column plus posterior hemitransverse fractures. Type C injuries are complete articular fractures with separation of the articular surface and are analogous to the both-column fractures described by Letournel. These are further subdivided into a high type, a low type and a

Table 33.3 Qualifiers of AO classification

Type	Description	Subtypes
α	Femoral head subluxation	α^1 Anterior subluxation
		α^2 Medial subluxation
		α^3 Posterior subluxation
§	Femoral head dislocation	$\S^1$ Anterior dislocation
		$\S^2$ Medial dislocation
		$\S^3$ Posterior dislocation
χ	Acetabular surface	χ^1 Chondral lesion
		χ^2 Impacted fracture
δ	Femoral head surface	δ^1 Chondral lesion
		δ^2 Impacted fracture
		δ^3 Osteochondral fracture
		ε^1 Intra-articular fragment requiring excision
		$\varnothing^1$ Undisplaced acetabular fracture

type which involves the sacroiliac joint. Further fracture characteristics can be added as qualifiers in order to guide prognosis (Table 33.3).

Special considerations in the elderly

The fracture patterns described by both Letournel and Tile typically relate to younger patients who have been involved in high energy trauma. Elderly patients with osteoporotic bone are more likely to present with atypical fracture patterns which do not necessarily conform to either of the described classification systems. In their study of 1309 acetabular fractures, Ferguson et al. reported that displaced fractures of the anterior column were significantly more common in the elderly population compared with

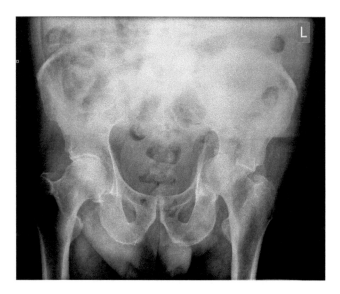

Figure 33.2 Central fracture-dislocation of the left femoral head with quadrilateral plate injury and articular impaction.

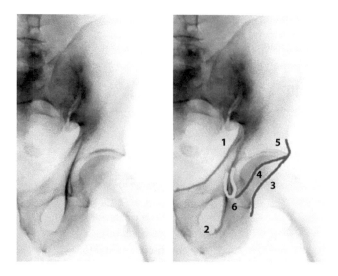

Figure 33.3 Radiographic landmarks.

younger patients (64% vs 43%).[7] Overall, elementary fractures were less common than associated fractures with complex both-column fractures occurring most frequently. Features specific to the elderly population were a separate quadrilateral plate component and roof impaction in the anterior fractures and comminution and marginal impaction in posterior wall fractures. Similarly, Ochs et al. found in a large trauma database study that there were more anterior wall, anterior column and anterior column with posterior hemitransverse fracture types in patients over 60 years of age.[12] In addition, central fracture-dislocations of the femoral head with medial displacement of the quadrilateral plate are more common in the elderly population and are frequently encountered in combination with associated fracture types (Figure 33.2).[13]

These observations can be explained by the presence of osteoporotic bone in the elderly cohort. As the severity of osteoporosis increases, characteristics such as comminution, impaction and loss of articular cartilage are more commonly encountered. These features are recognized as being poor prognostic indicators and correlate with worse clinical outcomes. Many of the complex fracture patterns frequently seen in the geriatric population are not easily defined by any current classification system. However, in the presence of good bone quality, more typical fracture patterns as seen in younger patients can be expected and therefore, the Letournel system can be reliably utilized.

RADIOLOGY

The diagnosis of fractures of the acetabulum is primarily radiological as elderly patients who present following a fall from standing height are at risk of multiple fractures of the pelvis and proximal femur. Therefore, plain radiography including an initial anteroposterior view of the pelvis and

affected hip is mandatory. A lateral view of the proximal femur should also be taken in order to avoid overlooking a concurrent femoral neck fracture. Inlet and outlet pelvic views are also warranted if pelvic ring or sacral injuries are suspected. There are *six* important landmarks on the anteroposterior radiograph of the pelvis that are relevant to acetabular anatomy. These help identify the fracture lines and guide classification (Figure 33.3). They are:

- The iliopectineal line (1) – this represents the arcuate line and runs along the inner aspect of the pelvic brim from the greater sciatic notch to the pubic symphysis. A break in this line signifies a fracture to the anterior column.
- The ilioischial line (2) – also known as Kohler's line, this is formed by the posterior aspect of the quadrilateral surface of the ilium and extends from the greater sciatic notch vertically down to the inner aspect of the obturator foramen. A break in this line represents a fracture to the posterior column.
- The posterior and anterior walls (3 and 4, respectively) – these are usually seen with the anterior wall superimposed over the posterior wall which projects more laterally due to normal acetabular anteversion. An abnormality of either landmark indicates a wall fracture. If the lines demarcating the edge of the two walls 'cross-over' then this may indicate a retroverted acetabulum due to pre-existing hip dysplasia.
- The roof of the acetabulum (5) – also known as the dome or 'sourcile', this being French for 'eyebrow'. This radiographic marker represents the subchondral area of the weight-bearing portion of the superior acetabulum. A roof arc angle of greater than 46 degrees confirms the presence of an intact weight-bearing surface.[14]
- The radiographic teardrop (6) – this is formed by a condensation of the innominate bone at the inferior end of the acetabulum and is normally U shaped. It consists of medial and lateral limbs. The medial limb is formed by the anteroinferior portion of the quadrilateral plate and

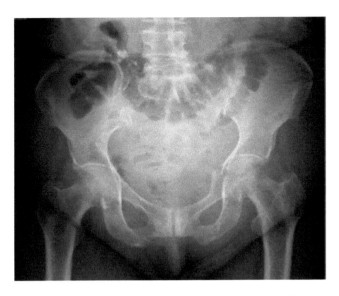

Figure 33.4 Anteroposterior view of a transverse left acetabular fracture in an elderly patient.

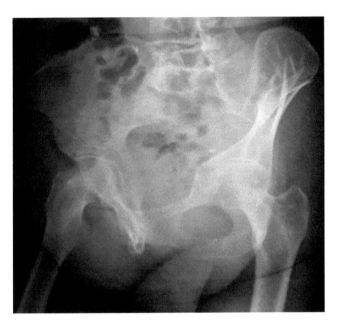

Figure 33.5 Obturator oblique view of a transverse left acetabular fracture.

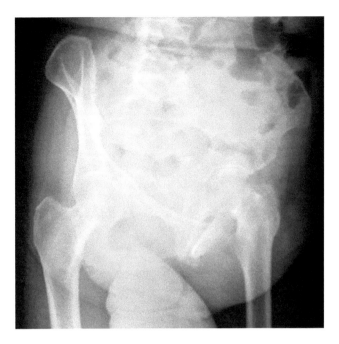

Figure 33.6 Iliac oblique view of a transverse left acetabular fracture.

is continuous with the ilioischial line. The lateral limb is continuous with the floor of the acetabulum superiorly and represents the inferior aspect of the anterior wall.

Judet et al. also recommended the use of additional obturator and iliac oblique views following identification of an acetabular fracture on the initial anteroposterior radiograph (Figure 33.4).[8] The obturator oblique view (Figure 33.5) is taken by rolling the patient into 45 degrees of internal rotation thereby raising the injured side. This shows the obturator foramen *en face* and allows clearer imaging of the anterior column, the posterior wall and part of the iliac wing. The iliac oblique view (Figure 33.6) is taken by rolling the patient into 45 degrees of external rotation thereby

raising the uninjured side. This shows the iliac wing *en face* and allows clearer imaging of the posterior column and the anterior wall. By convention, the beam is centred on the pubic symphysis so that both acetabuli can be visualized. Therefore, an obturator oblique view of one acetabulum will also show an iliac oblique view of the contralateral side on the same film and vice versa. Careful evaluation of all three of these acetabular views can help to identify the bony fragments and classify the fracture pattern. An important feature is the 'spur sign' (Figure 33.7) which is pathognomonic of a both-column fracture with associated medial displacement of the hip joint and is classically seen on the obturator oblique view.[15] A fragment of ilium remains attached to the sacroiliac joint but is separated from the fractured acetabulum resulting in a characteristic appearance. The 'gull sign' (Figure 33.8) is a double density also usually seen on plain radiography and represents marginal impaction of the superomedial joint surface. This sign has been associated with poorer outcomes following internal fixation of acetabular fractures in elderly patients.[16]

Further imaging in the form of CT scanning with 2–3 mm intervals is nearly always recommended, but especially when operative management of displaced fractures is being considered. Not only does this provide more detail with respect to fracture anatomy, but it also offers multiplanar imaging which can be extremely useful when planning surgical reconstruction. Furthermore, small intra-articular fragments can be more accurately identified and this may highlight the need for operative intervention. Due to the additional detail provided, other critical features can be defined and assessed with greater precision, for example, extent of fracture comminution, available bone stock, marginal impaction of the articular surface and concurrent

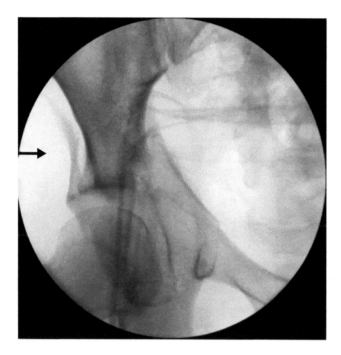

Figure 33.7 Spur sign.

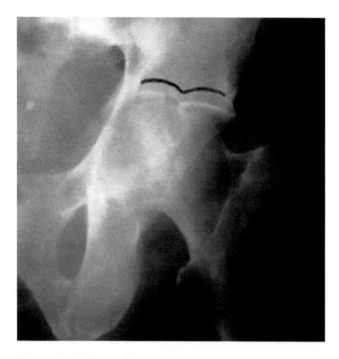

Figure 33.8 The 'gull' sign.

occult fractures of the pelvis and proximal femur. Where possible, three-dimensional reformatting is recommended and can assist in preoperative planning for internal fixation. Unless pathological fractures of the acetabulum or pelvic girdle are suspected, magnetic resonance imaging is not routinely advocated in the primary assessment of fractures of the acetabulum. However, it may have a role in detecting insufficiency fractures in the presence of normal plain radiographs.

TREATMENT

Initial treatment

Although elderly patients are less likely to experience high energy trauma than younger patients, they have a significantly higher rate of mortality and morbidity due to the presence of pre-existing medical disease, reduced cardiopulmonary function and altered physiological response mechanisms. Therefore, careful attention to detail must be paid during the initial assessment and work-up of these patients. As with all forms of trauma, the primary evaluation of elderly patients with suspected fractures of the acetabulum begins with a thorough history and physical examination. Specifically, details regarding the mechanism of injury, localization of pain and associated injuries must be obtained. In addition, a complete review of the patient's past medical history and current prescriptive medications must be performed as this will provide essential information in order to guide initial resuscitation manoeuvres and definitive management. There is great variation in the level of physical activity, functional demands and expectations from treatment among elderly patients and it is important not make any assumptions which may become central to surgical decision-making. Information about their social circumstances, accommodation, pre-injury mobility status, level of home care support and driving ability must be obtained. Many of these patients will have an element of chronic cognitive impairment and may therefore be unable to offer this information or even comply with assessment. Every effort must be made to obtain missing details from other relevant sources, for example, hospital notes, general practitioner records and care home records. Finally, a high index of suspicion with respect to safeguarding issues must be maintained, particularly if there are any discrepancies between the history and subsequent evaluation.

The physical examination of these patients should follow a systematic approach similar to the expected standards of assessing patients with hip fractures. Close inspection of the affected limb should be performed to evaluate the presence of deformity, swelling, bruising or degloving injury. This should also include an assessment of pressure sore areas and lower leg skin as many of these patients will have concurrent pre-tibial lacerations which may impact on subsequent traction. Palpation of the bony extremities can target areas for detailed radiographic review but unnecessary movements of the affected limb must be kept to a minimum to avoid pain. A complete neurovascular assessment must be performed and clearly documented. A general physical examination should also be conducted in order to avoid missing any concurrent pathology. This includes documentation of the Glasgow Coma Scale score, a full cardiorespiratory and abdominal examination, a skeletal survey and an assessment of cognitive function with the Abbreviated Mental Test Score. In the presence of multiple or high energy trauma, Advanced Trauma and Life Support guidelines should be followed.

Initial treatment measures must include adequate oxygenation, ensuring sufficient analgesia and administering careful fluid resuscitation. Initial laboratory investigations must involve routine serum blood tests to include a full blood count, urea and electrolytes, liver function tests, coagulation profile and blood group analysis. If there is gross haemodynamic instability, urgent cross-matching will be required for blood transfusion. Initially, cardiorespiratory evaluation must be performed with an electrocardiogram and chest X-ray with additional tests conducted if required, for example, echocardiography and lung function testing. Urinalysis can exclude the presence of urinary sepsis which must be treated if symptomatic. As discussed previously, the standard radiological assessment of acetabular fractures includes an anteroposterior view of the pelvis and two orthogonal views of the painful hip with subsequent imaging performed as required. The majority of elderly patients with acetabular fractures will require hospital admission and the affected limb should be immobilized in traction for pain control and fracture reduction. These patients commonly have extremely frail skin on their lower leg so this is typically best achieved with skeletal traction rather than skin traction. This can usually be performed in the emergency department under local anaesthesia. However, associated femoral head dislocations require emergent closed reduction under general anaesthesia and this is best accomplished in the operating theatre during which traction pins can be placed. Prophylaxis against venous thromboembolism is recommended and can be administered via low molecular weight heparin.

Deciding upon the most appropriate definitive management strategy in this complex patient group is challenging and many controversies exist with respect to treatment modality, timing of surgical intervention, surgical approach and implant selection. Multiple factors must be taken into consideration when determining treatment. These can be broadly divided into patient factors, fracture factors and surgical factors. Patient factors include level of physical activity, medical comorbidity, level of cognitive function and individual expectations from treatment. Fracture factors include the amount of displacement, the level of comminution, available bone stock for reconstruction and insufficiency or pathological fractures. Surgical factors include surgical approach, level of local expertise in internal fixation and/or complex primary arthroplasty, implant accessibility and theatre availability.

Non-operative treatment

The main indication for non-operative management of acetabular fractures in elderly patients is the presence of a stable, concentrically reduced fracture not involving the weight-bearing surface. Fractures are considered to be stable when they meet the following criteria *outside of traction*:

- Undisplaced fractures
- Minimally displaced fractures, that is, less than 2 mm of displacement

- Fractures of the acetabular walls where stability of the hip can be maintained
- Both-column fractures where secondary congruence has been obtained between the femoral head and the acetabular fragments; despite malunion of the ilium an acceptable functional outcome can still be expected[17]
- Insufficiency fractures.

As long as the fracture is stable and the joint remains congruent out of traction, the patient can be successfully managed non-operatively, for example, anterior wall fractures involving less than 20% of the articular surface, low anterior column fractures, low transverse fractures or low T-fractures. In addition, patients presenting with significant medical comorbidities may be deemed unsuitable for anaesthesia due to the excessively high risks of mortality. Along with non-ambulatory patients, these patients would also be candidates for non-operative treatment. This traditionally involves a period of bed rest followed by early and progressive mobilization. A knee extension brace can also be used in the short-term to prevent flexion of the hip. Prolonged bed rest with skeletal traction typically results in acceptable clinical and radiological outcomes in younger patients.[18] However, poorer outcomes can be expected in elderly patients due to an increased morbidity and mortality associated with lengthy immobilization and hospital in-patient stay. Therefore, in this patient group, only a short period of bed rest is advised. If prolonged traction is required to allow fracture healing, operative measures should be employed. In addition, certain fracture patterns associated with elderly patients are often impossible to reduce through closed measures, for example, quadrilateral plate fractures. These patients should be considered candidates for surgical intervention unless there are significant medical contraindications.

Following bed rest, early mobilization of the hip joint should be started as soon as pain subsides in order to prevent stiffness and muscle wasting. Functional physiotherapy includes gradually increasing the patient's weight-bearing status over a period of 3–6 months. This protocol should be individualized according to patient-specific requirements and capabilities. Caution should be used in patients with significant osteoporosis as their fractures may take more time to heal and therefore they may require a more gradual rehabilitation. Once mobile out of bed with assistance, plans can be made for discharge to an appropriate rehabilitation facility where more resources are available for further physical and occupational therapy. Prophylaxis against venous thromboembolism should be continued according to local guidelines or until the patient is fully mobile out of hospital. Regular radiographic follow-up every 1–2 weeks is mandatory in order to confirm bony union and guide rehabilitation. If there are minimal concerns regarding joint congruency and fracture displacement, radiographs can be taken less regularly, that is, at 4–6-week intervals for the first 3 months.

Most published studies on the clinical and functional outcomes of non-operative treatment of acetabular fractures involve a heterogeneous group of patients of varying age. However, a few small case series evaluating these injuries in elderly patients have shown that around one-third of patients experience unsatisfactory clinical and functional outcomes from non-operative treatment.[19,20] Factors that were shown to increase the rates of failure include the presence of osteoporosis, associated femoral head fractures, delayed diagnosis, inadequate radiographs, inappropriate traction and premature weight bearing.[20] Therefore, in elderly patients presenting with stable fractures, congruent hip joints and an intact weight-bearing dome or with life-threatening medical contraindications to surgery, non-operative treatment is correctly indicated. Provided adequate analgesia is achieved, this can also be extended to non-ambulatory patients with more displaced or unstable fracture patterns.

Operative treatment

The indications for operative treatment of geriatric acetabular fractures in patients who are usually ambulatory and are deemed medically fit for anaesthesia and surgery are:

- Fractures with more than 2 mm of displacement
- An incongruent hip joint
- Hip joint instability
- Fractures affecting the weight-bearing surface, that is, roof arc angle less than 46 degrees
- Associated femoral head dislocation or femoral neck fracture.

In general, the goals of managing these patients are to restore the congruity of the articular surface, alleviate pain, allow early mobilization and maximize long-term functional outcomes. These can be achieved through a variety of well established techniques and the decision as to which

to offer the patient is based on several factors as previously discussed. This challenging decision is best taken using a multidisciplinary team approach involving orthopaedic surgeons with expertise in acetabular reconstructive surgery and revision arthroplasty, geriatric physicians and anaesthetists. Surgical options currently include open reduction and internal fixation (ORIF), acute total hip replacement (THR) with or without ORIF and delayed THR. The advantages and disadvantages of these options are summarized in Table 33.4.

Open reduction and internal fixation

ORIF of acetabular fractures allows an anatomic restoration of the joint surface while preserving the femoral head. By restoring joint congruity, the risk of developing post-traumatic osteoarthritis is reduced and even in this eventuality, preservation of the patient's native bone stock should allow the use of primary THR implants. However, the presence of osteoporosis, fracture comminution, associated femoral head fractures and pre-existing osteoarthritis may result in altered bone quality that makes stable internal fixation a major operative challenge. Hence, there is a significant risk of construct failure and/or collapse of the hip joint in the elderly population. This type of surgical fixation is clearly complex and time consuming so patients must be medically robust enough to tolerate lengthy operating times with potentially significant blood loss. Typically, a partial weight-bearing regimen is required postoperatively which the patient must be unable to comply with. Therefore, indications for ORIF are the presence of a fracture pattern amenable to fixation through a single non-extensile exposure without performing a trochanteric osteotomy or disrupting the abductor musculature, adequate bone quality for fixation, an intact femoral head and that reconstruction can be performed in a reasonable surgical time.[21] Surgery should generally be performed as soon as the patient has been medically optimized although it may be detrimental

Table 33.4 Surgical options

	ORIF	Acute THR	Delayed THR
Advantages	Restores joint congruency	Single-stage surgery	Avoids complex internal fixation
	Minimizes risk of developing osteoarthritis	Immediate mobilization	Allows time for medical optimization and/or other injuries to be treated
	Preservation of bone stock, that is, femoral head	Avoids risk of failed internal fixation and secondary collapse	Salvage for failed internal fixation
		Prevents delayed THR	
Disadvantages	Challenging due to poor bone quality	Complex surgery	Technically challenging
	Requires compliance with partial weight bearing	Often requires combined ORIF	Abnormal anatomy
	Long operating times	May need tertiary referral	Residual pelvic deformity
	Blood loss	Greater operating times, blood loss and heterotopic ossification compared to delayed THR	Retained implants
			Prior heterotopic ossification
			Loss of bone stock
			Revision implants needed

Note: ORIF, open reduction and internal fixation; THR, total hip replacement.

to over delay due to the risks associated with prolonged recumbency.

Internal fixation can be achieved through standard open or percutaneous surgical approaches and is performed under fluoroscopic guidance to ensure hardware does not penetrate the hip joint. Standard open approaches provide much better visualization of fracture fragments and can therefore allow for a more complete reduction with application of internal fixation devices under direct vision. This is important so as to avoid any aberrant positioning of bone screws which may result in visceral injury with potentially fatal consequences. Percutaneous techniques allow for better pain relief and faster recovery. Proponents argue that an anatomic reduction of the joint surface is not mandatory in elderly patients for satisfactory function.[22] However, these techniques are highly specialized and are often difficult to achieve particularly with displaced fracture patterns resulting from more high energy trauma. There remains a significant risk of developing post-traumatic osteoarthritis with incomplete reduction and this may be unacceptable in active individuals.

Choice of approach depends on the 'personality' of the fracture and is guided by preoperative CT imaging. Generally, posterior column fractures are best visualized through the posterior Kocher-Langenbeck approach. This is also advantageous in allowing access for revision surgery if subsequent THR is indicated. Anterior column fractures are best treated with the anterior ilioinguinal approach but this carries a risk of injury to the femoral and lateral femoral cutaneous nerves. The anterior intrapelvic or Stoppa approach provides good access for quadrilateral plate fractures but care must be taken to identify and ligate the corona mortis in order to prevent massive bleeding. While the extensile iliofemoral approach allows greater visualization of both columns, it is associated with greater morbidity and a high incidence of heterotopic ossification and is therefore best avoided in elderly patients.

The most commonly used implants include a combination of stainless steel pelvic reconstruction plates and screws. Although locking plates enhance construct rigidity in osteoporotic bone, currently these are of limited value as the locking holes often have a fixed angle and do not allow for accurate placement into the natural bony contours of the pelvis. Newer titanium designs incorporating multidirectional locking screws are available but biomechanical testing has revealed similar construct rigidity when compared to standard methods.[23] Buttress plates are the most frequently applied fixation method for isolated wall fractures as these limit the shear forces that are commonly encountered during ambulation. Spring plates for buttressing comminuted posterior wall fractures used in combination with reconstruction plates provide a durable option.[24] Column fractures typically require the use of contoured reconstruction plates with large diameter periarticular screws which can be used to compress or hold sizeable fracture fragments. Usually lag screws have little compressive effect in osteoporotic bone and require adjunctive neutralization plates. Smaller articular fragments can be held with Kirschner wires, smooth bioabsorbable pins,

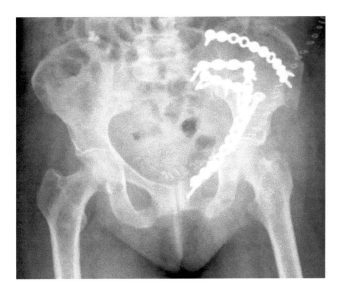

Figure 33.9 ORIF of a transverse left acetabular fracture using reconstruction plates and a periarticular screw.

mini-fragment plates and suture anchors. In the presence of gross comminution, bone graft, bone cement or synthetic calcium phosphate may be required. As many of the fractures experienced by the elderly are more complex type injuries, usually a combination of techniques is required (Figure 33.9). This highlights the need for meticulous preoperative planning and CT imaging.

The results of ORIF of acetabular fractures in the elderly population have not been as extensively investigated as in younger patients and as a result there are few published studies. Helfet et al. reported on 18 elderly patients who underwent ORIF via either an ilioinguinal approach or a Kocher-Langenbeck approach.[21] All but one were considered to have a successful result with acceptable functional outcomes by 2 years. There were two cases of pulmonary embolism which resolved with anticoagulation therapy. Anglen et al. published their results of 48 patients with displaced fractures requiring ORIF.[16] Difficulty in obtaining an anatomic reduction was experienced in 39% of patients which correlated closely with radiographic outcomes. However, functional outcomes were generally very good and were similar to age-matched controls. Jeffcoat et al. reported on 41 patients treated with ORIF via an ilioinguinal approach. They found that the use of a limited two-window approach was associated with a significant reduction in blood loss and operative time compared to the standard three-window approach.[25]

Laflamme et al. investigated the outcome of 21 patients with medially displaced quadrilateral plate fractures treated with an infrapectineal buttress plate via a Stoppa approach.[26] An anatomic reduction was achieved in only 52.4% of cases with the gull sign correlating closely with a poor outcome. There was one traumatic injury to the obturator nerve and two patients had temporary weakness of the hip adductors postoperatively. Archdeacon et al.[27] also reported on 39 patients with quadrilateral plate fractures stabilized with a combination of pelvic brim and infrapectineal plates via an ilioinguinal or Stoppa approach. By 3 years, 56% had a good-to-excellent functional outcome, 46% had a good-to-excellent radiographic outcome and 19% required a THR. Percutaneous fixation of acetabular fractures in geriatric patients has also been researched. Gary et al. reported acceptable short-term functional outcomes in a series of 79 patients treated with percutaneous reduction and fixation.[28] However, a quarter of patients required a THR by a mean of 1.4 years.[29]

Acute total hip replacement

In general, the indications for acute THR over ORIF in the elderly include severe femoral head injury, concomitant femoral neck fracture, significant posterior wall injury, severe acetabular impaction, the need for an extensile approach for ORIF, severe osteoporosis or comminution which prevents stable internal fixation, pathological fractures and pre-existing symptomatic osteoarthritis. Advantages of acute THR are that it offers single-stage surgery, allows immediate mobilization, avoids the risks of failed internal fixation and also prevents the need for delayed THR. However, this is a complex primary arthroplasty procedure due to distorted soft tissue and bony anatomy and can be technically very challenging. Furthermore, in order to achieve adequate fixation of the acetabular component either some inherent fracture stability is required or combined internal fixation is needed (Figure 33.10). Other options include the use of revision THR acetabular reconstruction techniques, for example, uncemented jumbo cups, highly porous metal augments, antiprotrusion cages or roof reinforcement rings. An experienced surgical team to include well practiced pelvic trauma and arthroplasty surgeons is required due to the complexity of surgery. If this is not available locally, then tertiary referral is advised.

The priority for internal fixation in this setting is the posterior column followed by the posterior wall. If this is not possible due to the extent of comminution, then fragments of the posterior wall can be removed and reconstructed using the femoral head as a structural autograft.[30] A posterior Kocher-Langenbeck surgical approach is often utilized as this facilitates both THR and fracture fixation. In this age group, standard metal-on-polyethylene bearing surfaces are sufficient and are also cost effective. Uncemented acetabular components with the option for supplementary screw fixation may be advised over cemented implants due to the risk of cement escape. The femoral component can be chosen according to canal geometry, bone quality and surgeon's preference. Larger heads should be used to help reduce the risk of instability. Postoperatively, partial weight bearing is routinely advised to allow fracture healing and bony ingrowth. Standard arthroplasty precautions must be taken with respect to postoperative mobilization in order to prevent early dislocation and component loosening.

The results of acute THR with combined ORIF have recently been well summarized in a systematic review by De Bellis et al.[31] Across the reviewed studies, satisfactory clinical outcomes were reported through a variety of validated hip function scoring systems. In addition, nearly all patients returned to walking but many required additional support in the form of a supplementary walking aid. Since this study, Malhotra et al. have reported equally satisfactory clinical and radiological results in 15 elderly patients using an uncemented THR with a malleable titanium acetabular cage allowing customizable screw fixation.[32] Most recently, Rickman et al. reported on their technique of combined acute THR and plate stabilization of both columns followed by early mobilization.[33] All patients were fully weight bearing by 1 week and all fractures had healed by 6 months with no evidence of component migration. Tidermark et al. reported the results of acute THR without concurrent internal fixation in a series of 10 patients in whom the acetabular component was supported by an antiprotrusion cage and autologous bone graft.[34] By a mean of 38 months, all components were stable with no signs of loosening and all patients were walking independently but with a slightly increased need for walking aids.

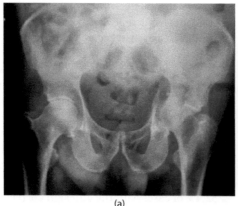
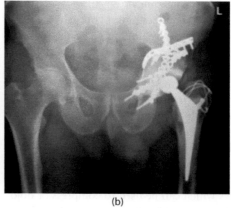

(a) (b)

Figure 33.10 Acute total hip replacement (THR) in combination with open reduction and internal fixation (ORIF) of a left acetabular fracture. **(a)** Left acetabular fracture with central dislocation. **(b)** Acute total hip replacement in combination with open reduction and internal fixation.

Delayed total hip replacement

Delayed THR for geriatric acetabular fractures can be performed for post-traumatic osteoarthritis following unsuccessful non-operative or operative management. An argument for applying this strategy early is that it avoids the need for complex internal fixation which can be unpredictable for certain fracture types, for example, marginal impaction, posterior wall comminution. Delaying surgery can also allow time for medical optimization and recuperation following a major traumatic event. There may also be other more significant injuries which require prioritization. The main disadvantage of this option is that THR following acetabular fracture is technically more difficult and is associated with longer operating times and greater blood loss. Challenges include residual pelvic deformity, non-union, malunited fractures, retained implants, heterotopic bone formation, previous scars, previous neurological injury and bone loss, particularly of the medial wall of the acetabulum.

The principles behind delayed THR are analogous to revision arthroplasty in the presence of acetabular bone loss. The extent of bone loss must be defined and classified using CT imaging. Infection must always be considered and investigated appropriately with baseline serum inflammatory markers and joint aspiration. Previous hardware and heterotopic bone can be selectively removed if interfering with the acetabular component and this should be performed during the time of THR to avoid multiple operations. However, a two-stage procedure may be required if positive microbial cultures are obtained. Further heterotopic bone formation can be suppressed with the use of prophylactic non-steroidal anti-inflammatory medication and/or radiation therapy although this may affect fixation of the acetabular component. In order to restore bone stock for the adequate fixation of the acetabular component, a variety of techniques are available including the use of structural bulk allografts, the application of a mesh and impaction bone grafting, jumbo uncemented acetabular components, highly porous metal augments and cup-cage constructs. This requires careful consideration as providing adequate fixation for the acetabular component is essential in preventing further morbidity. Cemented acetabular components have been associated with failure rates of up to 50% at 10 years and should therefore be avoided.[35]

The results of delayed THR following acetabular fracture have been well documented and satisfactory clinical results and functional improvements can be expected. With modern implants and techniques, clinical outcomes are similar to those of primary THR for non-traumatic conditions. However, it is important to note that most of the published studies investigating delayed THR do not differentiate between elderly and younger patients. Ranawat et al. reported a series of 32 patients with a mean age of 52 years who underwent delayed uncemented THR.[36] The 5-year survival rate with revision, loosening, dislocation or infection as the end point was 79% but survival for aseptic acetabular loosening alone was 97%. Revision surgery correlated with a non-anatomic restoration of the hip centre and a history of previous infection. Recently, Lai et al. published their results of delayed uncemented THR in a series of 31 patients with a mean age of 50 years and reported a survival rate of 100% with revision surgery or radiographic acetabular loosening as the end point.[37] Prior treatment had no effect on clinical outcome but patients treated with previous ORIF had longer surgical times and greater blood loss than those treated non-operatively due to soft tissue scarring, heterotopic ossification, hardware removal and the complexity of reconstruction. Compared to acute THR, Sermon et al. reported better functional outcomes in 121 elderly patients treated with delayed THR but noticed higher rates of heterotopic ossification and revision surgery due to instability and infection.[38] Most recently, Makridis et al. performed a systematic review of 654 patients and found that the 10-year survival rate of the acetabular component with loosening, osteolysis or revision as the end point was 81% in those who had acute THR compared to 76% in patients who had delayed THR.[39] However, in both studies the differences between the groups were not statistically significant.

COMPLICATIONS

Open reduction and internal fixation

The overall mortality rate following surgical treatment of acetabular fractures in the elderly has been reported as 19.1% with non-fatal complications seen in 39.8% by 5 years.[40] Elderly patients are at greater risk of major systemic complications, such as venous thromboembolism, myocardial infarction, chest infection and cerebrovascular accident, than younger patients due to pre-existing medical comorbidities and reduced physiological reserves. Appropriate medical optimization including venous thromboembolism prophylaxis can reduce these risks but patients must be counselled appropriately. In general, predictors of a poor outcome following ORIF include increasing age, osteoporosis, comorbidity, femoral head injury, comminuted posterior wall fracture, fracture extension into the subchondral roof, the gull sign, timing of surgery, quality of reduction and surgeon experience.[16,41-44]

Local complications following ORIF include delayed wound healing, infection, non-union, malunion, failure of fixation, post-traumatic osteoarthritis and injury to nerves, vessels and visceral organs. Wound healing problems and infection have an increased incidence in the geriatric population and therefore dietary supplements are advised to ensure adequate nutrition. Severe osteopenia and fracture comminution can predispose to non-union and fixation failure with subsequent malunion. This can lead to functional deterioration and a rapid progression of osteoarthritis requiring THR. A recent systematic review involving 415 acetabular fractures in elderly patients with a mean age of 71.8 years revealed a conversion to THR rate of 23.1% by 4 years.[37] Geriatric patients are also at increased risk of nerve injury due to the presence of concurrent spinal stenosis. Therefore, great care must be taken during soft tissue exposure and retraction of the posterior structures of the hip. Traction injury to the sciatic nerve can be prevented by keeping the hip extended and the knee flexed during surgery. Vascular injury is also more likely in the elderly due to the presence of atherosclerosis and this may result in vessel wall rupture or thrombosis. This again highlights the need for careful soft tissue retraction. The use of intraoperative fluoroscopy allows visualization of screw placement and can reduce the likelihood of intra-abdominal penetration.

Total hip replacement

De Bellis et al. reported complication rates following acute THR in a systematic review of six studies involving 206 patients.[31] Overall, systematic complications were seen in five patients (2.4%) and comprised of four cases of deep vein thrombosis and one case of transient ischaemic attack. Local complications were minor wound problems (1%), heterotopic ossification (up to 40%) and postoperative dislocation (up to 14%). Chémaly et al. reported a similar incidence of heterotopic ossification (38%) following acute THR for acetabular fractures. They also noted that patients who underwent surgery early after injury had a fourfold increased chance of developing this complication and more than twice the blood loss and operating times than those who had delayed THR.[45] The highest revision rate has been reported by Sarkar et al. (42%) together with the highest prevalence of radiographic loosening (21%).[46] However, the majority of THR procedures in this series were performed using cement which has consistently shown high rates of early failure.[35] The use of uncemented acetabular components can reliably give low rates of aseptic loosening similar to THR performed electively.[32-34]

Weber et al. published their results in 66 patients in whom THR was performed for post-traumatic osteoarthritis following previous ORIF for acetabular fracture.[47] The mean age of the patients at the time of THR was 52 years. Cemented acetabular components were used in 44 hips and uncemented acetabular components were used in 22 hips. By 9.6 years, 17 patients (25.8%) required revision THR. Of these, 16 revisions were performed for aseptic loosening of one or both components. The 10-year survival rate with revision due to aseptic loosening as the end point was 78% for the THR as a whole, 87% for the acetabular component and 84% for the femoral component. None of the uncemented acetabular components demonstrated radiographic loosening. Predictors of requiring revision for aseptic loosening were cemented acetabular components, age under 50 years, bodyweight over 80 kg and combined residual segmental and cavitatory acetabular deficiency.

REFERENCES

1. Mears DC. Surgical treatment of acetabular fractures in elderly patients with osteoporotic bone. *J Am Acad Orthop Surg* 1999;7(2):128–41.

2. Walsh KA, Bruza JM. Review: Hospitalization of the elderly. *Ann Long-Term Care* 2007;5(11):18–23.

3. Lohe F, Eckstein F, Sauer T, Putz R. Structure, strain and function of the transverse acetabular ligament. *Acta Anat* 1996;157:315–23.

4. Berst MJ, El-Khouri GY. Acetabular insufficiency fractures. *Emerg Radiol* 2000;7(2):98–102.

5. Wright RW, Schwartz HS. Pathologic acetabular fractures: New concepts in surgical management. *Semin Arthroplasty* 1994;5(2):95–105.

6. Laird A, Keating JF. Acetabular fractures: A 16-year prospective epidemiological study. *J Bone Joint Surg Br* 2005;87(7):969–73.

7. Ferguson TA, Patel R, Bhandari M, Matta JM. Fractures of the acetabulum in patients aged 60 years and older: An epidemiological and radiological study. *J Bone Joint Surg Br* 2010;92(2):250–7.

8. Judet R, Judet J, Letournel E. Fractures of the acetabulum: Classification and surgical approaches for open reduction. *J Bone Joint Surg* 1964;46A(8):1615–47.

9. Letournel E. Acetabulum fractures: Classification and management. *Clin Orthop Relat Res* 1980;(151):81–106.

10. Ohashi K, El-Khoury GY, Abu-Zahra KW, Berbaum KS. Interobserver agreement for Letournel acetabular fracture classification with multidetector CT: Are standard Judet radiographs necessary? *Radiology* 2006;241(2):386–91.

11. Tile T. Fractures of the acetabulum. *Orthop Clin North Am* 1980;11:481–506.

12. Ochs BG, Marintschev I, Hoyer H, Rolauffs B, Culemann U, Pohlemann T, Stuby FM. Changes in the treatment of acetabular fractures over 15 years: Analysis of 1266 cases treated by the German Pelvic Multicentre Study Group (DAO/DGU). *Injury* 2010;41(8):839–51.

13. White G, Kanakaris NK, Faour O, Valverde JA, Martin MA, Giannoudis PV. Quadrilateral plate fractures of the acetabulum: An update. *Injury* 2013;44(2):159–67.

14. Chuckpaiwong B, Suwanwong P, Harnroongroj T. Roof-arc angle and weight-bearing area of the acetabulum. *Injury* 2009;40(10):1064–6.

15. Johnson TS. The spur sign. *Radiology* 2005;235(3):1023–4.

16. Anglen JO, Burd TA, Hendricks KJ, Harrison P. The "gull sign": A harbinger of failure for internal fixation of geriatric acetabular fractures. *J Orthop Trauma* 2003;17(9):625–34.

17. Tile M, Helfet DL, Kellam JF. *Fractures of the Pelvis and Acetabulum*, 3rd ed. Lippincott, Philadelphia, 2003.

18. Sen RK, Veerappa LA. Long-term outcome of conservatively managed displaced acetabular fractures. *J Trauma* 2009;67:155–9.

19. Matta JM, Anderson LM, Epstein HC, Hendricks P. Fractures of the acetabulum: A retrospective analysis. *Clin Orthop* 1986;205:241–50.

20. Spencer RF. Acetabular fractures in older patients. *J Bone Joint Surg Br* 1989;71B:774–6.

21. Helfet DL, Borrelli J, DiPasquale T, Sanders R. Stabilization of acetabular fractures in elderly patients. *J Bone Joint Surg Am* 1992;74:753–765.

22. Miller AN, Prasarn ML, Lorich DG, Helfet DL. The radiological evaluation of acetabular fractures in the elderly. *J Bone Joint Surg Br* 2010;92(4):560–4.

23. Culemann U, Holstein JH, Köhler D, Tzioupis CC, Pizanis A, Tosounidis G, Burkhardt M, Pohlemann T. Different stabilisation techniques for typical acetabular fractures in the elderly—A biomechanical assessment. *Injury* 2010;41(4):405–10.

24. Richter H, Hutson JJ, Zych G. The use of spring plates in the internal fixation of acetabular fractures. *J Orthop Trauma* 2004;18(3):179–81.

25. Jeffcoat DM, Carroll EA, Huber FG, Goldman AT, Miller AN, Lorich DG, Helfet DL. Operative treatment of acetabular fractures in an older population through a limited ilioinguinal approach. *J Orthop Trauma* 2012;26(5):284–9.

26. Laflamme GY, Hebert-Davies J, Rouleau D, Benoit B, Leduc S. Internal fixation of osteopenic acetabular fractures involving the quadrilateral plate. *Injury* 2011;42(10):1130–4.

27. Archdeacon MT, Kazemi N, Collinge C, Budde B, Schnell S. Treatment of protrusio fractures of the acetabulum in patients 70 years and older. *J Orthop Trauma.* 2013;27(5):256–61.

28. Gary JL, VanHal M, Gibbons SD, Reinert CM, Starr AJ. Functional outcomes in elderly patients with acetabular fractures treated with minimally invasive reduction and percutaneous fixation. *J Orthop Trauma* 2012;26(5):278–83.

29. Gary JL, Lefaivre KA, Gerold F, Hay MT, Reinert CM, Starr AJ. Survivorship of the native hip joint after percutaneous repair of acetabular fractures in the elderly. *Injury* 2011;42(10):1144–51.

30. Sierra RJ, Mabry TM, Sems SA, Berry DJ. Acetabular fractures: The role of total hip replacement. *Bone Joint J* 2013;95-B(11 Suppl A):11–16.

31. De Bellis UG, Legnani C, Calori GM. Acute total hip replacement for acetabular fractures: A systematic review of the literature. *Injury* 2014;45(2):356–61.

32. Malhotra R, Singh DP, Jain V, Kumar V, Singh R. Acute total hip arthroplasty in acetabular fractures in the elderly using the Octopus System: Mid term to long term follow-up. *J Arthroplasty* 2013;28(6):1005–9.

33. Rickman M, Young J, Trompeter A, Pearce R, Hamilton M. Managing acetabular fractures in the elderly with fixation and primary arthroplasty: Aiming for early weightbearing. *Clin Orthop Relat Res* 2014;472(11):3375–82.

34. Tidermark J, Blomfeldt R, Ponzer S, Söderqvist A, Törnkvist H. Primary total hip arthroplasty with a Burch-Schneider antiprotrusion cage and autologous bone grafting for acetabular fractures in elderly patients. *J Orthop Trauma* 2003;17(3):193–7.

35. Romness DW, Lewallen DG. Total hip arthroplasty after fracture of the acetabulum: Long-term results. *J Bone Joint Surg Br* 1990;72-B:761–4.

36. Ranawat A, Zelken J, Helfet D, Buly R. Total hip arthroplasty for posttraumatic arthritis after acetabular fracture. *J Arthroplasty* 2009;24(5):759–67.

37. Lai O, Yang J, Shen B, Zhou Z, Kang P, Pei F. Midterm results of uncemented acetabular reconstruction for posttraumatic arthritis secondary to acetabular fracture. *J Arthroplasty* 2011;26(7):1008–13.

38. Sermon A, Broos P, Vanderschot P. Total hip replacement for acetabular fractures. Results in 121 patients operated between 1983 and 2003. *Injury* 2008;39(8):914–21.

39. Makridis KG, Obakponovwe O, Bobak P, Giannoudis PV. Total hip arthroplasty after acetabular fracture: Incidence of complications, reoperation rates and functional outcomes: Evidence today. *J Arthroplasty* 2014;29(10):1983–90.

40. Daurka JS, Pastides PS, Lewis A, Rickman M, Bircher MD. Acetabular fractures in patients aged >55 years: A systematic review of the literature. *Bone Joint J* 2014;96-B(2):157–63.

41. Matta JM. Fractures of the acetabulum: Accuracy of reduction and clinical results in patients managed operatively within three weeks of the injury. *J Bone Jt Surg* 1996;78(A):1632–45.

42. Saterbak AM, Marsh JL, Nepola JV, Brandser EA, Turbett T. Clinical failure after posterior wall acetabular fractures: The influence of initial fracture patterns. *J Orthop Trauma* 2000;14(4):230–7.

43. Giannoudis PV, Grotz MR, Papakostidis C, Dinopoulos H. Operative treatment of displaced fractures of the acetabulum. A meta-analysis. *J Bone Joint Surg Br* 2005;87(1):2–9.

44. Zha GC, Sun JY, Dong SJ. Predictors of clinical outcomes after surgical treatment of displaced acetabular fractures in the elderly. *J Orthop Res* 2013;31(4):588–95.

45. Chémaly O, Hebert-Davies J, Rouleau DM, Benoit B, Laflamme GY. Heterotopic ossification following total hip replacement for acetabular fractures. *Bone Joint J* 2013;95-B(1):95–100.

46. Sarkar MR, Wachter N, Kinzl L, Bischoff M. Acute total hip replacement for displaced acetabular fractures in older patients. *Eur J Trauma* 2004;5:296–304.

47. Weber M, Berry DJ, Harmsen WS. Total hip arthroplasty after operative treatment of an acetabular fracture. *J Bone Joint Surg Am* 1998;80(9):1295–305.

34

Intracapsular proximal femoral fractures

KJELL MATRE AND JAN-ERIK GJERTSEN

INTRODUCTION

Based on the current literature and estimates, the absolute number of hip fractures is expected to increase dramatically over the coming decades. By the year 2050, it is estimated that the total number of hip fractures world wide will exceed 6 million annually.[1] For the individual patient a hip fracture may cause short- and long-term pain, impaired function and reduced quality of life. Up to 50% of the patients will not regain their pre-injury mobility, independent living may no longer be possible, and the mortality is high.

Intracapsular femoral neck fractures represent 60% of all hip fractures.[2] These fractures have been one of the most extensively investigated and well-documented topics in the orthopaedic literature. However, we still do not know the best treatment for each patient and there are no generally accepted guidelines on how to manage these injuries. In recent years the treatment has shifted towards the increased use of arthroplasty and a reduction in fixation. Which patients, if any, should still have their fractures fixed? And if this is still a valid option, have we found the ideal implant and method of fixation? Treating a displaced femoral neck fracture in an elderly patient with an arthroplasty is no longer controversial. But how do we define 'an elderly patient'? Furthermore, what type of arthroplasty should be used, and should this be a cemented or uncemented procedure? Many options are available, but there are no clear answers to these questions.

EPIDEMIOLOGY

Hip fracture incidence varies considerably both between and within countries and continents. In Europe, there is a higher hip fracture incidence in northern Scandinavian countries compared to Mediterranean countries in the south. A similar difference is found between North and South America and between countries in Asia. In Oslo, the capital of Norway, the highest hip fracture incidence ever published was found in 1988/89 (124/100,000 annually for patients aged ≥50 years).[3] These numbers also represent a 50% increased hip fracture risk in Oslo compared to rural areas in the same country. The importance of increasing age, female gender, comorbidities, smoking, low body mass index (BMI) and previous osteoporotic fractures for hip fracture risk is well known. Further, the importance of sunlight and vitamin D and calcium for bone health is well established, as are the positive effects of physical activity. Genetic and ethnic differences also play an important role in the individual risk of sustaining a hip fracture.

In Norway, the average hip fracture patient is 80 years old and 72% of patients are female.[2] In parts of the world where life expectancy is much lower, geriatric fractures are, for obvious reasons, less of an issue. However, life expectancy is expected to increase considerably in developing countries and the elderly population in Asia and Western countries will multiply over the coming decades. These demographic changes, despite being indicators of improved health status and better living conditions, will also bring major challenges. Providing adequate healthcare services for future generations and a rapidly growing number of elderly patients will be demanding. However, several recent studies from Western countries have actually found a decline in hip fracture incidence, for women in particular.[4–6] Whether this reflects better health in general, a reduction in osteoporotic fractures secondary to medication, or other reasons, is not clear.

CLASSIFICATION

Femoral neck fractures have traditionally been classified as intracapsular or extracapsular fractures. Several classification systems have been designed to grade intracapsular fractures, based on anatomical location (subcapital or transcervical), displacement of the fracture (Garden and AO/OTA) or the angle of the fracture (Pauwels). Many authors suggest that the most reliable classification of intracapsular femoral neck fractures, both clinically and in scientific papers, is simply to divide the fractures into displaced and non-displaced.

Garden classification

The Garden classification was first described in 1961 and still is the most commonly used classification system for intracapsular fractures.[7] The fractures are divided into four groups based on the type and degree of displacement on the anteroposterior (AP) radiograph (Figure 34.1). A Garden I fracture is an incomplete fracture with an intact medial calcar and valgus impaction. A Garden II fracture is a complete but undisplaced fracture. A Garden III fracture is a complete fracture with incomplete displacement, where the trabecular lines in the proximal fragment are in varus relative to those in the distal fragment and in the acetabulum. A Garden IV fracture is a complete fracture with complete displacement.

A major drawback with the Garden classification is that it has been found to have poor reliability.[8-10] Several authors have advocated a simplification of the classification into non-displaced (Garden I and II) and displaced (Garden III and IV) fractures, which increases the reliability.[9-11] Studies have found this simplification sufficient for clinical use, with no benefit conferred when subdividing the undisplaced and displaced fractures further.[12,13] Accordingly, the simplified Garden classification is clinically relevant and is extensively used in treatment guidelines and scientific papers.

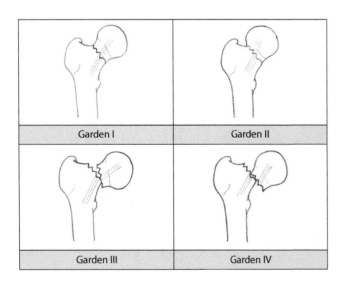

Figure 34.1 Garden classification.

Pauwels classification

The Pauwels classification was described in 1935.[14] This classification uses the inclination angle between the fracture line and the horizontal line on the AP radiograph to identify three subtypes of femoral neck fractures (Figure 34.2). Pauwels type I fractures have an angle of less than 30 degrees, in type II fractures the angle is 30–50 degrees and in type III the angle is larger than 50 degrees. The shearing stress over the fracture increases with increasing fracture angle at the expense of compression forces. Pauwels consequently suggested that the greater the angle of the fracture, the greater the probability of nonunion and failure following internal fixation. However, this association has not been supported in the literature.[15] There are several problems related to the use of Pauwels classification. First, to measure the fracture angle is difficult because the femur may be rotated. Second, the interpretation of the classification system in the literature has frequently been wrong.[16] Finally, the reliability of Pauwels classification has been reported as fair.[17]

AO classification

The AO (Arbeitsgemeninschaft für Osteosynthesefragen) has developed a comprehensive classification system for femoral neck fractures according to their severity and complexity in subtypes 31 B1 to 31 B3.[18] Type B1 comprises subcapital fractures with impaction or slight displacement,

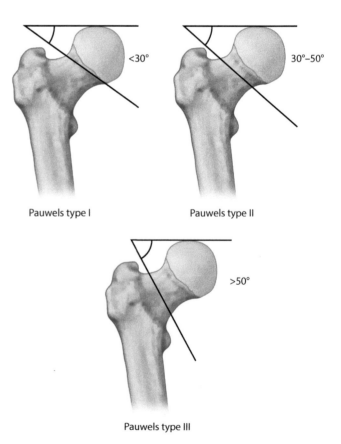

Figure 34.2 Pauwels classification.

the transcervical fractures are defined as subtype B2 and the displaced subcapital fractures are defined as subtype B3. The AO classification has, however, not been used frequently either clinically or for research purposes, probably due to its complexity.

CLINICAL ASSESSMENT

The clinical assessment of these patients can be difficult due to cognitive impairment and occult causes for the fall that may have precipitated the fracture. The patient should be assessed with a complete history and physical examination. A collateral history from family members or carers can be invaluable. The history should clearly determine both the mechanism of injury, as well as for any medical causes that have led to the presentation, e.g. arrhythmia or stroke. Be sure to establish if the patient has had a prolonged lie prior to presentation, as this can lead to a raised CK level and renal failure.

The medical and drug history should identify all preexisting comorbidities and medications, including anticoagulants that may need to be adjusted perioperatively. An understanding of the patient's baseline cognitive and functional status is essential.

The classic presenting features of a neck of femur fracture are hip pain, inability to weight bear and a shortened and externally rotated leg. The neurovascular status of the limb should be assessed, as well as the presence of any associated injuries. Please also see the perioperative care section below.

Imaging

Imaging should include an AP X-ray of the pelvis and a lateral view of the affected hip. Advanced imaging such as a bone scan, CT or MRI may be required when the diagnosis is in doubt or when a pathological fracture is suspected.

TREATMENT

The treatment of intracapsular femoral neck fractures should be individualized. Generally, and well supported in the literature, displaced femoral neck fractures in the elderly should be treated with an arthroplasty, and no longer with closed reduction and internal fixation.[19–31] This will reduce pain, improve function and substantially lower the number of surgical complications and subsequent need for reoperations. This trend, which shifted over the past few decades from internal fixation to arthroplasty, is also reflected in data from the Norwegian Hip Fracture Register (NHFR) (Figure 34.3). It is, however, less clear which type of arthroplasty is best, and whether arthroplasties should be cemented or not. Furthermore, it remains controversial which fractures and patients may still be treated with an internal fixation. Finally, several implants for internal fixation are optional, and there is no clear consensus as to which implant should be preferred. The decision-making should be evidence based on the patient's physiological age, functional status and a detailed analysis of the fracture pattern.

Non-operative treatment

In general, all intracapsular fractures of the proximal femur in the elderly should be treated surgically. Fractures left untreated will either have an increased risk of secondary displacement or, if primarily displaced, will cause unacceptable pain, and appropriate nursing or mobilization of the

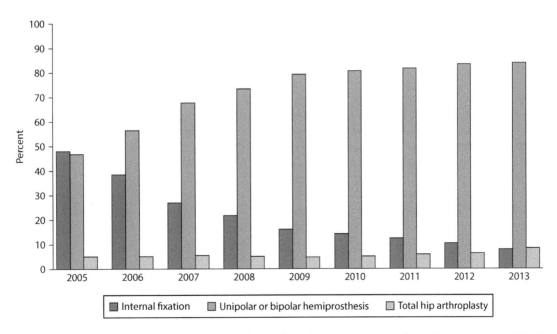

Figure 34.3 Time trends in the treatment of displaced femoral neck fractures. (Data from The Norwegian Hip Fracture Register, Annual Report 2014.)

patient will be impossible. The mortality for these patients is high.

Conservative treatment of valgus impacted or undisplaced femoral neck fractures (Garden I and II) in younger patients may have a good prognosis and acceptable rates of secondary displacement, but much higher complication rates must be expected in the elderly.[32,33] In their study of 115 patients with undisplaced femoral neck fractures, Shuqiang et al. found a strong correlation between secondary displacement and age, whereas fracture instability was independent of gender, American Society of Anesthesiologists (ASA) grade and Pauwels angle.[33] For patients in their seventh and eighth decade, a 48% secondary dislocation rate was found. Raaymakers found a similar correlation with age in a study of undisplaced fractures in 311 patients.[32] For healthy patients <70 years of age, a 7% secondary dislocation rate was found, while 41% of the patients older than 70 years had a secondary fracture dislocation. Additionally, fracture instability was also found to be negatively influenced by comorbidities, and for patients older than 70 years of age with more than one concomitant disease the failure rate increased to 83%.

There are, however, exceptions where non-operative treatment might be considered even in the elderly. When patients are so unwell that they are not expected to survive surgery, non-operative management might be justified. Non-operative treatment should include early mobilization, and only a short bed rest if required for pain relief. Non-weight-bearing would be preferable, but if this is not possible, weight bearing as tolerated should be accepted. If pain does not subside over time, if ambulation is not possible and certainly if fracture displacement is apparent, surgical treatment should be recommended. Treating acute hip fractures conservatively with bed rest for several weeks or months should no longer be an alternative. In our practice, non-operative treatment for any kind of femoral neck fracture is very unusual, and we do not recommend it.

Internal fixation

For young patients with displaced intracapsular femoral neck fractures the goal is to preserve the native femoral head, and closed reduction and internal fixation of the fracture are generally recommended. In the elderly, however, recent literature would suggest that displaced femoral neck fractures should be treated with an arthroplasty.[19-31] Compared to internal fixation, an immediate hip replacement for elderly patients will predictably reduce pain, speed up recovery, improve function and substantially lower the surgical complication rate and subsequent need for reoperations.

UNDISPLACED FRACTURES

Some 15–20% of all hip fractures are valgus impacted or undisplaced intracapsular femoral neck fractures (Garden I and II). Regardless of age and functional status of the patient, internal fixation is usually considered a good treatment option for these fractures. Percutaneous or mini-invasive surgical techniques using cannulated screws, or alternatively a sliding hip screw (SHS), are the most commonly used methods.[34] Parker et al. compared 346 patients treated with cannulated screws for *undisplaced* intracapsular fracture to a matched group of patients treated with a hemiarthroplasty for *displaced* intracapsular fractures.[35] They reported an increased risk of reoperation after treatment with cannulated screws compared to hemiarthroplasty, but internal fixation resulted in less perioperative complications, better functional outcome and a lower 1-year mortality. They concluded that internal fixation should be the treatment of choice for all undisplaced femoral neck fractures, even for elderly patients. Sikand et al. came to the same conclusion in their study. They found a higher mortality rate after hemiarthroplasties but more reoperations in the internal fixation group.[36]

Nevertheless, despite this apparent consensus on treatment, and a relatively good prognosis, mechanical failure, avascular necrosis, nonunion and hardware related pain may cause reoperation rates of 11–27% after internal fixation of undisplaced fractures.[35,37–41] In addition, the studies defining current treatment standards for undisplaced hip fractures were mostly based on old and uncemented prostheses with well-documented inferior results. Today, these prostheses should probably no longer be used. The results in favour of internal fixation in such studies should therefore be interpreted with caution.

A recent observational study from the NHFR found that patients with undisplaced fractures treated with cannulated screws had a poorer clinical outcome and a significantly higher reoperation rate after 1 year compared to a similar group of patients treated with contemporary hemiarthroplasties for displaced femoral neck fractures.[39] These data suggest that there might be a potential for improving results after undisplaced femoral neck fractures by using hemiarthroplasty. Another study from the NHFR could not find any significant difference in 1-year mortality comparing internal fixation (IF) and hemiarthroplasty (HA) in displaced fractures.[25]

Hui et al. suggested hemiarthroplasty as the preferred treatment for undisplaced fractures in patients older than 80 years.[42] They found a 31% reoperation rate for undisplaced fractures in patients older than 80 years treated with an SHS, whereas patients younger than 80 years had a significantly better prognosis (7% reoperation rate). Similarly, patients greater than 80 years with displaced fractures treated with a hemiarthroplasty had a 7% reoperation rate. In their study, mortality was not different between treatment groups.

To our knowledge no randomized clinical trial comparing IF and HA for undisplaced fractures has been published. The evidence in the current literature is inconsistent and limited, and the role of primary arthroplasty in the treatment of undisplaced femoral neck fractures in the elderly remains unclear. More studies, preferably large randomized trials, are required before the extended use of arthroplasty in elderly patients with undisplaced femoral neck fractures might be established as a common treatment. These studies should also take into account the health economic aspects of treatment.

DISPLACED FRACTURES

In general, closed reduction and internal fixation is no longer recommended for displaced femoral neck fractures in the elderly. These fractures are best treated with an arthroplasty and will be discussed later in this chapter.

However, some healthy elderly people remain very active, and their activity level, bone stock and biological age may be comparable to people much younger. Having an arthroplasty might be incompatible with their lifestyle and expectations of remaining highly active. In an effort to preserve a high functional level, even at the expense of an increased risk of mechanical failure, nonunion and avascular necrosis, closed reduction and internal fixation might be justified for these particular patients. Unless a perfect reduction of the fracture is obtained, a primary arthroplasty should be the treatment of choice for these patients.

IMPLANTS

The type of implant for internal fixation of femoral neck fractures is still a matter of discussion. It has not yet been proven whether cannulated screws or an SHS, with or without an antirotation screw, is the better implant.[43,44] Previous studies have not been sufficiently powered to give a definitive answer, and even meta-analyses have so far been unable to detect any major difference in outcome between these two implants. A summary of the results from 30 randomized trials comparing different implants in more than 6000 patients with femoral neck fractures concluded that the existing evidence does not clearly support one type of cannulated screw or pin over another.[44] Even though cannulated screws may result in a shorter operative time and less blood loss, and fractures treated with an SHS may have less avascular necrosis, long-term clinical outcomes and complication rates are comparable. Most of the relevant literature on these implant issues is not up-to-date. The question of whether there are clinically relevant differences between cannulated screws and a SHS device is currently being addressed in a large randomized multicenter and multinational clinical trial.[45]

Several new implants have been invented in recent years with the aim of improving results after internal fixation of femoral neck fractures, including various angular stable implants, as well as hydroxyapatite coated or augmented implants. So far, it remains to be proven in larger series whether these new implants will outperform traditional methods. Results after internal fixation of femoral neck fractures seem to be more dependent on fracture type, patient characteristics, quality of reduction and implant position than on the implant itself. In lateral or basocervical femoral neck fractures, where the calcar support for the cannulated screw is no longer intact, alternative methods such as the SHS are preferred.

PROGNOSIS AND SURGICAL TECHNIQUE

Increasing age, high ASA grade, cognitive impairment and pre-fracture domicile are established predictors of a poorer outcome, including nonunion and mechanical failure after internal fixation of femoral neck fractures. Unfortunately, these factors cannot be influenced. However, the quality of the reduction and the implant position are also important predictors, and these factors can be optimized.

Fracture reduction

Nonunion and mechanical failures correlate with fracture type and the quality of fracture reduction. Garden stated in his classic paper from 1961 that poor reduction is almost synonymous with nonunion, and that a good reduction greatly improves the outcome.[7] Yang et al. found a threefold increased risk of mechanical failure after internal fixation of displaced intracapsular hip fractures compared to undisplaced fractures. Fractures inadequately reduced had an 18 times higher rate of failure compared to those anatomically reduced.[46] Although the results regarding poor outcome are heterogeneous, all studies agree on the importance of a perfect reduction on mechanical failure and reoperation rates in intracapsular hip fractures. Accordingly, anatomical reduction should always be the goal, but a minor valgus position of the femoral head might be accepted. A varus reduction should be avoided as this is a more unstable configuration with shearing instead of compressive forces across the fracture.

Undisplaced fractures may have a posterior tilt of the femoral head in the lateral view. Palm et al. have described a method to measure the posterior tilt of the femoral head in the lateral plane and found a 1-year reoperation rate of 56% for fractures with more than 20 degrees of posterior tilt, as compared to 14% for those with a posterior tilt of less than 20 degrees.[40] Comparable results have also been found in other studies,[38,47] but Lapidus et al., in a review of 382 undisplaced femoral neck fractures, did not find any prognostic value of the posterior tilt measurement.[48] For younger patients we suggest trying to reduce any major dorsal angulation by careful distraction and internal rotation of the leg, but certainly not at the cost of displacing the fracture. Without any reduction, achieving a desirable position for the cannulated screws and thereby sufficient fracture stability may be difficult. Whenever a fracture cannot be satisfactorily reduced, a prosthesis should be the treatment of choice. In elderly patients, fractures with posterior tilt greater than 20 degrees should probably be treated as displaced fractures.

Implant position

The position of the implant is important. Regardless of the number of cannulated screws used, the key position of the first screw is low and central in the femoral head and neck. This screw should have direct calcar support and the threads should be anchored in the subchondral bone (Figure 34.4). This gives the cannulated screw the best three-point fixation

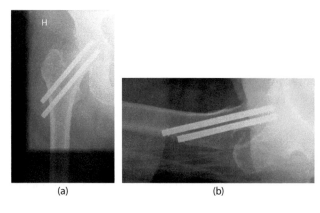

(a)   (b)

Figure 34.4 Internal fixation with two cannulated screws. **(a)** Anteroposterior (AP) and **(b)** lateral views of the right hip.

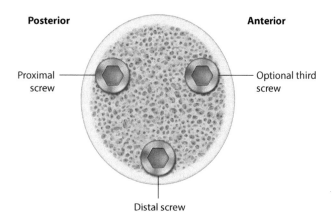

Figure 34.5 Configuration of cannulated screws.

and support for the fracture reduction. The second screw is placed parallel to, and as far away as possible from the first screw (in the AP view). Still, this screw should be anchored in the posterior part of the femoral head and neck for the best purchase in the bone. To provide three-point support, the second screw should rest on the (posterior) cortex. If three screws are used, two of the screws should be placed in the positions described above. The third screw should be placed anterior in the femoral head and neck fragment, thus creating an inverted triangle together with the two other screws (Figure 34.5). For the fracture to settle, and enabling compression without rotation, it is crucial that the screws are parallel. If, for instability reasons, more screws are felt to be required, an arthroplasty should be performed.

Whereas three screws seem to be the most common fixation in most countries, two parallel screws are most frequently used in Scandinavia. The number or type of screws does not seem to have any major influence on outcome. Less attention has been paid to the position of the femoral head and neck screw in an SHS device in femoral neck fractures. A centre–centre position in the AP and lateral plane, as described for intertrochanteric fractures,[49] is probably the best for intracapsular femoral neck fractures. Alternatively, the position might be slightly more caudal, at least when an

extra antirotation screw is added. This would be the case for basocervical fractures, fractures with a vertical fracture line, or fractures with comminution causing inherent instability.

Arthroplasty

HEMIARTHROPLASTY

The main indication for hemiarthroplasty is a displaced femoral neck fracture. Historically, prostheses with well-documented inferior clinical results, such as uncemented Austin-Moore and Thompson prostheses, have been used as treatment for hip fractures. Contemporary prostheses have been more commonly used over the last decade.[50,51] When performing a hemiarthroplasty, femoral stems that have performed well in total hip replacement should be preferred whenever possible.

Treatment with hemiarthroplasty has been compared to internal fixation in several studies (Table 34.1). Treatment with hemiarthroplasties reduces the number of complications and reoperations compared to internal fixation.[23–31] The functional results with contemporary hemiarthroplasties have also been found to be superior to internal fixation.[23–25,31]

Studies comparing old, uncemented Austin-Moore hemiprostheses and internal fixation have not reported such differences, indicating that these prostheses are inferior and should no longer be used.[27,28,30,52] From an economic point of view, hemiarthroplasties are preferable to internal fixation. The initial lower cost associated with internal fixation compared to hemiarthroplasties is outweighed by subsequent costs related to more reoperations and readmissions after internal fixation later on.[55,56] Based on the current literature, modern hemiarthroplasties appear to outperform internal fixation for displaced femoral neck fractures in elderly patients.

A hemiprosthesis can be either uni- or bipolar (Figure 34.6). Several studies have compared the results of bipolar and unipolar prosthesis. The results are summarized in Table 34.2. Unipolar and bipolar hemiarthroplasties seem to have equivalent short-term clinical results. The main concern with unipolar prostheses is the risk of acetabular erosion causing pain and impaired hip function, with some suggesting their use should be limited to very elderly patients with low demands and a relatively short life expectancy. The severity of erosion correlates with age, the level of physical activity and the duration of follow-up.[64,65] Increasing erosion over time may cause acetabular protrusion that has been found to be present in up to 16% of unipolar prostheses 10 years postoperatively.[66]

Bipolar prostheses have been found to reduce the risk of acetabular wear due to the dual-bearing system.[59,60] One disadvantage of bipolar hemiarthroplasties is that polyethylene wear may increase the risk of loosening of the prosthesis or interprosthetic dislocation.[67] Two large register based studies have found increased risk of

Table 34.1 Overview of studies comparing clinical results after hemiarthroplasty (HA) and internal fixation (IF)

Study (year)	Number of patients	Follow-up	Reoperation HA	Reoperation IF	Quality of life (EQ-5D) HA	Quality of life (EQ-5D) IF	Harris Hip Score (HHS) HA	Harris Hip Score (HHS) IF
Ravikumar and Marsh (2000)[30][a]	290	13 years	24%	33%	NI	NI	62	55
Parker et al. (2002)[28][a]	455	3 years	5%	40%	NI	NI	NI	NI
Blomfeldt et al. (2005)[52][a]	60	2 years	13%	33%	0.06	0.20	NI	NI
Keating et al. (2006)[26][a]	307	2 years	5%	39%	0.53	0.55	NI	NI
Frihagen et al. (2007)[23][a]	222	2 years	10%	42%	0.72	0.61	71	67
Gjertsen et al. (2008)[25][b]	4335	1 year	3%	23%	0.60	0.51	NI	NI
Hedbeck et al. (2013)[53][a]	60	2 years	3%	23%	0.25	0.11	NI	NI
Stoen et al. (2014)[54][a]	222	6 years	10%	43%	0.34	0.54	66	66

Note: EQ-5D: 0 = health state similar to death, 1 = best possible health state; HHS: 0 = worst possible hip function, 100 = best possible hip function. NI, not investigated.
[a] Randomized controlled study.
[b] Observational study.

Table 34.2 Overview of studies comparing clinical results of bipolar versus unipolar hemiarthroplasties

Study	Number of patients	Follow-up	Revision Unipolar HA	Revision Bipolar HA	Erosion Unipolar HA	Erosion Bipolar HA
Calder et al. (1996)[57][a]	250	1.6/1.9 years	–	–	2%	0%
Raia et al. (2003)[58][a]	115	1 year	3.3%	0%	NI	NI
Jeffcote et al. (2010)[59][a]	52	2 years	3.7%	4.2%	RSA: 1.5 mm	RSA: 0.6 mm
Hedbeck et al. (2011)[60][a]	120	1 year	5%	10%	20%	5%
Leonardsson et al. (2012)[61]	23,509	1.5 years	2.5%	3.5%	–	–
Enocson et al. (2012)[62]	830	3.1 years	7.3%	6%	0.5%	0.5%
Inngul et al. (2013)[63][a]	120	2 years	5%	13%	19%	14%

Note: HA, hemiarthroplasty; NI, not investigated; RSA, radiostereometric analysis.
[a] Randomized controlled study.

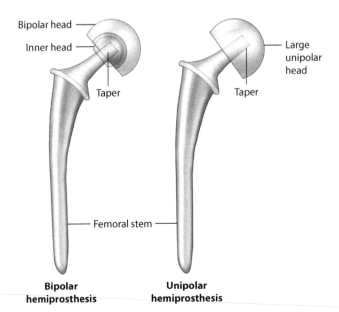

Figure 34.6 Unipolar and bipolar hemiprostheses.

revisions after bipolar hemiarthroplasties, in particular due to infection and periprosthetic fracture in the oldest patients.[61,68] There is no evidence in the current literature in favor of bipolar hemiprostheses regarding clinical outcome in the year following surgery. However, most studies comparing unipolar and bipolar prostheses have a short follow-up.[57–60,62,63,69–73] Some studies, with longer follow-up, have found better quality of life in patients with a bipolar prosthesis.[59,63,72]

For active elderly patients, with a longer life expectancy, a bipolar hemiarthroplasty may reduce the risk of erosion and improve function over time and could be used even if it is more costly. A unipolar prosthesis is certainly appropriate for the oldest and less active patients.

TOTAL HIP ARTHROPLASTY

Total hip arthroplasty (THA) is a well-documented treatment for displaced femoral neck fractures in healthy and independently mobile patients with no cognitive impairment.[19,26,30,65,74–78] For patients with systemic disease affecting the hip joint, such as rheumatoid arthritis, a THA should be considered as primary treatment for a femoral neck fracture. Compared to both internal fixation and hemiarthroplasties, THAs in cognitively fit patients demonstrate superior patient reported outcomes, including less pain, improved quality of life, and better hip function and walking ability.[19,26,75–80] The results of studies comparing THAs with internal fixation are summarized in Table 34.3. Fewer reoperations are reported after THA compared to internal fixation.

Table 34.4 summarizes the results of studies comparing the results of hemiarthroplasties and THAs. According to three meta-analyses, the total risk of reoperation is doubled following hemiarthroplasty versus THA.[81,83] A THA provides good and predictable long-term outcome but at the cost of an increased risk of early dislocation compared to a hemiarthroplasty.[81,83,84] Dislocation is twice as common following THAs when compared to hemiarthroplasties.[81–83] Age, cognitive impairment and a posterior

approach are factors associated with a higher dislocation rate.[85–88] To minimize the risk of dislocation the use of larger heads is recommended.[85] The use of dual mobility cups may further reduce the risk of dislocation and should be taken into account for patients at particularly high risk of dislocation.[89–91]

Compared to a hemiarthroplasty, a THA clearly represents greater surgical trauma for patients with a longer operation time and increased blood loss. Even so, no differences in the number of general complications or in mortality have been found.[81–83] Finally, THA is more expensive than a hemiarthroplasty. However, taking into account the improved long-term implant survival, superior functional outcome and a superior independence for patients who have received a THA, the costs appear to be justified.

Based on the recent literature, a total hip replacement for displaced femoral neck fractures in elderly, cognitively fit patients is a safe procedure with acceptable complication rates and good long-term outcome. A THA should be the

Table 34.3 Overview of studies comparing clinical results after total hip arthroplasty (THA) and internal fixation (IF)

Study (year)	Number of patients	Follow-up	Reoperation		Quality of life (EQ-5D)		Harris Hip Score (HHS)	
			THA	IF	THA	IF	THA	IF
Ravikumar and Marsh (2000)[30 a]	290	13 years	24%	33%	NI	NI	62	55
Blomfeldt et al. (2005)[19 a]	102	4 years	4%	47%	0.61	0.54	NI	NI
Keating et al. (2006)[26 a]	307	2 years	5%	39%	0.53	0.55	NI	NI
Chammout et al. (2012)[21 a]	100	17 years	23%	53%	NI	NI	84	76
Wani et al. (2014)[22 a]	100	1.5 years	0%	20%	NI	NI	94	91
Cao et al. (2014)[20 a]	285	5 years	10%	34%	NI	NI	89[b]	58[b]

Note: EQ-5D: 0 = health state similar to death, 1 = best possible health state; HHS: 0 = worst possible hip function, 100 = best possible hip function. NI, not investigated
[a] Randomized controlled study.
[b] Proportion of patients with HHS between 80 and 100.

Table 34.4 Overview of studies comparing clinical results after total hip arthroplasty (THA) and hemiarthroplasty (HA)

Study (year)	Number of patients	Follow-up	Reoperation		Quality of life (EQ-5D)		Harris Hip Score (HHS)	
			THA	HA	THA	HA	THA	HA
Ravikumar and Marsh (2000)[30 a]	290	13 years	24%	33%	NI	NI	62	55
Keating et al. (2006)[26 a]	307	2 years	5%	39%	0.53	0.55	NI	NI
Blomfeldt et al. (2007)[79 a]	120	1 year	3%	0%	0.68	0.63	87	79
Hedbeck et al. (2011)[76 a]	120	4 years	5%	0%	0.68	0.57	NI	NI

Note: EQ-5D: 0 = health state similar to death, 1 = best possible health state; HHS: 0 = worst possible hip function, 100 = best possible hip function. NI, not investigated.
[a] Randomized controlled study.

first choice in healthy patients with good pre-functional status and limited comorbidities.

SURGICAL APPROACH

The surgical approach for hemiarthroplasty and THA has been a controversial subject. The direct lateral approach as described by Hardinge involves detaching the anterior part of the gluteus medius.[92] After this approach some patients develop deficiency of the abductors of the hip producing a painful Trendelenburg gait.[93] In the posterior approach the insertions of the short external rotators of the hip are divided.[94] In hip fracture patients re-attachment of the posterior capsule and/or the external rotators should be done to decrease the risk of dislocation.[88,95,96] Compared to the lateral approach, the posterior approach has been shown to more than double the risk of dislocation after hemiarthroplasties and to result in a sixfold increase in dislocations after THAs.[68,88,95,97] The lateral approach, on the contrary, is associated with an increased reoperation rate due to postoperative haematoma and infection.[68,97] Consequently, the overall number of reoperations after posterior and lateral approaches has been reported to be similar in two studies.[61,97]

The Watson-Jones anterolateral inter-muscular approach between the tensor fascia lata and gluteus medius muscles has recently become more popular.[98] Even if early recovery is faster, no advantages in long-term results have been found for this approach compared to the direct lateral approach.[99,100] The Watson-Jones approach is associated with a longer surgery time and larger variations in implant positioning indicating that there is a learning curve.[101]

The anterior Smith-Petersen approach between the sartorius and tensor fascia lata muscles is rarely used. It has been associated with more postoperative pain and increased operation time compared to the lateral approach.[102]

Minimal invasive surgery (MIS) has gained increasing popularity recently. Reduced visibility, increased soft tissue constraints on instruments, and loss of landmarks may be pitfalls that increase the risk of malpositioning of components during MIS. It is still controversial whether MIS should be performed for the treatment of hip fractures and the results of different studies comparing MIS with conventional surgery are ambiguous.[103–105]

The available approaches have their advantages and complications. There is little evidence supporting the superiority of one approach over another. The most important factor determining the result of the surgery is probably not the approach itself, but the experience of the surgeon.[102,106] When performing arthroplasty surgery, junior surgeons should always be assisted by senior surgeons with experience in arthroplasty surgery and the surgical approach that the surgeons are most familiar with should be used.

IMPLANTS AND FIXATION

One of the most important issues in arthroplasty surgery is fixation of the prosthesis. This part of the surgery is critical for implant survival. Unsatisfactory fixation increases the risk of early loosening of the prosthesis. The femoral stem and acetabular component can be a cemented or uncemented design (Figure 34.7). In the past, old uncemented stems with documented inferior results have been used in the treatment of elderly patients with femoral neck fractures. More recently contemporary stems with hydroxyapatite coating have been used. When using cemented stems most surgeons use antibiotic impregnated bone cement, which has been demonstrated to reduce the risk of infection.[107,108] Cemented stems have been associated with a reduced risk of reoperation, in particular due to periprosthetic fractures and infection, when compared to uncemented prostheses.[50,68,109–111] A reduced reoperation rate has also been found when only contemporary femoral stems were compared. In a large register based study of contemporary cemented and uncemented hemiarthroplasties, the 5-year implant survival was 95% for cemented stems, and 91% for uncemented stems. The uncemented stems had doubled the risk of reoperation when compared to cemented stems, in particular due to an increased risk of periprosthetic fracture.[50]

Periprosthetic femoral fractures are an established complication of uncemented and some cemented implants.[112] These fractures occur more frequently in the elderly osteoporotic patient.[113] There are concerns regarding the potential cardiopulmonary risks associated with the use of cemented prostheses. Minor or major adverse events occur and increased perioperative mortality has been found after insertion of cemented hemiarthroplasties compared to uncemented procedures.[114–116] The increased mortality is most pronounced in those with multiple comorbidities.[115]

Conversely, a large study from the National Hip Fracture Database in the United Kingdom has reported improved perioperative survival for patients treated with a cemented arthroplasty compared to uncemented procedures.[117] Serious intraoperative cardiopulmonary complications may be caused by the so-called bone cement

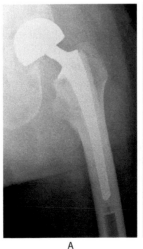
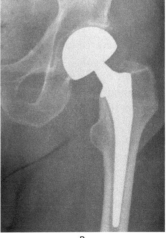

A   B

Figure 34.7 (a) Cemented and (b) uncemented femoral prostheses.

implantation syndrome.[118] When using cemented implants it is therefore crucial to optimize the patients before surgery, and anaesthetic input is essential to reduce cardiopulmonary complications. A bone-vacuum cementing technique has been shown to reduce the number of severe embolic events and could be considered for the frailest patients.[119,120] Downsizing the final femoral stem compared to the last reamer will also slightly decrease the cement pressure, which may be beneficial for these frail patients. Otherwise, for the more healthy patients (i.e. ASA grade 1–2),[121] modern cementing techniques, including high pressure lavage and insertion of an intramedullary distal plug, should be used to reduce the risk of implant loosening, although this is an infrequent reason for revision following hemiarthroplasty.

Based on the current literature, cemented implants appear superior with fewer surgical complications and reoperations. On the other hand, the cardiopulmonary side effects caused by bone cement implantation syndrome must be minimized. No matter which prosthesis and what fixation are preferred, the most important factor for a good surgical outcome is probably a good surgical technique.

Perioperative care

In order to reduce morbidity, mortality and complications, and to facilitate rapid recovery, a collaborative multidisciplinary approach is essential.[122–127] Femoral neck fractures should ideally be treated within 24 hours of presentation, and at latest within 48 hours after admission.[126,128–130] Still, some patients need optimization before surgery can be performed.[126] These patients should be assessed by experienced orthogeriatricians/physicians and anaesthesiologists prior to surgery. Delirium should be identified and treated, or even better, prevented where possible.[131] No studies have proven any benefit from preoperative traction, and this should not be used.[132] The preferred analgesics are paracetamol and additional opioids.[126] A peripheral nerve blockade, such as a fascia iliaca block, may provide effective analgesia and thereby reduce the need for opioids.[133]

Surgery is routinely performed using regional anaesthesia, or in selected cases general anaesthesia is used when this is contraindicated. No consensus exists as to which is the preferred or superior method.[132] However, there are concerns about neuraxial procedures in patients treated with newer oral anticoagulants due to the risk of bleeding.[134]

At present, there is no consensus regarding the optimal protocol for venous thromboembolism prophylaxis after hip fracture surgery.[132] At our institution we use prophylaxis with low molecular weight heparin initiated preoperatively. To reduce the risk of postoperative infections, prophylactic antibiotics are prescribed to all hip fracture patients, regardless of operative method.[107,135,136]

Surgery should be performed or supervised by an experienced surgeon in order to reduce reoperation rates.[126,137] Physiotherapists are essential in the early postoperative period and after discharge. The appropriate discharge destination is dictated by the patient's comorbidity, ambulatory ability and social support network, and by availability of rehabilitation facilities.[132] The goal of rehabilitation should be a rapid return to the pre-morbid level of function and to limit long-term disability.

Prevention

The importance of correct implant selection and well-performed surgical treatment in hip fracture care is indisputable. However, this will not prevent patients from sustaining a hip fracture. Consequently, a strategy to limit the hip fracture epidemic in the future is needed. The diagnosis and treatment of osteoporosis and falls prevention are the two key issues to be addressed. Strategies to identify patients at risk and well-documented preventive measures should be developed and subsequently implemented into daily practice.

Fracture liaison services (FLS), which represent a systematic approach to secondary fracture prevention, have been found to be cost-effective in preventing new fractures.[138] After introduction of FLS in Glasgow, the hip fracture rate was reduced by 7.3%, while at the same time, the rate increased by 17% in England.[139] Introducing effective falls prevention programs must be another major goal in the prevention of hip fractures, and hip protectors have been found to be effective when they are used.[140] Further research and product development should be encouraged, and methods to improve compliance need to be established.

Ultimately, the reasons why a patient falls are multifactorial. A detailed analysis and more knowledge about falls (when, where, why, how and in whom do they occur) is required to optimize the resources and to target interventions in the best way. To achieve these goals, major efforts and clear priorities from healthcare providers and society will be required. Improving elderly patients' balance, strength and general physical capacity would undoubtedly be beneficial, but how to achieve these goals, and how to assess the individual effects of different steps undertaken to reduce the number of falls, is a major challenge and needs to be explored.

Authors' preferred treatment

Our treatment of intracapsular femoral neck fractures has evolved over time. The patient factors to be addressed remain the same, but the indications for different treatment options, and to which patient each treatment should be offered, have changed.

Fracture displacement is the most important factor to address and in our opinion not only displacement in the AP view, but also displacement and angulation in the lateral view must be taken into account. Second, the patient's medical condition must be addressed. The patient's age, comorbidity, cognitive function, mobility, compliance and bone stock should be assessed before a decision can be made. Regardless of the chosen treatment for the individual

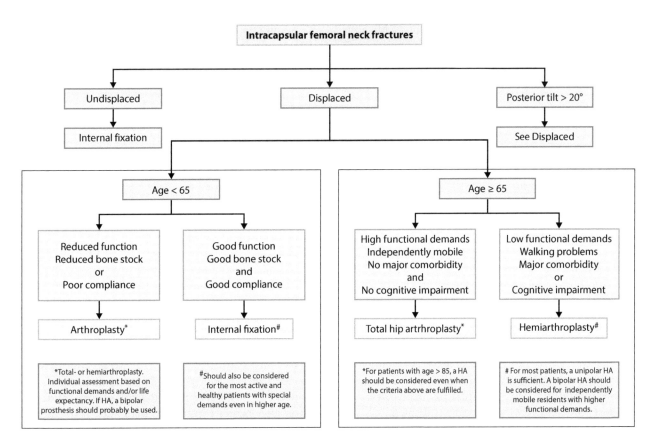

Figure 34.8 Authors' suggested algorithm.

patient, the perioperative treatment of all patients must be optimized as described earlier in this chapter. In general, we recommend surgical treatment for all femoral neck fractures in an elderly patient. Our treatment algorithm is summarized in Figure 34.8.

UNDISPLACED FRACTURES

The undisplaced femoral neck fracture is treated with internal fixation irrespective of age. We are aware of the common use of three screws placed in an inverted triangle in the femoral head and neck, but in our hands only two parallel cannulated screws are used for these fractures. In our opinion, it is not well documented that three screws are superior to two. We believe that a perfect reduction and the position of the screws are more important than the number of screws. To provide three-point support for both screws, the screws are positioned inferior and central in the AP view. In the lateral view the distal screw is positioned central and the proximal screw posterior. The older patient weight bears with crutches as tolerated. For the youngest patients we consider touch weight bearing if possible. Some fractures with no displacement on the AP view, but a posterior tilt of more than 20 degrees on the lateral view, have in the literature been shown to have inferior results when treated with internal fixation. In our opinion, these fractures should be treated as a displaced fracture.

DISPLACED FRACTURES IN YOUNGER PATIENTS

Displaced femoral neck fractures in healthy patients less than 65 years should in most cases be treated with closed reduction and internal fixation with two parallel screws. Special attention to achieve a good reduction is essential. If the fracture cannot be successfully reduced, an arthroplasty should be considered. Some patients, although young, may already have osteoporosis because of medical conditions, and their functional demands are low. For these patients we consider some form of arthroplasty. The type of prosthesis is based on individual assessment taking the patient's functional demands and life expectancy into consideration. We normally use a cemented bipolar hemiarthroplasty. In patients with poor compliance, such as alcohol abuse, a dual mobility total hip replacement may be used to reduce the risk of dislocation. Patients with a displaced femoral neck fracture and co-existing symptomatic hip osteoarthritis or rheumatoid arthritis are in our opinion best treated with a cemented THA.

DISPLACED FRACTURES IN OLDER PATIENTS

We prefer an arthroplasty for most patients above 65 years of age. The type of prosthesis selected is based on the patient's functional demands, walking ability, comorbidity, age and cognitive status. There is accumulating evidence in the literature that total hip replacements outperform hemiarthroplasties in the treatment of these fractures.

The healthiest, independently mobile patients with high functional demands should therefore be treated with a total hip replacement. In our practice we have no upper age limit for treating a patient with a total hip replacement, but we normally treat the oldest patients with a hemiarthroplasty even if the criteria above are fulfilled. We always use large metal prosthesis heads (32 mm) and a lateral approach to reduce the risk of dislocation. Most patients with femoral neck fractures, however, present with reduced function, low functional demands, walking problems, major comorbidity or cognitive impairment. For these patients, we prefer a cemented hemiarthroplasty. Until now, a bipolar hemiarthroplasty has been our favoured implant. As unipolar and bipolar hemiarthroplasties seem to have equivalent short-term clinical results, a unipolar hemiarthroplasty is probably sufficient for the oldest and less active patients. For the more active elderly patients, with a longer life expectancy, a bipolar hemiarthroplasty may reduce the risk of erosion and improve function over time. To reduce the risk of periprosthetic fractures, we recommend using well-documented cemented modern stems for all arthroplasties in elderly patients. However, to reduce the risk of bone cement implantation syndrome we normally reduce the size of the femoral stem and introduce it slowly. All patients treated with an arthroplasty progressively weight bear as tolerated.

POSTOPERATIVE FOLLOW-UP

We review all patients treated with an arthroplasty in the outpatient clinic 3 months postoperatively. The patients treated with internal fixation are reviewed 6 weeks postoperatively and are followed every 3 months until the fracture has healed.

Complications

Taking the nature of the fracture, the patient's age and frequent comorbidities into account, some complications are probably inevitable. The treatment of surgical complications, and even more important the prevention of such, is a challenge for orthopaedic surgeons. We believe careful and evidence-based selection of treatment modality, considering specific fracture and patient factors, together with attention to detail during surgery, may prevent surgical complications.

FIXATION FAILURE AND NONUNION

Two-thirds of all intracapsular femoral neck fractures are displaced (Garden III or IV), and most displaced fractures are currently treated with an arthroplasty.[141] Accordingly, nonunion and failure of internal fixation is less of a problem after a displaced femoral neck fracture in the elderly. However, internal fixation is the treatment of choice for undisplaced fractures, and for these 'stable' fractures, complication and reoperation rates of 11–27% are documented.[35,37–41]

Secondary fracture displacement and nonunion, implant failure and late avascular necrosis may occur. In this age group such complications will usually require the same treatment – a prosthetic hip replacement. In a study by Gjertsen et al., a prosthetic hip replacement was performed in 85% of the reoperations among patients treated with internal fixation for undisplaced fractures.[39] Occasionally, and after an otherwise successful healing process, removing an implant causing local pain might be justified. In elderly patients, a reoperation including revision internal fixation is rarely an option.

PROSTHESIS DISLOCATION

Dislocation is a well-documented complication after hip prosthesis surgery for fracture.[85,87,142,143] The risk of dislocation is most pronounced in the first year postoperatively.[144] Hip fracture patients treated with a THA have twice the risk of dislocation compared to osteoarthritis patients.[144] The rate of dislocation reported in the literature varies from 2% to 29%.[20,21,26,65,80,145,146] Increasing age, cognitive dysfunction and the posterior approach are associated with increased risk of dislocation.[85,86,88,95,97] The use of larger prosthesis heads or dual mobility cups decreases the risk of dislocation.[85,87,90,91,147] Furthermore, the risk of dislocation is 50% lower after hemiarthroplasties than after THA for femoral neck fractures.[81–83] Accordingly, to decrease the risk of revision in patients with a high risk of dislocation, a posterior approach should probably be avoided. Furthermore, prostheses with large heads, dual mobility cups or hemiarthroplasties should be considered.

Dislocations of THAs and unipolar hemiarthroplasties can normally be treated with closed reduction performed with sedatives or general anaesthesia. Closed reduction of a bipolar hemiarthroplasty is not always possible and an open reduction may be required. In 40% of patients with recurrent THA dislocations, revision surgery is performed.[148] Malposition of the implants is probably the most important cause of dislocation. This can best be investigated with a CT scan and a revision of the prosthesis should be performed if malposition is confirmed. A revision of the prosthesis normally includes an increase of offset, change of implant position or conversion to a dual mobility prosthesis.

INFECTION

Postoperative infection is probably the worst and most devastating complication after hip fracture surgery. Increasing age and comorbidity are factors associated with an increased risk of infection.[149] The incidence of infection after arthroplasty surgery has been reduced from 5–10% in the late 1960s to approximately 1% now. This is probably due to improved surgical technique, better perioperative treatment and antibiotic prophylaxis.[150,151] The use of antibiotic prophylaxis, both systemically and in bone cement, has been shown to reduce the risk of infection after hip replacement, and systemic antibiotic prophylaxis should be mandatory for all arthroplasties.[107,108]

Symptoms can vary from low grade pain, with or without other symptoms of infection, to the most dramatic cases of fulminant prosthetic joint infection with life-threatening sepsis. The diagnosis is made based on a combination of clinical symptoms, blood tests including inflammatory markers, radiological findings and microbiology/histopathological examination of peri-implant tissue and fluid. For equivocal cases, aspiration of the hip is indicated.

For hip arthroplasty, the treatment of an acute postoperative infection or an acute delayed infection (haematogenous) is in most cases irrigation and debridement with retention of the prosthesis. For chronic prosthesis infections, and for persistent infection after soft tissue debridement, a revision with exchange of the prosthesis should be performed. A one-stage revision can be an alternative for infections due to susceptible microbial pathogens in frail patients who are unlikely to tolerate further surgery. However, a two-stage revision with or without temporary implantation of an antibiotic-loaded spacer, followed by delayed reimplantation of the prosthesis, is seen as the gold standard by many and provides the lowest rate of recurrent infections. Antibiotic suppression alone may be an alternative when surgery presents a too high a risk in very old and frail patients.[152]

CONCLUSIONS

The proximal femoral fracture is the classic orthogeriatric fracture. In this group of old and frail patients, serious non-surgical complications are common, and the mortality is high. Elderly hip fracture patients have a 30-day mortality of approximately 10% and a 1-year mortality of 20–30%. The annual number of hip fractures will increase world wide and the management and care of elderly hip fracture patients now, and in the future, will be a major challenge for all healthcare systems. The diagnosis and treatment of osteoporosis and falls prevention are two main issues that need to be addressed.

It is essential to use a multidisciplinary approach for the management of these patients. Inevitably, enhanced focus on prevention and optimization of the treatment will be required. More research and interest in prevention, and less focus on surgical technique and implant related questions, should be a goal for the future. To identify patients at risk and to develop well-documented preventive measures, and subsequently implement these measures into daily life, is the mutual responsibility of politicians, society and healthcare professionals.

REFERENCES

1. Dennison E, Mohamed MA, Cooper C. Epidemiology of osteoporosis. *Rheum Dis Clin North Am* 2006;32:617–29.
2. Gjertsen JE, Engesaeter LB, Furnes O, Havelin LI, Steindal K, Vinje T, Fevang JM. The Norwegian Hip Fracture Register. Experiences after the first 2 years and 15,576 reported hips. *Acta Orthop* 2008;79(5):583–93.
3. Falch JA, Kaastad TS, Bohler G, Espeland J, Sundsvold OJ. Secular increase and geographical differences in hip fracture incidence in Norway. *Bone* 1993;14:643–5.
4. Brauer CA, Coca-Perraillon M, Cutler DM, Rosen AB. Incidence and mortality of hip fractures in the United States. *JAMA* 2009;302:1573–9.
5. Kannus P, Niemi S, Parkkari J, Palvanen M, Vuori I, Jarvinen M. Nationwide decline in incidence of hip fracture. *J Bone Miner Res* 2006;21:1836–8.
6. Lofthus CM, Osnes EK, Falch JA, Kaastad TS, Kristiansen IS, Nordsletten L, Stensvold I, Meyer HE. Epidemiology of hip fractures in Oslo, Norway. *Bone* 2001;29:413–18.
7. Garden RS. Low-angle fixation in fractures of the femoral neck. *J Bone Joint Surg Br* 1961;43-B:647–63.
8. Frandsen PA, Andersen E, Madsen F, Skjodt T. Garden's classification of femoral neck fractures. An assessment of inter-observer variation. *J Bone Joint Surg Br* 1988;70:588–90.
9. Scavenius M, Ibsen A, Rønnebech J, Aagaard H. Inter- and intra observer variation in the assessment of femoral neck fractures according to the Garden classification. *Acta Orthop Scand* 1996;67(Suppl. 267):29.
10. Van ED, Rhemrev SJ, Genelin F, Meylaerts SA, Roukema GR. The reliability of a simplified Garden classification for intracapsular hip fractures. *Orthop Traumatol Surg Res* 2012;98:405–8.
11. Thomsen NO, Jensen CM, Skovgaard N, Pedersen MS, Pallesen P, Soe-Nielsen NH, Rosenklint A. Observer variation in the radiographic classification of fractures of the neck of the femur using Garden's system. *Int Orthop* 1996;20:326–9.
12. Eliasson P, Hansson LI, Karrholm J. Displacement in femoral neck fractures. A numerical analysis of 200 fractures. *Acta Orthop Scand* 1988;59:361–4.
13. Parker MJ. Garden grading of intracapsular fractures: Meaningful or misleading? *Injury* 1993;24:241–2.
14. Pauwels F. *Der Schenkelhalsbruch. Ein mechanisches Problem*. Beilagheft Z. Orthop Chir. 63, F. Enke, Stuttgart, 1935.
15. Parker MJ, Dynan Y. Is Pauwels classification still valid? *Injury* 1998;29:521–3.
16. Bartonicek J. Pauwels' classification of femoral neck fractures: Correct interpretation of the original. *J Orthop Trauma* 2001;15:358–60.
17. Van ED, Roukema GR, Rhemrev SJ, Genelin F, Meylaerts SA. The Pauwels classification for intracapsular hip fractures: Is it reliable? *Injury* 2011;42:1238–40.

18. Muller ME. [Classification and international AO-documentation of femur fractures]. *Unfallheilkunde* 1980;83(5):251–9.

19. Blomfeldt R, Tornkvist H, Ponzer S, Soderqvist A, Tidermark J. Comparison of internal fixation with total hip replacement for displaced femoral neck fractures. Randomized, controlled trial performed at four years. *J Bone Joint Surg Am* 2005;87:1680–8.

20. Cao L, Wang B, Li M, Song S, Weng W, Li H, Su J. Closed reduction and internal fixation versus total hip arthroplasty for displaced femoral neck fracture. *Chin J Traumatol* 2014;17:63–8.

21. Chammout GK, Mukka SS, Carlsson T, Neander GF, Stark AW, Skoldenberg OG. Total hip replacement versus open reduction and internal fixation of displaced femoral neck fractures: A randomized long-term follow-up study. *J Bone Joint Surg Am* 2012;94:1921–8.

22. Wani IH, Sharma S, Latoo I, Salaria AQ, Farooq M, Jan M. Primary total hip arthroplasty versus internal fixation in displaced fracture of femoral neck in sexa- and septuagenarians. *J Orthop Traumatol* 2014;15(3):209–14.

23. Frihagen F, Nordsletten L, Madsen JE. Hemiarthroplasty or internal fixation for intracapsular displaced femoral neck fractures: Randomised controlled trial. *BMJ* 2007;335:1251–4.

24. Gjertsen JE, Vinje T, Lie SA, Engesaeter LB, Havelin LI, Furnes O, Fevang JM. Patient satisfaction, pain, and quality of life 4 months after displaced femoral neck fracture. A comparison of 663 fractures treated with internal fixation and 906 with bipolar hemiarthroplasty reported to the Norwegian Hip Fracture Register. *Acta Orthop* 2008;79(5):594–601.

25. Gjertsen JE, Vinje T, Engesaeter LB, Lie SA, Havelin LI, Furnes O, Fevang JM. Internal screw fixation compared with bipolar hemiarthroplasty for treatment of displaced femoral neck fractures in elderly patients. *J Bone Joint Surg Am* 2010;92-A:619–28.

26. Keating JF, Grant A, Masson M, Scott NW, Forbes JF. Randomized comparison of reduction and fixation, bipolar hemiarthroplasty, and total hip arthroplasty. Treatment of displaced intracapsular hip fractures in healthy older patients. *J Bone Joint Surg Am* 2006;88:249–60.

27. Parker MJ, Pryor GA. Internal fixation or arthroplasty for displaced cervical hip fractures in the elderly: A randomised controlled trial of 208 patients. *Acta Orthop Scand* 2000;71:440–6.

28. Parker MJ, Khan RJ, Crawford J, Pryor GA. Hemiarthroplasty versus internal fixation for displaced intracapsular hip fractures in the elderly. A randomised trial of 455 patients. *J Bone Joint Surg Br* 2002;84:1150–5.

29. Parker MJ, Gurusamy K. Internal fixation versus arthroplasty for intracapsular proximal femoral fractures in adults. *Cochrane Database Syst Rev* 2006;(4):CD001708.

30. Ravikumar KJ, Marsh G. Internal fixation versus hemiarthroplasty versus total hip arthroplasty for displaced subcapital fractures of femur—13 year results of a prospective randomised study. *Injury* 2000;31:793–7.

31. Roden M, Schon M, Fredin H. Treatment of displaced femoral neck fractures: A randomized minimum 5-year follow-up study of screws and bipolar hemiprostheses in 100 patients. *Acta Orthop Scand* 2003;74:42–4.

32. Raaymakers EL. The non-operative treatment of impacted femoral neck fractures. *Injury* 2002;33(Suppl. 3):C8–14.

33. Shuqiang M, Kunzheng W, Zhichao T, Mingyu Z, Wei W. Outcome of non-operative management in Garden I femoral neck fractures. *Injury* 2006;37:974–8.

34. Bhandari M, Devereaux PJ, Tornetta P, III, Swiontkowski MF, Berry DJ, Haidukewych G, Schemitsch EH, et al. Operative management of displaced femoral neck fractures in elderly patients. An international survey. *J Bone Joint Surg Am* 2005;87:2122–30.

35. Parker MJ, White A, Boyle A. Fixation versus hemiarthroplasty for undisplaced intracapsular hip fractures. *Injury* 2008;39(7):791–5.

36. Sikand M, Wenn R, Moran CG. Mortality following surgery for undisplaced intracapsular hip fractures. *Injury* 2004;35:1015–19.

37. Bjorgul K, Reikeras O. Outcome of undisplaced and moderately displaced femoral neck fractures. *Acta Orthop* 2007;78:498–504.

38. Conn KS, Parker MJ. Undisplaced intracapsular hip fractures: Results of internal fixation in 375 patients. *Clin Orthop Relat Res* 2004;(421):249–54.

39. Gjertsen JE, Fevang JM, Matre K, Vinje T, Engesaeter LB. Clinical outcome after undisplaced femoral neck fractures. *Acta Orthop* 2011;82:268–74.

40. Palm H, Gosvig K, Krasheninnikoff M, Jacobsen S, Gebuhr P. A new measurement for posterior tilt predicts reoperation in undisplaced femoral neck fractures: 113 consecutive patients treated by internal fixation and followed for 1 year. *Acta Orthop* 2009;80:303–7.

41. Rogmark C, Flensburg L, Fredin H. Undisplaced femoral neck fractures—No problems? A consecutive study of 224 patients treated with internal fixation. *Injury* 2009;40:274–6.

42. Hui AC, Anderson GH, Choudhry R, Boyle J, Gregg PJ. Internal fixation or hemiarthroplasty for undisplaced fractures of the femoral neck in octogenarians. *J Bone Joint Surg Br* 1994;76:891–4.

43. Watson A, Zhang Y, Beattie S, Page RS. Prospective randomized controlled trial comparing dynamic hip screw and screw fixation for undisplaced subcapital hip fractures. *ANZ J Surg* 2013;83:679–83.

44. Parker MJ, Stockton G. Internal fixation implants for intracapsular proximal femoral fractures in adults. *Cochrane Database Syst Rev* 2001;(4):CD001467.

45. Bhandari M, Sprague S, Schemitsch EH. Resolving controversies in hip fracture care: The need for large collaborative trials in hip fractures. *J Orthop Trauma* 2009;23(6):479–84.

46. Yang JJ, Lin LC, Chao KH, Chuang SY, Wu CC, Yeh TT, Lian YT. Risk factors for nonunion in patients with intracapsular femoral neck fractures treated with three cannulated screws placed in either a triangle or an inverted triangle configuration. *J Bone Joint Surg Am* 2013;95:61–9.

47. Clement ND, Green K, Murray N, Duckworth AD, McQueen MM, Court-Brown CM. Undisplaced intracapsular hip fractures in the elderly: Predicting fixation failure and mortality. A prospective study of 162 patients. *J Orthop Sci* 2013;18:578–85.

48. Lapidus LJ, Charalampidis A, Rundgren J, Enocson A. Internal fixation of Garden I and II femoral neck fractures: Posterior tilt did not influence the reoperation rate in 382 consecutive hips followed for a minimum of 5 years. *J Orthop Trauma* 2013;27:386–90.

49. Baumgaertner MR, Curtin SL, Lindskog DM, Keggi JM. The value of the tip-apex distance in predicting failure of fixation of peritrochanteric fractures of the hip. *J Bone Joint Surg Am* 1995;77:1058–64.

50. Gjertsen JE, Lie SA, Vinje T, Engesaeter LB, Hallan G, Matre K, Furnes O. More reoperations with uncemented hemiarthroplasties than with cemented hemiarthroplasties for the treatment of displaced femoral neck fractures. An observational study of 11,116 hemiarthroplasties reported to the Norwegian Hip Fracture Register. *J Bone Joint Surg Br* 2012;94(8):1113–19.

51. Leonardsson O, Garellick G, Karrholm J, Akesson K, Rogmark C. Changes in implant choice and surgical technique for hemiarthroplasty. 21,346 procedures from the Swedish Hip Arthroplasty Register 2005–2009. *Acta Orthop* 2012;83:7–13.

52. Blomfeldt R, Tornkvist H, Ponzer S, Soderqvist A, Tidermark J. Internal fixation versus hemiarthroplasty for displaced fractures of the femoral neck in elderly patients with severe cognitive impairment. *J Bone Joint Surg Br* 2005;87:523–9.

53. Hedbeck CJ, Inngul C, Blomfeldt R, Ponzer S, Tornkvist H, Enocson A. Internal fixation versus cemented hemiarthroplasty for displaced femoral neck fractures in patients with severe cognitive dysfunction: A randomized controlled trial. *J Orthop Trauma* 2013;27:690–5.

54. Stoen RO, Lofthus CM, Nordsletten L, Madsen JE, Frihagen F. Randomized trial of hemiarthroplasty versus internal fixation for femoral neck fractures: No difference at 6 years. *Clin Orthop Relat Res* 2014;472:360–7.

55. Frihagen F, Waaler GM, Madsen JE, Nordsletten L, Aspaas S, Aas E. The cost of hemiarthroplasty compared to that of internal fixation for femoral neck fractures. 2-year results involving 222 patients based on a randomized controlled trial. *Acta Orthop* 2010;81:446–52.

56. Rogmark C, Carlsson A, Johnell O, Sembo I. Costs of internal fixation and arthroplasty for displaced femoral neck fractures: A randomized study of 68 patients. *Acta Orthop Scand* 2003;74:293–8.

57. Calder SJ, Anderson GH, Jagger C, Harper WM, Gregg PJ. Unipolar or bipolar prosthesis for displaced intracapsular hip fracture in octogenarians: A randomised prospective study. *J Bone Joint Surg Br* 1996;78:391–4.

58. Raia FJ, Chapman CB, Herrera MF, Schweppe MW, Michelsen CB, Rosenwasser MP. Unipolar or bipolar hemiarthroplasty for femoral neck fractures in the elderly? *Clin Orthop Relat Res* 2003;(414):259–65.

59. Jeffcote B, Li MG, Barnet-Moorcroft A, Wood D, Nivbrant B. Roentgen stereophotogrammetric analysis and clinical assessment of unipolar versus bipolar hemiarthroplasty for subcapital femur fracture: A randomized prospective study. *ANZ J Surg* 2010;80:242–6.

60. Hedbeck CJ, Blomfeldt R, Lapidus G, Tornkvist H, Ponzer S, Tidermark J. Unipolar hemiarthroplasty versus bipolar hemiarthroplasty in the most elderly patients with displaced femoral neck fractures: A randomised, controlled trial. *Int Orthop* 2011;35(11):1703–11.

61. Leonardsson O, Karrholm J, Akesson K, Garellick G, Rogmark C. Higher risk of reoperation for bipolar and uncemented hemiarthroplasty. *Acta Orthop* 2012;83(5):459–66.

62. Enocson A, Hedbeck CJ, Tornkvist H, Tidermark J, Lapidus LJ. Unipolar versus bipolar Exeter hip hemiarthroplasty: A prospective cohort study on 830 consecutive hips in patients with femoral neck fractures. *Int Orthop* 2012;36(4):711–17.

63. Inngul C, Hedbeck CJ, Blomfeldt R, Lapidus G, Ponzer S, Enocson A. Unipolar hemiarthroplasty versus bipolar hemiarthroplasty in patients with displaced femoral neck fractures. A four-year follow-up of a randomised controlled trial. *Int Orthop* 2013;37:2457–64.

64. Phillips TW. Thompson hemiarthroplasty and acetabular erosion. *J Bone Joint Surg Am* 1989;71:913–17.

65. Baker RP, Squires B, Gargan MF, Bannister GC. Total hip arthroplasty and hemiarthroplasty in mobile, independent patients with a displaced intracapsular fracture of the femoral neck. A randomized, controlled trial. *J Bone Joint Surg Am* 2006;88:2583–9.

66. Wachtl SW, Jakob RP, Gautier E. Ten-year patient and prosthesis survival after unipolar hip hemiarthroplasty in female patients over 70 years old. *J Arthroplasty* 2003;18:587–91.

67. Figved W, Norum OJ, Frihagen F, Madsen JE, Nordsletten L. Interprosthetic dislocations of the Charnley/Hastings hemiarthroplasty. Report of 11 cases in 350 consecutive patients. *Injury* 2006;37:157–61.

68. Rogmark C, Fenstad AM, Leonardsson O, Engesaeter LB, Karrholm J, Furnes O, Garellick G, Gjertsen JE. Posterior approach and uncemented stems increases the risk of reoperation after hemi-arthroplasties in elderly hip fracture patients. *Acta Orthop* 2014;85:18–25.

69. Cornell CN, Levine D, O'Doherty J, Lyden J. Unipolar versus bipolar hemiarthroplasty for the treatment of femoral neck fractures in the elderly. *Clin Orthop Relat Res* 1998;(348):67–71.

70. Ong BC, Maurer SG, Aharonoff GB, Zuckerman JD, Koval KJ. Unipolar versus bipolar hemiarthroplasty: Functional outcome after femoral neck fracture at a minimum of thirty-six months of follow-up. *J Orthop Trauma* 2002;16:317–22.

71. Sabnis B, Brenkel IJ. Unipolar versus bipolar unce-mented hemiarthroplasty for elderly patients with displaced intracapsular femoral neck fractures. *J Orthop Surg (Hong Kong)* 2011;19:8–12.

72. Stoffel KK, Nivbrant B, Headford J, Nicholls RL, Yates PJ. Does a bipolar hemiprosthesis offer advantages for elderly patients with neck of femur fracture? A clinical trial with 261 patients. *ANZ J Surg* 2013;83:249–54.

73. Wathne RA, Koval KJ, Aharonoff GB, Zuckerman JD, Jones DA. Modular unipolar versus bipolar prosthesis: A prospective evaluation of functional outcome after femoral neck fracture. *J Orthop Trauma* 1995;9:298–302.

74. Abboud JA, Patel RV, Booth RE, Jr., Nazarian DG. Outcomes of total hip arthroplasty are similar for patients with displaced femoral neck fractures and osteoarthritis. *Clin Orthop Relat Res* 2004;(421):151–4.

75. Healy WL, Iorio R. Total hip arthroplasty: Optimal treatment for displaced femoral neck frac-tures in elderly patients. *Clin Orthop Relat Res* 2004;(429):43–8.

76. Hedbeck CJ, Enocson A, Lapidus G, Blomfeldt R, Tornkvist H, Ponzer S, Tidermark J. Comparison of bipolar hemiarthroplasty with total hip arthroplasty for displaced femoral neck fractures: A concise four-year follow-up of a randomized trial. *J Bone Joint Surg Am* 2011;93:445–50.

77. Johansson T, Jacobsson SA, Ivarsson I, Knutsson A, Wahlstrom O. Internal fixation versus total hip arthro-plasty in the treatment of displaced femoral neck fractures: A prospective randomized study of 100 hips. *Acta Orthop Scand* 2000;71:597–602.

78. Leonardsson O, Rolfson O, Hommel A, Garellick G, Akesson K, Rogmark C. Patient-reported outcome after displaced femoral neck fracture: A national survey of 4467 patients. *J Bone Joint Surg Am* 2013;95:1693–9.

79. Blomfeldt R, Tornkvist H, Eriksson K, Soderqvist A, Ponzer S, Tidermark J. A randomised controlled trial comparing bipolar hemiarthroplasty with total hip replacement for displaced intracapsular fractures of the femoral neck in elderly patients. *J Bone Joint Surg Br* 2007;89:160–5.

80. Tidermark J, Ponzer S, Svensson O, Soderqvist A, Tornkvist H. Internal fixation compared with total hip replacement for displaced femoral neck fractures in the elderly. A randomised, controlled trial. *J Bone Joint Surg Br* 2003;85:380–8.

81. Liao L, Zhao J, Su W, Ding X, Chen L, Luo S. A meta-analysis of total hip arthroplasty and hemiarthroplasty outcomes for displaced femo-ral neck fractures. *Arch Orthop Trauma Surg* 2012;132:1021–9.

82. Yu L, Wang Y, Chen J. Total hip arthroplasty versus hemiarthroplasty for displaced femoral neck frac-tures: Meta-analysis of randomized trials. *Clin Orthop Relat Res* 2012;470:2235–43.

83. Zi-Sheng A, You-Shui G, Zhi-Zhen J, Ting Y, Chang-Qing Z. Hemiarthroplasty vs primary total hip arthroplasty for displaced fractures of the femoral neck in the elderly: A meta-analysis. *J Arthroplasty* 2012;27:583–90.

84. Burgers PT, Van Geene AR, Van den Bekerom MP, Van Lieshout EM, Blom B, Aleem IS, Bhandari M, Poolman RW. Total hip arthroplasty versus hemi-arthroplasty for displaced femoral neck fractures in the healthy elderly: A meta-analysis and sys-tematic review of randomized trials. *Int Orthop* 2012;36:1549–60.

85. Bystrom S, Espehaug B, Furnes O, Havelin LI. Femoral head size is a risk factor for total hip luxation: A study of 42,987 primary hip arthroplas-ties from the Norwegian Arthroplasty Register. *Acta Orthop Scand* 2003;74:514–24.

86. Woolson ST, Rahimtoola ZO. Risk factors for dislocation during the first 3 months after pri-mary total hip replacement. *J Arthroplasty* 1999;14:662–8.

87. Berry DJ, von Knoch M, Schleck CD, Harmsen WS. Effect of femoral head diameter and opera-tive approach on risk of dislocation after primary total hip arthroplasty. *J Bone Joint Surg Am* 2005;87:2456–63.

88. Enocson A, Hedbeck CJ, Tidermark J, Pettersson H, Ponzer S, Lapidus LJ. Dislocation of total hip replacement in patients with fractures of the femoral neck. *Acta Orthop* 2009;80(2):184–9.

89. Adam P, Philippe R, Ehlinger M, Roche O, Bonnomet F, Mole D, Fessy MH. Dual mobility cups hip arthroplasty as a treatment for displaced fracture of the femoral neck in the elderly. A prospective, systematic, multicenter study with specific focus on postoperative dislocation. *Orthop Traumatol Surg Res* 2012;98:296–300.

90. Bensen AS, Jakobsen T, Krarup N. Dual mobility cup reduces dislocation and re-operation when used to treat displaced femoral neck fractures. *Int Orthop* 2014;38(6):1241–5.

91. Tarasevicius S, Busevicius M, Robertsson O, Wingstrand H. Dual mobility cup reduces dislocation rate after arthroplasty for femoral neck fracture. *BMC Musculoskelet Disord* 2010;11:175.

92. Hardinge K. The direct lateral approach to the hip. *J Bone Joint Surg Br* 1982;64:17–19.

93. Edmunds CT, Boscainos PJ. Effect of surgical approach for total hip replacement on hip function using Harris Hip scores and Trendelenburg's test. A retrospective analysis. *Surgeon* 2011;9:124–9.

94. Moore AT. The self-locking metal hip prosthesis. *J Bone Joint Surg Am* 1957;39-A:811–27.

95. Enocson A, Tidermark J, Tornkvist H, Lapidus LJ. Dislocation of hemiarthroplasty after femoral neck fracture: Better outcome after the anterolateral approach in a prospective cohort study on 739 consecutive hips. *Acta Orthop* 2008;79(2):211–17.

96. Tarasevicius S, Robertsson O, Wingstrand H. Posterior soft tissue repair in total hip arthroplasty: A randomized controlled trial. *Orthopedics* 2010;33:871.

97. Biber R, Brem M, Singler K, Moellers M, Sieber C, Bail HJ. Dorsal versus transgluteal approach for hip hemiarthroplasty: An analysis of early complications in seven hundred and four consecutive cases. *Int Orthop* 2012;36:2219–23.

98. Bertin KC, Rottinger H. Anterolateral mini-incision hip replacement surgery: A modified Watson-Jones approach. *Clin Orthop Relat Res* 2004;(429):248–55.

99. Martin R, Clayson PE, Troussel S, Fraser BP, Docquier PL. Anterolateral minimally invasive total hip arthroplasty: A prospective randomized controlled study with a follow-up of 1 year. *J Arthroplasty* 2011;26:1362–72.

100. Landgraeber S, Quitmann H, Guth S, Haversath M, Kowalczyk W, Kecskemethy A, Heep H, Jager M. A prospective randomized peri- and post-operative comparison of the minimally invasive anterolateral approach versus the lateral approach. *Orthop Rev (Pavia)* 2013;5:e19.

101. Mouilhade F, Matsoukis J, Oger P, Mandereau C, Brzakala V, Dujardin F. Component positioning in primary total hip replacement: A prospective comparative study of two anterolateral approaches, minimally invasive versus gluteus medius hemimyotomy. *Orthop Traumatol Surg Res* 2011;97:14–21.

102. Auffarth A, Resch H, Lederer S, Karpik S, Hitzl W, Bogner R, Mayer M, Matis N. Does the choice of approach for hip hemiarthroplasty in geriatric patients significantly influence early postoperative outcomes? A randomized-controlled trial comparing the modified Smith-Petersen and Hardinge approaches. *J Trauma* 2011;70:1257–62.

103. Park KS, Oh CS, Yoon TR. Comparison of minimally invasive total hip arthroplasty versus conventional hemiarthroplasty for displaced femoral neck fractures in active elderly patients. *Chonnam Med J* 2013;49:81–6.

104. Repantis T, Bouras T, Korovessis P. Comparison of minimally invasive approach versus conventional anterolateral approach for total hip arthroplasty: A randomized controlled trial. *Eur J Orthop Surg Traumatol* 2015;25(1)111–16.

105. Tsukada S, Wakui M. Minimally invasive intermuscular approach does not improve outcomes in bipolar hemiarthroplasty for femoral neck fracture. *J Orthop Sci* 2010;15:753–7.

106. Keene GS, Parker MJ. Hemiarthroplasty of the hip—The anterior or posterior approach? A comparison of surgical approaches. *Injury* 1993;24:611–13.

107. Engesaeter LB, Lie SA, Espehaug B, Furnes O, Vollset SE, Havelin LI. Antibiotic prophylaxis in total hip arthroplasty: Effects of antibiotic prophylaxis systemically and in bone cement on the revision rate of 22,170 primary hip replacements followed 0–14 years in the Norwegian Arthroplasty Register. *Acta Orthop Scand* 2003;74:644–51.

108. Espehaug B, Engesaeter LB, Vollset SE, Havelin LI, Langeland N. Antibiotic prophylaxis in total hip arthroplasty. Review of 10,905 primary cemented total hip replacements reported to the Norwegian Arthroplasty Register, 1987 to 1995. *J Bone Joint Surg Br* 1997;79:590–5.

109. Foster AP, Thompson NW, Wong J, Charlwood AP. Periprosthetic femoral fractures—A comparison between cemented and uncemented hemiarthroplasties. *Injury* 2005;36:424–9.

110. Langslet E, Frihagen F, Opland V, Madsen JE, Nordsletten L, Figved W. Cemented versus uncemented hemiarthroplasty for displaced femoral neck fractures: 5-year followup of a randomized trial. *Clin Orthop Relat Res* 2014;472:1291–9.

111. Viberg B, Overgaard S, Lauritsen J, Ovesen O. Lower reoperation rate for cemented hemiarthroplasty than for uncemented hemiarthroplasty and internal fixation following femoral neck fracture: 12- to 19-year follow-up of patients aged 75 years or more. *Acta Orthop* 2013;84:254–9.

112. Berry DJ. Epidemiology: Hip and knee. *Orthop Clin North Am* 1999;30(2):183–90.

113. Dorr LD, Glousman RF, Hoy AL, Vanis RF, Chandler R. Treatment of femoral neck fractures with total hip replacement versus cemented and noncemented hemiarthroplasty. *J Arthroplasty* 1986;1(1):21–8.

114. Costain DJ, Whitehouse SL, Pratt NL, Graves SE, Ryan P, Crawford RW. Perioperative mortality after hemiarthroplasty related to fixation method. *Acta Orthop* 2011;82:275–81.

115. Talsnes O, Vinje T, Gjertsen JE, Dahl OE, Engesaeter LB, Baste V, Pripp AH, Reikeras O. Perioperative mortality in hip fracture patients treated with cemented and uncemented hemiprosthesis: A register study of 11,210 patients. *Int Orthop* 2013;37(6):1135–40.

116. Yli-Kyyny T, Sund R, Heinanen M, Venesmaa P, Kroger H. Cemented or uncemented hemiarthroplasty for the treatment of femoral neck fractures? *Acta Orthop* 2014;85:49–53.

117. Costa ML, Griffin XL, Pendleton N, Pearson M, Parsons N. Does cementing the femoral component increase the risk of peri-operative mortality for patients having replacement surgery for a fracture of the neck of femur? Data from the National Hip Fracture Database. *J Bone Joint Surg Br* 2011;93:1405–10.

118. Donaldson AJ, Thomson HE, Harper NJ, Kenny NW. Bone cement implantation syndrome. *Br J Anaesth* 2009;102:12–22.

119. Engesaeter LB, Strand T, Raugstad TS, Husebo S, Langeland N. Effects of a distal venting hole in the femur during total hip replacement. *Arch Orthop Trauma Surg* 1984;103:328–31.

120. Pitto RP, Koessler M, Kuehle JW. Comparison of fixation of the femoral component without cement and fixation with use of a bone-vacuum cementing technique for the prevention of fat embolism during total hip arthroplasty. A prospective, randomized clinical trial. *J Bone Joint Surg Am* 1999;81:831–43.

121. American Society of Anaesthesiologists. New classification of physical status. *Anaesthesiology* 1963;24:111.

122. Vidan M, Serra JA, Moreno C, Riquelme G, Ortiz J. Efficacy of a comprehensive geriatric intervention in older patients hospitalized for hip fracture: A randomized, controlled trial. *J Am Geriatr Soc* 2005;53:1476–82.

123. Dy CJ, Dossous PM, Ton QV, Hollenberg JP, Lorich DG, Lane JM. Does a multidisciplinary team decrease complications in male patients with hip fractures? *Clin Orthop Relat Res* 2011;469:1919–24.

124. Kammerlander C, Roth T, Friedman SM, Suhm N, Luger TJ, Kammerlander-Knauer U, Krappinger D, Blauth M. Ortho-geriatric service—A literature review comparing different models. *Osteoporos Int* 2010;21:S637–46.

125. Pedersen SJ, Borgbjerg FM, Schousboe B, Pedersen BD, Jorgensen HL, Duus BR, Lauritzen JB. A comprehensive hip fracture program reduces complication rates and mortality. *J Am Geriatr Soc* 2008;56:1831–8.

126. National Institute for Health and Clinical Excellence. *The management of hip fractures in adults* (Clinical guideline CG124). NICE, 2011. https://www.nice.org.uk/guidance/cg124

127. Dy CJ, Dossous PM, Ton QV, Hollenberg JP, Lorich DG, Lane JM. The medical orthopaedic trauma service: An innovative multidisciplinary team model that decreases in-hospital complications in patients with hip fractures. *J Orthop Trauma* 2012;26:379–83.

128. Hamlet WP, Lieberman JR, Freedman EL, Dorey FJ, Fletcher A, Johnson EE. Influence of health status and the timing of surgery on mortality in hip fracture patients. *Am J Orthop (Belle Mead NJ)* 1997;26:621–7.

129. Orosz GM, Magaziner J, Hannan EL, Morrison RS, Koval K, Gilbert M, McLaughlin M, Halm EA, Wang JJ, Litke A, Silberzweig SB, Siu AL. Association of timing of surgery for hip fracture and patient outcomes. *JAMA* 2004;291:1738–43.

130. Zuckerman JD, Skovron ML, Koval KJ, Aharonoff G, Frankel VH. Postoperative complications and mortality associated with operative delay in older patients who have a fracture of the hip. *J Bone Joint Surg Am* 1995;77:1551–6.

131. National Institute for Health and Clinical Excellence. *Delirium: Diagnosis, Prevention and Management* (Clinical guideline CG103). NICE, 2010. https://www.nice.org.uk/guidance/cg103

132. Egol KA, Strauss EJ. Perioperative considerations in geriatric patients with hip fracture: What is the evidence? *J Orthop Trauma* 2009;23:386–94.

133. Foss NB, Kristensen BB, Bundgaard M, Bak M, Heiring C, Virkelyst C, Hougaard S, Kehlet H. Fascia iliaca compartment blockade for acute pain control in hip fracture patients: A randomized, placebo-controlled trial. *Anesthesiology* 2007;106:773–8.

134. Benzon HT, Avram MJ, Green D, Bonow RO. New oral anticoagulants and regional anaesthesia. *Br J Anaesth* 2013;111(Suppl. 1):i96–113.

135. Southwell-Keely JP, Russo RR, March L, Cumming R, Cameron I, Brnabic AJ. Antibiotic prophylaxis in hip fracture surgery: A metaanalysis. *Clin Orthop Relat Res* 2004;(419):179–84.

136. Gillespie WJ, Walenkamp GH. Antibiotic prophylaxis for surgery for proximal femoral and other closed long bone fractures. *Cochrane Database Syst Rev* 2010;(3):CD000244.

137. Palm H, Jacobsen S, Krasheninnikoff M, Foss NB, Kehlet H, Gebuhr P. Influence of surgeon's experience and supervision on re-operation rate after hip fracture surgery. *Injury* 2007;38:775–9.

138. Marsh D, Akesson K, Beaton DE, Bogoch ER, Boonen S, Brandi ML, McLellan AR, Mitchell PJ, Sale JE, Wahl DA. Coordinator-based systems for secondary prevention in fragility fracture patients. *Osteoporos Int* 2011;22:2051–65.

139. McLellan AR, Wolowacz SE, Zimovetz EA, Beard SM, Lock S, McCrink L, Adekunle F, Roberts D. Fracture liaison services for the evaluation and management of patients with osteoporotic fracture: A cost-effectiveness evaluation based on data collected over 8 years of service provision. *Osteoporos Int* 2011;22:2083–98.

140. Kannus P, Parkkari J, Niemi S, Pasanen M, Palvanen M, Jarvinen M, Vuori I. Prevention of hip fracture in elderly people with use of a hip protector. *N Engl J Med* 2000;343:1506–13.

141. Havelin LI, Furnes O, Engesaeter LB, Fenstad AM, Dybvik E. *The Norwegian Arthroplasty Register*. Annual report 2014. http://nrlweb.ihelse.net/Rapporter/Rapport2014.pdf

142. Lindberg HO, Carlsson AS, Gentz CF, Pettersson H. Recurrent and non-recurrent dislocation following total hip arthroplasty. *Acta Orthop Scand* 1982;53:947–52.

143. Mishra V, Thomas G, Sibly TF. Results of displaced subcapital fractures treated by primary total hip replacement. *Injury* 2004;35:157–60.

144. Gjertsen JE, Lie SA, Fevang JM, Havelin LI, Engesaeter LB, Vinje T, Furnes O. Total hip replacement after femoral neck fractures in elderly patients: Results of 8,577 fractures reported to the Norwegian Arthroplasty Register. *Acta Orthop* 2007;78(4):491–7.

145. Godoy MD, Iserson KV, Jauregui J, Musso C, Piccaluga F, Buttaro M. Total hip arthroplasty for hip fractures: 5-year follow-up of functional outcomes in the oldest independent old and very old patients. *Geriatr Orthop Surg Rehabil* 2014;5:3–8.

146. Johansson T. Internal fixation compared with total hip replacement for displaced femoral neck fractures: A minimum fifteen-year follow-up study of a previously reported randomized trial. *J Bone Joint Surg Am* 2014;96:e46.

147. Tarasevicius S, Robertsson O, Dobozinskas P, Wingstrand H. A comparison of outcomes and dislocation rates using dual articulation cups and THA for intracapsular femoral neck fractures. *Hip Int* 2013;23:22–6.

148. Daly PJ, Morrey BF. Operative correction of an unstable total hip arthroplasty. *J Bone Joint Surg Am* 1992;74:1334–43.

149. Ridgeway S, Wilson J, Charlet A, Kafatos G, Pearson A, Coello R. Infection of the surgical site after arthroplasty of the hip. *J Bone Joint Surg Br* 2005;87:844–50.

150. Charnley J. Postoperative infection after total hip replacement with special reference to air contamination in the operating room. *Clin Orthop Relat Res* 1972;87:167–87.

151. Gaine WJ, Ramamohan NA, Hussein NA, Hullin MG, McCreath SW. Wound infection in hip and knee arthroplasty. *J Bone Joint Surg Br* 2000;82:561–5.

152. Parvizi J, Adeli B, Zmistowski B, Restrepo C, Greenwald AS. Management of periprosthetic joint infection: The current knowledge: AAOS exhibit selection. *J Bone Joint Surg Am* 2012;94:e104.

35

Extracapsular proximal femur fractures

PAUL M. LAFFERTY

INTERTROCHANTERIC FRACTURES

Introduction

Hip fractures are associated with mortality, impaired function and decreased quality of life. The 1-year mortality rate after a hip fracture is approximately 20%, with men, patients more than 75 years old and patients in nursing homes at higher risk.[1,2] Among patients who were living independently prior to a hip fracture, only about half are able to walk unaided after a fracture,[3,4] and many ultimately require care in a long-term facility. The goal of hip fracture treatment is to decrease pain and return patients to their prefracture level of function.

Intertrochanteric hip fractures are extracapsular fractures of the proximal femur involving the area between the greater and lesser trochanters. Such fractures that extend into the area distal to the lesser trochanter are described as having a subtrochanteric component. The intertrochanteric region has an abundant blood supply, which makes fractures in this area much less susceptible to osteonecrosis and nonunion than femoral neck fractures. It is important to distinguish intertrochanteric fractures from fractures that occur just proximal to the intertrochanteric line. These fractures, referred to as basicervical femoral neck fractures, are at greater risk for osteonecrosis (secondary to being intracapsular in some cases) and malunion. However, they may be treated with the same implants used for intertrochanteric fractures.

Internal fixation of intertrochanteric fractures is the mainstay of treatment, although prosthetic replacement is occasionally indicated. Challenges include the combination of often osteopenic or osteoporotic bone and the adverse biomechanics of many intertrochanteric fracture patterns. Other factors include pre-existing osteoarthritis, degree of fracture comminution and pre-existing medical comorbidities.

The literature regarding intertrochanteric fractures points to the difficulty in applying evidence based treatment algorithms. The current evidence is conflicting and does not always support the treatment modalities that are widely used in practice.

Incidence and etiology

Intertrochanteric hip fractures occur in approximately the same demographics as femoral neck fractures. There is a female:male ratio between approximately 2:1 and 8:1. Patients with femoral neck fractures tend to be slightly older than patient with intertrochanteric fractures. Fractures typically occur following a low energy fall from standing height in often osteoporotic patients.

Anatomy

OSSEOUS

The intertrochanteric area extends between the greater and lesser trochanters. It consists of dense trabecular bone. The calcar femorale is an area of dense bone that extends from the posteromedial aspect of the femoral shaft to the posterior portion of the femoral neck (Figure 35.1).

MUSCULAR

Several muscles originate or insert around the hip (Figure 35.2). These muscles account for the typical deformities encountered following injury.

Patient assessment

PHYSICAL EXAMINATION

The patient with a displaced intertrochanteric femur fracture will typically present with inability to ambulate following the fall, pain in the groin, lateral hip and/or buttocks and will have a shortened and externally rotated lower

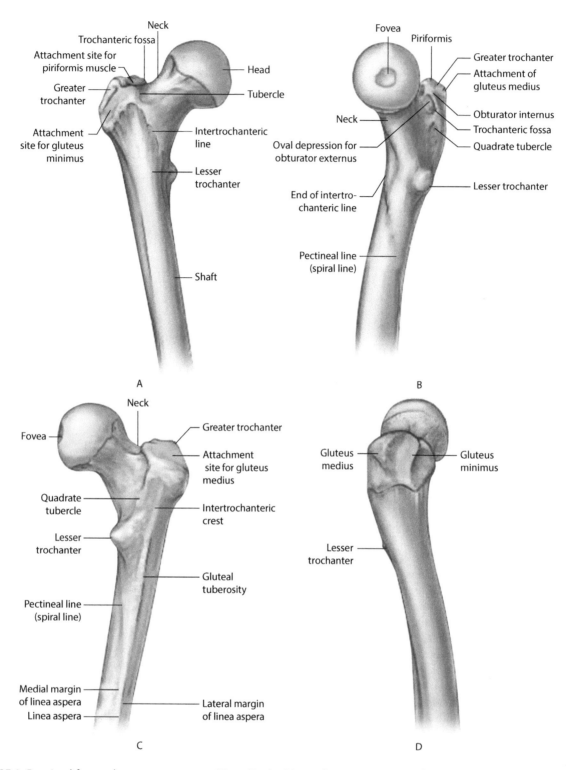

Figure 35.1 Proximal femoral osseous anatomy. (From Drake RL, et al. *Gray's Anatomy for Students*. 2nd ed. Philadelphia, PA: Churchill Livingstone/Elsevier; 2009.)

extremity. Neurovascular status should be carefully documented; however neurovascular injuries are rare in isolated intertrochanteric fractures.

RADIOGRAPHIC ASSESSMENT

Anteroposterior (AP) of the pelvis and AP and lateral views of the affected hip should be obtained in all cases. The contralateral hip on the AP pelvis is used to assist with preoperative planning, allowing the surgeon to ensure implants with appropriate neck-shaft angles are available. In cases where there is concern for subtrochanteric extension or when a long implant is being considered, full-length femur films should be obtained. In the case of suspected fracture with normal X-rays,

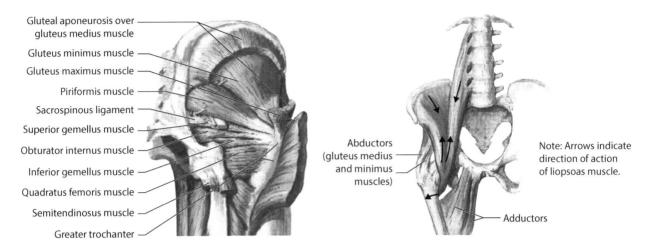

Gluteal aponeurosis over gluteus medius muscle
Gluteus minimus muscle
Gluteus maximus muscle
Piriformis muscle
Sacrospinous ligament
Superior gemellus muscle
Obturator internus muscle
Inferior gemellus muscle
Quadratus femoris muscle
Semitendinosus muscle
Greater trochanter

Abductors (gluteus medius and minimus muscles)

Note: Arrows indicate direction of action of lioposoas muscle.

Adductors

Figure 35.2 Proximal femoral muscular anatomy. Deforming forces affecting alignment of a proximal femoral fracture include the iliopsoas, short external rotators and hip abductors. (From Netter FH. *Atlas of Human Anatomy*. 4th ed. Philadelphia, PA: Saunders/Elsevier; 2006.)

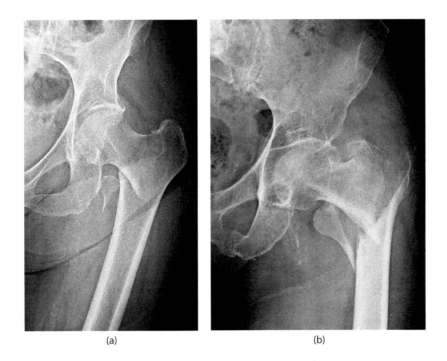

(a) (b)

Figure 35.3 Stable (a) and unstable (b) intertrochanteric fracture patterns. Note the minimal involvement of the medial calcar in (a) versus that seen in (b).

an MRI should be obtained to assess for nondisplaced fracture.

Traction-internal rotation views can be obtained to delineate between intertrochanteric and basicervical femoral neck fractures when necessary.

Classification

Most classification systems for intertrochanteric fractures have poor reliability and reproducibility. A simplified system to aid in evaluating treatment algorithms when assessing the literature is based on fracture stability, which is related to the condition of the posteromedial cortex. Fractures are considered stable in the absence of a comminuted posteromedial cortex, reverse obliquity and subtrochanteric extension.

Intertrochanteric fractures are typically classified as stable or unstable. Fractures are generally considered unstable when there is significant involvement of the medial calcar or lateral wall and when a reverse obliquity pattern or subtrochanteric extension is present (Figure 35.3). These fractures may also be classified according to the AO/OTA system (Figure 35.4).[5]

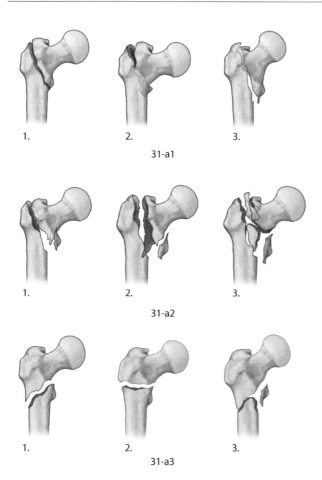

1.　　　2.　　　3.

31-a1

1.　　　2.　　　3.

31-a2

1.　　　2.　　　3.

31-a3

Figure 35.4 AO/OTA classification of intertrochanteric femur fractures. (From Rockwood CA, et al. *Rockwood and Green's Fractures in Adults*. 6th ed. Philadelphia, PA: Lippincott Williams & Wilkins; 2006.)

Management

NONOPERATIVE

Nonsurgical treatment of intertrochanteric hip fractures is usually reserved for patients with nondisplaced fractures discovered on MRI or comorbidities that place these patients at unacceptable risk from anaesthesia, the surgical procedure or both. Mortality from surgical treatment typically results from cardiopulmonary complications, thromboembolism and sepsis.[6]

Operative

Ten useful tips to consider when fixing intertrochanteric hip fractures are listed in Table 35.1.[7]

A strong case cannot be made in favor of specific surgical treatments for any type of hip fracture with use of the current randomized trial literature. Patient outcomes associated with different techniques produce only modest differences, if any. Any beneficial effect of one implant class over another appears to reach equivalence within 6 months after surgery. In addition, the literature often does not include important covariates that are essential in order to draw clinically

relevant conclusions about the effects of various treatments, given differences in baseline patient characteristics, fracture patterns and provider specific variables that affect treatment quality. The overall strength of the evidence in support of one treatment over another is low. The current randomized trial literature neither sufficiently nor consistently identifies fracture pattern subtypes enough to relate specific fracture patterns to non-mortality outcomes, particularly for intertrochanteric hip fractures. The inconsistency by which surgeons classify the AO/OTA 31A fracture subtypes as stable versus unstable across studies also substantially impedes comparison of results from orthopaedic randomized trials.[8]

Despite the lack of evidence supporting one fixation method over another, a dramatic change has occurred in surgeon preference for fixation devices, particularly among young orthopaedic surgeons and in training programs.[9] A review of the American Board of Orthopaedic Surgery Database found that the use of intramedullary devices increased from 3% in 1999 to 67% in 2006.[10] A comparative effectiveness study of Veterans Affairs hospital patients found that intramedullary nail use increased significantly from 1998 to 2005, but did not decrease perioperative mortality or comorbidity compared with standard plate-and-screw constructs. Additionally, this study and others have found wide geographic variation in implant selection.[10–12] Surgeons are clearly selecting implants on the basis of factors other than clinical outcomes evidence. Factors involved may include higher surgeon reimbursement for intramedullary nailing and the fact that surgeon reimbursement remains insulated from the treating hospital's burden of paying for the higher cost implant under the Medicare payment system.

IMPLANT SELECTION

While some early studies indicated better results with intramedullary nails for unstable fracture patterns,[13] more recent randomized trials and case series have failed to clearly define a benefit to utilizing intramedullary nails, reporting similar outcomes with higher costs compared with sliding hip screws.[14]

The implant decision is sometimes made after positioning the patient and reducing the fracture. Emergency department X-rays are often of suboptimal quality, so verification of the preoperative diagnosis using preoperative traction-internal rotation X-rays or evaluation of the fracture pattern in the operating room with image intensification is sometimes necessary. The stability of the fracture based on the integrity of the lesser trochanter and posteromedial buttress is an important factor. Fractures classified as unstable should be considered for intramedullary nails, whereas stable fractures can be treated adequately with a sliding hip screw. Lateral wall compromise is also critical. It has been found that compromised lateral femoral wall integrity is a significant predictor of reoperation. These patients may not be treated adequately with a sliding hip screw device and may benefit from intramedullary devices.[15] If in doubt about the number of parts and stability, a trochanteric stabilization plate can be added to the sliding hip screw or an intramedullary nail device can be utilized.

Table 35.1 Useful tips for fixing intertrochanteric hip fractures

Tip 1	Use the Tip-to-Apex Distance	• Useful intraoperative indicator of deep and central placement of lag screw in the femoral head, regardless of whether nail or a plate is used • Key measurement of accurate hardware placement • Ideal position for a lag screw in both planes is deep and central in the femoral head within 10mm of the subchondral bone • Tip-to-apex distance of <25mm shown to be generally predictive of a successful result; however, most traumatologists aim for a tip-to-apex distance of <20mm
Tip 2	No Lateral Wall, No Hip Screw	• Fractures involving lateral wall of the proximal femur are classified as either reverse obliquity fractures or transtrochanteric fractures and lack any osseous buttress • Use of sliding hip screws with these fracture types can cause medial translation of femoral shaft • Dr. Haidukewych and colleagues found 56% failure rate with use of sliding hip screw for reverse obliquity fractures of the proximal femur • Locking plates and 95° condylar blade-plates may function as prosthetic lateral cortices, but use with problematic proximal femur fractures has not been studied • IM nails seem to be superior to dynamic condylar screws for reverse obliquity fractures
Tip 3	Know the Unstable Intertrochanteric Fracture Patterns, and Nail Them	• Unstable interotrochanteric fractures should be treated with IM nail versus sliding hip screw due to more favorable biomechanics • Proximity to center of gravity allows resistance to high forces borne by device • Intramedullary positioning prevents shaft medialization, a common complication • There are 4 classic, unstable intertrochanteric fracture patterns: reverse obliquity fractures, transtrochanteric fractures, fractures with large posteromedial fragment, fractures with subtrochanteric extension • Note that a simple fracture of the lesser trochanter should not necessarily be defined as unstable • It is unknown how large the posteromedial fragment must be to be mechanically important • When there is doubt about the status of calcar, it is ideal to use IM nail
Tip 4	Beware of the Anterior Bow of the Femoral Shaft	• With age, the femoral diaphysis enlarges and femoral bow increases • The radius of curvature of an IM nail should ideally be ≤2 m • If resistance is encountered during insertion, always obtain a lateral radiograph of distal part of femur • Using a straight IM nail in a bowed osteopenic femur can cause impingement on the anterior femoral metaphyseal cortex • A nail that is impinging on the anterior cortex can produce an iatrogenic fracture during insertion • Locking screws in distal part of femur may also cause stress riser, leading to post-op fracture
Tip 5	When Using a Trochanteric Entry Nail, Start Slightly Medial to the Exact Tip of the Greater Trochanter	• Use a starting point that is slightly medial to the exact tip of the trochanter • Do not use reamers until they are well contained in proximal part of femur • These practices avoid gradual lateral enlargement of the pilot hole • Enlargement may cause more lateral placement of IM nail than desired, potentially resulting in varus reduction of proximal fragment or high lag-screw position in femoral head
Tip 6	Do Not Ream an Unreduced Fracture	• An intertrochanteric fracture must be reduced before reaming and passing of IM nail • It is not possible to perform manipulations with a reduction tool or IM nail once started in the proximal fragment, because the bone is too soft and the medullary canal is too large

(Continued)

Table 35.1 *(Continued)* Useful tips for fixing intertrochanteric hip fractures

		• Closed reduction using fluoroscopy is recommended
		• If closed reduction is not possible, percutaneous or mini-open reduction is recommended
		• A bone-hook along the lesser trochanter or percutaneous joysticks or clamps may be used without substantial stripping or evacuation
Tip 7	Be Cautious About the Nail Insertion Trajectory, and Do Not Use a Hammer to Seat the Nail	• It is crucial to achieve vertical trajectory with nail insertion
		• Insertion at an oblique angle can cause the nail to impact the soft bone, lead to oval entry, and lateral positioning
		• The nail should be inserted by hand with slight rotational motions
		• A mallet may be used to tap the jig for final seating
		• Use of a hammer may cause iatrogenic femoral fracture and is not recommended
		• If advancement is difficult without a hammer, there is an ulterior problem to identify
		• It is recommended to ream the canal to a diameter 1 mm larger than the diameter of the nail to be used
Tip 8	Avoid Varus Angulation of the Proximal Fragment—Use the Relationship Between the Tip of the Trochanter and the Center of the Femoral Head	• Varus and high lag-screw placement are associated with increased fixation failure frequency with both IM nails and sliding hip screws
		• In surgery, note that the tip of the greater trochanter and the center of the femoral head should be coplanar
		• Varus reduction: the center of the femoral head is distal to the tip of the greater trochanter
		• Valgus reduction: the center of the head is proximal to the greater trochanter
		• It is important to know the neck-shaft angle of the device being used – 130° neck-shaft configuration is common
		• Pre-op radiographs of the uninjured hip are useful for determining normal neck-shaft angle
Tip 9	When Nailing, Lock the Nail Distally if the Fracture is Axially or Rotationally Unstable	• Most unstable fractures of the proximal part of the femur require long IM nails and should be locked distally
		• Short nails can be associated with subsequent fracture in subtrochanteric area, despite smaller-diameter locking screws
		• Fragility fractures in elderly patients should be considered pathologic fractures and treated using long internal fixation devices to protect the entire bone
Tip 10	Avoid Fracture Distraction When Nailing	• Fracture malrotation and distraction are common when nails are used for fractures with transverse or reverse oblique configuration
		• A fracture locked in distraction has increased weight-bearing load on the device due to lack of osseous contact
		• Fixed distraction increases risk for nonunion and hardware failure
		• To eliminate distraction, traction on the lower limb should be released prior to insertion of the distal locking screws
		• Fluoroscopy should be used to confirm there is no bone-on-bone contact

Source: From Haidukewych GJ. Intertrochanteric fractures: ten tips to improve results. *J Bone Joint Surg Am.* 2009;91(3):712–9.

POSITIONING

The patient is positioned supine on the fracture table. The case can also be done on a radiolucent table in select cases (e.g. polytrauma) with or without the addition of a traction arc. The ipsilateral arm is secured across the chest to allow intramedullary nailing if necessary. The injured extremity is placed in traction. The well leg can be placed in either hemilithotomy or scissored position (Figure 35.5).

Prior to prepping and draping, the surgeon must ensure that adequate visualization and reduction can be achieved. Reduction is usually achieved by applying traction to regain length. Excessive traction can lead to pelvic rotation around the perineal post of the fracture table. Next comes internal rotation. The patella should point anteriorly. Abduction/adduction of the hip is then adjusted to ensure the fracture is not in varus. The reduction must be checked in both the AP and lateral with an image

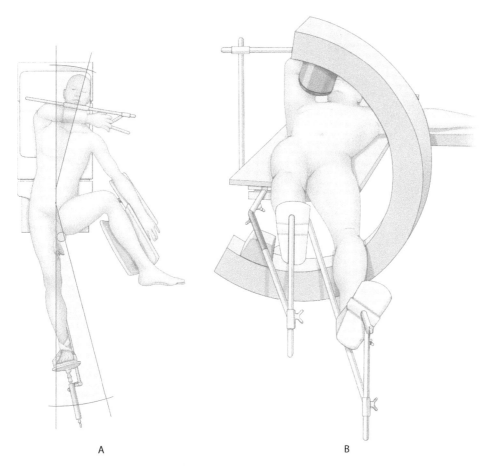

A   B

Figure 35.5 Positioning in hemilithotomy (a) and scissored (b). Note in both cases the torso has been shifted to the contralateral side to allow access to the greater trochanter for possible cephalomedullary nailing. (Copyright by AO Foundation, Switzerland. AO Surgery Reference. www.aosurgery.org)

intensifier. In case the closed reduction should fail, open reduction will be necessary.

SLIDING HIP SCREW

The lateral approach is used. The incision can be extended proximally to accommodate a trochanteric stabilizing plate. A straight incision is made parallel to the femoral axis. The fascia lata is incised in line with the skin incision and in line with its fibers. The vastus lateralis fascia is incised. The vastus lateralis muscle may be split in line with its fibers or elevated from the posterior leaflet of the fascia and retracted anteriorly. Elevating the vastus lateralis minimizes bleeding. To avoid bleeding, tie off or clip any perforating vessels encountered. A cob elevator is used to expose the footprint of the side plate. Bennett retractors are then placed anterior and posterior to the femur to allow visualization. If necessary for placement of a trochanteric stabilization plate or for open reduction of the fracture, the incision can be extended proximally to the greater trochanter. A pointed reduction clamp can be used to obtain reduction.

Choose the correct aiming device according to the neck-shaft angle as measured from the contralateral hip. Insert the guide wire through the aiming device and advance it into the subchondral bone of the head in a center-center position, stopping 10 mm short of the joint. Position it so that in the AP it is in the caudal half of the neck, and in the axial view in the center of the neck. Determine the length of the sliding hip screw with the help of the measuring device. Select a screw which is 10 mm shorter than the measured length. Adjust the cannulated triple reamer to the chosen length. Drill a hole for the screw and the plate sleeve. The correct screw is mounted on the handle and inserted over the guide wire. Do not push forcefully or you may distract the fracture. In patients with hard bone, it is best to use the tap to precut the thread for the screw. Otherwise the screw may not advance, and you may actually displace the fracture by rotating the proximal fragment as you attempt to insert the screw. The T-handle of the insertion piece should be parallel to the long axis of the bone to ensure the correct position of the plate. It been shown that maintaining tip-apex distance of 25 mm or less prevents screw cutout.[15–17]

Place the selected plate and slide it over the guide wire and mate it correctly with the screw. Then push it in over the screw and seat it home with the impactor. Fix the plate to the femoral shaft with an appropriate number and size of plate holding cortical screws. Finally, compression can be

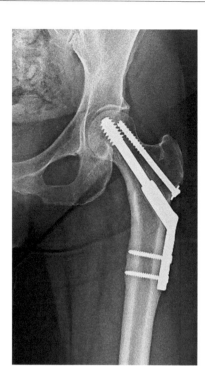

Figure 35.6 Healed intertrochanteric femur fracture. A derotation screw was added as injury was felt to be a transitional variant (intertrochanteric/basicervical femoral neck variant).

achieved by placing the compression screw. If there is concern that the fracture is a transitional type (basicervical), a derotation screw may be added (Figure 35.6).

CEPHALOMEDULLARY NAILING

It is important to ensure that the ipsilateral greater trochanter is accessible. To accomplish this, rotate the torso 10–15 degrees to the contralateral side when possible. Intramedullary nails for A-type proximal femur fractures enter through the top of the greater trochanter. However, the precise entry point in the greater trochanter depends on the design of the nail.

Make your skin incision in line with the femoral shaft axis and about 5 cm proximal to the tip of the trochanter. Split the fascia in line with the incision. Split the gluteal muscles in line with the fibers. Place the guide wire just lateral to the tip of the greater trochanter on the AP and in line with the middle of the femoral neck on the lateral. Insert the guide wire into the femoral shaft and check its position using the image intensifier. Ideally, the guide wire's position in the femoral shaft should be central and deviate slightly lateral proximally according to the degree of the lateral bend of the implant in the AP plane. In the lateral view it must be in line with the middle of the femoral neck. Insert the protection sleeve with its trocar over the guide wire and push it through the soft tissues until it abuts against the greater trochanter. Then withdraw the trocar and insert an appropriate drill bit over the guide wire. Ream out the trochanteric area.

Ream by hand or with an awl in osteoporotic patients to avoid damage to the fragile trochanteric metaphyseal bone. In patients with good quality bone, use power reaming. Remove the guide wire after reaming. If the fracture passes through the guidewire entry site, a medially directed force applied to the lateral trochanteric region along with slow advancement of the power reamer helps prevent diastasis of the fracture site by displacing the greater trochanteric segment(s) laterally. This allows proper creation of a channel for the nail, so that its insertion does not distract the fracture and produce varus deformity. Avoiding varus deformity is important to improve fixation and to preserve functionally important anatomy. In most patients the nail, mounted on the insertion device, can be inserted manually. Use the image intensifier as a help and insert the nail to such a depth that it will allow the cephalomedullary fixation to be placed through the middle of the femoral neck.

Mount the aiming arm for the cephalomedullary fixation onto the insertion device. Make a small skin incision at the appropriate place. Insert the drill sleeve assembly through the aiming device and advance it through the soft tissues to the lateral cortex. If you are using a device that takes a column screw, the ideal position of the guide wire in the AP plane is in line with the axis of the neck and slightly in the lower half. In the lateral view it must be in line with the axis of the neck. The guide wire is inserted subchondrally into the femoral head. Its tip should end 5 mm proximal of the joint. Check under image intensification that the femoral neck screw protrudes slightly over the lateral cortex. The cephalomedullary fixation has to be locked with the set screw device. Following this, the compression feature of the device can be used to compress the fracture site. Finally, distal interlocking is performed. With short nails, the radiolucent targeting guide is used. With long nails, distal interlocking screws are inserted using perfect circles techniques through percutaneous incisions (Figure 35.7).

EXTERNAL FIXATION

This technique is useful in special circumstances. A level I prospective randomized study compared pertrochanteric external fixation (PF) with sliding hip screw in 100 consecutive patients. The authors utilized a specially designed Pertrochanteric Fixator (Orthofix, Verona, Italy), which places two threaded half pins into the femoral neck at 110–130 degrees to a subchondral location and two self-drilling half pins into the proximal femur at a 90-degree angle. The authors found that use of PF resulted in significantly less blood loss, shorter operating times, reduced pain, shorter length of stay, earlier mobilization and reduced mechanical complications ($P < 0.001$). Superficial infection was more common with PF ($P < 0.001$). No differences were found in healing, mortality or functional outcomes.[18]

PROSTHETIC REPLACEMENT

Prosthetic hip replacement generally has not been considered a primary treatment option and is usually reserved for revision situations. Unlike femoral neck fractures, which retain some of the femoral neck in addition to the abductor mechanism, intertrochanteric fractures involve more

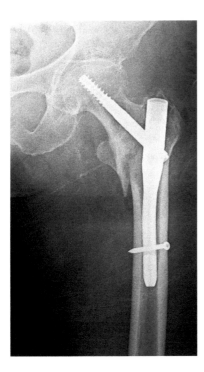

Figure 35.7 Unstable intertrochanteric fracture from the patient in Figure 35.3 stabilized with a short cephalo-medullary nail.

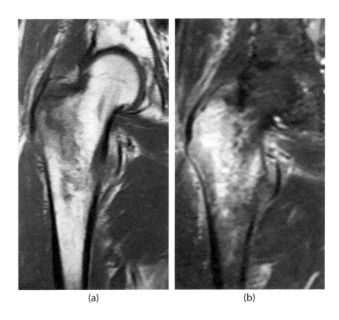

(a)   (b)

Figure 35.8 T1 (a) and STIR (b) MRI images of a nondisplaced intertrochanteric femur fracture.

distal femoral bone, and often the greater trochanter and the abductor are not attached to the proximal femur. In this setting, prosthetic replacement requires a more complex surgical procedure with potentially higher morbidity. In the patient with pre-existing symptomatic degenerative arthritis, primary prosthetic replacement may be the best option. It can also be considered for intertrochanteric fractures with severe comminution in severely osteoporotic bone in which internal fixation methods are unlikely to be successful. Calcar-replacing implants are typically required.

A randomized prospective level I study of unstable intertrochanteric fractures in elderly patients comparing long-stem cementless calcar-replacement hemiarthroplasty with a proximal femoral nail (PFN) found no significant differences between the two groups in terms of functional outcomes, hospital stay, time to weight bearing or risk of complications. However, surgical time, blood loss, need for blood transfusions and mortality rates were all significantly lower in the PFN group.[19]

In another level I study, hemiarthroplasty was compared with the sliding hip screw. No significant difference was found between surgical time, wound complications or mortality rates. However, the hemiarthroplasty group was reported to have higher transfusion rates.[20]

Special circumstances

NONDISPLACED FRACTURES

As in the case of nondisplaced femoral neck fractures, nondisplaced intertrochanteric fractures are best identified using MRI. Once discovered, treatment is controversial, as patients have been treated successfully with both operative and nonoperative approaches (Figure 35.8).

REVERSE OBLIQUITY AND TRANSVERSE FRACTURES

These are true intertrochanteric fractures. They are classified according to the fracture pattern. The fracture line passes between the greater and lesser trochanters, above the lesser trochanter medially and below the crest of the vastus lateralis laterally (Figure 35.9).

Reverse oblique fractures often have a typical displacement because of the pull of the abductors, which abducts and flexes the proximal fragment. Be careful in determining the distal extension of the fracture line as nondisplaced fracture lines can propagate distally into the femoral shaft.

Although some studies suggest that these fractures can be treated effectively with sliding hip screws,[21] and some studies have reported similar failure rates with sliding hip screws and intramedullary nails,[22] other studies have reported failure rates of up to 80% when these fracture patterns are treated with sliding hip screws.[23] Although a biomechanical study demonstrated that with anatomic reduction and bone contact a 135-degree hip screw, 95-degree hip screw and intramedullary hip screw performed equally, when a gap was created, the intramedullary hip screw was significantly stiffer with a greater load to failure than the other two implants.[24] Also, a randomized prospective study comparing intramedullary nails and 95-degree hip screws found that patients treated with intramedullary nails had shorter operative times, fewer blood transfusions and shorter hospital stays with significantly fewer implant failures and nonunions compared to those treated with the 95-degree hip screw.[25] Several other studies have demonstrated excellent results with low complication rates when these fractures are treated with cephalomedullary devices.[26]

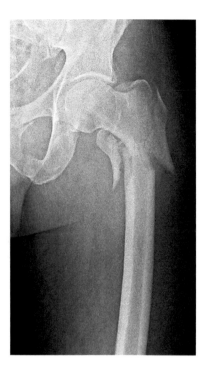

Figure 35.9 Reverse oblique intertrochanteric femur fracture.

Postoperative management

Although surgeons make decisions regarding weight bearing on a case-by-case basis, overall the literature supports immediate weight bearing after internal fixation of appropriately selected extracapsular hip fractures. Immediate weight bearing has demonstrated benefits in patient balance and mobility, which may decrease morbidity and promote greater independence. Patients without dementia can safely be advised to bear weight as tolerated after operative treatment of intertrochanteric femur fractures. Computerized weight bearing and gait analysis has demonstrated that these patients will autoregulate and voluntarily limit loading of the injured limb.[27]

Koval et al. reported the outcomes of a large cohort of elderly patients who were allowed to bear weight immediately and followed for ≥1 year. The authors reported on 208 patients who had stable or unstable intertrochanteric femur fractures, all of which were managed with sliding hip screws. The rate of revision for loss of fixation was 2.9%, in all cases because of femoral head lag screw cutout.[28] Herrera et al. reported on 551 intertrochanteric femur fractures in elderly patients (average age 82.8 years) who were treated with a short cephalomedullary nail and allowed to bear weight immediately after the procedure. The authors reported a 1.4% rate of screw cutout and a 4% rate of collapse into secondary varus >10 degrees at final follow-up.[29]

COMPLICATIONS

Maintaining a tip-apex distance of 25 mm or less can prevent screw cutout.[17] It has been found that, after adjusting for tip-apex distance and screw position, A3 fractures are at more risk for cutout than A1 fractures.[16] Helical blades have also been found to cutout of the femoral head at a low rate.[30] Compromised lateral femoral wall integrity has been found to be a significant predictor of reoperation in patients treated with sliding hip screw devices.[15] There have also been several reports of helical blade advancement into the pelvis.[31] Breakage of cephalomedullary nails at the lag screw site has also been reported (Figure 35.10).

SALVAGE

Most intertrochanteric hip fracture nonunions occur in older patients with poor proximal bone quality and fail by implant cutout from the femoral head. The decision to perform revision internal fixation versus prosthetic replacement is based on patient characteristics, fracture pattern, remaining bone quality and status of the hip joint. Arthroplasty has been found to be an effective salvage procedure with most patients experiencing good pain relief and functional improvement and a low complication rate. Arthroplasty allows earlier patient mobilization and is thus advantageous for rehabilitation (Figure 35.11).[32]

When hip arthroplasty is performed for salvage of failed intertrochanteric fractures, specific technical considerations must be addressed. The initial decision is whether to perform a total hip arthroplasty or a hemiarthroplasty. It is not uncommon for the cutout of the previous internal fixation to cause secondary damage to the hip joint. Usually, in this circumstance or in patients with markedly severe preexisting arthritis, a total hip arthroplasty is performed. With well-preserved articular cartilage, hemiarthroplasty may be considered. The same advantages and disadvantages of hemiarthroplasty versus total hip arthroplasty discussed for salvage of femoral neck nonunion also pertain to intertrochanteric nonunion.

Defects from previous internal fixation devices on the lateral femoral shaft create stress risers that can lead to intraoperative fracture of the femur, particularly with torsion. Preliminary dislocation of the hip before hardware is removed may reduce femur fracture risk in these hips, which often are quite stiff and can require much force to dislocate. Frequently, broken screws are present.

Most patients with failed intertrochanteric fracture fixation have bone loss below the standard resection level for a routine, primary total hip arthroplasty. Therefore, many need a calcar-replacing implant to restore leg length and hip stability. To prevent the chance of subsequent fracture when using longer stems, it is considered wise to bypass screw holes in the femur by two cortical diameters. Additionally, it has been found that arthroplasty following failed fixation with intramedullary implants leads to a high risk of greater trochanteric fracture and nonunion.[33] Successful femoral component fixation can be obtained with either cemented or cementless implants.

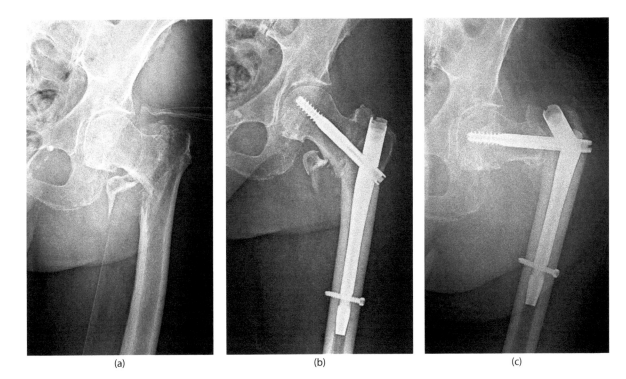

(a)　　　　　　　　　　(b)　　　　　　　　　　(c)

Figure 35.10 Unstable intertrochanteric femur fracture (a) fixed with cephalomedullary nail (b) which went on to failure (c).

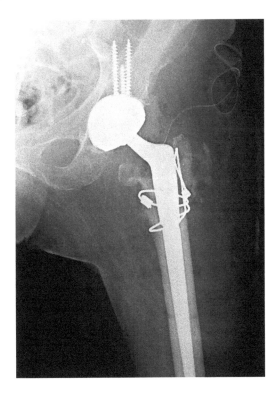

Figure 35.11 The patient in Figure 35.9 who went on to be revised to a total hip arthroplasty following failure.

Outcomes

PAIN AND FUNCTION

The literature on pain and functional outcomes for patients with intertrochanteric hip fractures is sparse. Randomized controlled trials suggest that neither plate-and-screw implants nor intramedullary nails produce superior patient outcomes. Several studies found that intramedullary nails were associated with more pain but earlier improvements in weight bearing and mobility. However, these improvements were short-lived, returning to nonsignificance within several months to one year postoperatively. Five level I studies suggested that patients regain equal ambulatory status regardless of fixation type. However, two level I and two level II studies concluded that intramedullary devices expedite return to pretreatment ambulatory function. It is important to note that many current studies have not separated stable from unstable patterns when assessing ambulatory status.[34] Cochrane reviews have supported plate-and-screw devices as superior to intramedullary nails for both stable and unstable intertrochanteric hip fractures, largely because of persistently higher complication rates with intramedullary nail procedures rather than any device advantage for functional outcomes.[35] There is some evidence that plate-and-screw devices are associated with higher complication rates in unstable AO/OTA 31 A3 fractures.[8] Conversely, in simple two-part AO/OTA 31 A1 fractures, intramedullary devices have been found to have a higher reoperation rate within 1 year and at 3 years postoperatively. Rates of reoperation for fixation failure were similar, however reoperation due to peri-implant fracture and implant related pain were statistically significantly higher in the intramedullary nail group.[36]

Observational studies assessing short-term functional outcomes found that younger patient age and higher prefracture levels of function were consistent predictors of functional recovery as measured by the ability to live independently, perform activities of daily living or independent activities of daily living, and mobility. Other predictors of functional recovery included lower American Society of Anesthesiologists (ASA) scores, living in the community at the time of the hip fracture, and having a femoral neck rather than an intertrochanteric hip fracture. The same general pattern of the influence of patient predictors was found for longer-term function after hip fracture. Observational studies that controlled for fracture type found similar functional results to those studies that excluded fracture type from the final analysis.

Rarely, patients will sustain ipsilateral femoral shaft and intertrochanteric fractures. A retrospective study was completed of 26 such patients treated with either a reconstruction nail or a sliding hip screw and retrograde nail. It was found that for most outcome measures, there were no significant differences in functional outcome scores between the two treatment groups.

MORTALITY

No significant differences in mortality have been found in multiple randomized clinical trials in mortality among patients treated with various plate-and-screw models compared with each other, different intramedullary nail models compared with each other, plate-and-screw devices compared with intramedullary nails for all intertrochanteric fracture types, plate-and-screw devices compared with intramedullary nails for unstable intertrochanteric hip fractures, or internal fixation compared with hemiarthroplasty for unstable intertrochanteric hip fractures.

However, compared with randomized clinical trials, observational studies provide more information about the relationship of patient factors and fracture type with outcomes. For short-term (3–6-month) mortality, increasing age, increased comorbidities and lower prefracture function have been found to be associated with higher mortality following hip fracture in general. Age, male sex, heart failure and an intertrochanteric fracture were associated with higher 10-year mortality. However, there were no differences in mortality by fracture type within 2 years after hip fracture.[8]

The relationship between 90-day mortality and provider volume has also been examined. The risk of inpatient mortality was found to be higher in patient having surgery anywhere but at the highest volume centers. Beyond 30 days postoperatively, the increased risk of mortality persisted only among patients managed at the lowest volume hospitals. However, the authors stated that the findings did not indicate a need to direct patients with routine hip fractures exclusively to high volume centers, although they stated the higher mortality rates found in the lowest volume centers warrant further investigation.[37]

LENGTH OF STAY

A retrospective cohort study of 4432 patients aged 70 or older comparing extramedullary and intramedullary implants was performed using the American College of Surgeons National Surgical Quality Improvement Program (ACS NSQIP) database. A total of 1612 (36.4%) were treated with an extramedullary implant and 2820 (63.6%) with an intramedullary implant. The rates of the composite outcomes 'serious adverse events' and 'any adverse events' did not differ by implant type. The mean postoperative length of stay was shorter for patients treated with an intramedullary implant compared with those treated with an extramedullary implant (5.4 compared with 6.5 days; $P < 0.001$). Operation time, operating room time and the rate of hospital readmission did not differ by implant type. These results reinforce the results of previous randomized trials, demonstrating little difference in rates of general surgical adverse events between implant types. However, the study does present an important departure from previous trials in its finding that patients treated with intramedullary implants have, on average, a shorter postoperative length of stay (by 1.1 days). The authors speculated that these findings may negate the perceived excess cost associated with intramedullary treatment.[38]

SUBTROCHANTERIC FRACTURES

Introduction

Subtrochanteric fractures of the femur that are caused by low energy trauma are less common than other proximal femoral fractures, but they occur in a similar population of elderly individuals. Subtrochanteric femur fractures are defined as fractures occurring between the lesser trochanter and the junction of the proximal and middle thirds of the femoral shaft. These fractures may extend proximally into the piriformis fossa or distally into the isthmus of the femur. The proximal extension of the fracture is variable and may include fracture patterns combined with intertrochanteric and femoral neck fractures. These patterns are often collectively referred to as 'pertrochanteric' fractures to reflect the complex combination of fractures involved. Regardless of associated fractures, the common element of all subtrochanteric femoral fractures is extension of the fracture to the level of the lesser trochanter, leaving a short proximal fragment. Subtrochanteric fractures may be misinterpreted as intertrochanteric fractures. Failure to identify the subtrochanteric fracture extension may lead to difficulties with reduction and improper selection of fixation, which could lead to implant failure.

Anatomy

OSSEOUS

The proximal femur consists of the femoral head and neck as well as the greater trochanter and lesser trochanters (Figure 35.1).[39] The calcar is a sheet of bone along the posteromedial aspect of the proximal femur, beginning just distal to the lesser trochanter and extending proximally to the posteroinferior femoral neck.

MUSCULAR

The iliacus and psoas major muscles comprise the iliopsoas group. The psoas major is a large muscle that runs from the bodies and discs of the L1–L5 vertebrae, joins with the iliacus via its tendon and connects to the lesser trochanter of the femur. The iliacus originates on the iliac fossa of the ilium. Together these muscles are commonly referred to as the iliopsoas.

The abductors consist of the gluteal muscles and include the gluteus maximus, gluteus medius and gluteus minimus. They cover the lateral surface of the ilium. The gluteus maximus, which forms most of the muscle of the buttocks, originates primarily on the ilium and sacrum and inserts on the gluteal tuberosity of the femur as well as the iliotibial tract. The gluteus medius and gluteus minimus originate anterior to the gluteus maximus on the ilium and both insert on the greater trochanter of the femur.

The short external rotators consist of the obturator externus and internus, the piriformis, the superior and inferior gemelli, and the quadratus femoris. These six originate at or below the acetabulum of the ilium and insert on or near the greater trochanter of the femur (Figure 35.2).[40]

Biomechanics

The medial calcar is subjected to significant compressive forces. It has been found that a 200 lb man generates forces up to 1,200 lb/in² on the medial aspect of the femur, 1–3 inches distal to the lesser trochanter. Because of these stresses, the subtrochanteric area of the proximal femur is composed of very dense cortical bone that is very difficult to fracture, especially in young patients.

Mechanism of Injury

It has long been recognized that a bimodal age distribution exists for subtrochanteric femoral fractures. The first peak occurs in younger trauma patients who sustain the fracture from a high energy mechanism of injury. The second peak occurs in elderly patients with osteoporotic bone and deteriorated calcar strength. These patients are usually injured from a ground level fall and may develop the same problems associated with other hip fractures, such as loss of independence and ambulation, pneumonia, sepsis and death.

Subtrochanteric femoral fractures also may occur after previous proximal femoral surgical procedures often performed on elderly patients. Cannulated screws placed distal to the lesser trochanter for treatment of femoral neck fractures create a stress riser in the lateral femoral cortex, which can lead to fracture.[41] When placing three cannulated screws to stabilize a femoral neck fracture, the inverted triangle pattern (i.e. triangle apex distal) is less likely to be associated with a subsequent subtrochanteric femoral fracture than when the base of the triangle is distal (i.e. triangle apex proximal).[42] Fractures can also occur following core decompression for osteonecrosis or following removal of a sliding hip screw and side plate.

Classification

RUSSELL-TAYLOR

This system describes the fracture pattern in a practical fashion based on mechanical stability and fracture extension. The binary points include the extension of the fracture into the piriformis fossa (types I and II) and the comminution of the lesser trochanter (types A and B) (Figure 35.12).

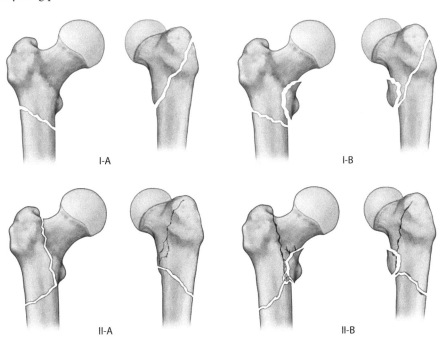

I-A I-B

II-A II-B

Figure 35.12 Russell-Taylor classification of subtrochanteric femur fractures. (From Rockwood CA, et al. *Rockwood and Green's Fractures in Adults*. 6th ed. Philadelphia, PA: Lippincott Williams & Wilkins; 2006.)

AO/OTA

This system is detailed and is useful for research purposes. However, many feel it is too cumbersome for routine communication (Figure 35.13).

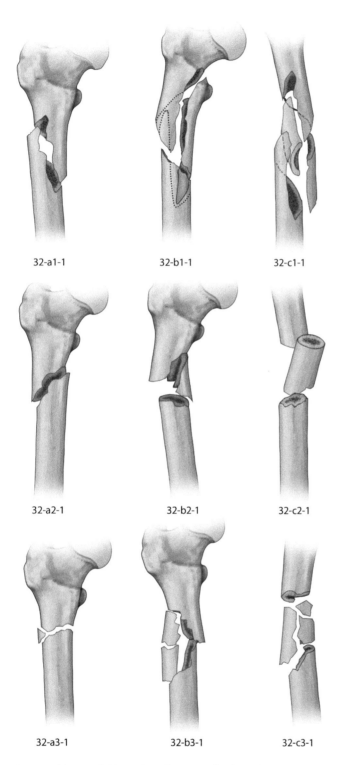

32-a1-1   32-b1-1   32-c1-1

32-a2-1   32-b2-1   32-c2-1

32-a3-1   32-b3-1   32-c3-1

Figure 35.13 AO/OTA classification of subtrochanteric fractures. (From Rockwood CA, et al. *Rockwood and Green's Fractures in Adults*. 6th ed. Philadelphia, PA: Lippincott Williams & Wilkins; 2006.)

Diagnosis

PHYSICAL EXAMINATION

The patient with subtrochanteric femoral fracture presents with a shortened and externally rotated lower extremity. The proximal fragment is usually flexed and abducted from the effects of the iliopsoas and gluteal muscles, respectively. The proximal fragment can be buttonholed through the quadriceps musculature. The distal fragment is typically shortened, adducted and externally rotated secondary to the pull of the quadriceps and hamstrings, adductors, and gluteals and short external rotators, respectively. Crepitance may be noted with movement of the extremity, and the soft tissue envelope is often swollen and tense. Although rare, the patient should be assessed for signs of thigh compartment syndrome. A thorough neurovascular examination must be completed. A secondary survey must be performed to assess for associated injuries, as low energy falls may result in multiple fractures in the osteoporotic elderly patient.

Initial management

Application of immediate traction may minimize fracture related blood loss via tamponade effect by decreasing the potential space within the zone of injury. Traction can also lessen the pain associated with these injuries. Immediate traction may be applied at the scene of the injury by utilizing commercially available lower extremity traction devices. This may be converted to skeletal traction with a distal femoral traction pin placement. Subtrochanteric femurs typically align best in 90/90 traction due to the flexed position the proximal fragment assumes due to the pull of the iliopsoas.

Surgical management

Definitive fixation should be performed in an expedient manner provided that the appropriate resources are available. More importantly, the patient should be adequately resuscitated, and the surgical team should be made aware of the potential for additional significant blood loss during surgery, much of which may be unseen due to minimally invasive approaches. The physiologic second hit of a major operation, combined with substantial blood loss, may be too traumatizing for some severely injured patients; a damage-control procedure to initially stabilize the patient may be indicated, with definitive fixation delayed for 3–5 days.[43]

PATIENT POSITIONING

Fracture table

The fracture table with in-line traction has typically been the operating table of choice for subtrochanteric femoral fractures. The patient is positioned in either the supine (Figure 35.5) or lateral (Figure 35.14) position. The lateral position is advantageous in obese patients. Additionally, lateral positioning can allow gravity to aid in reduction by countering the tendency of the fracture to assume a varus alignment.

Radiolucent table

The patient can be positioned supine, in the so-called sloppy lateral position (supine position with sandbag or large bump under the affected hip) or lateral decubitus (using a hip positioner or a sandbag) (Figure 35.15).

Intraoperative imaging

Fluoroscopic images are easily obtained in any of the above scenarios. The fluoroscopy unit is brought in from the contralateral side. It is crucial that prior to prepping and draping the surgeons ensure that all necessary views can be reliably obtained.

Implant selection

INTRAMEDULLARY DEVICES

General considerations

Intramedullary devices have become the implant of choice for many surgeons who treat subtrochanteric fractures. These can be either piriformis or trochanteric entry. No significant differences have been found between entry points. The entry point should be selected based on the surgeon's

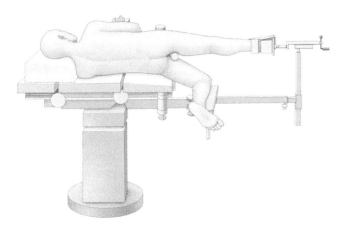

Figure 35.14 Lateral position on the fracture table. (Copyright by AO Foundation, Switzerland. AO Surgery Reference. www.aosurgery.org).

comfort level. Another factor that must be considered is radius of curvature of the nail. The femoral bow increases with patient age. The radius of curvature differs among commercially available nails and may be greater than the patient's radius of curvature. This mismatch can result in perforation of the anterior cortex distally.[44]

Reduction

Before placing the reaming guidewire down the canal, the surgeon must ensure that the fracture is adequately reduced and that all deformity is recognized and corrected. This reduction must be maintained throughout the reaming process. The nail will not reduce the fracture. If the femur is reamed with the fracture malreduced, the final reduction will be malreduced and unsatisfactory. This can lead to failure of fixation.

A number of methods may be employed to maintain reduction. Traction establishes length. External rotation of the distal fragment is required to align it with the proximal fragment, which is externally rotated. Restoration of femoral length, alignment and rotation should be assessed by judging the alignment of the reduced fragments or by comparison with the contralateral intact femur. Bumps and padded mallets may assist with correction of procurvatum and varus. If closed methods fail, percutaneous methods can be employed, such as a bone hook and ball spike pusher. If percutaneous methods fail, open clamp assisted reduction may be employed. Open reduction techniques have been found to be successful when applied appropriately. The viability of the medial femoral fragments is critical. These fragments should be handled with great care to minimize soft tissue dissection and avoid iatrogenic injury.[45] When assessing the adequacy of the reduction, the surgeon should strive for perfection. However, 10 degrees of angulation or 1 cm of shortening is common in difficult subtrochanteric fractures.

STANDARD NAILING

A subtrochanteric femoral fracture can be stabilized with standard first generation interlocking nails if it has an intact proximal fragment large enough for the nail and locking screw to control securely (Figure 35.16). The only

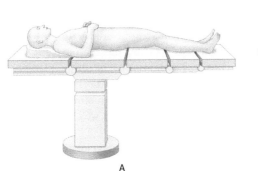

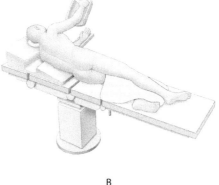

A   B

Figure 35.15 Supine (a) and lateral (b) positions with leg draped free on a radiolucent table. (Copyright by AO Foundation, Switzerland. AO Surgery Reference. www.aosurgery.org).

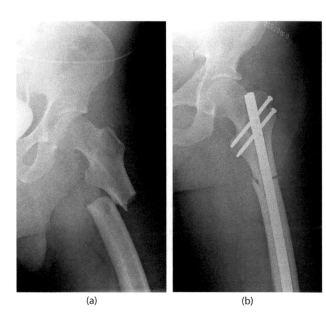

(a)   (b)

Figure 35.16 Subtrochanteric femur facture **(a)** stabilized with a standard intramedullary nail **(b)**. Cephalomedullary nails need not be used if adequate bone stock remains proximally to accommodate standard interlocking screws.

firm contact the fixation has with this fragment with antegrade insertion is the cortical entry point in the piriformis fossa and the purchase of the interlocking bolts. Therefore, if there is concern for proximal fracture extension, another implant should be chosen. Failure to stabilize the proximal fragment adequately results in failure of fixation with loss of reduction, usually consisting of a combination of procurvatum and varus. Antegrade nailing remains the treatment of choice for the vast majority of subtrochanteric femur fractures. However, retrograde femoral nailing may be an effective treatment option for some subtrochanteric fractures in a selected group of patients, such as polytrauma and morbidly obese patients. Good results with union rates up to 99% have been reported using standard intramedullary nails inserted either antegrade or retrograde to treat subtrochanteric femoral fractures.

RECONSTRUCTION NAILING

Reconstruction nails are nails which have proximal interlocking that engages the femoral neck and head. This feature allows the nail to better secure the proximal fragment because of the increased contact with the bone in the femoral neck and head. Reconstruction nails can be used to stabilize all patterns of subtrochanteric fractures, including those with extension to the lesser trochanter and piriformis fossa.

It is important to recognize that the starting point for reconstruction fixation must be more anterior than the point for standard antegrade nails. The axis of the femoral neck lies anterior to the axis of the femoral shaft on the lateral view. Placing the nail more anteriorly in the proximal fragment allows the proximal screws to assume a straighter

path into the femoral neck and head rather than being directed from posterolateral to anteromedial. Caution must be exercised however, as hoop stresses created by moving the starting point anteriorly away from the piriformis fossa could potentially burst the proximal fragment.[46]

CEPHALOMEDULLARY NAILS

Cephalomedullary nails are frequently employed in subtrochanteric fractures and have become the implant of choice for many surgeons (Figure 35.7). These devices have an apex-medial bend in the proximal aspect of the nail to allow the nail to easily traverse the intramedullary canal. Cephalomedullary nails have a large proximal diameter and employ screws or blades that engage the bone in the femoral neck. This makes them suitable for treating essentially all variants of subtrochanteric fractures, regardless of extension proximally.[47-49]

Entry points can vary based on implant design. The correct entry point on the greater trochanter has been investigated and it was found that the best starting point was at the tip of the greater trochanter. A slightly medial starting point was an acceptable alternative, but starting laterally on the greater trochanter invariably led to a varus malreduction. In placing the nail, it is also important to establish the correct anterior-to-posterior position on the greater trochanter so that the screws will be in line with the axis of the femoral neck.[46]

95-DEGREE ANGLED PLATES

For many years, 95-degree angled plate implants have been used to stabilize subtrochanteric femoral fractures (Figure 35.17). These implants are available in both 95-degree compression screw plate options and 95-degree blade plate options. Before intramedullary fixation techniques were described, the 95-degree angled implants were often the devices of choice in these injuries. Many of the early advances in stabilizing difficult proximal femoral fractures were in large part the result of the successful deployment of the 95-degree condylar blade plate.

The surgical technique for the 95-degree condylar blade plate is very challenging. These plates must be inserted precisely in all three planes (axial, sagittal and coronal). Many surgeons found that using this device was a difficult experience. An advantage of the 95-degree condylar screw plate compared with the 95-degree condylar blade plate is that the construct can be adjusted in the sagittal plane after the compression screw has been placed. As a result, this device has less potential for error in placement, particularly in the sagittal plane. Good results have been reported in subtrochanteric femoral fractures treated with the 95-degree condylar screw plate as well as with the 95-degree condylar blade-plate.[50,51]

Similar to the management of subtrochanteric fractures with intramedullary devices, minimally invasive and indirect reduction techniques should be used when possible. Maintenance of the biology of the fracture environment is imperative when using the 95-degree condylar screw plate.

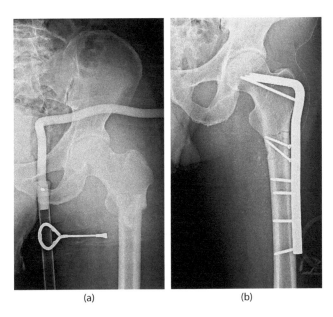

(a)   (b)

Figure 35.17 Subtrochanteric femur fracture (a) stabilized with lag screws and a 95-degree blade plate (b).

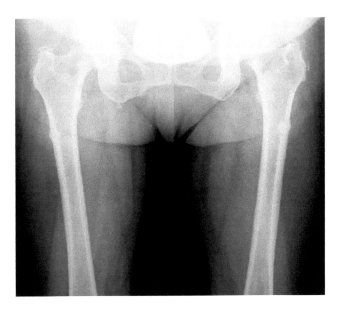

Figure 35.18 Bilateral bisphosphonate associated subtrochanteric femur fractures. (From Yoon RS, et al. *Orthopedics* 2010;33(4):267–70.)

PROXIMAL FEMUR LOCKING PLATE

Both formal open as well as minimally invasive fixation of subtrochanteric fractures can also be accomplished with a proximal femur locking compression plate. In both approaches, preservation of biology with indirect reduction techniques when possible should be employed. Again, maintenance of the biology of the fracture environment is imperative. High union rates have been observed with low complication rates with this implant.[52]

Special circumstances

OPEN FRACTURES

Open subtrochanteric fractures are rare but do occur in high-energy situations. The intermediate objectives are prevention of infection, fracture stabilization and soft tissue coverage. Immediate stabilization may consist of external fixation or definitive fixation depending on local and systemic patient factors. As these goals are interdependent, a coordinated treatment plan with early surgical intervention is required. Coordination of the reconstructive procedures with rehabilitation of the injured muscle is mandatory to obtain maximal possible function.

STRESS/INSUFFICIENCY FRACTURES AND ATYPICAL FRACTURES

Treatment of stress and insufficiency fractures and atypical ('bisphosphonate') fractures are approached in a similar manner. A number of case reports and series have identified a subgroup of atypical fractures of the femoral shaft associated with bisphosphonate use, which can be bilateral (Figure 35.18).[53] However, a population based study did not support this association. A secondary analysis was performed using the results of three large, randomized

bisphosphonate trials. The occurrence of fracture of the subtrochanteric or diaphyseal femur was very rare, even among women who had been treated with bisphosphonates for as long as 10 years. There was no significant increase in risk associated with bisphosphonate use, but the study was underpowered for definitive conclusions.[54] However, a more recent study over a 7-year study period found that a subgroup consisting of postmenopausal women who had been receiving continuous bisphosphonate therapy for ≥5 years had an increased risk for subtrochanteric or femoral shaft fractures. Intermediate or short-term use was not associated with increased risk.[55] This has led some physicians to recommend a 'bisphosphonate holiday' after 5 years or conversion to another agent.

If fracture does occur, surgical fixation is indicated. When incomplete fractures are found, a decision regarding treatment approach needs to be made. Nonoperative management consists of modified weight bearing based on pain with close follow-up. If the 'dreaded black line' appears on X-ray, it may be an indication for conversion to operative treatment. Rarely an incomplete fracture is found contralateral to a completed fracture. It has been found that a higher percentage of patients treated surgically became asymptomatic and demonstrated radiographic evidence of healing earlier than those treated nonsurgically. Surgical intervention was found to be effective for relief of symptoms when treating incomplete bisphosphonate related femur fractures. Patients should be counseled as to the risks but also potential benefits of prophylactic surgery.[56]

Postoperative management

Weight bearing is advanced based on the treating surgeon's impression of the stability achieved at the time of definitive fixation and the patient's ability to comply with instructions. Transverse patterns are typically amenable to immediate weight bearing to tolerance, while comminuted, spiral and oblique patterns typically have weight bearing restricted to varying degrees. Immediate range of motion to tolerance is begun of the hip, knee and ankle. Follow-up visits with new X-rays are performed at 2, 6, 12, 24 and 52 weeks.

The relatively high incidence of deep vein thrombosis seen in conjunction with fracture of the proximal femur should be kept in mind. Both mechanical and chemical prophylaxis should be considered while the patient is in-house, based on the clinical situation. Outpatient deep vein thrombosis prophylaxis is typically continued for 4–6 weeks based on patient mobilization.

Complications

LOSS OF FIXATION AND MALUNION

Subtrochanteric malunion has been defined as shortening >1 cm, 10-degree angulation in any plane, or rotational malalignment <15 degrees. Many Russell-Taylor IB subtrochanteric femoral fractures are reduced in varus. The importance of achieving appropriate reduction and stable fixation in subtrochanteric fractures cannot be overemphasized. Ensuring anatomic alignment of the fracture decreases the possibility of fixation failure (Figure 35.19). Choosing the appropriate implant and utilizing the implant correctly in a well-reduced fracture is the best way to maximize the chance of a good result.

The limited, often osteoporotic bone available for fixation in the proximal femur in elderly patients coupled with tremendous forces acting on the subtrochanteric region contribute to the loss of fixation seen in subtrochanteric femoral fractures. Secondary to the multiple deforming

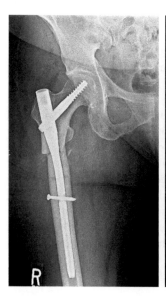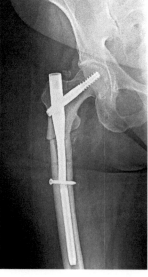

Figure 35.19 Failure of cephalomedullary nail. Postoperative AP view (a). Failure of implant via breakage of nail at interlocking screw hole. Varus malreduction may have contributed to implant breakage (b).

muscle forces that affect the fracture fragments, the proximal fragment can remain flexed (resulting in apex anterior malreduction), abducted (resulting in varus malreduction) and externally rotated (resulting in internal malrotation). Obtaining appropriate reduction and maintaining control of the proximal fragment at all times is absolutely critical during reaming and nail placement.

NONUNION

Nonunion is unusual in the management of subtrochanteric femoral fractures. However, nonunion is problematic when it does occur. Excessive soft tissue stripping, placement and reckless handling of the medial fragments may contribute to nonunion by devascularizing the bone fragments. When nonunion does occur, hardware often eventually fails if the patient continues to bear weight. This leads to the need for revision fixation. Malreduction and poor fixation can also contribute to nonunions.

Prior to revision, a CT scan and inflammatory markers (erythrocyte sedimentation rate, C-reactive protein and CBC with differential) should be obtained. A screening metabolic evaluation should also be completed, including vitamin D, calcium and intact PTH at minimum, with additional tests and formal referral to endocrinology obtained when indicated. Additionally, bone scans can be considered in cases where osteomyelitis is suspected. The patient's overall medial status should be optimized, including optimizing nutritional status, controlling comorbidities (specifically diabetes, with HgA1c <8 ideally) and smoking and alcohol cessation.

OUTCOMES

Subtrochanteric fractures caused by low energy trauma are similar to other proximal femoral fractures with a high mortality rate during the first year after the injury. As with other proximal femoral fractures in the elderly, there was an increased level of social dependence, an increase in the use of walking aids, and a reduction in mobility among survivors.

When executed properly, excellent outcomes can be achieved following management of subtrochanteric femur fractures with a variety of implants. Trochanteric-entry cephalomedullary nails are currently the mainstay of fixation for most orthopaedic surgeons who treat subtrochanteric femur fractures, with acceptable rates of perioperative complications, favourable functional outcomes and high union rates with low rates of complications.

A systematic review comparing intramedullary and extramedullary fixation of subtrochanteric fractures was performed using a search of MEDLINE (1950 to June 2007), CINAHL (1982 to June 2007) and EMBASE (1980 to June 2007). Three level I and nine level IV studies were identified and used in the systematic review of outcomes for intramedullary and extramedullary fixation for subtrochanteric fractures. The study found that there is grade B evidence that operative time is reduced and that fixation failure is reduced with the use of intramedullary implants for subtrochanteric fractures. The authors suggested future studies should perform subgroup analysis according to the type of population sampled (i.e. young versus elderly) and subtrochanteric fracture type.[57]

In a study of 302 patients who sustained low energy subtrochanteric fractures, the authors found that at 1 year, 74 (24.5%) patients had died and 17 (5.6%) had been lost to follow-up. The remaining 211 (69.9%) patients who were followed were evaluated with regard to functional outcome and postoperative complications during the first year after injury. As with other proximal femoral fractures in the elderly, there was an increased level of social dependence, an increase in the use of walking aids and a reduction in mobility among survivors. Although 88 (41.7%) of the 211 patients who were evaluated at 1 year after the injury had some degree of hip discomfort, only two described the pain as severe and disabling. Reoperation for the treatment of implant- or fracture-related complications was required in 27 (8.9%) of the 302 patients, however, only 18 of those patients required nail revision, corresponding with a 1-year nail-revision rate of 7.1%. Of the 250 patients who survived for 6 months after the injury, five (2%) had a nonunion that was confirmed at the time of surgical exploration.[49]

REFERENCES

1. Roche JJ, Wenn RT, Sahota O, Moran CG. Effect of comorbidities and postoperative complications on mortality after hip fracture in elderly people: Prospective observational cohort study. *BMJ* 2005;331(7529):1374.

2. Endo Y, Aharonoff GB, Zuckerman JD, Egol KA, Koval KJ. Gender differences in patients with hip fracture: A greater risk of morbidity and mortality in men. *J Orthop Trauma* 2005;19(1):29–35.

3. Koval KJ, Skovron ML, Aharonoff GB, Zuckerman JD. Predictors of functional recovery after hip fracture in the elderly. *Clin Orthop Relat Res* 1998;(348):22–8.

4. Koval KJ, Skovron ML, Aharonoff GB, Meadows SE, Zuckerman JD. Ambulatory ability after hip fracture. A prospective study in geriatric patients. *Clin Orthop Relat Res* 1995; (310):150–9.

5. Rockwood CA, Green DP, Bucholz RW. *Rockwood and Green's Fractures in Adults.* 6th ed. Philadelphia: Lippincott Williams & Wilkins; 2006.

6. Parker MJ, Handoll HH. Conservative versus operative treatment for extracapsular hip fractures. *Cochrane Database Syst Rev* 2000;(2):CD000337.

7. Haidukewych GJ. Intertrochanteric fractures: Ten tips to improve results. *J Bone Joint Surg Am* 2009;91(3):712–19.

8. Butler M, Forte ML, Joglekar SB, Swiontkowski MF, Kane RL. Evidence summary: Systematic review of surgical treatments for geriatric hip fractures. *J Bone Joint Surg Am* 2011;93(12):1104–15.

9. Forte ML, Virnig BA, Eberly LE, Swiontkowski MF, Feldman R, Bhandari M, et al. Provider factors associated with intramedullary nail use for intertrochanteric hip fractures. *J Bone Joint Surg Am* 2010;92(5):1105–14.

10. Anglen JO, Weinstein JN, American Board of Orthopaedic Surgery Research Committee. Nail or plate fixation of intertrochanteric hip fractures: Changing pattern of practice. A review of the American Board of Orthopaedic Surgery Database. *J Bone Joint Surg Am* 2008;90(4):700–7.

11. Radcliff TA, Regan E, Cowper Ripley DC, Hutt E. Increased use of intramedullary nails for intertrochanteric proximal femoral fractures in veterans affairs hospitals: A comparative effectiveness study. *J Bone Joint Surg Am* 2012;94(9):833–40.

12. Forte ML, Virnig BA, Kane RL, Durham S, Bhandari M, Feldman R, et al. Geographic variation in device use for intertrochanteric hip fractures. *J Bone Joint Surg Am* 2008;90(4):691–9.

13. Utrilla AL, Reig JS, Munoz FM, Tufanisco CB. Trochanteric gamma nail and compression hip screw for trochanteric fractures: A randomized, prospective, comparative study in 210 elderly patients with a new design of the gamma nail. *J Orthop Trauma* 2005;19(4):229–33.

14. Jones HW, Johnston P, Parker M. Are short femoral nails superior to the sliding hip screw? A meta-analysis of 24 studies involving 3,279 fractures. *Int Orthop* 2006;30(2):69–78.

15. Palm H, Jacobsen S, Sonne-Holm S, Gebuhr P, Hip Fracture Study Group. Integrity of the lateral femoral wall in intertrochanteric hip fractures: An important predictor of a reoperation. *J Bone Joint Surg Am* 2007;89(3):470–5.

16. De Bruijn K, den Hartog D, Tuinebreijer W, Roukema G. Reliability of predictors for screw cutout in intertrochanteric hip fractures. *J Bone Joint Surg Am* 2012;94(14):1266–72.

17. Baumgaertner MR, Curtin SL, Lindskog DM, Keggi JM. The value of the tip-apex distance in predicting failure of fixation of peritrochanteric fractures of the hip. *J Bone Joint Surg Am* 1995;77(7):1058–64.

18. Vossinakis IC, Badras LS. The external fixator compared with the sliding hip screw for pertrochanteric fractures of the femur. *J Bone Joint Surg Br* 2002;84(1):23–9.

19. Kim SY, Kim YG, Hwang JK. Cementless calcar-replacement hemiarthroplasty compared with intramedullary fixation of unstable intertrochanteric fractures. A prospective, randomized study. *J Bone Joint Surg Am* 2005;87(10):2186–92.

20. Stappaerts KH, Deldycke J, Broos PL, Staes FF, Rommens PM, Claes P. Treatment of unstable peritrochanteric fractures in elderly patients with a compression hip screw or with the Vandeputte (VDP) endoprosthesis: A prospective randomized study. *J Orthop Trauma* 1995;9(4):292–7.

21. Willoughby R. Dynamic hip screw in the management of reverse obliquity intertrochanteric neck of femur fractures. *Injury* 2005;36(1):105–9.

22. Brammar TJ, Kendrew J, Khan RJ, Parker MJ. Reverse obliquity and transverse fractures of the trochanteric region of the femur; a review of 101 cases. *Injury* 2005;36(7):851–7.

23. Haidukewych GJ, Israel TA, Berry DJ. Reverse obliquity fractures of the intertrochanteric region of the femur. *J Bone Joint Surg Am* 2001;83-A(5):643–50.

24. Kuzyk PR, Lobo J, Whelan D, Zdero R, McKee MD, Schemitsch EH. Biomechanical evaluation of extramedullary versus intramedullary fixation for reverse obliquity intertrochanteric fractures. *J Orthop Trauma* 2009;23(1):31–8.

25. Sadowski C, Lubbeke A, Saudan M, Riand N, Stern R, Hoffmeyer P. Treatment of reverse oblique and transverse intertrochanteric fractures with use of an intramedullary nail or a 95 degrees screw-plate: A prospective, randomized study. *J Bone Joint Surg Am* 2002;84-A(3):372–81.

26. Chou DT, Taylor AM, Boulton C, Moran CG. Reverse oblique intertrochanteric femoral fractures treated with the intramedullary hip screw (IMHS). *Injury* 2012;43(6):817–21.

27. Koval KJ, Sala DA, Kummer FJ, Zuckerman JD. Postoperative weight-bearing after a fracture of the femoral neck or an intertrochanteric fracture. *J Bone Joint Surg Am* 1998;80(3):352–6.

28. Koval KJ, Friend KD, Aharonoff GB, Zukerman JD. Weight bearing after hip fracture: A prospective series of 596 geriatric hip fracture patients. *J Orthop Trauma* 1996;10(8):526–30.

29. Herrera A, Domingo J, Martinez A. Results of osteosynthesis with the ITST nail in fractures of the trochanteric region of the femur. *Int Orthop* 2008;32(6):767–72.

30. Lenich A, Mayr E, Ruter A, Mockl C, Fuchtmeier B. First results with the trochanter fixation nail (TFN): A report on 120 cases. *Arch Orthop Trauma Surg* 2006;126(10):706–12.

31. Frank MA, Yoon RS, Yalamanchili P, Choung EW, Liporace FA. Forward progression of the helical blade into the pelvis after repair with the Trochanter Fixation Nail (TFN). *J Orthop Trauma* 2011;25(10):e100–3.

32. Haidukewych GJ, Berry DJ. Hip arthroplasty for salvage of failed treatment of intertrochanteric hip fractures. *J Bone Joint Surg Am* 2003;85-A(5):899–904.

33. Exaltacion JJ, Incavo SJ, Mathews V, Parsley B, Noble P. Hip arthroplasty after intramedullary hip screw fixation: A perioperative evaluation. *J Orthop Trauma* 2012;26(3):141–7.

34. Kaplan K, Miyamoto R, Levine BR, Egol KA, Zuckerman JD. Surgical management of hip fractures: An evidence-based review of the literature. II: Intertrochanteric fractures. *J Am Acad Orthop Surg* 2008;16(11):665–73.

35. Parker MJ, Handoll HH. Gamma and other cephalocondylic intramedullary nails versus extramedullary implants for extracapsular hip fractures in adults. *Cochrane Database Syst Rev* 2005;(4):CD000093.

36. Matre K, Havelin LI, Gjertsen JE, Espehaug B, Fevang JM. Intramedullary nails result in more reoperations than sliding hip screws in two-part intertrochanteric fractures. *Clin Orthop Relat Res* 2013;471(4):1379–86.

37. Forte ML, Virnig BA, Swiontkowski MF, Bhandari M, Feldman R, Eberly LE, et al. Ninety-day mortality after intertrochanteric hip fracture: Does provider volume matter? *J Bone Joint Surg Am* 2010;92(4):799–806.

38. Bohl DD, Basques BA, Golinvaux NS, Miller CP, Baumgaertner MR, Grauer JN. Extramedullary compared with intramedullary implants for intertrochanteric hip fractures: Thirty-day outcomes of 4432 procedures from the ACS NSQIP database. *J Bone Joint Surg Am* 2014;96(22):1871–7.

39. Drake RL, Vogl W, Mitchell AWM. *Gray's Anatomy for Students*. 2nd ed. Philadelphia, PA: Churchill Livingstone/Elsevier; 2009.

40. Netter FH. *Atlas of Human Anatomy*. 4th ed. Philadelphia, PA: Saunders/Elsevier; 2006.

41. Kloen P, Rubel IF, Lyden JP, Helfet DL. Subtrochanteric fracture after cannulated screw fixation of femoral neck fractures: A report of four cases. *J Orthop Trauma* 2003;17(3):225–9.

42. Oakey JW, Stover MD, Summers HD, Sartori M, Havey RM, Patwardhan AG. Does screw configuration affect subtrochanteric fracture after femoral neck fixation? *Clin Orthop Relat Res* 2006;443:302–6.

43. Lasanianos NG, Kanakaris NK, Giannoudis PV. Intramedullary nailing as a 'second hit' phenomenon in experimental research: Lessons learned and future directions. *Clin Orthop Relat Res* 2010;468(9):2514–29.

44. Ostrum RF, Levy MS. Penetration of the distal femoral anterior cortex during intramedullary nailing for subtrochanteric fractures: A report of three cases. *J Orthop Trauma* 2005;19(9):656–60.

45. Afsari A, Liporace F, Lindvall E, Infante A Jr, Sagi HC, Haidukewych GJ. Clamp-assisted reduction of high subtrochanteric fractures of the femur. *J Bone Joint Surg Am* 2009;91(8):1913–18.

46. Ostrum RF, Marcantonio A, Marburger R. A critical analysis of the eccentric starting point for trochanteric intramedullary femoral nailing. *J Orthop Trauma* 2005;19(10):681–6.

47. Menezes DF, Gamulin A, Noesberger B. Is the proximal femoral nail a suitable implant for treatment of all trochanteric fractures? *Clin Orthop Relat Res* 2005;439:221–7.

48. Starr AJ, Hay MT, Reinert CM, Borer DS, Christensen KC. Cephalomedullary nails in the treatment of high-energy proximal femur fractures

in young patients: A prospective, randomized comparison of trochanteric versus piriformis fossa entry portal. *J Orthop Trauma* 2006;20(4):240–6.

49. Robinson CM, Houshian S, Khan LA. Trochanteric-entry long cephalomedullary nailing of subtrochanteric fractures caused by low-energy trauma. *J Bone Joint Surg Am* 2005;87(10):2217–26.

50. Pai CH. Dynamic condylar screw for subtrochanteric femur fractures with greater trochanteric extension. *J Orthop Trauma* 1996;10(5):317–22.

51. Yoo MC, Cho YJ, Kim KI, Khairuddin M, Chun YS. Treatment of unstable peritrochanteric femoral fractures using a 95 degrees angled blade plate. *J Orthop Trauma* 2005;19(10):687–92.

52. Saini P, Kumar R, Shekhawat V, Joshi N, Bansal M, Kumar S. Biological fixation of comminuted subtrochanteric fractures with proximal femur locking compression plate. *Injury* 2013;44(2):226–31.

53. Yoon RS, Beebe KS, Benevenia J. Prophylactic bilateral intramedullary femoral nails for bisphosphonate-associated signs of impending subtrochanteric hip fracture. *Orthopedics* 2010;33(4):267–70.

54. Black DM, Kelly MP, Genant HK, Palermo L, Eastell R, Bucci-Rechtweg C, et al. Bisphosphonates and fractures of the subtrochanteric or diaphyseal femur. *N Engl J Med* 2010;362(19):1761–71.

55. Park-Wyllie LY, Mamdani MM, Juurlink DN, Hawker GA, Gunraj N, Austin PC, et al. Bisphosphonate use and the risk of subtrochanteric or femoral shaft fractures in older women. JAMA 2011;305(8):783–9.

56. Egol KA, Park JH, Prensky C, Rosenberg ZS, Peck V, Tejwani NC. Surgical treatment improves clinical and functional outcomes for patients who sustain incomplete bisphosphonate-related femur fractures. *J Orthop Trauma* 2013;27(6):331–5.

57. Kuzyk PR, Bhandari M, McKee MD, Russell TA, Schemitsch EH. Intramedullary versus extramedullary fixation for subtrochanteric femur fractures. *J Orthop Trauma* 2009;23(6):465–70.

36

Femoral diaphyseal fractures

JOYCE S.B. KOH AND TET SEN HOWE

INTRODUCTION

The femur is the longest and strongest bone in the human body. Fractures of the shaft of the femur are usually thought to be due to high velocity injuries, primarily after motor vehicle accidents or after falls from a height. There is increasing awareness that in the elderly these fractures are of an osteoporotic nature.[1,2] As opposed to fractures in younger groups, they typically involve females above the age of 70, usually with minimal trauma. This group of people requires the same detailed workup as any other osteoporotic fracture.

There is also a small subset of fractures in the elderly that are due to malignancy and metabolic bone diseases as well as stress fractures. These, although rare, must be considered in all cases despite innocuous-looking X-rays. Where appropriate, additional blood tests and imaging must be ordered.

There is a paucity of well-conducted studies in the elderly femoral shaft fracture. What little evidence we have suggests that they have approximately the same mortality and morbidity as a hip fracture in a patient of the same age. With a rising age distribution in most developed countries, these fractures are likely to increase in incidence as well as absolute numbers.

The vast majority of these fractures are treated surgically except in the very medically unfit. In general they should be treated along similar principles as hip fractures with the aim of allowing early weight bearing and rehabilitation.

EPIDEMIOLOGY OF FEMORAL FRACTURES IN THE ELDERLY

Femoral fractures exhibit a bimodal distribution. This epidemiological pattern has been demonstrated by numerous authors including Singer and Hedlund.[3,4] While the average incidence has been estimated at 1–1.33 fractures per 10,000 population per year, Singer has shown that cases clustered around the 15–34-year-old age group [incidence of 1.64–3.73 per 10,000 population] and started to peak again after 70 years of age [incidence of 2.3–37.14 per 10,000 population] in femoral shaft fractures presenting to the Royal Infirmary of Edinburgh from 1992 to 1993.[3] Chapter 1 in this book shows that currently 69.9% of all patients who present to the Royal Infirmary of Edinburgh with femoral diaphyseal fractures are ≥65 years of age with 84% of females being ≥65 years of age.

In addition to the bimodal distribution, a gender specific pattern of presentation has also been demonstrated by Singer[3] and Hedlund.[4] Singer's younger cohort clustered in male patients while the older cohort involved a far higher proportion of female patients.[3] In another Swedish cohort spanning 1998–2004, men had a younger median age (27 years, IQR 12–68),[5] whereas women had a far higher median age (79 years, IQR 62–86),[5] similar to those sustaining osteoporotic hip fractures. Analysis showed that 54% of the admissions were females and 46% males in this cohort.[5]

Although much attention has been focused on the epidemiological trends, prevention and management of proximal femoral fractures, diaphyseal femoral fractures in the elderly may carry an equivalent impact. Comparing a cohort in the 1950s to one in the 1970s and early 1980s, Bengnér and co-authors noted that the risk of low energy femoral shaft fractures had increased in elderly women.[6] These patients may be more frail and require more healthcare resources as evidenced by up to 85% of patients presenting with low energy femoral fractures having multiple comorbidities, with a length of hospital stay (15 days) equivalent or even longer than that of osteoporotic hip fracture cohorts. With a rapidly aging population in most developed countries, we are likely to see an increasing trend in the presentation of elderly diaphyseal femoral fractures which will place a strain on healthcare systems.

A decline in hip fracture incidence (600/100,000 person-years to 400/100,000 person-years) has been observed from 1996 to 2006 in national discharge and medical claims data in the United States, possibly as a result of aggressive preventive measures for osteoporotic fractures. In contrast, subtrochanteric, femoral shaft and lower femoral fracture rates remained stable, although at far lower rates of 20 per 100,000 person-years. Similar trends but lower rates were observed in males than females.[2]

CLASSIFICATION AND MECHANISM OF INJURY

There is no specific classification for elderly femoral diaphyseal fractures. The AO/OTA classification still remains the most common classification system used to categorize these fractures. In the AO/OTA classification, type A fractures are simple fractures and include spiral fractures (A1), oblique fractures (A2) and transverse fractures (A3). Type B fractures are wedge fractures and include spiral wedges (B1), bending wedges (B2) and fragmented wedges (B3). Type C fractures are complex fractures with the C1 group containing all spiral fractures, the C2 group all segmental fractures and the C3 group all comminuted fractures. In type A and B fractures the suffix 0.1 represents a fracture in the subtrochanteric zone, with 0.2 used for the middle zone and 0.3 for the distal zone. In type C fractures the suffixes 0.1 though 0.3 represent increasing bone damage.

It is important to distinguish high energy osteoporotic fractures from low energy fractures that happen to occur in the elderly. A small percentage of femoral diaphyseal fractures in the elderly result from polytrauma, usually as a result of motor vehicle accidents. These elderly patients sustaining a femoral fracture in a high energy injury behave like younger patients with a similar injury except that they have less physiological reserves. They also may have a more prolonged rehabilitation period and more trouble coping with rehabilitation.

Low energy osteoporotic femoral diaphyseal fractures

An AO/OTA A1 spiral fracture involving the middle third of the femoral shaft was reported as the most common pattern in low energy femoral shaft fractures in the mid-1990s

(Figure 36.1a). These fractures were closed with no or minimal comminution.[7] Such fractures are believed to occur as a result of a twisting force in osteopenic bone. Two-thirds of the patients had at least one local or general factor weakening the mechanical strength of the bone. In the majority of these patients, the femoral fracture is an isolated injury with no associated injuries.[7]

Age-related bone loss together with weakening of bone stock and quality from associated comorbid conditions contribute to the majority of these fractures. Aging also goes hand-in-hand with other pathophysiological changes and conditions that can predispose to femoral shaft fractures. They can be broadly classified into stress fractures arising from structural or biochemical abnormalities, pathological fractures from metastatic or primary bone diseases, metabolic disorders affecting the bone and periprosthetic fractures.

Atypical femoral fractures

An interesting shift in the pattern of femoral diaphyseal fractures in the elderly began to emerge in the mid-2000s. In contrast to the spiral pattern previously reported, these fractures had a transverse or short oblique configuration.[8] (AO/OTA A3 configuration), with characteristic beaking and a medial spike of varying length and hardly any comminution (Figure 36.1b). These almost pathognomonic features

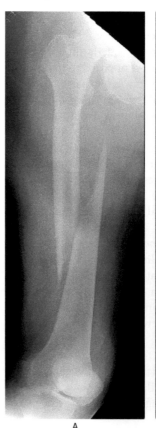
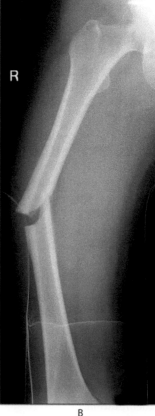

A   B

Figure 36.1 (a) Osteoporotic fracture with spiral pattern. (b) An atypical femoral fracture (AFF).

have formed the basis of the American Society for Bone and Mineral Research (ASBMR) Task Force criteria for the definition of atypical femoral fractures (AFFs), a term implying deviation from the usual characteristics of the typical spiral or oblique osteoporotic femoral shaft fracture.

Unlike the usual osteoporotic fractures which are usually seen in the middle third but can occur anywhere along the femoral shaft, AFFs are clustered around the subtrochanteric region[8] and the femoral shaft.[8] They are rarely seen beyond the middle third of the shaft[8] and they almost exclusively involve the tensile stress regions of the femur. These fractures usually occur as a result of low energy falls but some are actually atraumatic. Approximately 30–50% are bilateral[8] They are generally believed to originate from a lateral cortical stress fracture which manifests as localized cortical thickening,[8] and the presence of a 'dreaded black line' across the area of thickening in association with prodromal thigh pain has been shown to be associated with a high risk of complete fracture.[9] An initial lack of awareness of this condition among clinicians has led to the misdiagnosis of spinal stenosis or arthrosis of the hip or knee with referred pain even with radiological evidence of the stress lesion. Often these patients are thought to have osteoarthritis of the knee and a total knee replacement done for the wrong reasons (Figure 36.2).

These unusual features, in the presence of a known history of prolonged bisphosphonate therapy[8] have caused surgeons to postulates that the AFF is a stress fracture arising from oversuppression of bone turnover by bisphosphonate therapy.

Femoral stress fractures in the elderly

Stress fractures may occur as a result of physiological bowing and severe varus secondary to end-stage arthrosis. Age-related changes in femoral morphology, in conjunction with stiffness from knee arthrosis, can result in stress fractures along the femoral shaft (Figure 36.3). A resultant medialization of body weight transfer due to femoral bowing[10] and increasing knee varus can lead to tensile failures along the lateral cortex of the femoral shaft.

Pathological fractures

Pathological fractures can occur due to metastatic disease from a distant tumour or from a primary tumour arising from the bone, the most common being multiple myeloma.

METASTATIC DISEASE

Pathological fractures from metastatic bone disease, though uncommon, are encountered with increasing frequency in the young-old (reported median age of 63 years) due to improving survivorship in cancer patients. The skeleton is the third most frequent location for metastases, and cancers arising from the breast, prostate, lungs, thyroid and kidneys are known to commonly metastasize to bone, with breast cancer being the most common primary tumour. The femur is the most common long bone to be affected by bony

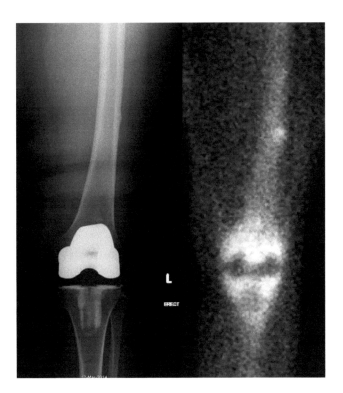

Figure 36.2 An atypical femoral fracture diagnosed as osteoarthritis of the knee with a total joint replacement done. The bone scan shows a typically hot spot on the lateral cortex.

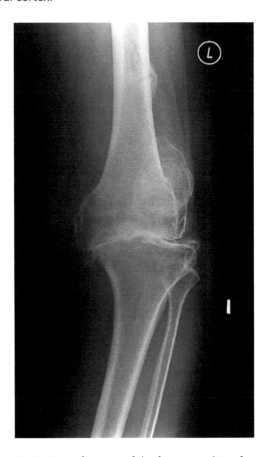

Figure 36.3 Stress fracture of the femur resulting from osteoarthritis with resulting varus and stiffness of the knee.

metastasis (44%)[11] with the upper third involved in 50% of cases. These fractures are consistently missed in a small number of patients and where there is an index of suspicion, additional imaging and investigations should be ordered as necessary. A large majority of these fractures are treated by closed nailing and often no biopsy is taken.

An impending pathological fracture of the femur is an indicator for prophylactic stabilization. The Mirel scoring system gives an estimate of fracture risk based on four parameters: the site and size of the lesion, the type of lesion and the degree of pain. Metastatic fractures are discussed further in Chapter 16.

MYELOMA

Myloma has become increasingly common in this age group and is often missed due to a low index of suspicion leading to delayed treatment and further morbidity from subsequent fractures. As many good treatment options are currently available, failure to make an early diagnosis can severely impact the patient's long-term outcome.

METABOLIC BONE DISEASE

Many elderly patients have associated comorbidities that can result in metabolic bone disease. Common conditions include end-stage renal disease, Paget's disease (Figure 36.4), vitamin D deficiency, malnutrition and hypoparathyroidism. An endocrinological consultation may be warranted in suspicious cases.

Periprosthetic and peri-implant fractures

The increasing incidence of arthroplasty procedures for degenerative hip and knee conditions is posing unique challenges with fractures occurring around the implants. Reported incidences of 1.1% after primary hip arthroplasty and 4.0% after revision arthroplasty, based on the Mayo Clinic Joint Registry,[12] have been recorded. The average age is 68.1 years with a male:female ratio of 1:2. Interactions between the native bone and implant may influence the fracture pattern and interfere with healing or the placement of other fixation devices, and the long-term presence of the device may even change the structure of the bone and increase risk of fracture. Duncan and Masri developed the Vancouver classification according to location, implant stability and degree of bone loss to account for this complex interplay of factors and provide an algorithm facilitating treatment of these fractures. Periprosthetic fractures are discussed in Chapter 17.

Polytrauma in the elderly

As life expectancy increases in developed nations, trauma centres are projected to see an increasing load of elderly patients sustaining femoral fractures as a result of polytrauma. In cohorts matched for sex, age, Injury Severity Score (ISS) and comorbidities, the presence of a femoral fracture led to an increased number of complications, longer

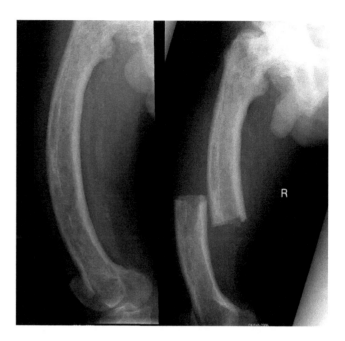

Figure 36.4 An 80-year-old patient with Paget's disease with subsequent bowing and a 'chalkstick' fracture.

total hospital length of stay, more discharges to rehabilitation centres, more accompanying long bone fractures and an increased likelihood of surgery. However, there was no difference in length of ICU stay or in-hospital, 6-month and 1-year mortality between patients with and without femoral fractures.[13] Polytrauma in the elderly is discussed in Chapter 14.

ASSOCIATED INJURIES

Femoral neck fractures are associated with femoral shaft fractures in 1–9% of cases. Up to 15–50%[14] of these ipsilateral fractures may be missed unless specifically looked for. Femoral fractures can also have extensions to the supracondylar or intra-articular region of the distal femoral, thus limiting common treatment options such as the intramedullary nail. Careful scrutiny of radiographs of the entire femur prevent any unnecessary perioperative surprises!

Low energy femoral fractures tend to occur in isolation. An exception is seen in AFFs where contralateral involvement may result in bilateral femoral shaft fractures. A full radiographic assessment of the contralateral femur is advocated once an AFF is diagnosed.

DIAGNOSIS

The diagnosis of a fracture of the shaft of the femur is usually relatively straightforward. A plain X-ray will reveal the type and pattern of these fractures in the large majority of these fractures. However, it is vital to obtain high quality films. In large people, the standard X-ray plates may not be able to cover the ends of the femur or one end may be over-penetrated or under-penetrated. In these cases, the hip and/or knee should have a separate well centred X-ray. Both the hip and knee should be scrutinized for associated fractures.

As most osteopenic fractures in the elderly are caused by a twisting force, many of these cases result in a spiral fracture pattern that extends distally. The distal extension is often missed if not looked for and may result in suboptimal fracture fixation with a plate or nail that is too short (Figure 36.5). If in doubt, additional imaging including CT scans and/or MRI studies should be obtained.

ASSESSMENT AND PREPARATION FOR SURGERY

This group of elderly patients should be rapidly worked up and surgery performed expeditiously. Most studies show that morbidity and mortality parallel those of hip fractures.[15] We recommend a similar workup, if possible in conjunction with a geriatrician and an anaesthetist. All patients should be treated as any patient with a femoral shaft fracture, with routine arterial blood gas and/or pulse oximetry monitoring, especially in the first 24 hours.

Elderly patients have a lower tolerance for blood loss and should receive crystalloid and colloid volume replacement and blood transfusions earlier than younger patients. All elderly patients should receive limb and chest physiotherapy upon admission to reduce respiratory complications and bedsores. We recommend a limb immobilizer or simple traction for pain relief if the delay until surgery is short. In cases where the time to surgical treatment is prolonged, we recommend a balanced form of traction using a skeletal traction pin inserted through the distal femur. The recommended traction weight is 15% of body weight.

TREATMENT

The aim of surgery is to restore the patient to walking and a normal lifestyle as soon as possible. Very few patients are treated non-operatively, the exception sometimes being very sick patients with a high anaesthetic risk. However we find that even bedridden patients benefit from surgery as it makes nursing, transfer and activities of daily living much easier to perform. For this reason, nailing is the treatment of choice in femoral diaphyseal fractures in the elderly. The majority of patients will undergo a closed intramedullary nailing procedure as soon as they are fit on the next operating list. We recommend against operating in the middle of the night on an emergency basis unless the patient has been fully worked up and an experienced operating team is available. Where possible, the surgical procedure should be done within 24 hours.[16]

Simultaneous hip and shaft fractures

Associated hip fractures are treated differently than in younger patient where priority is towards preservation of blood supply of the femoral head. In elderly patients, hip fractures, especially unstable ones, do not necessarily receive priority in treatment. A hip replacement may be

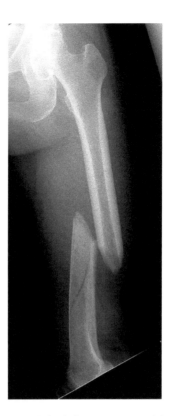

Figure 36.5 Femoral shaft fracture in an elderly patient with minimally displaced spiral extension.

done for the hip and the femoral fracture treated independently. In some cases femoral plating is warranted. If this is the case we recommend the use of locked plates.

INTRAMEDULLARY NAILING IN ELDERLY FEMORAL SHAFT FRACTURES

Advantages

An intramedullary nail is a load sharing device. This construct allows early ambulation and weight bearing. When done in a closed fashion, there is much less disruption of the soft tissue envelope and the fracture haematoma. The widespread use of locking nails has removed many of the problems associated with shortening and rotational stability. Although these benefits are important in all patients, they are particularly important in the elderly and in patients with osteoporotic bone where other constructs fail more often. Nailing of the femur spans the entire bone and is of particular importance in pathological fractures.

Disadvantages

Nailing of the femur takes a longer time, requires a higher level of surgical expertise and is associated with a significant level of radiation. In the elderly, nailing may be made more difficult by bowing of the femur. A severely bowed femur is a relative contraindication to femoral nailing.

Indications

Intramedullary nailing has become the default option so that nowadays the surgeon has to look for a reason not to perform this operation. The newer generation of nails have more locking options, stronger bolts and are more anatomical. They have extended the indications for nailing to include fractures in the proximal and distal metaphyseal regions of the femur. A long intramedullary nail to span the entire femur is particularly recommended in AFF. These fractures are generally thought to have slower healing times, may occur in contiguous locations in the same femur and are prone to stress risers.

Antegrade intramedullary nailing

Antegrade intramedullary nailing has become the procedure of choice in diaphyseal fractures.

Preoperative planning is an essential aid to a smooth, trouble-free surgery. When in doubt, the other femur should be X-rayed to assess both femoral bow and canal size. The hip should be scrutinized for an occult hip fracture.

Femoral nailing can be performed supine, with or without a traction table, or in a lateral position. We recommend a traction table if there is a shortage of skilled assistants as it allows better control of patient positioning. Femoral nailing done without a traction table has the advantage of a lower incidence of traction injury to the groin as well as a reduced likelihood of neuropraxia and compartment syndrome in the other leg. Small sized elderly patients, especially women, may have a narrow femoral canal. It is critical to preoperatively measure the isthmus of the femur (taking into account the degree of magnification) and ensure that an appropriate sized nail is available. Very narrow femoral canals are a relative contraindication to nailing and a plate should be used instead.

There is currently no strong evidence to show the advantage of either a piriformis entry point or a trochanteric entry point.[17] A trochanteric entry point is easier in obese patients and there may be fewer problems with nail insertion and less disturbance of the hip abductor mechanism but it is associated with a higher risk of iatrogenic medial wall comminution and varus malalignment. There is also a possibility of eccentrically reaming out the lateral femoral wall, especially if the starting point is too lateral. Newer nail designs with a lateral proximal bend have minimized these problems. The piriformis entry point is more collinear with the femoral shaft but may be more difficult to access.

Whatever entry point is used, this is the most critical part of the procedure and we recommend that this part of the nailing procedure be done with great care and that the optimum starting point be found and used. This will avoid many problems later in the procedure.

Reamed nailing provides a better fit, more stability and higher union rates even when the nail is locked. The amount of reaming done depends on the specific type of nail that is used. As a general principle, the femoral medullary cavity should be minimally reamed if there is an optimum entry point and normal femoral morphology. In such instances, only the region around the isthmus needs to be reamed. Reaming provides autogenous bone graft to the fracture site and this may improve union rates.[18] If the surgeon runs into difficulties however, over-reaming the medullary canal and using a slender nail allows the procedure to be completed without catastrophic problems, but with a slightly less robust construct.

There is currently a mismatch between the radius of curvature of commercially available nails and the anterior bow of the femur. The available nails generally have a larger radius of curvature compared to the average femur. In most mid-shaft femoral fractures, this results in a slight loss of the anterior bow but this is a relatively minor problem. Prophylactic nailing of unbroken femora in tumour cases may risk the nail impinging on the anterior cortex of the femur (Figure 36.6).

Another problem with this group of patients is that they may also have severe femoral bowing in the coronal plane. This may make them unsuitable for an intramedullary nailing procedure. Trochanteric entry point nails have a proximal bow in the opposite direction which accentuates the problem (Figure 36.7). In minor bowing cases a straight nail, designed for a piriformis entry point, may be used with a trochanteric staring point to minimize the risk of damage to the femur. This technique combined with over-reaming of the medullary canal and the use of a smaller more flexible nail allows nailing of coronally bowed femurs. AFFs may have an endosteal shelf (Figure 36.8) that causes eccentric reaming. Occasionally there is a complete shelf that needs to be drilled to re-establish medullary canal continuity.

We recommend the use of locked nails in all cases to prevent shortening. Careful assessment of the rotation of the leg should be made before completing the locking to avoid postoperative residual rotational deformity. We recommend the use of a long nail which reaches the superior pole of the patella or the distal femoral physeal scar. After completion of the procedure, an assessment of limb length and rotation should be made to exclude gross malalignment and rotation problems before the patient is woken.

Retrograde nailing

There is little literature on the use of retrograde nailing in the elderly. The indications remain the same as in a younger patient. The main indication in the elderly population would be a femoral shaft fracture associated with an ipsilateral hip fracture. This method allows for the optimal treatment of each fracture without compromising fixation of either one. Retrograde nails have also been used successfully in periprosthetic fractures of the distal femur with an open intercondylar box system. We do not recommend retrograde nailing in AFFs of the femoral shaft as the proximal portion of the nail terminates in the subtrochanteric region where these fractures most often occur.

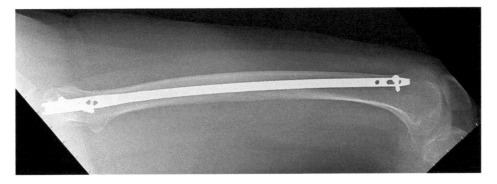

Figure 36.6 The radius of curvature of most femoral nails is greater than the anterior bow of the femur, resulting in anterior impingement in nailing incomplete or pathological fractures.

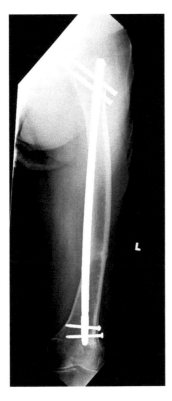

Figure 36.7 Superimposed diagram of a trochanteric entry point nail on a bowed femur showing curvature of the nail and the femur shaft in opposite directions.

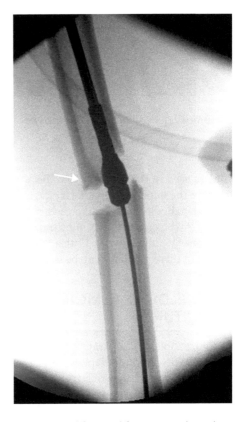

Figure 36.8 Atypical femoral fracture with endosteal shelf causing eccentric reaming.

Pathological fractures

The femur is a common site for metastatic disease in the elderly. All X-rays should be scrutinized with a high index of suspicion. If there is any doubt, further imaging investigations should be done to exclude a pathological fracture. The other femur should also be X-rayed. The studies need not be complete before the operation is undertaken as early stabilization of the femur has benefits that outweigh a lengthy investigative delay. We recommend biopsy of the lesion at the time of surgery with a long biopsy punch (Figure 36.9). This provides a higher yield, and better tissue, for histology than reamings, although reaming tissue should also

be sent for histology.[19] If there is any suspicion of tumour involvement near the proximal femur, we recommend the use of a reconstruction nail, with bolts passed through the femoral neck into the femoral head. After nailing, the entire femur should be irradiated.

Pitfalls and outcomes of nailing

Most large series show excellent results associated with the use of intramedullary nailing with union rates consistently above 95% and infection rates less than 1%. However there remain problems with limb rotation, and to a lesser degree, limb length. Angular deformities are a problem

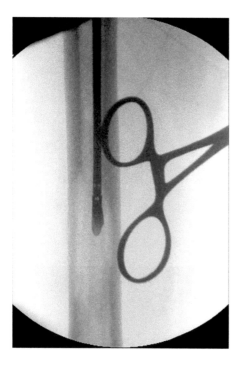

Figure 36.9 Biopsy punch for localized biopsy of the femur.

when nailing is used in the proximal and distal regions of the femur where the flare of the medullary cavity results in a loose fit of the nail which allows increasing deformity. A blocking screw can be used here to limit the nail to the central portion of the medullary cavity. With adequate care and expertise, most of these problems can be minimized.

PLATING IN ELDERLY FEMORAL SHAFT FRACTURES

The original principles of accurate reduction and rigid internal fixation of femoral diaphyseal fractures with plates have given way to that of relative stability for functional mobilization which requires the use of an intramedullary device as discussed in the previous section.

Although intramedullary nailing of elderly femoral shaft fractures is the current standard of care in most instances, plate osteosynthesis for femoral shaft fracture remains an important technique in the surgical management of femoral shaft fractures under certain circumstances.

Advantages

Open plating of femoral shaft fractures enables one to visualize the bone directly and hence achieve a more anatomical reduction of the fracture fragments, something which is largely recognized to be unnecessary in diaphyseal injuries except if there are fracture extensions into articular and periarticular regions. It should also be remembered that there is a potentially increased risk of iatrogenic femoral neck and distal femoral fractures from nail entry points

and eccentrically placed locking bolts in nails in the elderly because of the osteoporotic nature of the bone. It may also be impossible to insert an intramedullary nail into a femur with severe bowing in the coronal plane or if the femoral anatomy has been distorted by a previous malunion, whereas a plate can be contoured to fit the local anatomy.

Disadvantages

The need for an extensive surgical approach with the resultant soft tissue stripping, soft tissue insult and blood loss is less tolerated by an elderly patient. Also stress shielding of the bone spanned by the plate can result in stress fractures at the junction of the last screw hole and the adjacent bone. In addition, plate fixation of femoral diaphyseal fractures in osteopenic bone poses additional challenges in terms of screw pull-out and early loss of fixation. In the event of delayed union, the plate, being a load-bearing device, will cause stress transmission at the screw–bone interface, thus increasing the chance of pull-out in an already compromised screw purchase in poorer quality bone.

Indications

While intramedullary nailing has largely been established as the mainstay of surgical stabilization for femoral shaft fractures, plating may be advantageous in situations where intramedullary nailing is not technically feasible or poses potential physiological hazards to the patient. These include:

- Geriatric polytrauma with concomitant head trauma or pulmonary compromise
- Open fracture with a vascular injury where there is a need for exploration and repair
- Excessively narrow intramedullary canals
- Fractures in the presence of a previous malunion
- Severely bowed femora
- Fracture extension to the metaphyseal or intra-articular region
- Periprosthetic or peri-implant fractures
- Augmentative plating in femoral non-unions after intramedullary nailing
- Ipsilateral femoral neck and shaft fractures
- Fracture location in the proximal or distal femoral shaft
- Lack of availability of the equipment necessary for intramedullary nailing.

Evolution of femoral diaphyseal plating

Plating for femoral shaft fracture has undergone a paradigm shift with better understanding of soft tissue biology, diaphyseal bone healing and the biomechanics of diaphyseal plating.

Appreciation of the importance of the soft tissue and its contribution to periosteal blood supply and successful fracture healing has led to the concept of bridge plating

(Figure 36.10a) with careful tissue dissection, epi-periosteal exposure of bone, and indirect reduction of fractures to minimize stripping and devascularization of bone fragments.[20] Reduced soft tissue dissection also leads to less quadriceps tethering and improved knee range of motion. Routine bone grafting of the medial cortical defect as advocated in the 1980s is no longer advocated[21] as the reduced soft tissue dissection has obviated the need for a vascular stimulus. Plate construction and design has also evolved to optimize biological healing. Limited contact dynamic compression plates now allow for improved blood supply to the periosteum of the plated bone segment. Titanium plates have improved biological compatibility compared with stainless steel plates.

To optimize the biomechanics of plate and screw fixation in osteopenic bone, longer plates relative to the fracture length are thought to be particularly important.[21,22] This increases the lever arm of the plate. Oblique screws at either ends of the plate have also been described as another means to optimize fixation strength.[22] To avoid a longer exposure required for longer plate insertion, a minimally invasive plate osteosynthesis (MIPO) technique can be used proximally and distally with screws inserted percutaneously. Optimal siting of screws (Figure 36.10a) along the plate as opposed to filling every screw hole along the length of the plate (Figure 36.10b) has also been suggested. It is suggested that three screws are placed in each segment, with one screw at the end of the plate (preferably directed obliquely), one screw near the fracture site and a middle screw to improve torsional stability of the bone implant construct.[22] The use of unicortical screws at the periphery of the plate and multiple interfragmentary lag screws outside of the plate has been largely abandoned.

The wave plate (Figure 36.11) concept has been successfully used to tackle non-unions and re-fractures along the femoral shaft. Its use is associated with better preservation of periosteal blood supply and a biomechanically advantageous lever arm from the fracture site. When used in comminuted fractures, it encourages secondary bone healing with abundant callus formation. Another advantage is the capacity to apply periosteal bone graft at the fracture site.[23]

Locking plate and screws

The introduction of the locking compression plate (LCP) has revolutionized the management of diaphyseal fractures and may confer some advantages in the management of osteoporotic femoral shaft fractures. Depending on the application and resultant construct of the locked plate and screws, they provide different biological environments for healing.

An LCP may still be used as a compression plate for a simple femoral diaphyseal fracture. The initial screws are placed in the standard compressive fashion and additional locking screws may improve pull-out strength in osteoporotic bone. While conventional plate and screw constructs resist fracture fragment motion by the resultant friction generated by compressing plate to bone, a locking

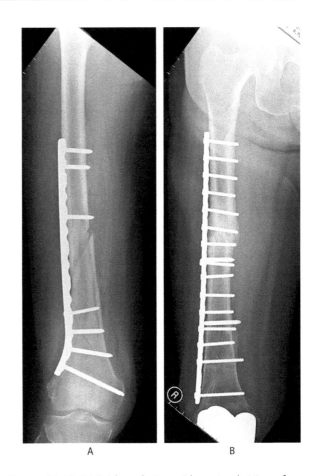

A   B

Figure 36.10 (a) Bridge plating with optimal siting of screws. (b) Excessive use of screws.

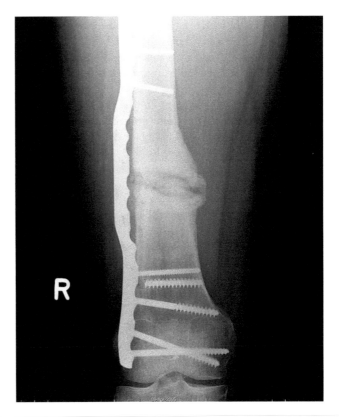

Figure 36.11 Wave plate.

plate-screw construct resists this motion via the engagement of the locking screw head in the plate. Although the pull-out strength for both conventional and locking screws from the bone is similar, this force is used more efficiently in a locked screw as it does not have to pull the plate to the bone. This has obvious advantages in treating an osteoporotic fracture.

In osteoporotic bone, locked plates may increasingly be indicated for diaphyseal/metaphyseal fractures where there is potential limitation in spanning the shorter segment. Locked plating in this instance has been shown to improve fixation strength under axial loading. However, fixation strength in bending and torsion is reduced compared to conventional plating. Adding one bicortical locked screw to an otherwise unicortical construct is recommended to improve torsional strength.[24]

An LCP construct is also indicated when bridging severely comminuted fractures. The plate serves as an 'internal fixator' device rather than a compression plate. In such a construct where there is minimal or no contact between the fracture site and the plate, placement of the innermost screws as close as practicable to the fracture should reduce potential failure in dynamic loading.[25] Construct rigidity is usually offset by the smaller interfragmentary strain within a comminuted fracture as opposed to that encountered in simple fracture patterns. Longer plate lengths are also advocated to improve overall axial stiffness.[25]

LCP construct rigidity and working length

While there is potential advantage in the improved pull-out strength of locked screws, there has always been concern that the LCP system creates a highly rigid construct detrimental to the degree of micromotion necessary for bone healing. This is relevant in a simple fracture where a similar deforming force will subject the fracture site to more strain compared to a comminuted fracture.

To moderate the rigidity of the LCP construct, the 'working length' concept has been suggested. The working length is defined as the distance between the screws in the proximal and distal segment closest to the fracture site (Figure 36.12). Axial stiffness and torsional rigidity are mainly influenced by the working length. By omitting one locking screw on either side of the fracture, the construct became almost twice as flexible in both compression and torsion. In terms of the number of screws per segment, more than three screws per fragment does little to increase axial stiffness, nor do four screws increase torsional rigidity.[25] In simple osteoporotic fractures, the rigidity can be reduced to optimize callus formation by increasing the working length, that is, by omitting the two screws adjacent to the fracture site.

Hybrid constructs combining the use of locking and non-locking screws have also increasingly been advocated to decrease the overall construct rigidity. Biomechanical studies showed that the hybrid construct was 7% stronger in bending, 42% stronger in torsion and 7% weaker in axial

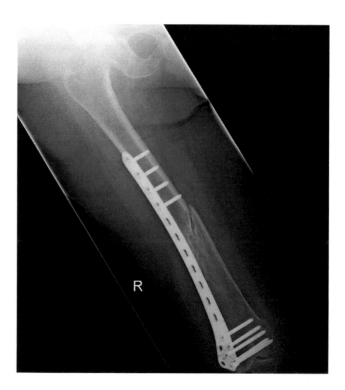

Figure 36.12 Plate with long working length.

compression compared to a pure locking screw construct. The small decrease in axial strength is likely to be well tolerated with protected weight bearing and hence, the hybrid construct may be of benefit in osteoporotic fixation.[26] Another study advocated the use of a non-locking screw at the end of a locking construct to reduce the risks of a peri-implant fracture in osteoporotic diaphyseal fractures by reducing the stress concentration at the end of the plate.[27]

Plating in peri-implant and periprosthetic fractures

Periprosthetic femoral fractures have been shown to be increasing with the increasing number of hip and knee arthroplasties in an active elderly cohort worldwide. They pose unique challenges due to the presence of an implant which interferes with securing either the proximal or distal segment of the fracture. Treatment should be individualized on the basis of the location of the fracture relative to the implant, the stability of the prosthesis and the presence or absence of associated bone loss.

Management commences with fracture classification and the Vancouver classification for femoral fractures around femoral components is an example of a well-accepted classification system that guides surgical decision-making. Proper preoperative planning and templating is paramount to ensure that proper instrumentation, implants and the necessary skills are available to avoid intraoperative problems.

Plating can be applied to most periprosthetic fractures of stable implants around the proximal femur [around hip stems] and the distal femur in periprosthetic fractures in the femoral component of total knee arthroplasties. The fracture pattern, simple or comminuted, will dictate the specific plating technique, compression plating or bridge plating. The development of indirect reduction techniques and an array of peri-articular plates allowing for secure cable placement, locking screw constructs and variable angle screw placement has enhanced the capability to secure sufficient stability in the segment of bone with the implant for early mobilization and fracture healing.

In general, broad large-fragment plates with offset holes to secure fixation around the stem of an intramedullary prosthesis with sufficient length allowing for overlap of as much of the intramedullary implant by at least six or even eight holes are currently advocated.[28] In osteoporotic bone, a longer plate that can be placed close to the end of the bony metaphysis instead of the metadiaphyseal junction is also advocated to avoid a potential stress riser.[28] Other steps include contouring of the implant for better coronal plane reduction, provisional fixation of the implanted segment with cables and locked screws, and reduction of the other fragment by a compression screw followed by additional locked screws to enhance fixation. Comparing locked plates and conventional cable plates, locked plates showed stiffer constructs in axial loading and torsion, and a greater potential for catastrophic failure.[29]

In the absence of femoral stem loosening and bone loss (Vancouver B1 fractures), a systematic review has shown that the use of additional strut allografts leads to increased deep infection rates and time to union.[30] See Chapter 17 for further information about periprosthetic fractures.

Pitfalls and outcomes in plating

Most studies involving plating of femoral shaft fractures have shown worse results compared with intramedullary nailing. The most common complications include infection, malunion, delayed union, non-union, pain from hardware and loss of knee motion from soft tissue scarring and shortening.

Early experience in compression plating of the femoral shaft showed implant loosening in 6–11% of cases, non-union in 2–8% and infection in 0–7%. Böstman et al.[31] demonstrated a substantially higher number of major complications occurring in patients treated with femoral plating as opposed to intramedullary nailing in 378 patients with 381 femur fractures treated in the 1980s.

In osteoporotic bone, screw pull-out with loss of fixation used to be the most common mode of implant failure. The introduction of locking plate technology has largely circumvented this problem but has led to other modes of failure such as delayed unions from over-rigid constructs, peri-implant fractures from stress risers at the end of the plate-screw construct, screw breakages and plate deformation and breakages.

Rozbruch et al. showed improvements in outcome with new biological internal fixation.[21] Another later series showed no difference between open plating with emphasis

on preservation of soft tissue integrity and submuscular plating of femoral shaft fractures, with a 2.5% incidence of non-union and a 5% incidence of infection.[32] The drop in infection rates and improved union rates in recent literature may be a result of our current understanding of fracture biology with improved emphasis on soft tissue preservation and less invasive techniques of fracture stabilization. Increasingly, geriatric traumatologists are advocating spanning femoral fixations (from the trochanters to the condyles) with long plates to avoid stress risers in osteoporotic bone (Figure 36.13).

More recent literature detailing the use of locked plates in femoral diaphyseal fractures tends to involve subtrochanteric fractures, distal femoral fractures or periprosthetic and peri-implant fractures. The latter are a challenge to treat both in terms of the physiological condition of the patients who tend to be elderly with multiple comorbidities as well as the difficulties in securing fixation around the periprosthetic region. Polyaxial locking implants, an off-shoot of the recent LCP technology, have been associated with up to 14% complication rates in minimally invasive treatment of complex osteoporotic femoral fractures.[33] In another cohort comprising entirely of periprosthetic and peri-implant

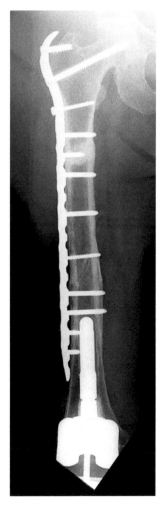

Figure 36.13 Plate spanning the entire femur for a periprosthetic fracture.

fracture fixations, major surgical site related complications required five surgical revisions (12.1%) to be performed out of 41 patients for early seroma (one case), plate breakages (two cases) and ligamentous instability and problems with soft tissue balancing of the patella (one case).[34] Time to union was quoted as 4–6 months.[34] Hence, peri-implant and periprosthetic fractures are still fraught with complications and outcome remains guarded even with current technology.

CONCLUSION

The management of femoral shaft fractures in the elderly with osteoporotic bone is challenging. Data on timing of surgery, morbidity and mortality and overall benefit from surgery remain scarce. General principles suggest expedient surgery to minimize complications from prolonged immobilization. Intramedullary nailing remains the method of choice. However significant advances have been made with locking plate technology which can be used in some patients who are unsuitable for an intramedullary nailing procedure. If used appropriately this method also yields a reasonable percentage of good to excellent results. These challenging injuries will increase as the population ages, and clinicians must learn to recognize and manage difficult osteoporotic fractures.

REFERENCES

1. Kanis JA, Oden A, Johnell O, Jonsson B, de Laet C, Dawson A. The burden of osteoporotic fractures: A method for setting intervention thresholds. *Osteoporos Int* 12 (2001):417–427.
2. Nieves JW, Bilezikian JP, Lane JM, Einhorn TA, Wang Y, Steinbuch M, Cosman F. Fragility fractures of the hip and femur: Incidence and patient characteristics. *Osteoporos Int* 21 (2010):399–408.
3. Singer BR, McLauchlan GJ, Robinson CM, Christie J. Epidemiology of fractures in 15,000 adults: The influence of age and gender. *J Bone Joint Surg Br* 80 (1998):243–248.
4. Hedlund R, Lindgren U. Epidemiology of diaphyseal femoral fractures. *Acta Orthop Scand* 57 (1986):423–427.
5. Weiss RJ, Montgomery SM, Al Dabbagh Z, Jansson KA. National data of 6409 Swedish inpatients with femoral shaft fractures: Stable incidence between 1998 and 2004. *Injury* 40 (2009):304–308.
6. Bengnér U, Ekbom T, Johnell O, Nilsson BE. Incidence of femoral and tibial shaft fractures. Epidemiology 1950–1983 in Malmö, Sweden. *Acta Orthop Scand* 61 (1990):251–254.
7. Salminen S, Pihlajamäki H, Avikainen V, Kyrö A, Böstman O. Specific features associated with femoral shaft fractures caused by low-energy trauma. *J Trauma* 43 (1997):117–122.
8. Shane E, Burr D, Abrahamsen B, Adler RA, Brown TD, Cheung AM, et al. Atypical subtrochanteric and diaphyseal femoral fractures: Second

report of a task force of the American Society for Bone and Mineral Research. *J Bone Miner Res* 29 (2014):1–23.
9. Koh JS, Goh SK, Png MA, Kwek EB, Howe TS. Femoral cortical stress lesions in long-term bisphosphonate therapy: A herald of impending fracture? *J Orthop Trauma* 24 (2010):75–81.
10. Oh Y, Wakabayashi Y, Kurosa Y, Ishizuki M, Okawa A. Stress fracture of the bowed femoral shaft is another cause of atypical femoral fracture in elderly Japanese: A case series. *J Orthop Sci* 19(4) (2014):579–586.
11. Narazaki DK, de Alverga Neto CC, Baptista AM, Caiero MT, de Camargo OP. Prognostic factors in pathologic fractures secondary to metastatic tumors. *Clinics (Sao Paulo)* 61 (2006):313–320.
12. Berry DJ. Management of periprosthetic fractures: The hip. *J Arthroplasty* 17(4 Suppl 1) (2002):11–13.
13. Patel KV, Brennan KL, Davis ML, Jupiter DC, Brennan ML. High-energy femur fractures increase morbidity but not mortality in elderly patients. *Clin Orthop Relat Res* 472 (2014):1030–5.
14. Nork SE. Fractures of the shaft of the femur. In: Bucholz RW, Heckman JD, Court-Brown CM, eds. *Rockwood and Green's Fractures in Adults* (6th Ed.). Lippincott Williams & Wilkins: Philadelphia, 2006:1845–1914.
15. DeCoster TA, Miller RA. Closed locked intramedullary nailing of femoral shaft fractures in the elderly. *Iowa Orthop J* 23 (2003):43–45.
16. Bone LB, Johnson KD, Weigelt J, Scheinberg R. Early versus delayed stabilization of femoral fractures. A prospective randomized study. *J Bone Joint Surg Am* 71 (1989):336–340.
17. Ricci WM, Gallagher B, Haidukewych GJ. Intramedullary nailing of femoral shaft fractures: Current concepts. *J Am Acad Orthop Surg* 17 (2009):296–305.
18. Canadian Orthopaedic Trauma Society. Reamed versus unreamed intramedullary nailing of the femur: Comparison of the rate of ARDS in multiple injured patients. *J Orthop Trauma* 20 (2006):384–387.
19. Zhan X, Takano AM, Kesavan S, Howe TS. Laparoscopic grasper for intramedullary biopsy: A technique to improve tissue sampling. *Singapore Med J* 55(8) (2014):e116–e118.
20. Wenda K, Runkel M, Degreif J, Rudig L. Minimally invasive plate fixation in femoral shaft fractures. *Injury* 28(Suppl 1) (1997):A13–A19.
21. Rozbruch SR, Müller U, Gautier E, Ganz R. The evolution of femoral shaft plating technique. *Clin Orthop Relat Res* 354 (1998):195–208.
22. Stoffel K, Stachowiak G, Forster T, Gächter A, Kuster M. Oblique screws at the plate ends increase the fixation strength in synthetic bone test medium. *J Orthop Trauma* 18 (2004):611–616.

23. Ring D, Jupiter JB, Sanders RA, Quintero J, Santoro VM, Ganz R, Marti RK. Complex nonunion of fractures of the femoral shaft treated by wave-plate osteosynthesis. *J Bone Joint Surg Br* 79 (1997):289–294.

24. Fitzpatrick DC, Doornink J, Madey SM, Bottlang M. Relative stability of conventional and locked plating fixation in a model of the osteoporotic femoral diaphysis. *Clin Biomech (Bristol, Avon)* 24 (2009):203–209.

25. Stoffel K, Dieter U, Stachowiak G, Gächter A, Kuster MS. Biomechanical testing of the LCP—How can stability in locked internal fixators be controlled? *Injury* 34 (Suppl 2) (2003):B11–B19.

26. Doornink J, Fitzpatrick DC, Boldhaus S, Madey SM, Bottlang M. Effects of hybrid plating with locked and nonlocked screws on the strength of locked plating constructs in the osteoporotic diaphysis. *J Trauma* 69 (2010):411–417.

27. Bottlang M, Doornink J, Byrd GD, Fitzpatrick DC, Madey SM. A nonlocking end screw can decrease fracture risk caused by locked plating in the osteoporotic diaphysis. *J Bone Joint Surg Am* 91 (2009):620–627.

28. Ricci WM, Bolhofner BR, Loftus T, Cox C, Mitchell S, Borrelli J Jr. Indirect reduction and plate fixation, without grafting, for periprosthetic femoral shaft fractures about a stable intramedullary implant. Surgical technique. *J Bone Joint Surg Am* 88 (2006):275–282.

29. Fulkerson E, Koval K, Preston CF, Iesaka K, Kummer FJ, Egol KA. Fixation of periprosthetic femoral shaft fractures associated with cemented femoral stems: A biomechanical comparison of locked plating and conventional cable plates. *J Orthop Trauma* 20 (2006):89–93.

30. Moore RE, Baldwin K, Austin MS, Mehta S. A systematic review of open reduction and internal fixation of periprosthetic femur fractures with or without allograft strut, cerclage, and locked plates. *J Arthroplasty* 29 (2014):872–876.

31. Böstman O, Varjonen L, Vainionpää S, Majola A, Rokkanen P. Incidence of local complications after intramedullary nailing and after plate fixation of femoral shaft fractures. *J Trauma* 29 (1989):639–645.

32. Zlowodzki M, Vogt D, Cole PA, Kregor PJ. Plating of femoral shaft fractures: Open reduction and internal fixation versus submuscular fixation. *J Trauma* 63 (2007):1061–1065.

33. El-Zayat BF, Zettl R, Efe T, Krüger A, Eisenberg F, Ruchholtz S. [Minimally invasive treatment of geriatric and osteoporotic femur fractures with polyaxial locking implants (NCB-DF®)]. *Unfallchirurg* 115 (2012):134–144.

34. Ruchholtz S, El-Zayat B, Kreslo D, Bücking B, Lewan U, Krüger A, Zettl R. Less invasive polyaxial locking plate fixation in periprosthetic and peri-implant fractures of the femur—A prospective study of 41 patients. *Injury* 44 (2013):239–248.

37

Distal femoral fractures

ELEANOR DAVIDSON AND CHARLES M. COURT-BROWN

INTRODUCTION

Surgeons have understood the complexities of treating distal femoral fractures in the elderly for many years, but it has only been in the last 30 years that different fixation techniques and their outcome have been examined in detail. Wade and Okinaka[1] in 1959 reported on 23 patients with supracondylar femoral fractures, of which 18 were in women and the majority were in their eighth decade. They stated that the predisposing causes of fracture were osteoporosis, pre-existing disabilities of the hip and knee and other medical comorbidities.

The majority of their patients were managed non-operatively with skeletal traction, but they observed that internal fixation was often required for displaced intercondylar or 'shattered' fractures. They noted that the mortality and the time patients spent in hospital were very similar in both patient groups, although they thought that patients treated surgically often had greater comorbidities. They favoured using a blade plate for operative management, but they also used intramedullary nailing.

One might ask how much has changed since Wade and Okinaka's study?[1] Chapter 1 shows that the prevalence of osteoporotic fractures has increased with greater life expectancy and it seems likely that many of the elderly patients who present with distal femoral fractures will be even less fit than 50–60 years ago. Surgical techniques have essentially remained the same, although blade plates have largely been replaced by locking plates, which are now often inserted through a submuscular approach, and the intramedullary nails available today are superior to the Küntscher nails used by Wade and Okinaka.[1] In addition, primary arthroplasty is often used nowadays to treat distal femoral fractures. One problem which has occurred since Wade and Okinaka's classic study is that of periprosthetic distal femoral fractures. These are becoming progressively more common.

EPIDEMIOLOGY

Kolmert and Wulff[2] analyzed the epidemiology of distal femoral fractures in Malmö, Sweden, in 1969–1976. They stated that distal femoral fractures accounted for 4% of all femoral fractures and had an incidence of $5.1/10^5$/year in patients >16 years of age. They pointed out that 84% of fractures occurred in patients >50 years of age and that in patients >60 years of age, 87% occurred in females. In their group of 135 patients, 19% had had impaired function in both legs and 42% had impaired function in the affected leg because of disease or previous fractures.

Analysis of fracture epidemiology in Edinburgh, Scotland, in a 1-year period in 2010/2011 shows that distal femoral fractures still account for 4% of femoral fractures, but their incidence in patients ≥16 years of age was $7/10^5$/year suggesting that the incidence of distal femoral fractures has increased in the last 30–40 years. In Chapter 1 distal femoral fractures were shown to comprise 0.9% of fractures in patients aged ≥65 years and 1.2% of fractures in patients aged ≥80 years. Their incidence in males and females aged ≥65 years was $8.4/10^5$/year and $30.1/10^5$/year, respectively, with the equivalent incidences in the 80+ year group being $20.1/10^5$/year and $64.0/10^5$/year. They have a type II pattern (see Chapter 1) with increasing age between 65 and 90+ years correlating with increasing fracture incidence in females but not in males. To permit a more detailed assessment of the epidemiology of distal femoral fractures in the elderly, a 15-year study of all distal femoral fractures admitted to the Royal Infirmary of Edinburgh between 1996 and 2010 was undertaken. The Royal Infirmary is the only hospital admitting trauma in a population of about 520,000 adults aged ≥16 years. During this period 392 patients were admitted of whom 271 (69.1%) were ≥65 years of age. The average age of all patients who presented with a distal femoral fracture was 69.3 years. The average ages of the patients who presented with AO/OTA type A, B and C fractures were 74.3 years, 59.2 years and 62.9 years, respectively, indicating a higher prevalence of high energy type B and C fractures in younger patients. The average age of patients who presented with distal femoral periprosthetic fractures was 78.7 years.

A total of 186 (68.3%) patients aged ≥65 years presented with AO/OTA type A supracondylar fractures, while 31 patients (11.6%) presented with type B condylar fractures and 54 patients (20.1%) had type C intercondylar fractures.

Figure 37.1 shows the fracture distribution curves of the different types of distal femoral fracture. The overall distribution curves show a marked increase in fracture incidence in females aged >85 years, whereas the incidence in males is much lower and tends to decline after 80 years of age.

Figure 37.1 shows that the fracture distribution curves for type A supracondylar fractures are virtually identical to the overall fracture distribution curves, emphasizing the importance of this fracture in the elderly population. However, the fracture distribution curves for type B and type C fractures are different. Elderly females show the same increasing incidence with increasing age, but in type B fractures the incidence in males declines after 85 years and in type C fractures the incidence declines after 70 years of age. In the 15-year study there were no intercondylar fractures in males aged >80 years. This suggests increasing male frailty compared with elderly females. Periprosthetic fractures have similar fracture distribution curves to type B and C fractures with an increasing fracture incidence in older females and a decline in incidence in males over 80 years of age.

Overall, 92.9% of patients aged ≥65 years in the 15-year study sustained their fracture as a result of a standing fall, with a further 3.7% having a spontaneous fracture. It is interesting to observe that there were no metastatic distal femoral fractures, although 8.7% of patients aged 50–64 years who presented with distal femoral fractures in the same time period had metastatic fractures. Only 1.5% of distal femoral fractures in the ≥65-year-old group occurred as a result of high energy injuries with 25% of these following a fall from a height and 75% following a road traffic accident.

Both Wade and Okinaka[1] and Kolmert and Wulff[2] pointed out that many elderly patients who present with distal femoral fractures will often be infirm and in poor health. This continues to be the case and analysis of the data in the 15-year study shows that only 64.9% of patients lived at home, 9.7% were in residential care and the remaining 25.4% were in a nursing home or a hospital when they sustained their fracture. Only 22.4% of the patients walked normally without aids prior to the fracture. A further 28% used one or two walking sticks, 28.7% used a walking frame and 15.7% were in a wheelchair. The remaining 3.7% were bed bound. The older age of the patients with the distal femoral periprosthetic fractures probably accounts for the fact that while 67.7% lived at home, only 16.6% walked without aids.

OPEN FRACTURES

Open distal femoral fractures are very rare in the elderly population. A review of the 271 distal femoral fractures treated in the 15-year period showed that only six (2.2%) were open. There were five (2.7%) open supracondylar fractures, one (3.2%) open condylar fracture and no open intercondylar fractures. The overall incidence of open fractures in the ≥65-year-old patients was $0.4/10^5$/year with $0.2/10^5$/year being recorded in males and $0.6/10^5$/year in females. There were no Gustilo[3] type IIIb fractures confirming the low energy nature of these fractures in the elderly. There were three Gustilo type I, one Gustilo type II and two Gustilo type IIIa fractures. Four followed a fall and two resulted from road traffic accidents.

CLASSIFICATION

A number of classification systems have been devised, but the one that is used by most surgeons nowadays is the AO/OTA classification which was originally proposed by Müller et al.[4] In this classification the first number refers to the femur (3), the second number refers to the location within the femur (3) and the letters A, B and C refer to the type of fracture. A is an extra-articular fracture, B is a partial articular fracture and C is a complex articular fracture. The subsequent numbers 1–3 refer to the morphology of the fracture with 0.1 to 0.3 detailing the morphology more precisely. The AO/OTA classification is given in Table 37.1 and an illustration of the fracture types is shown in Figure 37.2. An example of an AO/OTA 33A3.2 distal femoral fracture is shown in Figure 37.3.

ANATOMY

The supracondylar area of the femur is the area between the femoral condyles and the junction of the metaphysis with the femoral diaphysis. It comprises the distal 15 cm of the femur. The shaft of the femur is almost cylindrical, but at the lower end it broadens into two curved condyles (Figure 37.4a). The distal femur is trapezoidal and is narrower anteriorly than posteriorly. Medially there is an angle of inclination of about 25 degrees. Anteriorly the two condyles form a joint for articulation with the patella. Posteriorly they are separated by a deep intercondylar fossa that gives attachment to the cruciate ligaments. The lateral epicondyle arises from the lateral condylar surface and gives rise to the lateral, or fibular, collateral ligament. Distal to the lateral epicondyle is an oblique groove for the popliteus tendon. The medial epicondyle gives attachment to the medial, or tibial, collateral ligament and the abductor magnus tendon inserts into the adductor tubercle. When the distal femur fractures, the pull of the quadriceps and hamstrings leads to limb shortening and

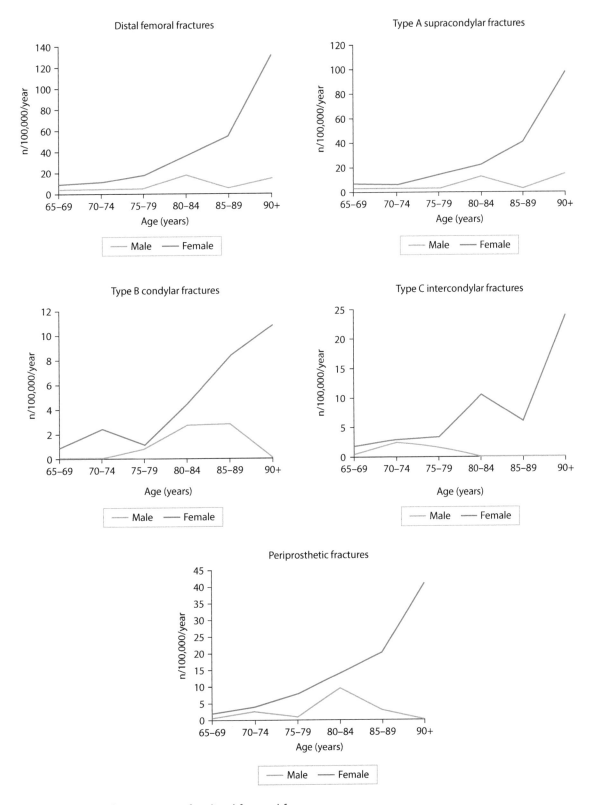

Figure 37.1 Fracture distribution curves for distal femoral fractures.

a varus deformity. The pull of the gastrocnemius, which arises from the lateral and medial femoral condyles, leads to apex posterior angulation. This is shown in Figure 37.3.

The nerves and arteries at risk following distal femoral fracture and reconstructive surgery are shown in Figure 37.4b. The popliteal artery and vein run through the popliteal fossa which also contains the tibial nerves. The common peroneal nerve, the other terminal branch of the sciatic nerve, arises just above the popliteal fossa and descends along the lateral border of the fossa. It runs over the lateral head of the gastrocnemius and around the neck of the fibula before it divides into the superficial and deep peroneal nerves.

Table 37.1 AO/OTA classification of distal femoral fractures

33A Extra-articular fractures

A1 Simple articular fractures
A1.1 Apophyseal
A1.2 Metaphyseal oblique or spiral
A1.3 Metaphyseal transverse

A2 Metaphyseal wedge fractures
A2.1 Intact lateral or medial wedge
A2.2 Fragmented lateral wedge
A2.3 Fragmented medial wedge

A3 Metaphyseal complex
A3.1 Intermediate split segment
A3.2 Irregular, limited to metaphysis
A3.3 Irregular, extending to diaphysis

33B Partial articular fractures

B1 Lateral condyle, sagittal
B1.1 Simple, through notch
B1.2 Simple, through weight bearing surface
B1.3 Multifragmentary

B2 Medial condyle, sagittal
B2.1 Simple, through notch
B2.2 Simple, through weight bearing surface
B2.3 Multifragmentary

B3 Frontal
B3.1 Anterior and lateral flake fracture
B3.2 Unilateral posterior (lateral or medial)
B3.3 Bicondylar posterior

33C Complete articular fractures

C1 Articular simple, metaphyseal simple
C1.1 T or Y shaped, slight displacement
C1.2 T or Y shaped, marked displacement
C1.3 T shaped, epiphyseal

C2 Articular simple, metaphyseal multifragmentary
C2.1 Intact wedge, lateral or medial
C2.2 Fragmented wedge, lateral or medial
C2.3 Complex

C3 Multifragmentary
C3.1 Metaphyseal simple
C3.2 metaphyseal multifragmentary
C3.3 Metaphysio-diaphyseal multifragmentary

Source: Müller ME, et al. *The Comprehensive Classification of Fractures of Long Bones.* Springer, Berlin, 1990.

SURGICAL APPROACHES

Lateral approach

This is probably the most commonly used approach to the distal femur. It can be undertaken with the patient placed supine or laterally. The skin incision is along the mid-lateral line of the femoral diaphysis. Distally it is curved anteriorly to over the centre of the lateral condyle. The iliotibial band is incised

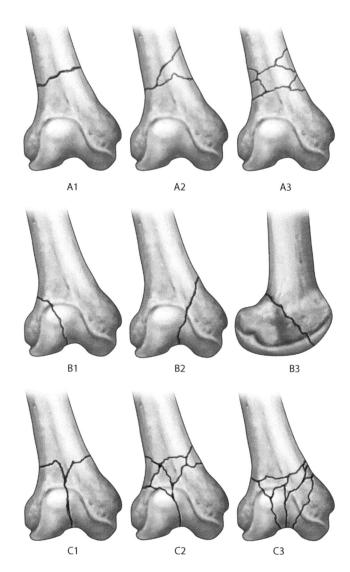

Figure 37.2 The different types of distal femoral fractures as defined by the AO/OTA classification. (From Müller ME, et al. *The Comprehensive Classification of Fractures of Long Bones.* Springer, Berlin, 1990.)

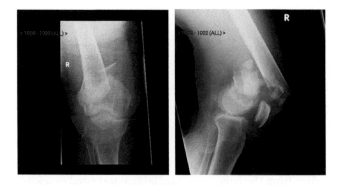

Figure 37.3 Anteroposterior and lateral X-rays of an AO/OTA A3.2 distal femoral fracture. Note the marked metaphyseal comminution and posterior displacement of the distal fragments.

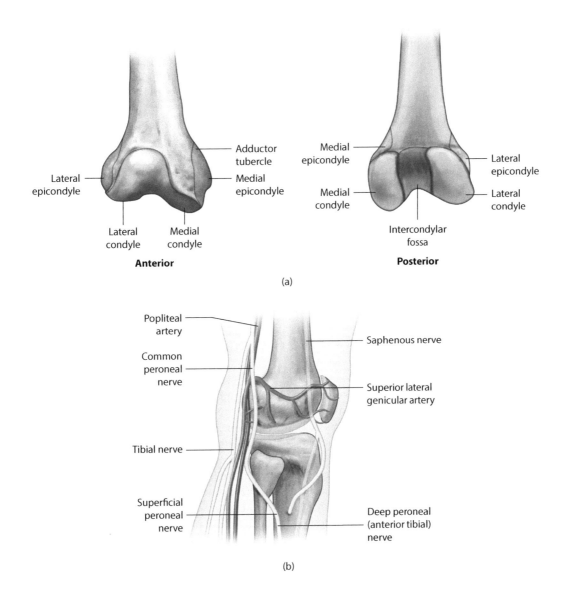

Figure 37.4 **(a)** Anatomy of the distal femur. **(b)** Anatomy of the blood vessels and nerves at risk during surgery.

and the vastus lateralis elevated from the linear aspera and the femur. If necessary a lateral arthrotomy can be undertaken to facilitate treatment of type B or type C fractures.

Minimally invasive lateral approach

This approach has become more popular in recent years as it is associated with less soft tissue stripping. It employs a shortened skin incision which measures 5–6 cm and is confined to the area of the lateral condyle and distal metaphysis. The iliotibial band is incised and the distal femur exposed. The plate is slid in submuscularly and small proximal stab incisions used to insert the screws under radiological control.

Medial approach

This is used for open reduction and fixation of medial condylar fractures. The skin incision is in the line of the tendon of adductor magnus. The adductor tubercle is identified and

the tendon is followed proximally, but it should be remembered that the femoral vessels pierce the adductor magnus 10–12 cm above the knee joint. The vastus medialis is retracted and the distal femur is exposed. Care should be taken to stay anterior to the medial collateral ligament and to avoid damage to the medial meniscus.

Approach for retrograde intramedullary nailing

A longitudinal midline skin incision is made 2 cm distal to the inferior pole of the patella. The patella tendon is retracted laterally and the medial tissues are dissected. A guide wire can now be inserted medial to the patella. The anatomical landmark is the Blumensaat line, which corresponds to the roof of the intercondylar notch. Care should be taken not to damage the posterior cruciate ligament and the articular cartilage. If preferred, an anteromedial incision can be used and if a type C fracture is to be treated, some surgeons prefer an anterolateral approach.

TREATMENT

As has already been pointed out, the treatment methods that can be used for distal femoral fractures have changed little in 50–60 years,[1] although there has been considerable improvement in plate and nail design, with locking plates now being preferred by most surgeons. Arthroplasty is also a new treatment method which seems to be gaining in popularity. The role of non-operative management has changed considerably. It is salutary to note that in 1984 the second edition of Rockwood and Green recommended that closed treatment was suitable for many distal femoral fractures, particularly if they occurred in older patients.[5] Traction was still extensively used despite the fact that earlier publications had shown that internal fixation tended to give better results.[5-7] It is always difficult to know how popular different treatment methods are and the assumption must be nowadays that most patients are treated by internal fixation or arthroplasty if they are older. To investigate this we analyzed the types of treatment employed during the 15-year study of distal femoral fractures in the elderly undertaken in the Royal Infirmary of Edinburgh. This is shown in Table 37.2. We were surprised that 30% of the patients were treated non-operatively. No traction was used, but it is clear that many patients with undisplaced or minimally displaced fractures were treated with a cast or brace. Table 37.2 shows that the patients treated non-operatively were the least fit patients with only 10% able to walk without aids and only 50% living at home. It is probable that a number of elderly patients with distal femoral fractures were considered too unfit for surgery. Table 37.2 also shows that intramedullary nailing became popular in the early 2000s, but the advent of more modern plates is reflected by a higher prevalence of plating from 2003 onwards. About 40% of elderly patients were treated by plating.

Non-operative management

As has already been stated, most surgeons nowadays would reserve non-operative management for undisplaced or minimally displaced fractures or for patients who are considered pre-terminal and too ill for surgical intervention. The most recent papers comparing traction with operative management favour surgery. Healy and Brooker[8] analyzed 17 patients treated by skeletal traction and stated that only four (23.5%) had good results. Butt et al.[9] undertook a prospective controlled trial comparing the use of traction with a dynamic condylar screw in patients >60 years of age. They demonstrated excellent or good results in 53% of the operated group and 31% of the non-operated group. There were more complications and a longer hospitalization time in the non-operated group and they strongly favoured surgical treatment.

Nowadays there is no place for skeletal traction and non-operative management for fitter older patients should be

reserved for undisplaced or minimally displaced fractures. Unfortunately, as yet, there are no studies analyzing the results of non-operative management in patients who present with displaced or minimally displaced fractures.

Plating

Once plating became established as a principal method of treatment for distal femoral fractures, most of the literature dealt with the use of blade plates or dynamic condylar screws and plates. Schatzker[7] should be credited with describing how these plates should be used. He analyzed the results of the treatment of 35 patients, 30 of whom had been treated with a blade plate. He showed that when the principles of rigid internal fixation were adhered to, 71% of patients achieved good or excellent results compared with 21% if rigid internal fixation was not achieved. He particularly showed that poor results followed the use of poor fixation methods in elderly patients. Ostrum and Geel[10] achieved 87% good and excellent results using a dynamic condylar screw and plate and pointed out that 66.6% of the failures occurred in elderly osteoporotic women.

In recent years, the blade plate and the dynamic condylar screw and plate have largely been replaced with locking plates which are either monoaxial or polyaxial (Figure 37.5). In addition, surgeons have tended to use more 'biological' incisions with submuscular placement of these plates. Most of the studies on the use of these plates have been carried out in level 1 trauma centres and accordingly many of the patients in these studies are younger patients with high energy injuries. However, there are some papers that have documented the results of plating in older patients.

The use of the less invasive stabilization system (LISS) plate in the treatment of distal femoral fractures was analyzed in a systematic review by Smith et al.[11] They analyzed 663 patients with 694 fractures in 21 studies. The average age was 58.7 years (16–101 years). As with all systematic reviews, the authors found it difficult to analyze all aspects of the use of the LISS plate but they documented 19% loss of reduction, 6% delayed or non-union and 5% implant failure. They pointed out that the majority of complications occurred in papers published before 2005.

Hoffmann et al.[12] studied 111 patients with distal femoral fractures that were treated with locked plating. The average age was 54 years (18–95) and 40.5% of the fractures were open, demonstrating that many of the fractures were high energy fractures in younger patients. The patients were treated in two level 1 trauma centres and only 36.9% of the fractures followed a low energy fall. The authors documented that 74.8% of the fractures healed after the index procedure, but 91% eventually united. Submuscular minimally invasive surgery was associated with a lower prevalence of non-union. They found that hardware failure was related to non-union and that fractures above total knee arthroplasty had a significantly greater rate of failed hardware with the worst clinical outcomes. They showed that 75.7% of the patients had acceptable flexion with reduced

Table 37.2 Analysis of the method of treatment of 271 patients aged ≥65 years who presented with distal femoral fractures to the Royal Infirmary of Edinburgh between 1996 and 2010

	Prevalence (%)				
	Non-operative	Plate	Nail	Arthroplasty	Other
Year					
1996	21.7	47.8	13.0	8.7	8.7
1997	41.2	17.6	23.5	17.6	0
1998	47.9	7.1	14.3	0	21.4
1999	23.5	41.2	17.6	0	17.6
2000	25.0	25.0	37.5	6.3	6.3
2001	40.0	15.0	35.0	5.0	5.0
2002	22.7	22.7	22.7	31.8	0
2003	28.6	42.9	21.4	7.1	0
2004	20.0	66.6	6.7	6.7	0
2005	30.0	20.0	10.0	30.0	10.0
2006	40.0	50.0	10.0	0	0
2007	11.1	72.2	5.6	5.6	5.6
2008	34.8	43.5	13.0	8.7	0
2009	30.0	40.0	5.0	15.0	10.0
2010	21.0	68.4	5.3	5.3	0
Total	29.5	39.1	16.0	10.8	5.2
Average age	83.1	82.2	78.0	85.2	84.9
Residence					
Home (%)	50.6	75.8	76.9	61.5	57.2
Residential home (%)	40.5	12.1	4.7	3.8	7.1
Nursing home/hospital (%)	8.9	12.1	18.6	34.6	35.7
Walking ability					
Normal (%)	10.1	29.3	32.6	15.4	35.7
Sticks (%)	25.3	29.3	32.6	26.9	28.6
Frame (%)	27.8	31.3	20.9	38.5	21.4
Wheelchair (%)	27.8	9.1	13.9	15.4	7.1
Bedbound (%)	8.9	1.0	–	3.8	7.1

Note: The average age, place of domicile and walking ability are shown. The 'Other' column includes nine patients treated with screws for condylar fractures, two amputations and three patients who died before treatment. The 'Nail' column includes both antegrade and retrograde nails.

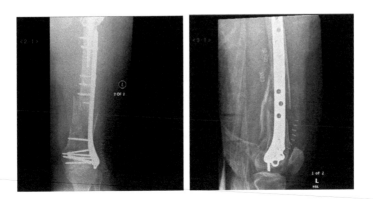

Figure 37.5 An AO/OTA A3.3 distal femoral fracture treated with a monoaxial locking plate.

flexion being associated with advanced age and periprosthetic fractures. Overall outcome was not related to age, but they reported that poor outcome was related to the patient's body mass index (BMI) and to periprosthetic fractures. The overall outcome was not related to whether open surgery or submuscular surgery was performed. In a further study, Hanschen et al.[13] compared monoaxial and polyaxial plates in four trauma centres in Germany. They found that knee flexion was better after polyaxial plating, although the difference did not reach statistical significance. There was no other difference between the plates.

The role of modern plating systems in the management of distal femoral fractures has also been questioned by Vallier and Immler.[14] They compared the 95-degree-angled blade plate with the locking condylar plate. They showed that complications occurred in 10% of patients treated with blade plates compared with 35% of patients treated with locking condylar plates. The complications included deep infection, non-unions and malunions. The complications were more common in females and the average age of the patients who developed complications was 63.9 years, compared with 52.8 years in those patients who did not. They found more complications in older patients with lower energy injuries and in those treated with a locking condylar plate, especially in type A fracture patterns and in females. They pointed out that modern plates are substantially more expensive than the previous generation of plates, but did not seem to produce better results.

Forster et al.[15] also compared the results of several different types of plates with other methods of treating distal femoral fractures. The study was undertaken before the use of polyaxial plates, but a review of the literature showed that angled blade plates were associated with good or excellent results in 52–85% of cases compared with dynamic condylar screws and plates (71–74%) and monoaxial plates (72–88%). The prevalence of non-union, malunion and infection was similar.

There are a number of studies that have selectively examined the role of plating in older patients. The results of four studies[16–19] are shown in Table 37.3. All used monoaxial or polyaxial locking plates and all gave individual results for their patients. Two studies only examined older patients[18,19] with the other two studies including patients of all ages.[16,17] Table 37.3 indicates clearly that virtually all distal femoral fractures in older patients occur in low energy falls, whereas most younger patients sustain high energy injuries. It is clear that the prevalence of excellent and good results in older patients after low energy injuries is virtually identical to that in younger patients after high energy injuries, suggesting that Vallier and Immler[14] were correct in stating that older patients fare less well after treatment of equivalent injuries. The two papers dealing exclusively with older patients[18,19] had relatively few complications with two cases of loosening in 40 patients. The overall prevalence of non-union was 5%.

The prevalence and causes of non-union in distal femoral fractures have been addressed in a number of studies. Smith et al.,[11] in their study of 694 fractures, stated that the prevalence of delayed or non-union was 5.8%. Hoffmann et al.[12] documented a non-union prevalence of 18% in the 111 patients that they studied but it is clear that they were mostly treating high energy fractures and 40.5% of their fractures were open. Rodriguez et al.[20] had a 9.9% infection rate in 283 fractures treated in three trauma centres. They stated that obesity, open fractures, infection and the use of stainless steel plates were inherent risk factures, but age, gender and the AO/OTA classification were not risk factors for non-union. Most elderly distal femoral fractures are low energy injuries and a non-union rate of 5% is probably accurate.

Table 37.3 Results from studies where individual patient results for knee function have been published

		Cause of fracture (%)		Knee function (%)	
	No.	Falls	High energy	Excellent/ good	Fair/ poor
Syed et al.[16] (≥65 years)	11	100	0	100	0
Syed et al.[16] (<65 years)	7	14.3	85.7	28.6	71.4
Erhardt et al.[17] (≥65 years)	9	66.6	33.3	44.4	55.6
Erhardt et al.[17] (<65 years)	16	18.7	68.8	93.8	6.2
Doshi et al.[18] (≥65 years)	24	100	0	79.2	20.8
Wong et al.[19] (≥65 years)	16	93.8	6.2	62.5	37.5
All studies (≥65 years)	60	93.3	6.7	73.3	26.7
All studies (<65 years)	23	17.4	82.6	73.9	26.1

Note: Syed et al.[16] used a monoaxial plate, an open lateral approach and the Hospital for Special Surgery (HSS) knee score. Erhardt et al.[17] used a polyaxial plate, a minimally invasive approach and the HSS score. Doshi et al.[18] used a monoaxial plate, a minimally invasive approach and the Knee Society Score. Wong et al.[19] used a monoaxial plate, a minimally invasive approach and the Oxford Knee Score.

There were no infections reported in elderly patients in the four studies[16–19] in Table 37.3, although Smith et al.[11] reported a prevalence of 3.9% in 21 studies of young and older patients.

Intramedullary nailing

Intramedullary nailing of distal femoral fractures was popularized after locked nailing became the treatment method of choice for femoral diaphyseal fractures. Prior to that unlocked nails had been used,[1] but surgeons frequently had to use cerclage wires to stabilize fractures. Small diameter flexible nails such as Rush pins, Ender nails or Zickel nails[21] were used, but they did not provide rigid fixation and an additional cast or brace was often required. However, good results were reported and Forster et al.[15] reported good or excellent results in 72–84% of patients, with a non-union rate of 2%. They did, however, stress that knee stiffness was a problem.

Most studies of intramedullary nailing of distal femoral fractures have used a locked supracondylar nail inserted through the knee joint (Figure 37.6). Table 37.2 shows that the technique became more popular in the late 1990s, but in recent years it has been superseded by monoaxial and polyaxial plating. However, the literature concerning intramedullary nailing concentrates more on fractures in the elderly than does the plating literature, and the impression is that many surgeons believe that nailing is a more useful technique in elderly and infirm patients.

Papadokostakis et al.[22] reviewed the literature concerning retrograde nailing of distal femoral fractures. As with the plating literature, this type of study obviously includes patients of all ages. The authors showed that the average infection rate associated with retrograde nailing was 1.4% and the union rate was 96.9%. The average range of knee motion was 105 degrees and 16.5% of patients complained of knee pain. The re-operation rate was 17%, and 5.2% of patients had a malunion.

There have been a number of studies investigating the use of retrograde nailing in elderly distal femoral fractures. The results of six studies[23–28] are shown in Table 37.4. The results highlight the relative frailty of this patient group with 14% of the patients dying before union was achieved. However, Table 37.4 shows that this elderly group achieved reasonable

knee mobility and the complication rate was low. There were no infections and a non-union rate of 4%. Malunion was clearly an issue, but in most cases it was simply accepted in this elderly group of patients.

In their study Dunlop and Brenkel[25] analyzed outcome. At 6 months they had 85% excellent or satisfactory results in their surviving patients. They documented that 60% of patients came from their own home and 50% of these patients were discharged home. The average length of stay in the acute ward was 19 days. There were no deaths following the surgery, but 29% of the patients died within a year.

The alternative nailing procedure is antegrade nailing. A recent study of 30 patients showed good results using this technique.[29] The average age of the patients was 48.7 years, but the authors documented the results in all patients, and in the seven patients who were aged ≥60 years who were not lost to follow-up, six had excellent results and one had a good result. The average range of knee motion was 103 degrees. They used the technique for both AO/OTA type A and type C fractures, although all of the type C fractures were C1 fractures. If this technique is to be used for type C fractures, distal interfragmentary screws must be inserted prior to nail insertion.

In their analysis of all methods of treating distal femoral fractures, Forster el al.[15] showed that the literature stated that supracondylar nails were associated with good or excellent results in 69–91% of cases, compared with 72–88% for monoaxial plates. The non-union and infection rates were identical, but there was a slightly higher rate of malunion with nails. Markmiller et al.[30] prospectively compared supracondylar nailing and monoaxial plating in AO/OTA type A and C fractures. The two groups of patients had virtually identical results with 87.5% of both groups having good or excellent results. The only difference was that the use of monoaxial plating was associated with a higher prevalence of malalignment.

The literature shows that excellent results can be achieved with intramedullary nailing of distal femoral fractures. In the elderly type A and simple type C fractures can be expected to have good results and at the moment there is no evidence that plating or nailing is associated with superior results.

Arthroplasty

The difficulty of treating distal femoral fractures in elderly patients, who already have significant medical and social comorbidities and not infrequently also have significant osteoarthritis of the knee, stimulated surgeons to treat some fractures by excision of the distal femur and insertion of a prosthesis (Figure 37.7). This was first undertaken by Wolfgang in 1982[31] who described the use of a total knee replacement in a patient with a supracondylar fracture and rheumatoid arthritis. The first series was reported by Bell et al.[32] They used a hinged knee replacement in 13 patients who presented with AO/OTA type A and type C fractures. The results were excellent. The patients were mobile at an

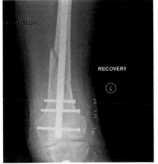
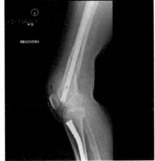

Figure 37.6 The use of a retrograde intramedullary nail to treat an A2.1 distal femoral fracture.

Table 37.4 Results of studies examining the use of retrograde nailing for the treatment of distal femoral fractures in the very elderly

	No.	Died before follow-up	Average age (years)	AO/OTA type A (%)	Knee ROM (degrees)	Nonunion (%)	Malunion (%)	Infection (%)
Janzing et al.[23]	26	2	82	83.3	?	0	?	0
Gynning and Hansen[24]	30	9	82	62.1	90–130	7.1	?	0
Dunlop and Brenkel[25]	31	5	82	80.6	?	7.7	?	0
Kumar et al.[26]	16	1	82	100	100	6.2	>19	0
El-Kawy et al.[27]	23	2	75	78.3	100 (6 weeks)	0	39	0
Kim et al.[28]	13	0	79	100	116	0	7.7	0

Note: ROM, range of motion.

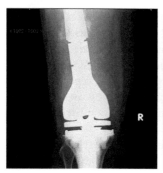 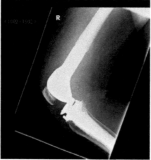

Figure 37.7 The distal femoral fracture shown in Figure 37.3 treated by primary arthroplasty.

average of 4 days after surgery and they were only in the acute ward for an average of 8 days. There were no infections and the only complications were a patella tendon rupture at 15 months and loosening of a prosthesis after 5 years.

In a later study from the same institution,[33] 54 fractures treated with a knee arthroplasty were examined. The authors made the point that the patients were socially dependent and poorly mobile. The average age was 82 years and only 14% could walk without assistance. Given their significant medical and physical problems, the patients did well and only seven required a further procedure. There was one deep infection (1.9%), which resulted in an amputation, and four (7.7%) patients sustained a periprosthetic fracture. The poor physical condition of this group of patients was highlighted by the median survival time which was 1.7 years. Survival analysis showed that mortality in the first year was 41.1%. This rose to 82% after 5 years. The authors concluded that with appropriate patient selection the prosthesis had a high probability of surviving as long as the patient!

Most recent studies have confirmed the success of primary arthroplasty in the treatment of distal femoral fractures. Parratte et al.[34] analyzed 26 patients and reported one postoperative death and one deep infection. Of the 23 patients who were followed up, 19 returned to their preoperative domicile and the mean active knee flexion was 99 degrees. Similar results were demonstrated by Choi et al.[35] who treated 88 patients with an average age of 77 years.

They had no postoperative deaths or infections and they commented that at final follow-up the mean range of knee movement was 114 degrees.

It is likely that arthroplasty will become more popular as patients age and surgeons are keen to undertake definitive surgery in a frail population. The literature shows that while surgeons used to favour hinged prostheses, a wide range of prostheses are now being used. It is recommended that if arthroplasty is to be used, it should be in older patients with pre-existing osteoarthritis. The technique should be used with caution if there is a pre-existing hip implant, as periprosthetic fracture is a recorded complication.

External fixation

External fixation has been demonstrated to be useful in the management of distal femoral fractures in younger patients. Hoffmann et al.[12] treated 26.1% of distal femoral fractures, which were subsequently treated with a locked plate, with primary external fixation. They stated that 38.5% of the fractures were open. There are reports of external fixation being used successful as definitive treatment,[36] but not in elderly patients. Currently external fixation is not recommended for treatment of distal femoral fractures in older patients.

Periprosthetic fractures

A review of the periprosthetic distal femoral fractures that were admitted to the Royal Infirmary of Edinburgh between 1996 and 2010 shows that in patients aged ≥65 years, the overall incidence was $6.6/10^5$/year, the incidence in males being $2.5/10^5$/year and in females $9.4/10^5$/year. Analysis of the ≥80-year-old population shows that the overall incidence of periprosthetic fractures rises to $16.1/10^5$/year, the incidence being $6.3/10^5$/year in males and $20.7/10^5$/year in females. In the 65+ group the majority of periarticular distal femoral fractures (58.8%) were associated with a previously inserted knee prosthesis, 20.6% with a hip prosthesis and 13.4% with a fracture implant. In the remaining 7.2% of patients there were implants in both the hip and knee. In this group of patients 93% of the periprosthetic fractures were supracondylar, 3.5% were condylar and 3.5% were intercondylar.

The treatment of periprosthetic distal femoral fractures is obviously not dissimilar to that of non-periprosthetic fractures. Table 37.2 shows that patients who present with periprosthetic distal femoral fractures tend to be slightly older and frailer than those who present with non-periprosthetic fractures. In our 15-year study only 61.5% lived at home and only 15.4% could walk without walking aids. It is likely that the incidence of periprosthetic fractures will rise in the future and it may well be that patients with distal femoral periprosthetic fractures become even less fit over the next few decades. It is likely that treatment methods will evolve accordingly.

The most commonly used classification system for supracondylar periprosthetic fractures is that of Lewis and Rorabeck[37] (Table 37.5). It is a simple classification which is based on fracture displacement and the stability of the prosthesis in the distal femur. In a review of the management of periprosthetic fractures, Johnston et al.[38] drew attention to the importance of defining the exact fracture morphology in relation to the proximal end of the femoral prosthesis. They also emphasized the importance of determining whether the distal femoral fragment(s) provided adequate bone for screw insertion. Johnston et al.[38] also published a list of risk factors associated with periprosthetic fractures of the knee (Table 37.6).

As with all distal femoral fractures, the initial management of periprosthetic fractures was either non-operative or with flexible intramedullary fixation, such as Rush nails. Herrera et al.[39] in a systematic review of 415 acute distal femoral fractures above a knee arthroplasty showed that non-operative management was associated with a non-union rate of 12%, a deep infection rate of 0.8% and 18% of patients required a secondary procedure. Nowadays few surgeons would use non-operative management for displaced periprosthetic fractures and, as with non-periprosthetic fractures, it should be reserved for undisplaced periprosthetic fractures where the implant is stable or for patients who are too unwell to tolerate a major surgical procedure.

The use of blade plates and dynamic condylar screw plates has been shown to be effective in the management of periprosthetic fractures. Healy et al.[8] treated 20 periprosthetic distal femoral fractures with a variety of plates. They

bone grafted 15 patients and achieved union in 18 patients. Other authors have not been as successful, probably because of the frailty of the patients and the significant osteopenia of the affected femur.

In recent years polymethylmethacrylate, autografts and allografts have been used to supplement conventional plating systems but, as with non-periprosthetic fractures, attention has turned to modern plating systems and to intramedullary nailing. Large et al.[40] compared locked plates with non-locked plates and intramedullary nailing in the management of 52 periprosthetic fractures. They felt that locked plates were associated with better knee flexion, a reduced prevalence of malunion and non-union, and fewer re-operations. However, in their systematic review of 415 cases, Herrera et al.[39] showed that while locked plates had better results than conventional plating, the results were not as good as intramedullary nailing. The nonunion rate following locked plating was 5.3% with a fixation failure rate of 3.5%, a deep infection rate of 5.3% and a secondary procedure rate of 8.8%. The equivalent figures for intramedullary nailing were 1.5%, 1.5%, 0% and 4.6%. Horneff et al.[41] undertook a retrospective comparative study of retrograde nailing and locked plating of periprosthetic distal femoral fractures. The two groups of patients had a similar average age and BMI. The authors examined time to union, time to full weight bearing and the requirement for revision surgery. They showed that locked plating was associated with a higher union rate 36 weeks after surgery and a lower rate of revision surgery. They concluded that locked plating was better than intramedullary nailing.

In a second retrospective comparative study, Meneghini et al.[42] compared locked plating and intramedullary nailing in 91 patients. In this study intramedullary nailing patients fared better than those treated with a plate. Intramedullary nailing was associated with 9% non-union, compared with 19% non-union or delayed union in the locked plate group. However, the intramedullary nail group demonstrated a lower level of ambulation than the locked plate group and the authors suggested that there was a surgical bias towards using nails in more sedentary, less mobile, patients.

Table 37.5 Classification of supracondylar periprosthetic fractures

Type	Description
1	Undisplaced fracture; prosthesis intact
2	Displaced fracture; prosthesis intact
3	Displaced or undisplaced fracture; prosthesis loose or failing

Source: Lewis PL, Rorabeck CH. Periprosthetic fracture. In Engh GA, Rorabeck CH (eds.). *Techniques of Revision Surgery*. Williams & Wilkins, Philadelphia, PA, 1997.

Table 37.6 Risk factors associated with periprosthetic fractures around the knee

Osteopenia
Female sex
Chronic steroid use
Increasing age
Osteolysis
Infection
Implant wear/loosening
Stiff knee
Anterior femoral notching
Neurological abnormalities
Revision knee arthroplasty

Source: Johnston AT, et al. *Knee* 2012; 19(3): 156–62.

Another method of management of distal femoral periprosthetic fractures is distal femoral replacement. This is indicated in patients who have poor bone stock, significant fracture comminution and loose or damaged prosthetic components. Mortazavi et al.[43] examined 22 revision arthroplasties in 20 patients with an average age of 69.5 years. They followed up 16 patients and stated that the patient satisfaction rate was high and that 61.1% of their results were excellent. Five patients required secondary surgery. Jassim et al.[44] reviewed distal femoral replacements in 11 patients who were significantly older. They had an average age of 81 years and all had medical comorbidities and impaired pre-operative mobility. Predictably the results were less good than in the younger cohort of patients analyzed by Mortazavi et al.,[43] but postoperative complications were reasonable and most patients fared well.

MORTALITY

The literature clearly shows that, like patients who present with proximal femoral fractures, many elderly patients who have distal femoral fractures are frail and infirm. This is confirmed in Table 37.2. The overall mortality during the 15-year study was 19.5% at 3 months, 25% at 6 months and 32% at 1 year. This is very similar to the mortality after proximal femoral fractures. Kammerlander et al.[45] examined 43 patients with a mean age of 80 years and found that 51.2% had had previous fractures and 30.2% sustained further fractures in the follow-up period of 5.3 years. They used the Barthel Index to measure the patients' ability to undertake daily activities of living and found it to be very similar to the score seen in proximal femoral fracture patients. Their in-hospital mortality was 4.6%, the 1-year mortality was 18.4% and the 3-year mortality was 39.1%. Before the fracture only 65.1% of patients lived at home.

Streubel et al.[46] found similar results in a cohort of 92 consecutive patients >60 years of age with low energy fractures. They documented the 30-day, 6-month and 1-year mortality as 6%, 18% and 25%, respectively, and found that the overall mortality for non-periprosthetic fractures was 30% with a 46% mortality in patients who presented with periprosthetic fractures, indicating that these are a frailer group of patients. This is confirmed in Table 37.2 which shows that the only patients frailer than those with periprosthetic fractures were those with fractures that were treated non-operatively. They demonstrated that the mortality rates were similar to those seen in patients with proximal femoral fractures.

SUGGESTED TREATMENT

The majority of patients who present with distal femoral fractures are elderly and infirm. The literature suggests that their social and medical comorbidities are not dissimilar to those seen in patients with proximal femoral fractures. We believe that both sets of patients should be treated in a similar fashion with rapid surgery being undertaken as soon as the patient is fit for an anaesthetic. Non- or minimally displaced fractures can be treated non-operatively, but it must be stressed that little is known about the outcome of this method of treatment. A number of patients will be too ill to undergo surgery and in a small minority of patients, the severity of the fracture and the poor physical state of the patient will mean that an above knee amputation may have to be performed.

Shulman et al.[47] compared the quality of life and the functional outcomes in older and younger patients with similarly treated distal femoral fractures. They analyzed 57 patients dividing them into those aged ≥65 years and those aged <65 years. All patients were treated with nail or plate fixation. The union rate at 6 months was similar. They stated that the elderly patients had slightly worse knee movement but the difference was not statistically significant. The older group also had poorer functional scores although there was no difference in emotional or mobility indices. They felt that age should not be used as a determinant in deciding against operative treatment. This work is supported by the results shown in Table 37.3 where it is apparent that the results of treating the elderly with low energy injuries are not dissimilar from the results of treating high energy injuries in younger patients.

In recent years the introduction of modern plating systems has meant that most patients will be treated using a monoaxial or polyaxial plate. There is little evidence that these plates give better results than the last generation of plates, but it seems unlikely that their use will be discontinued. If plating is used there is no demonstrable difference between the results from using a monoaxial or a polyaxial plate. It is recommended that a submuscular approach is used, rather than an open approach.

There is evidence that retrograde intramedullary nailing provides somewhat better results in the very elderly and it is associated with fewer complications. There are, however, no precise indications for the use of a locked plate or a retrograde nail and the implant that is used will depend on the preference of the surgeon. We believe that primary arthroplasty should be considered in elderly patients who already have significant osteoarthritis of the knee. The results in the literature are good and surgeons should remember that with the high mortality associated with these fractures the failure rate of the prosthesis is low, although periprosthetic fractures can occur.

REFERENCES

1. Wade PA, Okinaka AJ. The problem of the supracondylar fracture of the femur in the aged person. *Am J Surg* 1959; 97: 499–510.
2. Kolmert L, Wulff K. Epidemiology and treatment of distal femoral fractures in adults. *Acta Orthop Scand* 1982; 53: 957–62.

3. Gustilo RB, Anderson JT. Prevention of infection in the treatment of 1035 open fractures of long bones: Retrospective and prospective analysis. *J Bone Joint Surg Am* 1976; 58: 453–8.

4. Müller ME, Nazarian S, Koch P, Schatzker J. *The Comprehensive Classification of Fractures of Long Bones*. Springer, Berlin, 1990.

5. Hohl M. Fractures and dislocations of the knee, Part 1: Fractures about the knee. In: Rockwood CA, Green DP (eds.). *Fractures in Adults*, 2nd ed. JB Lippincott, Philadelphia, PA, 1984, pp. 1429–44.

6. Brown A, D'Arcy JC. Internal fixation for supracondylar fractures of the femur in the elderly patient. *J Bone Joint Surg Br* 1971; 53-B: 420–4.

7. Schatzker J, Lambert DC. Supracondylar fractures of the femur. *Clin Orthop Rel Res* 1979; 138: 77–83.

8. Healy WL, Brooker AF. Distal femoral fractures. *Clin Orthop Rel Res* 1983; 174: 166–71.

9. Butt MS, Krikler SJ, Ali MS. Displaced fractures of the distal femur in elderly patients. *J Bone Joint Surg Br* 1995; 77-B: 110–14.

10. Ostrum RF, Geel C. Indirect reduction and internal fixation of supracondylar femur fractures without bone graft. *J Orthop Trauma* 1995; 4: 278–84.

11. Smith TO, Hedges C, MacNair R, Schankat K, Wimhurst JA. The clinical and radiological outcomes of the LISS plate for distal femoral fractures: A systematic review. *Injury* 2009; 40: 1049–63.

12. Hoffmann MF, Jones CB, Sietsema DL, Tornetta P, Koenig SJ. Clinical outcomes of locked plating of distal femoral fractures in a retrospective cohort. *J Orthop Surg Res* 2013; 8: 13.

13. Hanschen M, Aschenbrenner IM, Fehske K, Kirchhoff S, Keil L, Holazpfel BM, Winkler S, et al. Mono- versus polyaxial locking plates in distal femur fractures: A prospective randomized multicentre clinical trial. *Int Orthop* 2014; 38: 857–63.

14. Vallier HA, Immler W. Comparison of the 95-degree angled blade plate and the locking condylar plate for the treatment of distal femoral fractures. *J Orthop Trauma* 2012; 26: 327–32.

15. Forster MC, Komarsamy B, Davison JN. Distal femoral fractures: A review of fixation methods. *Injury* 2006; 37: 97–108.

16. Syed AA, Agarwal M, Giannoudis PV, Matthews SJE, Smith RM. Distal femoral fractures: Long-term outcome following stabilization with the LISS. *Injury* 2004; 35: 599–607.

17. Erhardt JB, Vincenti M, Pressmar J, Kuelling FA, Spross C, Gebhard F, Roederer G. Mid term results of distal femoral fractures treated with a polyaxial locking plate: A multi-center study. *Open Orthop J* 2014; 8: 34–40.

18. Doshi HK, Wenxian P, Burgula MV, Murphy DP. Clinical outcomes of distal femoral fractures in the geriatric population using locking plates with a minimally invasive approach. *Geriatr Orthop Surg Rehabil* 2013; 4: 16–20.

19. Wong M-K, Leung F, Chow SP. Treatment of distal femoral fractures in the elderly using a less-invasive plating technique. *Int Orthop* 2005; 29: 117–20.

20. Rodriguez EK, Boulton C, Weaver MJ, Herder LM, Morgan JH, Chacko AT, Appleton PT, Zurakowski D, Vrahas MS. Predictive factors of distal femoral fracture nonunion after lateral locked plating: A retrospective multicenter case-control study of 283 fractures. *Injury* 2014; 45: 554–9.

21. Marks DS, Isbister ES, Porter KM. Zickel supracondylar nailing for supracondylar femoral fractures in elderly or infirm patients. *J Bone Joint Surg Br* 1994; 76-B: 596–601.

22. Papadokostakis G, Papakostidis C, Dimitriou R, Giannoudis PV. The role and efficacy of retrograde nailing for the treatment of diaphyseal and distal femoral fractures: A systematic review of the literature. *Injury* 2005; 36: 813–822.

23. Janzing HMJ, Stockman B, Van Damme G, Rommens P, Broos PLO. The retrograde intramedullary supracondylar nail: An alternative in the treatment of distal femoral fractures in the elderly. *Arch Orthop Trauma Surg* 1998; 118: 92–5.

24. Gynning JB, Hansen D. Treatment of distal femoral fractures with intramedullary supracondylar nails in elderly patients. *Injury* 1999; 30: 43–6.

25. Dunlop DG, Brenkel IJ. The supracondylar intramedullary nail in elderly patients with distal femoral fractures. *Injury* 1999; 30: 475–84.

26. Kumar A, Jasani V, Butt MS. Management of distal femoral fractures in elderly patients using retrograde titanium supracondylar nails. *Injury* 2000; 31: 199–73.

27. El-Kawy S, Ansara S, Moftah A, Shalaby H, Varughese V. Retrograde femoral nailing in elderly patients with supracondylar fracture femur; is it the answer for a clinical problem? *Int Orthop* 2007; 31: 83–6.

28. Kim J, Kang S-B, Nam K, Rhee SH, Won JW, Han H-S. Retrograde intramedullary nailing for distal femur fracture with osteoporosis. *Clin Orthop Surg* 2012; 4: 307–12.

29. Kulkarni SG, Varshneya A, Kulkarni GS, Kulkarni MG, Kulkarni VS, Kulkarni RM. Antegrade interlocking nailing for distal femoral fractures. *J Orthop Surg* 2012; 20: 48–54.

30. Markmiller M, Konrad G, Südkamp N. Femur-LISS and distal femoral nail for fixation of distal femoral fractures. *Clin Orthop Rel Res* 2004; 426: 252–7.

31. Wolfgang GL. Primary total knee arthroplasty for intercondylar fracture of the femur in a rheumatoid patient. *Clin Orthop Rel Res* 1982; 171: 80–2.

32. Bell KA, Johnstone AJ, Court-Brown CM, Hughes SPF. Primary knee arthroplasty for distal femoral fractures in elderly patients. *J Bone Joint Surg Br* 1992; 74-B: 400–2.

33. Appleton P, Moran M, Houshian S, Robinson CM. Distal femoral fractures treated by hinged total knee replacement in elderly patients. *J Bone Joint Surg Br* 2006; 88-B: 1065–70.

34. Parratte S, Bonnevialle P, Pietu G, Saragaglia D, Cherrier B, Lafosse JM. Primary total knee arthroplasty in the management of epiphyseal fracture around the knee. *Orthop Traumatol Surg Res* 2011; 97: S87–94.

35. Choi N-Y, Sohn J-M, Cho S-G, Kim S-C, In Y. Primary total knee arthroplasty for simple distal femoral fractures in elderly patients with knee osteoarthritis. *Knee Surg Rel Res* 2013; 25: 141–6.

36. Ali F, Saleh M. Treatment of isolated complex distal femoral fractures by external fixation. *Injury* 2000; 31: 139–46.

37. Lewis PL, Rorabeck CH. Periprosthetic fracture. In: Engh GA, Rorabeck CH (eds.). *Techniques of Revision Surgery*. Williams & Wilkins, Philadelphia, PA, 1997.

38. Johnston AT, Tsiridis E, Eyres KS, Toms AD. Periprosthetic fractures in the distal femur following total knee replacement: A review and guide to management. *Knee* 2012; 19(3): 156–62.

39. Herrera DA, Kregor PJ, Cole PA, Levy BA, Jönsson A, Zlowodzki M. Treatment of acute distal femur fractures above a total knee arthroplasty. *Acta Orthop* 2008; 79: 22–7.

40. Large TM, Kellam JF, Bosse MJ, Sims SH, Althausen P, Masonis JL. Locked plating of supracondylar periprosthetic femur fractures. *J Arthroplasty* 2008; 23: 115–20.

41. Horneff JG, Scolaro JA, Jafari SM, Mirza A, Parvizi J, Mehta S. Intramedullary nailing versus locked plating for treating supracondylar periprosthetic femur fractures. *Orthopedics* 2013; 36: e561–6.

42. Meneghini RM, Keyes BJ, Reddy KK, Maar DC. Modern retrograde intramedullary nails versus periarticular locked plates for supracondylar femur fractures after total knee arthroplasty. *J Arthroplasty* 2014; 29: 1478–81.

43. Mortazavi SM, Kurd ME, Bender B, Post Z, Parvizi J, Purtill JJ. Distal femoral arthroplasty for the treatment of periprosthetic fractures after total knee arthroplasty. *J Arthroplasty* 2010; 25: 775–80.

44. Jassim SS, McNamara I, Hopgood P. Distal femoral replacement in periprosthetic fracture around total knee arthroplasty. *Injury* 2014; 45: 550–3.

45. Kammerlander C, Riedmüller P, Gosch M, Zegg M, Kammerlander-Knauer U, Schmid R, Roth T. Functional outcome and mortality in geriatric distal femoral fractures. *Injury* 2012; 43: 1096–101.

46. Streubel PN, Ricci WM, Wong A, Gardner MJ. Mortality after distal femur fractures in elderly patients. *Clin Orthop Rel Res* 2011; 469: 1188–96.

47. Shulman BS, Patsalos-Fox B, Lopez N, Konda SR, Tejwani NC, Egol KA. Do elderly patients fare worse following operative treatment of distal femur fractures using modern techniques? *Geriatr Orthop Surg Rehab* 2014; 5: 27–30.

38

Patellar fractures

OLIVIA C. LEE AND MARK S. VRAHAS

INTRODUCTION

The patella is the largest sesamoid bone in the human body. It serves as the fulcrum of the extensor mechanism between the quadriceps and patellar tendons. The patella shifts the moment arm of the quadriceps anteriorly thereby increasing the efficiency of the extension force. Fractures of the patella most commonly occur following a simple fall in the elderly, with open fractures rare. In the elderly patient, fractures can also occur around a total knee arthroplasty or could be due to a pathological lesion.

The primary goal of management in the elderly patient is to regain function. Treatment is guided by bone quality, fracture pattern, physical examination, as well as the patient's functional status and medical comorbidities. Options for treatment include non-operative management, open reduction internal fixation, partial patellectomy and in rare cases total patellectomy.

EPIDEMIOLOGY

Patellar fractures represent about 1% of all fractures,[1,2] with an incidence in the elderly of 0.5 per 1000 from a national database of patients the over the age of 65 years.[3] The risk of patellar fracture is about 3.5 times higher in women than men. There is conflicting data on whether each decade of life adds further risk of a patellar fracture.[3] In a study of patellar fractures in 68 patients over the age of 65, Shabat et al.[4] demonstrated that 66% had a comminuted fracture pattern and 85% of fractures were associated with disruption of the extensor mechanism requiring surgical fixation.

Associated injuries may include hip dislocations, knee ligamentous injuries, femoral neck or shaft fractures and distal femur or proximal tibia fractures.[2,3] Fractures can also occur after total knee arthroplasty, anterior cruciate ligament (ACL) graft harvesting or due to a pathological lesion. Primary patellar tumours are exceedingly rare, with predominantly case reports and small series in the literature. Benign tumours are more common than malignant, with a giant cell tumour being the most commonly reported lesion.[5]

Mechanism of injury

Fractures of the patella can be caused by either a direct blow or indirectly through eccentric contraction of the quadriceps. The most common mechanism of injury in the elderly is a simple low energy fall from standing height.[1] The subcutaneous position of the patella increases the chance of direct trauma and open injury. Open patellar fractures are rare, and more frequent following a high energy injury such as a motor vehicle collision. Open fractures are more likely to have associated injuries and a higher Injury Severity Score (ISS).

Periprosthetic fractures

The overall prevalence of total knee arthroplasty in the United States is estimated to be 4.2% in those over 50 years of age, with increasing prevalence in each decade of life. The estimated number of patients who have had a total knee arthroplasty in the United States alone is over 4 million.[6] Patellar fractures may be the most common periprosthetic fracture after total knee arthroplasty with a very large range of reported prevalence ranging from 0.05% to 21%.[7-10] The true prevalence of periprosthetic patellar fracture is likely below 1%. However, given the large numbers of current and future total knee arthroplasty patients, periprosthetic patellar fractures will continue to become more common in the elderly population.

Patellar fractures are much more common after total knee arthroplasty (TKA) when the patella is resurfaced.[11] Factors that have been shown to increase the risk of fracture after resurfacing are the number of previous surgeries, preoperative mechanical limb malalignment, postoperative patellar tendon length and patellar post-resection thickness.[12]

CLASSIFICATION

The commonly utilized classification systems for patellar fractures are descriptive in nature. Fractures can be broadly described as non-displaced or displaced. Displacement has been defined as articular step-off of greater than 2 mm and/or fragment separation of greater than 3 mm.[13–16] The degree of displacement is associated with the severity of medial and lateral retinacular damage. Displaced fractures with disruption of the extensor mechanism are often treated surgically given the inferior outcomes associated with non-operative treatment.[16]

Non-displaced and displaced fractures are further categorized by location and pattern of fracture. Patellar fracture descriptions by location and pattern may be predictive of the injury mechanism. Several common descriptive patterns of fracture are shown in Figure 38.1. Pattern descriptors include transverse, vertical, stellate and multifragmented. These patterns may be non-comminuted or comminuted. Elderly patients are more likely to sustain comminuted fractures of the patella.[4,17] Location descriptors include proximal pole, distal pole or osteochondral. Osteochondral fractures are typically seen in younger patients.

The Orthopaedic Trauma Association (OTA) classification system designates the patella as location 34. This classification divides patella fractures into the standard A-type extra-articular, B-type partial articular, vertical, and C-type complete articular, non-vertical.[18] There is no prognostic outcome data for the OTA classification system; however, it is useful for the purposes of research.

Anatomical considerations

The patella is a triangular bone that resides within the quadriceps femoris tendon. It is convex and is covered by a continuation of the quadriceps tendon anteriorly. The superior three-fourths of the posterior patella is covered by thick articular cartilage. The distal anterior apex of bone serves as the origin of the patellar tendon. The posterior surface of the patella is divided into two major medial and lateral facets separated by a large vertical ridge. The medial and lateral facets are divided transversely by two smaller ridges, creating superior, intermediate and inferior facets. A smaller vertical ridge at the medial edge of the posterior patella separates the medial facet from the small facet.[1]

The patella typically forms from a single ossification center. There is anomalous ossification in approximately 3% of the population causing a bipartite or tripartite patella. One or two irregular fragments with smooth cortical edges are seen at the superolateral corner of the patella. This anomaly is more common bilaterally.[19] This developmental variation should not be mistaken for an acute fracture (Figure 38.2).

The vascular supply of the patella has been of interest due to the risk of osteonecrosis and the prevalence of anterior knee pain after injury. Scapinelli[20] described the extraosseous and intraosseous vascular supply of the patella. The extraosseous system is an anastomotic ring comprised of the supreme genicular, medial superior genicular, medial inferior genicular, lateral superior genicular, lateral inferior genicular and anterior tibial recurrent arteries. The intraosseous arteries are organized into two separate systems. The first are the mid-patellar vessels that enter the patella from the anterior surface. The second are the polar vessels that enter the patella from the distal pole, between the patellar tendon and the articular cartilage. Given this vascular arrangement, the proximal pole of the patella is at risk of devascularization following fracture (Figure 38.3).[20,21]

CLINICAL ASSESSMENT

The patient should be evaluated with a complete history and physical examination. A history of direct trauma to the knee or eccentric load and subsequent knee pain should

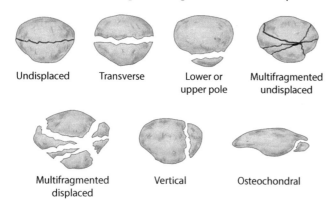

Undisplaced   Transverse   Lower or upper pole   Multifragmented undisplaced

Multifragmented displaced   Vertical   Osteochondral

Figure 38.1 Patellar fracture patterns.

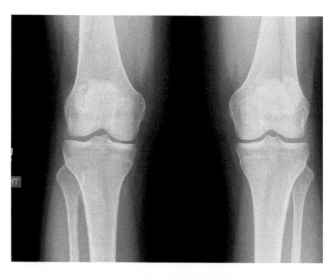

Figure 38.2 Standing bilateral knee radiographs demonstrating a right-sided tripartite patella and a left-sided bipartite patella.

alert the clinician to a possible extensor mechanism injury. A large hemarthrosis may be present depending on the injury to the retinaculum. Removal of the hemarthrosis and injection of local anesthetic can help facilitate further physical examination testing, although the literature to support this is limited. Patients can often retain a portion of their active extension in the setting of a patella fracture if the medial and/or lateral retinaculum is intact. In this setting, an extension lag is often seen. With a patellar fracture and complete rupture of the retinaculum, the patient will have no ability to actively extend the knee and perform a straight leg raise.

The subcutaneous patella should be palpated and examined for tenderness, crepitus or separation of fracture fragments if possible. Any lacerations, abrasions and contusions must be carefully examined for possible open injury. A saline load test can be performed with an intra-articular injection of 150 mL of sterile saline when in doubt, with extravasation of fluid from the wound or soft tissue seen.[22]

Imaging

Patellar fractures should be evaluated using anteroposterior, lateral and sunrise X-ray views. The superimposed distal femur may make interpretation of the anteroposterior (AP) view difficult. The lateral view allows a profile view of the patella demonstrating displacement and articular incongruity. The axial view is helpful for vertical and osteochondral fracture patterns (Figure 38.4). Further advanced imaging such as bone scan, CT or MRI are rarely needed. However, there may be a role for advanced imaging when evaluating for stress fractures in osteoporotic elderly patients or other pathologic lesions of the patella.[5,23]

TREATMENT

The treatment goals of patellar fracture management in the elderly are to restore prior functional level, maintain function of the extensor mechanism and restore articular congruence. The choice of fracture treatment depends on the fracture pattern, physical examination findings and the patient's functional status and medical comorbidities. In the elderly, it is also important to consider age, bone quality, surgical risk and the ability to maintain weight bearing and range of motion restrictions.

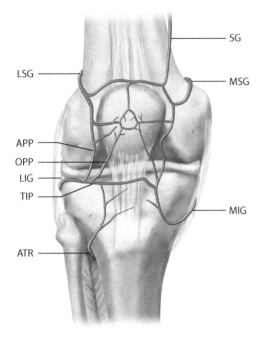

Figure 38.3 Arterial supply of the patella with the extraosseous geniculate system and intraosseous system. APP, ascending parapatellar artery; ATR, anterior tibial recurrent artery; LIG, lateral inferior genicular artery; LSG, lateral superior genicular artery; MIG, medial inferior genicular artery; MSG, medial superior genicular artery; OPP, oblique prepatellar artery; SG, supreme genicular artery; TIP, transverse infrapatellar artery. (Reprinted with permission from Scapinelli R. *J Bone Joint Surg Br* 1967;49(3):563–570.)

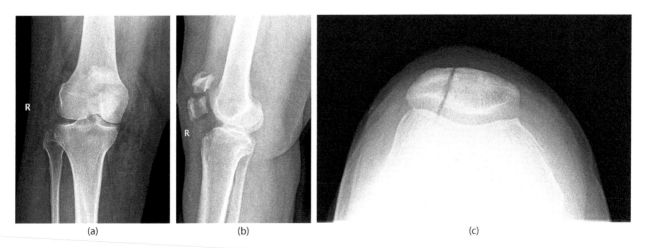

Figure 38.4 Anteroposterior (AP) **(a)** and lateral **(b)** views of a displaced transverse patellar fracture. Sunrise view of a vertical patellar fracture **(c)**.

Efforts should be made to preserve as much of the patella as possible. However, in cases of severe comminution, part or all of the patella may have to be excised. Options for treatment include non-operative treatment, open reduction internal fixation, partial patellectomy and total patellectomy.

Non-operative

Non-displaced fracture patterns are amenable to non-operative treatment. Fractures may be transverse, stellate or vertical. There should be no more than 3 mm of fracture fragment separation or 2 mm of articular incongruity, and there should be an intact extensor mechanism on physical exam.

Patients are immobilized with the knee held in extension for 4–6 weeks. This can be done with a cylinder or long leg cast, a hinged knee brace or a knee immobilizer. Weight bearing is allowed as tolerated with the knee in the extended position. Straight leg raising exercises may be initiated within several days.

Casts must be changed if there is any concern for skin compromise. The lighter hinged knee braces or knee immobilizers may be better tolerated by the elderly. However, the patient must reliably wear the brace as directed with the knee locked in extension for ambulation. After evidence of healing is noted, a program of strengthening and active motion is initiated. Typically the knee is allowed to flex in a staged manner. This can be done with a hinged knee brace, which can continue to be locked in extension for ambulation until the quadriceps strength and patella healing allow for a pain-free straight leg raise. One such protocol would be to allow flexion from 0 to 30 degrees after 6 weeks of extension. The amount of flexion can then be advanced by 30 degrees every 2–3 weeks thereafter with careful follow-up to ensure no further displacement. Elderly patients may require a closely monitored physical therapy regimen to maximize strength and motion.

Non-operative management may be appropriate for patients with displaced fractures in the face of significant medical comorbidities. These patients can be allowed to ambulate and initiate range of motion once their pain allows. Pritchett[24] reported a series of 18 patients with patellar fractures displaced greater than 1 cm managed non-operatively. Twelve surviving patients were followed for 2 years. At follow-up, no patients had severe pain and nine patients had only minimal or moderate activity restrictions.

Operative

For displaced fractures and patients unable to perform a straight leg raise, operative intervention is routinely required. Generally, greater than 2 mm of displacement and/or articular incongruity are defined as displacement. The preferred open approach is a longitudinal midline incision centred over the patella. This approach can be extended proximally to the quadriceps tendon and distally to the tibial tubercle as needed. Percutaneous and external fixation methods have also been described.[25–27] These techniques may be useful in cases of severe soft tissue damage.

OPEN REDUCTION INTERNAL FIXATION

Large, displaced vertical fracture fragments can be treated with lag screw fixation alone. For transverse or comminuted patterns, various techniques have been described consisting of wire fixation in cerclage or tension band configurations. These techniques have been evaluated biomechanically and clinically. The modified anterior tension band wire technique has been found to provide a superior fracture stability compared to other wiring techniques.[2,13,15,28,29] The force across the patella during flexion causes apex anterior angulation. The anterior tension band allows conversion of the tension force to a compressive force at the articular surface of the patella. A cerclage wire or cancellous screws may be added for additional stability, especially in the face of comminution.[29,30] Further studies have shown increased stability, decreased complications and good clinical outcomes when the tension band wire is threaded through cannulated screws.[13,31]

Modified anterior tension band wiring

Although Benjamin et al.[32] showed screw fixation alone to be adequate for transverse fractures in patients with adequate bone, fixation in the elderly requires more stable fixation. Modified anterior tension band wiring remains the treatment of choice for transverse, non-comminuted patellar fractures with good bone stock. After incision, fracture edges are exposed and cleaned of hematoma and soft tissue. The knee joint should be thoroughly irrigated. A provisional reduction can be performed and held with reduction forceps to evaluate reduction. The reduction of the articular surface should be palpated through the retinacular tear. If the tear is too small, longitudinal medial or lateral arthrotomies can be performed as described by Carpenter et al.[13] and Gardner et al.,[33] respectively. Subsequently, 1.6 mm K-wires or 4.0 mm cancellous screws can be placed in a vertical, parallel manner to maintain the reduction and to anchor the cerclage wire. The reduction can also be taken down to allow the K-wires to be passed in a retrograde manner through the fracture site. A 14- or 16-gauge angiocatheter or equivalent is then passed through the patellar and quadriceps tendon adjacent to the patella, posterior to the tips of the K-wires. This minimizes the soft tissue between the cerclage wire and the bone. An 18-gauge wire is then passed through the catheter in a circular or a crossed figure-of-eight pattern. After ensuring reduction of the articular surface, the wire is then tightened. When using a figure-of-eight pattern, the medial and lateral loops should be tightened symmetrically. The proximal ends of the K-wires are then bent, twisted to face posteriorly around the cerclage wire and then buried into the proximal patella. The excess distal ends of the K-wires are then cut (Figure 38.5).[34]

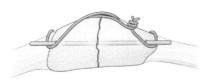
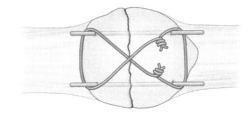

Figure 38.5 Modified anterior tension band construct. (Reprinted with permission from Archdeacon M, Sanders R. Patella fractures and extensor mechanism injuries. In: Browner B, Levine A, Jupiter J, Trafton P, Krettek C, editors. *Skeletal Trauma*. 4th Edition. Philadelphia, PA: Saunders; 2009. pp. 2131–2166.)

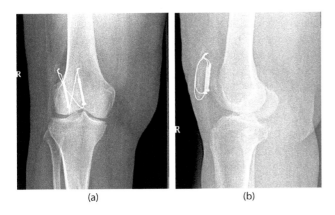

(a)   (b)

Figure 38.6 Tension band through cannulated screws on anteroposterior (AP) **(a)** and lateral **(b)** radiographs of the knee.

Care must be taken to close any retinacular tears. This is done routinely with figure-of-eight sutures placed in an interrupted fashion. These sutures may be placed and temporarily clamped prior to final reduction of the patellar fracture. The retinacular sutures can then be tied after final irrigation of the knee joint.

Miller et al.[35] reported a higher incidence of failure in elderly patients when constructs utilize wires alone. The modified anterior tension band can be supplemented in several ways. Fortis et al.[36] showed biomechanically increased compression forces when supplementing the modified anterior tension band technique with a cerclage wire in a cadaver model. The modified anterior tension band technique can also be used in conjunction with cannulated compression screws which mitigate the effect of fracture displacement in extension and the osteoporotic bone.[13,31] In this technique, partially threaded cannulated 4.0 mm screws are placed in lag fashion over longitudinal parallel K-wires. The screws are left short within the patella to prevent stress on the tension band wire at the screw tips. The 18-gauge wire is threaded through the cannulated screws in loops or a figure-of-eight pattern symmetrically tightened through medial and lateral loops (Figure 38.6).

In the face of a comminuted transverse fracture, the bony fragments may require removal or fragment specific fixation prior to using the above techniques. Individual lag screws, K-wires or cerclage wiring may be needed to secure comminuted fragments which can be salvaged. Palpation and direct evaluation of the articular surface is required to

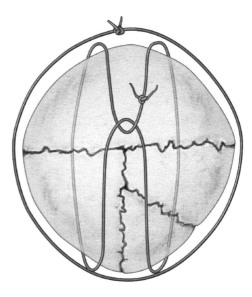

Figure 38.7 Lotke anterior tension band with cerclage wiring. (Reprinted with permission from Lotke PA, Ecker ML. *Clin Orthop Relat Res* 1981;(158):180–184.)

ensure congruence. Arthrotomy extension can facilitate the reduction and fixation of these comminuted fractures. The tension band technique can then be utilized as described.

Lotke anterior tension band with cerclage wiring

Lotke and Ecker[17] describe an alternate technique which can be utilized for severely comminuted stellate fractures. These fractures may not have fragments large enough to anchor a modified anterior tension band. An 18-gauge cerclage wire is placed around the patella adjacent to the bone. Subsequently, 2.0 mm K-wires are used to drill longitudinal parallel tracts through the reduced patella approximately 1 cm from the medial and lateral edges of bone. The two ends of an 18- or 20-gauge wire are passed distally through the K-wire holes forming a loop. One free proximal end of the wire is fed through the distal loop. The proximal ends are secured together and tightened (Figure 38.7).

Suture fixation

The use of a non-absorbable polyester suture can be considered instead of the standard stainless steel wire. A non-absorbable polyester suture was compared with a standard stainless steel wire using a cadaveric biomechanical model in the modified anterior tension band and the Lotke anterior tension band configurations. There were no failures of the suture or wire models tested to 1000 cycles.[37] A clinical study comparing wire fixation in 21 patients versus suture fixation in 16 patients revealed a 38% re-operation rate and 14% infection rate in the stainless steel wire group compared with a 6% re-operation and no infections in the suture group.[38] Using suture obviates the complications of broken wires, which is of particular importance in the elderly patient when comorbidities and skin quality make wound healing potentially problematic. This combined with a potentially decreased re-operation rate make suture fixation a reasonable alternative to the standard wire fixation methods. Care must be taken to maintain the principles of close apposition to the patellar bone and to ensure adequate suture tensioning.

PARTIAL PATELLECTOMY

Non-comminuted polar fractures with significant bone stock of the polar fragment or comminuted polar fractures which can be reduced adequately may be fixed using the modified anterior tension band or Lotke anterior tension band with cerclage techniques as described. Separate vertical wiring and the use of a basket plate have also been described to preserve inferior polar fragments with clinical success.[39–41] These techniques may allow for earlier range of motion and preservation of patellar height. All efforts should be made to preserve large articular fragments. However, if the polar fragment cannot be salvaged, a partial patellectomy can be performed with effective results. Although results are poor with >40% removal of the patella,[15] Saltzman et al.[42] reported on a group of 40 patients who underwent partial patellectomy. The mean strength of the quadriceps in this group was 85% of the contralateral extremity and good or excellent results were observed in 78% of patients.

Although partial patellectomy decreases the contact area of the patellofemoral joint and increases the joint contact pressure, Marder et al.[43] demonstrated that anterior reattachment of the patellar tendon significantly decreases these contact pressures. This anterior attachment site more accurately restores the native anatomy.

Comminuted, unsalvageable polar fractures can be managed with partial patellectomy treated as a quadriceps or patellar tendon avulsion injury. For partial patellectomy of the inferior pole, the remaining superior patellar fragment is prepared to form a transverse surface. Three evenly spaced parallel holes are drilled in the fragment exiting superiorly. A heavy, non-absorbable suture is used in a running locking stitch such as a Krakow. This stitch is placed moving inferiorly along one edge of the tendon and then superiorly up the center of the tendon. This is repeated with a second suture on the opposite edge of the tendon. The suture ends are subsequently passed through the three drill holes with the two center sutures passing through the central hole. These sutures are then tied with the knee in hyperextension and the tendon edge approximating the fractured portion of the patella. This repair is often

supplemented and protected with a wire or heavy suture passed through the tibial tubercle and around the proximal patella (Figure 38.8).

PATELLECTOMY

Complete patellectomy can lead to decreased efficiency of the extensor mechanism. Extension after patellectomy requires a 30% increase in quadriceps force[44] and several studies have demonstrated around a 50% loss of quadriceps strength post patellectomy.[45,46] All efforts should be made to preserve a fragment of bone if articular congruity can be maintained. However, patellectomy is an option for unreconstructable patellar fractures or for specific circumstances such as failed fixation, tumour or infection.

The patellar fragments and unhealthy tendon are removed and the remaining extensor apparatus is then primarily repaired. Removal of the patella effectively lengthens the extensor mechanism and therefore repair must include imbrication of the remaining tendon or an extensor lag will result. The knee is taken through a range of motion and tension should be evident at 90 degrees of flexion.[16]

Should insufficient tendon remain, a quadriceps turndown can be performed. This will also provide some prepatellar soft tissue if needed. One common method was described by Shorbe and Dobson[47] using an inverted V-plasty of the quadriceps tendon. The apex of the V is located 2.5 inches proximal to the free edge. The limbs extend distally 2 inches leaving half an inch of tendon

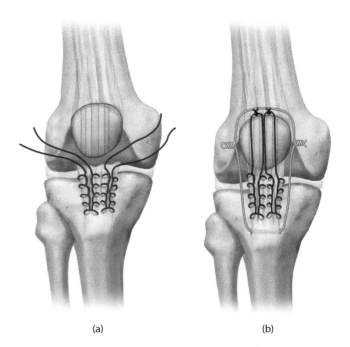

(a)   (b)

Figure 38.8 Patellar tendon repair to the remaining patella. (a) Two heavy non-absorbable sutures are placed in Krakow fashion through the tendon. Three parallel drill holes are placed through the patella. (b) The sutures are passed through the drill holes and tied with the knee in hyperextension and with tendon–bone contact. This can be reinforced with a protective cerclage wire or suture.

continuous with the retinaculum. The corners of the V may be reinforced with suture as needed. The apex is then folded distally and sutured into the proximal portion of the patellar tendon. The remaining quadriceps tendon is repaired as are all retinacular edges (Figure 38.9).

For large defects without sufficient quadriceps tendon, Gallie and Lemesurier[48] described a method of utilizing a free fascial or tendinous strip graft. With the knee extended, the post-debridement defect is measured. A 1.5 cm thick strip of fascia lata twice the length of the defect plus 2 inches is obtained. It is rolled along its length and sutured to itself. This graft is then woven through the remaining quadriceps tendon or muscle, passed through the patellar tendon, and then sewn to itself.[16,34]

Gunal et al.[49] found improved strength and subjective functional outcomes when patellectomy was combined with vastus medialis obliquus advancement. In this technique, the patellectomy defect is closed longitudinally and then the vastus medialis obliquus is advanced distally and laterally over the defect (Figure 38.10).

Periprosthetic patellar fracture

Treatment of patellar fractures after TKA can be guided by three main criteria: integrity of the extensor mechanism, fixation status of the patellar implant and quality of the remaining bone.[9] Stress fractures, fractures with intact extensor mechanism and well-fixed implants can usually be treated non-operatively with good outcomes.[9,50] Hozack et al.[50] found that non-displaced fractures of the patella

following TKA were best treated non-operatively and displaced fractures without extensor lag could also be treated nonoperatively.

Ortiguera and Berry[9] recommend treatment based on their classification system (Table 38.1). Type I fractures have a stable implant and preserved extensor mechanism and are treated non-operatively. Type II fractures have a stable implant and disrupted extensor mechanism. These are treated with extensor mechanism repair with partial patellectomy, complete patellectomy or open reduction internal fixation of the fracture. Type III fractures are those with an unstable implant and are further subdivided into type IIIa (good patellar bone stock) and type IIIb (poor patellar bone stock). These are managed operatively if symptomatic. Type IIIa fractures are treated by patellar component revision or removal of the component and patelloplasty. Type IIIb fractures are treated with component removal and partial or complete patellectomy. All of the operative interventions in these groups of patients were associated with high rates of complications, re-operations and residual symptoms.

Postoperative management and rehabilitation

Fixation should be examined intraoperatively to evaluate for the amount of flexion that can be immediately tolerated. Postoperative range of motion protocols have varied from immediate continuous passive motion to cast immobilization.[31,51] Weight bearing is usually initiated immediately and it is recommended that motion be initiated at least by 6 weeks after surgery.[52] Typically range of motion is limited completely or to less than 30 degrees at least until wound healing. Activity is then guided by wound healing, stability of the extensor mechanism and stability of the repair. When the extensor mechanism has remained longitudinally intact,

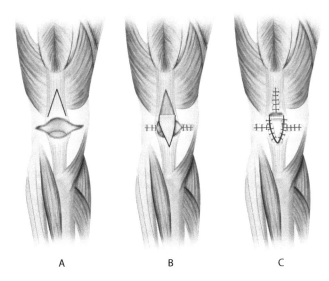

A   B   C

Figure 38.9 Shorbe and Dobson quadriceps tendon inverted V-plasty (a). Patellar resection with residual transverse defect in the extensor mechanism. The medial and lateral retinacula are first repaired. (b) An inverted V-shaped flap of quadriceps tendon is turned distally to repair the remaining central defect. (c) The flap is then sutured in place, covering and reinforcing the defect. (Adapted from Shorbe and Dobson. *J Bone Joint Surg Am* 1958;40-A(6):1281–4 (Figure 2).)

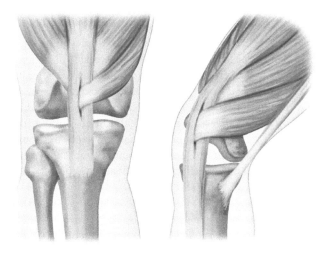

Figure 38.10 Gunal vastus medialis obliquus advancement supplementation of patellectomy. (Reprinted with permission from Gunal I, et al. *J Bone Joint Surg Br* 1997;79(1):13–16.)

Table 38.1 Classification and treatment recommendations for patellar fracture after total knee arthroplasty

Fracture type	Description	Treatment
I	Implant intact Extensor mechanism intact	Non-operative
II	Implant intact Extensor mechanism disrupted	Extensor mechanism repair with partial/complete patellectomy or ORIF
IIIa	Implant loose Good bone stock	If symptomatic: patellar component revision or component resection arthroplasty
IIIb	Implant loose Poor bone stock	If symptomatic: patellar component removal with patelloplasty or complete patellectomy

Source: Adapted from Ortiguera CJ, Berry DJ. *J Bone Joint Surg Am* 2002;84-A(4):532–540.

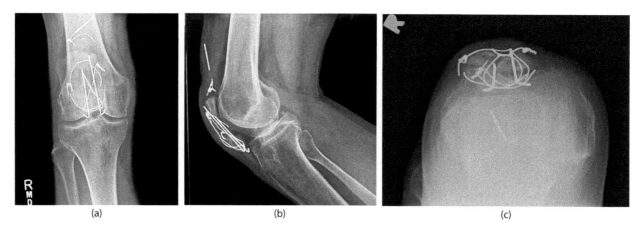

(a) (b) (c)

Figure 38.11 Loss of fixation with failure of hardware on anteroposterior (AP) **(a)**, lateral **(b)**, and sunrise **(c)** radiographs of the knee.

motion can be advanced relatively quickly. However, the majority of these injuries require more stringent protection of the repairs.

Two studies by Shabat et al.[4,51] have focused exclusively on rehabilitation in the elderly following operative intervention. In both studies, patients were immobilized in cylinder casts at 10 degrees of flexion for the first 4–6 weeks. All patients received physical therapy after discontinuation of the casts. In the series of 14 operatively managed octogenarians, all were able to achieve flexion greater than 100 degrees and all rated their function as not limited or almost not limited. The conclusion was made that immobilization may be appropriate for the comminuted and osteoporotic fractures of the elderly without adverse effects on the final outcome.

Complications

Several studies have reported fair to poor functional results in 19–69% of patients after an operatively managed patellar fracture with 28% of patients dissatisfied with their knee function.[2,15,53] A meta-analysis by Dy et al.[54] of 24 studies (737 patellar fractures) revealed that after open reduction internal fixation of patellar fractures, the estimated rates

are 33.6% for re-operation, 3.2% for infection and 1.9% for nonunion. These rates were not significantly influenced by age, gender, operative technique or the date of publication.

LOSS OF REDUCTION

Smith et al.[55] found a 22% rate of loss of reduction greater than 2 mm when using a modified anterior tension band (MATB) technique with early range of motion. It is unclear whether protected range of motion would have prevented these complications. Miller et al.[35] noted a 12% failure rate in a group of 109 patients with operatively managed patellar fractures. Factors that predicted failure were older patient age and the use of K-wires in a tension band construct. The use of other types of hardware (screws, wires) in a tension band fashion was not found to correlate with failure. Revision fixation is recommended if the fracture fragments separate by more than 3–4 mm or cause articular incongruity of more than 3 mm[16,34] (Figure 38.11).

NONUNION

The overall rate of nonunion in patellar fractures ranges from 2.4% to 12.5% in the literature.[16,56] This includes non-operatively and operatively managed fractures. Operative management was found to have a 1.9% rate of nonunion.[54] Open fractures and transverse fracture patterns may be at increased risk for nonunion.[57]

Klassen and Trousdale[56] reported on a series of 20 patients with delayed union or nonunion of patellar fractures treated initially non-operatively (n=12) and operatively (n=8). Patients were recommended for surgery if symptomatic. It was found that minimally symptomatic nonunions could be managed non-operatively, although these fractures did not ultimately unite. Operative management of non-unions was found to achieve union with some improvement of function. Patients recommended for non-operative management and those recommended for operative management who underwent surgery had a statistically significant difference in improvement compared to those recommended for surgery who refused.

INFECTION

The meta-analysis rate of infection in operatively managed patellar fractures was 3.2%[54] with rates ranging from 0% to 12.8%. Infection rates were higher in open fractures and in immunocompromised patients.[55,58] Superficial infections may necessitate oral antibiotics, wound care or prominent hardware removal after fracture healing. Devitalized soft tissue and any unstable fixation must be removed. Stable fixation in the presence of deep infection or osteomyelitis may be retained after aggressive debridement and with the use of culture specific intravenous antibiotics. All efforts should be made to preserve any remaining patella, although patellectomy may be required to control infection. Flaps may be necessary for adequate soft tissue coverage.

SYMPTOMATIC HARDWARE

Rates of symptomatic hardware have ranged from 0% to 60%, with many of these patients requiring hardware removal.[17,31,52,58,59] Symptomatic hardware can be broken or intact. Miller et al.[35] found the only predictor for hardware removal was increasing follow-up time. After fracture healing, hardware can be removed if symptomatic. There have been case reports of migrating broken hardware from the patella to the popliteal fossa and the right ventricle of the heart.[60,61] These cases prompt consideration of hardware removal for broken wires or periodic radiographs to evaluate for migration.

STIFFNESS

Stable fixation of patellar fractures should allow for early range of motion. If immobilization is required or chosen for the initial 4–6 weeks, Shabat et al.[4,51] have shown that functional range of motion can be regained with physical therapy. If stiffness does not improve after a course of therapy, manipulation under anaesthesia can be considered. This must be performed carefully to prevent soft tissue rupture or failure of fixation. Should manipulation not achieve adequate range of motion, arthroscopic lysis of adhesions can be considered in severe cases. Epidural anesthesia, continuous passive motion and frequent physical therapy can be used in conjunction with surgery. Quadricepsplasty can be considered if stiffness

persists at the 9- to 12-month postoperative period, although in the elderly this will likely be used sparingly.

POSTTRAUMATIC ARTHRITIS

Long terms rates of patellofemoral arthritis after patella fractures have ranged from 16% to 70% following non-operative and operative management.[1,62] Sorensen[62] noted a 70% prevalence of patellofemoral arthritis at the fractured patella. However, 30% of patients also had radiographic patellofemoral arthritis on the contralateral non-fractured knee and all patients were either asymptomatic or had mild symptoms. Most patellofemoral arthritis can be managed with physical therapy, quadriceps strengthening and non-steroidal anti-inflammatory medications. Intra-articular injections and total knee arthroplasty can be considered in the appropriate patient.

CONCLUSIONS

Fractures of the patella most commonly occur following a low energy simple fall in the elderly, with comminuted fractures more frequently seen. In the elderly patient, we are likely to see an increasing number of fractures around a total knee arthroplasty.

It is important to consider both the patient and fracture characteristics when managing these injuries in the elderly patient. Although it is optimal to restore the articular surface and extensor mechanism for displaced fractures, potential complications of surgical intervention must be considered. More data is required on the long-term outcome of these injuries following both operative and non-operative intervention in the elderly patient. Important outcomes to consider are patient reported outcomes along with complication and re-operation rates.

REFERENCES

1. Bostrom A. Fracture of the patella. A study of 422 patellar fractures. *Acta Orthop Scand Suppl* 1972;143:1–80.
2. Levack B, Flannagan JP, Hobbs S. Results of surgical treatment of patellar fractures. *J Bone Joint Surg Br* 1985;67(3):416–419.
3. Baron JA, Karagas M, Barrett J, Kniffin W, Malenka D, Mayor M, et al. Basic epidemiology of fractures of the upper and lower limb among Americans over 65 years of age. *Epidemiology* 1996;7(6):612–618.
4. Shabat S, Mann G, Kish B, Stern A, Sagiv P, Nyska M. Functional results after patellar fractures in elderly patients. *Arch Gerontol Geriatr* 2003;37(1):93–98.
5. Bhagat S, Sharma H, Bansal M, Reid R. Presentation and outcome of primary tumors of the patella. *J Knee Surg* 2008;21(3):212–216.
6. Weinstein AM, Rome BN, Reichmann WM, Collins JE, Burbine SA, Thornhill TS, et al. Estimating the burden of total knee replacement in the United States. *J Bone Joint Surg Am* 2013;95(5):385–392.

7. Sheth NP, Pedowitz DI, Lonner JH. Periprosthetic patellar fractures. *J Bone Joint Surg Am* 2007;89(10):2285–2296.

8. Keating EM, Haas G, Meding JB. Patella fracture after post total knee replacements. *Clin Orthop Relat Res* 2003;(416):93–97.

9. Ortiguera CJ, Berry DJ. Patellar fracture after total knee arthroplasty. *J Bone Joint Surg Am* 2002;84-A(4):532–540.

10. Reed MR, Farhan MJ, Chaudhuri C. Patellar stress fracture: A complication of knee joint arthroplasty without patellar resurfacing. *J Arthroplasty* 1999;14(3):383–385.

11. Parvizi J, Kim KI, Oliashirazi A, Ong A, Sharkey PF. Periprosthetic patellar fractures. *Clin Orthop Relat Res* 2006;446:161–166.

12. Seo JG, Moon YW, Park SH, Lee JH, Kang HM, Kim SM. A case-control study of spontaneous patellar fractures following primary total knee replacement. *J Bone Joint Surg Br* 2012;94(7):908–913.

13. Carpenter JE, Kasman RA, Patel N, Lee ML, Goldstein SA. Biomechanical evaluation of current patella fracture fixation techniques. *J Orthop Trauma* 1997;11(5):351–356.

14. Braun W, Wiedemann M, Ruter A, Kundel K, Kolbinger S. Indications and results of nonoperative treatment of patellar fractures. *Clin Orthop Relat Res* 1993;(289):197–201.

15. Bostman O, Kiviluoto O, Nirhamo J. Comminuted displaced fractures of the patella. *Injury* 1981;13(3):196–202.

16. Harris R. Fractures of the patella and injuries to the extensor mechanism. In: Bucholtz R, Heckman J, Court-Brown C, editors. *Rockwood and Green's Fractures in Adults.* 6th ed. Philadelphia, PA: Lippincott Williams & Wilkins; 2006. pp. 1969–1997.

17. Lotke PA, Ecker ML. Transverse fractures of the patella. *Clin Orthop Relat Res* 1981;(158):180–184.

18. Marsh JL, Slongo TF, Agel J, Broderick JS, Creevey W, DeCoster TA, et al. Fracture and dislocation classification compendium—2007: Orthopaedic Trauma Association classification, database and outcomes committee. *J Orthop Trauma* 2007;21(10 Suppl):S1–133.

19. Todd TW, McCally WC. Defects of the patellar border. *Ann Surg* 1921;74(6):775–782.

20. Scapinelli R. Blood supply of the human patella. Its relation to ischaemic necrosis after fracture. *J Bone Joint Surg Br* 1967;49(3):563–70.

21. Lazaro LE, Wellman DS, Klinger CE, Dyke JP, Pardee NC, Sculco PK, et al. Quantitative and qualitative assessment of bone perfusion and arterial contributions in a patellar fracture model using gadolinium-enhanced magnetic resonance imaging: A cadaveric study. *J Bone Joint Surg Am* 2013;95(19):e1401–7.

22. Nord RM, Quach T, Walsh M, Pereira D, Tejwani NC. Detection of traumatic arthrotomy of the knee using the saline solution load test. *J Bone Joint Surg Am* 2009;91(1):66–70.

23. Apple JS, Martinez S, Allen NB, Caldwell DS, Rice JR. Occult fractures of the knee: Tomographic evaluation. *Radiology* 1983;148(2):383–387.

24. Pritchett JW. Nonoperative treatment of widely displaced patella fractures. *Am J Knee Surg* 1997;10(3):145–7; discussion 147–8.

25. Ma YZ, Zhang YF, Qu KF, Yeh YC. Treatment of fractures of the patella with percutaneous suture. *Clin Orthop Relat Res* 1984;(191):235–241.

26. Wardak MI, Siawash AR, Hayda R. Fixation of patella fractures with a minimally invasive tensioned wire method: Compressive external fixation. *J Trauma Acute Care Surg* 2012;72(5):1393–1398.

27. Liang QY, Wu JW. Fracture of the patella treated by open reduction and external compressive skeletal fixation. *J Bone Joint Surg Am* 1987;69(1):83–89.

28. Weber MJ, Janecki CJ, McLeod P, Nelson CL, Thompson JA. Efficacy of various forms of fixation of transverse fractures of the patella. *J Bone Joint Surg Am* 1980;62(2):215–220.

29. Burvant JG, Thomas KA, Alexander R, Harris MB. Evaluation of methods of internal fixation of transverse patella fractures: A biomechanical study. *J Orthop Trauma* 1994;8(2):147–153.

30. Curtis MJ. Internal fixation for fractures of the patella. A comparison of two methods. *J Bone Joint Surg Br* 1990;72(2):280–282.

31. Berg EE. Open reduction internal fixation of displaced transverse patella fractures with figure-eight wiring through parallel cannulated compression screws. J Orthop Trauma 1997;11(8):573–576.

32. Benjamin J, Bried J, Dohm M, McMurtry M. Biomechanical evaluation of various forms of fixation of transverse patellar fractures. *J Orthop Trauma* 1987;1(3):219–222.

33. Gardner MJ, Griffith MH, Lawrence BD, Lorich DG. Complete exposure of the articular surface for fixation of patellar fractures. *J Orthop Trauma* 2005;19(2):118–123.

34. Archdeacon M, Sanders R. Patella fractures and extensor mechanism injuries. In: Browner B, Levine A, Jupiter J, Trafton P, Krettek C, editors. *Skeletal Trauma.* 4th ed. Philadelphia, PA: Saunders; 2009. pp. 2131–2166.

35. Miller MA, Liu W, Zurakowski D, Smith RM, Harris MB, Vrahas MS. Factors predicting failure of patella fixation. *J Trauma Acute Care Surg* 2012;72(4):1051–1055.

36. Fortis AP, Milis Z, Kostopoulos V, Tsantzalis S, Kormas P, Tzinieris N, et al. Experimental investigation of the tension band in fractures of the patella. *Injury* 2002;33(6):489–493.

37. Patel VR, Parks BG, Wang Y, Ebert FR, Jinnah RH. Fixation of patella fractures with braided polyester suture: A biomechanical study. *Injury* 2000;31(1):1–6.

38. Gosal HS, Singh P, Field RE. Clinical experience of patellar fracture fixation using metal wire or non-absorbable polyester—A study of 37 cases. *Injury* 2001;32(2):129–135.

39. Yang KH, Byun YS. Separate vertical wiring for the fixation of comminuted fractures of the inferior pole of the patella. *J Bone Joint Surg Br* 2003;85(8):1155–1160.

40. Kastelec M, Veselko M. Inferior patellar pole avulsion fractures: Osteosynthesis compared with pole resection. *J Bone Joint Surg Am* 2004;86-A(4):696–701.

41. Matejcic A, Puljiz Z, Elabjer E, Bekavac-Beslin M, Ledinsky M. Multifragment fracture of the patellar apex: Basket plate osteosynthesis compared with partial patellectomy. *Arch Orthop Trauma Surg* 2008;128(4):403–408.

42. Saltzman CL, Goulet JA, McClellan RT, Schneider LA, Matthews LS. Results of treatment of displaced patellar fractures by partial patellectomy. *J Bone Joint Surg Am* 1990;72(9):1279–1285.

43. Marder RA, Swanson TV, Sharkey NA, Duwelius PJ. Effects of partial patellectomy and reattachment of the patellar tendon on patellofemoral contact areas and pressures. *J Bone Joint Surg Am* 1993;75(1):35–45.

44. Kaufer H. Mechanical function of the patella. *J Bone Joint Surg Am* 1971;53(8):1551–1560.

45. Sutton FS, Jr, Thompson CH, Lipke J, Kettelkamp DB. The effect of patellectomy on knee function. *J Bone Joint Surg Am* 1976;58(4):537–540.

46. Watkins MP, Harris BA, Wender S, Zarins B, Rowe CR. Effect of patellectomy on the function of the quadriceps and hamstrings. *J Bone Joint Surg Am* 1983;65(3):390–395.

47. Shorbe HB, Dobson CH. Patellectomy; repair of the extensor mechanism. *J Bone Joint Surg Am* 1958;40-A(6):1281–1284.

48. Gallie WE, Lemesurier AB. The late repair of fractures of the patella and of rupture of the ligamentum patellae and quadriceps tendon. *J Bone Joint Surg Am* 1927;9(1):47–54.

49. Gunal I, Taymaz A, Kose N, Gokturk E, Seber S. Patellectomy with vastus medialis obliquus advancement for comminuted patellar fractures: A prospective randomised trial. *J Bone Joint Surg Br* 1997;79(1):13–16.

50. Hozack WJ, Goll SR, Lotke PA, Rothman RH, Booth RE, Jr. The treatment of patellar fractures after total knee arthroplasty. *Clin Orthop Relat Res* 1988;(236):123–127.

51. Shabat S, Folman Y, Mann G, Gepstein R, Fredman B, Nyska M. Rehabilitation after knee immobilization in octogenarians with patellar fractures. *J Knee Surg* 2004;17(2):109–112.

52. Carpenter JE, Kasman R, Matthews LS. Fractures of the patella. *Instr Course Lect* 1994;43:97–108.

53. Hung LK, Chan KM, Chow YN, Leung PC. Fractured patella: Operative treatment using the tension band principle. *Injury* 1985;16(5):343–347.

54. Dy CJ, Little MT, Berkes MB, Ma Y, Roberts TR, Helfet DL, et al. Meta-analysis of re-operation, nonunion, and infection after open reduction and internal fixation of patella fractures. *J Trauma Acute Care Surg* 2012;73(4):928–932.

55. Smith ST, Cramer KE, Karges DE, Watson JT, Moed BR. Early complications in the operative treatment of patella fractures. *J Orthop Trauma* 1997;11(3):183–187.

56. Klassen JF, Trousdale RT. Treatment of delayed and nonunion of the patella. *J Orthop Trauma* 1997;11(3):188–194.

57. Nathan ST, Fisher BE, Roberts CS, Giannoudis PV. The management of nonunion and delayed union of patella fractures: A systematic review of the literature. *Int Orthop* 2011;35(6):791–795.

58. Torchia ME, Lewallen DG. Open fractures of the patella. *J Orthop Trauma* 1996;10(6):403–409.

59. Catalano JB, Iannacone WM, Marczyk S, Dalsey RM, Deutsch LS, Born CT, et al. Open fractures of the patella: Long-term functional outcome. *J Trauma* 1995;39(3):439–444.

60. Choi HR, Min KD, Choi SW, Lee BI. Migration to the popliteal fossa of broken wires from a fixed patellar fracture. *Knee* 2008;15(6):491–493.

61. Biddau F, Fioriti M, Benelli G. Migration of a broken cerclage wire from the patella into the heart. A case report. *J Bone Joint Surg Am* 2006;88(9):2057–2059.

62. Sorensen KH. The late prognosis after fracture of the patella. *Acta Orthop Scand* 1964;34:198–212.

39

Proximal tibial fractures

MATTHEW D. KARAM AND J. LAWRENCE MARSH

INTRODUCTION

In North America as our population ages, an increasing number of elderly patients (see Chapter 1) sustain injuries including tibial plateau fractures. Unfortunately, there is a relative paucity of evidence based, high quality literature reporting on treatment techniques and outcomes for patients in this age group who sustain tibial plateau fractures. The majority of studies on proximal tibia fractures stratify the analysis based upon fracture or type of treatment without assessment of the elderly as a subgroup. Given this lack of published information, treatment recommendations in this chapter are often extrapolated from studies on tibial plateau fractures without age or bone quality stratification combined with opinions based on our personal experience.

Proximal tibia fractures are complex injuries and the presence of osteoporosis or osteopenia complicates management. Even low energy injuries lead to greater fracture comminution than would occur in patients with normal bone stock.[1] Given the relative frailty of the bone there is an increased risk of secondary displacement with both operative and non-operative management. Even with modern implant designs and fixation techniques the effectiveness of operative treatment in maintaining reduction is decreased in the setting of compromised bone stock. Additionally, elderly patients do not tolerate prolonged periods of non-weight bearing or immobilization.

Despite these difficulties in the treatment of elderly patients who sustain proximal tibia fractures, the treatment may be less intensive and in some cases easier than some other osteoporotic peri-articular fractures involving the lower extremity. For instance, non-operative treatment and mobilization is possible for many patterns of injury. In contrast, patients who sustain distal femur fractures or hip fractures require surgical management prior to mobilization. When surgery is chosen less invasive surgical approaches and implants are often possible in the proximal tibia. The knee tolerates joint incongruity to a greater extent than the hip joint.[2] Despite articular incongruity and radiographic evidence of posttraumatic osteoarthritis it is not uncommon for patients to remain relatively asymptomatic and function well, as long as the overall alignment of the limb is maintained.[3] For these reasons in elderly patients with osteoporosis and a tibial plateau fracture, it is often appropriate to minimize extensive, invasive soft tissue compromising surgical approaches and focus on preserving mechanical alignment of the limb while minimizing the risk for complications.

In this chapter we use elderly age, poor bone quality, osteoporosis and osteopenia relatively interchangeably since there is substantial overlap in these conditions. The epidemiology, evaluation and approach to treatment of these challenging injuries will be covered.

EPIDEMIOLOGY

Proximal tibia fractures occur throughout the entire spectrum of patient age, from young patients who sustain physeal injuries to the most elderly patients where low energy mechanisms can lead to a variety of different fracture patterns. Multiple studies have demonstrated that the highest incidence of tibial plateau fractures is in the fifth decade of life followed by the fourth and six decades.[4,5] There are also gender differences, with men typically having a higher incidence in the second, third and fourth decades, often due to higher energy mechanisms. Women have an increasing incidence of tibial plateau fractures with age, often peaking in the seventh decade.[5] It is in this population that osteoporotic proximal tibia fractures are most commonly encountered and lower energy mechanisms start to predominate.[5,6]

While the specific incidence of tibial plateau fractures complicated by osteoporosis remains difficult to elucidate, such fractures are felt to be increasingly common. Previous studies have demonstrated that approximately 30–40% of all tibial plateau fractures may have some degree of underlying osteoporosis or osteopenia.[5,6] Given the increasing population of elderly individuals and with improved techniques for assessing osteoporosis, a focused study might demonstrate that this is a conservative estimate.

CLASSIFICATION

Fractures of the tibial plateau represent a diverse and complex group of injuries. There are many different mechanisms of injury with varying degrees of radiographic displacements and associated soft tissue injuries. These varied injuries require different evaluation and treatment techniques, yet all remain classified as fractures of the tibial plateau. Nowhere is this variation more apparent than in elderly patients, where injury patterns span the spectrum from severe high energy bicondylar fracture dislocation patterns resulting from motor vehicle accidents to low energy valgus loading fractures with joint impaction.

The two most commonly used classification schemes for tibial plateau fractures are the Schatzker classification[6] and the AO/OTA classification.[7] These classifications are utilized for elderly patients and have similar relevance to when they are used in younger patients with tibial plateau fractures.

The relative incidence of tibial plateau fractures varies in patients with osteoporosis or osteopenia compared to that of patients who have normal bone. The lateral split depression fracture (Schatzker II, 41-B) is the most common fracture pattern in patients with osteoporosis or osteopenia.[3] In a patient with compromised bone stock, a valgus load leads mainly to overloading of the lateral plateau and a split depression fracture, whereas in an individual with normal bone in some cases a bone contusion or medial ligamentous injury may occur as a result of the better structural integrity of the subchondral bone. Likewise a pure split fracture (Schatzker I) is rare in patients with osteoporosis because structural integrity of the bone is requisite for this pattern. As opposed to younger patients with normal bone stock, bicondylar fracture patterns in the elderly may occur without high-energy mechanisms. When they do occur significant comminution and cancellous bone loss or impaction lead to difficulties in subsequent surgical management.[8–10] Crushing, loss of bone stock and small soft articular fragments with metaphyseal comminution are common features of these patterns in elderly patients (Figure 39.1).

TREATMENT

Evaluation

Associated injuries to the soft tissues, including open wounds, compartment syndrome and vascular injuries, may all be associated with high-energy tibial plateau

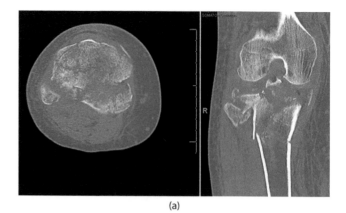

(a)

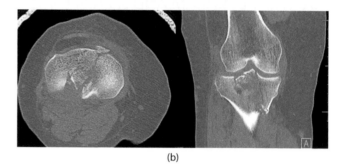

(b)

Figure 39.1 (a) Axial and coronal CT images of a 72-year-old woman who sustained a closed bicondylar tibial plateau fracture. (b) Axial and coronal CT images of a 38-year-old woman who sustained a tibial plateau fracture involving both condyles. Note that despite similar injury mechanisms there is significantly more metaphyseal comminution and cancellous bone impaction in the older woman (a).

fractures.[11,12] High energy fracture patterns may occur from relatively low energy trauma in patients with osteoporosis or osteopenia so these associated injuries must be considered and the patient carefully evaluated even when the mechanism is a simple fall.

Although not clearly documented in the literature, vascular injuries may be more common in severe injury patterns because of less compliance of potentially calcified vessels[13] (Figure 39.2). In elderly patients the soft tissue envelope may be less resilient and more poorly vascularized. For this reason careful assessment of the soft tissues prior to surgical approaches is equally or more important than in younger patients. The soft tissue envelope in elderly patients with osteoporotic fractures may be less tolerant of extensive surgical approaches.

Ligamentous injuries about the knee are commonly associated with tibial plateau fractures.[14,15] For example, in lateral split depression injuries or local lateral compression fractures from a valgus load on the knee, a common injury pattern in the elderly population, a medial collateral ligament (MCL) injury may occur. However the incidence of MCL injury is generally thought to be higher in patients with normal bone stock since osteopenic bone protects ligamentous structures about the knee, as failure occurs through the bone rather than soft tissue.[3]

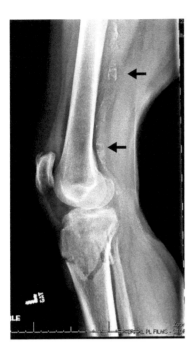

Figure 39.2 Lateral radiograph of an 89-year-old man with a bicondylar tibial plateau fracture. Vascular calcifications (black arrow) can be easily seen.

The physical exam is important and should be similar to that for other patients with tibial plateau fractures. This includes inspection of the soft tissues as well as a detailed neurovascular examination, both of which are critical for determining subsequent treatment strategies. Stability testing or ligamentous examination may be appropriate in low energy type fracture patterns when considering non-operative management, as mechanical stability and limb alignment are important for a satisfactory outcome.[16] Sometimes just assessing limb alignment in the supine position is helpful in assessing likely deformity without surgical treatment.

Radiographic assessment and work-up of tibial plateau fractures is similar regardless of bone quality. This includes anteroposterior (AP), lateral and caudal or plateau view radiographs. Radiographs of adjacent joints including the hip and ankle may be indicated. When surgical management is considered, a CT scan of the injured extremity will assist with surgical planning. MRI may identify associated soft tissue injuries to menisci and ligaments but we do not routinely use it in all plateau fractures. In elderly patients we would rarely obtain an MRI since the need to assess and treat ligament and meniscal injuries is less. We could find no specific study addressing the treatment of intra-articular or periarticular soft tissue injuries of the knee in elderly or osteoporotic patients.

General considerations

The treatment of proximal tibia fractures in elderly patients with osteoporosis requires several considerations that can lead to different treatment techniques than what would be chosen for younger patients with good bone stock. Patients who are elderly or those with decreased bone stock from osteoporosis are more likely to have lower functional demands than those with normal stock. Additionally, complications occurring in elderly or infirm patients are particularly problematic. For these reasons less aggressive treatment techniques, including non-operative treatment, are often more appropriate than in younger or more active patients with a commensurate injury. The literature supports numerous surgical and non-surgical techniques that can achieve satisfactory outcomes after tibial plateau fractures in both young patients and in those who have underlying osteoporosis or osteopenia.[3,10,17] Given this finding, a surgeon can be reassured that a potentially less aggressive surgical strategy may yield an acceptable outcome.

In deciding on treatment the surgeon should strongly consider those factors that lead to favourable outcomes. Central to this is avoiding limb malalignment. Malalignment greater than 10 degrees tends to alter the weight-bearing axis and predispose to an unfavourable prognosis. Like malalignment, ongoing instability in the knee is also poorly tolerated and attempts should be made to minimize it.[5] Persistent intra-articular displacement is felt to be an important predictor of prognosis; however tolerances of residual articular displacement remain difficult to fully elucidate.[18] This remains an area of ongoing controversy in both healthy and osteoporotic bone.[16,19,20] Less aggressive treatment techniques designed only to maintain or restore limb alignment may be preferable to interventions designed to perfectly reduce the injured articular surface. When functional demands are very low, even limb alignment becomes less important. A modest deformity in a non-ambulatory patient will have little functional or cosmetic significance.

When possible, early joint motion for tibial plateau fractures should be instituted and indeed this is felt to be one of the main advantages of surgical management.[19,21–24] It should be noted, however, that tibial plateau fractures treated non-operatively tolerate 4–6 weeks of immobilization without negative consequences.[25]

There is a clear association between poor patient outcomes and operative complications such as infection, wound breakdown and neurologic injury, so whenever possible these should be avoided.[11,26] Complications may require prolonged and difficult treatment particularly in injuries that result from higher energy mechanisms.

Nonoperative treatment

Nonoperative treatment of tibial plateau fractures may be an option in elderly patients. Unlike some fractures in other areas of the body including the hip or distal femur, prolonged skeletal traction is not required for non-operative management. Patients may be mobilized with a simple splint or brace without significant difficulty. Surgery may therefore be reserved for those cases where predictable improvements in ultimate knee function may be achieved. Given the increased risks of complications and difficulties of surgical management in elderly patients with poor bone stock, the indications for nonoperative treatment in this patient population are increased.[25] For those individuals who have lateral split depression type fractures without significant valgus instability, treatment would consist of early knee range of motion and protected weight bearing with a lightweight maneuverable soft brace (Figure 39.3). Generally progression to full weight bearing may begin at 6 weeks following injury. Most commonly, clinical symptoms including pain and significant swelling recede and patients are able to return to full baseline function within several months following the initial injury. Often when patients have unstable injury patterns such as valgus instability, more rigid immobilization in a formal cast may be considered. This however has to be weighed against the decreased mobilization and the potential need for increased nursing support. Segal and colleagues have shown that weight bearing in a cast-type brace may be allowed with the expectation of no greater than 2 mm of increased displacement.[27] With increased initial displacement of the fracture and in bicondylar fracture patterns, non-operative management often results in malalignment and less satisfactory outcomes.[25]

In higher energy injury patterns, such as bicondylar tibial plateau fractures or in fractures with predictable instability greater than 10 degrees or in those where satisfactory limb alignment cannot be achieved, skeletal traction may be considered; however, in such patients prolonged immobility or bed rest is often poorly tolerated, and operative management may be more appropriate.[28] Traction with a spanning fixator will usually be preferable.[29]

Indications for operative treatment

As with all patients who undergo operative management of displaced tibial plateau fractures, but particularly in those with compromised bone quality, many factors must be considered prior to surgery. It is clear that elderly patients undergoing surgical management, including reduction and fixation, have worse outcomes than those patients who are otherwise healthy and have normal bone stock.[6,30] These less than satisfactory results may in part result from a higher rate of postoperative settling or collapse of the articular surface and decreased stability of implants used to hold fracture fragments. Other considerations include the risks of anaesthesia as well as the continued potential for decreased mobility even with successful operative management. Despite these potential risks, there are patients who will clearly benefit from thoughtful and carefully planned and executed surgical intervention. As in many situations, a surgical plan must be individualized based on the patient, fracture pattern and the quality of bone. Likewise, a patient's baseline functional demands and ultimate expectations must be also carefully considered. When limb malalignment is predicted with non-operative management in patients with split lateral depression fractures with significant articular depression, baseline valgus

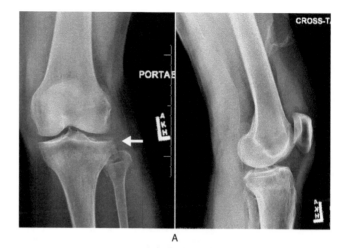

A

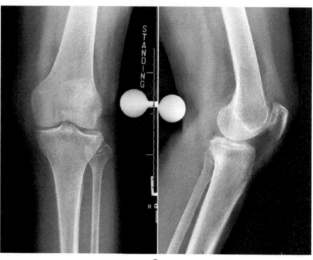

B

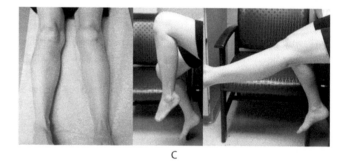

C

Figure 39.3 (a) Anteroposterior (AP) and lateral radiograph of 66-year-old woman who sustained a twisting injury to her left knee (note fracture line, white arrow). (b) Standing AP and lateral radiograph 8 weeks following injury. (c) Clinical photographs of the patient's limb alignment, knee flexion and knee extension. The patient had 6 weeks of protected weight bearing with a hinged knee orthotic; range of motion was unrestricted when not ambulating.

deformity or bicondylar fracture patterns with large initial displacements, surgery should be contemplated.[25] When surgery is chosen, some newer techniques may have particular advantages in patients with poor bone stock. These include percutaneous insertion techniques that are less damaging to the soft tissues and locking plate and screw constructs that provide improved fixation and in some cases avoid more damaging soft tissue approaches, including extensile and dual approaches. Additionally, calcium phosphate cement may maintain articular elevation to a greater extent than autogenous graft.[31] The use of external fixation with limited internal fixation may allow for control of coronal alignment, while at the same time minimizing surgical soft tissue dissections that can potentially lead to catastrophic complications.[32] Spanning external fixation may be used in selected difficult fracture problems as a definitive treatment with or without limited internal fixation.

In the following sections we will review surgical treatment techniques for specific tibial plateau fracture patterns in the elderly patient population.

Operative treatment

SPLIT DEPRESSION LATERAL PLATEAU FRACTURES

The most common tibial plateau fracture in the elderly population is the split depression lateral plateau fracture[3] (Figure 39.4). Given that continued displacement may lead to unacceptable valgus alignment in this fracture pattern, surgery may be considered. For purposes of preoperative planning a CT scan may help to precisely localize the depression. A CT scan also allows further characterization of the fracture lines, rotations and translations of fracture fragments.

The surgical approach utilized for reduction and internal fixation of a split depression lateral plateau fracture is the same as that utilized for patients with normal bone, however direct articular visualization through a submeniscal arthrotomy is less necessary in the elderly patient population. Indirect assessment of reduction through the use of fluoroscopy is preferred in our practice, particularly in elderly osteoporotic patients where the goal is not perfect articular congruity. Additional approaches including the use of a percutaneous plate and screw placement guide may be considered to minimize surgically induced soft tissue trauma (Figure 39.5).

The approach begins with an anterolateral surgical incision at or around Gerdy's tubercle and in line with the tibial shaft. Careful dissection should be made with consideration for subsequent wound closure and includes gentle skin and subcutaneous tissue retraction, clear identification of the underlying fascia and when possible fascial incisions made slightly off the anterior tibial crest so as to allow an appropriate layered closure. Articular impaction may be elevated with the use of surgical instruments such as a hemostat or bone tamp from below the depressed articular fragment(s); the articular surface during surgical elevation should be visualized with fluoroscopic imaging both in the AP and lateral views. Comparison views of the opposite knee are often helpful in assessing the reduction of the lateral joint. Elevation of a lateral split depression fracture, particularly in an elderly patient with poor bone

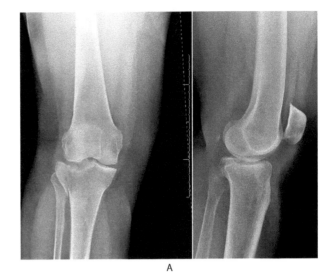

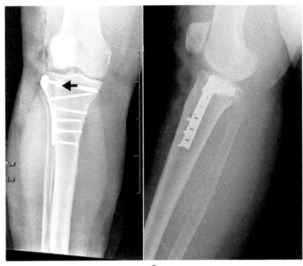

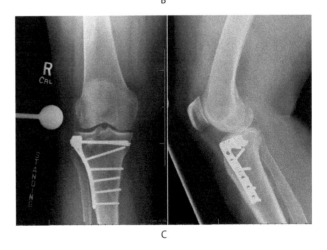

Figure 39.4 (a) Anteroposterior (AP) and lateral radiograph of an isolated lateral split depression fracture in a 72-year-old woman. (b) Postoperative AP and lateral radiograph of the knee (note the use of calcium phosphate bone void filler, black arrow). (c) AP and lateral standing radiograph 18 months postoperatively demonstrating maintenance of articular reduction. The patient was ambulating without pain.

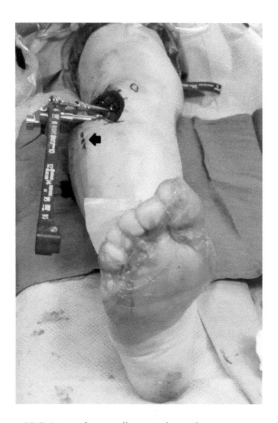

Figure 39.5 Note the small anterolateral incision, use of a percutaneous guide, and three distal incisions for percutaneous screw placement (solid black arrow). Targeting devices, as illustrated, may be used to decrease surgical soft tissue dissection.

stock, commonly leaves a void in the subchondral cancellous bone. A variety of bone void fillers may be utilized to backfill this void including calcium phosphate cement or allograft chips. The compressive strength of calcium phosphate cement and resistance to articular subsidence compare favourably to those of autograft.[31] These non-autogenous void fillers should be used in an attempt to decrease the surgical morbidity of harvesting autografts, such as from the iliac crest.

In general after reduction, osteoporotic split lateral depression tibial plateau fractures require buttress plate fixation as well as subchondral rafting screws for support. A variety of plate constructs are available, including pre-contoured proximal tibial plates with a variety of non-locking and locking screw options. No evidence currently exists for the use of locking screws in split depression plateau fractures. The plate functions to buttress the weak lateral wall and to restore lateral side stability through compression; this important function is facilitated with non-locking screws and is prevented with locking screws.[33]

BICONDYLAR OR METAPHYSEAL DIAPHYSEAL DISRUPTION FRACTURES

Bicondylar tibial plateau fractures represent a higher energy spectrum of injury. They are often seen in a younger patient population with normal bone stock. However, they do occur

in elderly patients with compromised bone stock and can lead to significant intra-articular comminution, fracture displacement and compromised soft tissues with small difficult to fix fracture fragments, all of which may contribute to more difficult management decisions.

Aggressive surgical treatment of these injuries may lead to more complications as compared to a similar treatment strategy in younger and healthier patients. While dual incision and medial, lateral and posterior plating techniques have increased in popularity for bicondylar tibial plateau fractures in a younger patient population,[34] in more elderly patients these choices should be made only after careful consideration of the soft tissue injury, the degree of osteopenia, the fracture pattern, and the comorbidities and functional demands of the patient (Figure 39.6). A poor clinical outcome with failing dual plates placed at 180 degrees in an elderly patient is a formidable reconstruction problem. In general, a secondary total knee replacement will require a staged surgical approach including hardware removal followed by total knee replacement weeks or months later (Figure 39.7).

Often slightly more conservative choices than dual plating are possible. When a predominantly medial tibial plateau fracture pattern is encountered and leads to significant shortening and displacement of the tibial shaft with respect to the distal femur, a medial approach with medial antiglide plating may be appropriate (Figure 39.8).

The surgical approach utilized is a longitudinal surgical incision in the interval posterior to the pes anserine tendons and anterior to the medial head of the gastrocnemius. This approach and plate position often has good soft tissue coverage even in the setting of soft tissue trauma.[35] Another possibility for predominately lateral patterns with a medical condyle fracture is to utilize lateral fixed angle plating only for these bicondylar tibial plateau fractures in elderly patients with poor bone stock. The lateral implant can be applied through a single anterior lateral surgical approach, often with the use of a percutaneous guide with limited soft tissue dissection (Figure 39.9). In these cases fixed angle locking screws are of great benefit to prevent varus from off axis bending forces. In this instance, priorities of surgical management should include restoring the overall mechanical alignment of the limb and supporting the subchondral surface. The ability to control the fracture with a lateral locking plate alone will depend on the characteristics of the medial plateau fracture. Coronal splits resulting in a separate posteromedial fragment and metaphyseal comminution are fracture characteristics that make lateral fixation only more difficult. Small degrees of subsequent varus collapse may be preferable to dual plating and dual incisions, given that functional demands are often less and secondary total knee arthroplasty if necessary would be much less complicated. When concerns persist over varus collapse, a medial external fixator may augment medial support and prevent subsequent varus deformity and be preferable to dual plates.

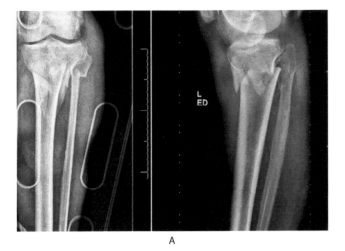

A

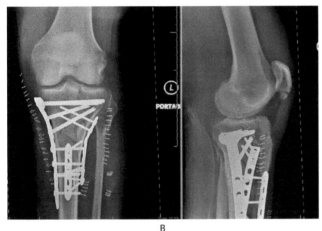

B

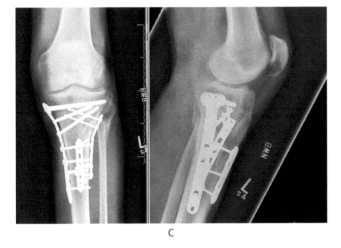

C

Figure 39.6 (a) Anteroposterior (AP) and lateral radiograph of an 81-year-old man who sustained a closed bicondylar tibial plateau fracture following a motor vehicle accident. (b) Postoperative AP and lateral radiographs following dual incision open reduction and internal fixation. (c) AP and lateral radiograph 8 months postoperatively demonstrating maintenance of limb alignment and articular reduction. The patient reported ambulating with only occasional pain in the left knee.

External fixation may be used as the definitive treatment for tibial plateau fractures[12,21]; however, clinical studies typically include all patients and do not specifically review those with osteoporosis. Ali et al. did however report that load to failure in an osteoporotic bicondylar tibial plateau was similar using either dual plating or external fixation techniques.[9] The advantages of external fixation include minimal soft tissue disruption, maintenance of mechanical alignment and the ability to separately place percutaneous screws for reduction of the articular surface.

A bicondylar tibial plateau fracture in patients with poor bone stock and significant comminution of the proximal tibia and articular surface may make definitive management with external fixation in the proximal tibia difficult. This is in part due to ongoing fracture instability despite external fixation pins and pins or wires traversing joint depressions that communicate with the joint. Generally pins or wires should be placed as far from the joint as possible and still obtain proximal fixation. Reports of septic arthritis from pin tract inoculation of the knee joint raise concern and allow only a subset of bicondylar patterns to be amenable to this technique.[21]

When there is a large zone of soft tissue injury, fracture displacement and difficult to fix osteopenic fragments in complex bicondylar tibial plateau fractures, joint spanning external fixation as definitive treatment may be an appropriate alternative (Figure 39.10). This technique avoids the zone of injury, is compatible with limited articular reduction, restores length and overall alignment and allows the patient to mobilize. The downside is that this technique will usually not completely restore proximal tibial anatomy and requires a period of joint immobility. Imperfect anatomy may be acceptable in some patients and the immobilization may be well tolerated in the majority of patients for as long as 6 weeks, and satisfactory restoration of knee mobility is the norm.[21] In an elderly patient some loss of knee mobility may be a satisfactory trade-off if complications are avoided in a very difficult fracture pattern.

RESULTS

Loss of reduction is always a concern after operative fracture treatment. In patients with tibial plateau fractures who have poor bone stock, some re-displacement of proximal tibia fractures is relatively common. A stereophotogrammetric analysis identified re-displacement on average of 2.8 mm in three out of five cases of operatively managed tibial plateau fractures that underwent elevation of depressed bone fragment, bone grafting, placement of cancellous bone screws.[36] Displacement after non-operative treatment is also common. While re-displacement after operative or non-operative management of tibial plateau fractures is a cause for concern and is relatively common in elderly patients, little correlation between radiographic displacement and ultimate functional outcome has been noted. Rasmussen[16] could find

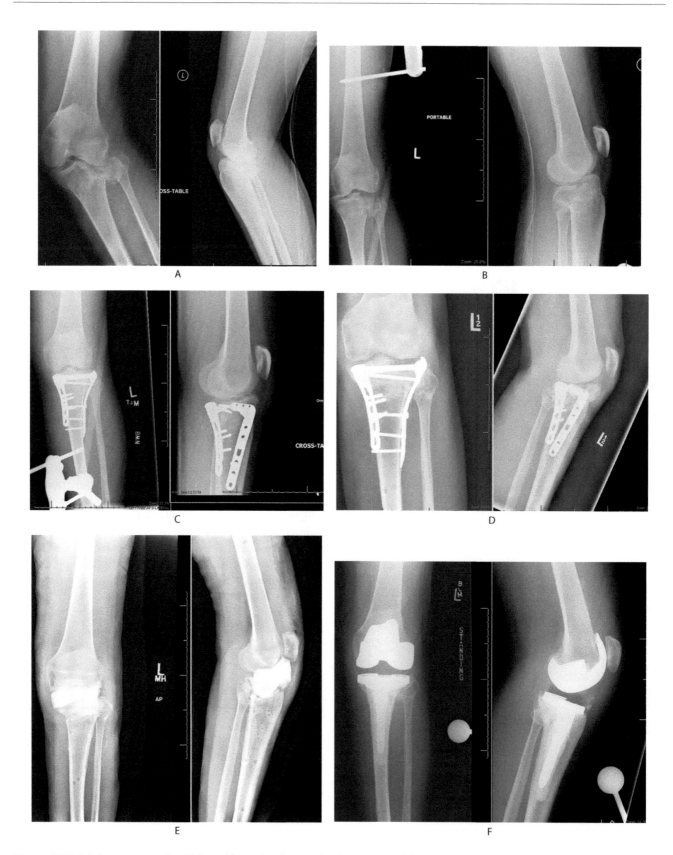

Figure 39.7 (a) Anteroposterior (AP) and lateral radiograph of a 69-year-old woman who fell from a ladder on to her left knee. (b) AP and lateral radiographs following placement of a spanning external fixator on the night of injury. (c) AP and lateral radiograph following internal fixation through dual incisions (note external fixator remained on for 4 weeks postoperatively). (d) AP and lateral radiograph at 6 months with draining lateral sinus and persistent pain with weight bearing. (e) AP and lateral radiograph after removal of hardware, debridement and placement of antibiotic cement spacer. (f) AP and lateral radiograph of knee following total knee arthroplasty 14 months after injury.

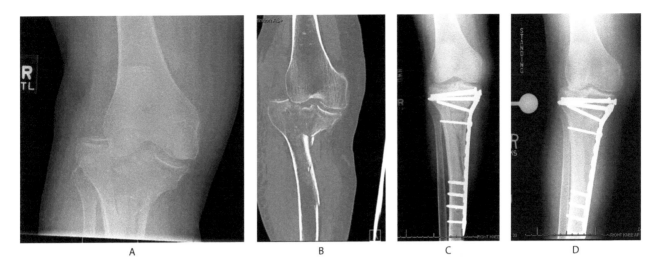

Figure 39.8 (a) Anteroposterior (AP) radiograph of an 82-year-old woman with a medial tibial plateau fracture dislocation. Note the significant osteoporosis and shortening of the proximal tibia shaft. (b) Coronal CT scan demonstrating the intact lateral cortical surface and significant medial-sided comminution and displacement. (c) AP radiograph at 1 month and (d) standing AP radiograph at 1-year follow-up visit. Despite some settling of the lateral joint surface, the patient was ambulating pain free at pre-injury baseline.

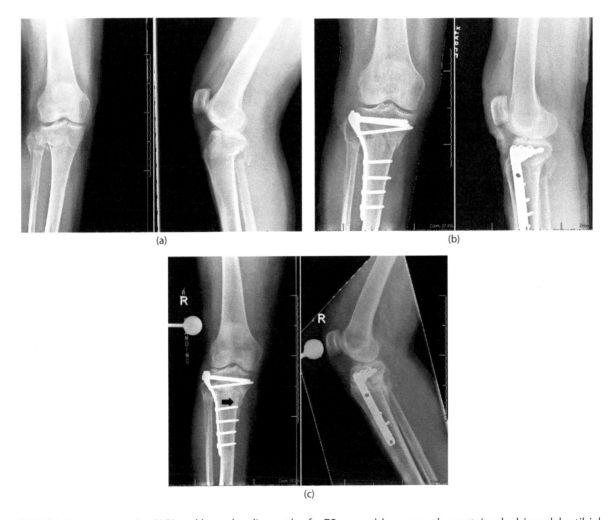

Figure 39.9 (a) Anteroposterior (AP) and lateral radiograph of a 70-year-old woman who sustained a bicondylar tibial plateau fracture after a fall from standing height. (b) AP and lateral radiograph after operative management consisting of limited incision and lateral only internal fixation. (c) AP and lateral standing radiograph; note some subsidence with bridging medial callous (black arrow) and slight shift to varus alignment, which is an acceptable result to avoid dual plating.

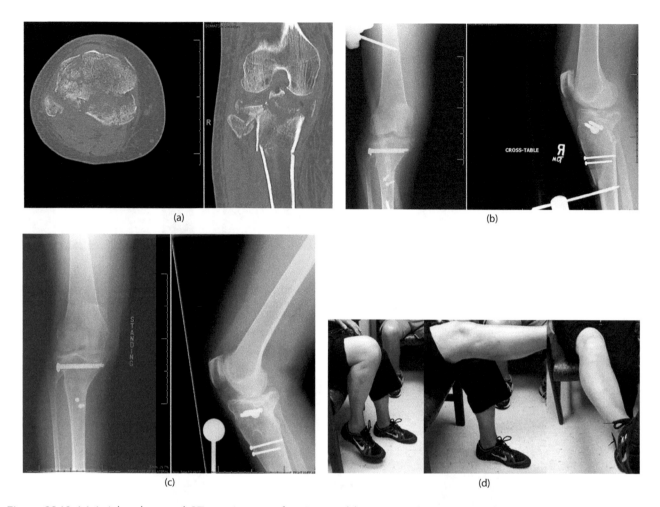

Figure 39.10 **(a)** Axial and coronal CT scan images of a 72-year-old woman with a comminuted bicondylar tibial plateau fracture associated with a significant closed soft tissue injury. **(b)** AP and lateral radiograph 8 weeks postoperatively of the knee treated with limited internal fixation and definitive knee spanning external fixation. **(c)** AP and lateral standing radiograph 3 years after injury. **(d)** Clinical photos of the patient's knee flexion and extension. The patient ambulates several miles daily with minimal discomfort. This case illustrates that acceptable results are possible with less invasive techniques without perfect anatomic restoration of the plateau.

no correlation between radiographic measurements and function. Additionally, Honkonen was unable to correlate the amount of articular step-off with function.[5] Angular malalignment however does appear to correlate with long-term results. Lansinger et al. in their 20-year follow-up noted a 90% rate of good to excellent outcomes in patients with less than 10-degree knee instability in full extension.[19] This data is particularly important when considering patients with poor bone stock who more commonly have late displacement in both operative and nonoperative settings.

There are few studies that specifically focus on proximal tibia fractures in an osteoporotic or elderly patient population. Biyani et al. noted that there was no correlation between the appearance of knee radiographs and clinical outcome in a group of patients who underwent surgical management and were over 65 years of age.[3] They noted good to excellent results in 23 out of 32 patients who underwent formal open reduction and internal fixation. Importantly these patients also had no serious complications. Multiple studies have included elderly patients treated with either operative or non-operative

management in clinical series and have either demonstrated no difference or worse clinical outcomes as compared to the remainder of a younger patient cohort.[18,30,37]

Total knee replacement following tibial plateau fracture is relatively uncommon and serves as an indicator that profound loss of knee function is rare after most tibial plateau fractures.[18,29,38] A recent study of 8,426 patients who had undergone fixation of a tibial plateau fracture and a matched control population demonstrated a rate of total knee replacement of 7.3% at 10 years, representing a 5.3-fold increased likelihood compared with controls.[37] When total knee replacement is utilized following failed management of tibial plateau fracture, improvements in pain and function are usually achieved but the rate of perioperative complications remains high (21%).[29]

Given these reports it is clear that a direct correlation between radiographic appearances and functional outcome cannot be made in patients with underlying osteoporosis. Consequently, when patients who are elderly or osteoporotic sustain a tibial plateau fracture, decision-making should be guided by treatment that considers comorbidities and functional demands and emphasizes minimizing complications and maintaining limb alignment.

CONCLUSION

In conclusion, osteoporosis and osteopenia complicate nearly one-third of tibial plateau fractures. The most common fracture pattern encountered in these patients is a split lateral depression fracture, but severe and difficult to manage bicondylar patterns also occur.

The tibial plateau fracture, unlike other major osteoporotic fractures of the lower extremity (hip and distal femur), may be treated with non-operative techniques. Non-operative treatment may lead to an acceptable functional result, while minimizing risks associated with surgical management. Operative treatment follows techniques recommended in patients with normal bone stock but should emphasize more limited approaches while focusing on limb alignment rather than perfect articular reduction. Locking plates, limited surgical approaches, calcium phosphate cement and select use of spanning external fixation are all useful tools in tibial plateau fractures in patients with osteoporosis. The surgeon should be aware that re-displacement or continued displacement of fractures beyond the initial radiograph occurs more commonly in osteoporotic or osteopenic patients than in patients with similar patterns but with normal bone stock.

REFERENCES

1. Foltin E. Osteoporosis and fracture patterns. A study of split-compression fractures of the lateral tibial condyle. *Int Orthop* 1988;12(4):299–303.
2. McKinley TO, Rudert MJ, Koos DC, Brown TD. Incongruity versus instability in the etiology of posttraumatic arthritis. *Clin Orthop Relat Res* 2004;(423):44–51.
3. Biyani A, Reddy NS, Chaudhury J, Simison AJ, Klenerman L. The results of surgical management of displaced tibial plateau fractures in the elderly. *Injury* 1995;26(5):291–7.
4. Rasmussen PS, Sorensen SE. Tibial condylar fractures—Non-operative treatment of lateral compression fractures without impairment of knee-joint stability. *Injury* 1973;4(3):265–71.
5. Honkonen SE. Indications for surgical treatment of tibial condyle fractures. *Clin Orthop Relat Res* 1994;(302):199–205.
6. Schatzker J, McBroom R, Bruce D. The tibial plateau fracture. The Toronto experience 1968–1975. *Clin Orthop Relat Res* 1979;(138):94–104.
7. Marsh JL, Slongo TF, Agel J, Broderick JS, Creevey W, DeCoster TA, et al. Fracture and dislocation classification compendium—2007: Orthopaedic Trauma Association classification, database

and outcomes committee. *J Orthop Trauma* 2007;21(10 Suppl):S1–133.
8. Krappinger D, Struve P, Smekal V, Huber B. Severely comminuted bicondylar tibial plateau fractures in geriatric patients: A report of 2 cases treated with open reduction and postoperative external fixation. *J Orthop Trauma* 2008;22(9):652–7.
9. Ali AM, Saleh M, Eastell R, Wigderowitz CA, Rigby AS, Yang L. Influence of bone quality on the strength of internal and external fixation of tibial plateau fractures. *J Orthop Res* 2006;24(11):2080–6.
10. Ali AM, Burton M, Hashmi M, Saleh M. Treatment of displaced bicondylar tibial plateau fractures (OTA-41C2&3) in patients older than 60 years of age. *J Orthop Trauma* 2003;17(5):346–52.
11. Barei DP, Nork SE, Mills WJ, Henley MB, Benirschke SK. Complications associated with internal fixation of high-energy bicondylar tibial plateau fractures utilizing a two-incision technique. *J Orthop Trauma* 2004;18(10):649–57.
12. Canadian Orthopaedic Trauma Society. Open reduction and internal fixation compared with circular fixator application for bicondylar tibial plateau fractures. Results of a multicenter, prospective, randomized clinical trial. *J Bone Joint Surg Am* 2006;88(12):2613–23.
13. Levy BA, Zlowodzki MP, Graves M, Cole PA. Screening for extremity arterial injury with the arterial pressure index. *Am J Emerg Med* 2005;23(5):689–95.
14. Gardner MJ, Yacoubian S, Geller D, Suk M, Mintz D, Potter H, et al. The incidence of soft tissue injury in operative tibial plateau fractures: A magnetic resonance imaging analysis of 103 patients. *J Orthop Trauma* 2005;19(2):79–84.
15. Delamarter RB, Hohl M, Hopp E Jr. Ligament injuries associated with tibial plateau fractures. *Clin Orthop Relat Res* 1990;(250):226–33.
16. Rasmussen PS. Tibial condylar fractures. Impairment of knee-joint stability as an indication for surgical treatment. *J Bone Joint Surg Am* 1973;55(7):1331–50.
17. Katsenis D, Athanasiou V, Megas P, Tyllianakis M, Lambiris E. Minimal internal fixation augmented by small wire transfixion frames for high-energy tibial plateau fractures. *J Orthop Trauma* 2005;19(4):241–8.
18. Keating JF. Tibial plateau fractures in the older patient. *Bulletin* 1999;58(1):19–23.
19. Lansinger O, Bergman B, Korner L, Andersson GBJ. Tibial condylar fractures—A 20-year follow-up. *J Bone Joint Surg Am* 1986;68A(1):13–19.
20. Schwartsman R, Brinker MR, Beaver R, Cox DD. Patient self-assessment of tibial plateau fractures in 40 older adults. *Am J Orthop* 1998;27(7):512–19.

21. Marsh JL, Smith ST, Do TT. External fixation and limited internal fixation for complex fractures of the tibial plateau. *J Bone Joint Surg Am* 1995;77(5):661–73.

22. Burri C, Bartzke G, Coldewey J, Muggler E. Fractures of the tibial plateau. *Clin Orthop Relat Res* 1979;(138):84–93.

23. Gausewitz S, Hohl M. The significance of early motion in the treatment of tibial plateau fractures. *Clin Orthop Relat Res* 1986;(202):135–8.

24. Gaston P, Will EM, Keating JF. Recovery of knee function following fracture of the tibial plateau. *J Bone Joint Surg Br* 2005;87(9):1233–6.

25. DeCoster TA, Nepola JV, el-Khoury GY. Cast brace treatment of proximal tibia fractures. A ten-year follow-up study. *Clin Orthop Relat Res* 1988;(231):196–204.

26. Ruffolo MR, Gettys FK, Montijo HE, Seymour RB, Karunakar MA. Complications of high-energy bicondylar tibial plateau fractures treated with dual plating through 2 incisions. *J Orthop Trauma* 2015;29(2):85–90.

27. Segal D, Mallik AR, Wetzler MJ, Franchi AV, Whitelaw GP. Early weight bearing of lateral tibial plateau fractures. *Clin Orthop Relat Res* 1993;(294):232–7.

28. Apley AG. Fractures of the lateral tibial condyle treated by skeletal traction and early mobilisation; a review of sixty cases with special reference to the long-term results. *J Bone Joint Surg Br* 1956;38-B(3):699–708.

29. Weiss NG, Parvizi J, Trousdale RT, Bryce RD, Lewallen DG. Total knee arthroplasty in patients with a prior fracture of the tibial plateau. *J Bone Joint Surg Am* 2003;85-A(2):218–21.

30. Rademakers MV, Kerkhoffs GM, Sierevelt IN, Raaymakers EL, Marti RK. Operative treatment of 109 tibial plateau fractures: Five- to 27-year follow-up results. *J Orthop Trauma* 2007;21(1):5–10.

31. Russell TA, Leighton RK, Alpha-BSM Tibial Plateau Fracture Study Group. Comparison of autogenous bone graft and endothermic calcium phosphate cement for defect augmentation in tibial plateau fractures. *J Bone Joint Surg Am* 2008;90A(10):2057–61.

32. Hall JA, Beuerlein MJ, McKee MD, Canadian Orthopaedic Trauma Society. Open reduction and internal fixation compared with circular fixator application for bicondylar tibial plateau fractures. Surgical technique. *J Bone Joint Surg Am* 2009;91(Suppl 2 Pt 1):74–88.

33. Anglen J, Kyle RF, Marsh JL, Virkus WW, Watters WC 3rd, Keith MW, et al. Locking plates for extremity fractures. *J Am Acad Orthop Surg* 2009;17(7):465–72.

34. Barei DP, Nork SE, Mills WJ, Coles CP, Henley MB, Benirschke SK. Functional outcomes of severe bicondylar tibial plateau fractures treated with dual incisions and medial and lateral plates. *J Bone Joint Surg Am* 2006;88(8):1713–21.

35. Georgiadis GM. Combined anterior and posterior approaches for complex tibial plateau fractures. *J Bone Joint Surg Br* 1994;76(2):285–9.

36. Ryd L, Toksvig-Larsen S. Stability of the elevated fragment in tibial plateau fractures. A radiographic stereophotogrammetric study of postoperative healing. *Int Orthop* 1994;18(3):131–4.

37. Wasserstein D, Henry P, Paterson JM, Kreder HJ, Jenkinson R. Risk of total knee arthroplasty after operatively treated tibial plateau fracture: A matched-population-based cohort study. *J Bone Joint Surg Am* 2014;96(2):144–50.

38. Mehin R, O'Brien P, Broekhuyse H, Blachut P, Guy P. Endstage arthritis following tibia plateau fractures: Average 10-year follow-up. *Can J Surg* 2012;55(2):87–94.

40

Tibia and fibula diaphyseal fractures

LEELA C. BIANT AND CHARLES M. COURT-BROWN

INTRODUCTION

Many fractures are increasing in incidence because of an expanding population and a higher proportion of elderly people in the population. This, however, is not true of fractures of the tibia and fibula. In 2000 Court-Brown and Caesar[1] recorded that tibial diaphyseal fractures accounted for 1.9% of all adult fractures in a defined population in the United Kingdom. However, between 2010 and 2011 tibial fractures only accounted for 1% of fractures in the same population.[2]

The relatively rapid decline in the prevalence of tibial fractures together with an increased interest in fragility fractures, such as those of the proximal femur, proximal humerus and distal radius, has meant that the literature dealing with tibial fractures in the elderly is somewhat deficient. There are virtually no papers discussing the management of tibial fractures in the elderly, and to allow us to write this chapter we have used data from three databases constructed over a 13–15-year period in Edinburgh, Scotland. The first is a consecutive series of 187 tibial fractures, in patients aged ≥65 years, collected over a 13-year period. This database has been used to establish the type of fracture presenting to surgeons and their reasons for the choice of treatment method. The second database was one of 233 patients used by Clement et al.[3] to identify the complications of tibial fractures in the elderly and the reasons for their occurrence, and the third database consisted of 484 consecutive open fractures in the elderly, collected over a 15-year period,[4] from which we were able to study the characteristics of open tibial fractures in the elderly. During this 15-year period there were 48 open tibial fractures in patients ≥65 years of age.

Tibial fractures have always interested orthopaedic surgeons. The older arguments promoting non-operative management have largely disappeared[5] and most surgeons now use surgical management, usually intramedullary nailing.[6,7] The high prevalence of open fractures and high energy fractures in the elderly means that treatment can be difficult and there is a relatively high complication rate. In this chapter we will analyse the epidemiology of tibial fractures in the elderly aged ≥65 years and the super-elderly aged ≥80 years. We will also analyse why surgeons choose particular treatment methods and how successful these methods are. In addition we will also present a brief section on fibular fractures in the elderly that are not associated with proximal tibial or ankle fractures.

EPIDEMIOLOGY

There is no doubt that fragility fractures such as proximal humeral fractures and distal radial fractures are increasing in incidence in elderly patients,[2] but fractures of the tibial diaphysis are decreasing in incidence. A review of the tibial diaphyseal fractures treated in the Royal Infirmary of Edinburgh in 1991 showed that the incidence was $24.4/10^5$/year. This fell to $13.5/10^5$/year in 2010/2011. The incidence in males fell from $37.2/10^5$/year to $20.1/10^5$/year and in females it fell from $13.5/10^5$/year to $7.3/10^5$/year.[2] This is shown in Figure 40.1.

One might expect the incidence in younger patients to fall because of improved industrial and workplace safety legislation and drink driving laws. However, a review of the incidence of tibial diaphyseal fractures in the ≥65-year-old group and ≥80-year-old group shows that the overall incidence of tibial diaphyseal fractures has declined. This is mainly seen in women (Figure 40.1). Figure 40.1 shows that the incidence in males is essentially unchanged, but this is not the case in women. In 1991 the incidence in ≥65-year-old women was 56.1/10⁵/year. This declined to 27.5/10⁵/year in 2000 and to 6/10⁵/year in 2010/2011.[2] The equivalent figures for the ≥80-year-old population were 97.9/10⁵/year, 47.4/10⁵/year and 13.5/10⁵/year. In ≥80-year-old men there were no fractures in 1991 and the incidences in 2000 and 2010/2011 were very similar at 13.7/10⁵/year and 10.5/10⁵/year.[2]

The question arises as to why tibial diaphyseal fractures in the elderly are declining in incidence. Chapter 1 (Table 1.6) shows that tibial diaphyseal fractures in the elderly are usually caused by a standing fall or are high energy injuries caused by road traffic accidents. It shows that more tibial diaphyseal fractures are caused by high energy injuries than any other fracture in the elderly. This does not appear to have changed in the last 20 years. Analysis of tibial diaphyseal fractures in the elderly in 1991 shows that 34.5% were caused by road traffic accidents and that 90% of these were in pedestrians. A further 58.6% were caused by falls, which is similar to the 68.8% seen in 2010/2011.[2] It would seem that while the incidence of tibial diaphyseal fractures in the elderly has reduced considerably, particularly in women,

the prevalence of the two main causes of fractures has not changed very much. One might postulate that improved road safety measures have caused fewer elderly women to be struck by cars, but there would seem to be no good reason for the decline in fall related fractures when this is not the case in other fractures.

However, increased frailty is obviously a factor as fracture incidence is greater in ≥80-year-old women than in ≥65-year-old women (Chapter 1 and Table 1.5). It should be remembered that tibial diaphyseal fractures are not fragility fractures[1] and if an elderly person falls he or she is more likely to sustain a proximal femoral, proximal humeral or distal radial fracture. It may be that the falls that cause tibial diaphyseal fractures are somewhat different. There may be more energy involved in these falls, but we think it likely that the fall often involves a rotational force on the tibial diaphysis which causes the spiral fractures that are commonly seen in the elderly.

Open fractures

Open tibial fractures are very common in the elderly. Table 1.6 in Chapter 1 shows that in a recent 2-year study period 43.8% of the fractures in the ≥65-year-old group were open. One might expect that the open fractures would be caused by high energy injuries, but 36.4% of the fall related fractures were open, highlighting the problems associated with the poor quality soft tissues in the elderly and the subcutaneous location of the tibia. Tables 1.7 and 1.8 in Chapter 1 also show that the problems related to poor soft tissues are more common in women. In the 15-year analysis of open fractures, 48.6% of open tibial fractures in women aged ≥65 years were Gustilo[8,9] type III in severity. Women aged ≥80 years had a similar prevalence of Gustilo type III fractures, but in men aged ≥65 years the prevalence of Gustilo type III fractures was only 7.7% and there were no Gustilo type III fractures in men aged ≥80 years. This suggests increasing male frailty, as presumably men ≥80 years of age are less active than women.

Tables 1.7 and 1.8 in Chapter 1 give the combined incidences of open fractures of the tibia and fibula, expressed as x/10⁶/year, but analysis shows that of the 48 open fractures of the tibia and fibula treated in the 15-year period, 46 were open tibial fractures and two were isolated open fibular fractures.[4] This indicates an incidence of open tibial fractures of 3.1/10⁵/year in ≥65-year-old patients and 4.4/10⁵/year in ≥80-year-old patients. The equivalent figures for open fibular fractures are 0.1/10⁶/year and 0.2/10⁶/year, confirming their rarity.

Of the 48 patients who presented with an open tibial or fibular fracture, 25 (52.1%) were isolated injuries. In the remaining 23 (47.9%) patients the average Injury Severity Score (ISS) was 18 and altogether 8 (16.7%) had an ISS ≥16. All of these patients were pedestrians struck by a motor vehicle. Open fractures are discussed in Chapter 13.

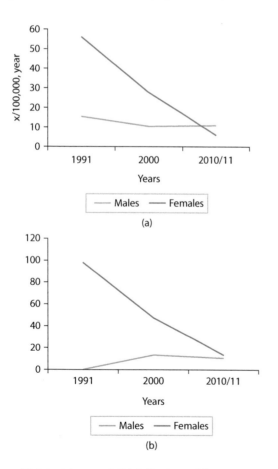

Figure 40.1 Incidence of tibial diaphyseal fractures over a 20-year period in patients aged ≥65 years **(a)** and ≥80 years **(b)**.

Insufficiency fractures

Insufficiency fractures occur as a result of repetitive normal loading on abnormal bone that has decreased resistance. Obviously all osteopenic and osteoporotic fractures can be considered to be insufficiency fractures, but these fractures usually require a defined injury mechanism, this commonly being a fall. In a number of fractures in the elderly there is no causative mechanism and we have referred to these as insufficiency fractures. An analysis of the 187 consecutive elderly tibial fractures in patients ≥65 years of age showed that eight (4.3%) were insufficiency fractures. All of these fractures occurred in women and the average age was 72.5 years. The incidence of tibial insufficiency fractures in ≥65-year-old women was $1.1/10^5$/year and in ≥80-year-old women it was $0.4/10^5$/year. An example of a tibial insufficiency fracture is shown in Figure 40.2.

By far the most common site of insufficiency fractures in elderly patients is the thoracolumbar spine and studies have shown that 25–30% of post-menopausal women have insufficiency fractures.[10,11] A study from France showed that pelvic and sacral insufficiency fractures are relatively common.[12] The investigators also found that insufficiency fractures occurred in the tibia (Figure 40.2), femoral head, femoral neck and femoral diaphysis. A review of the location of the fractures in the tibia showed that the majority were transverse distal diaphyseal fractures, but the authors also reported a tibial plateau fracture, a proximal tibial diaphyseal fracture (Figure 40.2) and four longitudinal insufficiency fractures. A recent case report has shown that, like femoral insufficiency fractures, tibial insufficiency fractures can follow the use of bisphosphonate therapy.[13]

Metastatic fractures

Metastatic fractures of the tibia in the elderly population are rare and only two (1.1%) occurred in the 13-year study, giving an overall incidence of about $0.2/10^5$/year in the ≥65-year-old group. One was caused by a metastasis from an adenocarcinoma and the other by a metastasis from a malignant melanoma. Metastatic fractures are discussed in detail in Chapter 16.

Periprosthetic fractures

In the study of 187 patients aged ≥65 years there were three periprosthetic tibial fractures (Figure 40.3) with an average age of 69.7 years. This indicates that the incidence of periprosthetic tibial fractures is about $0.2/10^5$/year. The rarity of tibial periprosthetic fractures means that there is very little information about them in the literature. In a series of 102 fractures from the Mayo Clinic[14] it was estimated that 0.4% of the knee arthroplasties undertaken in a 25-year period in the Mayo Clinic developed a periprosthetic tibial fracture. Periprosthetic fractures are discussed in Chapter 17.

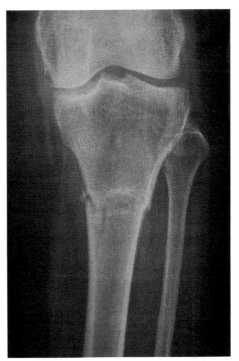
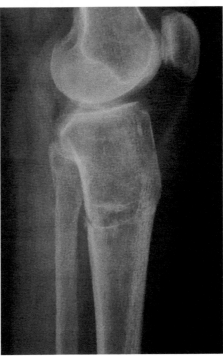

Figure 40.2 A proximal tibial diaphyseal insufficiency fracture.

CLASSIFICATION

The classification system most commonly used for tibial diaphyseal fractures is the AO/OTA[15] system. The basic fracture types delineated by this classification system are shown in Figure 40.4. Type A fractures are simple fractures with A1 fractures being spiral fractures, A2 fractures being oblique fractures with an angle ≥30 degrees and

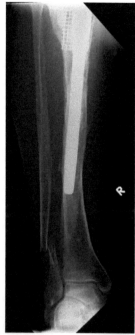

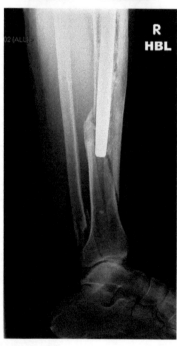

Figure 40.3 A periprosthetic tibial diaphyseal fracture after a knee arthroplasty.

A3 fractures being oblique fractures with an angle of <30 degrees. Type B fractures are wedge fractures with B1 fractures having a spiral wedge, B2 fractures a bending wedge and B3 fractures a fragmented wedge. Type C fractures are complex fractures with C1 fractures having a spiral morphology. C2 fractures are segmental fractures and C3 fractures are irregular, comminuted fractures. The suffix .X is used to define an associated fibular fracture in type A and B fractures. Thus .1 means that the fibula is intact, .2 means that the fibular fracture is not at the same level as the tibial fracture and .3 means that it is at the same level. In type C

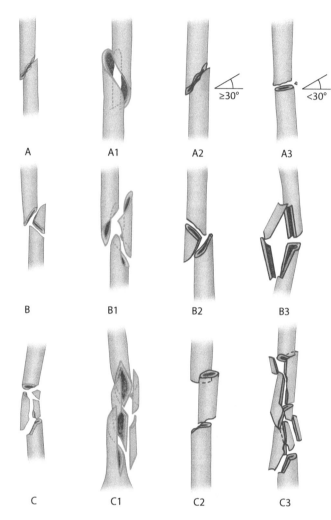

Figure 40.4 The AO/OTA classification of tibial diaphyseal fractures. (Redrawn from *J Orthop Trauma* 1996;10(Suppl):1–154.)

fractures the suffixes .1, .2, and .3 detail the amount of damage to the diaphysis.

FRACTURE MORPHOLOGY

Analysis of the fracture morphology in the ≥65-year-old group shows that 64.4% were AO/OTA[15] type A fractures, 15.6% were type B and 20% were type C fractures. The equivalent figures in the ≥80-year-old group were 58.8%, 11.8% and 29.4%. With increased aging and increased frailty the prevalence of more severe fractures increases. However, further analysis shows that 53.3% of tibial fractures have an A1 or B1 morphology and that 91.7% of these fractures followed a fall. This strongly suggests a rotational component to the force that causes a fall related tibial diaphyseal fracture.

TREATMENT

As with all tibial diaphyseal fractures, the treatment methods most commonly used by the majority of surgeons treating the elderly are non-operative management, intramedullary nailing, external fixation and plating. Occasionally a primary amputation may be undertaken.

In recent years most surgeons have moved from non-operative management of tibial diaphyseal fractures to operative treatment with intramedullary nailing being the preferred method for closed fractures[6] and most open fractures.[7] Plating has become less popular, particularly in the elderly, as in the past plates were associated with relatively high rates of implant failure, non-union and infection. Recently monoaxial and polyaxial locking plates have been introduced and many surgeons are now using minimally invasive plating techniques to try to minimize these complications. As yet there is no information about how useful monoaxial or polyaxial locking plating techniques are in elderly patients with tibial diaphyseal fractures.

To try to determine the reason for undertaking a particular treatment method in the elderly, we analysed the reasons for selection of the different treatment methods used in the 187 patients that have already been detailed. We found that 64.7% of the patients were treated with intramedullary nailing, 20.3% were treated non-operatively, 12.8% were treated with external fixation and 1.1% had a primary amputation. One patient (0.5%) was treated with a dynamic compression plate and one patient died prior to treatment.

Intramedullary nailing

Over the past 20–25 years intramedullary nailing has become the standard method of treating closed tibial fractures and most open fractures in adults.[5–7] The results are better than achieved with other methods of treatment. We believe that it is the preferred technique for treating tibial diaphyseal fractures in the elderly. It is a relatively simple treatment that allows the patients to mobilize fully weight bearing, as they are able to do so. Clearly in elderly patients, it is very important to facilitate mobilization by allowing patients to weight bear as soon as possible.

The technique of intramedullary tibial nailing, using a locked nail, is well documented. Nailing can be undertaken on a nailing table or freehand on a standard surgical table. It is, however, vital to reduce the fracture and the use of a nailing table facilitates this. Most surgeons use a longitudinal incision over the patellar tendon and either go through the tendon or retract the tendon. An anterior hole is made in the proximal tibia about half way between the tibial tuberosity and the knee joint. A blunt reamer is passed through the proximal metaphysis and a guidewire is then passed over the fracture site so that it is in the middle of the distal tibia on anteroposterior and lateral fluoroscopic views. Failure to place the guidewire in the middle of the distal tibia increases the risk of fracture malposition, particularly in distal tibial diaphyseal or metaphyseal fractures.

The tibia is then reamed to allow the passage of an intramedullary nail. In older patients the intramedullary canal is wider than in younger patients and an 11–13 mm nail is often required. The intramedullary canal should be reamed to 1–2 mm more than the proposed nail diameter. The length of the nail is assessed. The nail is inserted taking care to ensure that the fracture is reduced. Appropriate locking screws are then inserted. It should be remembered that many tibial diaphyseal fractures in the elderly are distal or proximal in location and have a spiral morphology and static locking will often be required. An example of a distal tibial diaphyseal fracture treated with an intramedullary nail is shown in Figure 40.5.

Postoperative mobilization and weight bearing should be encouraged. Clearly this will depend on the general health of the patient and whether they have any significant

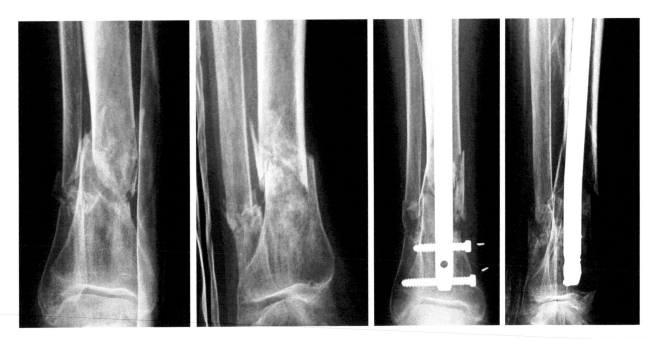

Figure 40.5 Intramedullary nailing of a tibial diaphyseal fracture in a 76-year-old woman.

comorbidities. The other relevant fact is that a proportion of patients will have other fractures which may preclude the use of crutches or other walking aids. In fall related fractures a number of the co-existing fractures will be in the upper limbs making the use of walking aids difficult.

There is little information about the success of tibial intramedullary nailing in the elderly. However Clement et al.[3] reviewed 233 elderly tibial fractures and they noted that in the fractures treated with intramedullary nailing there was a 7.3% non-union rate, together with a 5.7% malunion rate and a 4.9% deep infection rate. There was also a 1.6% amputation rate (Table 40.1). This study also showed that there was a 16% mortality rate at 120 days and a 22% mortality rate at 1 year in elderly patients treated with intramedullary nailing.

Non-operative management

While we believe that intramedullary nailing is the preferred method for treating tibial fractures in the elderly, we accept that other methods will need to be used. Whichever method is used should ideally facilitate postoperative mobilization and non-operative management should only be used if there are good reasons to avoid surgery. Table 40.2 shows the reasons why non-operative management was preferred in 38 (20.3%) elderly patients during the 13-year study period. The most common reason was that the

fractures were undisplaced or very minimally displaced and the surgeon was prepared to allow the patient to weight bear postoperatively. A similar number of patients were non-ambulant prior to the fracture. The majority of these patients had dementia, but others had other comorbidities such as rheumatoid arthritis or multiple sclerosis. A further 15.8% of the patients presented with an insufficiency fracture and 11.6% were considered to be unfit for surgery. One (2.6%) patient had a tibial deformity secondary to a previous fracture that prevented intramedullary nailing.

Clement et al.[3] showed that the use of non-operative management in the elderly was associated with a 26.4% malunion rate, but there were no non-unions or infections (Table 40.1). The 120-day mortality was 12% with a 36% mortality at 1 year. Presumably the absence of a non-union relates to the high prevalence of undisplaced and insufficiency fractures and the high mortality related to the age of the cohort and the fact that many patients had significant severe comorbidities prior to the fracture.

External fixation

External fixation is in widespread use for the management of high energy severe open fractures in younger patients, but there is little information about its use in elderly patients. Its use needs to be considered with care because the elderly patient will not be able to weight bear postoperatively and

Table 40.1 The prevalence of complications in elderly patients

	Nonunion (%)	Malunion (%)	Infection (%)	Amputation (%)
Overall	9.9	17.1	6.9	3.0
Age				
≥65 years	12.2	17.2	9.3	2.9
≥80 years	6.4	17.0	3.2	3.2
Gender				
Male	9.5	14.3	12.7	3.2
Female	10.0	18.2	4.7	2.9
Fracture type				
AO type A	3.2	12.2	2.4	0.8
AO type B	17.2	25.9	6.9	5.2
AO type C	17.3	19.2	17.3	5.8
Closed	5.5	17.1	3.0	0
Open	20.3	17.4	15.9	10.1
Treatment				
IM nail	7.3	5.7	4.9	1.6
Cast	0	26.4	0	1.6
Ex fix	13.8	37.9	10.3	0

Source: From Clement ND, et al. *Bone Joint J* 2013;95-B:1255–62.
Note: Ex fix, external fixation; IM, intramedullary.

Table 40.2 The reasons why non-operative management or external fixation was chosen to treat tibial diaphyseal fractures in the elderly

Treatment method			
Non-operative		External fixation	
Undisplaced or minimally displaced fracture	36.8%	Proximal fracture extension	25.0%
Non-ambulant patient	34.2%	Damage control/ severe open fracture	25.0%
Insufficiency fracture	15.8%	Distal fracture extension	20.8%
Not fit for surgery	11.5%	Knee arthroplasty	12.5%
Tibial deformity	2.7%	Infected skin	8.3%
		Narrow intramedullary canal	4.2%

external fixation requires considerable postoperative nursing and medical care which may interfere with the elderly patient being able to return to his or her domicile.

Table 40.2 shows that 45.8% of fractures in which external fixation was used were either very proximal or distal. It has already been pointed out that more than 50% of tibial diaphyseal fractures in the elderly have a spiral configuration and the surgeons favoured external fixation because the spiral fracture was too proximal or distal to permit straightforward intramedullary nailing. The other main reason for the use of external fixation was if the open fracture was very severe or the patient was badly injured and the surgeon wished to practice damage control surgery. Three patients (12.5%) had knee arthroplasties and two (8.3%) had significant skin sepsis on presentation. One (4.2%) patient had a very narrow intramedullary canal.

Clement et al.[3] showed that external fixation was associated with a 14% non-union rate, a 38% malunion rate and a 10% deep infection rate in elderly patients (Table 40.1). All of these parameters are higher than those associated with intramedullary nailing, but analysis shows that 37.5% of the fractures treated with external fixation were open fractures, compared with 14% of fractures treated with intramedullary nailing. The 120-day mortality for externally fixed tibial fractures in the elderly was 17% and the 1-year mortality was 20%.

Plating

Plating was formerly a very popular method of treating tibial diaphyseal fractures in younger patients but it was associated with relatively high non-union and infection rates and it was largely replaced by intramedullary nailing in the 1980s and 1990s. However, the recent introduction of monoaxial and polyaxial locked plates and percutaneous, or minimally invasive, surgery has rekindled an interest in tibial plating, particularly in the distal tibia where it is perceived that fracture alignment is more difficult to achieve with an intramedullary nail. There is no data relating to the use of diaphyseal plates in the elderly, but there are circumstances when a plate might be used, and in the cohort of 187 patients a dynamic compression plate was used to stabilize a distal diaphyseal periprosthetic fracture. There are other circumstances when plating might be used in the tibial diaphysis and an example

is shown in Figure 40.6 where a previous tibial fracture had been treated non-operatively and the resulting non-union prevented nailing. A locking plate was used.

The rationale behind percutaneous plating of the distal tibia is that there is less damage to the soft tissues and therefore improved vascularity, bone union and patient function. Locking plates were designed for improved fixation in osteoporotic bone, but there has been no evidence that they are more effective than older plates in the proximal humerus,[16] distal femur[17] and ankle.[18]

There have been a number of studies comparing plating and nailing of distal tibial fractures. The fractures that have been studied are predominantly distal diaphyseal fractures, rather than metaphyseal fractures. Guo et al.[19] found that patients treated with nails had more pain, but better function, alignment and foot and ankle scores than patients treated with a locking plate. Overall they advocated the use of intramedullary nailing.

Vallier et al.[20] compared nailing and plating in a study that was mainly of high energy injuries in younger patients. They found similar results, but that intramedullary nailing was associated with a higher rate of malalignment than plates. Xue et al.[21] undertook a meta-analysis comparing intramedullary nailing and plating and showed that intramedullary nailing was associated with better function and a lower infection rate, although, like Vallier et al.,[20] they demonstrated a lower malunion rate with plating. Overall it is likely that intramedullary nailing is better than plating, particularly if care is taken to correctly reduce the fracture prior to the nail being introduced. There are no studies specifically dealing with elderly patients, but logically it would seem that intramedullary nailing is a better technique for the management of tibial diaphyseal fractures in this group.

Amputation

The requirement for primary amputation is rare, but there are a number of indications which are shown in Table 40.3. One might think that it would be rarely required in the elderly, but there is a relatively high prevalence of high energy injuries and if the patient is unfit an amputation may be required to save the patient's life. In addition, the surgeon must consider the extent of any potential later reconstructive

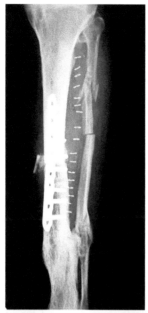

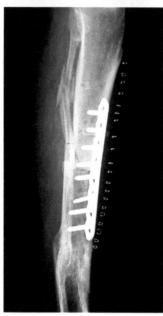

Figure 40.6 A locking plate used to treat a tibial diaphyseal fracture in an elderly patient. The previous malunion prevented nailing.

surgery and whether the patient will tolerate it. In older patients a severe leg injury may well mean that the patient is confined to a wheelchair anyway and an amputation may well simplify the treatment to the patient's benefit.

MANAGEMENT OF OPEN FRACTURES

As with younger patients the treatment of open fractures in the elderly involves careful management of the soft tissues and stabilization of the fracture. During the initial debridement care must be taken to assess the degree of skin degloving which often occurs in older patients (Figure 40.7). Care must be taken to resect all degloved skin back to bleeding

Table 40.3 Indications for primary amputation in elderly patients who present with a tibial fracture

Warm ischaemia time of >6 hours in a non-viable limb

Irreparable vascular injury with no collateral flow on arteriography

Severe crushing injury with minimal viable tissue

Presence of severe comorbidities or diseases where lengthy surgical procedures could endanger life

Presence of severe multisystem injuries where salvage may lead to multiple organ dysfunction syndrome (MODS) and death

Tissue damage is so severe that limb function will be better with a prosthesis

Very extensive metastasis or primary tumour

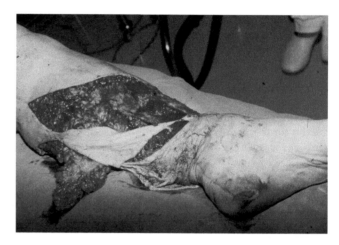

Figure 40.7 A Gustilo type IIIa open fracture in an elderly patient. Note the extensive degloving.

dermis. Soft tissue cover involves the same techniques as used in younger patients. These are discussed in Chapter 13. In the 48 open fractures treated in elderly patients in the 15-year period in Edinburgh, 56.2% did not require plastic surgery, 12.5% required split skin grafting and 31.2% required flap cover.

The choice of implant is usually an intramedullary nail or external fixation. Intramedullary nailing is recommended for fractures up to Gustilo type IIIa in severity. There is no evidence as to whether intramedullary nailing or external fixation is preferable in Gustilo type IIIb fractures in the elderly. However, surgeons should be aware of the problems of a prolonged operating time in a severely injured elderly patient and external fixation, using damage control techniques, may well be useful in this group of patients, although if primary intramedullary nailing can be used it may reduce the risk of later infection and the number of surgical procedures that the elderly patient may require. Primary amputation has been discussed (Table 40.3) and this should be considered in severely injured elderly patients and in most Gustilo type IIIc fractures, particularly if there is extensive associated soft tissue injury.

MANAGEMENT OF INSUFFICIENCY FRACTURES

Insufficiency fractures are usually diagnosed with standard anteroposterior and lateral radiographs (Figure 40.2), but if there is clinical suspicion, without radiological evidence, of an insufficiency fracture, CT and MRI scanning may be used. The majority of tibial insufficiency fractures can be treated non-operatively,[12] but in the series of 187 tibial fractures treated in Edinburgh over 13 years, two (25%) were treated by intramedullary nailing because of displacement.

MANAGEMENT OF PERIPROSTHETIC FRACTURES

Tibial periprosthetic fractures are usually classified using the system developed by Felix et al.[14] Type I fractures are condylar fractures of the tibial plateau which are either depression or split fractures. Type II fractures are metaphyseal or proximal diaphyseal fractures of the tibia around the stem of the implant. Type III fractures are distal to the implant stem and type IV fractures are avulsion fractures of the tibial tuberosity. An example of a type III tibial periprosthetic fracture is shown in Figure 40.3. The fractures are further subdivided according to the adequacy of fixation of the prosthesis and the timing of the fracture. Type A fractures occur with a well-fixed prosthesis while type B fractures occur with a loose prosthesis. Type C fractures are intraoperative fractures.

Felix et al.[14] recorded that 59.8% of tibial periprosthetic fractures were type I, 21.6% were type II, 16.7% were type III and only 2% were type IV. They also found that 81.4% of tibial periprosthetic fractures were postoperative fractures and that 62.6% of patients who presented with postoperative fractures had no history of trauma.

Treatment depends on the fixation of the prosthesis. If the prosthesis is stable, a brace and protected weight bearing is often adequate. If there is tibial displacement, internal or external fixation will be required and if the prosthesis is loose revision arthroplasty will be needed.

SUGGESTED TREATMENT

Where possible we believe that intramedullary nailing should be used to treat tibial fractures in the elderly. Table 40.1 shows that the results are better than those associated with other techniques. However in patients that are unfit for surgery or who are non-ambulant and have multiple or severe pre-fracture comorbidities non-operative management is the obvious method of management. The mortality rate in this group of patients is unknown but it must be very high. If the patient is badly injured or has a severe open fracture the surgeon may use an external fixator particularly if the patient has pre-operative medical comorbidities and the surgeon wishes to use damage control techniques. If the patient presents with a proximal or distal spiral fracture which makes nailing difficult, an external fixator or polyaxial locking plate may be indicated. Primary amputation should be considered if the conditions listed in Table 40.3 exist.

COMPLICATIONS

Clement et al.[3] analysed the complications that arose in the management of 233 tibial diaphyseal fractures in patients ≥65 years of age. Their results are shown in Table 40.1.

Non-union

The fracture non-union rate for patients ≥65 years of age is about 10% (Table 40.1). This is higher than many surgeons might expect, but it should be remembered that there is a high prevalence of high energy fractures and open fractures in a population with more infirmity and medical and social comorbidities than is seen in a younger population. The infection rate is lower in the ≥80-year-old patients, but the prevalence of high energy fractures is lower in this group.

There is a clear relationship between fracture morphology and the prevalence of non-union. AO/OTA[15] type A fractures have a much lower non-union rate than AO/OTA type B and C fractures (Table 40.1). Predictably the nonunion rate in closed fractures is much less than in open fractures and is very similar to the rate seen in a younger population. The infection rate associated with open fractures is about 20%, which is considerably higher than seen in younger patients with tibial diaphyseal fractures. Court-Brown showed that the overall infection rate in 247 nailed open tibial diaphyseal fractures of all Gustilo types, in all ages, was 7.7%.[7] This again emphasizes the difficulties surgeons face in having to treat older patients with more comorbidities.

Aseptic non-union treated initially by intramedullary nailing is managed by exchange nailing.[22] There are many studies showing excellent results in younger patients, but very little information exists about the results of exchange nailing in older patients. There is no reason to believe that the results are not equivalent and a study by Swanson et al.[23] of 46 aseptic tibial non-unions included five patients aged ≥60 years. The results in these patients were equivalent to the younger patients. Exchange nailing is widely practised and merely involves removing the nail, reaming the intramedullary canal by a further 1–2 mm and then inserting a larger nail, usually without cross screws unless the fracture is very proximal or distal. The procedure is osteogenic and the results are excellent. Exchange nailing, using a reamed nail, has been shown to facilitate union in bone defects up to 2 cm in length, which involve up to 50% of the circumference, in aseptic nonunions.

Table 40.1 shows that there were no nonunions in the patients treated with a cast in the 233 fractures reported by Clement et al.[3] We believe that this is because of the high mortality in this group of patients. However if a nonunion does occur, its management depends on whether there is any deformity in the tibia. The best treatment is intramedullary nailing, but this may have to be done using an open technique if the tibia requires to be straightened. The literature shows that good results can be achieved.[24] If the fracture is very proximal or distal, surgeons may prefer to plate the non-union and use supplementary bone graft or a bone graft substitute. The best treatment of non-unions in plated fractures is also intramedullary nailing. This technique has been shown to be successful and supplementary bone grafting is rarely required.[25]

The treatment of tibial non-unions following external fixation is more difficult because of the relatively high prevalence of pin tract infections in the elderly. If infection is present it should be treated by appropriate bone and soft tissue resection followed by fixation with an intramedullary nail or an external fixator with soft tissue cover and bone grafting being undertaken as required. Brinker and O'Connor[26] documented the use of the Ilizarov method of treating tibial non-unions in older patients. They treated 23 patients with an average age of 72.8 years. Four patients either died or were lost to follow-up and 56.2% of the remaining patients had excellent or very good results. All 20 patients who completed treatment returned to full weight bearing but in infected non-unions a frame was worn for an average of 426 days, compared with 244 days in uninfected non-unions.

Non-unions have a devastating effect on patients and it is the duty of the surgeon undertaking the primary surgery and early subsequent fracture treatment to try to minimize the nonunion rate in a population that often has significant social and medical problems already. Brinker et al.[27] analysed the effect of non-union and concluded that there was a significant effect on physical health, mental health and pain. They concluded that the impact of tibial non-union on physical health was comparable with the reported impact of end-stage hip arthrosis and worse than congestive cardiac failure. Antonova et al.[28] also examined the sequelae of non-union and showed that they were associated with the use of substantial healthcare resources.

Malunion

Table 40.1 shows that there is a relatively high malunion rate in the ≥65-year-old and ≥80-year-old group. Further analysis shows that this is because over 25% of cast managed patients and about 40% of patients treated with an external fixator had a malunion. In the study referred to in Table 40.1[3] malunion was defined as >5 degrees of angulation or rotational deformity or >1 cm of shortening. It is questionable as to how important minor degrees of malunion are in this elderly population. Many of the cast managed patients were non-ambulant, had dementia or had significant other comorbidities and a malunion would not have been a problem for them. Even in fitter elderly patients minor degrees of malunion are unlikely to be a significant problem. However, Table 40.1 does show that where intramedullary nailing is used primarily, it is associated with a lower prevalence of malunion.

Infection

Table 40.1 shows that the overall infection rate in the 233 elderly patients documented by Clement et al.[3] was 6.9%. This is higher than in the overall adult population. Court-Brown analysed the infection rate of 1106 closed and open adult tibial fractures treated by intramedullary nailing and found an overall infection rate of 3.1%.[7] It is interesting to observe that the infection rate in the ≥80-year-old group is lower than in the ≥65-year-old group. This may be because there are fewer high energy injuries in this group (Chapter 1, Table 1.6), although the prevalence of Gustilo type III fractures is very similar in both groups. Another explanation is that the ≥80-year-old group may simply be fitter than the ≥65-year-old group. This may also be reflected in the higher incidence of infection in male patients compared with female patients. Not unexpectedly the infection rate was higher in open fractures than in closed fractures and as with non-union and malunion, the results of intramedullary nailing are better than the results of external fixation, although this may simply reflect that a number of the patients with severe open tibial fractures were treated with external fixation.

The treatment of infection in the elderly is the same as for younger patients with the proviso that severe osteomyelitis in patients with dementia or non-ambulant patients, or in those with significant comorbidities who might not survive multiple operative procedures, might best be treated by amputation. The treatment of infection involves soft tissue and bone debridement, fracture stabilization, soft tissue reconstruction and bone reconstruction. It can be very time consuming and difficult for the patients and amputation may be the preferred option in some patients.

Compartment syndrome

Compartment syndrome is relatively unusual in older patients. There is very limited information about compartment syndrome in elderly patients, but Clement et al.[3] documented a 2.6% prevalence in ≥65-year-old patients. The severity of compartment syndrome in this group of patients is illustrated by the fact that in this series 50% of the compartment syndromes were complicated by deep infection and 16.6% by skin necrosis. Compartment syndrome is discussed in detail in Chapter 6.

AMPUTATION

Table 40.1 shows that the amputation rate in the 233 patients detailed by Clement et al.[3] was 3%. This rose to 10.1% in open fractures. As has already been discussed in the section dealing with infection, amputation may well be the preferred option in elderly infirm patients, patients with dementia or non-ambulant patients. Many elderly patients will not tolerate, or indeed survive, a prolonged management protocol involving multiple operations and surgeons should remember that a number of elderly patients will not walk again after sustaining a severe tibial fracture complicated by infection.

FIBULAR FRACTURES

Isolated fractures of the fibula are rare. Most fractures of the fibula are associated with fractures of the tibial plateau or ankle fractures. In younger patients they are more common in males and are often caused by a direct blow.[2] Analysis of the data used in Chapter 1 shows that there were eight isolated fractures of the fibula in ≥65-year-old patients in the 2-year period that was examined. The incidence of fibular fractures in the ≥65-year-old group was $4.1/10^5$/year and in the ≥80-year-old group it was $3.9/10^5$/year. The male/female ratio was 37/63 and 62.5% occurred as a result of a fall. The remaining fractures occurred as a result of a direct blow (12.5%), a road traffic accident (12.5%) or a golf injury (12.5%). The analysis showed that 75% of the fractures were in the proximal fibula and the remaining 25% were in the diaphysis. Open fibular fractures are extremely rare and their incidence has been given in the section dealing with the epidemiology of open fractures. The treatment of isolated fibular fractures in the elderly is almost always non-operative. If there is significant displacement the fracture should be reduced and plated.

REFERENCES

1. Court-Brown CM, Caesar B. Epidemiology of adult fractures: A review. *Injury* 2006;37:691–7.
2. Court-Brown CM. The epidemiology of fractures and dislocations. In: Court-Brown CM, Heckman JD, McQueen MM, Ricci WM, Tornetta P, eds. *Rockwood and Green's Fractures in Adults.* 8th ed. Philadelphia, PA: Lippincott Williams & Wilkins, 2014, pp. 59–108.
3. Clement ND, Beauchamp NJF, Duckworth AD, McQueen MM, Court-Brown CM. The outcome of tibial diaphyseal fractures in the elderly. *Bone Joint J* 2013;95-B:1255–62.
4. Court-Brown CM, Biant LC, Clement ND, Bugler KE, Duckworth AD, McQueen MM. Open fractures in the elderly: The importance of skin ageing. *Injury* 2015;46(2):189–94.
5. Hooper GJ, Keddell RG, Penny ID. Conservative management or closed nailing for tibial shaft fractures: A prospective randomised trial. *J Bone Joint Surg Br* 1991;73-A:83–5.
6. Court-Brown CM, Christie J, McQueen MM. Closed intramedullary tibial nailing: Its use in closed and type I open fractures. *J Bone Joint Surg Br* 1990;72-B:605–11.
7. Court-Brown CM. Reamed intramedullary tibial nailing: An overview and analysis of 1106 cases. *J Orthop Trauma* 2004;18:96–101.
8. Gustilo RB, Anderson JT. Prevention of infection in the treatment of 1025 open fractures of long bones: Retrospective and prospective analysis. *J Bone Joint Surg Am* 1976;58-A:453–8.
9. Gustilo RB, Mendoza RM, Williams DM. Problems in the management of type III (severe) open fractures: A new classification of type III open fractures. *J Trauma* 1984;24:742–6.
10. El Moghraoui A, Morjane F, Nouijai A, Achemlal L, Bezza A, Ghozlani I. Vertebral fracture assessment in Moroccan women: Prevalence and risk factors. *Maturitas* 2009;62:171–5.
11. Ven den Berg M, Verdiik NA, van den Bergh JP, Geusens PP, Talboom-Kamp EP, Leusink GL, Pop VJ. Vertebral fractures in women aged 50 years and older with clinical risk factors for fractures in primary care. *Maturitas* 2011;70:74–9.
12. Soubrier M, Dubost J-J, Boisgard S, Sauvezie B, Gaillard P, Michel JL, Ristori J-M. Insufficiency fracture: A survey of 60 cases and review of the literature. *Joint Bone Spine* 2003;70:209–18.
13. Breglia MD, Carter JD. Atypical insufficiency fracture of the tibia associated with long-term bisphosphonate therapy. *J Clin Rheumatol* 2010;16:76–8.
14. Felix NA, Stuart MJ, Hanssen AD. Periprosthetic fractures of the tibia associated with total knee arthroplasty. *Clin Orthop Rel Res* 1997;345:113–24.
15. Fracture and dislocation compendium: Orthopaedic Trauma Association Committee for Coding and Classification. *J Orthop Trauma* 1996;10(Suppl):1–154.
16. Jost B, Spross C, Grehn H, Gerber C. Locking plate fixation of the proximal humerus: Analysis of complications, revision strategies and outcome. *J Shoulder Elbow Surg* 2013;22:542–9.
17. Vallier HA, Immler W. Comparison of the 95-degree angled blade plate and the locking condylar plate for the treatment of distal femoral fractures. *J Orthop Trauma* 2012;26:327–32.
18. Schepers T, Van Lieshout EMM, De Vries MR, Van der Elst M. Increased rates of wound complications with locking plates in distal fibular fractures. *Injury* 2011;42:1125–9.
19. Guo JJ, Tang N, Yang HL, Tang TS. A prospective, randomized trial comparing closed intramedullary nailing with percutaneous plating in the treatment of distal metaphyseal fractures of the tibia. *J Bone Joint Surg Br* 2010;92-B:984–8.
20. Vallier HA, Cureton BA, Patterson BM. Factors influencing functional outcomes after distal tibial shaft fractures. *J Orthop Trauma* 2012;26:178–83.
21. Xue X-H, Yan SG, Cai X-Z, Shi M-M, Lin T. Intramedullary nailing versus plating for extra-articular distal tibial metaphyseal fracture: A systematic review and meta-analysis. *Injury* 2014;45:667–76.
22. Court-Brown CM, Keating JF, Christie J, McQueen MM. Exchange intramedullary nailing. Its use in aseptic tibial non-union. *J Bone Joint Surg* 1995;77-B:407–11.

23. Swanson EA, Garrard EC, O'Connor DP, Brinker MR. The results of a systematic approach to exchange nailing for the treatment of aseptic tibial nonunions. *J Orthop Trauma* 2015;29(1):28–35.

24. Richmond J, Colleran K, Borens O, Kloen P, Helfet DL. Nonunions of the distal tibia treated by reamed intramedullary nailing. *J Orthop Trauma* 2004;18:603–10.

25. Wu CC. Reaming bone grafting to treat tibial shaft nonunion after plating. *J Orthop Surg* 2003;11:16–21.

26. Brinker MR, O'Connor DP. Outcomes of tibial nonunion in older adults following treatment using the Ilizarov method. *J Orthop Trauma* 2007;21:634–42.

27. Brinker MR, Hanus BD, Sen M, O'Connor DP. The devastating effects of tibial nonunion on health-related quality of life. *J Bone Joint Surg Am* 2013;95:2170–6.

28. Antonova E, Kim Le T, Burge R, Mershon J. Tibia shaft fractures: Costly burden of nonunions. *BMC Musculoskelet Disord* 2013;14:42.

41

Distal tibial fractures

PAUL S. WHITING AND WILLIAM T. OBREMSKEY

INTRODUCTION

As the proportion of elderly individuals increases due to longer average life expectancies, fracture incidence in this population is on the rise. In addition to decreasing bone mineral density (BMD), multiple explanations have been proposed for the increased incidence of fractures in the aging population including 'frailty', a condition defined by a diminished capacity to perform activities of daily living and often characterized by inactivity and weight loss.[1] Other risk factors for osteoporotic fractures include vitamin D deficiency, malnutrition, chronic inflammatory conditions, physical deconditioning and poor balance.[1]

Although much less common than the classic fragility fractures of the proximal femur, pelvis, proximal humerus and distal radius, fractures of the distal tibia and fibula in the elderly most commonly result from similar mechanisms of injury – ground level falls. Measurements of BMD obtained from the tibial diaphysis and epiphysis have been shown to predict clinical fracture risk as accurately as BMD measurements obtained from the hip or lumbar spine, substantiating the fact that osteopenia and osteoporosis are manifest in the entire skeleton.[2]

EPIDEMIOLOGY

Although the majority of recent literature examining changes in the incidence of fragility fractures has focused on the classic fragility fractures described above, Court-Brown et al. have recently published a detailed epidemiologic analysis of fractures in patients 65 years of age and older.[3] In this series of 4,786 fractures that occurred over 24 months of data collection, only 16 (0.33%) occurred in the distal tibia, representing an overall incidence of 8.2 per 100,000 population per year (3.9 in males and 11.0 in females). Of the 16 distal tibia fractures, 15 occurred as the result of low energy falls, and one occurred spontaneously (Court-Brown CM, personal communication). Unlike with many other fragility fractures, the incidence of distal tibia fractures did not increase significantly with advancing age (Table 41.1).

CLASSIFICATION

Fractures of the distal tibia and fibula are characterized using two main classification systems. The Rüedi and Allgöwer system, first published in 1968 in German[4] but subsequently translated and published in English in 1969,[5] is a relatively simple descriptive classification system that divides intra-articular fractures of the distal tibia into three types. Non-displaced intra-articular fractures are classified as type I fractures. Type II fractures involve displacement of the distal tibial articular surface without significant comminution. Type III fractures are displaced intra-articular fractures with significant comminution, often involving articular impaction.

The AO/OTA classification system divides fractures of the distal tibia into three main types: extra-articular (type a), partial articular (type b) and complete articular (type c) as depicted in Figure 41.1.[6] Fractures in each type are then classified on the basis of fracture comminution into one of three groups, each of which can be further subdivided into three subgroups based upon other fracture characteristics. With its 27 resultant fracture types, the AO/OTA classification system is a comprehensive descriptive system designed to include all possible fractures of the distal tibia, both extra-articular and intra-articular.

While Martin et al.[7] demonstrated better interobserver reliability with the AO/OTA classification system (kappa = 0.60) than with the Rüedi and Allgöwer system

Table 41.1 Distal tibia fracture incidence per 100,000 population in individuals aged 65 and above, grouped in 5-year age ranges, with P values calculated between groups

	Age						
	65–69	70–74	75–79	80–84	85–89	90+	P value
Men	3.9	4.6	0	0	16.7	0	0.67
Women	17.7	13.1	4.2	5.3	8	30.4	0.87

Source: Courtesy of Charles Court-Brown MD.

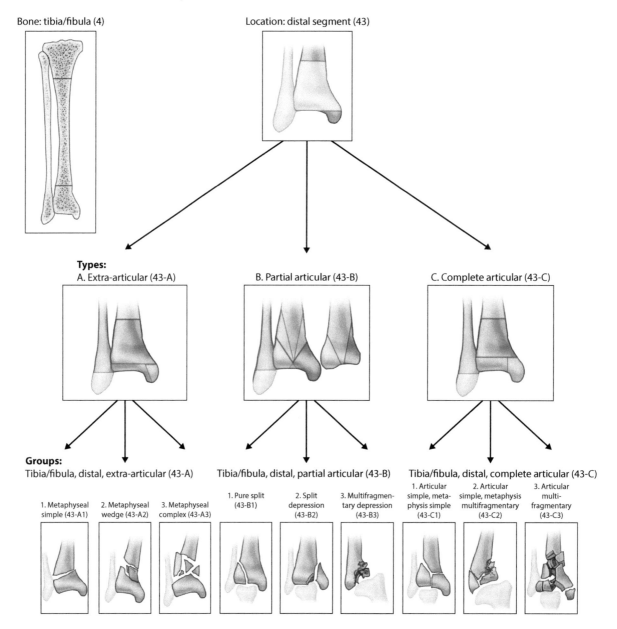

Figure 41.1 AO/OTA Classification System for Distal Tibia and Fibula Fractures. (Reproduced with permission from Marsh JL et al. *J Orthop Trauma.* 2007; 21(10 Suppl): S1–133.)

(kappa = 0.46), Swiontkowski et al.[8] showed that the interobserver reliability of the AO/OTA classification system was highest for determining fracture type (A, B or C, kappa = 0.57) and lower for fracture group (kappa = 0.43) and subgroup (kappa = 0.41). Despite only achieving moderate overall interobserver reliability scores, both of these systems can be useful clinically (for effective communication among healthcare workers, determining an appropriate treatment plan and preoperative planning) and for research purposes.

TREATMENT

Multiple treatment options exist for fractures of the distal tibia in the elderly. Radiographs of the entire tibia and ankle are required for a complete assessment of the fracture pattern and bone quality. A key determination to make is whether the fracture is extra-articular or intra-articular. If intra-articular extension is present or suspected, advanced imaging with computed tomography may assist in further characterization of the fracture, including any articular incongruity, impaction or comminution.

Although the majority of distal tibia fractures in the elderly occur as the result of low-energy mechanisms of injury, a careful assessment of the soft tissue envelope is essential. The degree of soft tissue injury, presence of open wounds or chronic venous stasis, baseline cellulitis and location of any previous surgical scars must be noted when considering both operative and non-operative treatment options. Likewise, patient comorbidities (such as diabetes, cardiovascular disease and peripheral vascular disease) and risk factors for wound complications (such as smoking, poor nutrition and immunosuppression) must be identified and optimized prior to any proposed surgical intervention. Finally, a patient's functional demands, including ambulatory status, level of independence and support system must be considered in the development of an individualized treatment plan.

Non-operative treatment

Non-operative treatment was used almost exclusively for treatment of extra-articular fractures of the distal tibia through the 1960s. Although evidence based guidelines for tibial alignment do not exist, acceptable criteria for non-operative management have included fracture shortening of less than 1 cm, less than 5 degrees of valgus and 0 degrees of varus, less than 10 degrees of angulation in the sagittal plane and 5–10 degrees of external rotation and no internal rotation.[9] In a series of more than 700 tibial shaft fractures which included proximal, mid-shaft and distal fractures, Nicoll reported a malunion rate of only 8.6%.[10] However, Coles and Gross reported a 31.7% rate of malunion, a 13.1% rate of delayed union and a 4.1% rate of non-union in their systematic review of the prospective literature, which identified 145 tibial fractures treated non-operatively.[11] High rates of associated ankle and knee stiffness (25% in Nicoll's series) have also been reported with non-operative treatment.

Sarmiento popularized the functional brace for the closed treatment of proximal, diaphyseal and distal tibia fractures. In a large case series of 450 distal tibia fractures treated with the functional brace, Sarmiento and Latta reported a non-union rate of only 0.9%.[12] Less than 10% of patients had an angular deformity greater than 6 degrees in any plane, and varus deformity was more commonly seen in the setting of an intact fibula. Two-thirds of patients healed with less than 5 degrees of deformity in any plane, and 90% healed with a deformity of less than 8 degrees. An average of 5.1 mm of shortening was reported, and 94.2% of patients healed with less than 12 mm of shortening. Mean fracture shortening did not change from injury to fracture union, leading the authors to conclude that axially unstable distal tibia fractures do not undergo further shortening when treated non-operatively in a functional brace. These favorable results are comparable to the results achieved in Sarmiento's even larger case series of over 1000 closed diaphyseal tibia fractures treated with the functional brace, with union occurring in over 99%.[13]

Non-operative management of intra-articular fractures of the distal tibia has proven to be less successful. In a small case series of 19 pilon fractures, Ayeni reported good clinical outcomes in 11 Rüedi and Allgöwer type I fractures treated non-operatively but universally poor clinical outcomes in the three type II fractures treated non-operatively.[14] Kellam and Waddell classified 26 pilon fractures into two groups based on fracture pattern (rotational versus compressive).[15] For both groups, clinical results after non-operative treatment were inferior to those obtained with surgical treatment, and non-operative treatment was only successful in rotational injuries that did not displace over the course of treatment. Based on these and other case series, non-operative treatment is best reserved for non-displaced intra-articular distal tibia fractures that are unlikely to displace during cast immobilization. In addition, non-operative management may still be the preferred method of treatment for certain elderly patients with intra-articular distal tibia fractures. Non-ambulatory patients (including those with quadriplegia or paraplegia), patients with absolute contraindications to surgical treatment (critical aortic stenosis or other unstable cardiopulmonary conditions) and those with limited functional capacity (dementia/Alzheimer) or metabolic bone diseases such as osteogenesis imperfecta may be best served with non-surgical treatment (Figure 41.2).

External fixation

External fixation is a useful technique for provisional fixation of distal tibia fractures in the setting of significant open wounds or severe soft tissue swelling. Multiple techniques of external fixation can be utilized including thin-wire, half-pin and hybrid constructs (combining thin wires and half pins). Although anatomically 'safe corridors' have been described for thin-wire fixation in the distal tibia, a cadaveric study in which surgeons familiar with such corridors each placed two thin wires in the distal tibia demonstrated that 55% of wires impaled at least one tendon that crossed the ankle joint.[16] Other structures at risk with thin wire fixation were the saphenous vein, superficial peroneal nerve and superior capsular reflection of the ankle joint, which extended an average of 32 mm above the medial malleolus and 21 mm above the anteromedial joint line.

External fixation is generally less successful than other methods of fixation in the definitive treatment of distal tibia fractures. In a prospective comparative trial at multiple level 1 trauma centers, Richards et al. assessed outcomes after fixation of intra-articular distal tibia fractures treated by delayed open reduction internal fixation (ORIF) versus

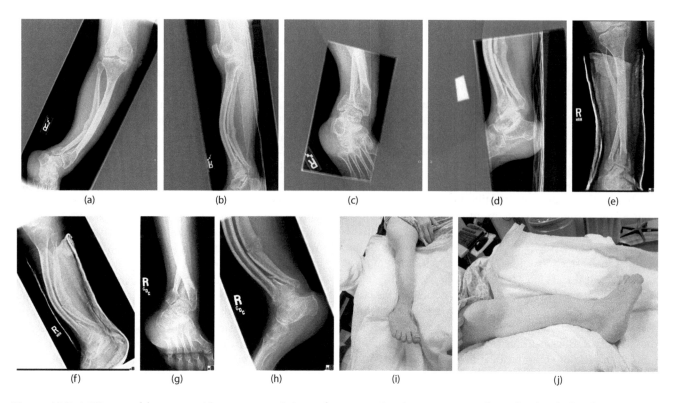

Figure 41.2 A 55-year-old woman with osteogenesis imperfecta sustained an extra-articular right distal tibia fracture in a motor vehicle collision. Anteroposterior (AP) and lateral views of the tibia **(a,b)** and ankle **(c,d)** are shown. Based on the patient's non-ambulatory status and poor bone quality, non-operative management was chosen and a short-leg splint was applied **(e,f)**. X-rays at 16 weeks after injury showed abundant callus formation and healing **(g,h)**. The patient was able to return to her baseline level of function, using the right lower extremity for transfers. Clinical photos **(i,j)** demonstrate alignment satisfactory for her required level of mobility.

definitive external fixation.[17] External fixation was associated with a significantly higher rate of delayed union or non-union (22.2% vs 3.7%, $P = 0.05$), and the ORIF group had significantly better Short Form-36 (SF-36) physical function scores at 6 months and Iowa Ankle Scores at 6 and 12 months. There were no differences between groups in preoperative patient or fracture characteristics, quality of articular reduction or rates of deep infection.

Plate fixation

In the 1970s, plate fixation began to supplant non-operative treatment as the preferred method of managing distal tibia fractures. Multiple anatomic locations in the distal tibia are amenable to plate fixation. Lee et al. retrospectively reviewed 88 patients with distal tibia fractures treated with an anterolateral plate (n = 49) or a medial plate (n = 39).[18] The authors found no difference in rates of operative time, fracture union, malunion, ankle range of motion or functional outcomes, but medial plating was associated with a higher rate of hardware complications and total complications.

Concerns for wound infection and hardware prominence have led to the development of techniques for plate insertion that both minimize disruption of the fracture environment and limit the extent of additional injury to the often tenuous soft tissue envelope of the distal tibia.

Minimally invasive plate osteosynthesis (MIPO) involves making relatively small periarticular incisions through which the distal-most aspect of the plate is positioned appropriately on the bone. Submuscular (extraperiosteal) dissection is then performed with relatively atraumatic instruments in order to 'slide' the plate proximally. Proximal holes in the plate are filled in a percutaneous manner with stab incisions and often a counter-incision over the proximal end of the plate. Bloomstein et al. have described a helpful technique for percutaneous plate application.[19] Using a suture tied to the proximal portion of the plate enables manipulation of both poles of the plate, which assists in achieving anatomic plate positioning while simultaneously avoiding soft tissue stripping. The MIPO technique can be utilized in a variety of clinical scenarios in which the soft tissue envelope is at risk.

Collinge et al. evaluated clinical outcomes in 26 high-energy distal tibia fractures with minimal or no intra-articular extension treated with minimally invasive medial plating.[20] There were two cases of loss of fixation (8%), and all but one case achieved acceptable alignment, defined as shortening <1 cm and angulation <5 degrees in any plane. Risk factors for healing problems included significant fracture comminution, bone loss and high-grade open fractures, and 35% of patients required secondary procedures to achieve union. Nonetheless, SF-36 functional outcomes scores had returned to normal in 81% of patients at 2 years.

More recently, Collinge and Protzman reported functional outcomes in 38 patients with distal tibia fractures treated with a hybrid MIPO technique (using locking and non-locking screws above and below the fracture).[21] Fracture union was achieved in all cases, malalignment and loss of fixation each occurred in one patient (3%), and two patients (6%) required secondary procedures to achieve union. Good to excellent functional outcomes on the American Orthopaedic Foot and Ankle Surgeons' (AOFAS) and Olerud and Molander scales were attained by 30 of 38 patients (79%), and mean SF-36 scores were only significantly diminished in the physical function domain when compared to normative data. In a similar study, Oh et al. reported 100% union in 21 distal tibia fractures treated with MIPO.[22] There were no cases of sagittal or coronal malalignment >5 degrees, and only one case of malrotation (10 degrees of internal rotation) occurred. Outcomes in elderly distal tibia fractures treated with MIPO are more likely to approximate those of the latter two studies, which represented a spectrum of low and high-energy injuries with an age range of 17–82 years.

As MIPO has gained popularity, some concern has arisen regarding injury to neurovascular structures at risk with the various surgical approaches to the distal tibia. Wolinsky and Lee performed a cadaveric study to investigate the relationships between an anterolateral distal tibia plate and important neurovascular structures in the lower leg.[23] Using a pre-contoured anterolateral plate designed for minimally invasive submuscular application and percutaneous proximal fixation, the authors identified the superficial peroneal nerve in all 10 cadaveric specimens in the distal wound and concluded that this structure is not at risk. The neurovascular pedicle consisting of the deep peroneal nerve along with the anterior tibial artery and vein lies posterior to the plate proximally but courses anteriorly, crossing over the plate in a consistent region 4–11 cm proximal to the ankle joint, placing them at risk in this location.

In a similar study, Ozsoy et al. investigated the anatomic structures at risk when performing MIPO medially.[24] The saphenous nerve and great saphenous vein were most at risk over holes 4, 5 and 6 of the Synthes 3.5/4.5 mm locking compression distal tibial metaphyseal plate and over holes 3, 5 and 8 of the Synthes 3.5 mm locking compression medial distal tibial plate with tab. In order to minimize injury to these neurovascular structures, the authors recommended using careful dissection down to the plate, atraumatic placement of drill sleeves and protection of the soft tissues during screw insertion. Mirza et al. also investigated the risk of injury to the saphenous nerve and vein with the medial MIPO technique.[25] Percutaneous placement of smooth Kirschner wires (K-wires) in each hole of the plate caused injury to both structures in every specimen in a reproducible region 2.0–4.7 cm proximal to the tip of the medial malleolus. This study also assessed risk of injury to the superficial peroneal nerve with percutaneous lateral plating of the fibula. The nerve, which was found to exit the lateral compartment fascia an average of 11.5 cm proximal to the tip of the lateral malleolus, was injured in only one of 10 specimens.

Soft tissue considerations such as open wounds, previous scars, extensive swelling or fractures blisters often preclude one or more anatomic approaches to the distal tibia. In such settings, the surgeon must be familiar with multiple surgical approaches and options for fixation. Sheerin et al. reported a technique for fixation of distal tibia fractures with significant anteromedial soft tissue compromise.[26] Using a 90-degree cannulated blade plate applied through a posterolateral approach, the authors achieved primary union in 14 of 15 cases; in one case of delayed union, the fracture healed after compression plating with bone grafting. Another useful technique for fixation of distal tibia and fibula fractures in the setting of severe anteromedial soft tissue injury is trans-syndesmotic fixation through the fibula, as described by Sciadini et al.[27] In this technique, a 3.5 mm locking compression plate is placed on the posterolateral surface of the fibula after fracture reduction has been performed. Fixation is then extended into the tibia by means of long trans-syndesmotic screws placed through the plate and the fibula (Figure 41.3). Having already passed through two fibular cortices, these screws function as angular stable screws, and together the fibula and plate act as a bridge plate construct for the distal tibia fracture. The authors reported good results with this technique in six patients with minimum follow-up of 14 months (Figure 41.3).

Intramedullary nail fixation

Nork et al. reported excellent outcomes following intramedullary nailing of 36 distal tibia fractures (located within 5 cm of the ankle joint) using two or three distal interlocking screws.[28] Acceptable radiographic alignment (<5 degree angulation in any plane) was achieved and maintained in 92% of fractures, and union occurred in all 30 patients who completed follow-up, although three patients (10%) required a staged autograft procedure due to significant traumatic bone loss. Functional outcome scores at 2 years were available for 35% of patients, and SF-36 functional outcomes scores did not differ from normative values in seven of the eight subsets (physical function remained decreased) of this tool. Average Musculoskeletal Function Assessment (MFA) scores at 2 years were better than previously published average MFA scores following isolated knee, leg or ankle injuries. Wysocki et al.[29] achieved acceptable alignment (<5 degrees in any plane, <1 cm shortening) in 25 of 27 distal tibia fractures treated with an intramedullary nail by using a two-pin external fixator ('travelling traction') during nail passage and locking. Alternatively, a femoral distractor can be used for this same purpose.

Obremskey and Medina investigated rates of malalignment in distal third tibia fractures treated by intramedullary nailing by community orthopaedic surgeons versus orthopaedic trauma specialists.[30] Angular malalignment of more than 5 degrees occurred in 23% of fractures treated by community orthopaedic surgeons compared with only 5% of fractures treated by orthopaedic trauma surgeons ($P < 0.05$). Patients with malaligned

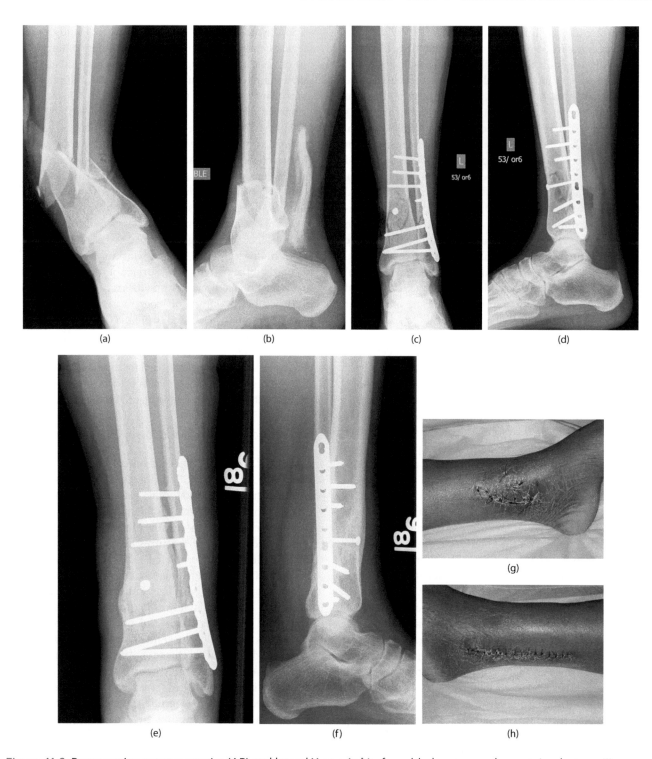

Figure 41.3 Preoperative anteroposterior (AP) and lateral X-rays **(a,b)** of an elderly woman who sustained a type IIIa open distal tibia and fibula fracture with a large medial wound. Trans-syndesmotic fibular plating was carried out through a posterolateral approach to provide fixation of both fractures through a favourable soft tissue envelope **(c,d)**. AP and lateral X-rays 6 months after fixation **(e,f)** show healing of the fractures with excellent alignment. Uncomplicated healing of the medial traumatic wound and the posterolateral surgical incision were achieved **(g,h)**. (Courtesy of Marcus Sciadini MD.)

fractures had significantly higher bodily pain scores on the Musculoskeletal Outcomes Data Evaluation and Management System (MODEMS) scale than patients with well-aligned fractures. The MODEMS program was launched in the late 1990s by the American Academy of Orthopaedic Surgeons in order to develop standardized assessment criteria and measurement instruments related to the musculoskeletal system. Although the program achieved early success, it never garnered the critical mass of subscribers necessary to become economically viable and financially successful. However, the efforts of the MODEMS program helped set standards for quality in clinical outcomes research on the musculoskeletal system.

Extension of the fracture line from the distal tibial diaphysis into the articular surface is not necessarily a contraindication to intramedullary nail fixation. Konrath et al. reported union in 19 of 20 distal tibia fractures (95%) treated with lag screw fixation of the intra-articular extension followed by intramedullary nailing.[31] Excellent alignment was also achieved in 19 of 20 cases.

Fixation of the fibula in the setting of tibial intramedullary nailing remains a topic of controversy in the management of distal tibia fractures. In a retrospective review of 72 distal tibia and fibula fractures treated with intramedullary nailing of the tibia with or without fibular fixation, Egol et al. found that fibular fixation was associated with maintenance of reduction 12 weeks post-surgery.[32] Loss of reduction occurred in only 4% of cases in which fibular

fixation was performed compared with 13% of cases without fibular fixation. The advantages of fibular fixation must be weighed against the risk of an additional incision in an elderly patient who might have poor healing potential due to peripheral vascular disease, chronic venous stasis or an extremely thin and fragile soft tissue envelope.

Surgeons must consider all options to formulate a plan to attain and maintain limb alignment. An unusual option for a very distal fracture in a patient with a poor soft tissue envelope over a distal tibia fracture is a retrograde hindfoot fusion nail. Due to the necessity of sacrificing the subtalar and ankle joints, this option should be used only as a last resort for displaced fractures where a distal incision is not feasible or advisable (Figure 41.4). However, previous surgery of the ipsilateral limb and unfavourable soft tissue conditions may also preclude certain options for fixation, making non-traditional fracture constructs such as a hindfoot fusion nail more appropriate (Figure 41.5).

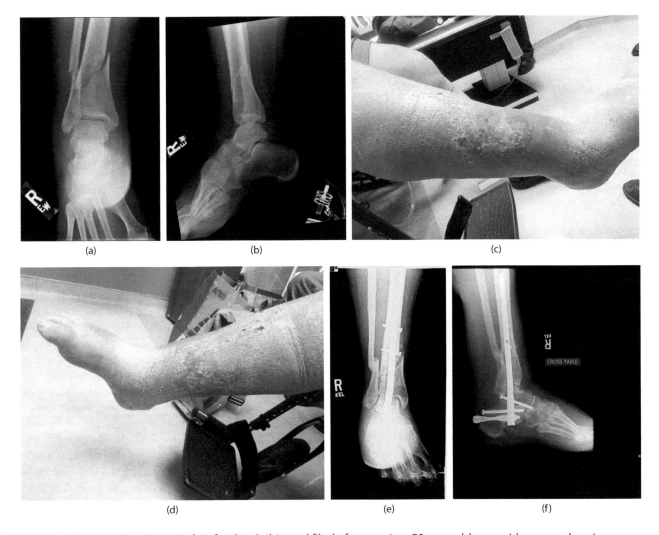

(a) (b) (c)

(d) (e) (f)

Figure 41.4 Preoperative X-rays **(a,b)** of a distal tibia and fibula fracture in a 58-year-old man with severe chronic venous stasis disease and circumferential pitting oedema with ulceration **(c,d)**. The patient also had a history of chronic ipsilateral tibio-talar instability. This fracture was managed with a hindfoot nail to address both problems. X-rays at 12 weeks show evidence of complete fibular healing and bridging callus of the tibia **(e,f)**.

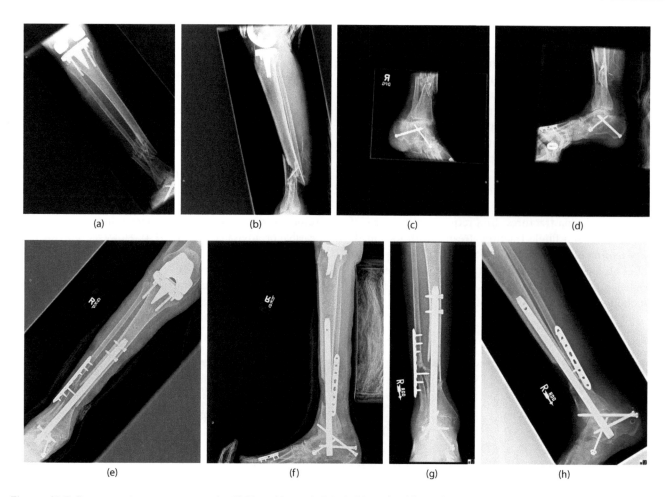

Figure 41.5 Preoperative anteroposterior (AP) and lateral tibia **(a,b)** and ankle **(c,d)** X-rays show a type IIIa open, commi-nuted distal tibia and fibula fracture with intra-articular extension in a 77-year-old woman with severe rheumatoid arthritis and a history of previous ipsilateral subtalar fusion and total knee arthroplasty. The patient desired limb salvage. Given her poor bone quality and unfavourable soft tissue envelope, management of this injury with a hindfoot fusion nail was determined to be preferable to preservation of the tibiotalar joint. Staged management included initial spanning external fixation with antibiotic beads. Definitive management included fibular fixation followed by ankle fusion with a hindfoot fusion nail. Immediate postoperative AP and lateral images **(e,f)** show satisfactory limb alignment. AP and lateral X-rays taken 8 months later demonstrate maintenance of alignment and no hardware complications **(g,h)**.

Biomechanics

Numerous biomechanical studies of distal tibia and fibula fractures have been conducted, investigating a variety of parameters pertinent to these fractures. The majority of these studies have used cadaveric specimens of advanced age or synthetic specimens that represent osteoporotic bone. The biomechanical impact of fixation of associated fibula fractures has been a controversial subject in the lit-erature. In a cadaveric model, Weber et al. tested the effect of fibular fixation (with either a plate and screw construct or an Enders intramedullary nail) on the stability of a tib-ial shaft fracture model.[33] Age of the specimens was not reported. Fibular fixation of either variety led to significant decreases in motion at the tibial fracture site when the tibia was stabilized with an external fixator but not with an intra-medullary nail. This study suggests that fibular fixation is not necessary if stable intramedullary nail fixation of the tibia is achieved, but it may add significantly to construct

stability if tibial fixation is less rigid. Kumar et al. corrobo-rated these findings in another cadaveric study using elderly specimens (average age 75 years).[34] The authors determined that fibular fixation in the setting of intramedullary nailing of distal tibia fractures resulted in only a small increase in rotational stability at the initial torque testing point but not with additional torque. The importance of fibular fixation in elderly distal tibia and fibula fractures was investigated further in a cadaveric study by Attal et al. (average speci-men age 78 years). Multidirectional distal locking of a tibial intramedullary nail without fibular plating was found to be significantly more stable rotational than conventional dis-tal tibial interlocking with fibular fixation.[35] The authors concluded that multidirectional distal locking renders fib-ular fixation largely unnecessary unless it is required as a reduction tool.

In a cadaveric model of distal tibia fractures with and without a concurrent fibula fracture, Strauss et al. tested the construct stability of a locked plate versus an intramedullary nail in a variety of loading scenarios.[36] Cadaveric specimen age ranged from 45 to 63 years. The locked plating construct proved to be significantly stiffer in anterior, central and posterior axial loading, while the intramedullary nail construct was stiffer in anterior to posterior and posterior to anterior cantilever bending. There was no difference between constructs in medial or lateral vertical loading or torsional loading. The presence of a concurrent fibula fracture produced significantly greater displacements at the fracture site and decreased torsional stiffness in both constructs, and the locking plate was significantly stiffer than the nail under these circumstances.

In a cadaveric study investigating the effect of blocking screws on the stability of elderly distal tibia fractures (average specimen age 67) stabilized with an intramedullary nail, Krettek et al. noted a 57% decrease in deformation of the bone-implant construct with the addition of blocking screws to the distal tibial metaphysis.[37] Since the addition of blocking screws appears to increase the primary stability of distal tibial fractures stabilized by intramedullary nailing, this technique may have some utility in the treatment of distal tibia fractures in elderly patients, in whom poor bone quality amplifies the need for strong metaphyseal fixation. Gorczyca et al. used a cadaveric study to test the biomechanical impact of removing 1 cm from the distal tip of a tibial nail.[38] There were no differences in stiffness to compression, torsion or compression-bending loads between the modified and unmodified nails, suggesting that very distal fractures (at least 4 cm from the ankle joint) can be successfully nailed with this simple nail modification. The redesign of many tibial nails to achieve improved fixation in very proximal or very distal fractures has largely made such modifications unnecessary. An important secondary finding of the study was the fact that fixation strength using either nail was not sufficient to resist moderate compression-bending loads, suggesting that distal tibia fractures stabilized with intramedullary nails require protected weight bearing until fracture callus provides additional stability. Although the average specimen age was not reported, this conclusion is even more applicable to the elderly, in whom poorer bone stock renders distal fixation much more tenuous.

In a biomechanical study of elderly distal fibula fractures, Dunn et al. investigated the impact on stability of adding supplemental fixation in the form of three quadricortical screws inserted through the distal fibula into the distal tibia after primary fixation with a plate and intramedullary K-wires.[39] In matched cadaveric specimens, the addition of three trans-syndesmotic screws significantly decreased axial deformation and increased mean stiffness, strength at 30 degrees external rotation and strength at failure. In another biomechanical study of osteoporotic distal fibula fractures, construct stability was tested in matched cadaveric legs with or without injection of a calcium sulfate and calcium phosphate composite graft into drill holes prior to screw insertion.[40] The authors reported

decreased displacement and increased load and energy to failure in the augmented constructs compared to non-augmented constructs. However, whether the findings of these studies represent clinically significant differences and may permit, as the authors suggest, earlier weight bearing after ankle fracture fixation in the elderly requires further clinical investigation.

Hoenig et al. performed a biomechanical investigation to compare four methods of fixation – standard plating, locked plating, standard intramedullary nailing and angular stable nailing – in extra-articular distal tibia fractures with an intact fibula.[41] Cadaveric specimens were obtained from individuals aged 61–97 years at the time of death, and average BMD was equivalent in all four groups. In axial loading, both intramedullary nailing constructs demonstrated increased stiffness, load and energy to failure compared with locking plate fixation, which in turn demonstrated greater stiffness, load and energy to failure compared with standard plating. Although the angular stable nailing constructs failed earlier than standard nailing constructs, the difference was not significant. Since all intramedullary nailing specimens and seven of eight locked plate specimens survived initial and cyclical loading (determined to simulate body weight for a 71.4 kg person), the authors concluded that intramedullary nailing and locked plating provide stable fixation in distal extra-articular tibia fractures. In a similar study, Hoegel et al. tested four methods of fixation – reamed intramedullary nailing, unreamed nailing, unreamed angular stable nailing and locked plating – in synthetic tibiae with a 10 mm fracture gap.[42] All intramedullary nail constructs demonstrated significantly less motion at the fracture gap compared to the locked plate construct, but only the reamed nail achieved significantly greater stiffness to axial compression. All nail constructs achieved greater torsional stiffness compared with the locking plate, and the reamed nail again outperformed both unreamed constructs. Gueorguiev et al. also studied the impact of angular stable distal interlocking on the stability of intramedullary nailing constructs for distal tibia fractures.[43] There was no difference to medial–lateral and anterior–posterior bending or number of cycles to failure between constructs. However, angular-stable distal interlocking was associated with a statistically significant decrease in fracture gap motion in axial compression compared with standard interlocking.

Interpreted together, biomechanical data have tended to prove that reamed intramedullary nail fixation and locking plate fixation both provide stiffness adequate to stabilize metaphyseal fractures of the distal tibia to enable fracture healing. Intramedullary nailing appears to possess a slight advantage in overall construct stiffness compared to locked plating, and the ideal type of distal interlocking remains somewhat controversial. Fixation of concurrent fibular fractures tends to increase the overall construct stability regardless of the method of tibial fixation, although multidirectional distal tibial interlocking may render this added stability unnecessary.

OUTCOMES

Comparison of treatments

In a systematic review of 1125 extra-articular distal tibia fractures published in 2005, Zelle et al. reported pooled outcomes data for fractures treated non-operatively and operatively with intramedullary nailing or plate fixation.[44] Overall, there was a 2.4% rate of non-union and 14.3% rate of malunion. While the non-randomized, non-comparative, pooled data showed a significantly lower rate of non-union with non-operative treatment versus intramedullary nailing, the nail group had a significantly higher proportion of open fractures than the non-operative group (28.1% vs 1%, P<0.001) (Table 41.2). At the time of data collection for this study, there had been no prospective randomized trials comparing non-operative to operative treatment or different methods of operative fixation.

Vallier et al. retrospectively reviewed 113 distal tibia fractures 4–11 cm from the tibial plafond treated with an intramedullary nail or a medial plate.[45] Angular malalignment >5 degrees in any plane occurred in 29% of patients treated with intramedullary nailing and only 5.4% of patients treated with plating (P=0.003). Secondary procedures were more common after intramedullary nailing than plating (23.7% vs 13.5%, P=0.033). Intramedullary nailing also resulted in a non-significant trend toward higher rates of delayed or nonunion (12% vs 2.7%, P=0.10) compared with plating. In addition, there was a significantly higher rate of tibial non-union in patients who had concurrent fibular fixation (14% vs 2.6%, P=0.04) regardless of the method of tibial fixation used.

In the last 10 years, multiple randomized controlled trials have been performed to assess radiographic and clinical outcomes following intramedullary nailing and plate fixation of distal tibia fractures. Im et al. randomized 78 consecutive fractures of the distal tibia to closed reduction and intramedullary nailing versus ORIF with an anterolateral plate, 64 of which were available for 2-year follow-up.[46] Intramedullary nailing was associated with significantly

shorter operative time (72 vs 89 minutes, P = 0.02), decreased infection rate (2.9% vs 23.3%, P = 0.03) and improved ankle dorsiflexion (14 vs 7 degrees, P = 0.001), whereas plating was associated with more anatomic reduction (average angulation of 0.9 vs 2.8 degrees, P = 0.01). There were no differences in time to union or Olerud and Molander functional ankle score between groups.

Guo et al. randomized 85 patients with metaphyseal distal tibia fractures to treatment with a reamed intramedullary nail or a locked compression plate applied using a MIPO technique.[47] All fractures healed by 12 months, and there were no significant differences between groups in time to union, alignment, pain score, mean AOFAS score or proportion with wound complications. Compared to percutaneous plating, IM nailing was associated with significantly shorter operative time (81.2 vs 97.9 minutes, P = 0.001) and fluoroscopy time (2.1 vs 3.0 minutes, P = 0.001).

Vallier et al. randomized 104 extra-articular distal tibia fractures to treatment with a reamed, locked IM nail or a standard large fragment medial plate.[48] There were no significant differences between groups in rates of deep infection, non-union or secondary procedures. However, there was a significantly higher incidence of primary angular malalignment in the IM nailing group compared with the plating group (23% vs 8.3%, P=0.02). Interestingly, of the 13 fractures nailed in a malaligned position, 11 (85%) did not have fixation of the associated fibula fracture. In their discussion, the authors reported combined outcomes from the current trial and a previous retrospective comparative study performed at their institution. In this combined analysis, IM nailing was associated with higher rates of non-union (9.8% vs 3.5%, P=0.04) and malunion (27.3% vs 12.9%, P=0.006) compared with plating.

Using this same prospective patient population, Vallier et al. investigated factors influencing functional outcomes after operative fixation of distal tibia fractures.[49] At minimum 12-month follow-up, there were no significant differences in rates of malunion, secondary procedures, ongoing narcotic requirement, ankle or knee pain, Foot Function Index (FFI) or MFA scores between the plating

Table 41.2 Rates of non-union, infection, malunion and secondary surgical procedures for non-operative treatment, IM nailing and plate fixation of distal tibia fractures

Treatment	N	Non-union (95% CI)	Infection (95% CI)	Malunion (95% CI)	Revision surgery (95% CI)
Non-operative	521	1.3% (0.7% to 2.7%)	NA	15.0% (12.2% to 18.3%)	4.3% (1.4% to 11.7%)
IM nail	489	5.5% (3.7% to 8.1%)	4.3% (2.6% to 7.0%)	16.2% (16.0% to 20.0%)	16.4% (12.7% to 21.2%)
Plate	115	5.2% (2.4% to 10.9%)	2.6% (0.9% to 7.4%)	13.1% (8.0% to 20.8%)	8.7% (4.8% to 15.3%)
Total	1125	3.4% (2.5% to 4.7%)	3.9% (2.5% to 6.9%)	16.1% (14.0% to 18.6%)	12.8% (10.1% to 16.1%)

Source: Adapted from Zelle BA, et al. J Orthop Trauma. 2006; 20(1): 76–9.
Note: IM, intramedullary.

and nailing groups. Both knee and ankle pain were present in 27% of patients treated with nails compared to 15% treated with plates, a trend that did not reach statistical significance (P=0.08). Overall, 95% of individuals employed at the time of injury had returned to work at final follow-up, although 31% had modified their work activities due to their injury. Mauffrey et al. also sought to investigate the functional outcomes after operative fixation of distal tibia fractures by means of a pilot study in which 24 patients with extra-articular distal tibia fractures were randomized to IM nailing or plating.[50] After 6 months, there was a difference of 13 points in the Disability Rating Index (DRI, the primary outcome measure) favoring IM nailing. Although a difference of this magnitude is more than one and a half times the minimum clinically significant difference (MCID) on the DRI instrument, this difference failed to reach statistical significance with the number of patients and length of follow-up. The expected outcomes in patients older than 65 years have not been published. Results would be expected to be poorer than those reported in younger patients.

COMPLICATIONS

Non-union

In the prospective study by Vallier et al.,[48] primary union occurred in 100% of closed fractures, but open fractures had a 15% rate of non-union. An analysis of over 400 operatively treated tibial shaft fractures identified independent risk factors for delayed or non-union to include distal fracture location, open wounds greater than 5 cm and a postoperative gap at the fracture site.[51] Open fractures with a skin wound greater than 5 cm had the greatest impact on predicted union rates, with a relative risk of 5.7 for delayed or non-union versus closed fractures. Multiple options exist for management of distal tibial non-union. As is the case for primary fracture fixation, multiple patient and fracture related factors must be considered in selecting the appropriate treatment plan. Richmond et al. reported their results from treatment of 32 non-unions of the distal tibia with reamed, locked IM nailing.[52] Of 32 fractures, 29 healed after an average of 3.5 months, and the remaining three united after dynamization (two) or exchange nailing (one). Of four patients with positive intra-operative cultures, only two patients required nail removal after union, and none developed chronic osteomyelitis at final follow-up. Chin et al. published a series of 13 distal tibia non-unions treated with a 90-degree cannulated blade plate, all of which achieved radiographic and clinical union at an average of 15.6 weeks.[53] No secondary procedures were required to achieve union, and all patients were ambulatory without assistive devices at final follow-up.

Infection

Infected non-unions of the distal tibia present an even greater challenge to the treating surgeon. Traumatic injury to the already thin soft tissue envelope in this region often leaves limited reconstructive options. Dhar et al. reported a case series of 12 infected non-unions of the distal tibia in patients older than 55 treated with acute docking over a distance up to 2.5 cm.[54] Average limb shortening at final follow-up was 1.8 cm, and good to excellent radiographic and functional outcomes were obtained in 11 of the 12 cases. If other reconstructive options have failed, docking appears to be a reasonable salvage procedure to consider.

Reoperation

Sathiyakumar et al. conducted a retrospective review of 93 patients who underwent open reduction and medial plating of extra-articular or partial articular distal tibia fractures to identify factors influencing reoperation.[55] Overall, 35.5% of patients required at least one reoperation (28.6% of closed injuries and 45.9% of open injuries, P = 0.12). Patients with open injuries were significantly more likely to undergo reoperation for non-union, whereas patients with closed injuries were more likely to undergo reoperation for painful/prominent hardware.

REFERENCES

1. Suh TT and Lyles KW. Osteoporosis considerations in the frail elderly. *Curr Opin Rheumatol.* 2003; 15: 481–6.
2. Popp AW, Senn C, Franta O, Krieg MA, Perrelet R and Lippuner K. Tibial or hip BMD predict clinical fracture risk equally well: Results from a prospective study in 700 elderly Swiss women. *Osteoporos Int.* 2009; 20: 1393–9.
3. Court-Brown CM, Clement ND, Duckworth AD, Aitken S, Biant LC and McQueen MM. The spectrum of fractures in the elderly. *Bone Joint J.* 2014; 96-B: 366–72.
4. Ruedi T, Matter P and Allgower M. [Intra-articular fractures of the distal tibial end]. *Helv Chir Acta.* 1968; 35: 556–82.
5. Rüedi TP and Allgöwer M. Fractures of the lower end of the tibia into the ankle-joint. *Injury.* 1969; 1: 92–9.
6. Marsh JL, Slongo TF, Agel J, et al. Fracture and dislocation classification compendium—2007: Orthopaedic Trauma Association classification, database and outcomes committee. *J Orthop Trauma.* 2007; 21: S1–133.
7. Martin JS, Marsh JL, Bonar SK, DeCoster TA, Found EM and Brandser EA. Assessment of the AO/ASIF fracture classification for the distal tibia. *J Orthop Trauma.* 1997; 11: 477–83.
8. Swiontkowski MF, Sands AK, Agel J, Diab M, Schwappach JR and Kreder HJ. Interobserver variation in the AO/OTA fracture classification system for pilon fractures: Is there a problem? *J Orthop Trauma.* 1997; 11: 467–70.

9. Petrisor BA, Bhandari M and Schemitsch E. *Tibial Shaft Fractures*. In: Bucholz RW, Heckman JD, Court-Brown CM, Tornetta P, eds. *Rockwood and Green's Fractures in Adults*. Philadelphia, PA: Lippincott Williams & Wilkins; 2010, pp. 1867–927.

10. Nicoll EA. Fractures of the tibial shaft. A survey of 705 cases. *J Bone Joint Surg Br*. 1964; 46: 373–87.

11. Coles CP and Gross M. Closed tibial shaft fractures: Management and treatment complications. A review of the prospective literature. *Can J Surg*. 2000; 43: 256–62.

12. Sarmiento A and Latta LL. 450 closed fractures of the distal third of the tibia treated with a functional brace. *Clin Orthop Relat Res*. 2004; (428): 261–71.

13. Sarmiento A, Sharpe FE, Ebramzadeh E, Normand P and Shankwiler J. Factors influencing the outcome of closed tibial fractures treated with functional bracing. *Clin Orthop Relat Res*. 1995; (315): 8–24.

14. Ayeni JP. Pilon fractures of the tibia: A study based on 19 cases. *Injury*. 1988; 19: 109–14.

15. Kellam JF and Waddell JP. Fractures of the distal tibial metaphysis with intra-articular extension—The distal tibial explosion fracture. *J Trauma*. 1979; 19: 593–601.

16. Vives MJ, Abidi NA, Ishikawa SN, Taliwal RV and Sharkey PF. Soft tissue injuries with the use of safe corridors for transfixion wire placement during external fixation of distal tibia fractures: An anatomic study. *J Orthop Trauma*. 2001; 15: 555–9.

17. Richards JE, Magill M, Tressler MA, Shuler FD, Kregor PJ and Obremskey WT. External fixation versus ORIF for distal intra-articular tibia fractures. *Orthopedics*. 2012; 35: e862–7.

18. Lee YS, Chen SH, Lin JC, Chen YO, Huang CR and Cheng CY. Surgical treatment of distal tibia fractures: A comparison of medial and lateral plating. *Orthopedics*. 2009; 32: 163.

19. Bloomstein L, Schenk R and Grob P. Percutaneous plating of periarticular tibial fractures: A reliable, reproducible technique for controlling plate passage and positioning. *J Orthop Trauma*. 2008; 22: 566–71.

20. Collinge C, Kuper M, Larson K and Protzman R. Minimally invasive plating of high-energy metaphyseal distal tibia fractures. *J Orthop Trauma*. 2007; 21: 355–61.

21. Collinge C and Protzman R. Outcomes of minimally invasive plate osteosynthesis for metaphyseal distal tibia fractures. *J Orthop Trauma*. 2010; 24: 24–9.

22. Oh CW, Kyung HS, Park IH, Kim PT and Ihn JC. Distal tibia metaphyseal fractures treated by percutaneous plate osteosynthesis. *Clin Orthop Relat Res*. 2003; (408): 286–91.

23. Wolinsky P and Lee M. The distal approach for anterolateral plate fixation of the tibia: An anatomic study. *J Orthop Trauma*. 2008; 22: 404–7.

24. Ozsoy MH, Tuccar E, Demiryurek D, et al. Minimally invasive plating of the distal tibia: Do we really sacrifice saphenous vein and nerve? A cadaver study. *J Orthop Trauma*. 2009; 23: 132–8.

25. Mirza A, Moriarty AM, Probe RA and Ellis TJ. Percutaneous plating of the distal tibia and fibula: Risk of injury to the saphenous and superficial peroneal nerves. *J Orthop Trauma*. 2010; 24: 495–8.

26. Sheerin DV, Turen CH and Nascone JW. Reconstruction of distal tibia fractures using a posterolateral approach and a blade plate. *J Orthop Trauma*. 2006; 20: 247–52.

27. Sciadini MF, Manson TT and Shah SB. Trans-syndesmotic fibular plating for fractures of the distal tibia and fibula with medial soft tissue injury: Report of 6 cases and description of surgical technique. *J Orthop Trauma*. 2013; 27: e65–73.

28. Nork SE, Schwartz AK, Agel J, Holt SK, Schrick JL and Winquist RA. Intramedullary nailing of distal metaphyseal tibial fractures. *J Bone Joint Surg Am*. 2005; 87: 1213–21.

29. Wysocki RW, Kapotas JS and Virkus WW. Intramedullary nailing of proximal and distal one-third tibial shaft fractures with intraoperative two-pin external fixation. *J Trauma*. 2009; 66: 1135–9.

30. Obremskey WT and Medina M. Comparison of intramedullary nailing of distal third tibial shaft fractures: Before and after traumatologists. *Orthopedics*. 2004; 27: 1180–4.

31. Konrath G, Moed BR, Watson JT, Kaneshiro S, Karges DE and Cramer KE. Intramedullary nailing of unstable diaphyseal fractures of the tibia with distal intraarticular involvement. *J Orthop Trauma*. 1997; 11: 200–5.

32. Egol KA, Weisz R, Hiebert R, Tejwani NC, Koval KJ and Sanders RW. Does fibular plating improve alignment after intramedullary nailing of distal metaphyseal tibia fractures? *J Orthop Trauma*. 2006; 20: 94–103.

33. Weber TG, Harrington RM, Henley MB and Tencer AF. The role of fibular fixation in combined fractures of the tibia and fibula: A biomechanical investigation. *J Orthop Trauma*. 1997; 11: 206–11.

34. Kumar A, Charlebois SJ, Cain EL, Smith RA, Daniels AU and Crates JM. Effect of fibular plate fixation on rotational stability of simulated distal tibial fractures treated with intramedullary nailing. *J Bone Joint Surg Am*. 2003; 85-A: 604–8.

35. Attal R, Maestri V, Doshi HK, et al. The influence of distal locking on the need for fibular plating in intramedullary nailing of distal metaphyseal tibiofibular fractures. *Bone Joint J*. 2014; 96-B: 385–9.

36. Strauss EJ, Alfonso D, Kummer FJ, Egol KA and Tejwani NC. The effect of concurrent fibular fracture on the fixation of distal tibia fractures: A laboratory comparison of intramedullary nails with locked plates. *J Orthop Trauma*. 2007; 21: 172–7.

37. Krettek C, Miclau T, Schandelmaier P, Stephan C, Mohlmann U and Tscherne H. The mechanical effect of blocking screws ("Poller screws") in stabilizing tibia fractures with short proximal or distal fragments after insertion of small-diameter intramedullary nails. *J Orthop Trauma*. 1999; 13: 550–3.

38. Gorczyca JT, McKale J, Pugh K and Pienkowski D. Modified tibial nails for treating distal tibia fractures. *J Orthop Trauma*. 2002; 16: 18–22.

39. Dunn WR, Easley ME, Parks BG, Trnka HJ and Schon LC. An augmented fixation method for distal fibular fractures in elderly patients: A biomechanical evaluation. *Foot Ankle Int*. 2004; 25: 128–31.

40. Panchbhavi VK, Vallurupalli S, Morris R and Patterson R. The use of calcium sulfate and calcium phosphate composite graft to augment screw purchase in osteoporotic ankles. *Foot Ankle Int*. 2008; 29: 593–600.

41. Hoenig M, Gao F, Kinder J, Zhang LQ, Collinge C and Merk BR. Extra-articular distal tibia fractures: A mechanical evaluation of 4 different treatment methods. *J Orthop Trauma*. 2010; 24: 30–5.

42. Hoegel FW, Hoffmann S, Weninger P, Buhren V and Augat P. Biomechanical comparison of locked plate osteosynthesis, reamed and unreamed nailing in conventional interlocking technique, and unreamed angle stable nailing in distal tibia fractures. *J Trauma Acute Care Surg*. 2012; 73: 933–8.

43. Gueorguiev B, Wahnert D, Albrecht D, Ockert B, Windolf M and Schwieger K. Effect on dynamic mechanical stability and interfragmentary movement of angle-stable locking of intramedullary nails in unstable distal tibia fractures: A biomechanical study. *J Trauma*. 2011; 70: 358–65.

44. Zelle BA, Bhandari M, Espiritu M, Koval KJ, Zlowodzki M and Evidence-Based Orthopaedic Trauma Working Group. Treatment of distal tibia fractures without articular involvement: A systematic review of 1125 fractures. *J Orthop Trauma*. 2006; 20: 76–9.

45. Vallier HA, Le TT and Bedi A. Radiographic and clinical comparisons of distal tibia shaft fractures (4 to 11 cm proximal to the plafond): Plating versus intramedullary nailing. *J Orthop Trauma*. 2008; 22: 307–11.

46. Im GI and Tae SK. Distal metaphyseal fractures of tibia: A prospective randomized trial of closed reduction and intramedullary nail versus open reduction and plate and screws fixation. *J Trauma*. 2005; 59: 1219–23; discussion 23.

47. Guo JJ, Tang N, Yang HL and Tang TS. A prospective, randomised trial comparing closed intramedullary nailing with percutaneous plating in the treatment of distal metaphyseal fractures of the tibia. *J Bone Joint Surg Br*. 2010; 92: 984–8.

48. Vallier HA, Cureton BA and Patterson BM. Randomized, prospective comparison of plate versus intramedullary nail fixation for distal tibia shaft fractures. *J Orthop Trauma*. 2011; 25: 736–41.

49. Vallier HA, Cureton BA and Patterson BM. Factors influencing functional outcomes after distal tibia shaft fractures. *J Orthop Trauma*. 2012; 26: 178–83.

50. Mauffrey C, McGuinness K, Parsons N, Achten J and Costa ML. A randomised pilot trial of "locking plate" fixation versus intramedullary nailing for extra-articular fractures of the distal tibia. *J Bone Joint Surg Br*. 2012; 94: 704–8.

51. Audige L, Griffin D, Bhandari M, Kellam J and Ruedi TP. Path analysis of factors for delayed healing and nonunion in 416 operatively treated tibial shaft fractures. *Clin Orthop Relat Res*. 2005; 438: 221–32.

52. Richmond J, Colleran K, Borens O, Kloen P and Helfet DL. Nonunions of the distal tibia treated by reamed intramedullary nailing. *J Orthop Trauma*. 2004; 18: 603–10.

53. Chin KR, Nagarkatti DG, Miranda MA, Santoro VM, Baumgaertner MR and Jupiter JB. Salvage of distal tibia metaphyseal nonunions with the 90 degrees cannulated blade plate. *Clin Orthop Relat Res*. 2003; (409): 241–9.

54. Dhar SA, Butt MF, Mir MR, Kawoosa AA, Sultan A and Dar TA. Draining infected non union of the distal third of the tibia. The use of invaginating docking over short distances in older patients. *Ortop Traumatol Rehabil*. 2009; 11: 264–70.

55. Sathiyakumar V, Thakore RV, Ihejirika RC, Obremskey WT and Sethi MK. Distal tibia fractures and medial plating: Factors influencing re-operation. *Int Orthop*. 2014; 38: 1483–8.

42

Ankle fractures

MURRAY D. SPRUIELL AND CYRIL MAUFFREY

INTRODUCTION

The current trend of an increasingly aging population associated with a more active lifestyle is changing the epidemiology of fractures, as well as altering healthcare costs and medical and surgical treatment strategies. The problems related to osteoporosis have become one of the priorities in most healthcare systems and considerable efforts have been made to reduce the financial burden associated with this ever-growing subgroup of patients. However, despite these efforts orthopaedic surgeons are faced with an epidemic of fragility fractures in a group of patients who wish to get back to their pre-injury level of activity as soon as possible. Both the equipment manufacturing industry and orthopaedic researchers have addressed this expanding market in an attempt to solve the problems of reduction and fixation of osteoporotic fractures. To complicate things further, patients with fragility fractures have poorer soft tissues and an increased prevalence of associated medical comorbidities that put them at risk of developing complications. They also have a lower physiological reserve making early mobilization more challenging.

This chapter reviews ankle fractures in older patients and focuses on the changing epidemiology, treatment strategies and surgical options when traditional treatment methods fail. We also review common complications as well as solutions that can be utilized to treat these fractures and prevent their occurrence.

EPIDEMIOLOGY

The age at which ankle fractures are defined as occurring in elderly patients varies, but it has tended to increase in more recent studies. Beauchamp et al.[1] defined it as 50 years in 1983, but Vioreanu et al.[2] defined it as 70 years in 2007. Many surgeons accept an age of ≥65 years as defining an elderly patient and ≥80 years as defining a super-elderly patient. However, we believe that it is important to consider the patients' physiological age as opposed to their chronological age, as patients' comorbidities often dictate treatment. We believe that strict reliance on an age range is often of little value.

Ankle fractures are the fourth most common fracture in the ≥65-year-old age group after proximal femoral, distal radial and proximal humeral fractures.[3] A review of the data presented in Chapter 1 shows that about 90% of ankle fractures in this group follow a standing fall and that only 3% are high energy injuries. A further 3% present with multiple fractures. In the super-elderly group there are fewer high energy injuries, but over 6% of patients have multiple fractures, confirming the relative frailty of this group. Overall ankle fractures in the ≥65-year-old group have a type IV pattern with a relatively constant incidence of fractures in females aged between 65–69 years and 90+ years, but a declining incidence in males (Chapter 1).

Review of the different fracture types in the series presented in Chapter 1 shows that 25.9% were AO/OTA type A fractures, 67.6% were type B fractures and 6.5% were type C fractures. In the super-elderly group the equivalent figures were 24.1%, 74.4% and 1.3%, indicating the reduction in prevalence of type C supra-syndesmotic fractures with increasing age. There were no type C ankle fractures in females 80 years or older and none in males aged 75 years or older.

Chapter 1 also shows that there is a relatively high incidence of open ankle fractures in females, and in females aged ≥65 years only open fractures of the distal radius and ulna and the finger phalanges had a higher incidence. About 57% of open fractures in females aged ≥65 years were Gustilo and Anderson[4] type III in severity. This rose to about 73% in the super-elderly group, confirming increasing patient frailty and the poorer condition of the soft tissues around the ankle in the aging patient.

There is evidence that the incidence of ankle fractures is increasing in the elderly population. Kannus et al.[5] looked at the epidemiology of ankle fractures in Finland between 1970 and 2000 and showed that the incidence of low velocity ankle fractures in patients aged ≥60 years was $57/10^5$/year in 1970 and $150/10^5$/year in 2000. In males it rose from $38/10^5$/year to $114/10^5$/year and in females it rose from $66/10^5$/year to $174/10^5$/year. This study only examined in-patients and therefore might have underestimated the incidence of ankle fractures, particularly in 1970 when less surgical treatment would have been undertaken.

An analysis of the equivalent figures in Edinburgh confirms that the incidence of ankle fractures in the elderly is increasing. In 2000 the incidence of ankle fractures in males aged ≥60 years was $83/10^5$/year. This rose to $107/10^5$/year in 2010/2011. The equivalent figures for females were $159/10^5$/year and $213/10^5$/year. In the super-elderly population the incidence of male ankle fractures rose from $55/10^5$/year in 2000 to $99/10^5$/year in 2010/2011. The equivalent figures for the super-elderly female group were $166/10^5$/year and $174/10^5$/year. This suggests that the males were more active and less frail in 2010/2011 than in 2000. It has been shown that smoking, polypharmacy and poor mobility are the factors that best predict ankle fractures in the elderly,[6] but it would be reasonable to suggest that as the elderly get fitter and the population ages, ankle fractures will continue to increase in incidence and have a significantly greater impact on society.

CLASSIFICATION

In general, the Lauge-Hansen[7] and AO/OTA[8] classifications are used to describe the different patterns of ankle fractures, although they are suboptimal for elderly patients as they are less likely to guide treatment than in a younger patient population. In addition, the classic fracture configurations that characterize different fracture subtypes in the Lauge-Hansen classification are not always seen in elderly patients. Poor bone quality and the consequences of lengthy osteoporosis medication can alter the classic fracture patterns that are seen in younger patients. However, there are, as yet, no classifications for ankle fractures in the elderly.

The Lauge-Hansen classification[7] is based on the position of the foot at the time of fracture (supination or pronation) and the direction of the deforming force (abduction, adduction, internal or external rotation). This gives four types of injury, these being supination external rotation (SER), pronation external rotation (PER), supination adduction (SA) and pronation abduction (PA). A number is then applied which refers to the progression through the stages of bone and soft tissue injury. The Lauge–Hansen classification is summarized in Table 42.1. The AO/OTA[8] classification is derived from the earlier Weber classification and is a morphological classification. Type A fractures occur below the level of the inferior tibio-fibular syndesmotic ligaments. A1 fractures are unifocal lateral lesions. In A2 fractures there is an associated medial malleolar fracture and in A3 fractures there is an associated posteromedial fracture. Type B fractures are trans-syndesmotic fractures. In B1 fractures there is an oblique or spiral distal fibular fracture. In B2 fractures there is an associated medial malleolar fracture and in B3 fractures there is an associated posterior malleolar fracture. Type C fractures are rare in the elderly. These are supra-syndesmotic fractures with C1 fractures having a simple fibular fracture with damage to the anterior tibio-fibular ligaments. In C2 fractures the fibular fracture is multifragmentary and in C3 fractures the fibular fracture is located in the proximal fibula.

In open fractures (Figure 42.1) the Gustilo and Anderson[4] classification is universally used, but it is not as predictive of outcome in the elderly as it is in younger patients. This is because of poorer skin quality and the state of the soft tissues. There is often difficulty in skin closure and soft tissue treatment can be a challenge because of the difficulties of surgery and the associated medical comorbidities in these patients. Open fractures in the elderly are discussed further in Chapter 13.

TREATMENT

The goals of treatment for this patient population are early mobilization and return to performing activities of daily living as the same comorbidities that may influence the mode of treatment can decompensate with a prolonged recovery and adversely affect patients' outcomes from a general health perspective. Regardless of the chosen mode of treatment, the surgeon must emphasize medical optimization during the healing phase. This includes encouraging adequate sun exposure, a healthy diet with adequate protein and calcium intake, avoidance of alcohol and tobacco, and perhaps even arranging follow-up with a primary care physician to direct and encourage the above interventions. Patients must be counselled about the diagnosis and treatment of osteoporosis and when required a DEXA scan should be ordered. Osteoporosis is diagnosed by the presence of a fragility fracture, or if bone mineral density of the spine, hip or wrist is less than 2.5 standard deviations from the reference mean (T score of −2.5 or less). The United States Preventative Services Task Force (USPSTF) provides recommendations for routine screening of women aged 65 years or greater. Additionally, the USPSTF recommends this screening to begin at age 60 in high risk females based on several clinical considerations (body weight <70 kg, smoking, weight loss, family history, alcohol/caffeine use and/or low calcium/vitamin D).[9]

Table 42.1 Lauge-Hansen classification of ankle fractures

Fracture severity	SER	SA	PER	PA
I	Anterior tibio-fibular sprain	Talofibular sprain or avulsion of distal fibula	Isolated medial malleolar fracture or deltoid ligament rupture	Isolated medial malleolar fracture or deltoid ligament rupture
II	Stable short oblique fracture of the distal fibula	Vertical medial malleolar and transverse distal fibular fracture. Possible medial plafond impaction	Anterior tibio-fibular ligament injury or fracture of Chaput's tubercule	Anterior tibio-fibular ligament injury or fracture of Chaput's tubercule
III	As for II with additional rupture of posterior tibio-fibular ligament or fracture of posterior tibial margin		Medial malleolar fracture or deltoid ligament injury with high fibular fracture	Transverse or laterally comminuted fibular fracture with medial malleolar fracture or deltoid ligament injury. Possible anterolateral tibial impaction
IV	Unstable short oblique fracture of the distal fibula with a medial malleolar fracture or a deltoid ligament rupture		As for III with posterior malleolar fracture or tibio-fibular ligament injury	

Note: PA, pronation abduction; PER, pronation external rotation; SA, supination adduction; SER, supination external rotation.

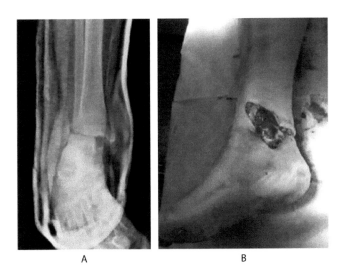

A   B

Figure 42.1 A 77-year-old woman who presented with an open Gustilo type II ankle fracture dislocation. **(a)** Anteroposterior (AP) radiograph of the ankle showing a lateral malleolar fracture. **(b)** Clinical photograph of the medial open wound exposing the medial malleolus.

NON-OPERATIVE MANAGEMENT

Non-operative management refers to the use of a cast or brace. It is often referred to as 'conservative' management due to the avoidance of surgical risk. However, one must appreciate that the use of casts or braces in the elderly population can result in adverse events. Diabetes and patients with frail skin are at risk of developing soft tissue damage, particularly if the cast or brace is poorly applied. Careful attention must be paid to provide extra padding over the bony prominences most at risk of skin damage, these being the medial and lateral malleoli and the heel. The cast should also be reinforced with more casting material in the elderly to avoid damage associated with weight bearing as it is often impractical for elderly patients to remain non-weight bearing.

Casts are often preferred to braces because of the ease of application and moulding. However, it should be remembered that plaster material undergoes an exothermic reaction that can severely burn patients. Lavalette demonstrated that increased plaster thickness, increased water temperature and unintentional insulation caused by placing a pillow beneath the splint during the setting process were all related to the generation of temperatures high enough to cause skin burns.[10] This is especially important in elderly patients as their fragile skin and comorbidities place them at increased risk. Halanski et al. recommend using water temperatures lower than 24°C to reduce the risk of thermal injury.[11] Splint material should be cut to the appropriate length and folding the splint material should be avoided. The splint should not be allowed to sit on a pillow or to have inadequate ventilation and it should not be over-wrapped with fibreglass casting material until it is completely cooled.[11]

The use of non-operative management in elderly patients with ankle fractures has changed in the last few decades. Beauchamp et al.[1] compared operative and non-operative management in 126 patients over 50 years of age between 1976 and 1979. They stated that operative fixation achieved better reduction, but there was a higher complication rate in females. They stressed that patient satisfaction was very similar. Salai et al.[12] stated that non-operatively managed patients had higher AOFAS scores after 3 years and that 33% of patients required hardware removal. They advocated the use of non-operative management if reduction could be maintained in a cast.

More recently Vioreanu et al.[2] analysed 40 patients with non-operatively managed ankle fractures. The average age was 78.6 years and 28 (70%) were independent. They reported that 27.5% of the patients subsequently required surgery and 17.2% required re-manipulation. Only 45% of the patients returned to their pre-fracture activity level. They compared the group with a similar cohort of patients that had been managed operatively and recorded that 72% of their patients returned to their pre-accident activity levels.

The recent literature indicates that non-operatively managed displaced ankle fractures in the elderly are associated with poorer results than operatively managed fractures. We suggest that non-operative management is only used for undisplaced fractures or if the physical state of the patient means that they cannot undergo surgery. If it is to be used for displaced fractures, serial radiographs should be obtained after reduction to look for secondary displacement.

OPERATIVE MANAGEMENT

Operative management for ankle fractures in the elderly is associated with better results, but the surgeon has a number of challenges which differ from those encountered in younger patients. The poorer bone quality can make the usual methods of fracture reduction and fixation more difficult. For example, serrated reduction forceps, which are often used to reduce fibular fractures, can easily cause increased comminution with minimal force. Restoring length and rotation can be quite difficult and surgeons may have to rely on more indirect methods of reduction. In addition, comminution of the fracture fragments can make fracture reduction very difficult and the use of lag screws impossible. There are a number of operative techniques that can be used to treat ankle fractures in the elderly.

Conventional plating

The standard technique used to treat ankle fractures in all ages is compression plating of the fibula with screw fixation of the medial malleolus and posterior malleolus, if required. In recent years different plates have been introduced, but compression plating and screw fixation remains in widespread use. The plates that are usually used are one-third tubular plates or dynamic compression plates. As has already been discussed, the results of plate fixation, combined with appropriate fixation of the medial and posterior malleoli, are better than those associated with non-operative management. A review of the results associated with plate fixation for

ankle fractures in the elderly is presented in Table 42.2.[2,13–19] It shows that the complications associated with plate fixation in the elderly range from 8% to 35%. The various studies in Table 42.2 list their complications differently but it should be understood that many of these complications are medical with deep venous thrombosis being a significant problem. Medical complications also occur in non-operative management. Table 42.2 shows that the surgical complications have a relatively low prevalence in elderly patients. The rates of deep infection, non-union and malunion are low and while the rate of superficial infection is higher, the papers indicate that it was usually successfully treated.

A number of studies have investigated functional outcome after plate fixation. Davidovitch et al.[16] used the AOFAS score to compare patients <60 years of age with those aged ≥60 years. They showed no overall difference over a 12-month period, but older patients did report greater functional limitation than younger patients at 3 months, 6 months and 12 months. At 12 months after fixation 7.4% of patients aged >60 years reported functional limitation compared with 29% of patients aged <60 years. In a more recent study, Little et al.[18] compared surgical treatment of SER IV ankle fractures (Table 42.1) in older and younger populations. They reported that despite the older patients having higher rates of diabetes and peripheral vascular disease, there were statistically better Foot and Ankle Outcome Scores in the geriatric population than in the younger population. They also reported that there was no significant difference in articular reduction, syndesmotic reduction, wound complications, postoperative infections or range of motion between the two groups. The literature suggests that 72–84% of elderly patients with ankle fractures return to their previous level of activity[14–19] and Pagliaro et al.[13] stated that 91% of patients were discharged home after initial fixation of the ankle fracture.

There is one study of plate fixation in the super-elderly.[17] In this study 92.3% of patients were treated with conventional one-third tubular plates or dynamic compression plates and the remaining 7.7% had a locking plate. Table 42.2 shows that, as with the ≥65-year-old group, most of the complications were medical and that the prevalence of surgical complications was very similar to those seen in the elderly group of patients. The 30-day mortality was 5.4%. This rose to 8.7% at 3 months and 12% at 1 year. Despite the patients advanced age, 86% had returned to their pre-injury mobility by 3–6 months.

Locking plates

In recent years there has been considerable interest in the use of monoaxial and polyaxial locking plates to treat osteoporotic fractures. When screw purchase is poor, a fixed angle construct needs to be employed (Figure 42.2). In conventional plates part of the force created by screw insertion creates friction between the plate and the bone with the remainder left to resist the forces of physiological loading, such as weight bearing. In locking plating none of the screw force is used to create friction between the plate

Table 42.2 Complications listed in recent papers discussing use of plates in management of ankle fractures in the elderly

Author(s) (year)	No	Age (years)	Complications (%)	Deep infection (%)	Superficial infection (%)	Non-union/ malunion (%)
Pagliaro et al. (2001)[13]	23	72	34.8	4.3	13.0	0
Srinivasan and Moran (2001)[14]	74	76	18.9	1.4	9.5	5.4
Makwana et al. (2001)[15]	36	66	8.3	0	1.5	0
Vioreanu et al. (2007)[2]	72	76.4	9.7	0	4.2	0
Davidovitch et al. (2009)[16]	34	68.9	20.6	2.9	2.9	2.9
Shivarathre et al. (2011)[17]	92	85.2	22.8	4.3	6.5	3.3
Little et al. (2013)[18]	27	≥65	29.6	3.7	7.4	7.4
Zaghloul et al. (2014)[19]	186	70.7	23.7	7.0	9.1	4.8
Total	544		20.6	3.9	7.3	3.7

Note: In all papers at least 70% of the patients were treated by conventional lateral plating techniques.

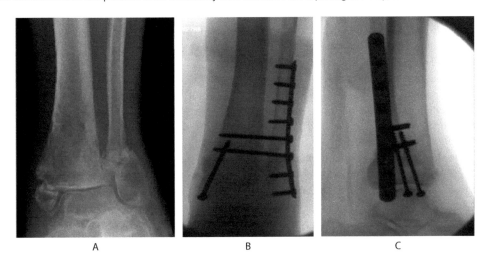

A B C

Figure 42.2 (a) An 82-year-old woman who developed symptomatic non-union following non-operative management of a bimalleolar ankle fracture. She was treated with a locked fibular plate and syndesmotic screw fixation through the plate. (b,c) Postoperative anteroposterior and lateral radiographs.

and the bone and thus the function of the construct is to resist physiological loading and maintain the alignment achieved at the time of fixation. In a cadaveric biomechanical model contoured locking plates for fibular fixation of osteoporotic bone were found to have higher torque to failure and maximal torque, compared with conventional non-locking methods.[20] In theory this fixed angle construct may be advantageous in the elderly who may be less capable of complying with weight-bearing restrictions. It is, however, worth noting that failure of fixation with locked constructs occurs differently than with conventional plates. Instead of screw loosening and implant failure with loss of reduction, locked constructs undergo catastrophic failure. Since the screws are screwed into the plate, the screws rarely loosen and instead the bone around the screws tends to fail. This can result in catastrophic failure of the entire construct with cut-out and intra-articular penetration.[21] Additionally, plate breakage can occur if there is insufficient working length or if non-locking screws are placed after locking screw insertion. Screw breakage may also occur below the plate due to the inability of the screws to loosen in response to repetitive axial loading.

In other locations the use of locking plates has not been shown to be advantageous and Vallier and Immler[22] have shown that in distal tibial fractures locking plates did not give better results than the previous generation of plates. Lynde et al.[23] compared the use of locking and non-locking plates in ankle fractures in patients aged ≥60 years. They found that locking plates were associated with a higher rate of hardware failure and revision surgery than non-locking plates, but the results were not statistically significant. However, locking plates were associated with a statistically significant increase in wound dehiscence. A similar study was undertaken by Schepers et al.[24] who showed that there was a statistically significant increase in wound complications associated with locking plates. They found an 8.3-fold increase in major complications in the locking plate group in which plate removal was required. Multivariate analysis showed the difference in wound complications remained significant after gender, patient age, smoking, diabetes, use of titanium, grade of surgeon or the classification of fracture was taken into account. It may well be that with lower profile locking plates the wound complications will diminish in the future, but at the moment there is little clinical evidence that locking plates confer any benefit over non-locking plates in the treatment of ankle fractures in the elderly.

Posterolateral plating

Posterolateral antiglide plating can also be used for fibular stabilization. There are several advantages to this method of fixation. If posterolateral plating is used there is better soft tissue cover and wound complications are less likely to occur. Several biomechanical studies have demonstrated improved fixation strength compared to lagged screw fixation and lateral plating using both conventional[25] and locking[26] plates. Posterolateral fixation is an excellent technique if the distal fragment is comminuted, and stable fixation is difficult, as fixation of the distal fragment is unnecessary with this technique. However, for additional stability the distal fragment may be fixed to the proximal fibular fracture by placing a lag screw through the plate (Figure 42.3). The most common complication of the technique is peroneal tendon irritation. The plate may need to be removed if this occurs. If a lag screw is placed through the plate, care should be taken to avoid screw head prominence which increases peroneal irritation.[25]

Little et al.[28] reviewed a series of 112 SER ankle fractures treated by posterolateral plating. They documented 4.4% deep infection and 1.8% superficial infection which compares with the results for lateral plating shown in Table 42.2. They had to remove the hardware in 7.1% of the patients because of pain. They also stressed the potential for damage to the superficial peroneal nerve in the lateral approach and they only had one (0.9%) case using the posterolateral approach. However, surgeons should be aware that the sural nerve is at risk with this approach.

Injectable cement or bone substitutes

Recently there has been interest in using injectable cement to improve screw purchase in osteoporotic bone. In a biomechanical study Motzkin et al. found improved pull-out strength when inserting cortical screws into fluid state polymethylmethacrylate (PMMA) or into solid state PMMA which was drilled and tapped after hardening.[29] Different types of cement have also been investigated. Larsson et al. found that injectable calcium phosphate cement improved pull-out strength in osteoporotic bone biomechanical models.[30] Collinge et al. compared PMMA with tricalcium phosphate cement and found comparable pull-out strength.[31] Panchbhavi et al. also found significantly greater purchase and load to failure using injectable calcium sulphate and calcium phosphate cements compared with non-augmented screw replacement.[32] Thus the use of resorbable cements may be an excellent option because of their improved biocompatibility compared with PMMA, while maintaining the goal of improved screw purchase and stable fixation. This technique can potentially allow for early return to weight bearing and better range of motion, but as yet there are few clinical results.

Tension band wiring

Tension band wiring is a classic technique employed to achieve direct bone healing of medial malleolar fractures. It is particularly useful in cases of comminuted fractures which are unable to accept 3.5 or 4.0 mm screws. In this technique Kirschner wires (K-wires) are directed proximally into the tibial metaphysis from the tip of the medial malleolus through as many fracture fragments as possible. The wires are passed distal to the main fracture line and typically two wires are used. A unicortical, partially threaded screw is placed obliquely into the distal tibial metaphysis proximal to the main fracture line. A 20-gauge wire is wrapped underneath the deltoid ligament and the K-wires distally and around the screw head proximally. Appropriate tension is applied to maintain fracture reduction (Figure 42.4). Biomechanical studies have demonstrated this technique to provide a stiffer construct than screw fixation alone.[33] It has been shown that it has twice the maximal load to failure.[34] However, it should be noted that these studies were not undertaken in osteoporotic bone models.

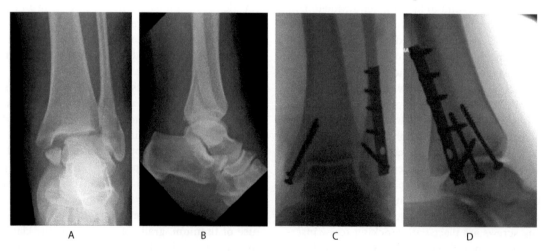

A   B   C   D

Figure 42.3 Supination external rotation (SER) type IV ankle fracture treated with posterolateral antiglide plating, with a lag screw through the plate reducing the distal fragment. **(a,b)** Preoperative radiographs; **(c,d)** postoperative result.

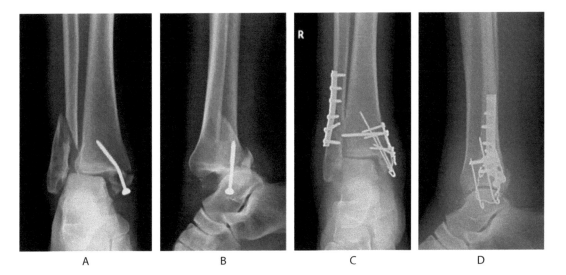

A	B	C	D

Figure 42.4 This patient sustained a trimalleolar ankle fracture through a lag screw placed 28 years earlier for a medial malleolus fracture. (a,b) Preoperative radiographs. Significant comminution of the medial malleolus necessitated tension band fixation. An antiglide one-third tubular plate was applied posteromedially for fixation of a large posterior fragment. (c,d) Postoperative radiographs.

Syndesmotic fixation

McKean et al. showed that the syndesmosis was not typically involved in osteoporotic ankle fractures as the ligamentous structures become stronger than the bone with increasing age.[35] It is somewhat analogous to paediatric ankle fractures associated with open physes. However, in cases without any apparent syndesmotic injury, some surgeons argue that the tibia-pro-fibular screw constructs should be employed to achieve better purchase and more stable fixation. This involves placing screws through the fibula into the tibia obtaining purchase in either three or four cortices rather than the standard bicortical fibular screw placement.

Intramedullary nailing

Intramedullary nailing of the fibula is a technique that minimizes soft tissue dissection and permits good fracture reduction and fixation. Unlocked intramedullary pins have been used for many years with good results. Pritchett[36] compared the use of Rush pins with standard lateral plating in a prospective randomized study. He found that 88% of elderly patients treated with Rush pins had good or fair functional results compared with 76% of patients treated with plates. He also found that full weight bearing was possible 6 weeks earlier if a Rush pin was used.

In a similar study, Lee et al.[37] compared the use of a Knowles pin with lateral plating. Both groups had an average age of at least 60 years. They found that the group treated with Knowles pins had significantly smaller skin incisions, shorter surgery time, shorter hospital stays, less symptomatic hardware and lower complication rates than the group treated by plating. An analysis of the complications showed that 13.3% of the plating group showed complications similar to those listed in Table 42.2. None of the groups treated with

a Knowles pin had complications. The authors recommended fibular nailing in elderly patients.

In recent years there has been increased interest in the use of locking fibular nails (Figure 42.5). Rajeev et al.[38] undertook a retrospective review of 24 patients treated with a locking fibular nail. The average age of the patients was 79 years. There were no intraoperative complications and the average time to fracture union was 8.7 weeks. There were no infections, non-unions or wound breakdowns. Twenty-one (87.5%) of the patients were discharged within 2 weeks and 18 (75%) had no pain on final follow-up.

Bugler et al.[39] undertook a similar study in 105 patients with an average age of 64.8 years. They recorded that 75% of the patients had pre-existing medical comorbidities. The authors analysed the merits of using a locking nail. In six patients nailed without locking screws, only 66% of the fractures had satisfactory stability. If distal locking screws were used, 96% of fractures were stable and if a supplementary proximal blocking screw was used, 93% of the fractures were stable. As a result of their experience with the locking system, the authors recommend the use of a distal locking screw and a screw placed across the syndesmosis (Figure 42.5). Both of the studies using locked fibular nailing had improved results when compared with the results of lateral plating shown in Table 42.2 and it seems logical to recommend fibular nailing, particularly for the very elderly and those patients with significant comorbidities.

Intramedullary fixation can also be employed using intramedullary screws or Kirschner wires (K-wires) for fibular fixation. This is a percutaneous technique and is particularly useful for elderly diabetic patients with low functional demands. The K-wires are left protruding through the skin and removed when the fracture has united. Figure 42.6 shows a case in which an elderly, obese patient with diabetes underwent closed reduction and percutaneous K-wire

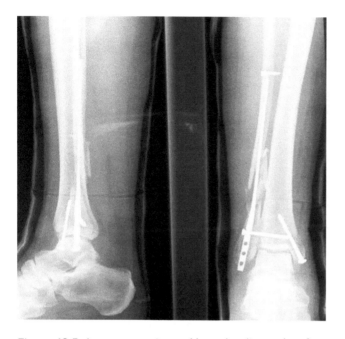

Figure 42.5 Anteroposterior and lateral radiographs of a Pronation Abduction type III (PAIII) injury with extensive fibular comminution. A locked fibular nail has been used with a trans-syndesmotic screw.

fixation because it was considered that there was a high risk of infection as a result of the poor soft tissues and patient cormorbidities.

External fixation

External fixation is often used for the staged management of severe ankle injuries which are not amenable to primary open reduction and internal fixation (Figure 42.7). These occur with open fractures or with severe soft tissue compromise. Occasionally external fixation may be used as a definitive mode of fixation. Our preferred method of external fixation involves the use of anterior tibial pins, transverse calcaneal pin placement and a delta frame. We also arrange the external fixator frame to avoid the patient having to rest their leg directly on the compromised skin.

Other techniques

Some ankle fractures, particularly those referred to tertiary referral centres, may not be amenable to fixation using the techniques that have been described. It is important for the

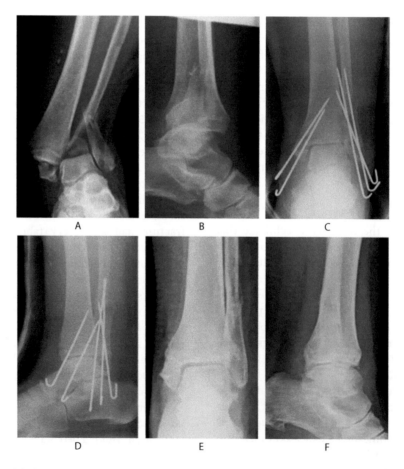

Figure 42.6 An 85-year-old obese osteoporotic woman with diabetes presented with a bimalleolar fracture dislocation of the ankle (a,b). She was treated by closed reduction and K-wire placement in the medial and lateral malleoli (c,d). The wires were removed when the fracture was healed. Good alignment and is demonstrated on the anteroposterior and lateral radiographs (e,f) taken 4 months after fixation. (Case courtesy of David Seligson.)

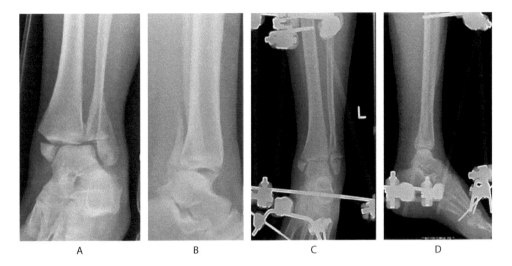

Figure 42.7 **(a,b)** Anteroposterior and lateral radiographs of an ankle fracture dislocation sustained 2 weeks earlier and left unreduced by another hospital. The swelling of the soft tissues did not permit open reduction internal fixation and the patient was placed in a temporary external fixator with forefoot pins to prevent equinus deformity **(c,d)**. Definitive fixation was performed 2 weeks later.

orthopaedic traumatologist to develop strategies to permit treatment of those patients with fractures which cannot be fixed with lateral plating, posterolateral plating, locking plates or intramedullary nails. These cases are usually associated with large wounds or significant skin compromise, but surgeons may also have to treat very osteoporotic patients, patients with neglected ankle fractures, postoperative infections or patients who present with malreduced or ununited ankle fractures.

Surgeons will have to use their judgement and experience to apply appropriate treatment methods. They will need to consider the fracture type, bone and soft tissue quality, the presence of infection, alignment and the stage of fracture healing.

Other factors will also influence the surgical strategy. These include patient compliance, associated comorbidities such as diabetes, the immune status of the patient, smoking and alcohol intake. There are a number of surgical techniques which may be used.

TRANSCALCANEAL PINNING

This technique can be used to correct talar translation and poor mechanical alignment in patients with delayed presentation of fibular fractures. It can also be used when the status of the skin is not amenable to a surgical incision. We have found that the technique is associated with a high complication rate, particularly infection, although this may represent selection bias. In this technique reduction of the fracture fragments is undertaken indirectly using manual traction in the same way as an acute fracture is reduced. Once reduction is achieved Steinmann pins or K-wires (Figure 42.8) are passed vertically upwards from the plantar aspect of the heel across the subtalar and ankle joint. This allows reduction to be maintained without disturbing the soft tissues around the ankle.

RETROGRADE TIBIOTALOCALCANEAL NAILING

Tibiotalocalcaneal (TTC) fusion with a retrograde nail is often described as a salvage procedure for ankle arthritis, Charcot arthropathy, avascular necrosis of the talus or failed total ankle replacement.[40] For patients who are not candidates for open reduction and internal fixation, primary fusion is a viable option. Retrograde nailing should also be considered for low demand patients as the requirement for future surgery to treat post-traumatic arthritis is removed and the patient can be rendered pain free with one operation (Figure 42.9).

TTC fusion is not without its complications! A systematic review of 33 cases, undertaken by Jehan et al.,[41] showed that the most common indications for the operation were inflammatory arthritis (22.6%), followed by neuropathic arthropathy (21.7%) and secondary osteoarthritis (21.6%). Only 1.2% of the patients in the study had a TTC fusion to treat a fracture. The main complications recorded in the study were metalwork problems (30.0%), non-union (23.8%), infection (15.1%) and delayed union (6.4%). The conclusions were that the technique was associated with a relatively high union rate, but it also had a high complication rate.

The same type of nail can be used to stabilize an ankle fracture in an elderly patient in the same way as has been described for Steinmann pins. Lemon et al.[42] described the use of an expandable calcaneotalotibial nail in 12 female patients with an average age of 84 years. The nail was placed through the calcaneus and talus into the tibial intramedullary canal. There were no intraoperative complications and all patients began weight bearing 1 day after surgery. There were no cases of delayed union, non-union or talar shift. Eleven of the patients returned to their pre-injury mobility and had no pain. The 1-year mortality was 16.7% and the 2-year mortality was 33.3%.

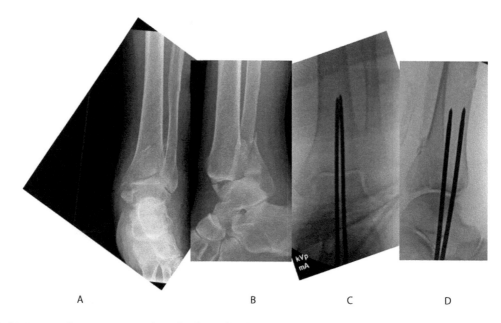

Figure 42.8 **(a,b)** A severely osteoporotic bimalleolar ankle fracture dislocation shown in a 70 years old diabetic patient. The state of the skin and the patient's comorbidities prevented us from performing an open reduction internal fixation and we elected to use transcutaneous pins through the calcaneus, talus and tibia to stabilize the ankle mortise **(c,d)**.

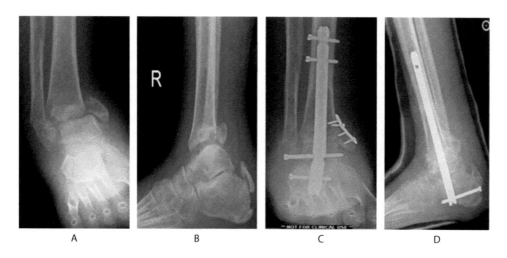

Figure 42.9 **(a,b)** A severe injury in an elderly woman showing a trimalleolar fracture, significant articular damage and a calcaneal tuberosity fracture. **(c,d)** An ankle fusion using a retrograde tibiotalocalcaneal nail was carried out.

Two other recent studies have shown similar results. Jonas et al.[43] undertook a retrospective study of 31 patients with a mean age of 77 years. All were weight bearing 1 day after surgery and the majority were discharged from hospital within 2 weeks. There were three (9.7%) periprosthetic fractures and two (6.5%) broken nails. The authors stressed that there was a risk of implant failure in more active patients. Al-Nammari et al.[44] treated 48 patients with a retrograde nail. There was one deep infection, four superficial infections and screw breakage occurred in three patients. They stressed that the main complications were medical, as shown in Table 42.2 for lateral plating, but they felt that the technique was very useful in the elderly frail patient.

The technique can be used with an interlocking nail augmented with an antibiotic coating. The use of an antibiotic coated cement interlocking nail in unsalvageable cases of infected, malreduced or ununited ankle fractures in poor hosts is useful. We have started using MRI compatible interlocking carbon fibre antibiotic nails for these indications (Figure 42.10). It allows MRI monitoring of the osteomyelitis when inflammatory markers are unreliable.[45]

OPEN FRACTURES

The literature contains very little information about the optimal treatment and prognosis of open ankle fractures in the elderly. We have already pointed out that open ankle

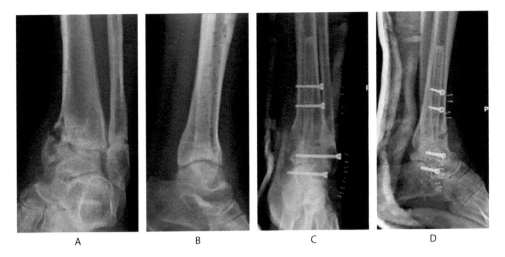

A   B   C   D

Figure 42.10 An unsalvageable osteomyelitic arthritic ankle fracture malunion (**a,b**) treated with a newly developed technique using a MR compatible carbon fibre retrograde antibiotic interlocked fusion nail (**c,d**). This allows MRI follow-up of the osteomyelitis.

fractures in the elderly (Figure 42.1) are more commonly seen than many other open fractures particularly in females and in patients aged ≥80 years. There is a high incidence of Gustilo type III fractures because of the poor state of the skin and soft tissues. The epidemiology of open fractures is discussed in Chapter 1.

The papers listed in Table 42.2 contain some information on the success of treating open ankle fractures in the elderly. These papers document information on 30 open fractures although in some studies only Gustilo type I fractures were included in the data. The results suggest that the management of open ankle fractures, particularly Gustilo type III fractures, is difficult and associated with a high complication rate. Zaghloul et al.[19] referred to 10 open fractures although they were not classified. They stated that 50% had minor complications and 10% had major complications. Srinivasan and Moran[14] included eight Gustilo type II fractures in their study, all for which were treated with split skin grafts. The implication is that the results were good. However, Pagliaro et al.[13] treated two Gustilo type II fractures and had one deep infection.

The most informative study is that of Vioreanu et al.[2] who treated six open ankle fractures in elderly patients during the time in which they undertook their study. There were four Gustilo type II low energy fractures and two Gustilo IIIa fractures following motor vehicle accidents. They recorded a high rate of deep infection with serious complications. One patient died and two had below knee amputations. This emphasizes a problem for the future with an increasing number of open fractures in poor quality tissue.

OUTCOME

Most surgeons have shown that elderly patients generally have good results if their ankle fractures are treated appropriately. Koval et al.[46] reported better outcome scores in elderly patients than in younger patients. However, most surgeons would accept that age is a predictor of outcome and older patients have worse functional outcomes than younger patients. We have reported mortality rates in a number of studies but Koval et al.[46] compared mortality rates following operative and non-operative management of 33,000 elderly Medicare patients who had undergone treatment for an ankle fracture. The analysis demonstrated that the overall mortality rate was significantly higher at all time points in those patients managed non-operatively compared with those who underwent operative fixation. The medical and operative complication rates were less than 2% in both cohorts. However, rehospitalization rates were higher in the operative group. The non-operative cohort may of course represent a sicker population.

The outcome and quality of life after surgically treated ankle fractures in patients ≥65 years of age was studied by Nilsson et al.[47] in Sweden. They used a number of scoring systems and questioned the patients regarding their pre-fracture physical status. At 1 year after fracture about 60% of the patients reported pain, swelling, problems when stair climbing and reduced activities of daily life. However, 40% rated their ankle function as good or very good at 6 months and 60% at 12 months. Of the patients who were physically active before injury only 43.9% had returned to their pre-injury activity level 1 year after fracture. However, the use of the Short Form-36 score showed that only females had a functional status that was below the age- and gender-matched normative data of the Swedish population.

CONCLUSIONS

1. Ankle fractures in the elderly are increasing in incidence and will represent an increasing problem for society over the next few decades.
2. The classifications that have been described for younger patients may not be applicable to fragility fractures around the ankle.

3. An elderly patient with an ankle fracture must be treated holistically. Consideration of their nutritional status, diabetes control, exposure to sunlight and adequate social support may improve their outcomes and reduce the risk of further fractures.

4. Patients with a fragility fracture around the ankle must be referred to their primary care provider for diagnosis, treatment and/or prevention of osteoporosis.[48]

5. Undisplaced ankle fractures can be treated in a cast, but casting does carry a high risk of skin complications.

6. The results of operative fixation for displaced ankle fractures are generally better than the results of non-operative fixation.

7. As yet there is no good clinical evidence that the results of locking plates are better than the results of one-third tubular or dynamic compression plates.

8. Intramedullary nailing of the fibula produces good results, particularly in elderly infirm patients.

9. The balance between a mild degree of malreduction using less invasive techniques against anatomical reduction with the risk of developing surgical site complications has yet to be defined.

10. It is important to have knowledge of bail-out strategies such as transcalcaneal pinning and retrograde nailing. These may be important in those patients who are not candidates for open reduction and internal fixation.

REFERENCES

1. Beauchamp CG, Clay NR, Thexton PW. Displaced ankle fractures in patients over 50 years of age. *J Bone Joint Surg Br* 1983;65(3):329–32.

2. Vioreanu M, Brophy S, Dudeney S, et al. Displaced ankle fractures in the geriatric population: Operative or non-operative treatment. *Foot Ankle Surg* 2007;13(1):10–14. doi:10.1016/j.fas.2006.06.004.

3. Court-Brown CM, Clement ND, Duckworth AD, et al. The spectrum of fractures in the elderly. *Bone Joint J* 2014;96-B(3):366–72. doi:10.1302/0301-620X.96B3.33316.

4. Gustilo RB, Anderson JT. Prevention of infection in the treatment of one thousand and twenty-five open fractures of long bones: Retrospective and prospective analyses. *J Bone Joint Surg Am* 1976;58:453–8.

5. Kannus P, Palvanen M, Niemi S, et al. Increasing number and incidence of low-trauma ankle fractures in elderly people: Finnish statistics during 1970–2000 and projections for the future. *Bone* 2002;31(3):430–3.

6. Zwipp H, Amlang M. [Treatment of fractures of the ankle in the elderly]. *Orthopade* 2014;43(4):332–8. doi:10.1007/s00132-013-2168-z.

7. Lauge N. Fractures of the ankle; analytic historic survey as the basis of new experimental, roentgenologic and clinical investigations. *Arch Surg* 1948;56(3):259–317.

8. Orthopaedic Trauma Association Committee for Coding and Classification. Fracture and dislocation compendium. *J Orthop Trauma* 1996;10(Suppl 1):1–154.

9. U.S. Preventive Services Task Force. *Osteoporosis: Screening Recommendations summary.* 2011. http://www.uspreventiveservicestaskforce.org/3rduspstf/osteoporosis/osteorr.htm (accessed 9 Dec 2015).

10. Lavalette R, Pope MH, Dickstein H. Setting temperatures of plaster casts. The influence of technical variables. *J Bone Joint Surg Am* 1982;64(6):907–11.

11. Halanski MA, Halanski AD, Oza A, et al. Thermal injury with contemporary cast-application techniques and methods to circumvent morbidity. *J Bone Joint Surg Am* 2007;89(11):2369–77. doi:10.2106/JBJS.F.01208.

12. Salai M, Dudkiewicz I, Novikov I, et al. The epidemic of ankle fractures in the elderly—Is surgical treatment warranted? *Arch Orthop Surg* 2000;120:511–13.

13. Pagliaro AJ, Michelson JD, Mizel MS. Results of operative fixation of unstable ankle fractures in geriatric patients. *Foot Ankle Int* 2001;22:399–402.

14. Srinivasan CMS, Moran CG. Internal fixation of ankle fractures in the very elderly. *Injury* 2001;342:559–63.

15. Makwana NK, Bhowal B, Harper WM, et al. Conservative versus operative treatment for displaced ankle fractures in patients over 55 years of age. *J Bone Joint Surg Br* 2001;83-B:525–9.

16. Davidovitch RI, Walsh M, Spitzer A, et al. Functional outcome after operatively treated ankle fractures in the elderly. *Foot Ankle Int* 2009;30:728–33.

17. Shivarathre DG, Chandran P, Platt SR. Operative fixation of unstable ankle fractures in patients aged over 80 years. *Foot Ankle Int* 2011;32:599–602.

18. Little MTM, Berkes MB, Lazaro LE, et al. Comparison of supination external rotation ankle Type IV fractures in geriatric versus nongeriatric populations. *Foot Ankle Int* 2013;34:512–17.

19. Zaghloul A, Haddad B, Barksfield R, et al. Early complications of surgery in operative treatment of ankle fractures in those over 60: A review of 186 cases. *Injury* 2014;45:780–3.

20. Zahn RK, Frey S, Jakubietz RG, et al. A contoured locking plate for distal fibular fractures in osteoporotic bone: A biomechanical cadaver study. *Injury.* 2012;43(6):718–25. doi:10.1016/j.injury.2011.07.009.

21. Tan SLE, Balogh ZJ. Indications and limitations of locked plating. *Injury.* 2009;40(7):683–91. doi:10.1016/j.injury.2009.01.003.

22. Vallier HA, Immler W. Comparison of the 95-degree angled blade plate and the locking condylar plate for the treatment of distal femoral fractures. *J Orthop Trauma* 2012;26:327–32.

23. Lynde MJ, Sautter T, Hamilton GA, et al. Complications after open reduction and internal fixation of ankle fractures in the elderly. *Foot Ankle Surg* 2012;18:103–7.

24. Schepers T, Van Lieshout EMM, De Vries MR, et al. Increased rates of wound complications with locking plates in distal fibular fractures. *Injury* 2011;42:1125–9.

25. Schaffer JJ, Manoli A, 2nd. The antiglide plate for distal fibular fixation. A biomechanical comparison with fixation with a lateral plate. *J Bone Joint Surg Am* 1987;69(4):596–604.

26. Minihane KP, Lee C, Ahn C, et al. Comparison of lateral locking plate and antiglide plate for fixation of distal fibular fractures in osteoporotic bone: A biomechanical study. *J Orthop Trauma* 2006;20(8):562–6. doi:10.1097/01.bot.0000245684.96775.82.

27. Weber M, Krause F. Peroneal tendon lesions caused by antiglide plates used for fixation of lateral malleolar fractures: The effect of plate and screw position. *Foot Ankle Int* 2005;26(4):281–5.

28. Little MTM, Berkes MB, Lazaro LE, et al. Complications following treatment of supination external rotation ankle fractures through the posterolateral approach. *Foot Ankle Int* 2013;34:523–9.

29. Motzkin NE, Chao EY, An KN, et al. Pull-out strength of screws from polymethylmethacrylate cement. *J Bone Joint Surg Br* 1994;76(2):320–3.

30. Larsson S, Stadelmann VA, Arnoldi J, et al. Injectable calcium phosphate cement for augmentation around cancellous bone screws: In vivo biomechanical studies. *J Biomech* 2012;45(7):1156–60.

31. Collinge C, Merk B, Lautenschlager EP. Mechanical evaluation of fracture fixation augmented with tricalcium phosphate bone cement in a porous osteoporotic cancellous bone model. *J Orthop Trauma* 2007;21(2):124–8.

32. Panchbhavi VK, Vallurupalli S, Morris R, et al. The use of calcium sulfate and calcium phosphate composite graft to augment screw purchase in osteoporotic ankles. *Foot Ankle Int* 2008;29(6):593–600. doi:10.3113/FAI.2008.0593.

33. Ostrum RF, Litsky AS. Tension band fixation of medial malleolus fractures. *J Orthop Trauma* 1992;6(4):464–8.

34. Johnson BA, Fallat LM. Comparison of tension band wire and cancellous bone screw fixation for medial malleolar fractures. *J Foot Ankle Surg* 1997;36(4):284–9.

35. McKean J, Cuellar DO, Hak D, et al. Osteoporotic ankle fractures: An approach to operative management. *Orthopedics* 2013;36(12):936–40. doi:10.3928/01477447-20131120-07.

36. Pritchett JW. Rush rods versus plate osteosynthesis for unstable ankle fractures in the elderly. *Orthop Rev* 1993;22:691–6.

37. Lee YS, Huang HL, Lo TY, et al. Lateral fixation of AO type-B2 ankle fractures in the elderly: The Knowles pin versus the plate. *Int Orthop* 2007;31:817–21.

38. Rajeev A, Senevirathna S, Radha S, et al. Functional outcomes after fibula locking nail for fragility fractures of the ankle. *J Foot Ankle Surg* 2011;50(5):547–50. doi:10.1053/j.jfas.2011.04.017.

39. Bugler KE, Watson CD, Hardie AR, et al. The treatment of unstable fractures of the ankle using the Acumed fibular nail: Development of a technique. *J Bone Joint Surg Br* 2012;94(8):1107–12. doi:10.1302/0301-620X.94B8.28620.

40. Rammelt S, Pyrc J, Agren P-H, et al. Tibiotalocalcaneal fusion using the hindfoot arthrodesis nail: A multicenter study. *Foot Ankle Int* 2013;34(9):1245–55. doi:10.1177/1071100713487526.

41. Jehan S, Shakeel M, Bing AJF, et al. The success of tibiotalocalcaneal arthrodesis with intramedullary nailing—A systematic review of the literature. *Acta Orthop Belg* 2011;77(5):644–51.

42. Lemon M, Somayaji HS, Khaleel A, et al. Fragility fractures of the ankle: Stabilisation with an expandable calcaneotalotibial nail. *J Bone Joint Surg Br* 2005;87-B(6):809–13. doi:10.1302/0301-620X.87B6.16146.

43. Jonas SC, Young AF, Curwen CH, et al. Functional outcome following tibio-talar-calcaneal nailing for unstable osteoporotic ankle fractures. *Injury* 2013;44:994–7.

44. Al-Nammari SS, Dawson-Bowling S, Amin A, et al. Fragility fractures of the ankle in the frail elderly patient. Treatment with a long calcaneotalotibial nail. *Bone Joint J* 2014;96-B:817–22.

45. Mauffrey C, Chaus GW, Butler N, et al. MR-compatible antibiotic interlocked nail fabrication for the management of long bone infections: First case report of a new technique. *Patient Saf Surg* 2014;8:14. doi:10.1186/1754-9493-8-14.

46. Koval KJ, Zhou W, Sparks MJ, et al. Complications after ankle fracture in elderly patients. *Foot Ankle Int* 2007;28(12):1249–55. doi:10.3113/FAI.2007.1249.

47. Nilsson G, Jonsson K, Ekdahl C, et al. Outcome and quality of life after surgically treated ankle fractures in patients 65 years or older. *BMC Musculoskelet Disord* 2007;8:127. doi:10.1186/1471-2474-8-127.

48. Farmer RP, Herbert B, Cuellar DO, et al. Osteoporosis and the orthopaedic surgeon: Basic concepts for successful co-management of patients' bone health. *Int Orthop* 2014;38(8):173.

43

Foot fractures

DOLFI HERSCOVICI, JR. AND JULIA M. SCADUTO

INTRODUCTION

One often pictures elderly patients sustaining foot fractures falling from a standing height or less due to decreased visual, auditory or proprioceptive input, loss of strength, an inability to recognize and avoid hazardous situations, or for medical reasons such as syncope, cerebral vascular accidents, arrhythmias, or as a side effect of medications.[1-3] However, the current elderly population is healthier, more mobile and much more active than previous generations. Although many exceed the national guidelines of moderate activity for at least 30 minutes per day,[4] there are still sizeable numbers of patients who fail to meet these recommendations. Given these variable levels of activity and physiology, one can expect injuries to range from simple toe fractures to severe foot trauma.[5-7]

There are some problems however, when addressing elderly foot trauma. First, most studies are retrospective and discuss polytraumas or common injuries rather than specific problem areas. Secondly, bony and soft tissue injuries are often grouped together.[8] Third, authors often describe the outcomes of all their patients rather than specifically targeting the elderly patient.[9] Fourth, there is the difficulty in classifying fractures. Concerns about classifications include inter- and intraobserver reliability, ease of application, whether classifications are prognostic enough to guide treatment, and a consistent criticism that classifications are often too complex and serve better as a research tool. To improve dialog, historical and recently developed comprehensive classification systems will be discussed together. Lastly, it is difficult to decide how to classify someone as elderly, since there is no consensus concerning the age at which a patient is considered 'elderly'.

Demetriades et al. recommended 70 years but were unable to draw any conclusions regarding the true impact of age.[10] Classifying someone according to their physiology may be more important than simply classifying by age, but this too can be confusing. What we are certain of is that more people are living past 65 and that by 2040 some 21% of the US population will be 65 years and older.[11]

How then do we manage foot fractures in the elderly? Do we withhold certain treatments because they are too expensive? Studies have already shown that the cost of managing fractures and dislocations of the foot and ankle in the 2011 US Medicare population was approximately US$3.5 billion.[12] Or do we withhold treatments due to expectations that the elderly will not do as well as nonelderly patients? This comes with the understanding that withholding treatment can produce avoidable complications, result in significant disabilities of the foot, create chronic pain conditions and lead to socioeconomic burdens on patients, their families and payer systems.

The decision driving treatment should be based primarily on the injury pattern and not solely on the patient's age. If surgery is anticipated a discussion should include preoperative medical evaluations and the use of adjunctive fixation, cement and locking plate technology. Given the advances in techniques and implants, this chapter will hopefully provide a rational approach for the physician tasked with managing foot fractures in the elderly patient.

EPIDEMIOLOGY

Evaluating the incidence of elderly foot fractures is difficult because recent studies have poorly defined an elderly patient, have looked only at low-energy injuries or have looked only at fractures occurring in elderly women.[13] In addition, foot trauma is often discussed presenting as a high- or low-energy injury rather than encompassing all foot injuries.[5,6,14–16] Finally, the only injuries mentioning specific incidences, evaluations and treatment of foot fractures in the elderly are those involving the calcaneus.[14–16]

A recent study using data from the National Electronic Injury Surveillance System (NEISS) describing the anatomic site, disease category, age and circumstance of injury, analyzed all patients presenting to an emergency department with a lower extremity injury.[9] Analysis of almost 120,000 reports from 1 January 2009 through 31 December 2009 revealed that the foot accounted for 15% of all lower extremity injuries with an additional 7% for toe injuries. In this study, the toe was the most common location (38%) for a fracture of the lower extremity with an additional 17% of lower extremity fractures located elsewhere in the foot. The authors also observed a correlation between increasing age and lower trunk fractures, allowing them to estimate the incidence of sustaining either a foot or toe fracture as 37 per 100,000/year (Table 43.1). Unfortunately, except for fractures of the toes, their findings did not segregate other anatomic locations of foot fractures nor did they specifically report the incidence of fractures in the elderly.

Currently, the best epidemiology on elderly foot fractures was presented in a 2-year review by Court-Brown et al.[7] Data on all patients presenting to the Royal Infirmary of Edinburgh, Scotland, were collected from July 2007 to June 2008 and again from September 2010 to August 2011. Identifying fractures that occurred in patients 65 and older, the authors segregated the injuries into those involving the calcaneus, talus, midfoot, metatarsals and toe phalanges. The study identified metatarsal fractures as the most common foot injuries, with a rate of 67.6 (range 25.4–114.6) per 100,000/year. Toes (phalanges) were the next most frequent fractures, with a reported incidence of 8.5 (range 0–15.5) per 100,000/year. In the remaining three other locations, the incidences were 0.5 per 100,000/year (range 0–1.2) for talus fractures, 2.9 (range 0–5.1) for midfoot fractures and 4.7 (range 0–7.9) for calcaneus fractures (Table 43.1).

Table 43.1 Incidence of foot fractures

	NEISS Study[9]	Court-Brown et al.[7]
Foot fractures	37/100,000	
Phalanges (range)	37/100,000	85/1,000,000 (0–15.5)
Metatarsals		67.6/100,000 (25.4–114.6)
Midfoot		2.9/100,000 (0–5.1)
Calcaneus		4.7/100,000 (0–7.9)
Talus		0.5/100,000 (0–1.2)

TALUS

The talus has no tendonous attachments and more than 60% of its surface is covered with articular cartilage. It is divided into a head, neck and body and articulates with the tibia, the fibular, the calcaneus and the navicular. The blood supply consists of an extraosseous and an intraosseous supply. The extraosseous supply arises from the dorsalis pedis, peroneal and posterior tibial arteries, with the latter two giving rise to the arteries to the tarsal sinus and the tarsal canal. The intraosseous supplies blood to the head, neck, the posterior talar tubercle and the medial talar body. The artery of the tarsal canal supplies most of the body while the artery of the dorsal pedis helps supply the head and neck.

Biomechanically, the talus links motion of the foot to the leg allowing gait to proceed from heel strike to toe lift. At the talocrural joint it allows dorsiflexion and plantar flexion. At the syndesmosis, during dorsiflexion, it produces external rotation of the fibula and internal rotation during plantar flexion. Through the subtalar joint, it contributes to flexion-abduction and extension-adduction of the hindfoot. It also contributes to pronation and supination as part of the transverse tarsal or Chopart's joint at the midfoot. Therefore, malalignment can compromise motion of the ankle, subtalar and transverse tarsal joints.

Classification

Fractures are described involving the talar neck, body, head, lateral and posterior processes or as producing an osteochondral injury. Historically, talar neck fractures have been classified using Hawkins' classification with the Canale–Kelly modification.[17] Type I are nondisplaced fractures, type II are displaced fractures with subluxation of the subtalar joint, type III are displaced fractures with subluxation or dislocations of the subtalar and tibiotalar joints and type IV describes a type III fracture with an associated talonavicular dislocation.

Historical classifications for fractures of the body are not as commonly recognized and none has gained acceptance because classifications often combine both neck and body fractures. To differentiate these fractures, Inokuchi et al. stated that fracture lines exiting anterior to the lateral process were considered neck fractures and a talar body fracture if it existed posterior to the lateral process.[18] Body fractures can also be described as osteochondral, coronal or sagittal shear, posterior tubercle, lateral process or crush fractures.

The Orthopaedic Trauma Association (OTA) compendium[19] has classified all talus fractures into three *simple* groups: A, B and C. Group A describes fractures involving the lateral or posterior processes, the talar head or those producing an avulsion fracture. Group B divides talar neck fractures into three patterns: nondisplaced, displaced with subluxation of the subtalar joint or displaced with subluxation of both the subtalar and tibiotalar joints. The latter two are subdivided into noncomminuted, comminuted or those involving the talar head. Group C divides body fractures into dome fractures, those affecting the subtalar joint and those involving both the subtalar and tibiotalar joints. All three are also subdivided into noncomminuted and comminuted patterns.

Nonoperative treatment: talus

Nondisplaced fractures are uncommon injuries. Any fracture demonstrating more than 1 mm of displacement should be diagnosed as being displaced. Use of computed tomography (CT) scans and/or magnetic resonance imaging (MRI) confirms whether a patient can be treated nonoperatively.

The authors' preferred method of nonoperative treatment is a below knee nonweight-bearing cast for 6 weeks. The patient is X-rayed again in 2–3 weeks and after 6 weeks is placed into a removable boot and begins therapy. The patient is nonweight-bearing for the first 12 weeks and is then advanced to full weight bearing over the next 6 weeks.

Operative treatment: talar neck

Preoperative planning should include the use of small and minifragment instruments and implants, small headless screws and poly-L-lactic acid (PLLA) bioabsorbable pins.

Most fractures are managed through a dual incision approach. The *anterolateral incision*, or Böhler approach, begins between the bases of the third and fourth metatarsals and extends towards Chaput's tubercle of the tibia. The superficial peroneal nerve is protected as it crosses the field (Figure 43.1) and the extensor retinaculum is divided exposing the extensor tendons. Retracting the tendons medially should allow one to see the tibial plafond, the dome, neck and head of the talus (Figure 43.2). The *medial incision* extends from the medial malleolus towards the tuberosity of the navicular, dorsal to the posterior tibial tendon (Figure 43.3). Working through both incisions allows visualization to determine whether an anatomic reduction has been obtained. Posterior and percutaneous approaches are rarely indicated because they do not allow for adequate visualization.

In fixation of closed fractures, there does not appear to be any difference whether they are treated before or after 6 hours.[20] However, fracture dislocations should be reduced urgently in order to avoid necrosis of the underlying soft tissues. Unless there is comminution, compression techniques should be used to manage these injuries. Kirschner pins (K-wires) should only be used for provisional fixation. Definitive fixation is achieved using countersink screws placed retrograde, through the head, or antegrade, through the body, in order to prevent impingement during ankle or foot motion.

The goal is to place at least two screws across the fracture (Figure 43.4). On the lateral side of the talus, the authors' preferred approach is a 2.7 or 3.5 mm cortical screw. This is placed either along the lateral border of the neck or through the lateral articular region of the talar head and

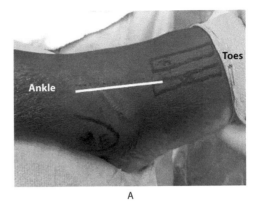

A

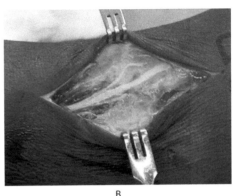

B

Figure 43.1 Anterolateral incision from the bases of the third to fourth metatarsals towards Chaput's tubercle (a). Superficial peroneal nerve lies beneath the skin incision (b).

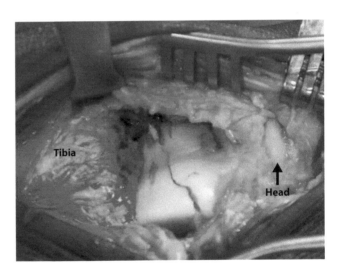

Figure 43.2 Deep dissection demonstrating the tibial plafond, dome, neck and head of the talus (black arrow).

is directed towards the posteromedial corner of the talar body. Medially, a retrograde 2.7 or 3.5 mm screw is placed through the inferomedial region of the talar head and directed towards the posterolateral corner of the talar body. Care should be taken to avoid screw penetration of the body posteriorly and the subtalar joint inferiorly.

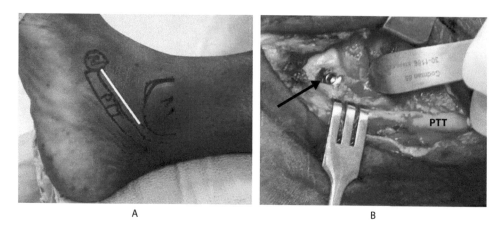

Figure 43.3 Approach from the medial malleolus to the navicular tuberosity (**a**). The deep dissection lies dorsal to the posterior tibial tendon (**b**). Note the countersunk screw through the head of the talus (arrow).

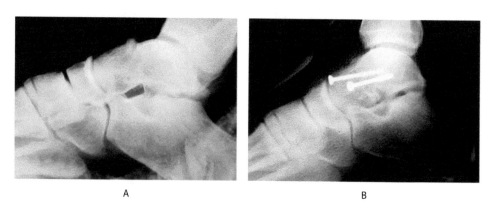

Figure 43.4 Pre- and postoperative lateral X-rays demonstrating a type II talar neck fracture (**a,b**).

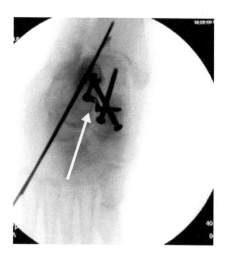

Figure 43.5 Canale view demonstrating a plate used to maintain talar neck length (arrow).

In the presence of comminution, compression technique should be avoided since it produces shortening of the neck and the medial column of the foot. Using transfixion (non-lag technique) screws or 2.4 or 2.0 mm minifragment plates is necessary in order to maintain length. If a plate is selected it can be safely placed along the lateral border of the neck, proximal to the head and distal to the lateral process, since this region is devoid of cartilage and will not interfere with any joint (Figure 43.5). It is also possible to place a very short plate along the medial border of the neck, proximal to the talar head and distal to the medial articular facet of the talus. Fluoroscopic views of the subtalar joint and neck can be used to gauge the reduction and length of the talus. For postoperative care see Table 43.2.

OUTCOMES AND COMPLICATIONS

Despite anatomic reduction, outcomes have demonstrated that significant functional impairment can be identified an average of 3 years post-fixation.[21] Factors such as patient's age, time to surgery and associated body fractures do not influence outcomes but comminution and dislocation or subluxation of the joint do.

Complications are divided into those occurring early and those occurring late. Early complications are due to malreduction of the fracture, often due to poor visualization of the fracture, medial compression of comminuted fractures, inadequate fixation of the fracture and early weight bearing. Late complications include delayed or nonunions, malunions, the development of osteonecrosis (avascular necrosis, AVN) and post-traumatic arthritis. Of these

Table 43.2 Postoperative management of foot fractures

	Week 1	Weeks 2–3	Weeks 3–12	Months 4–5	Month 6
Talus					
Head, neck, body, lateral process	Well-padded splint	Short leg NWB cast	Remove sutures, book, ROM therapy, NWB	Slowly advanced to WBAT[a]	Unrestricted activity
Calcaneus					
Tongue-type, intra-articular	Well-padded splint	Short leg NWB cast	Remove sutures, book, ROM therapy, NWB	Slowly advanced to WBAT	Unrestricted activity
Navicular	Well-padded splint	Short leg NWB cast	Remove sutures, book, ROM therapy, NWB, remove pins weeks 7–8	Slowly advanced to WBAT	Unrestricted activity
Cuboid	Well-padded splint	Short leg NWB cast	Remove sutures, book, ROM therapy, NWB, remove pins weeks 7–8	Slowly advanced to WBAT	Unrestricted activity
Cuneiforms	Well-padded splint	Short leg NWB cast	Remove sutures, book, ROM therapy, NWB, remove pins weeks 7–8	Slowly advanced to WBAT	Unrestricted activity
Metatarsals	Well-padded splint	Short leg NWB cast	Remove sutures, book, ROM therapy, NWB, remove pins weeks 7–8	Slowly advanced to WBAT	Unrestricted activity
Phalanges	Well-padded splint	Short leg NWB cast	Remove sutures, book, ROM therapy, remove pins week 6, WBAT	**Unrestricted Activity**	

Note: NWB, nonweight bearing; ROM, range of motion; WBAT, weight bearing as tolerated.

[a] While wearing a boot, this is obtained by having the patient press the foot down onto a scale: weeks 1–2, 25% body weight applied to foot; weeks 3–4, 50%; weeks 5–6, 75%, after week 6, WBAT.

AVN has received the most attention. Historically, AVN has been reported to occur in 60–100% of all patients. However, recent studies report an incidence of 36–40%, regardless of the time to definitive fixation.[20,21] Delayed unions or nonunions are relatively uncommon with a reported incidence of between 4% and 13%. They are often associated with a shortened talar neck and an adducted deformity of the forefoot, while malunions are often due to a missed fracture or loss of reduction. The most common late complication reported, however, is the development of post-traumatic arthritis, with studies reporting that 60–100% of patients will develop some arthritis in the ankle, subtalar or talonavicular joint.[20,21]

Operative treatment: talar body

Body fractures present as sagittal, coronal or horizontal patterns (Figure 43.6). To improve exposure, an osteotomy of the medial or lateral malleolus is often necessary. However, exposure to the lateral half of the talar body can also be facilitated using the Böhler approach. The medial incision begins proximal to the medial malleolus and extends distally (Figure 43.7). Once the medial malleolus is isolated, the authors' preference is for a chevron osteotomy with the apex proximal to the articular surface (Figure 43.8). This osteotomy provides stability so that pre-drilling is not necessary.

Starting with a small, oscillating saw, the osteotomy is completed using a flexible chisel. The medial malleolus is reflected distally, using the intact deltoid ligament as a hinge (Figure 43.9). If visualization is inadequate, a femoral distractor may be necessary to gain better access to the fracture.

Most fractures can be fixed using 2.7 or 3.5 mm screws, countersunk and placed perpendicular to the fracture line (Figure 43.10). If an adjacent osteochondral fragment is present, a PLLA pin or a small headless screw can also be used. For postoperative care see Table 43.2.

OUTCOMES AND COMPLICATIONS

Talar body fractures are significant injuries producing fair to poor outcomes. Open injuries and dislocations should be addressed emergently, however, neither the patient's age nor time to definitive fixation affects outcome.[21] What does affect outcomes is a malunion, AVN or post-traumatic arthritis. Malunions often result from inadequate visualization or poor reduction techniques, often after using closed, percutaneous methods (Figure 43.11). The development of AVN is seen with open fractures, those with significant comminution or associated talar neck fractures, with a reported incidence of 35–40%.[22]

The most common complication is the development of post-traumatic arthritis, often affecting the ankle and

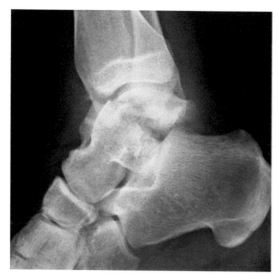
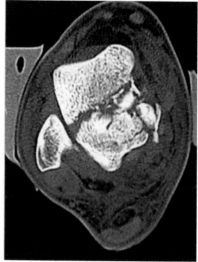

Figure 43.6 Lateral X-ray and an axial CT scan demonstrating a comminuted talar body fracture.

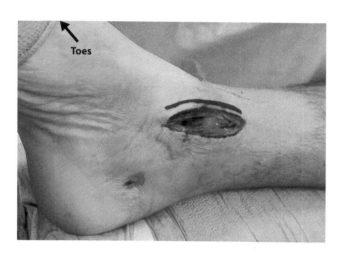

Figure 43.7 Medial approach to the ankle. The line indicates the position of the greater saphenous vein.

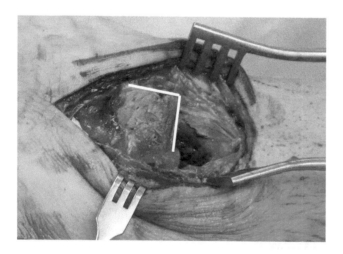

Figure 43.8 Chevron osteotomy has been completed using a flexible chisel.

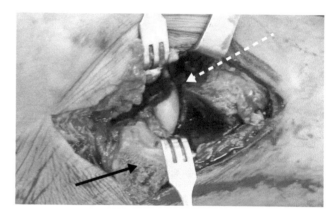

Figure 43.9 Deep dissection showing reflected medial malleolus (black arrow) and the talar body fracture (white dotted arrow). Visualization is improved with distraction.

subtalar joints. Historically, the incidence has approached 90% for the ankle and 50% for the subtalar joint. However, recent literature has shown an incidence of 65% for ankle joints and 35% for the subtalar joint.[22]

Operative treatment: lateral process fractures

Lateral process fractures are often overlooked and account for 24% of all body fractures. They result from acute ankle dorsiflexion combined with inversion of the foot. A large, displaced fracture can produce chronic ankle instability (Figure 43.12).

The fracture is approached with an incision across the sinus tarsi (Figure 43.13). To improve visualization, distraction of the joint is often necessary. If the fragment is a single large piece, fixation is obtained using one or two 2.0 mm screws (Figure 43.14). If comminuted, a 2.4 or 2.0

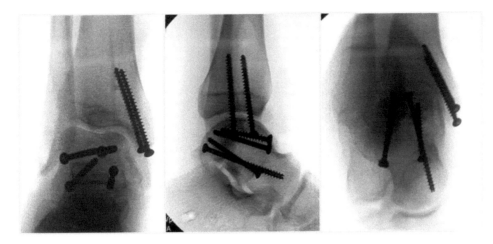

Figure 43.10 Anteroposterior (AP), lateral and Canale views demonstrating reduction of the talar body fracture and the osteotomy. Note the posterior screw below the articular surface.

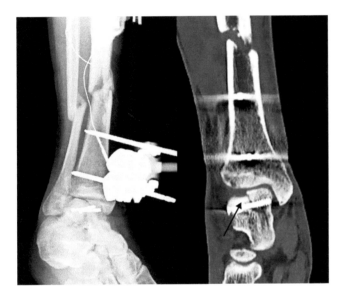

Figure 43.11 Oblique ankle X-ray and coronal CT scan demonstrating malreduction of a talar body, it was originally treated with two percutaneously placed screws (arrow).

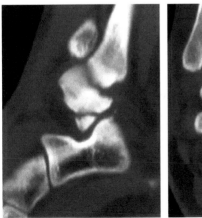
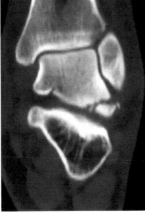

Figure 43.12 Sagittal and coronal CT scans demonstrating a lateral process fracture of the talus.

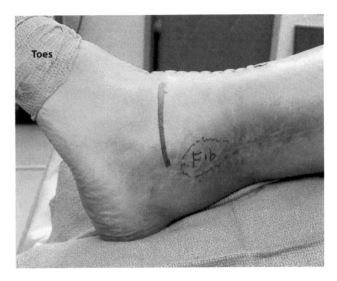

Figure 43.13 Surgical incision lies directly over the sinus tarsi and distal to the fibula.

locking plate is used to buttress the fracture. For postoperative care, see Table 43.2.

OUTCOMES AND COMPLICATIONS

Outcomes and complications can be attributed to inadequately treated or missed injuries. The complications associated with this injury consist of chronic lateral ankle instability, nonunions, the development of subtalar arthrosis and potential impingement of the ankle along the talofibular joint.

Operative treatment: talar head fractures

Talar head fractures represent 5–10% of all talar fractures and present as a compression, from impaction with the navicular, or an oblique fracture, also identified as a shearing pattern, due to significant abduction/adduction of the foot.

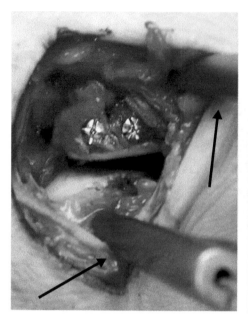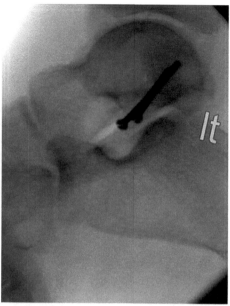

Figure 43.14 Fixation obtained using two 2 mm screws. Note pins used for joint distraction (arrows).

Displaced fractures are approached dorsally, medially, anterolaterally or, if necessary, through two incisions. Fixation is achieved with countersunk 2.4 or 2.0 mm screws and can be augmented with the use of PLLA pins for smaller osteochondral lesions. If fixation is deemed inadequate, the addition of a temporary transarticular pin, placed across the talonavicular joint, will increase stability. If impaction is identified, disimpaction and bone grafting may be needed to restore medial column stability. If excision is contemplated, at least 70% of the head should be retained. For postoperative care, see Table 43.2.

OUTCOMES AND COMPLICATIONS

Outcomes and complications are attributed to inadequate treatment or to missed injuries. Nonunions are exceedingly rare but a malreduction can result in the development of talonavicular arthritis, compromise the stability of the medial column of the foot, and affect other midtarsal joints. AVN occurs in about 10% of all cases.

CALCANEUS

The calcaneus is divided into a tuberosity, two processes and four articular surfaces. The two processes are the anterior process, near the cuboid facet, and a medial (sustentaculum tali) process, which supports the talar neck and part of the body. Of its four articular surfaces, three lie superiorly (anterior, middle and posterior facets) and articulate with the talus while the fourth is distal and articulates with the cuboid. The calcaneus is supplied by branches of the medial and lateral calcaneal arteries (branches of the posterior tibial and peroneal arteries), lateral and medial plantar arteries, arteries of the sinus tarsi and the tarsal canal, and directly from perforating arteries of the peroneal artery.

Biomechanically, at the subtalar joint the calcaneus allows flexion, extension, abduction and adduction. At the midfoot, it contributes to supination and pronation through the transverse tarsal or Chopart's joint. When a malunited varus position occurs it produces a flexed, supinated and rigidly adducted forefoot that restricts eversion. Immobility (fusion) at the subtalar joint can also affect motion at the talonavicular and calcaneocuboid joints but immobility of the calcaneocuboid joint produces less disability of the subtalar or talonavicular joints.[23]

Classification

Plain X-rays can be used to identify fractures of the tuberosity, the processes and the articular surfaces. Additionally, lateral X-rays can be used to measure intra-articular displacement using Böhler's angle and the crucial angle of Gissane (Figure 43.15). Böhler's angle, normally 20–40 degrees, describes collapse (impaction) of the posterior facet when the angle is described as either flat (zero) or has a negative value. It is defined with a line drawn from the highest point on the posterior-superior edge of the tuberosity towards the highest point on the posterior-superior edge of the posterior facet, intersecting a line drawn from the highest point on the anterior-superior edge of the anterior process. The crucial angle of Gissane supports the lateral process of the talus and also describes a fracture of the posterior facet when the angle is increased. It is formed by intersecting lines drawn along the subchondral bone of the anterior, middle and posterior facets.

Historically, lateral plain radiographs were used to describe two fracture patterns, based on relationship to the posterior facet. The first was the tongue-type pattern, where a vertical line extended plantar through the angle of Gissane and intersected a horizontal line exiting posteriorly

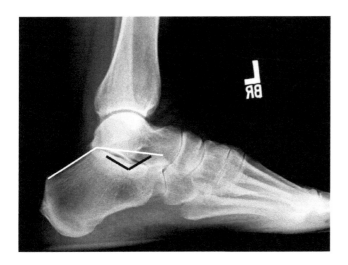

Figure 43.15 Lateral view demonstrating Böhler's angle (white line) and the angle of Gissane (black line).

into the tuberosity. The second was a joint depression, with the posterior facet not attached to the tuberosity. However, CT scans have significantly improved our ability to evaluate and understand intra-articular displacement.

Use of CT scans has led to the development of classifications, including four patterns (types I–IV) proposed by Sanders et al.,[24] based on coronal CT scans. Type I are nondisplaced fractures. Type II has two posterior facet fragments with three subtypes (A, B and C) describing, in descending alphabetical order, a more medially propagated pattern. Type III has three posterior facet fragments, with a centrally depressed segment, and the same three subtypes as type II. Type IV describes a comminuted posterior facet with four or more fragments. Although the degree of articular comminution is prognostic, there may be little intra- or interobserver agreement as to the subtype patterns.

The OTA compendium has divided *all calcaneal* fractures into types A, B and C. Type A describes fractures of the anterior process, sustentaculum tali or the tuberosity with further subdivision into noncomminuted (type 1) or comminuted (type 2) patterns. Type B describes non-articular body fractures and classifies them into those with or without comminution. Type C describes fractures involving the posterior facet and divides them into nondisplaced, two-part fractures, three-part fractures or those with four or more parts.[19]

Nonoperative treatment

Calcaneus fractures represent 2% of all fractures with displaced intra-articular fractures representing almost 75% of all calcaneal fractures. Fixation is demanding, the soft tissue envelope is vulnerable and such fractures have a complex anatomy and high rates of complications with and without surgery. Even with recent advancements, the management is still controversial and specific age bias and nonoperative approaches have been proposed in the elderly patient.[25]

Nonoperative treatment should be reserved for the non-displaced fracture. Other factors to consider when deciding to treat patients nonoperatively include significant medical comorbidities that preclude surgical intervention, chronic steroid dependency, bed or wheelchair bound patients, and peripheral vascular disease or those with a significant smoking history that would affect overall healing. The patient's age is not an indication for nonoperative care. In patients treated with nonoperative care, immobilization in a cast or splint should not exceed 3 weeks. This period of time will allow the soft tissue envelope to improve. The patient is then placed into a removable boot and begins therapy. The authors' preference is nonweight bearing for the first 12 weeks which is advanced to full weight bearing over the subsequent 6 weeks. Unrestricted activity is allowed at 5 months.

OUTCOMES AND COMPLICATIONS

If the decision is made to treat displaced intra-articular fractures nonoperatively, poor outcomes with significant complications can occur, resulting in difficult salvage of these injuries and problems with shoewear. Due to compression, the tuberosity fragment displaces laterally and superiorly, producing a malunited varus or valgus hindfoot. The calcaneus also widens leading to the development of painful bony exostoses and calcaneo-fibular impingement. Continued impaction decreases height and leads to talar declination and the potential for anterior impingement of the tibiotalar joint. This is in addition to the development of post-traumatic arthritis in the subtalar, lateral ankle, and calcaneocuboid joints (Figure 43.16).

These bony abnormalities then lead to impingement, entrapment or dislocation of the peroneal tendons and

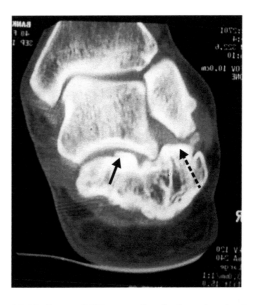

Figure 43.16 Coronal CT scan of a displaced malunited intra-articular calcaneus fracture treated nonoperatively. Note the flattened calcaneus, the irregular posterior facet (solid black arrow) and the malalignment and impingement of the talofibular joint (dotted black arrow).

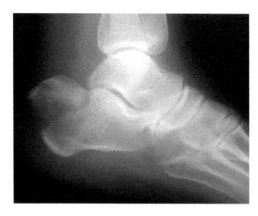
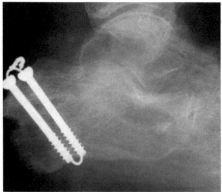

Figure 43.17 Lateral views of a tongue-type fracture fixed using percutaneous screws. Note the wire placed through the screws to prevent loss of fixation.

entrapment of the posterior tibial and sural nerves. Additionally, using a nonoperative approach for displaced tuberosity (tongue-type) fractures may result in pressure necrosis to the skin necessitating free tissue transfers or even amputation in a nonsalvageable extremity.

Operative treatment: tuberosity (tongue-type) fractures

Most are extra-articular fractures but some can have a remnant of posterior facet. Fixation is performed using either an open technique or, more commonly, percutaneous, with peritendonous placement of cannulated or non-cannulated screws. Adjunctive fixation, consisting of wires or fiber wire placed through cannulated screws, and may be necessary to prevent the screws from backing out of osteopenic bone (Figure 43.17). Postoperatively, the authors' preference is a splint with the foot in a plantar flexed position and recasted every 2 weeks to gradually increase dorsiflexion to a neutral position. For further postoperative care, see Table 43.2.

OUTCOMES AND COMPLICATIONS

Good to excellent outcomes can be expected with adequate reduction and fixation. Post-traumatic arthritis of the subtalar joint is rare. The most common complication is skin necrosis, resulting from prolonged pressure to the posterior skin. Therefore, fractures should be treated urgently. Nonunions are rare; however, failure of fixation or a malreduction of the fragment can occur, producing a flattened heel or an elevated fragment. Other complications can include entrapments or lacerations of the Achilles tendon or the sural nerve.

Operative treatment: articular fractures

The goals of operative treatment of articular fractures are to reconstruct the height, narrow the width, reconstruct the length, correct the deformity of the tuberosity and reduce the joint (Figure 43.18). This is performed through an extensile, lateral approach, developing a full-thickness

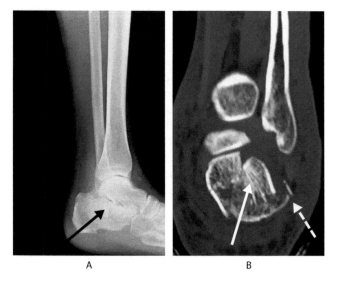

A   B

Figure 43.18 Lateral (a) and coronal (b) CT scan demonstrating impaction of the lateral one-third of the posterior facet (solid arrow) and the lateral wall (white dotted arrow).

fasciocutaneous flap with dissection deep to the peroneal tendons, exposing the posterior talocalcaneal and calcaneocuboid joints (Figure 43.19). The lateral wall is often removed and placed into saline on the back table.

To improve visualization, a 4.0 or 4.5 mm Schanz pin is placed into the tuberosity and is used to distract the fracture and correct the varus deformity of the body. Disimpaction and removal of the lateral third/half of the joint allows one to see the medial articular surface (Figure 43.19). After elevating the medial joint, the Schanz pin is used to reconstruct the calcaneal height, medialize the tuberosity and correct the varus deformity of the hindfoot. To hold this reduction, K-wires are placed from the tuberosity into the medial joint. The lateral articular segment is now replaced and provisional fixation is used to hold the posterior facet. Next is the reduction of the anterior process, which aids in the reduction of the angle of Gissane because the calcaneocuboid joint is attached to

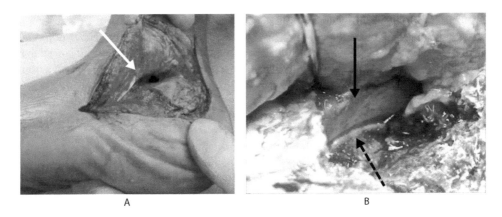

Figure 43.19 A full-thickness fasciocutaneous flap **(a)** has been developed through a lateral approach (white arrow). Removal of the lateral wall and joint exposes the talus (solid black arrow) and medial two-thirds of the posterior facet (dotted black line) **(b)**.

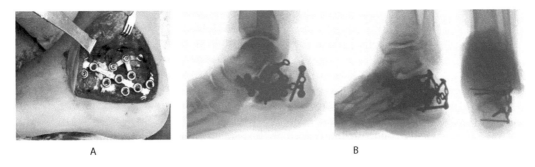

Figure 43.20 Post-reduction using a locked plate augmented with calcium sulfate bone graft **(a)**. Lateral, Broden's and Harris views demonstrating reduction **(b)**.

the angle of Gissane and, due to its dense nature, can be used for screw placement.

Once the height, length, width, varus deformity and the articular surface have been provisionally reduced, the lateral wall can be replaced. If there is a large defect this can be filled with synthetic bone graft. Definitive fixation is accomplished using 3.5, 2.7 or 2.0 mm screws, combined with low profile, preformed, locked calcaneal plates. Plates can be contoured and cut to ensure proper placement along the lateral border of the calcaneus (Figure 43.20). Final views should verify that no screws have been placed across a joint.

Closure is performed over a small drain, such as a quarter-inch Hemovac (Zimmer, Warsaw, Indiana), placed deep to the peroneal tendons. A 0 or 2-0 absorbable suture approximates the fasciocutaneous layer. The sutures are tagged and an assistant gently reduces the flap while the surgeon ties sutures from one end towards the other. The skin is closed using 3-0 or 4-0 nylon, with the knots placed on the posterior and inferior margins of the incision. The authors' preference is for a well-padded splint, admission for at least 23 hours, with the drain pulled prior to discharge. For postoperative care, see Table 43.2.

OUTCOMES AND COMPLICATIONS

In the elderly, internal fixation of calcaneal fractures has demonstrated healing rates approaching 97% with complications and outcomes equivalent to those of younger patients.[14,15] The only difference has been an increase in the development of post-traumatic arthritis of the subtalar joint, attributed to some pre-existing arthritis.[15] However, even with optimal treatment, complications can still occur.[14]

The most common soft tissue complications include dehiscence and wound edge necrosis. The incidence is 2% in closed fractures and commonly occurs at the apex of the incision. Risk factors include tobacco use, diabetes and an open injury. Although deep infections can occur, most wounds can often be managed with nonoperative approaches. If conservative measures fail, serial debridements, negative pressure therapy, intravenous antibiotics and the use of a free tissue transfer may be necessary. Other soft tissue complications include damage to the sural nerve, scarring of the tarsal tunnel and nonspecific heel pain. Bony complications consist of malreductions and the development of arthritis, similar to those identified with the nonoperative management of displaced fractures.

NAVICULAR

The navicular is horseshoe in shape with a proximal concavity articulating with the talar head and a distal kidney shape articulating with the cuneiforms. It provides for the calcaneonavicular portion of the bifurcate ligament and has the posterior tibial tendon insert onto its prominent tuberosity, before reaching the cuneiforms and cuboid. Dorsally it is supplied by the dorsalis pedis, plantarly by a medial plantar branch of the posterior tibial artery, and the tuberosity is supplied by a network of vessels.

Biomechanically, the navicular is the keystone for the medial longitudinal arch of the foot and contributes to pronation and supination of the foot as a function of the transverse tarsal and subtalar joints. If motion of the subtalar joint is affected it also limits motion at the talonavicular joint.[23]

Classification

Fractures are uncommon injuries. Historically, four types have been identified: cortical avulsion or dorsal lip fractures, stress fractures, fractures of the tuberosity and fractures of the body. Body fractures are the most severe and are often associated with other foot injuries. Sangeorzan et al.[25] described three patterns. In type I, the primary fracture line runs parallel to the sole of the foot, producing a large dorsal fragment but does not compromise the medial column of the foot. Type II is the most common with the fracture running from dorsolateral to plantarmedial, often with comminution. The major fragment lies medially or dorsomedially with comminution of the plantar fragment. There is often no disruption of the cuneonavicular joint, so the medial column of the foot remains intact. In type III, there is central or centrolateral comminution. The major fragment lies medially, disrupts both the cuneonavicular and the talonavicular joints and produces instability to the medial column of the foot.

The OTA compendium has proposed a *simple* approach to the classification of fractures of the navicular. They have divided all navicular fractures into one of two types: A, without comminution, and B, with comminution.[19]

Nonoperative treatment

Nonoperative care should be considered only for nondisplaced body fractures, cortical avulsions or minimally displaced tuberosity fractures. Fragments involving 20% of the articular surface, those with a greater than 1 mm step-off, or fractures producing talonavicular or naviculocuneiform instability or subluxation should be treated surgically.

Conservative management consists of a nonweight-bearing cast for 4 weeks. The patient is nonweight bearing for the first 12 weeks and gradually advanced to full weight bearing over the next 6 weeks. Unrestricted activity is allowed at the 5-month mark.

Operative treatment: tuberosity and body

Prefabricated 'navicular' plates are available, but small and minifragment locking implants or screws alone are sufficient to manage these injuries. Additionally, distraction, achieved either with a commercially available device or with something as simple as a small external fixator, allows visualization of the fracture.

The fracture can be approached medially, parallel and slightly dorsal to the posterior tibialis tendon, dorsally, between the tibialis anterior and extensor hallucis longus tendons, or through a combination of these approaches. Surgical management is divided into excisions and fixation. Excision of fragments is directed towards cortical avulsions or small tuberosity fractures, while fixation is directed towards body fractures. In large tuberosity fractures with at least 5 mm of displacement, early fixation rather than excision should be performed in order to avoid a progressive planovalgus deformity (Figure 43.21).

Stabilization of comminuted fractures can be difficult, even with locked minifragment implants. If fixation is tenuous, a transarticular fixation can be extended to the cuneiforms. In fractures with severe comminution, total excision of the navicular should be avoided since it will produce shortening of the medial column and malrotation of the forefoot. In these patients, external fixation supplemented with provisional K-wires should be used.[27] For postoperative care, see Table 43.2.

OUTCOMES AND COMPLICATIONS

Outcomes are related to the adequacy of the reduction. For displaced fractures treated nonoperatively, the prognosis is poor. Complications consist of malunions, AVN, post-traumatic arthritis, bony prominences, irritable implants, failure of fixation, subluxations and the development of progressive deformities. The causes leading to a malunion are early removal of implants and allowing weight bearing before adequate healing has occurred. Post-traumatic

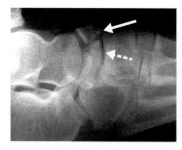
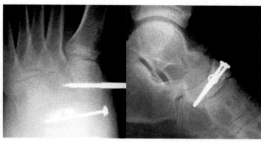

Figure 43.21 Lateral view demonstrating a comminuted navicular body fracture with a dorsal segment (solid arrow) and an impacted central portion (dotted arrow). Postoperative views (a) demonstrating reduction of the navicular (b).

arthritis can be minimized if at least 60% of the articular surface has been restored and, despite an adequate reduction, an AVN rate of 29% has been reported.[26,27]

CUBOID

In general, cuboid fractures account for half of all midfoot fractures with a reported incidence of 1.8 per 10,000 annually.[28] However, the true incidence in the elderly is unknown.[7] The cuboid is pyramid shaped with its base located medially and its apex laterally. It has five articular facets. Distally it articulates with the fourth and fifth metatarsals, proximally with the calcaneus, medially with the lateral cuneiform and posteromedially with the navicular. Its blood supply is from a plantar arterial rete and from the lateral and medial plantar arteries, with a contribution from the dorsal arterial rete.

Biomechanically, it is a spacer to the lateral column of the foot, with a loss of length producing a flatfoot deformity. With the talonavicular joint, it 'locks' and 'unlocks' the midtarsal region necessary for heel strike and toe lift.[29] Immobility (fusion) across the calcaneocuboid joint does not produce much disability to either the subtalar or talonavicular joints.[23]

Classification

Historical eponyms such as 'nutcracker fracture' have described injuries that compress the cuboid between the calcaneus and the metatarsals, but there are no accepted classifications. Currently, fractures are described as extra-articular or avulsion and intra-articular or compression. Extra-articular fractures are the most common, occur on the lateral aspect of the foot and do not disrupt the lateral column of the foot. Intra-articular fractures involve the entire body of the cuboid or just the articular surface of the tarsometatarsal (TMT) joint, leading to shortening or dorsal subluxation of the lateral column.

The OTA compendium has proposed a *simple* approach for classifying cuboid fractures. All fractures have been divided into two patterns: type A, without comminution, and type B, with comminution.[19]

Nonoperative treatment

Fractures are often non- or minimally displaced, and present as closed injuries. Fractures with little or no articular involvement or without changes to the morphology of the cuboid can be treated conservatively. This consists of a non-weight-bearing cast for 3–4 weeks followed by the use of a boot. The patient is allowed to weight bear once they have the boot and can progress to full weight bearing as tolerated. Unrestricted activity is allowed at the 5-month mark.

Operative treatment

Isolated injuries are rare and are often seen with injuries to the TMT joints. Fractures with a depressed articular fragment, comminution producing shortening of the lateral column, and any dislocations, subluxations or tenting of the skin should be managed surgically. Although prefabricated 'cuboid' plates are available, a locked, minifragment plate is sufficient to maintain the reduction. Preoperative planning should also include some type of distractor and the use of PLLA pins.

The incision begins near the calcaneocuboid joint and extends towards the base of the fourth metatarsal, dorsal to the peroneal tendons. After protecting the sural nerve, the extensor digitorum brevis is elevated and retracted dorsally while the peroneal tendons are retracted plantarly. Distraction is accomplished with pins placed into the calcaneus and the metatarsals. After bone grafting and provisional fixation, locking 2.4 or 2.0 mm plates can be used to maintain length and provide a buttress affect. If fixation is tenuous the external fixator can be left in place for another 2–4 weeks or transarticular pin fixation, across the calcaneus or metatarsals, can be used (Figure 43.22). For postoperative care, see Table 43.2.

OUTCOMES AND COMPLICATIONS

Approximately 60% of patients have very good results, with some demonstrating no limitations after 1 year.[30] Although operative and nonoperative treatments can lead to arthritis,

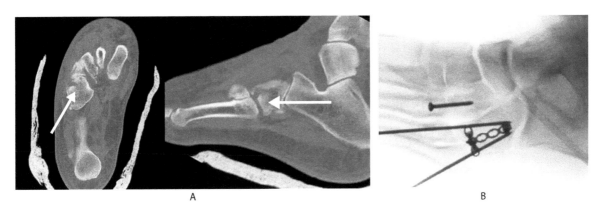

A   B

Figure 43.22 Axial and sagittal CT scans demonstrating an impacted distal cuboid fracture (a). Reduction obtained using a 2.0 mm locked plate (b). Note adjunctive fixation across unstable third, fourth and fifth tarsometatarsal (TMT) joints.

the majority of complications and long-term sequelae are often due to nonoperative care leading to intra-articular incongruity, residual lateral column shortening and forefoot abduction with a progressive planovalgus deformity. Additionally, the development of compartment syndrome has also been reported.[30]

CUNEIFORMS

The medial, middle and lateral cuneiforms are wedge-shaped bones forming the transverse arch of the foot. They are supplied by the dorsal arterial rete, with these supplemental arteries decreasing with age. Biomechanically, they provide stability to the medial column of the foot and contribute to the motion of the transverse arch. They allow for compressive forces on the convex (dorsal) side of the foot and tensile forces on the concave (plantar) side. They also contribute to a small amount of pronation-supination and flexion-extension through the TMT joints.

Classification

The true incidence is unknown since isolated fractures are uncommon. Injuries are the result of direct trauma and are described as medial, middle or lateral cuneiform fractures. Their most common presentation is either as an avulsion or as a nondisplaced fracture. Most fractures are identified as a component of the TMT (Lisfranc) joint.

The OTA compendium has proposed a *simple* approach in classifying cuneiform fractures. All fractures are described as affecting the medial, middle or lateral cuneiform and divided into type A, without comminution, and type B, with comminution.[19]

Nonoperative treatment

In nondisplaced or avulsion fractures the authors' preference is a nonweight-bearing cast for 4 weeks followed by a walking boot for an additional 4–6 weeks. Unrestricted activity is allowed at 4 months. Long-term complications rarely occur but consist of post-traumatic arthritis.

Operative treatment

Displaced fractures should be evaluated for midtarsal instability. The surgical approach is a dorsal incision from the first webspace towards the naviculocuneiform joint. A medial approach, for an isolated medial cuneiform fracture, can also be used but both approaches should develop a full-thickness fasciocutaneous flap. Fixation consists of a transarticular fixation to the other cuneiforms, the metatarsals or the navicular. With comminution, length can be achieved and maintained using a locked, minifragment plate placed dorsally across the naviculocuneiform or TMT joints. For postoperative care, see Table 43.2.

Outcomes are dependent on the anatomic reduction and residual joint instability. Those with anatomic reductions result in better outcome scores, a decrease in subjective complaints and a gait without significant abnormality.[31] Complications increase with the conservative care of displaced fractures and include vascular compromise, compartment syndrome and the development of bony prominences. Other complications include skin necrosis, infection, malunions, arthritis and implant irritability. Malunions are often due to screw breakage, inadequate fixation, early removal of implants or allowing weight bearing before adequate healing has occurred. Post-traumatic arthritis has been reported but is significantly decreased with an anatomic reduction.

METATARSALS AND LISFRANC INJURIES

Metatarsal fractures are the most common foot injuries in the elderly population[7] and are divided into head, shaft and base fractures. The bases form the transverse arch of the foot, with the apex occurring at the base of the second metatarsal, and all metatarsals are plantar flexed distally so that all five heads are located in the same horizontal plane. The first metatarsal is broader than the lesser four but is shorter than the second and the third metatarsals. All have tubercles attaching to ligaments or tendons, but only the fifth metatarsal has a recognized tuberosity. The blood supply to the second, third and fourth metatarsals is from a nutrient artery formed by the dorsal and lateral plantar arteries. The first dorsal and plantar metatarsal arteries and a superficial branch from the medial plantar artery supply the first metatarsal. The fifth metatarsal obtains its supply from dorsal and plantar metatarsal arteries, while the tuberosity is supplied by two additional arteries producing a radiate pattern.

Biomechanically, the first three metatarsals contribute to the medial column of the foot, the fourth and fifth to the lateral column. About one-third of the body weight is transmitted through the first metatarsal. The second and third TMT joints bear forces that are two to three times the force across the first or fourth/fifth TMT joints, while the third bears the most force at all loads and foot positions. However, the first, fourth and fifth TMT joints have a more active role in foot position than at a neutral position.[32] Significant displacement affects gait by producing mechanical impingement, transfer lesions, bony prominences and difficulties with shoewear.

Classification

Fractures are described as occurring in the head, shaft or base. However, they can also be described as injuries to the proximal, middle or distal thirds. Additionally, fractures to the fifth metatarsal have been classified as a styloid or avulsion (zone I) fracture, tuberosity or diaphyseal-metaphyseal region (type II) fracture or a diaphyseal (type III) fracture.[33] Lastly, when dislocations occur at the TMT joint they have been historically classified using Hardcastle's and Myerson's modifications.

The OTA compendium has classified fractures into three patterns. Type I are simple (transverse, oblique or spiral) noncomminuted diaphyseal fractures or any non-articular fracture (with or without comminution) of the proximal or distal ends. Type II are comminuted diaphyseal fractures presenting with a wedge of bone (spiral, bending or comminuted) or any partial articular fracture of the proximal or distal ends. The articular injuries are subclassified as avulsion or partial split, depression or split/depression fractures. Type III are comminuted diaphyseal fractures (segmental or complex comminuted) or complete comminution of the proximal or distal articular surfaces. The articular fractures are subclassified as simple articular pattern, simple articular with a comminuted metaphyseal pattern or a comminuted articular and metaphyseal pattern.[19]

Addressing TMT dislocations, the OTA compendium has classified these injuries into six subgroups, describing them from medial to lateral. The first five dislocations are described as affecting an isolated metatarsal (one through five) and its corresponding cuneiform or cuboid with the sixth group used to describe multiple dislocations.[19]

Nonoperative treatment

Injuries are usually the result of a direct blow to the foot, a twisting type of injury or a stress fracture. Isolated or multiple fractures, presenting without any displacement or deformity, can be treated conservatively. This consists of a nonweight-bearing cast, for severe pain, or a postoperative shoe or a boot, if weight bearing is tolerated. Displaced styloid avulsions, at the base of the fifth metatarsal, or displaced fractures 1.5 cm distal to the styloid (Jones fracture) can also be treated conservatively with a stiff soled shoe. It is extremely rare that fixation of avulsion or Jones fractures is necessary in the elderly population. Good outcomes are expected for these patients and unrestricted activity is allowed after the fourth month.

All displaced TMT injuries should be managed surgically. The only indication for treating patients nonoperatively is a medical condition that would preclude any surgical intervention.

Operative treatment

First metatarsal fractures and second through fifth injuries, with shortening, angular deformities, or changes in the weight distribution to the metatarsal heads, require fixation. Neck and shaft fractures can be managed using an open reduction antegrade/retrograde pinning technique. The approach is a longitudinal incision between the two bones being surgically managed. The pinning is first performed antegrade, through the head and exiting plantarly, and then retrograde into the proximal shaft (Figure 43.23). It is critical that for most patients a 2.0 mm K-wire is used to fill the medullary canal.

For displaced fractures of the first metatarsal, the use of a locking, minifragment plate may be needed to maintain length and the reduction. A medial or slightly dorsomedial incision over the first metatarsal can be used, after developing a full-thickness fasciocutaneous flap (Figures 43.24 and 43.25). For postoperative care see, Table 43.2.

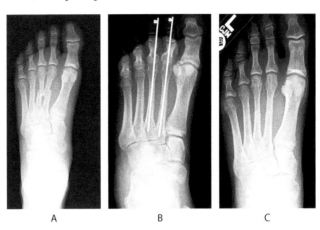

A   B   C

Figure 43.23 Anteroposterior (AP) views of plantar flexed and bayoneted second and third metatarsal fractures (a). Fixation achieved using 2.0 mm K-wires (b) and 4 months after fixation (c).

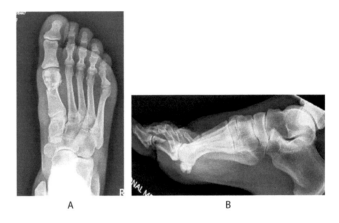

A   B

Figure 43.24 Anteroposterior (AP) (a) and lateral (b) views of a comminuted, plantar flexed first metatarsal fracture and nondisplaced second neck fracture.

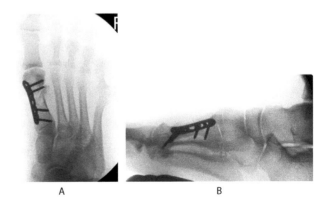

A   B

Figure 43.25 Fixation and length achieved using a locked 2.4 mm minifragment plate (a,b).

In displaced TMT injuries, there is consensus that the best outcomes are obtained with an anatomic reduction. Definitive fixation with K-wires should only be used to manage the fourth and fifth TMT joints. For a single, isolated first, second or third TMT injury, a percutaneously placed cannulated screw can be considered, provided that an anatomic reduction is obtained. If not, an open technique, using one incision placed over the first webspace at the level of the TMT joint with a second over the fourth metatarsal if necessary, should be used. For injuries presenting with comminution, a locked, dorsal plate can be placed across the joint to maintain length (Figure 43.26). For postoperative care, see Table 43.2.

OUTCOMES AND COMPLICATION

Good outcomes are expected when normal weight-bearing alignment has been restored. Early complications include infections, irritable implants and skin necrosis. Late complications consist of malunions, nonunions and post-traumatic arthritis. Malunions are due to poorly aligned metatarsals and can produce pain, disability and difficulty with shoewear. Nonunions are often due to loss of reduction, breakage of implants, early removal of implants or allowing weight bearing before adequate healing has occurred. In addition, metatarsophalangeal joint stiffness and post-traumatic arthritis at the base or the head have also been reported.

For TMT injuries, good outcomes can be expected with an anatomic reduction. Patients with nonanatomic reductions have higher levels of pain, gait abnormalities, difficulties with shoewear, more post-traumatic arthritis and significantly lower outcome scores.

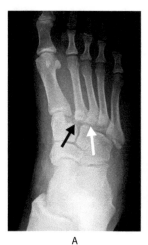 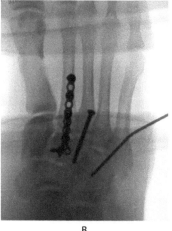

A   B

Figure 43.26 Anteroposterior (AP) view (a) demonstrating comminution of the base of the second metatarsal (black arrow) with dislocations of the second and third tarsometatarsal (TMT) (white arrow) joints and mild subluxation of the fourth and fifth joints. Fixation (b) achieved using a locked dorsal 2.4 mm plate across the second TMT joint, single screw fixation across the third TMT joint and a temporary K-wire to hold the fifth TMT joint.

PHALANGES

Phalangeal fractures are the second most common foot fracture in the elderly.[7] Anatomically, phalanges of the great toe are larger than those of the lesser toes. The proximal phalanges are the longest and most often injured. Circulation is through nutrient perforations with the proximal phalanges obtaining theirs from the dorsal digital arteries, the middle through plantar and dorsal digital arteries and the distal phalanges via a plantar supply.

Biomechanically, the toes contact the ground during 75% of the stance phase. During heel rise the generated force is through an oblique axis from the second through the fifth metatarsophalangeal joints. This is increased by forces from a transverse axis of the first and second metatarsophalangeal joints. Push-off is increased as the transverse axis moves towards the tips of the great toe and second toes, with toes three to five contributing to roll-over of the foot.

Classification

Historically, fractures describe the toe that is injured and then as occurring in proximal, middle or distal thirds or by describing fractures seen in the proximal or distal articular surfaces.

The OTA compendium has classified phalangeal fractures into three types. Type A fractures are simple (transverse, oblique or spiral) noncomminuted diaphyseal fractures or nonarticular fractures (with or without comminution) of the proximal or distal ends. Type B describes comminuted diaphyseal fractures presenting with a wedge of bone (spiral, bending or comminuted) or partial articular fractures of the proximal or distal ends. The articular fractures are subclassified as avulsion or partial split, depression or split/depression fractures. Type C describes comminuted diaphyseal fractures (segmental or complex comminuted) or articular fractures with complete comminution of the proximal or distal articular ends. The articular fractures are subclassified as simple articular, simple articular/comminuted metaphyseal or comminuted articular and metaphyseal fractures. In addition, modifiers describe specific toes. 'T' denotes the great toe and is further delineated as 1 (proximal) or 2 (distal phalanx), for example, T2 describes a distal phalanx fracture. 'N' is used for the second toe, 'M' for the middle toe, 'R' for the ring toe and 'L' for the little toe. The lesser toes are further subclassified 1 (proximal), 2 (middle) or 3 (distal phalanx).[19]

Nonoperative treatment

Fractures of the lesser toes are treated with buddy taping and a hard soled shoe. Fractures with some deformity can be managed with a closed reduction and a conservative approach but angular deformities should be corrected to prevent development of painful plantar pressures. Immediate weight bearing in a protective shoe is allowed and unrestricted activity is permitted at 3 months. Good

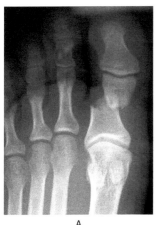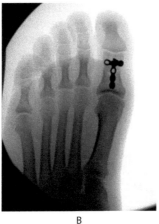

A   B

Figure 43.27 Anteroposterior (AP) view demonstrating a comminuted, bayoneted proximal phalanx fracture (a). Fixation achieved using a 2.0 mm locked plate (b).

outcomes can be expected as long as the general alignment is satisfactory.

Operative treatment

The primary indication is a displaced fracture of the proximal phalanx of the great toe. These include fracture dislocations, displacement of the distal condyles, shaft fractures with bayoneting or angular deformities unable to be managed closed. Simple pinning can be used but comminuted fractures may need a locked, minifragment implant (Figure 43.27). If overlapping of the lesser toes cannot be managed closed then an open reduction and pinning may be necessary. For postoperative care, see Table 43.2.

OUTCOMES AND COMPLICATIONS

Good outcomes can be expected and even some residual deformity does not seem to produce much disability. Complications include nonunions and malunions, which are symptomatic if they produce abnormal plantar pressure or irritability with shoewear. Joint stiffness and post-traumatic arthritis, from articular fractures, may also develop.

REFERENCES

1. Bloch F, Thibaud M, Duqué B, Brèque C, Riqaud AS, Kemoun G. Episodes of falling among elderly people: A systematic review and meta-analysis of social and demographic pre-disposing characteristics. *Clinics (San Paulo)* 2010;65:895–903.
2. Rossat A, Fatino B, Nitenberg C, Annweiler C, Poujol L, Herrmann FR, Beauchet O. Risk factors for falling in community-dwelling older adults: Which of them are associated with the recurrence of falls? *J Nutr Health Aging* 2010;14:787–791.
3. Kwan MM, Close JC, Wong AK, Lord SR. Falls incidence, risk factors, and consequences in Chinese older people: A systematic review. *J Am Geriatr Soc* 2011;59:536–543.
4. Paterson DH, Jones GR, Rice CL. Ageing and physical activity: Evidence to develop exercise recommendations for older adults. *Can J Pub Health* 2007;98:S69–108.
5. Keller JM, Sciadini MF, Sinclair E, O'Toole RV. Geriatric trauma: Demographics, injuries, and mortality. *J Orthop Trauma* 2012;26:e161–165.
6. Herscovici D Jr., Scaduto JM. Management of high-energy foot and ankle injuries in the geriatric population. *Geriatr Orthop Surg Rehabil* 2012;3:33–44.
7. Court-Brown CM, Clement ND, Duckworth AD, Aitken S, Biant LC, McQueen MM. The spectrum of fractures in the elderly. *Bone Joint J* 2014:96-B:366–372.
8. Sobhani S, Dekker R, Postema K, Dijkstra PU. Epidemiology of ankle and foot injuries in sports: A systematic review. *Scand J Med Sci Sports* 2013;23:669–686.
9. Lambers K, Ootes D, Ring D. Incidence of patients with lower extremity injuries presenting to US emergency departments by anatomic region, disease category, and age. *Clin Orthop Rel Res* 2010;470:284–290.
10. Demetriades D, Karaiskakis M, Velmahos G, Alo K, Newton E, Murray J, Asensio J, Belzberg H, Berne T, Shoemaker W. Effect on outcome of early intensive management of geriatric trauma patients. *Br J Surg* 2002;89:1319–1322.
11. Centers for Medicare & Medicaid Services, CMS Statistics Reference Booklet, 2013 edition. http://cms.hhs.gov/Research-Statistics-Data-and-Systems/Statistics-Trends-and-Reports/CMS-Statistics-Reference-Booklet/2013.html
12. Belatti DA, Phisitkul P. Economic burden of foot and ankle surgery in the US Medicare population. *Foot Ankle Int* 2014;35:334–340.
13. Hasselman CT, Vogt MT, Stone KL, Cauley JA, Conti SF. Foot and ankle fractures in elderly white women. *J Bone Joint Surg Am* 2003;85:820–824.
14. Gaskill T, Schweitzer K, Nunley J. Comparison of surgical outcomes of intra-articular calcaneal fractures by age. *J Bone Joint Surg Am* 2010;92:2884–2889.
15. Herscovici D Jr., Widmaier J, Scaduto JM, Sanders RW, Walling A. Operative treatment of calcaneal fractures in elderly patients. *J Bone Joint Surg Am* 2005;87:1260–1264.
16. Basile A. Operative versus nonoperative treatment of displaced intra-articular calcaneal fractures in elderly patients. *J Foot Ankle Surg* 2010;49:25–32.
17. Canale ST, Kelly FB. Fractures of the neck of the talus: Long term evaluation of seventy-one cases. *J Bone Joint Surg Am* 1978;60:143–156.

18. Inokuchi S, Ogawa K, Usami N. Classification of fractures of the talus: Clear differentiation between neck and body fractures. *Foot Ankle Int* 1996;17:748–750.

19. Marsh JL, Slongo TF, Agel J, Broderick JS, Creevey W, DeCoster TA, Prokuski L, et al. Fracture and Dislocation Compendium-2007. Orthopaedic Trauma Association Classification, Database and Outcomes Committee. *J Orthop Trauma* 2007;21(10 Suppl):S90–102, S125–8.

20. Lindvall E, Haidukewych G, DiPasquale T, Herscovici D Jr., Sanders R. Open reduction and stable fixation of isolated, displace talar neck and body fractures. *J Bone Joint Surg Am* 2004;86:2229–2234.

21. Vallier HA, Reichard SG, Boyd AJ, Moore TA. A new look at the Hawkins classification for talar neck fractures: Which features of injury and treatment are predictive of osteonecrosis? *J Bone Joint Surg Am* 2014;96:192–197.

22. Vallier HA, Nork SE, Benirschke SK, Sangeorzan BJ. Surgical treatment of talar body fractures. *J Bone Joint Surg Am* 2003;85:1716–1724.

23. Astion DJ, Deland JT, Otis JC, Kenneally S. Motion of the hindfoot after simulated arthrodesis. *J Bone Joint Surg Am* 1997;79:241–246.

24. Sanders R, Fortin P, DiPasquale T, Walling A. Operative treatment in 120 displaced intraarticular calcaneal fractures. Results using a prognostic computed tomography scan classification. *Clin Orthop Rel Res* 1993;290:87–95.

25. Buckley RE, Tough S, McCormack R, Pate G, Leighton R, Petrie D, Galpin R. Operative compared with nonoperative treatment of displaced intraarticular calcaneal fractures: A prospective, randomized, controlled multicenter study. *J Bone Joint Surg Am* 2002;84:1733–1744.

26. Sangeorzan BJ, Bernirscke SK, Mosca V, Mayo KA, Hansen ST. Displaced intra-articular fractures of the tarsal navicular. *J Bone Joint Surg Am* 1989;71:1504–1510.

27. Herscovici D Jr., Sanders R. Fractures of the tarsal navicular. *Foot Ankle Clin* 1999;4:587–601.

28. Court-Brown C, Zinna S, Ekrol I. Classification and epidemiology of midfoot fractures. *Foot* 2006;16:138–141.

29. Leland RH, Marymont JV, Trevino SG, Varner KE, Noble PC. Calcaneocuboid stability: A clinical and anatomic study. *Foot Ankle Int* 2001;22:880–884.

30. Weber M, Locher S. Reconstruction of the cuboid in compression fractures: Short to midterm results in 12 patients. *Foot Ankle Int* 2002;23:1008–1013.

31. Teng AL, Pinzur MS, Lomasney L, Mohoney L, Harvey R. Functional outcome following anatomic restoration of tarso-metatarsal fracture dislocation. *Foot Ankle Int* 2002;23:922–926.

32. Likin RC, Degnore LT, Pienkowski D. Contact mechanics of normal tarsometatarsal joints. *J Bone Joint Surg Am* 2001;83:520–528.

33. Dameron TB Jr. Fractures of the proximal fifth metatarsal: Selection the best treatment option. *J Am Acad Orthop Surg* 1995;3:110–114.

44

Soft tissue injuries

NICOLA MAFFULLI, ALESSIO GIAI VIA, ELEONORA PICCIRILLI AND FRANCESCO OLIVA

INTRODUCTION

Soft tissue injuries are common not only in young and active patients but also in older individuals. Rotator cuff injury, greater trochanter pain syndrome, anterior cruciate ligament rupture and Achilles tendon injury are debilitating problems both for older people who practice sporting activities and in everyday activities. In this chapter, these frequent conditions are described and evidence based treatment strategies are discussed.

ROTATOR CUFF INJURY

Rotator cuff tears (RCTs) are a frequent source of shoulder pain and disability in older patients. Since the first description of an RCT by Smith[1] in the *London Medical Gazette* in 1834, a wide variation in the prevalence of RCTs has been reported. Many studies have been conducted in symptomatic and asymptomatic patients, and imaging and cadaveric studies have been performed. Cadaver studies estimate the prevalence of full thickness tears ranging from 5% to 30%.[2] In 2006, a review of the cadaveric and imaging prevalence of RCTs[3] showed an overall prevalence of 23% in 4629 cadaveric shoulders. The prevalence of RCTs increases linearly with age from the third decade, increasing from 33% in the 40s to 55% in the 50s.[4]

Pathogenesis

The pathogenesis of RCTs is multifactorial and is still not completely clear.[4] Many theories have been proposed, and tears are traditionally classified into 'extrinsic' and 'intrinsic' (Table 44.1). Chronic impingement, as described by Neer in his chronic impingement syndrome

theory, is the best known extrinsic pathological factor in RCTs.[5] Excessive load, repetitive load or loads applied from different directions have been implicated in the process of tendinopathy. Other theories include localized hypoxia produced by tensile load, hyperthermic injury as the tendon heats up with exercise, tenocyte apoptosis, and cytokines or proteolytic enzymes released as a result of applied stress. The release of nitrous oxide has also been implicated in the tendinopathy process. Currently, RCTs are considered to be of multifactorial etiology, and the relative contributions of these factors remain to be determined.

Any process that impairs tissue healing may be implicated in rotator cuff disease. Nicotine exerts deleterious effects on tendon healing,[6] and smokers are less likely to respond favorably to cuff repair operations, with reduced postoperative function and satisfaction compared to nonsmokers.[7] In the current literature, factors such as patient age, sex and fatty muscle infiltration are highly correlated to the presence of RCTs and the prevalence of recurrence of tears.[4]

Many studies emphasize the importance of extracellular matrix (ECM) for the homeostasis of connective tissue. ECM is the substrate to which cells adhere, migrate and differentiate. ECM imparts information to cells and tissues by providing cell-binding motifs in its own proteins or by presenting growth factors and morphogens to the cells. Physiological and pathological modifications of the ECM seem to be the most important intrinsic factors involved in tendinopathies and tendon ruptures.[8] Transglutaminases (TGs) have been implicated in the formation of hard tissue development, matrix maturation and mineralization and have been shown to be down-regulated in human supraspinatus tendon ruptures.[9]

Table 44.1 Extrinsic and intrinsic theories about the pathogenesis of rotator cuff tears

Theory	Authors	Year
Extrinsic factors		
Chronic impingement syndrome	Neer	1972
Overuse	Codman, McMaster	1931, 1993
Multifactorial	Soslowsky	2004
Intrinsic factors		
Hypoperfusion theory	Uhthoff	1990
Degenerative theory	Sano	1999
Degeneration-microtrauma	Yadav	2009
Apoptotic theory	Yuan	2002
Extracellular matrix modifications	Riley	2002

Source: Via AG, et al. *Muscles Ligaments Tendons J* 2013;3:70–79.

The roles of hormonal and metabolic diseases have recently been investigated.[10] The relationship between thyroid disorders and shoulder pain has been suspected since the late 1920s[11] but has not been systematically investigated. The thyroid hormones, T3 and T4, play an essential role in the development and metabolism of many tissues and organs. Thyroxine is important for both collagen synthesis and ECM metabolism. A recent study demonstrated that thyroid hormone nuclear receptors are present in healthy and pathologic rotator cuff tendons, and that, in vitro, thyroid hormones enhance tenocyte growth and counteract apoptosis in healthy tenocytes isolated from tendon in a dose- and time-dependent manner.[12] Hypothyroidism causes accumulation of glycosaminoglycans in the ECM, which may, in turn, predispose to tendon calcification.[10] Diabetes is also a risk factor for RCTs.[13] In a study on asymptomatic subjects, age related rotator cuff tendon changes were more common in diabetic subjects.[14] Diabetic patients show a restricted shoulder range of motion, a higher prevalence of recurrent tears after surgical repair and a higher rate of complications and infections after open and arthroscopic repair of RCTs.[15] An association between obesity and RCTs has also been proposed.[16]

Physical examination

The clinical diagnosis is not always easy. Painful conditions of the long head of the biceps or the acromioclavicular joint may result in a high false positive rate. The clinical presentation of rotator cuff pathology is extremely variable. A recent review concluded that RCTs are frequently asymptomatic.[7] Such variation in clinical features remains unexplained. Physical examination should include inspection, palpation, the evaluation of active and passive range of motion and the execution of strength and provocative tests. Many specific clinical tests are available to test the muscles forming the rotator cuff. Patients with shoulder pain who test positive for supraspinatus weakness, weakness in external rotation and impingement have 98% chance of having an RCT. If none of these clinical features are present, the chance of having a tear decreases to 5%.[4]

Rotator cuff healing

Tendon healing is a complex and well-orchestrated series of physiological events involving synthesis, migration and degradation of ECM components. The ability of tendons to heal is controversial: tendon tissue can repair but not regenerate.[13] Tissue adjacent to an RCT (2.5 mm) appears to be histologically viable in both microvasculature and cellular synthesis of type I procollagen. Therefore, many authors advise avoiding wide excision of the edges of the torn rotator cuff before reattachment.[4] This is supported by the observation of Jost et al.[17] who, in a long-term follow-up after structural failure of rotator cuff repairs, observed compelling evidence that small reruptures have a potential to heal.

It is very important to provide the tendon with the best conditions to heal. The subacromial bursa seems to play an important role. In normal conditions, the subacromial bursa has three functions. It facilitates gliding between two layers of tissue, provides blood supply to the cuff tendons and provides cells and vessels to aid healing after surgical repair. Mobilization after repair promotes cellular activity, improves tensile properties and enhances gliding function. A fine balance exists between the progression of tendon healing and postoperative mobilization.

Treatment of rotator cuff tears

Both arthroscopic and mini-open techniques are effective for rotator cuff repair, but there is still considerable debate over the benefits of these procedures. Many improvements have been made since the first completely arthroscopic rotator cuff repair described by Johnson,[18] and arthroscopists state that the main advantages of all-arthroscopic repairs are less postoperative pain and shorter rehabilitation time. However, when the outcome of arthroscopic and mini-open repair are compared, no significant differences are found. Functional outcome, pain, range of motion and complications do not significantly differ between all arthroscopically repaired patients and those treated with mini-open repair in the first year after surgery.[19] Pearsall et al.[20] and Kim et al.,[21] in retrospective studies, found no differences in outcome for small and medium sized tears of the rotator cuff at mid-term follow-up. A systematic review showed decreased pain at short-term follow-up in patients treated arthroscopically.[22] However, massive tears remain difficult to treat arthroscopically, and the mini-open surgical technique could be a good choice in the elderly patient. Another difference between the two different methods is the re-tear rate, which is higher in patients treated arthroscopically at 24-month follow-up.[23] In reality, there is no evidence about which is the best treatment.

Irreparable RCTs in elderly patients are a challenging problem. There are several treatment options, but determining the correct treatment for each patient is difficult. Reverse shoulder arthroplasty (RSA) is an emerging solution for these patients in whom anatomic shoulder arthroplasty or hemiarthroplasty has failed. Many mid-term studies showed early encouraging results, and the first long-term studies show good survivorship. Favard et al.[24] retrospectively reviewed 527 arthroplasties in 506 patients and found 89% survivorship at 10 years. Similar results have been reported by Guery et al.,[25] who demonstrated deteriorating function and increasing pain after 6 years. Boileau et al.[26] reported improved shoulder function and restored active elevation in patients with cuff-deficient shoulders treated with RSA. Supported by these encouraging results, original indications for RSA were expanded. Originally, the reverse shoulder prostheses were designed for rotator cuff arthropathy, and massive RCTs with arthritis and massive irreparable RCTs were considered appropriate indications. Recently, displaced three- or four-part neck of humerus fractures in older patients, RCTs with fatty infiltration of infraspinatus or subscapularis muscles, sequelae of fracture, rheumatoid arthritis, revision arthroplasty and tumors are becoming common indications for RSA.[27] RSA combined with latissimus dorsi and teres major tendon transfer has been developed to improve external rotation and spatial control in patients with no functional teres minor and infraspinatus with early promising results.[28] However, a high rate of complications is still reported after RSA and progressive functional and radiographic deterioration continue to be of concern.[29] Scapular notching is one of the most important complications of RSA.[25]

Future perspectives

Several strategies have been proposed to enhance tendon healing. Recently research focused on regenerative therapies such as growth factors (GFs) and plasma rich platelet (PRP) which have become a popular treatment for tendon injuries. However, the efficacy of PRP treatment is highly controversial. In vitro studies showed that the addition of PRP to human tenocytes resulted in cell proliferation, collagen deposition, well-ordered angiogenesis and improved gene expression for matrix degrading enzymes and endogenous growth factors.[30,31] More recently, two studies demonstrated that PRP induced in vitro tendon mesenchymal stem cells (T-MSCs) to differentiate into active tenocytes, and that PRP has an anti-inflammatory function by suppressing the levels of prostaglandin E (PGE) biosynthetic pathway components (COX-1, COX-2 and PGE synthase-1 [PGES-1] expression) and PGE2 production.[32] These results have important clinical implications because high levels of PGE2 cause pain, decrease cell proliferation and collagen production and induce degenerative changes in rabbit

tendons.[33] But the same authors also reported that, even if PRP is able to induce the differentiation of T-MSCs into tenocytes under regular culture conditions, PRP injection in clinics may not be able to effectively reverse the degenerative conditions of late-stage tendinopathy.[34]

However, clinical studies do not report any substantial benefit using PRP for rotator cuff lesions. A few studies demonstrated that the application of PRP for large to massive rotator cuff repairs significantly improved structural outcomes with a decreased re-tear rate.[35] Gumina found that the platelet-leukocyte membrane improved structural repair integrity, but without improvement in functional outcome.[36] Other works did not report better results with the use of PRP. Randelli et al.[37] found that PRP reduces pain in the short term, making it possible to mobilize the patient earlier, but they did not find long-term improvement in functional scores. No differences in rotator cuff healing or improvements in function were found at 1-year follow-up.[38] No statistically significant difference in the recurrent tear rate between patients treated with or without the addition of PRP was found.[38] Castricini et al.[39] performed a randomized double blind controlled trial with 88 patients and there were no statistically significant differences at 16-month follow-up. They stated that the study does not support the use of PRP in small to medium sized RCTs. There results were confirmed in a further RCT by Rodeo et al.[40]

GREATER TROCHANTER PAIN SYNDROME

Lateral hip pain is a debilitating condition characterized by pain at or around the greater trochanter, which is the site of confluence of three bursae, the hip abductor-lateral thigh muscles and the iliotibial tract. It was originally described as trochanteric bursitis, but advanced imaging and surgical findings did not evidence a real bursal involvement and instead showed different disorders such as insertional tendinopathy, tendon tears or avulsion of the gluteus medius and gluteus minimus tendons.[41,42] External coxa saltans (snapping hip) is also related to greater trochanter pain. For these reasons, the term greater trochanteric pain syndrome (GTPS) is now used to better define this clinical condition.[41]

The incidence of GTPS is reported to be approximately 1.8 per 1000 patients per year, and it is more frequent in women (female:male ratio of 4:1) between 40 and 60 years old. It has been reported to affect 10–25% of the general population, and up to 35% in patients with leg length discrepancy and low back pain.[43] It is particularly frequent in road runners, exposed to increased friction over the iliotibial tract over the greater trochanter, but it occurs also in sedentary older patients. Acute trauma, osteoarthritis, rheumatoid arthritis, lumbosacral disorders and infections (especially tuberculosis) have to be excluded.

The diagnosis of GTPS is usually based on clinical findings. Plain radiographs are performed in all patients to exclude concomitant hip or knee joint disease.

Calcification may be detected at the site of insertion to the greater trochanter. MRI is useful to recognize partial and full tears of the gluteus medius and minimus tendons, tendon calcification and fatty muscle degeneration.

The optimal management for GTPS remains unclear. Conservative measures, including relative rest, nonsteroidal anti-inflammatories, ice, and supervised stretching and strengthening exercises are usually effective as the first-line management of GTPS. Home training programs seem to be effective, and good results and improvement in symptoms have been reported in 41% of patients at 4-month follow-up and in 80% of patients at 15 months.[42] The correction of training errors and modifying physical activities is also important, while leg length discrepancy was recently confirmed to be a risk factor for GTPS. Local corticosteroid injections are widely used in clinical practice, but there is no conclusive evidence on their effectiveness. Small observational studies suggest that corticosteroid injections provide good short-term outcomes, but symptom recurrence and incomplete pain relief are not uncommon. Furthermore, fluoroscopically assisted injections of corticosteroid and local anaesthetics have not resulted in better treatment outcomes.[42] Laser therapy and shock wave therapy are useful for the treatment of GTPS. A randomized controlled trial comparing different non-operative treatments reported that, even though the results of corticosteroid injections were significantly better than those of home training or shock wave therapy at 1-month follow-up, their effect quickly declined after 1 month. At 15-month follow-up, home training and shock wave therapy were more effective than corticosteroid injection, with success rates of 74%, 80% and 48%, respectively.[44] The authors concluded that the role of corticosteroid injection for GTPS should be reconsidered because it is significantly less successful than home training and shock wave therapy at long-term follow-up.

If conservative treatment fails, surgery is indicated. Several operative procedures, open and endoscopic, have been described for patients not responding to conservative treatment. In a study by Slawski and Howard, five active patients (seven hips) received longitudinal release of the iliotibial band and excision of the subgluteal bursa.[45] All patients were satisfied with the surgical results and returned to their pre-injury sporting level. Pain reduction has been reported after open trochanteric reduction osteotomy, tendon repair and reattachment of the medius gluteus. Endoscopic bursectomy has also been proposed with early improvements at 1-month follow-up. Minimally invasive procedures such as endoscopic repair techniques provided good short-term outcomes,[2] but further larger studies, with longer follow-up, are needed.[46]

ANTERIOR CRUCIATE LIGAMENT TEARS IN OLDER PATIENTS

The incidence of anterior cruciate ligament (ACL) tears in the United States is about 200,000 per year, with at least 50% of these patients undergoing arthroscopic reconstruction.

Although this procedure may reduce the progression of knee osteoarthritis in chronic ACL deficiency, the management of knee instability in older patients is debated. Satisfactory functional outcomes have been reported in patients older than 50 undergoing conservative management at long-term follow-up.[47] However, reduction in recreational activity level and increased chronic instability impair physical activities in older patients with a high functional activity level, and ACL reconstruction may be indicated.[48] The management of older patients with ACL tears depends on several specific factors, including age, occupation and desired activity level. In less active people with sedentary lifestyles, conservative management consisting of physical therapy and activity modification can provide successful outcomes, but surgery may be indicated in active patients participating in jumping or pivoting sports.[47]

Although the management of older patients with ACL insufficiency remains controversial, in the last few years surgical management of ACL deficiency has been increasingly advocated. A study comparing pre- and postoperative status showed that patients over 50 who underwent ACL reconstruction experienced improved postoperative clinical outcomes. Even if older patients show a lower return rate to pre-injury sport activity level, they seem to be subjectively more satisfied with the overall results than younger patients. Surgical expectations should be tailored to age and activity level. Surgical management in healthy subjects older than 40 years to prevent further secondary injuries and return to pre-injury sport activity performance status has been advocated by some authors.[49]

Even if age and time from injury to surgery have been considered as risk factors for osteoarthritis, they are not absolute contraindications to surgical management, and age itself is not a contraindication to ACL surgery. When faced with patients with ACL instability, physiological age, condition of the knee at the time of examination, life expectancy and activity levels are probably more important than chronologic age. The optimal treatment in adult patients with ACL tears should be planned after careful consideration of the patient's characteristics, their desire to return to activity and knee-specific comorbidities, especially meniscal pathology or osteoarthritis.

ACHILLES TENDON INJURY IN OLDER PATIENTS

Tendinopathy of the main body of the Achilles tendon (AT) affects both athletic and sedentary patients, and about 30% of patients do not participate in sports activities.[50] Acute AT rupture is a serious injury, with an incidence ranging from 6 to 18 per 100,000 subjects per year. Most (75%) acute ruptures occur during recreational activities in men between the ages of 30 and 40, and 25% of ruptures occur in sedentary patients.[51]

The pathogenesis of AT injuries is not completely clear. Metabolic diseases, such as diabetes mellitus,[52] hypercholesterolemia and obesity, seem to play a role.[53]

Hyperglycaemia may be a risk factor for tendinopathy because of non-enzymatic glycosylation processes which change collagen cross-links.[54]

Management of acute ruptures of the AT is still controversial. Operative management provides earlier functional rehabilitation, less calf atrophy and stronger pushoff than non-surgical treatment. Surgical treatment ensures a lower rerupture rate compared to non-operative treatment, which has been reported in up to 13% of patients treated conservatively.[55] A recent review article showed that surgical treatment results in higher costs and a 20-fold higher rate of complications, such as wound problems and superficial or deep infections, than conservative treatment.[56] On the other hand, recent well-conducted randomized controlled trials showed that conservative and open surgery management produce, in an unselected population, similar functional results. Willits et al. showed acceptable and similar outcomes in patients treated with accelerated functional rehabilitation for acute AT ruptures compared to patients who received operative repair.[57] However, the first group experienced a higher rerupture rate. Non-operative management using functional bracing with early mobilization has similar outcomes compared to open surgical treatment with regard to rerupture rate, range of motion and calf circumference.[58] The major advantage of conservative treatment is a lower rate of complications.[59] The risk of complications following surgery was 3.9-fold than in non-surgically treated patients, with an absolute risk increase of 15.8%.

Other concerns when dealing with elderly patients with AT rupture include the high incidence of comorbidities in this age group. Comorbidities can make it difficult for the patients to return to their previous state of activity and immobility in the elderly may progressively impair their general health status.

Minimally invasive AT repair has been successfully used to avoid these complications and it is becoming a well-accepted treatment. It provides many advantages, such as less iatrogenic damage to normal tissues, less postoperative pain, accurate opposition of the tendon ends, minimized surgical incisions and improved cosmesis. A recent systematic review reported a rate of superficial infections of 0.5% and 4.3% after minimally invasive and open surgeries, respectively. Deep infections did not occur in subjects who received minimally invasive repair.[56] Shorter hospitalization and average time to return to work were also found in the minimally invasive group. The indications were grossly comparable, and the functional outcomes were not significantly different between minimally invasive and open surgery. Although sural nerve injury has been reported as a potential complication of this kind of surgery, new techniques have minimized the risk of sural nerve damage. Good results have been reported in 27 patients with a mean age of 73 years.[60] All patients were able to bear weight fully on the affected limb by the eighth postoperative week. The rerupture rate was 7%, superficial infection managed with oral antibiotics occurred in 11% of cases, and 11% of patients experienced hypaesthesia over the area of distribution of

the sural nerve which resolved over 6 months in most cases. The authors concluded that percutaneous repair of the AT is a suitable option for patients older than 65 because it reduces the risk of rerupture compared to non-operative treatment, produces lower risk of other complications and provides similar outcomes compared to percutaneous repair in younger patients. Encouraging results have also been reported in diabetic patients, with a rate of superficial infection of 20%.[61] Hence, mini-invasive techniques are a proper alternative for AT repair in older patients, in particular in patients with comorbidities such as diabetes or vascular diseases with higher risk of infection and wound complications.

Percutaneous Achilles tendon repair: surgical technique

A 1-cm transverse incision is made over the defect using a size 11 blade. Four longitudinal stab incisions are made lateral and medial to the tendon 6 cm proximal to the palpable defect. Two further longitudinal incisions on either side of the tendon are made 4–6 cm distal to the palpable defect. Forceps are then used to mobilize the tendon from beneath the subcutaneous tissues. A 9 cm Mayo needle is threaded with two double loops of Number 1 Maxon, and this is passed transversely between the proximal stab incisions through the bulk of the tendon (Figure 44.1). The bulk of the tendon is surprisingly superficial. The loose ends are held with a clip. In turn, each of the ends is then passed distally from just proximal to the transverse Maxon passage through the bulk of the tendon to pass out of the diagonally opposing stab incision. A subsequent diagonal pass is then made to the transverse incision over the ruptured tendon. To prevent entanglement, both ends of the Maxon are held in separate clips. This suture is then tested for security by pulling with both ends of the Maxon distally. Another double loop of Maxon is then passed between the distal stab incisions through the tendon (Figure 44.2), and in turn through the tendon and out of the transverse incision starting distal to the transverse passage (Figure 44.3). The ankle is

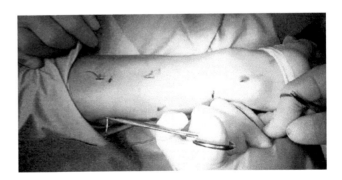

Figure 44.1 A 9 cm Mayo needle is threaded with two double loops of Number 1 Maxon, and this is passed transversely between the proximal stab incision through the bulk of the tendon.

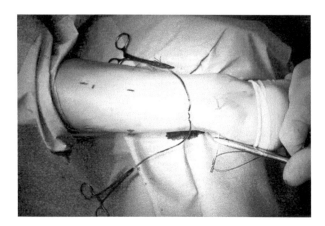

Figure 44.2 Another double loop of Maxon is then passed between the distal stab incision through the tendon.

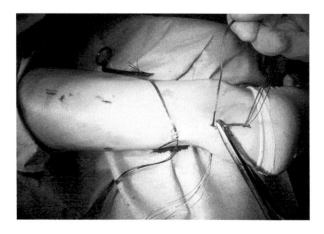

Figure 44.3 The double loop of Maxon is passed in turn through the tendon and out of the transverse incision starting distal to the transverse passage.

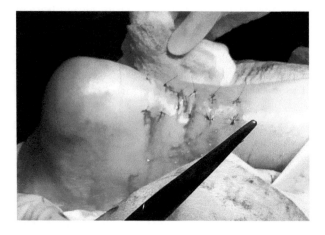

Figure 44.4 Final appearance of the surgical procedure.

held in full plantar flexion, and in turn opposing ends of the Maxon thread are tied together with a double throw knot, and then three further throws before being buried using the forceps. A clip is used to hold the first throw of the lateral side to maintain the tension of the suture.

We use 3-0 Vicryl sutures to close the transverse incision and Steri-Strips to close the stab incisions (Figure 44.4). A non-adherent dressing is applied. A full plaster cast is applied in the operating room with the ankle in physiologic equinus. The cast is split on both medial and lateral sides to allow for swelling. The patient is discharged on the same day of the operation.

CONCLUSIONS

Soft tissue injuries are common problems not only in young and active patients but also in older people. For RCTs, similar outcomes have been reported with all-arthroscopic repair treatment or mini-open repair, so a mini-open approach could be a valid option for older patients with a massive rotator cuff rupture and for lesions that are difficult to treat arthroscopically. We believe that treatment should be tailored to the individual patient. Promising results are reported with RSA for those patients who are not candidates for rotator cuff repair, but careful patient selection and attention to appropriate technique are required to reduce the current high rate of complications. Despite laboratory evidence of the positive effects of GFs in tendon healing, only well-conducted, appropriately powered randomized controlled trials, with adequate outcome measures and length of follow-up, will clarify whether GFs play a role in routine clinical practice.

GTPS is a complex syndrome, and many different causes may contribute to its pathogenesis. The effectiveness of the various treatment modalities needs to be tested in carefully conducted randomized controlled trials.

Older patients can achieve good outcomes after reconstruction of an ACL injury. However, the quality of currently available data is still limited and further well-designed studies are needed to determine long-term efficacy and to better inform our patients with regard to expected outcomes. AT rupture is a serious injury also in older patients. Non-operative management and mini-invasive techniques are suitable alternatives for AT repair in older patients, in particular in patients with comorbidities such as diabetes or vascular diseases with a higher risk of infection and wound complications.

REFERENCES

1. Smith JG. Pathological appearances of seven cases of injury of the shoulder joint with remarks. *London Med Gaz* 1834;14:280.
2. Lehman C, Cuomo F, Kummer FJ, Zuckerman JD. The incidence of full thickness rotator cuff tears in a large cadaveric population. *Bull Hosp Jt Dis* 1995;54:30–31.
3. Reilly P, Macleod I, Macfarlane R, Windley J, Emery R. Dead men and radiologists don't lie: A review of cadaveric and radiological studies of rotator cuff tear prevalence. *Ann R Coll Surg Engl* 2006;88:116–121.

4. Via AG, De Cupis M, Spoliti M, Oliva F. Clinical and biological aspects of rotator cuff tears. *Muscles Ligaments Tendons J* 2013;3:70–79.

5. Neer CS, 2nd. Anterior acromioplasty for the chronic impingement syndrome in the shoulder: A preliminary report. J Bone Joint Surg Am 1972;54:41–50.

6. Galatz LM, Silva MJ, Rothermich SY, Zaegel MA, Havlioglu N, Thomopoulos S. Nicotine delays tendon-to-bone healing in a rat shoulder model. *J Bone Joint Surg Am* 2006;88:2027–2034.

7. Mallon WJ, Misamore G, Snead DS, Denton P. The impact of preoperative smoking habits on the results of rotator cuff repair. *J Shoulder Elbow Surg* 2004;13:129–132.

8. Modesti A, Oliva F. All is around ECM of tendons!? *Muscles Ligaments Tendons J* 2013;3:1.

9. Tarantino U, Oliva F, Taurisano G, et al. FXIIIA and TGF-beta over-expression produces normal musculoskeletal phenotype in TG2-/-mice. *Amino Acids* 2009;36:679–684.

10. Oliva F, Berardi AC, Misiti S, Maffulli N. Thyroid hormones and tendon: Current views and future perspectives. Concise review. *Muscles Ligaments Tendons J* 2013;3:201–203.

11. Duncan WS. The relationship of hyperthyroidism to joint conditions. *JAMA* 1928;91:1779–1782.

12. Oliva F, Berardi AC, Misiti S, Verza Felzacappa C, Iacone A, Maffulli N. Thyroid hormones enhance growth and counteract apoptosis in human tenocytes isolated from rotator cuff tendons. *Cell Death Dis* 2013;4:e705.

13. Wildemann B, Klatte F. Biological aspects of rotator cuff healing. *Muscles Ligaments Tendons J* 2011;1:161–168.

14. Abate P, Schiavone C, Salini V. Sonographic evaluation of the shoulder in asymptomatic elderly subjects with diabetes. *BMC Musculoskel Disord* 2010;11:278.

15. Clement ND, Hallett A, MacDonald D, Howie C, McBirnie J. Does diabetes affect outcome after arthroscopic repair of the rotator cuff? *J Bone Joint Surg Br* 2010;92:1112–1117.

16. Wendelboe M, Hegmann KT, Gren LH, Alder SC, White GL Jr, Lyon JL. Associations between body-mass index and surgery for rotator cuff tendinitis. *J Bone Joint Surg Am* 2004;86:743–747.

17. Jost B, Zumstein M, Pfirrmann CW, Gerber C. Long-term outcome after structural failure of rotator cuff repairs. *J Bone Joint Surg Am* 2006;88:472–479.

18. Johnson LL. Rotator cuff. In: *Diagnostic and Surgical Arthroscopy of the Shoulder*, Johnson LL, ed. St. Louis, MO: Mosby; 1993, pp. 365–405.

19. van der Zwaal, Thomassen BJ, Nieuwenhuijse MJ, Lindenburg R, Swen JW, van Arkel ER. Clinical outcome in all-arthroscopic versus mini-open rotator cuff repair in small to medium-sized tears: A randomized controlled trial in 100 patients with 1-year follow-up. *Arthroscopy* 2013;29:266–273.

20. Pearsall AW 4th, Ibrahim KA, Madanagopal SG. The results of arthroscopic versus mini-open repair for rotator cuff tears at mid-term follow-up. *J Orthop Surg Res* 2007;2:24.

21. Kim SH, Ha KI, Park JH, Kang JS, Oh SK, Oh I. Arthroscopic versus mini-open salvage repair of the rotator cuff tear: Outcome analysis at 2 to 6 years' follow-up. *Arthroscopy* 2003;19:746–754.

22. Lindley K, Jones GL. Outcomes of arthroscopic versus open rotator cuff repair: A systematic review of the literature. *Am J Orthop (Belle Mead NJ)* 2010;39:592–600.

23. Zhang Z, Gu B, Zhu W, Zhu L, Li Q. Arthroscopic versus mini-open rotator cuff repair: A prospective, randomized study with 24-month follow-up. *Eur J Orthop Surg Traumatol* 2014;24(6):845–850.

24. Favard L, Lévigne C, Nerot C, et al. Reverse prostheses in arthropathies with cuff tear: Are survivorship and function maintained over time? *Clin Orthop Relat Res* 2011;469:2469–2475.

25. Guery J, Favard L, Sirveaux F, et al. Reverse total shoulder arthroplasty. Survivorship analysis of eighty replacements followed for 5 to 10 years. *J Bone Joint Surg Am* 2006;88:1742–1747.

26. Boileau P, Watkinson D, Hatzidakis AM, Hovorka I. Neer Award 2005: The Grammont reverse shoulder prosthesis: Results in cuff tear arthritis, fracture sequelae, and revision arthroplasty. *J Shoulder Elbow Surg* 2006;15(5):527–540.

27. Smithers CJ, Young AA, Walch G. Reverse shoulder arthroplasty. *Curr Rev Musculoskelet Med* 2011;4:183–190.

28. Boileau P, Rumian AP, Zumstein MA. Reversed shoulder arthroplasty with modified L'Episcopo for combined loss of active elevation and external rotation. *J Shoulder Elbow Surg* 2010;19:20–30.

29. Zumstein MA, Pinedo M, Old J, et al. Problems, complications, reoperations, and revisions in reverse total shoulder arthroplasty: A systematic review. *J Shoulder Elbow Surg* 2011;20(1):146–157.

30. Oliva F, Via AG, Maffulli N. Role of growth factors in rotator cuff healing. *Sports Med Arthrosc* 2011;19:218–226.

31. Yuan T, Zhang CQ, Wang JH. Augmenting tendon and ligament repair with platelet-rich plasma (PRP). *Muscles Ligaments Tendons J* 2013;3:139–149.

32. Wang JHC. Can PRP effectively treat injured tendons? *Muscles Ligaments Tendons J* 2014;4:35–37.

33. Khan MH, Li Z, Wang JH. Repeated exposure of tendon to prostaglandin-E2 leads to localized tendon degeneration. *Clin J Sport Med* 2005;15:27–33.

34. Zhang J, Wang JHC. PRP treatment effects on degenerative tendinopathy—An in vitro model study. *Muscles Ligaments Tendons J* 2014;4:10–17.

35. Jo CH, Shin JS, Lee YG, et al. Platelet-rich plasma for arthroscopic repair of large to massive rotator cuff tears: A randomized, single-blind, parallel-group trial. *Am J Sports Med* 2013;41:2240–2248.

36. Gumina S, Campagna V, Ferrazza G, et al. Use of platelet-leukocyte membrane in arthroscopic repair of large rotator cuff tears: A prospective randomized study. *J Bone Joint Surg Am* 2012;94:1345–1352.

37. Randelli P, Arrigoni P, Ragone V, Aliprandi A, Cabitza P. Platelet rich plasma in arthroscopic rotator cuff repair: A prospective RCT study, 2-year follow-up. *J Shoulder Elbow Surg* 2011;20:518–528.

38. Ruiz-Moneo P, Molano-Muñoz J, Prieto E, Algorta J. Plasma rich in growth factors in arthroscopic rotator cuff repair: A randomized, double-blind, controlled clinical trial. *Arthroscopy* 2013;29:2–9.

39. Castricini R, Longo UG, De Benedetto M, et al. Platelet-rich plasma augmentation for arthroscopic rotator cuff repair: A randomized controlled trial. *Am J Sports Med* 2011;39:258–265.

40. Rodeo SA, Delos D, Williams RJ, Adler R, Pearle AD, Warren RF. The effect of platelet-rich fibrin matrix on rotator cuff tendon healing: A prospective, randomized clinical study. Am J Sports Med 2012;40:1234–1241.

41. Ho GW, Howard TM. Greater trochanteric pain syndrome: More than bursitis and iliotibial tract friction. *Curr Sports Med Rep* 2012;11:232–238.

42. Del Buono A, Papalia R, Khanduja V, Denaro V, Maffulli N. Management of the greater trochanteric pain syndrome: A systematic review. *Br Med Bull* 2012;102:115–131.

43. Strauss EJ, Nho SJ, Kelly BT. Greater trochanteric pain syndrome. *Sports Med Arthrosc* 2010;18:113–119.

44. Rompe JD, Segal NA, Cacchio A, Furia JP, Morral A, Maffulli N. Home training, local corticosteroid injection, or radial shock wave therapy for greater trochanter pain syndrome. *Am J Sports Med* 2009;37:1981–1990.

45. Slawski DP, Howard RF. Surgical management of refractory trochanteric bursitis. *Am J Sports Med* 1997;25:86–89.

46. Govaert LH, van Dijk CN, Zeegers AV, Albers GH. Endoscopic bursectomy and iliotibial tract release as a treatment for refractory greater trochanteric pain syndrome: A new endoscopic approach with early results. *Arthrosc Tech* 2012;1:e161–e164.

47. Bogunovic L, Matava MJ. Operative and nonoperative treatment options for ACL tears in the adult patient: A conceptual review. *Phys Sportsmed* 2013;41:33–40.

48. Osti L, Papalia R, Del Buono A, Leonardi F, Denaro V, Maffulli N. Surgery for ACL deficiency in patients over 50. *Knee Surg Sports Traumatol Arthrosc* 2011;19:412–17.

49. Brown CA, McAdams TR, Harris AH, Maffulli N, Safran MR. ACL reconstruction in patients aged 40 years and older: A systematic review and introduction of a new methodology score for ACL studies. *Am J Sports Med* 2013;41:2181–90.

50. Rolf C, Movin T. Etiology, histopathology, and outcome of surgery in achillodynia. *Foot Ankle Int* 1997;18:565–569.

51. Maffulli N, Waterston SW, Squair J, et al. Changing incidence of Achilles tendon rupture in Scotland: A 15-year study. *Clin J Sport Med* 1999;9:157–160.

52. de Oliveira RR, Lemos A, de Castro Silveira PV, da Silva RJ, de Moraes SR. Alterations of tendons in patients with diabetes mellitus: A systematic review. *Diabet Med* 2011;28:886–95.

53. Oliva F, Via AG, Maffulli N. Physiopathology of intra-tendinous calcific deposition. *BMC Med* 2012;10:95.

54. Rosenthal AK, Gohr CM, Mitton E, Monnier VM, Burner T. Advanced glycation endproducts increase transglutaminase activity in primary porcine tenocytes. *J Invest Med* 2009;57:460–466.

55. Guillo S, Del Buono A, Dias M, et al. Percutaneous repair of acute ruptures of the tendo Achillis. *Surgeon* 2013;11:14–19.

56. Del Buono A, Volpin A, Maffulli N. Minimally invasive versus open surgery for acute Achilles tendon rupture: A systematic review. *Br Med Bull* 2014;109:45–54.

57. Willits K, Amendola A, Bryant D, et al. Operative versus nonoperative treatment of acute Achilles tendon ruptures: A multicenter randomized trial using accelerated functional rehabilitation. *J Bone Joint Surg Am* 2010;92:2767–2775.

58. Ebinesan AD, Sarai BS, Walley GD, Maffulli N. Conservative, open or percutaneous repair for acute rupture of the Achilles tendon. *Disabil Rehabil* 2008;30(20–22):1721–1725.

59. Maffulli N, Longo UG, Denaro V. Complications after surgery or nonoperative treatment for acute Achilles tendon rupture. *Clin J Sport Med* 2009;19:441–442.

60. Maffulli N, Longo UG, Ronga M, Khanna A, Denaro V. Favorable outcome of percutaneous repair of achilles tendon ruptures in the elderly. *Clin Orthop Relat Res* 2010;468:1039–1046.

61. Maffulli N, Longo UG, Maffulli GD, Khanna A, Denaro V. Achilles tendon ruptures in diabetic patients. *Arch Orthop Trauma Surg* 2011;131:33–38.

45

Sports injuries in the elderly

MARC TOMPKINS, ROBBY SIKKA AND DAVID FISCHER

BACKGROUND

Sports injuries in the elderly commonly involve either fracture or soft tissue injuries, such as ligament and tendon injuries. Fractures have been extensively covered in previous chapters, so this chapter will focus on soft tissue injuries. There is scant literature specifically on the elderly athlete, but we will discuss injuries in multiple areas of the extremities. We have chosen pathologies that have at least a modicum of studies in an older population. Also, defining what is elderly, particularly when it comes to sports, is somewhat a matter of personal discretion, so rather than focus on a specific age cutoff in this chapter, we have focused more on the aging athlete.

Before discussing specific injuries, however, it is important to be mindful that although these injuries may occur during athletic participation, it is the changing environment and structure of the ligaments and tendons with age that place them at increased risk for injury.[1] Age related changes to the soft tissues also have implications for treatment options and outcomes.[1]

With age, tendons undergo changes at the cellular level with fewer cells per muscle unit and a change in the composition of the extracellular matrix.[2] The healing ability on a cellular level and cell response is then compromised.[3] On a macroscopic scale, tendons become more stiff and less able to respond normally to mechanical load.[4] In addition, the blood supply to tendons can change over time.[5,6] Some tendons such as the rotator cuff or Achilles tendon already have watershed areas of poor blood supply at baseline.[7,8] All of these changes put tendons at risk for frank injury or to tendinopathic and degenerative changes, which ultimately can result in frank rupture of the tendon or can affect the ability of the tendon to heal.[9]

Ligaments are similar in that they also need to resist load, generally tensile. Ligaments also change over time making them less elastic and able to resist load.[10,11] Similar to tendons, there are age related changes on the cellular level as well, with less cellularity and alterations in the extracellular matrix.[12,13] In addition, there are changes to microarchitecture such as more disorganization of collagen fibres.[14] Finally, aging ligaments may also have vascular changes. These age-related changes put ligaments at risk for rupture and affect the ability of the ligaments to heal.

In addition to tendon and ligament changes other important structures, such as muscle and bone, are experiencing age related changes, which can have an impact on the stresses to which tendons and ligaments are exposed. Muscle, for example, will have decreased mass, decreased turnover and healing capacity and change in fiber distribution and innervation.[15] These lead to functional changes in the muscle and, consequently, changing requirements of tendons and ligaments.

Simple commonsense strategies may help prevent some injuries in older adults. It is recommended that older adults have a pre-exercise evaluation, especially if they intend to begin exercising after a period of primarily sedentary lifestyle.[16] Increases in activity duration or intensity should be gradual over time.[17] Warm-up and cool-down periods, or the use of ice or heat, may be beneficial; however, the evidence for this is weak.[18] Evidence is also weak for stretching; however, it may be most beneficial after a workout.[19]

OUR EXPERIENCE AND SCOPE OF THE PROBLEM

At our institution, which is a dedicated outpatient orthopaedic facility, we see many aging athletes. We have searched our database to identify the top 50 ICD-9 and CPT codes both for patients over the age of 60 and for those over the age of 65 and effectively they are similar between the two. The most common problems for these patients are arthritis, spine issues, hand and wrist issues, and fractures. Common pathologies treated by orthopaedic sports medicine physicians are infrequent in the list, the most dominant being rotator cuff and anterior cruciate ligament (ACL) injuries.

We expect these pathologies, including sports related pathologies, to increase with aging populations. There was a significant increase in birth rate in many countries following the end of World War II, particularly in Western countries, which has brought about significant increases in the aging population. In the United States, this is the baby boomer generation, which totals over 75 million people.[20] Baby boomers began turning 65 years old in the year 2011, and their average life expectancy continues to rise, with estimates of between 80 and 85 years for this generation.[20] In Britain, one sixth of the population is currently over 65 years, and this is expected to rise to one in four, with an estimate of 19 million people over the age of 65 by 2050.[21] As they age this generation is experiencing better health, which is improving relative to previous generations, so we expect that they will remain more active, resulting in more sports related pathologies in this population. According to the Outdoor Foundation, recreational activity participation in adults over the age of 50 may be as high as 50% and maintained at 30–40% for adults over 65.[22] For older adults, the CDC recommends 150 minutes of moderately strenuous aerobic activity each week and muscle building activity on 2 or more days each week.[23]

ACHILLES TENDON

The aging Achilles tendon strongly demonstrates all the above tendon changes. It has also been shown to have a change in reflex with a decrease in motoneuronal excitability.[24] As a mature athlete is attempting to be active, these changes in Achilles architecture and function mean the Achilles is less able to respond to athletic demands and possibly can place the tendon more at risk for rupture. How best to manage Achilles tendon ruptures has become even more complicated with recent systematic reviews suggesting similar results between surgical intervention and an accelerated rehabilitation program.[25–27] Therefore, indications for surgery are not exactly clear but should consider the patient's overall activity level before injury and desired level of functional return. At our institution, the majority of elderly patients with Achilles ruptures are not active in athletics, but rather seek a return to normal daily activities. In our experience, these patients generally do well with a non-operative approach with accelerated rehabilitation, supporting the findings of Soroceanu et al.[25] and van der Eng et al.[26]

For those patients who do undergo surgery, the literature suggests generally good results as well (Table 45.1). In particular, percutaneous repair has been analysed in the elderly. In a cohort of 27 patients over the age of 65 years, Maffulli et al. demonstrated an improvement in the postoperative

Achilles tendon Total Rupture score (ATRS) compared with the preoperative score and all patients were weight bearing by the eighth week.[28] Carmont et al. also found improvement in the ATRS within the first year following percutaneous repair.[29] Their data included five patients greater than the age of 65 who demonstrated similar or better results to their younger counterparts. In a study looking at both open and percutaneous Achilles repair involving 434 patients over the age of 60, the results were also good with the patients returning to their pre-injury activities and a mean American Orthopaedic Foot and Ankle Society (AOFAS) score of 93.1 points.[30] It should be noted, however, that there are reports of complications. Nestorson et al. demonstrated just that with complications in 11 of 25 patients older than 65 years; comorbidities, however, were common in their patient population.[31] To date, no studies have looked at return to sports. Most studies would suggest while patients may see improvement compared to their preoperative functional state, there is not a return to pre-injury function following Achilles tendon rupture, regardless of treatment option.[28–31]

ANTERIOR CRUCIATE LIGAMENT

In general, anterior cruciate ligament reconstruction (ACL-R) has been shown to produce good results in an older population (Table 45.2). Studies looking only at older patients report good outcomes scores, return of function and improved stability.[32–37] Blyth et al. demonstrated an improvement in International Knee Documentation Committee (IKDC), Lysholm, Cincinnati and Tegner scores, as well as on examination, in a group of 30 patients over the age of 50 at mean follow-up of 46 months.[35] In studies directly comparing younger and older patients, there are similar findings between the groups. Osti et al. compared 20 patients over the age of 50 and 20 patients under the age of 30 and found similar improvement on physical examination and in IKDC and Lysholm scores with no difference between groups for final scores.[38] In our own patient population, we evaluated 19 consecutive patients over the age of 50. The majority (90%) returned to the same level of sports participation, but more slowly than younger patients with a mean of 11 months for the older patients to return; there were no failures.[39]

Many studies in older populations have also looked at ACL graft options. Generally, studies have demonstrated good results regardless of graft choice including patellar tendon (BTB), hamstring (HT) and allograft options.[34,36,40–42] Struewer et al. directly compared BTB and HT autografts and, at 2 years, found no differences between groups for IKDC, Tegner and Lysholm scores or for grading of osteoarthritis.[40] Barrett et al. compared allograft BTB with autograft BTB and demonstrated good improvements for both groups.[41] It was noted, however, that allograft patients returned to sports sooner, but had a higher risk of failure.[41]

Kinugasa et al.[43] performed second look arthroscopy on 102 patients of all ages and found those over the age of 50 demonstrated less robust healing of the ACL HT autograft;

Table 45.1 Clinical outcomes following Achilles tendon repair involving cohorts of patients aged 60 years and older

Authors	Year	Study level	Number of patients	Average age	Purpose	Key points
Carmont et al.[29]	2013	IV	73	45.5	Evaluate the outcome of patients managed by percutaneous repair. Assess the effects of time between injury and surgery and age.	There was marked improvement in function between 3 and 6 months following surgery, with continuing but less steep improvement up to 1 year after surgery. The presence of a complication other than re-rupture did not affect end-stage outcome. The complication rate was 13.5%. There was no significant difference in outcomes for those undergoing early (≤48 hours) compared with late surgery or between those <65 and those >65 years of age.
Cretnik et al.[30]	2010	IV	13	67.9	Report the incidence and outcome of operatively treated Achilles tendon ruptures in an elderly population.	Seven had open repair under spinal anaesthesia and seven percutaneously under local anaesthesia. There were no major complications in either group. One patient in the percutaneous group had transient sural nerve injury and one patient in the open group had a superficial infection. All of the patients returned to their previous activities, four of them with some limitations. The average AOFAS score was 93.1 points.
Maffulli et al.[28]	2010	IV	27	73.4	Review outcomes in patients older than 65 who underwent percutaneous repair of the Achilles tendon.	All patients were able to bear weight fully on the affected limb by the eighth postoperative week. Percutaneous repair of the Achilles tendon is a suitable option for patients older than 65, producing similar outcomes when compared to percutaneous repair in younger patients of previous reports.
Nestorson et al.[31]	2000	IV	25	Median 71	Analyse function after Achilles tendon rupture in patients older than 65 years comparing operative and non-operative management.	14 treated surgically and 10 treated non-surgically. Surgical complications included 1 re-rupture, 3 superficial infections, 1 injury to the sural nerve and 2 patients with adhesions between the tendon and the skin. Non-surgical complications included 4 re-ruptures, 1 fibular nerve injury, 1 superficial infection and 1 deep venous thrombosis.

Note: AOFAS, American Orthopaedic Foot and Ankle Society.

clinical outcomes were comparable. The literature does suggest, not surprisingly, that worse outcome are achieved in the face of more advanced degenerative change. Blyth et al., at medium-term follow-up, found poor outcome scores in patients with Outerbridge grade 3 or 4 degenerative changes present at time of surgery.[35] Interestingly, Kim et al.

found cartilage degenerative associated pain with activity improved with ACL-R; the patients' pain at rest was no different following ACL-R.[44]

The indications for ACL-R are evolving. As the aging population increases and remains active, it is expected we will see more ACL injuries in older patients. There is a

Table 45.2 Clinical outcomes in anterior cruciate ligament reconstruction for patients aged 50 years and older

Authors	Year	Study level	Number of patients	Average age	Graft type	Outcomes
Osti et al.[38]	2011	II	20	56	Did not report	Comparable clinical outcomes were seen in middle-aged patients and in patients under 30 years of age. Physiological age, condition of the knee, life expectancy and activity level are more important than chronological age.
Arbuthnot et al.[37]	2010	IV	14	60	9 BPTB and 5 hamstring autograft	ACL reconstruction in this population restored knee stability, improved postoperative function, and allowed a return to increased activity level but less than pre-injury activity level.
Dahm et al.[33]	2008	IV	35 knees in 34 patients	57	23 BPTB allograft and 12 BPTB autograft	Postoperatively, patients had improvement in 3 functional outcomes scores and 94% of knees were stable. Graft failure requiring revision occurred in 9%.
Trojani et al.[34]	2008	IV	18	57	18 hamstring tendon	There were no graft failures, and all patients were satisfied with the operation and reported no instability. Previous meniscectomy resulted in worse outcomes.
Blyth et al.[35]	2003	II	31 knees in 30 patients	54.5	10 BPTB autograft and 21 hamstring autograft	Poor results, as determined by three outcomes scores, were associated mainly with advanced articular degenerative changes (Outerbridge grade 3 or 4) seen at the time of reconstruction. All patients reported improved stability and overall function of the knee.

Note: ACL, anterior cruciate ligament; BPTB, bone-patellar tendon-bone.

paucity of studies evaluating operative versus non-operative options in this population, so who would likely benefit from an ACL-R is not always clear. It does appear, however, that patients who wish to remain active, particularly those involved in cutting and pivoting activities, do well with ACL-R.[45] Care of these patients, therefore, warrants careful assessment of the patient's activity goals and engaged conversation with the patients regarding both operative and non-operative management of ACL injury, and the associated rehabilitation is required.

MENISCUS

The number of patients undergoing treatment for meniscal injuries in the older population is increasing. Thorlund et al. reported the incidence of arthroscopic meniscal procedures in Denmark almost doubled between 2000 and 2011.[46] The largest relative increase (i.e. a threefold increase in incidence rate) occurred in patients older than 55. Abrams et al. reported on the number of meniscectomies and meniscal repairs in this population subset, and noted there has been an increase in the number of isolated meniscectomies performed in the United States over the past 7 years without

a concomitant increase in meniscal repairs over the same time frame.[47] From 2006 to 2011, the authors noted a 4.7% rise in meniscectomies versus a 3.2% decline in meniscal repairs in patients aged 55–64. In patients older than 64 there was a 1.3% decline in meniscectomy and no meniscal repairs using a large patient database for the USA. Some of this increase is likely simply due to the increasing number of people in the elderly population.

Meniscal lesions in the aging population can be acute and/or traumatic, degenerative or both. Degenerative tears frequently occur in the absence of a distinct trauma but in the presence of other structural joint changes characteristic of knee osteoarthritis.[48,49] Thus, there is often a constellation of knee structural abnormalities characteristic of knee osteoarthritis, such as meniscal tearing, osteophytes, bone marrow lesions and cartilage damage. This set of findings is often noted on both radiographs and MRI examination of both asymptomatic and painful knees of middle-aged and older patients.[48,50] Other studies have shown a high incidence of meniscal tears even in asymptomatic knees.[48,51–53] However, elderly patients may also have minimal degenerative change in the knee but consistent evidence of meniscal tear on history, examination and MRI.[54–56]

Given the low rates of meniscal repair in the aging population, this section will focus on meniscal debridement in older individuals. When to perform arthroscopic partial meniscectomy in this population is hotly debated. Several randomized controlled trials (RCTs) published in the past decade have failed to show long-term benefit of arthroscopic interventions over and above that of placebo surgery, physiotherapy alone or physiotherapy combined with other medical treatments for patients with advanced osteoarthritis of the knee[57-60] (Table 45.3). Poorer clinical outcome after meniscectomy has been associated with greater severity of cartilage loss, bone marrow oedema in the same compartment as the meniscal tear greater severity of meniscal extrusion, greater overall severity of joint degeneration, a meniscal root tear and a longer meniscal tear at preoperative MR imaging.[61] For patients with minimal change or mild arthritis, the results of partial meniscectomy appear to be more positive.[54-56,62-64] In particular, early return to activity and early outcomes are reported to be good.[54,62] The results generally deteriorate over time, but in some patients partial meniscectomy may have beneficial long-term effects.[55,62]

The literature on partial meniscectomy surgery in the aging population emphasizes the need for careful patient selection. The appropriate patient can have very good results from partial meniscectomy, but poorly chosen patients can have poor results or be made worse following surgery. It is up to the physician to identify which patients' symptoms, exam findings and imaging findings are more likely due to a meniscal tear versus other problems such as degenerative change.

PROXIMAL HAMSTRING

Injuries to the proximal common hamstring tendon origin are rare but may be seen in the active elderly population. These injuries may be partial or complete tendinous avulsions. Complete avulsions are generally acute injuries, and partial tears of the hamstring origin are more insidious in onset. Delay in diagnosis can complicate management of these injuries when patients present months after injury.

Historically, management of this injury has been controversial. Non-operative management of these injuries, regardless of the type of injury, does not always yield acceptable clinical outcomes. Sallay et al. reported 'persistent and significant functional impairment' in a series of 12 patients with avulsion injuries managed non-operatively.[65] There are limited series reported in the literature characterizing surgical outcomes of either acute or chronic complete avulsions. Surgical repair of acute avulsions, however, has shown good to excellent results. Late repairs of complete avulsions are more difficult and outcomes are variable but have shown promising results in recent series (Table 45.1). Studies have not delineated results specifically in active older patients;

Table 45.3 Randomized trials comparing arthroscopic partial meniscectomy with non-operative interventions

Author	Year	Age (years) and entry criteria	Treatment modalities	Mean age (SD)	Outcomes
Moseley et al.[66]	2002	<75, OA	Arthroscopic lavage vs arthroscopic partial meniscectomy and debridement vs placebo surgery	51.2 (10.5) 53.6 (12.2) 52 (11.1)	No difference at 24-month follow-up
Herrlin et al.[58]	2007	45–64, OA grade 0 or 1	Arthroscopic partial meniscectomy+exercise vs exercise	54 57	No difference in KOOS scores at 6-month follow-up
Herrelin et al.[67]	2013	45–64, OA grade 0 or 1	Arthroscopic partial meniscectomy+physical and medical therapy vs exercise	54 57	No difference in KOOS scores at 60-month follow-up
Kirkley et al.[59]	2008	≥18, OA grade ≥2	Arthroscopic partial meniscectomy+physical and medical therapy vs physical and medical therapy	58.6 (10.2) 60.6 (9.9)	No difference in WOMAC scores at 24-month follow-up
Katz et al.[63]	2013	≥45, OA on MRI	Arthroscopic partial meniscectomy+physical therapy	59.0 (7.9) 57.8 (6.8)	No difference in WOMAC scores at 6 months
Yim et al.[57]	2013	No age criteria, OA grade 0 or 1	Arthroscopic partial meniscectomy+home exercise program vs combined supervised and home rehabilitation program	54.9 (10.3) 57.6 (11.0)	No difference in Lysholm score at 24 months
Sihvonen et al.[60]	2013	35–65, OA grade 0 or 1	Arthroscopic partial meniscectomy vs placebo surgery	52 (7) in both groups	No difference in Lysholm score, WOMET score or knee pain after exercise at 12-month follow-up

Note: KOOS, Knee injury and Osteoarthritis Outcome Score; OA, osteoarthritis; WOMAC, Western Ontario and McMaster Universities Index; WOMET, Western Ontario Meniscal Evaluation Tool.

however, some have included these patients as part of their study population and are discussed below.

In direct repairs of both acute and chronic tears, Birmingham et al. found that nearly all of their 23 patients returned to at least 95% of their pre-injury activity level.[68] Hamstring strength and endurance were also found to be improved.[68] Also in a series of both acute and chronic direct repairs in 72 injuries, Wood et al. noted an average strength of 84% and endurance of 89% for their entire cohort as compared to the contralateral leg.[69] They also noted that with a greater delay to surgery, there was more sciatic nerve involvement, postoperative restrictions and slower return to function.[69] Folsom et al. reported a series of acute and chronic repairs. The delayed repairs were performed using Achilles allograft.[70] They reported no statistically significant difference in the hamstring strength or hamstring to quadriceps ratios between acute primary repairs and chronic repairs with allograft. Over 90% of patients were satisfied in both groups.[70]

The authors have evaluated our own experience with these injuries in the active aging population, including a consecutive series of seven patients who presented in a delayed fashion and had all attempted a period of non-operative management including physical therapy with no improvement in outcome.[71,72] Patients who were older than 50 took 11 months to return to sport compared to an average of 7.8 months in a cohort of patients aged 20-30. Six patients had anatomic reattachment of the common hamstring tendon to the ischial tuberosity with suture anchors, and one required Achilles tendon allograft interposition. There were no intraoperative complications. Isokinetic testing at an average of 21.6 months postoperatively (range, 12–36 months) demonstrated average strength and power of 87% and 87%, respectively, compared to the normal contralateral side.[71,72]

In summary, avulsion injuries of the proximal common hamstring origin are uncommon. Diagnosis may be delayed, thereby complicating treatment. Operative intervention is not always the ideal option, but in patients with both acute and chronic complete tendinous avulsions with persistent symptoms or deficits, primary direct repair should be considered. In chronic, irreparable avulsions, Achilles tendon allograft interposition may be used to restore the common hamstring tendon to its anatomic origin with a satisfactory functional outcome.

DISTAL BICEPS

There are no studies evaluating distal biceps ruptures specifically in an elderly population; however, we know that distal biceps ruptures do occur in this population.[73] This discussion will, therefore, cover a number of studies looking at outcomes following distal biceps rupture that include patients in their 50s, 60s and 70s. The ruptures often occur during eccentric contraction, which may include sports activity.[73]

There are many studies looking at operative outcomes of both acute and chronic ruptures. Generally, repair of acute ruptures demonstrates good results in terms of both strength return and functional outcomes tools, including the Disabilities of the Arm, Shoulder and Hand (DASH) and the American Shoulder and Elbow Surgeons (ASES) scores.[74–76] The surgeon must be aware of possible complications such as posterior interosseous nerve palsy or radioulnar synostosis. Chronic ruptures can also have good results with operative fixation in terms of both strength return and outcomes scores including the DASH, ASES and Mayo Elbow Performance Score (MEPS).[77–79] It appears repairs in chronic ruptures can be done well with either direct repair or using allograft tissue.[77–80] Schneider et al. even looked at outcomes in patients who sustained ruptures in bilateral biceps and demonstrated good results from operative intervention.[76]

There are few studies comparing operative to non-operative intervention, particularly in the elderly population, so the indications for operative intervention are evolving. Freeman et al. evaluated a cohort of non-operative patients, ranging in age from 35 to 74 years, and found generally good results.[81] They compared their cohort to historical operative controls and found the biggest difference to be a deficit in supination for the non-operative patients.[81] Other areas of debate in distal biceps repair have not been evaluated in an elderly population, such as single incision versus two incisions. In a study that included elderly patients, Grewal et al. found no significant differences between single or two incisions.[74]

ROTATOR CUFF

While rotator cuff tears are not associated specifically with sports injury, they can occur from athletic participation and are a condition managed by orthopaedic sports medicine physicians, among other providers, and therefore we feel rotator cuff tears warrant discussion. In addition, rotator cuff tears represent a quintessential tendon pathology related to aging since we know rotator cuff tear incidence is associated with increasing age.[82]

The effect of aging on the rotator cuff is well documented. In a histological study comparing cadaveric specimens at different ages, Brewer et al. demonstrated that with age there is degeneration of the intrasubstance of the rotator cuff and the tendon attachment to the bone.[83] In addition, there is decreased cellularity and vascularity. Tempelhof et al. evaluated a population of 411 asymptomatic shoulders and demonstrated there is an increasing incidence of rotator cuff tears in asymptomatic patients with age.[84] Fehringer et al. and Hattrup demonstrated that tear size also increases with age.[85,86]

As related to age, debate remains regarding management of rotator cuff tears. Likely because of the complex interplay of factors affecting clinical decision-making, there are surprisingly few studies looking at operative compared to non-operative intervention for rotator cuff tears, and the results are conflicting.[87–90] While not universally true, operative intervention is often recommended for medium to large sized tears in active patients.[91–94]

Numerous studies have evaluated clinical outcomes after operative intervention, including those specifically in older patients[86,95–102] (Table 45.4). Generally operative

Table 45.4 Clinical outcomes following rotator cuff repair for patients 60 years and older

Authors	Year	Study level	Number of patients	Average age	Purpose	Key points
Rhee et al.[95]	2014	III	238	N/A	Evaluate clinical and structural outcomes of cuff repairs in patients aged >70 years and <70 years.	There were no significant differences in clinical outcomes between patients aged 60–69 and those >70. The re-tear rate was higher with increasing intraoperative tear size but not with increasing age.
Robinson et al.[105]	2013	IV	68	77	Evaluate clinical and sonographic outcome of arthroscopic rotator cuff repair in patients aged ≥70 years and determine factors associated with re-tear.	Contrary to the above study, re-tear free survival was associated with age at operation. Male gender was associated with a higher score at 1 year. Arthroscopic rotator cuff repair can be a successful operation in patients aged ≥70 years.
Djahangiri et al.[102]	2012	IV	44	69	Review the results of cuff repair in patients >65 years old and identify factors predicting outcome.	In patients older than 65 years who do not respond to conservative treatment, repair of symptomatic single-tendon rotator cuff tears has good success.
Charousset et al.[103]	2010	IV	88	70	Assess tendon healing and clinical results of cuff tears repaired arthroscopically in patients aged 65 years or older.	Significant functional improvement can be seen from arthroscopic repair in patients aged 65 years or older. This was especially noted when the tear was isolated to the supraspinatus tendon.
Verma et al.[97]	2010	IV	39	75.3	Evaluate outcomes of arthroscopic rotator cuff repair in patients aged 70 years or older.	In carefully selected patients aged 70 years or older, there was a low complication rate and improvement in pain and function following arthroscopic cuff repair for symptomatic full-thickness rotator cuff tears.
Rebuzzi et al.[100]	2005	IV	64	67.7	Analyse results by age, tear size and type of suture repair of arthroscopic cuff repair in patients older than 60 years.	Regardless of age, tear size and type of suture repair, arthroscopic rotator cuff repair resulted in good outcomes in a large percentage of cases. The best results with margin convergence using side-to-side sutures were achieved in patients older than 65 years.
Grondel et al.[98]	2001	IV	92	70.4	Evaluate efficacy of cuff repair in patients >62 years old.	Overall, 87% of patients had good or excellent results. Including 3 patients who needed to be revised, 98% of patients were satisfied with their result.
Worland et al.[99]	1999	IV	69	75	Evaluate results obtained in patients older than 70 years treated with open surgical repair for massive ruptures of the cuff tendons.	In open rotator cuff repair for massive tears, good tendon to bone repair and satisfactory outcomes were achieved in roughly 80% of patients.

outcomes are good; however, the effect of age on outcomes is also still being defined. When comparing a group of patients in their 60s to a group 70 and older, Rhee et al. demonstrated improvements in University of California-Los Angeles (UCLA), Constant and visual analog scale (VAS) scores, with no difference between groups.[95] Hattrup, however, demonstrated overall positive results, but there were fewer excellent results in patients over the age of 65.[86] Although the specific surgical technique is debatable, studies have demonstrated satisfactory results in both open and arthroscopic rotator cuff repairs. In a population of patients with massive rotator cuff tears, Worland et al. demonstrated an improvement in UCLA scores and good patient satisfaction with open repairs in patients over 70 years.[99] Rebuzzi et al., in an early study of arthroscopic rotator cuff repairs, demonstrated an improvement in UCLA score in older patients.[101] In more recent studies, Osti et al. and Verma et al. have corroborated positive arthroscopic results demonstrating improvements in UCLA, SF-36, ASES and Simple Shoulder Test scores.[96,97]

Interestingly, healing of the rotator cuff does not necessarily correlate with outcome. Patients with healed rotator cuffs following surgery tend to have superior outcomes to those who fail to heal.[102,103] Patients with non-healing tendons, however, can also do well following surgery.[102,103] In a systematic review, Lambers Heerspink et al. found that age is a factor in rotator cuff healing.[104] Both Oh et al. and Charousset et al. provided evidence of this when, using computed tomography arthrograms, they found less reliable healing in older patients, particularly as it related to tear size prior to surgery.[101,103] Despite the demonstrably less reliable healing in older patients, Djahangiri et al. and Robinson et al. had acceptable rates of rotator cuff healing as evaluated by ultrasonography.[102,105] This literature suggests that operative intervention can be beneficial in appropriately chosen patients.

CONCLUSION

Aging athletes generally can return to sports following sports related injury. For many of the more common orthopaedic sports related injuries, the indications for operative intervention are still being defined. Not all patients require operative intervention for the diagnoses discussed above, but careful patient selection for operative procedures can result in good outcomes, including return to satisfactory function and activity level. As our population ages, and more people continue to be active into later years in life, it is important for providers to have an understanding of these considerations.

REFERENCES

1. McCarthy, M.M. and J.A. Hannafin. The mature athlete: Aging tendon and ligament. *Sports Health*, 2014; 6(1): 41–8.

2. Ippolito, E., et al. Morphological, immunochemical, and biochemical study of rabbit Achilles tendon at various ages. *J Bone Joint Surg Am*, 1980; 62(4): 583–98.

3. Arnoczky, S.P., M. Lavagnino, and M. Egerbacher. The mechanobiological aetiopathogenesis of tendinopathy: Is it the over-stimulation or the understimulation of tendon cells? *Int J Exp Pathol*, 2007; 88(4): 217–26.

4. Plate, J.F., et al. Normal aging alters in vivo passive biomechanical response of the rat gastrocnemius-Achilles muscle-tendon unit. *J Biomech*, 2013; 46(3): 450–5.

5. Yang, X., et al. The volume of the neovascularity and its clinical implications in Achilles tendinopathy. *Ultrasound Med Biol*, 2012; 38(11): 1887–95.

6. Yu, J.S., et al. Correlation of MR imaging and pathologic findings in athletes undergoing surgery for chronic patellar tendinitis. *AJR Am J Roentgenol*, 1995; 165(1): 115–18.

7. Codman, E.A., and I.B. Akerson. The pathology associated with rupture of the supraspinatus tendon. *Ann Surg*, 1931; 93(1): 348–59.

8. Stein, V., et al. Quantitative assessment of intravascular volume of the human Achilles tendon. *Acta Orthop Scand*, 2000; 71(1): 60–3.

9. Hannafin, J.A. and T.A. Chiaia. Adhesive capsulitis. *Clin Orthop Rel Res*, 2000; 372: 95–109.

10. Woo, S.L., et al. Tensile properties of the human femur-anterior cruciate ligament-tibia complex. The effects of specimen age and orientation. *Am J Sports Med*, 1991; 19(3): 217–25.

11. Noyes, F.R., and E.S. Grood. The strength of the anterior cruciate ligament in humans and Rhesus monkeys. *J Bone Joint Surg Am*, 1976; 58(8): 1074–82.

12. Wang, I.E., et al. Age-dependent changes in matrix composition and organization at the ligament-to-bone insertion. *J Orthop Res*, 2006; 24(8): 1745–55.

13. Stolzing, A., et al. Age-related changes in human bone marrow-derived mesenchymal stem cells: Consequences for cell therapies. *Mech Ageing Dev*, 2008; 129(3): 163–73.

14. Hasegawa, A., et al. Anterior cruciate ligament changes in the human knee joint in aging and osteoarthritis. *Arthritis Rheum*, 2012; 64(3): 696–704.

15. Siparsky, P.N., D.T. Kirkendall, and W.E. Garrett, Jr. Muscle changes in aging: Understanding sarcopenia. *Sports Health*, 2014; 6(1): 36–40.

16. Concannon, L.G., M.J. Grierson, and M.A. Harrast. Exercise in the older adult: From the sedentary elderly to the masters athlete. *PM R*, 2012; 4(11): 833–9.

17. Elsawy, B. and K.E. Higgins. Physical activity guidelines for older adults. *Am Fam Physician*, 2010; 81(1): 55–9.

18. U.S. Department of Health and Human Services. 2008 Physical Activity Guidelines for Americans. 2008. http://www.health.gov/paguidelines/guidelines/ (accessed 26 January 2015).

19. Collins, S. WebMD Feature. The Truth about Stretching. Find out the best ways to stretch and the best times to do it. http://www.webmd.com/fitness-exercise/guide/how-to-stretch (accessed 26 January 2015).

20. Ortman, J.M., V.A. Velkoff, and H. Hogan. An aging nation: The older population in the United States. In: U.S Department of Commerce, ed. Washington, DC: U.S. Census Bureau; 2014, p. 28.

21. Cracknell, R. *The Ageing Population.* London: House of Commons Library Research; 2010, p. 1.

22. Outdoor Foundation. 2013 Outdoor Recreation Participation Report. 2013. http://www.outdoorfoundation.org/research.participation.2013.html

23. Centers for Disease Control and Prevention. How much physical activity do older adults need? Physical Activity is Essential to Healthy Aging. http://www.cdc.gov/physicalactivity/everyone/guidelines/olderadults.html (accessed 27 January 2015).

24. Chung, S.G., et al. Aging-related neuromuscular changes characterized by tendon reflex system properties. *Arch Phys Med Rehabil*, 2005; 86(2): 318–27.

25. Soroceanu, A., et al. Surgical versus nonsurgical treatment of acute Achilles tendon rupture: A meta-analysis of randomized trials. *J Bone Joint Surg Am*, 2012; 94(23): 2136–43.

26. van der Eng, D.M., et al. Rerupture rate after early weightbearing in operative versus conservative treatment of Achilles tendon ruptures: A meta-analysis. *J Foot Ankle Surg*, 2013; 52(5): 622–8.

27. Wallace, R.G., G.J. Heyes, and A.L. Michael. The non-operative functional management of patients with a rupture of the tendo Achillis leads to low rates of re-rupture. *J Bone Joint Surg Br*, 2011; 93(10): 1362–6.

28. Maffulli, N., et al. Favorable outcome of percutaneous repair of Achilles tendon ruptures in the elderly. *Clin Orthop Relat Res*, 2010; 468(4): 1039–46.

29. Carmont, M.R., et al. Functional outcome of percutaneous Achilles repair: Improvements in Achilles tendon total rupture score during the first year. *Orthop J Sports Med*, 2013; 1(1): 2325967113494584.

30. Cretnik, A., R. Kosir, and M. Kosanovic. Incidence and outcome of operatively treated Achilles tendon rupture in the elderly. *Foot Ankle Int*, 2010; 31(1): 14–18.

31. Nestorson, J., et al. Function after Achilles tendon rupture in the elderly: 25 patients older than 65 years followed for 3 years. *Acta Orthop Scand*, 2000; 71(1): 64–8.

32. Kuechle, D.K., et al. Allograft anterior cruciate ligament reconstruction in patients over 40 years of age. *Arthroscopy*, 2002; 18(8): 845–53.

33. Dahm, D.L., et al. Reconstruction of the anterior cruciate ligament in patients over 50 years. *J Bone Joint Surg Br*, 2008; 90(11): 1446–50.

34. Trojani, C., et al. Four-strand hamstring tendon autograft for ACL reconstruction in patients aged 50 years or older. *Orthop Traumatol Surg Res*, 2009; 95(1): 22–7.

35. Blyth, M.J., et al. Anterior cruciate ligament reconstruction in patients over the age of 50 years: 2- to 8-year follow-up. *Knee Surg Sports Traumatol Arthrosc*, 2003; 11(4): 204–11.

36. Khan, R.M., et al. Anterior cruciate ligament reconstruction in patients over 40 years using hamstring autograft. *Knee Surg Sports Traumatol Arthrosc*, 2010; 18(1): 68–72.

37. Arbuthnot, J.E. and R.B. Brink. The role of anterior cruciate ligament reconstruction in the older patients, 55 years or above. *Knee Surg Sports Traumatol Arthrosc*, 2010; 18(1): 73–8.

38. Osti, L., et al. Surgery for ACL deficiency in patients over 50. *Knee Surg Sports Traumatol Arthrosc*, 2011; 19(3): 412–17.

39. Steubs, T., et al. ACL reconstruction in patients over 50: Outcomes at an ambulatory surgery center. American Association of Orthopaedic Surgeons Annual Meeting; March 23, 2013, 2013; Chicago, IL.

40. Struewer, J., et al. Isolated anterior cruciate ligament reconstruction in patients aged fifty years: Comparison of hamstring graft versus bone-patellar tendon-bone graft. *Int Orthop*, 2013; 37(5): 809–17.

41. Barrett, G., D. Stokes, and M. White. Anterior cruciate ligament reconstruction in patients older than 40 years: Allograft versus autograft patellar tendon. *Am J Sports Med*, 2005; 33(10): 1505–12.

42. Barber, F.A., J. Aziz-Jacobo, and F.B. Oro. Anterior cruciate ligament reconstruction using patellar tendon allograft: An age-dependent outcome evaluation. *Arthroscopy*, 2010; 26(4): 488–93.

43. Kinugasa, K., et al. Effect of patient age on morphology of anterior cruciate ligament grafts at second-look arthroscopy. *Arthroscopy*, 2011; 27(1): 38–45.

44. Kim, S.J., et al. Anterior cruciate ligament reconstruction improves activity-induced pain in comparison with pain at rest in middle-aged patients with significant cartilage degeneration. *Am J Sports Med*, 2010; 38(7): 1343–8.

45. Brown, C.A., et al. ACL reconstruction in patients aged 40 years and older: A systematic review and introduction of a new methodology score for ACL studies. *Am J Sports Med*, 2013; 41(9): 2181–90.

46. Thorlund, J.B., K.B. Hare, and L.S. Lohmander. Large increase in arthroscopic meniscus surgery in the middle-aged and older population in Denmark from 2000 to 2011. *Acta Orthop*, 2014; 85(3): 287–92.

47. Abrams, G.D., et al. Trends in meniscus repair and meniscectomy in the United States, 2005–2011. *Am J Sports Med*, 2013; 41(10): 2333–9.

48. Englund, M., et al. Incidental meniscal findings on knee MRI in middle-aged and elderly persons. *N Engl J Med*, 2008; 359(11): 1108–15.

49. Englund, M., et al. Meniscal tear in knees without surgery and the development of radiographic osteoarthritis among middle-aged and elderly persons: The Multicenter Osteoarthritis Study. *Arthritis Rheum*, 2009; 60(3): 831–9.

50. Guermazi, A., et al. Prevalence of abnormalities in knees detected by MRI in adults without knee osteoarthritis: Population based observational study (Framingham Osteoarthritis Study). *BMJ*, 2012; 345: e5339.

51. Zanetti, M., et al. Patients with suspected meniscal tears: Prevalence of abnormalities seen on MRI of 100 symptomatic and 100 contralateral asymptomatic knees. *AJR Am J Roentgenol*, 2003; 181(3): 635–41.

52. Boks, S.S., et al. Magnetic resonance imaging abnormalities in symptomatic and contralateral knees: Prevalence and associations with traumatic history in general practice. *Am J Sports Med*, 2006; 34(12): 1984–91.

53. Englund, M., et al. Effect of meniscal damage on the development of frequent knee pain, aching, or stiffness. *Arthritis Rheum*, 2007; 56(12): 4048–54.

54. Barrett, G.R., S.H. Treacy, and C.G. Ruff. The effect of partial lateral meniscectomy in patients > or = 60 years. *Orthopedics*, 1998; 21(3): 251–7.

55. Matsusue, Y. and N.L. Thomson. Arthroscopic partial medial meniscectomy in patients over 40 years old: A 5- to 11-year follow-up study. *Arthroscopy*, 1996; 12(1): 39–44.

56. Menetrey, J., O. Siegrist, and D. Fritschy. Medial meniscectomy in patients over the age of fifty: A six year follow-up study. *Swiss Surg*, 2002; 8(3): 113–19.

57. Yim, J.H., et al. A comparative study of meniscectomy and nonoperative treatment for degenerative horizontal tears of the medial meniscus. *Am J Sports Med*, 2013; 41(7): 1565–70.

58. Herrlin, S., et al. Arthroscopic or conservative treatment of degenerative medial meniscal tears: A prospective randomised trial. *Knee Surg Sports Traumatol Arthrosc*, 2007; 15(4): 393–401.

59. Kirkley, A., et al. A randomized trial of arthroscopic surgery for osteoarthritis of the knee. *N Engl J Med*, 2008; 359(11): 1097–107.

60. Sihvonen, R., et al. Arthroscopic partial meniscectomy versus sham surgery for a degenerative meniscal tear. *N Engl J Med*, 2013; 369(26): 2515–24.

61. Kijowski, R., et al. Arthroscopic partial meniscectomy: MR imaging for prediction of outcome in middle-aged and elderly patients. *Radiology*, 2011; 259(1): 203–12.

62. Jaureguito, J.W., et al. The effects of arthroscopic partial lateral meniscectomy in an otherwise normal knee: A retrospective review of functional, clinical, and radiographic results. *Arthroscopy*, 1995; 11(1): 29–36.

63. Katz, J.N., et al. Surgery versus physical therapy for a meniscal tear and osteoarthritis. *N Engl J Med*, 2013; 368(18): 1675–84.

64. Lyman, S., et al. Surgical decision making for arthroscopic partial meniscectomy in patients aged over 40 years. *Arthroscopy*, 2012; 28(4): 492–501.e1.

65. Sallay, P.I., et al. Hamstring muscle injuries among water skiers. Functional outcome and prevention. *Am J Sports Med*, 1996; 24(2): 130–6.

66. Moseley JB, O'Malley K, Petersen NJ, Menke TJ, Brody BA, Kuykendall DH, Hollingsworth JC, Ashton CM, Wray NP. A controlled trial of arthroscopic surgery for osteoarthritis of the knee. *N Engl J Med*, 2002; 347(2):81–8.

67. Herrlin SV, Wange PO, Lapidus G, Hållander M, Werner S, Weidenhielm L. Is arthroscopic surgery beneficial in treating non-traumatic, degenerative medial meniscal tears? A five year follow-up. *Knee Surg Sports Traumatol Arthrosc*, 2013;21(2):358–64.

68. Birmingham, P., et al. Functional outcome after repair of proximal hamstring avulsions. *J Bone Joint Surg Am*, 2011; 93(19): 1819–26.

69. Wood, D.G., et al. Avulsion of the proximal hamstring origin. *J Bone Joint Surg Am*, 2008; 90(11): 2365–74.

70. Folsom, G.J. and C.M. Larson. Surgical treatment of acute versus chronic complete proximal hamstring ruptures: Results of a new allograft technique for chronic reconstructions. *Am J Sports Med*, 2008; 36(1): 104–9.

71. Sikka, R., et al. Injuries to the common hamstring origin: Operative treatment. American Orthopaedic Association/Canadian Orthopaedic Association Annual Meeting; June 5, 2008; Quebec City, Quebec, Canada.

72. Sikka, R., et al. Injuries to the common hamstring origin: Operative treatment. American Academy of Orthopaedic Surgeons Annual Meeting; March 6 2008; San Francisco, CA.

73. Safran, M.R. and S.M. Graham. Distal biceps tendon ruptures: Incidence, demographics, and the effect of smoking. *Clin Orthop Relat Res*, 2002; (404): 275–83.

74. Grewal, R., et al. Single versus double-incision technique for the repair of acute distal biceps tendon ruptures: A randomized clinical trial. *J Bone Joint Surg Am*, 2012; 94(13): 1166–74.

75. Davison, B.L., W.D. Engber, and L.J. Tigert. Long term evaluation of repaired distal biceps brachii tendon ruptures. *Clin Orthop Relat Res*, 1996; (333): 186–91.

76. Schneider, A., et al. Bilateral ruptures of the distal biceps brachii tendon. *J Shoulder Elbow Surg*, 2009; 18(5): 804–7.

77. Snir, N., et al. Clinical outcomes after chronic distal biceps reconstruction with allografts. *Am J Sports Med*, 2013; 41(10): 2288–95.

78. Bosman, H.A., M. Fincher, and N. Saw. Anatomic direct repair of chronic distal biceps brachii tendon rupture without interposition graft. *J Shoulder Elbow Surg*, 2012; 21(10): 1342–7.

79. Morrey, M.E., et al. Primary repair of retracted distal biceps tendon ruptures in extreme flexion. *J Shoulder Elbow Surg*, 2014; 23(5): 679–85.

80. Cross, M.B., et al. Single-incision chronic distal biceps tendon repair with tibialis anterior allograft. *Int Orthop*, 2014; 38(4): 791–5.

81. Freeman, C.R., et al. Nonoperative treatment of distal biceps tendon ruptures compared with a historical control group. *J Bone Joint Surg Am*, 2009; 91(10): 2329–34.

82. Tokish, J.M. The mature athlete's shoulder. *Sports Health*, 2014; 6(1): 31–5.

83. Brewer, B.J. Aging of the rotator cuff. *Am J Sports Med*, 1979; 7(2): 102–10.

84. Tempelhof, S., S. Rupp, and R. Seil. Age-related prevalence of rotator cuff tears in asymptomatic shoulders. *J Shoulder Elbow Surg*, 1999; 8(4): 296–9.

85. Fehringer, E.V., et al. Full-thickness rotator cuff tear prevalence and correlation with function and co-morbidities in patients sixty-five years and older. *J Shoulder Elbow Surg*, 2008; 17(6): 881–5.

86. Hattrup, S.J. Rotator cuff repair: Relevance of patient age. *J Shoulder Elbow Surg*, 1995; 4(2): 95–100.

87. Kukkonen, J., et al. Treatment of non-traumatic rotator cuff tears: A randomised controlled trial with one-year clinical results. *Bone Joint J*, 2014; 96-B(1): 75–81.

88. Fucentese, S.F., et al. Evolution of nonoperatively treated symptomatic isolated full-thickness supraspinatus tears. *J Bone Joint Surg Am*, 2012; 94(9): 801–8.

89. Merolla, G., et al. Conservative management of rotator cuff tears: Literature review and proposal for a prognostic. Prediction Score. *Muscles Ligaments Tendons J*, 2011; 1(1): 12–19.

90. Coghlan, J.A., et al. Surgery for rotator cuff disease. *Cochrane Database Syst Rev*, 2008; (1): CD005619.

91. Galatz, L.M., et al. The outcome and repair integrity of completely arthroscopically repaired large and massive rotator cuff tears. *J Bone Joint Surg Am*, 2004; 86-A(2): 219–24.

92. Kim, H.M., et al. Relationship of tear size and location to fatty degeneration of the rotator cuff. *J Bone Joint Surg Am*, 2010; 92(4): 829–39.

93. Yamaguchi, K., et al. The demographic and morphological features of rotator cuff disease. A comparison of asymptomatic and symptomatic shoulders. *J Bone Joint Surg Am*, 2006; 88(8): 1699–704.

94. Mall, N.A., et al. Symptomatic progression of asymptomatic rotator cuff tears: A prospective study of clinical and sonographic variables. *J Bone Joint Surg Am*, 2010; 92(16): 2623–33.

95. Rhee, Y.G., N.S. Cho, and J.H. Yoo. Clinical outcome and repair integrity after rotator cuff repair in patients older than 70 years versus patients younger than 70 years. *Arthroscopy*, 2014; 30(5): 546–54.

96. Osti, L., et al. Comparison of arthroscopic rotator cuff repair in healthy patients over and under 65 years of age. *Knee Surg Sports Traumatol Arthrosc*, 2010; 18(12): 1700–6.

97. Verma, N.N., et al. Outcomes of arthroscopic rotator cuff repair in patients aged 70 years or older. *Arthroscopy*, 2010; 26(10): 1273–80.

98. Grondel, R.J., F.H. Savoie, 3rd, and L.D. Field. Rotator cuff repairs in patients 62 years of age or older. *J Shoulder Elbow Surg*, 2001; 10(2): 97–9.

99. Worland, R.L., et al. Repair of massive rotator cuff tears in patients older than 70 years. *J Shoulder Elbow Surg*, 1999; 8(1): 26–30.

100. Rebuzzi, E., et al. Arthroscopic rotator cuff repair in patients older than 60 years. *Arthroscopy*, 2005; 21(1): 48–54.

101. Oh, J.H., et al. Effect of age on functional and structural outcome after rotator cuff repair. *Am J Sports Med*, 2010; 38(4): 672–8.

102. Djahangiri, A., et al. Outcome of single-tendon rotator cuff repair in patients aged older than 65 years. *J Shoulder Elbow Surg*, 2013; 22(1): 45–51.

103. Charousset, C., et al. Arthroscopic repair of full-thickness rotator cuff tears: Is there tendon healing in patients aged 65 years or older? *Arthroscopy*, 2010; 26(3): 302–9.

104. Lambers Heerspink, F.O., et al. Specific patient-related prognostic factors for rotator cuff repair: A systematic review. *J Shoulder Elbow Surg*, 2014; 23(7): 1073–80.

105. Robinson, P.M., et al. Rotator cuff repair in patients over 70 years of age: Early outcomes and risk factors associated with re-tear. *Bone Joint J*, 2013; 95-B(2): 199–205.

Index

For Product Safety Concerns and Information please contact
our EU representative GPSR@taylorandfrancis.com Taylor & Francis
Verlag GmbH, Kaufingerstraße 24, 80331 München, Germany

T - #0301 - 160425 - C696 - 279/216/31 - PB - 9780367574659 - Gloss Lamination